American Cancer Society Textbook Of Clinical Oncology

SECOND EDITION

The *American Cancer Society Textbook of Clinical Oncology* is available through local offices of your American Cancer Society. To obtain a copy, please consult your telephone directory for the office serving your area or call 1-800-ACS-2345.

This book will be published in Spanish through a joint effort of the Pan American Health Organization, the National Cancer Institute, and the American Cancer Society and will be available in the fall of 1995. To obtain copies, contact:

Pan American Health Organization
Publications Marketing Program
525 Twenty-third Street, NW
Washington, D.C. 20037
FAX: (202)338-0869
Phone: (202)293-8130

AMERICAN CANCER SOCIETY TEXTBOOK OF

CLINICAL ONCOLOGY

SECOND EDITION

Gerald P. Murphy, MD

Walter Lawrence, Jr., MD

Raymond E. Lenhard, Jr., MD

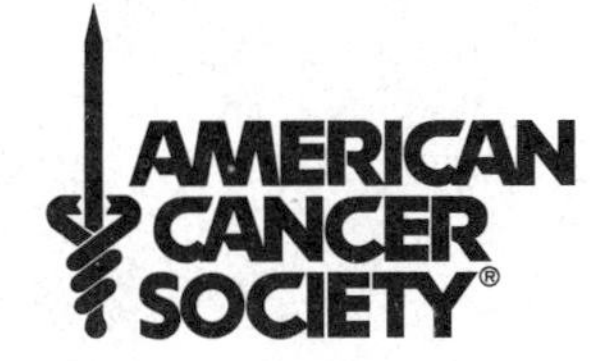

The American Cancer Society, Inc., Atlanta, Georgia 30329

Published 1995. First edition 1991
Printed in the United States of America

98 97 96 95 5 4 3 2 1

Library of Congress Cataloging-in-Publication Data
American Cancer Society textbook of clinical oncology / [edited by]
Gerald P. Murphy, Walter Lawrence, Jr., Raymond E. Lenhard, Jr. –
2nd ed.
p. cm.
Includes bibliographical references and index.
ISBN 0-944235-10-7
1. Cancer. 2. Oncology. I. Murphy, Gerald Patrick. II. Lawrence, Walter, 925- III. Lenhard, R.E. (Raymond E.) IV. American Cancer Society. V. Title: Textbook of clinical oncology.
[DNLM: 1. Neoplasms. QZ 200 A5127 1995]
RC261.A677 1995
616.99'4—dc20
DNLM/DLC 95-132
for Library of Congress CIP

CONTENTS

PREFACE

Health-care providers are the front line in the fight against cancer. Screening for early detection of the disease and counseling patients about healthy lifestyles and risk reduction are critical steps in cancer control, and it is the health-care provider, in partnership with the patient, who is in the best position to accomplish this.

The *American Cancer Society Textbook of Clinical Oncology* was conceived and produced as a source of information on the multiple aspects of cancer that will enable providers to adopt practices to encourage cancer prevention and early detection and to offer state-of-the-art treatment for the disease. The textbook was designed as a comprehensive resource for medical and nursing students as well as for primary care physicians, nurses, and other clinicians who are part of the medical care team in cancer. It offers immediate information and clinical strategies and also serves as a bridge to more specialized textbooks and to the medical literature. Although this textbook is directed at generalists in the various health professions, it will also serve as a resource for those specializing in the oncology field.

The *American Cancer Society Textbook of Clinical Oncology* is the outcome of the collaborative efforts of a team of American Cancer Society volunteers who donated their time and talents to this project. Their commitment and dedication made possible this second edition (the first edition was published in 1991). For both editorial board members and chapter authors this was entirely a volunteer effort for which they received no payment or honoraria.

It is equally important to note that the generous financial contributions of individuals throughout the United States to the American Cancer Society made possible the typesetting, printing, and distribution of this textbook.

It was both these contributions of financial and volunteer resources that enabled the Society to render this service to the education of health-care providers and, ultimately, to those who will benefit most from this text: cancer patients and their families.

Gerald P. Murphy, MD
Walter Lawrence, Jr., MD
Raymond E. Lenhard, Jr., MD

PREFACE TO THE FIRST EDITION

The *American Cancer Society Textbook of Clinical Oncology* is the product of the combined efforts of 50 of the leading cancer experts in the United States. The Society assembled this distinguished group of authors to create a new, more comprehensive text for medical students and for physicians working in, or interested in, oncology; a text that addresses not only the treatment of the disease, but also the related issues that are keys to a multidisciplinary approach to cancer care.

In the time that has elapsed since the publication of the last edition of this text's predecessor, *Clinical Oncology: A Multidisciplinary Approach*, the body of knowledge relative to cancer has grown dramatically. The range of issues affecting the cancer patient has expanded, and there has been an explosion in biological knowledge as it relates to cancer treatment. A medical text was needed that would take into account this rapid growth in the science of treatment as well as how clinical issues relate to research. Thus, the American Cancer Society felt that a more comprehensive treatment of the various forms of the disease was required rather than a revision of our former oncology text. For this reason, the American Cancer Society undertook publication for the first time of its own new textbook, one that would embrace the entire body of knowledge relative to oncology and the issues critical to cancer control.

In addition to timely, in-depth discussions of the pathology, etiology, and nature of cancer, the scope of this new text has been broadened to reflect the increased specialization within medicine and the team approach to patient care. And, in keeping with the emerging understanding that health care must be a partnership between physicians and patients, theories of lifestyle factors and preventive measures have been addressed, as have the areas of social work, sexuality, and rehabilitation.

Because of the skill and knowledge of our authors and their broad base of experience in both research and clinical practice, it is our anticipation that the American Cancer Society Textbook of Clinical Oncology will be recognized as a definitive work in oncology, one that will be of great educational value to medical students, physicians, and nurses in the United States and elsewhere.

ACKNOWLEDGEMENTS

The editors wish to express our appreciation to the authors who so generously donated their time and expertise to create this textbook. We would also like to thank Larry Garfinkel, past American Cancer Society Vice President for Epidemiology, for volunteering his help in reviewing and updating statistics throughout the book, and our managing editor, Rosemarie Perrin, of the American Cancer Society National Home Office, who shepherded this project from its inception to its completion. We are also grateful to the editorial board of the textbook whose members volunteered their time to come together and plan this new edition.

INTRODUCTION: THE AMERICAN CANCER SOCIETY

The American Cancer Society is the nationwide community-based voluntary health organization dedicated to eliminating cancer as a major health problem by preventing cancer, saving lives from cancer, and diminishing suffering from cancer through research, education, and service.

The Society originated in 1913 with a group of 10 physicians and five laymen who met in New York City to found the American Society for the Control of Cancer. Its stated purpose at that time was to "disseminate knowledge concerning the symptoms, treatment, and prevention of cancer; to investigate conditions under which cancer is found; and to compile statistics in regard thereto." This organization was later renamed the American Cancer Society and is today one of the oldest and largest voluntary health agencies in the United States.

Today's Society includes over two million volunteers and is governed by an elected board of directors from throughout the United States, half of whom are members of the medical and scientific professions and half, lay members. The Society is a community-based organization made up of thousands of local volunteer leaders who form the connection between the community and the Society's national programs in cancer prevention, early cancer detection, and service to cancer patients and their families.

EDITORIAL BOARD

1

CANCER STATISTICS AND TRENDS

Lawrence Garfinkel, MA

Statistical data play an integral role in evaluating the scope of the cancer problem and the results of cancer control efforts. The data can show which sites of cancer are increasing or decreasing over time, as well as subgroups such as age, sex, or ethnic origin that are showing the greatest statistical changes. Plotting these changes can suggest subjects for research efforts. Trends in cancer rates are also used to evaluate the results of educational programs in local areas, in individual states, or throughout the nation. International differences in rates may also suggest subjects for further research.

The most important cancer data sources come from mortality statistics, published annually in the United States by the National Center for Health Statistics of the Department of Health and Human Services. The most recent reports are published about three years prior to the current year.[1] Mortality rates are computed according to the number of deaths per 100,000 population as estimated by the Census Bureau.

Data on incidence (the number of new cases reported in a year) are not published for the entire country. Although many states have their own registries to report cases, the figures most often used come from the SEER (Surveillance, Epidemiology, and End Results) program of the National Cancer Institute (NCI). This population-based program covers four states, Puerto Rico, and five metropolitan areas and constitutes an estimated 12% of all cancer cases in the US.[2]

The National Cancer Data Base was organized by the American College of Surgeons Commission on Cancer and was funded by the American Cancer Society beginning in 1989. It collects standardized data on cancer incidence from hospitals throughout the US on stages of disease, types of treatment, and effects of treatment. For example, in 1992, data were collected from hospitals representing 40% of all cancer cases in the US. Annual reports on different sites furnish important information on patterns and trends in cancer treatment.

Estimates of the number of new cases and deaths in 1994, by sex and site, are made by American Cancer Society (ACS) staff by projecting trends from published mortality and incidence data.[3]

Leading Causes of Death

Heart disease is the most common cause of death in the US, and accounts for 33.5% of all deaths. The next most common is cancer. While death rates from heart disease, stroke, and other diseases have been decreasing over the past generation, the percentage of deaths due to cancer rose from 16.8% in 1967 to 23.5% in 1990.

Prevalence of Cancer

Cancer is a disease of aging: 67% of cancer deaths occur after the age of 65. As the US population ages, cancer death rates must be statistically adjusted for age before we can observe trends and make appropriate comparisons. The age-adjusted cancer death rate per 100,000 population was 143 in 1930; 152 in 1940; 157 in 1950; and 174 in 1990. The major cause of the increase was lung cancer (Fig 1-1). If lung cancer deaths were excluded, the cancer death rate would show no increase in males and a long-term decrease in females.

The ACS estimates that in the 1980s, more than 4.5 million Americans died of cancer. In addition, there were nearly 9 million new cases and about 12 million people were under medical care for cancer. About 33% of Americans now living (about 89 million) will develop cancer if present rates continue. More than 8 million living Americans have had a history of the disease, and the diagnosis was made 5 or more years ago in about 5 million. Most of these 5 million patients are considered to be cured of cancer.

Lawrence Garfinkel, MA, Special Consultant in Epidemiology and Statistics, American Cancer Society, New York, New York

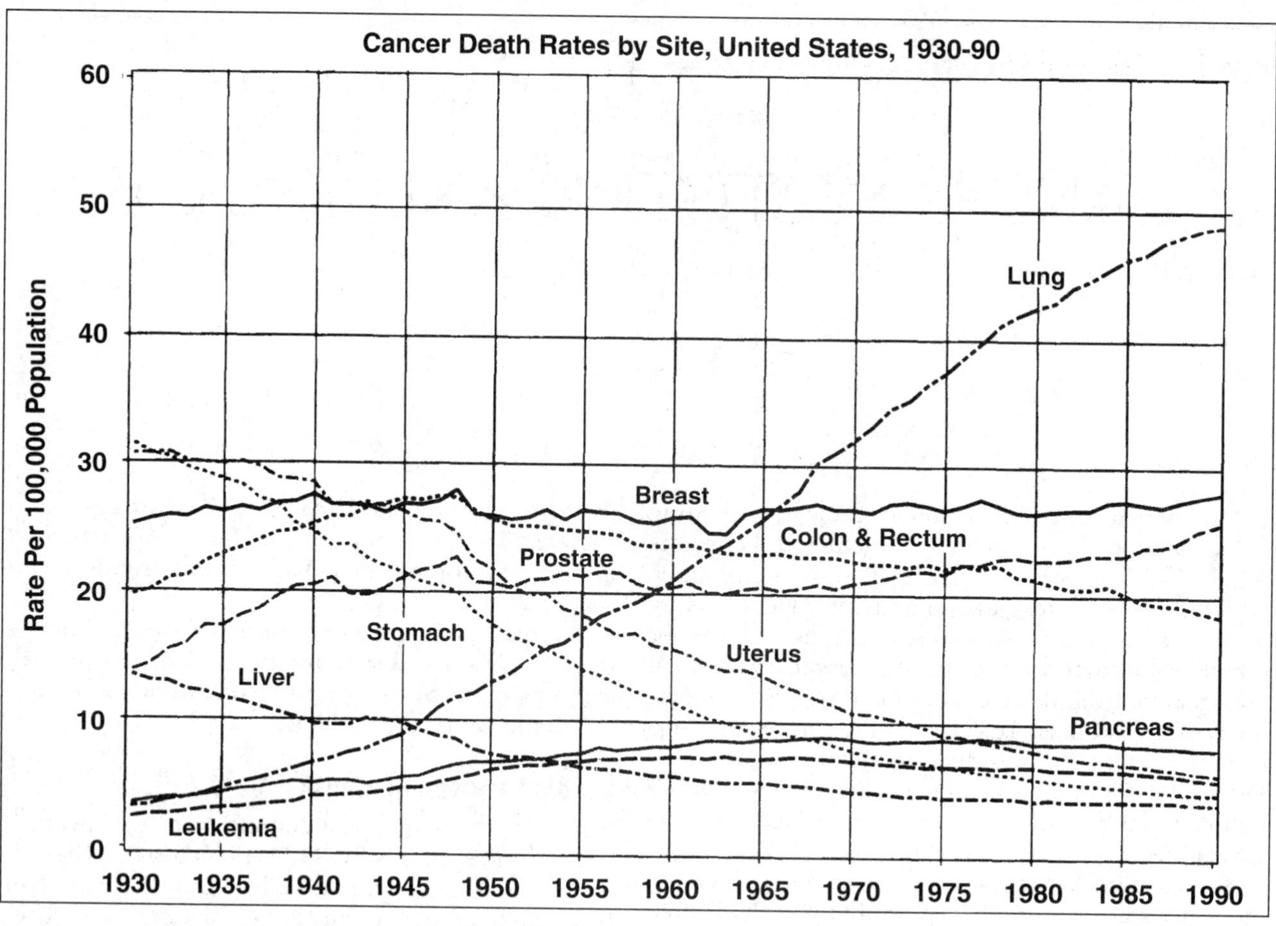

Fig 1-1. Cancer Death Rates by Site, United States 1930-90. Rates are adjusted to the age distribution of the 1970 census population. Sources of Data: National Center for Health Statistics and Bureau of the Census, United States. Note: Rates are for both sexes combined except breast and uterus (female population only) and prostate (male population only).

Survival Rates

Survival rates from cancer—that is, those who are alive 5 years after diagnosis—were 1 in 5 in the 1930s, 1 in 4 in the 1940s, and 1 in 3 in the 1960s. In recent years, 4 of 10 patients have survived 5 years: this is the observed survival rate. In terms of normal life expectancy (when other causes of death are taken into account), 53% are alive after 5 years: this is called the relative survival rate, and is the figure customarily used.

Racial and Economic Factors

Mortality and incidence rates are rising more in blacks than in whites. For example, during a 30-year period, the cancer death rate among black males rose 66%, compared with 21% in white males. Among females there was a 10% increase in blacks and virtually no change in whites. Five-year survival rates from cancer are 16% lower in blacks than in whites.

It has become evident that poor people have higher overall cancer rates. The differences in cancer death rate between blacks and whites can be attributed, in large part, to the relatively higher percentage of socioeconomically disadvantaged among blacks. Poor Americans, regardless of race, have a 10% to 15% lower 5-year survival.[4]

Statistics for Different Cancer Sites

Cancer is a family of diseases. The following discussion characterizes the mortality, morbidity, and survival data for cancers of selected sites. Estimates of the number of new cases and deaths in the US in 1994, by site and sex, are shown in Table 1-1. Survival rates appear in Table 1-2. Trends in cancer mortality rates from 1930 through 1990 are shown in Fig 1-1.

Lung

This is the most common site of cancer in both mortality and incidence, with an estimated 153,000 deaths and 172,000 new cases in 1994. Lung cancer mortality rates rose rapidly, from 7 per 100,000 population in 1940 to 50 per 100,000 in 1990. Mortality rates in men increased greatly from 1940 to 1979; in the 1980s the

Table 1-1. Estimated New Cancer Cases and Deaths, United States—1994*

	Estimated New Cases			Estimated Deaths		
	Both Sexes	Male	Female	Both Sexes	Male	Female
All sites	1,208,000	632,000	576,000	538,000	283,000	255,000
Buccal cavity & pharynx **(Oral)**	29,600	19,800	9,800	7,925	5,150	2,775
Lip	3,300	2,800	500	75	50	25
Tongue	6,000	3,800	2,200	1,750	1,100	650
Mouth	11,100	6,600	4,500	2,100	1,200	900
Pharynx	9,200	6,600	2,600	4,000	2,800	1,200
Digestive organs	233,300	123,100	110,200	121,450	64,550	56,900
Esophagus	11,000	8,000	3,000	10,400	7,800	2,600
Stomach	24,000	15,000	9,000	14,000	8,400	5,600
Small intestine	3,600	2,000	1,600	950	500	450
Large intestine } **(Colon-Rectum)**	107,000	52,000	55,000	49,000	24,000	25,000
Rectum } **(Colon-Rectum)**	42,000	23,000	19,000	7,000	3,800	3,200
Liver and biliary passages	16,100	8,800	7,300	13,200	7,200	6,000
Pancreas	27,000	13,000	14,000	25,900	12,400	13,500
Other and unspecified digestive	2,600	1,300	1,300	1,000	450	550
Respiratory system	189,000	112,800	76,200	158,200	97,900	60,300
Larynx	12,500	9,800	2,700	3,800	3,000	800
Lung	172,000	100,000	72,000	153,000	94,000	59,000
Other and unspecified respiratory	4,500	3,000	1,500	1,400	900	500
Bone	2,000	1,100	900	1,075	600	475
Connective tissue	6,000	3,300	2,700	3,300	1,600	1,700
Melanoma of skin	32,000	17,000	15,000	6,900	4,300	2,600
Breast	183,000	1,000	182,000	46,300	300	46,000
Genital organs	283,400	208,100	75,300	63,725	38,525	25,200
Cervix uteri } **(Uterus)**	15,000	—	15,000	4,600	—	4,600
Corpus and unspecified } **(Uterus)**	31,000	—	31,000	5,900	—	5,900
Ovary	24,000	—	24,000	13,600	—	13,600
Other and unspecified genital, female	5,300	—	5,300	1,100	—	1,100
Prostate	200,000	200,000	—	38,000	38,000	—
Testis	6,800	6,800	—	325	325	—
Other and unspecified genital, male	1,300	1,300	—	200	200	—
Urinary organs	78,800	55,000	23,800	21,900	13,800	8,100
Bladder	51,200	38,000	13,200	10,600	7,000	3,600
Kidney and other urinary	27,600	17,000	10,600	11,300	6,800	4,500
Eye	1,750	950	800	250	125	125
Brain and central nervous system	17,500	9,600	7,900	12,600	6,800	5,800
Endocrine glands	14,450	4,150	10,300	1,725	750	975
Thyroid	13,000	3,400	9,600	1,025	400	625
Other endocrine	1,450	750	700	700	350	350

Continued

Table 1-1 *Continued.* Estimated New Cancer Cases and Deaths, United States—1994*

	Estimated New Cases			Estimated Deaths		
	Both Sexes	Male	Female	Both Sexes	Male	Female
Leukemia	28,600	16,200	12,400	19,100	10,500	8,600
Lymphocytic leukemia	12,500	7,300	5,200	5,700	3,300	2,400
Granulocytic leukemia	11,400	6,200	5,200	7,500	4,100	3,400
Other and unspecified leukemia	4,700	2,700	2,000	5,900	3,100	2,800
Other blood and lymph tissues	65,600	35,900	29,700	32,550	17,100	15,450
Hodgkin's disease	7,900	4,400	3,500	1,550	900	650
Non-Hodgkin's lymphoma	45,000	25,000	20,000	21,200	11,200	10,000
Multiple myeloma	12,700	6,500	6,200	9,800	5,000	4,800
All other and unspecified sites	43,000	24,000	19,000	41,000	21,000	20,000

*Excludes basal and squamous cell cancers and in situ carcinomas except bladder. Carcinoma in situ of the uterine cervix accounts for about 55,000 new cases annually, carcinoma in situ of the female breast accounts for about 25,000 new cases annually, and melanoma carcinoma in situ accounts for about 8,000 new cases annually. Overall, about 100,000 new cases of carcinoma in situ of all sites of cancer are diagnosed each year.

Basal cell and squamous cell skin cancers account for more than 700,000 new cases annually. About 2,300 nonmelanoma skin cancer deaths occurred in 1994.

Incidence estimates are based on rates from NCI SEER program 1988-90.

rate of increase has been less. Five-year age-specific mortality rates in younger men (under age 55) have actually decreased. In women a rapid increase, comparable to the increase observed in men in the 1940s, was seen starting in the mid-1960s. This reflects the fact that women began smoking cigarettes later than did men. In addition, women who started smoking in the 1940s were reaching ages, 30 and 40 years later, when cancer is more prevalent.

Incidence rates published by SEER show a decrease in lung cancer in men from 86.5 per 100,000 in 1984 to 79.6 per 100,000 in 1990, after a steady rise since 1973. In women the incidence rate continues to increase, from 18.2 per 100,000 in 1973 to 40.7 per 100,000 in 1990.

Overall, only 13% of lung cancer patients—12% of males and 16% of females—survive 5 or more years after diagnosis. The survival rate is 46% for cases detected when the disease is localized, but only 16% of lung cancers are detected that early.

Table 1-2. Five-Year Survival Rates* for Selected Sites by Stage

Size	All Stages %	Local %	Regional %	Distant %
Oral	53	78	42	19
Colon-rectum	58	89	58	6
Pancreas	3	8	4	2
Lung	13	46	13	1
Melanoma	84	92	55	14
Female breast	79	93	72	18
Cervix uteri	67	90	52	13
Corpus uteri	83	94	69	27
Ovary	39	88	36	17
Prostate	77	92	82	28
Bladder	79	91	46	9
Kidney	55	86	57	10

*Adjusted for normal life expectancy. This chart based on cases diagnosed in 1983-87, followed through 1990.

Source: Cancer Statistics Branch, National Cancer Institute

Colon and Rectum

Cancer of the colon and rectum is second only to lung cancer in both incidence and mortality. Estimates for 1994 are 149,000 new cases (107,000 colon and 42,000 rectum) and 56,000 deaths. The mortality rate has shown a decline, mostly for rectal cancer, while the incidence rate has risen about 0.5% from 1973 to 1990. The incidence rate in males (59.7 per 100,000) is higher than in females (41.2 per 100,000).

The overall 5-year survival for colon and rectal cancer is 56%. However, colon cancer 5-year survival improves to 92% and rectal cancer to 85% when the disease is diagnosed at a localized stage. Survival rates for colon cancer increased from 42% in the early 1960s to 59% in recent years. For the same period, rectal cancer survival rates increased from 37% to 57%.

Breast

It is estimated that 182,000 new cases of breast cancer occurred in 1994. About one in nine women will develop breast cancer at some time during their lives, assuming life expectancy to age 85.

Breast cancer mortality rates have been fairly stable during the past 60 years: about 27 per 100,000 population. Incidence rates were stable for many years; however, there was a 32% increase from 1980 to 1987 (85 vs 112.3 per 100,000). During the same period, there has been a rapid increase in the percent of women who have mammograms,[5] and the two increases may be related. Since 1987, incidence rates have leveled off.

The 5-year survival rate is 79% for all patients, but 93% for cases diagnosed at an early stage. This trend was reflected in the results of the Breast Cancer Detection Demonstration Program (BCDDP), a study of 280,000 asymptomatic women offered annual mammograms for a 5-year period. BCDDP reported overall 5-year survival of 87%.[6]

Prostate

About 200,000 new cases were diagnosed in 1994. The incidence rate increased by 3.3% per year from 1973 to 1990, and has accelerated in recent years. About 1 in 8 men will develop prostate cancer sometime during their lifetimes. It has the highest incidence in men, after skin cancer. About 38,000 deaths are estimated for 1994, making it the second leading cause of cancer death in men. Eighty-seven percent of cases are diagnosed at age 65 and older. The incidence rate in 1990 was 128.9 per 100,000, about double the rate in 1973. Mortality rates increased 23% from 1973 to 1990. Many believe the increase in incidence is attributable to greater use of prostate-specific antigen and other diagnostic tools, such as transrectal ultrasound and digital-rectal examinations, as well as invasive procedures, such as transurethral prostatic resections.

Prostate cancer is much more common in blacks than in whites; incidence rates in 1990 were 163.6 and 128.5 per 100,000, respectively. Five-year survival rates have increased during the past 30 years from 50% to 78%. Fifty-eight percent of cases are diagnosed when in a localized stage, which has a 5-year survival rate of 92%.

Uterus (Cervix and Endometrium)

The ACS estimates that in 1994 there were 15,000 new cases of cervical cancer. Incidence and mortality rates for cervical cancer have decreased steadily over the last several decades but have increased in recent years in women under age 50. By 1990 incidence was 8.7 per 100,000. Much of the decrease has been associated with widespread use of the Pap test. While cervical cancer incidence has been decreasing, cases diagnosed as carcinoma in situ of the cervix have been increasing and are now more common than invasive cases, especially in women under age 50. An estimated 4,600 deaths from cervical cancer were projected for 1994. The mortality rate in 1990 was 3.0 per 100,000. The endometrial cancer incidence rate in 1990 was 21.2 per 100,000 and the mortality rate was 3.5 per 100,000. About 31,000 new cases are estimated for 1994 along with 5,900 deaths. Incidence and mortality rates for endometrial cancer have also been decreasing, about 3% annually for the past 30 years. Cervical cancer incidence is nearly twice as high in blacks as in whites; endometrial cancer incidence is 1.5 times as high in whites as in blacks.

The 5-year survival rate for invasive cervical cancer is 67% overall, but 90% for cases diagnosed at an early stage. The survival rate for carcinoma in situ of the cervix is virtually 100%. The 5-year survival figures for endometrial cancer are 83% for all cases and 94% for cases diagnosed as localized.

Ovary

Ovarian cancer accounts for 4% of all cancers in women. In 1994 an estimated 24,000 new cases were diagnosed and about 13,600 women died of the disease. The incidence rate (14.9 per 100,000 in 1990) has changed little over the years. The mortality rate (7.8 per 100,000) has decreased slightly. When treated early, 88% of patients survive 5 or more years. However, the 5-year survival rate is 41%, because only 23% of ovarian cancers are diagnosed early.

Oral Cavity

An estimated 29,600 new cases of cancer of the buccal cavity and pharynx were diagnosed in 1994, and an estimated 7,925 deaths were expected. The incidence rate for oral cancer (10.4 per 100,000 in 1990) has not shown much change during the past 15 years. The mortality rate (3.0 per 100,000) has decreased slightly in the past 15 years. Five-year survival rates average 52%, but vary considerably for different sites: lip, 90%; mouth, 53%; tongue, 42%; and pharynx, 32%. Incidence rates are 2.5 times as high in males as in females, and 1.5 times higher in blacks than in whites.

Bladder

Bladder cancer accounted for about 51,200 new cases in 1994, about 7% of all cancers in males, and 2% of cases in females. It is the fourth most common cancer in men and ninth most common in women. The overall incidence rate in 1990 was 16.7 per 100,000. Incidence was four times as high in males (29.2 per 100,000) as in females (7.5), and nearly twice as high in whites (17.9) as in blacks (10.1). The mortality rate was 3.3 per 100,000.

Mortality rates for both sexes have been decreasing.

The overall 5-year survival rate is 79%. When diagnosed early, bladder cancer is associated with 91% survival; when diagnosed in a regional stage, the rate is 46%; as a distant stage, it is 9%.

Pancreas

Pancreatic cancer is the fifth leading cause of cancer death. About 27,000 new cases occurred in the US in 1994 and about 25,900 patients died of the disease. It is about 1.6 times more common in blacks than in whites. Pancreatic cancer incidence and mortality rates have been fairly stable since the early 1970s. The incidence rate in 1990 was 9.1 per 100,000; the death rate, 8.3 per 100,000.

Survival rates for cancer of the pancreas are poor. Only 3% of patients survive 5 years. Nine percent of cases are diagnosed in a localized stage; of these, only 8% survive 5 years.

Leukemia

An estimated 28,600 new cases will occur in 1994—about half acute and half chronic—and there will be 19,100 deaths. Each year, leukemia strikes many more adults (26,000) than children (2,600). Among adults the most common types are acute myeloid leukemia (AML) (24% of cases) and chronic lymphocytic leukemia (30%). Among children, acute lymphoblastic leukemia (ALL) is most common (77%). The incidence rate in 1990 for leukemia was 9.2 per 100,000; the mortality rate, 6.2 per 100,000.

The overall 5-year survival rate is 38%, mainly because of poor survival for AML. During the past 30 years, however, there has been a dramatic improvement in survival of patients with ALL. In the early 1960s about 4% of white patients with ALL survived five years. This increased to 28% in the 1970s and to 52% in the 1980s. In some medical centers, optimum treatment has raised survival of children with ALL to 72%.

Stomach

In 1930 stomach cancer was the most common type of cancer; by 1994 it ranked 12th. An estimated 24,000 new cases and 14,000 deaths occurred in 1994. During the past 30 years, mortality rates have decreased 61% in males and 65% in females. The reason for the decline is not known; some suspect a correlation with changes in the national diet. Survival rates are low, only 18%. In cases diagnosed as localized, the 5-year survival rate is 56%.

Skin

The ACS estimates that more than 700,000 new cases of skin cancer occurred in 1994, most of them highly curable basal or squamous cell carcinoma. Malignant melanoma strikes about 32,000 persons a year and causes 6,900 deaths. In 1990 the incidence rate for melanoma was 9.7 per 100,000. The rate of increase in incidence is one of the highest among cancers: about 4% per year. The mortality rate in 1990 was 2.2 per 100,000. The 5-year survival rate for patients with malignant melanoma is 84%.

Other Sites

Kidney cancer, with 27,600 new cases and 11,300 deaths, has shown a 32% increase in mortality during the past 30 years. The incidence of non-Hodgkin's lymphoma (NHL) has also increased rapidly: from 8.5 per 100,000 in 1973 to 14.9 in 1990 (60%). It accounted for 45,000 new cases and 21,200 deaths in 1992. Hodgkin's disease (about 7,900 new cases and 1,550 deaths in 1994) is another cancer in which survival rates have improved greatly, from 40% in the early 1960s to 78% in recent years. Testicular cancer accounted for only 6,800 new cases and an estimated 325 deaths in 1994. Improvement in survival for cancer of the testis has been dramatic, from 63% in the 1960s to 93% in recently diagnosed cases.

Childhood Cancers

About 8,000 new cases of childhood cancer (in children under the age of 15) were estimated in 1994 and about 1,500 deaths, about one third from leukemia. Cancer is the main cause of death due to disease in children aged 1 to 14. Mortality has decreased from 8.3 per 100,000 in 1950 to 3.3 in 1990. Five-year survival rates vary according to site: for bone cancer, it is 58%; neuroblastoma, 57%; brain and central nervous system, 60%; Wilms' tumor, 88%; Hodgkin's disease, 88%; and acute lymphocytic leukemia, 72%.

Geographic Comparisons

The overall cancer death rate in the US is 174 per 100,000. It varies among states from a low of 124 in Utah to a high of 230 in the District of Columbia. Cancer death rates are generally higher in New England and the mid-Atlantic states, and lower in the West and Southwest.

Cancer mortality rates vary even more among countries. Colorectal cancer is four times higher in Luxembourg than in Greece. Stomach cancer is six times higher in Japan than in the US. Esophageal cancer in northern Iran is 10 times higher than in Israel. Liver cancer is 100 times more common in parts of Africa than in England. In general, the highest rates are in the more developed European countries. Mortality rates associated with lung, breast, colon, and rectal cancers are higher in more developed countries, and rates associated with cervical and stomach cancers are high in Third World countries. Japan has relatively low death rates for breast, colon, and rectal cancers but high stomach cancer death rates. Lung cancer death rates in Japan are rising rapidly (Table 1-3).

Table 1-3. Cancer Around the World, 1988-91. Age-standardized Death Rates* per 100,000 Population for Selected Sites for 46 Countries

Country	All Sites		Oral		Colon and Rectum		Prostate
	Male	Female	Male	Female	Male	Female	Male
United States	164.4 (24)	110.6 (11)	3.7 (29)	1.3 (12)	16.7 (20)	11.4 (19)	16.8 (17)
Argentina††	151.8 (29)	97.6 (26)	4.0 (26)	0.9 (35)	13.7 (31)	9.3 (33)	13.1 (29)
Australia†	164.0 (25)	102.2 (22)	4.7 (20)	1.3 (13)	21.5 (9)	14.7 (9)	17.2 (15)
Austria	172.3 (18)	106.9 (19)	5.9 (16)	0.9 (33)	22.4 (6)	14.2 (11)	16.7 (18)
Bulgaria	139.0 (37)	84.2 (38)	3.8 (28)	0.6 (45)	15.1 (25)	10.7 (26)	7.8 (39)
Canada#	170.8 (21)	110.6 (12)	4.4 (22)	1.3 (14)	17.8 (17)	12.0 (17)	16.9 (16)
Chile††	140.8 (36)	109.4 (14)	2.3 (39)	0.6 (44)	7.0 (40)	6.0 (41)	13.1 (28)
China††+	154.1 (27)	87.3 (35)	2.5 (36)	1.2 (17)	7.9 (39)	6.5 (40)	—
Costa Rica††	166.6 (22)	108.6 (16)	3.2 (31)	1.0 (25)	6.6 (42)	6.7 (39)	19.6 (5)
Cuba#	129.8 (39)	95.6 (28)	5.6 (19)	2.0 (3)	10.2 (36)	11.4 (20)	18.7 (7)
Czechoslovakia#	232.8 (2)	121.0 (8)	9.0 (6)	2.0 (26)	30.7 (1)	17.0 (4)	13.6 (26)
Denmark	179.5 (11)	139.8 (1)	4.0 (27)	1.4 (9)	22.8 (5)	17.5 (3)	18.1 (10)
Ecuador†	83.6 (45)	85.2 (37)	0.7 (46)	0.7 (40)	2.7 (46)	4.1 (45)	11.1 (32)
England and Wales	179.2 (12)	125.7 (6)	2.9 (33)	1.2 (18)	20.2 (12)	13.7 (14)	16.6 (20)
Finland	154.1 (28)	90.6 (32)	2.3 (40)	0.8 (39)	12.2 (35)	8.6 (36)	17.5 (12)
France#	200.7 (5)	88.1 (34)	13.6 (3)	1.3 (15)	17.3 (19)	10.3 (27)	17.3 (13)
Germany, Fed.##	177.9 (13)	108.3 (17)	6.3 (13)	1.0 (22)	21.1 (10)	15.2 (6)	15.9 (21)
Greece#	144.3 (34)	77.5 (43)	1.6 (44)	0.6 (46)	6.8 (41)	5.5 (42)	8.1 (38)
Hong Kong††	175.1 (16)	91.0 (31)	14.5 (2)	4.4 (2)	14.8 (29)	10.7 (25)	2.6 (45)
Hungary	246.5 (1)	131.5 (3)	14.7 (1)	1.7 (5)	29.0 (2)	18.1 (2)	15.7 (22)
Iceland	147.6 (32)	114.6 (10)	2.1 (42)	1.0 (27)	14.9 (27)	10.8 (24)	19.4 (6)
Ireland#	174.9 (17)	127.5 (4)	4.4 (24)	1.0 (28)	23.2 (4)	15.1 (7)	17.6 (11)
Israel††	115.5 (42)	98.7 (24)	1.0 (45)	0.7 (42)	14.4 (30)	11.9 (18)	8.6 (37)
Italy††	192.3 (10)	99.2 (23)	6.3 (11)	1.0 (23)	15.6 (21)	10.3 (28)	11.5 (31)
Japan	150.2 (30)	76.7 (44)	2.3 (41)	0.6 (43)	15.1 (24)	9.7 (32)	3.8 (44)
Luxembourg	197.6 (8)	109.4 (15)	10.1 (5)	1.4 (10)	21.8 (7)	12.4 (16)	16.6 (19)
Malta	144.0 (35)	92.5 (30)	3.6 (30)	1.6 (6)	13.5 (32)	10.0 (31)	9.1 (35)
Mauritius	85.0 (44)	62.3 (46)	4.6 (21)	1.8 (4)	5.0 (44)	4.1 (44)	5.3 (42)
Mexico#	83.5 (46)	79.7 (42)	2.0 (43)	0.7 (41)	3.3 (45)	3.1 (46)	10.6 (33)
Netherlands#	195.3 (9)	109.8 (13)	2.8 (35)	1.0 (32)	17.9 (16)	13.3 (15)	18.3 (9)
New Zealand††	171.9 (19)	126.8 (5)	4.3 (25)	1.4 (8)	25.7 (3)	20.5 (1)	18.7 (8)
Northern Ireland	176.6 (14)	122.3 (7)	2.8 (34)	1.0 (31)	21.5 (8)	14.8 (8)	15.4 (23)
Norway#	148.2 (31)	102.2 (21)	3.1 (32)	1.1 (20)	20.0 (13)	14.2 (10)	21.7 (2)
Poland	203.5 (4)	107.8 (18)	6.2 (14)	1.0 (24)	14.9 (26)	10.2 (29)	9.8 (34)
Portugal	145.9 (33)	86.6 (36)	5.7 (18)	0.8 (37)	15.3 (22)	10.1 (30)	14.5 (25)
Puerto Rico#	125.5 (41)	75.1 (45)	7.9 (7)	1.4 (7)	9.6 (38)	7.4 (37)	17.3 (14)
Romania	135.3 (38)	83.8 (39)	5.7 (17)	1.0 (29)	9.7 (37)	7.2 (38)	7.1 (40)
Scotland	198.5 (6)	137.1 (2)	4.4 (23)	1.3 (11)	20.6 (11)	15.2 (5)	14.9 (24)
Singapore#	175.3 (15)	103.9 (20)	12.9 (4)	4.4 (1)	19.1 (14)	14.0 (13)	4.2 (43)
Spain††	166.3 (23)	80.8 (41)	6.3 (12)	0.8 (38)	13.2 (34)	9.2 (35)	12.9 (30)
Sweden††	129.4 (40)	98.1 (25)	2.4 (38)	0.8 (36)	14.9 (38)	11.1 (21)	20.4 (3)
Switzerland	171.1 (20)	97.2 (27)	6.6 (10)	1.2 (16)	18.2 (15)	10.9 (23)	22.5 (1)
Uruguay#	204.7 (3)	116.6 (9)	6.0 (15)	0.9 (34)	17.7 (18)	14.1 (12)	19.9 (4)
USSR#	198.3 (7)	94.5 (29)	7.4 (8)	1.0 (30)	15.2 (23)	10.9 (22)	6.3 (41)
Venezuela††	92.7 (43)	83.7 (40)	2.4 (37)	1.1 (19)	5.7 (43)	5.2 (43)	13.3 (27)
Yugoslavia#	158.4 (26)	90.2 (33)	6.9 (9)	1.0 (21)	13.4 (33)	9.3 (34)	8.9 (36)

Continued

Table 1-3 *Continued.* Cancer Around the World, 1988-91. Age-standardized Death Rates* per 100,000 Population for Selected Sites for 46 Countries

	Lung		Breast	Uterus		Stomach		Leukemia	
Country	Male	Female	Female	Cervix	Other	Male	Female	Male	Female
United States	57.1 (10)	24.7 (2)	22.4 (16)	2.6 (31)	2.6 (33)	5.2 (46)	2.3 (46)	6.3 (8)	3.8 (9)
Argentina††	39.2 (30)	5.8 (38)	20.9 (19)	4.6 (16)	6.5 (5)	12.8 (26)	5.6 (29)	4.6 (33)	3.3 (28)
Australia†	45.1 (25)	12.8 (15)	20.7 (21)	3.1 (29)	1.7 (44)	8.4 (41)	3.6 (44)	6.1 (11)	3.8 (10)
Austria	45.1 (24)	9.0 (20)	22.0 (17)	2.9 (30)	5.1 (9)	16.7 (19)	8.2 (15)	5.4 (21)	3.5 (24)
Bulgaria	40.3 (29)	6.3 (36)	15.6 (31)	4.1 (22)	6.0 (7)	19.8 (11)	10.7 (9)	4.5 (36)	2.9 (43)
Canada#	57.3 (9)	20.6 (6)	23.9 (12)	2.3 (37)	2.5 (35)	8.0 (42)	3.4 (45)	6.2 (10)	3.9 (8)
Chile††	21.1 (40)	5.8 (39)	12.5 (39)	12.5 (2)	2.4 (38)	35.2 (3)	13.6 (6)	3.9 (42)	3.3 (32)
China††+	34.0 (33)	14.5 (13)	4.6 (46)	4.2 (21)	—	32.6 (5)	15.7 (4)	4.1 (40)	3.3 (27)
Costa Rica††	17.5 (43)	6.4 (34)	12.9 (38)	10.4 (3)	3.5 (22)	54.7 (1)	22.8 (1)	6.2 (9)	4.9 (1)
Cuba#	39.0 (32)	14.3 (14)	14.8 (33)	6.2 (9)	7.3 (4)	7.3 (45)	3.8 (42)	4.6 (32)	3.6 (16)
Czechoslovakia#	74.4 (2)	8.3 (22)	19.8 (22)	5.6 (11)	5.7 (8)	19.7 (12)	8.9 (12)	6.7 (4)	4.3 (4)
Denmark	51.9 (15)	23.9 (3)	27.7 (4)	5.3 (12)	3.5 (23)	7.8 (43)	4.2 (41)	6.8 (3)	4.1 (5)
Ecuador†	6.9 (46)	2.8 (46)	5.6 (45)	5.8 (10)	13.7 (1)	26.9 (6)	19.2 (2)	3.7 (45)	3.2 (33)
England and Wales	57.0 (11)	20.5 (7)	28.7 (1)	4.4 (18)	2.5 (34)	12.5 (29)	5.1 (31)	5.3 (24)	3.3 (31)
Finland	47.8 (21)	6.6 (33)	17.0 (28)	1.7 (43)	2.6 (31)	13.0 (25)	7.0 (23)	5.2 (25)	3.0 (38)
France#	46.8 (22)	5.0 (41)	19.7 (23)	1.8 (40)	4.0 (17)	9.1 (38)	3.6 (43)	6.1 (13)	3.7 (15)
Germany, Fed.##	48.7 (19)	7.8 (26)	21.9 (18)	3.6 (25)	3.2 (25)	14.9 (21)	7.7 (17)	5.9 (14)	3.7 (13)
Greece#	49.8 (17)	6.9 (32)	15.2 (32)	1.3 (45)	3.0 (26)	9.6 (36)	4.9 (34)	5.7 (16)	3.4 (25)
Hong Kong††	54.2 (14)	23.3 (5)	8.6 (41)	3.9 (23)	1.4 (45)	11.5 (31)	5.3 (30)	3.8 (43)	2.7 (45)
Hungary	76.4 (1)	14.9 (12)	22.6 (15)	6.8 (7)	5.0 (11)	24.0 (8)	10.2 (10)	7.2 (1)	4.6 (2)
Iceland	30.8 (34)	23.8 (4)	23.7 (13)	2.6 (34)	1.8 (42)	18.1 (15)	7.7 (18)	4.9 (29)	3.1 (37)
Ireland#	47.9 (20)	19.2 (8)	27.8 (3)	3.2 (27)	2.9 (27)	12.0 (30)	5.9 (27)	6.1 (12)	3.7 (12)
Israel††	24.5 (38)	7.9 (24)	23.0 (14)	1.4 (44)	2.2 (39)	7.7 (44)	4.2 (40)	6.4 (7)	4.5 (3)
Italy††	58.9 (8)	7.3 (28)	20.8 (20)	0.9 (46)	5.1 (10)	18.2 (14)	8.6 (13)	6.7 (5)	4.0 (7)
Japan	30.1 (36)	8.0 (23)	6.3 (44)	1.8 (41)	2.4 (37)	34.9 (4)	15.5 (5)	4.3 (38)	2.8 (44)
Luxembourg	62.9 (7)	8.8 (21)	25.4 (10)	3.2 (28)	4.5 (14)	11.3 (32)	4.3 (38)	6.7 (6)	3.6 (21)
Malta	42.2 (28)	3.7 (44)	28.1 (2)	1.9 (39)	3.8 (20)	14.9 (22)	6.1 (26)	5.4 (22)	3.6 (17)
Mauritius	18.9 (42)	5.1 (40)	6.7 (43)	3.6 (24)	7.4 (3)	12.7 (27)	7.2 (21)	3.5 (46)	2.3 (46)
Mexico#	16.5 (45)	5.9 (37)	8.1 (42)	15.9 (1)	2.6 (32)	10.5 (35)	7.6 (19)	3.8 (44)	3.0 (40)
Netherlands#	71.2 (4)	10.2 (17)	26.8 (7)	2.5 (35)	2.5 (36)	13.1 (23)	5.0 (33)	5.6 (18)	3.5 (23)
New Zealand††	44.4 (27)	17.3 (11)	27.0 (6)	4.5 (17)	2.8 (28)	8.8 (40)	4.7 (35)	7.2 (2)	4.1 (6)
Northern Ireland	55.4 (12)	17.8 (9)	26.5 (8)	3.5 (26)	2.0 (41)	12.6 (28)	6.7 (25)	4.5 (34)	3.2 (34)
Norway#	30.3 (35)	10.3 (16)	19.2 (24)	4.3 (19)	2.8 (29)	11.0 (34)	5.0 (32)	4.9 (28)	3.3 (30)
Poland	70.4 (5)	9.7 (19)	15.7 (30)	7.9 (6)	4.0 (16)	23.1 (9)	8.2 (14)	5.8 (15)	3.6 (18)
Portugal	26.0 (37)	4.4 (43)	17.8 (26)	2.3 (36)	4.9 (12)	24.9 (7)	12.0 (7)	5.0 (27)	3.7 (14)
Puerto Rico#	19.5 (41)	7.0 (31)	14.2 (35)	2.6 (32)	3.5 (21)	11.0 (33)	4.5 (36)	4.8 (30)	3.5 (22)
Romania	39.1 (31)	6.4 (35)	14.8 (34)	10.3 (4)	3.9 (18)	18.2 (13)	7.1 (22)	4.5 (35)	3.0 (39)
Scotland	71.3 (3)	28.3 (1)	27.1 (5)	4.6 (15)	2.1 (40)	13.1 (24)	5.9 (28)	4.4 (37)	3.1 (35)
Singapore#	50.6 (16)	17.5 (10)	12.9 (37)	6.4 (8)	1.8 (43)	20.3 (10)	10.8 (8)	4.2 (39)	3.0 (41)
Spain††	45.2 (23)	3.4 (45)	17.1 (27)	1.7 (42)	3.8 (19)	15.0 (20)	6.9 (24)	5.3 (23)	3.4 (26)
Sweden††	23.4 (39)	9.9 (18)	18.2 (25)	2.2 (38)	2.7 (30)	8.9 (39)	4.5 (37)	5.1 (26)	3.3 (29)
Switzerland	44.9 (26)	7.2 (29)	24.3 (11)	2.6 (33)	3.3 (24)	9.6 (37)	4.2 (39)	5.6 (17)	3.6 (20)
Uruguay#	55.0 (13)	4.6 (42)	26.4 (9)	4.7 (14)	6.4 (6)	17.0 (18)	7.3 (20)	5.5 (20)	3.8 (11)
USSR#	63.6 (6)	7.1 (30)	13.6 (36)	5.2 (13)	4.4 (15)	36.8 (2)	16.0 (3)	5.5 (19)	3.6 (19)
Venezuela††	16.5 (44)	7.9 (25)	9.6 (40)	9.7 (5)	7.9 (2)	17.1 (17)	9.5 (11)	4.0 (41)	3.1 (36)
Yugoslavia#	48.9 (18)	7.3 (27)	15.9 (29)	4.2 (20)	4.6 (13)	18.0 (16)	7.8 (16)	4.7 (31)	3.0 (42)

Note: Figures in parentheses are order of rank within site and sex group. †1988 only. ††1988-1989 only. #1988-1990 only. ##1989-1990 only. *Rates are age-adjusted to the WHO world standard population. +Oral cancer mortality rate includes nasopharynx only.

References

1. *Vital Statistics of the United States.* Washington, DC: US Public Health Service, National Center for Health Statistics; 1934-1990.

2. Miller BA, Ries LAG, Hankey BF, et al. SEER Cancer Statistics Review: 1973-1990. Bethesda, Md: National Cancer Institute. 1993. NIH publication no 93-2789.

3. Boring CC, Squires TS, Tong T, Montgomery S. Cancer statistics, 1994. *CA Cancer J Clin.* 1994;44:7-26.

4. Freeman HP. Cancer in the economically disadvantaged. *Cancer.* 1989;64(suppl):324-334.

5. Gallup Organization. *The 1987 Survey of Public Awareness and Use of Cancer Detection Tests.* Princeton, NJ: The Gallup Organization; 1988.

6. Seidman H, Gelb SK, Silverberg E, et al. Survival experience in the Breast Cancer Detection Demonstration Project. *CA Cancer J Clin.* 1987;37:258-290.

2

CAUSES OF CANCER

John H. Weisburger, PhD, MD (hon), Gary M. Williams, MD

All cancers have causes. Discovering these causes may spare future generations preventable cancer.

Many major diseases no longer threaten human life and well-being because of prevention—the definitive cure. In the field of cancer causation, similar successes have been achieved.

The link between cancer in humans and occupational exposure first came to public and professional attention with the discovery of scrotal cancer in chimney sweeps and urinary bladder cancer in chemical industry workers. Subsequently, a number of industrial chemicals were found to produce cancer in humans (Table 2-1).[1] During the 1940s, the heavy exposure of shipyard and insulation workers in the United States to asbestos fibers led to a low but definite incidence of mesothelioma, that even today claims about 400 lives per year. More important, such industrial workers who were also cigarette smokers had a high risk of cancer of the lung. Such cases are now becoming mortality statistics, even though exposure occurred decades ago during hazardous working conditions that have since been corrected.

Because the history of research in cancer causation has documented cancer induced by exposure to certain chemicals in the workplace, environmental pollution is thought by many to be a major cause of many forms of cancer. Yet, careful research over the past 30 years has failed to prove this supposition. According to current estimates, no more than 5% of all cancers, but more likely a lesser percentage, can be traced directly to occupational or environmental exposure.[2-4] Observations show that anywhere in the world, lifestyle and lifestyle-related behavior are more likely to cause or promote cancer development. For the most part, this progress has been made not by determining what type of carcinogen, eg, benzo(a)pyrene or 4-aminobiphenyl, would yield what type of cancer, but rather by starting with a specific neoplastic disease and elucidating the etiologic factors and environmental conditions associated with its development. In other words, an organ-site basis for research has disclosed the major causative factors of specific cancers (Table 2-2). In many instances, the associated factors are not single chemicals or substances, but complex lifestyle-related mixtures with distinct characteristics that act through well-defined mechanisms.

Prior to a review of this field, it will be useful to briefly explore (1) the mechanisms of carcinogenesis as a basis for delineating and classifying risk factors, and (2) the methods for detecting carcinogens in the broadest sense. It is fairly certain that neoplastic disease stems from a somatic mutation. Once the genetic factors of a cell system undergo a change, the damage is generally irreversible after several cell duplication cycles. Environmental chemicals and ionizing radiation, as well as lifestyle factors, have been demonstrated to react with chromosomes and especially DNA, a reaction with important functional consequences.

Other agents display no evidence of interaction with DNA. Such nongenotoxic chemicals, which nevertheless demonstrate an enhancing effect in cancer causation under a variety of conditions in vitro, in animal models, or in man, may operate by promoting mechanisms or other epigenetic effects (Table 2-3). Most chemicals that cause cancer in humans are of the DNA-reactive type, but some epigenetic agents have also led to cancer (Table 2-1). Thus, it is important to define the specific factors associated with each type of human cancer and determine which have genotoxic properties, and which promoting or otherwise enhancing agents also play a role (Table 2-4). Cancer prevention depends on a careful evaluation of the genotoxic and promoting factors in each type of cancer, and inhibition of their often complex actions.

For example, the chief cause of cancer of the

John H. Weisburger, PhD, MD (hon), Senior Member, Director Emeritus, American Health Foundation, Valhalla, New York

Gary M. Williams, MD, Director, Medical Sciences, American Health Foundation, Valhalla, New York

Table 2-1. Chemicals and Mixtures Judged to be Carcinogenic to Humans by the International Agency for Research on Cancer

DNA-Reactive	
Aflatoxins	Coal tars
4-Aminobiphenyl	Cyclophosphamide
2-Aminonaphthalene	Melphalan
5-Azacytidine	MOPP (nitrogen mustard, vincristine, procarbazine, and prednisone)
Benzidine	Nickel and nickel compounds
Betel quid with tobacco	Phenacetin-containing analgesic mixtures
N,N-bis(2-Chloroethyl)-2-aminonaphthalene	Soot
bis (Chloromethyl) ether	Sulfur mustard
1,4-Butanediol dimethanesulfonate (Myleran)	Triethylenethiophosphoramide (thiotepa)
Chlorambucil	Tobacco smoke and products
1-(2-Chloroethyl)ether (methylcyclohexyl)-1-nitrosourea	Treosulphan
Hexavalent chromium compounds	Vinyl chloride
Epigenetic	
Azathioprine	Oral contraceptives
Cyclosporin A	Steroidal estrogens
Unclassified	
Alcoholic beverages	Shale oils
Arsenic and arsenic compounds	Untreated and mildly treated mineral oils
Benzene	

From International Agency for Research on Cancer.[1] The table does not include processes or fibers. The classification is according to Williams and Weisburger.[3]

glandular stomach appears to be a DNA-reactive chemical, as demonstrated by studies of migrants relocating from high- to low-risk areas of the world who maintain their risk,[5] and from animal models, in which a few doses of a gastric carcinogen lead eventually to the occurrence of gastric cancer. On the other hand, while tobacco smoke contains a number of genotoxic carcinogens, lung cancer stems largely from the presence of nongenotoxic, cytotoxic enhancing factors.[6] On cessation of smoking, the effect of these enhancing factors is reversible, and individuals who stop smoking have a progressively lower risk of lung cancer (Table 2-5). Research in models for breast cancer, in which the level as well as type of dietary fat plays an important promoting role, has demonstrated that lowering the fat level and modifying the type reduce the extent of mammary carcinogenesis.[7] The Women's Intervention Nutrition Study uses a low-fat (20% of total calories) dietary regimen to establish whether a lower risk for breast cancer would result, a likely outcome based on current concepts.[8]

Table 2-2. Documentation in the Elucidation of the Etiology of Human Cancers

I. Epidemiology
   A. Geographic pathology
   B. Migrant populations
   C. Special populations
   D. Time trends

II. Laboratory studies
   A. Metabolic and biochemical epidemiology (population studies)
   B. Model studies in animals
   C. Model studies in cell and organ cultures
   D. Definition of mechanisms

III. Development and validation of hypotheses
   A. Established risk factors and their mode of action
   B. Suspected risk factors and their possible role

Table 2-3. Classes of Carcinogenic Chemicals

Type of Agent	Mode of Action	Example
A. Genotoxic		
1. Activation-independent	Electrophile, organic compound, interacts with DNA	Ethylene imine; bis (chloromethyl) ether; alkylating agents
2. Activation-dependent (procarcinogen)	Requires conversion through metabolic activation by host or in vitro to type 1 (above) agent	Vinyl chloride, benzo(a)pyrene, 2-naphthylamine, 2-amino-3-methyl-imidazo[4,5-*f*]-quinoline dimethylnitrosamine
3. Activation-independent (inorganic)	Not directly genotoxic, leads to changes in DNA by selective alteration in fidelity of DNA replication; can block DNA repair	Nickel, chromium, arsenic cadium*
B. Epigenetic		
4. Solid-state carcinogen	Usually affects only mesenchymal cells and tissues; physical form vital; exact mechanism unknown, but may increase cell cycling and generation of hydroxy radicals	Polymer or metal foils; asbestos
5. Hormone	Mainly alters endocrine system balance and differentiation: often acts as promoter; usually not genotoxic	Estradiol, diethylstilbestrol, amitrole
6. Immunosuppressor	Mainly stimulates "virally induced," transplanted, or metastatic neoplasms; usually not genotoxic	Azathioprine, antilymphocytic serum, cyclosporin A
7. Peroxisome proliferator	Increases generation of hydroxy radicals, overloading cellular defenses	Clofibrate, diethylhexylphthalate
8. Cytotoxin	Not genotoxic or carcinogenic; above specific dosages, kills cells, increases regeneration and cell cycling, can cause inflammation and generate active oxygen	Butylated hydroxyanisole; nitrilotriacetate; carbon tetrachloride
9. Promoter	Not genotoxic or carcinogenic, but enhances effect of type 1 or type 2 agent, often increases cell cycling; induces enzymes like ornithine decarboxylases or blocks phosphatases	Phorbol esters, phenols, bile acids, sodium saccharin

*Some metal ions react with DNA, but others may involve epigenetic mechanisms, such as changes in fidelity of DNA polymerases.

Thus, human cancers involve genotoxic carcinogens and, depending on the tissue affected, powerful enhancing and promoting factors. These factors will be discussed on the basis of either organ site (Table 2-6) or mechanism of action of carcinogens, promoters, and inhibitors in lifestyle-related etiologic mechanisms (Table 2-7).

Well-controlled multidisciplinary studies of the causes of major diseases have disclosed the main factors contributing to premature death or disability from coronary heart disease, stroke, and major types of cancer.[2,4,5,7,9] The causative factors for these chronic diseases are interrelated, and effective, simultaneous control can be achieved by research-based reduction of these factors. Since cancer is, in effect, many distinct diseases, confusion can ensue unless a detailed analysis is made to delineate the elements causing, or enhancing the risk for, each kind of cancer.

Table 2-4. Types of Agents Associated with the Etiology of Human Cancers

Problems or questions to be resolved for each type of cancer:

I. Nature of genotoxic carcinogens or mixtures: can be chemical, viral, or associated with radiation
II. Nature of any nongenotoxic promoting or enhancing stimulus: can be chemical or viral
III. Amount, duration of exposure, and potency of each kind of agent
IV. Possibility of inhibition of the action of agents under I or II above

Effective prevention requires identification of the real causes of each type of cancer.

Time trends, worldwide incidence, and mortality figures for diverse cancers, the altered risk of migrants moving from areas of high to low incidence, and the analysis of data obtained under controlled conditions in animal models provided clues to the etiology of each major human cancer (Table 2-8). Leads were developed further by laboratory research groups who, by studying the risk factors under highly controlled experimental conditions, gained insight into the underlying mechanisms, which, in turn, could be validated through a multidisciplinary team approach. "Spontaneous" changes in disease incidence or mortality, such as the decline of gastric cancer in the US over the past 50 years, have also provided clues as to etiology.[5,10-14] Through such approaches, it has been established that cancer, for the most part, stems from elements of lifestyle (Table 2-9).[15]

The term *lifestyle,* as used here, refers to certain self-imposed habits practiced by the individual, such as cigarette smoking and other tobacco use, as well as to prevailing dietary customs. In the Western world, dietary patterns have led to a high rate of coronary heart disease and specific types of cancer (eg, of the breast, colon, and pancreas), and, to some extent, to hypertension and stroke. In Japan, particularly the northern region, the traditional diet has conveyed a high risk for hypertensive disease, stroke, and distinct kinds of cancer (eg, of the stomach, esophagus, and liver). This pattern also occurs in parts of Latin America, although the underlying mechanism may differ. Frequent alcohol use bears on cancer causation at specific target organs such as liver or rectum. If an individual smokes and consumes alcohol frequently, he or she may be at risk for cancer of the mouth or esophagus.

The medical practitioner will be helped by insight into disease mechanisms because recurrence may be minimized. Modern medicine needs to take advantage of the achievements of research, the subject of this chapter, to reduce "recalls" in the medical field. Good medical management includes advising patients and the general public of effective means of cancer prevention.

Mechanisms of Carcinogenesis

The concept that chemicals can induce cancer by a variety of modes of action is derived from an understanding of the complex processes of carcinogenesis.[3,16,17] A series of essential steps appear to be involved in cancer causation and development (Fig 2-1). Neoplastic conversion begins with production of an altered DNA in the cell by attack from a reactive form of carcinogen or the effective generation of hydroxy radicals. This reaction, in turn, leads to mutation of specific genes, proto-oncogenes, and tumor suppressor genes, which translate to abnormal properties of the cells bearing such altered genes. Recognition of these effects, in turn, has provided the basis for determining through specific rapid, efficient, and economical in vitro bioassays whether a given substance might induce a mutation in prokaryotic or

Table 2-5. Irreversibility or Reversibility of Carcinogenesis as a Function of Mechanism of Action

Type of Cancer	Type and Mode of Action of Carcinogen	Reversibility	Evidence
Glandular stomach	Genotoxic from salted, pickled foods	Poor	Migrant studies: maintenance of risk in migrants
Lung	Small amounts of genotoxic carcinogens: polycyclic aromatic hydrocarbons and nicotine-derived nitrosamines. Large amounts of epigenetic cytotoxic enhancing agents: phenols, catechols, terpenes	Good	People who stop smoking have progressively lower risk

Table 2-6. Types of Cancer Associated with Tobacco Use

Organ	Additional Factors
Oral cavity, Upper gastrointestinal tract, respiratory tract	Alcohol, chewing tobacco, inadequate nutrition
Lung	Asbestos, mineral and radioactive dusts, air pollution
Pancreas	High-fat diet, heterocyclic amines, others?
Kidneys, bladder	Diet (high protein)
Cervix	Human papillomavirus; poor nutritional status

eukaryotic cell systems.[3,18] Advantage can also be taken of the presence of enzyme systems performing DNA repair to provide complementary effective test systems to outline the possible DNA reactivity of chemicals.[19] When a specific chemical displays properties of reacting with DNA,[20] inducing mutations and DNA repair in a number of cell systems, it is designated DNA-reactive or genotoxic. Most human carcinogens are genotoxic (Table 2-1); some agents such as the hormone diethylstilbestrol (DES) or estradiol may give rise to genotoxic products. Thus, the determination that a given product is reliably genotoxic signals a potential cancer risk to man, given appropriate dosage and chronicity of exposure.

During cellular metabolism, reactive oxygen, hydroxy radicals, or hydrogen peroxide can be generated. There are endogenous defense mechanisms, such as catalase-destroying hydrogen peroxide, superoxide dismutase, or glutathione peroxidase (in turn involving glutathione [GSH], or sulfhydryl amino acids), that neutralize reactive oxygen. Exogenous antioxidants, vitamins C and E, and sources of GSH aid in the disposition of reactive species. However, modification of DNA with formation of nucleotides containing 8-hydroxydeoxyguanine (8-OHdG) can occur, especially in the presence of carcinogens.[6,21] 8-OHdG also can be eliminated, a form of DNA repair. A specific case is that of methylating and ethylating agents, yielding the key O^6-alkylguanines, that can be repaired by a specific enzyme system operating under stoichiometric (mole for mole) conditions, transferring the O^6-methyl group to an SH-residue on the methyltransferase.[22] Many actions of methylating or alkylating carcinogens of this type have been clarified by understanding this kind of repair mechanism.

The consequences of DNA-carcinogen interactions are being intensively explored in terms of protooncogene and tumor suppressor gene mutations, which can be measured by highly specific and sensitive polymerase chain reaction techniques.[6,17,23-28] The results can serve as diagnostic tools and guides to prognosis.

Table 2-7. Nutritionally Linked Cancers

Site	Carcinogen From	Promoter		Inhibitors
		From	Mechanism	
Esophagus	Pickled, salted foods; alcohol	Alcohol	Carcinogen activation	Yellow-green vegetables, tea
Stomach	Pickled, smoked foods; nitrate	Salt, *H pylori*	Atrophic gastritis	Yellow-green vegetables, tea
Liver	Mycotoxins, nitrosamines, Senecio alkaloids, hepatitis antigen	Hepatitis antigen Alcohol	Cytotoxicity Cytotoxicity	Vaccine
Colon	Fried foods	Fats	Bile acids	Bran fiber, calcium ions, vegetables
Rectum	Fried foods	Fats, alcohol	Bile acids, cytotoxicity	Bran fiber, calcium ions, vegetables
Breast	Fried foods	Fats	Hormonal balances	Vegetables, fruits
Prostate	Fried foods? Hydroxy radicals?	Fats	Hormonal balances	Vegetables, fruits
Endometrium and ovary	Hydroxy radicals?	Fats	Obesity, estrogen	Vegetables, fruits

Table 2-8. Factors and Possible Mechanisms in Main Epithelial Cancer Causation and Prevention

Disease	Risk Factors	Mechanism	Protective Elements	Mechanism
Lung cancer	Cigarette smoking	Complex mixture of genotoxic carcinogens, polycylic aromatic hydrocarbons, tobacco-specific nitrosamines, and risk-determining enhancing, promoting agents; asbestos, air pollutants and dietary fats have strong cocarcinogenic effect	Yellow-green vegetables	Retinoids, β-carotene, other inhibitors
	Occupational	Polycyclic hydrocarbons, coal gas, bis(chloromethyl) ether, bis(chloroethyl)sulfide, arsenic, nickel, and chromate ores, asbestos		
Oral cancer	Smoking; tobacco or betel chewing; smoking plus alcohol	Carcinogens in tobacco (mainly tobacco-specific nitrosamines), betel nut	Yellow-green vegetables	Retinoids, β-carotene, other inhibitors
Kidney cancer	Smoking; high protein diets; other factors unknown; obesity	Carcinogens from tobacco, unknown mechanisms; fat cells produce estrogens as possible carcinogens; cell cycling	Water intake?	Dilution?
			Weight control/loss	Lowers excessive nonphysiologic estrogen level
Bladder cancer	Bilharzia; schistosomiasis	Carcinogens unknown; hydroxy radicals? increased cell proliferation enhances risk	Yellow-green vegetables	?
	Smoking; high protein diets	Unknown (arylamines? tobacco nitrosamines?)	Yellow-green vegetables	Retinoids
	Occupational	Chronic high-dose arylamines	High water intake	Dilution
Endocrine-related cancers (prostate, breast, ovary)	Total dietary fat (saturated + ω-6-poly-unsaturated lipids)	Complex multieffector elements: hormonal balances, membrane and intracellular effectors, hydroxy radicals	Monounsaturated oil (olive)	Neutral action on hormone metabolism
			ω-3 poly-unsaturated oils	Protective effect in hormone metabolism
			Medium-chain triglycerides	Caloric equivalent to carbohydrate
			Cereal fiber and pectin	Affects enterohepatic cycling of hormones
			Phytoestrogens; soy	Protective effect in hormone action and metabolism
	Fried, broiled meats	Source of heterocyclic aromatic amines (HCA)	Soyprotein/antioxidants; tryptophan/proline	Inhibit formation of HCA
			Microwave cooking	Does not form HCA (lower temperature)

Continued

Table 2-8 *Continued.* Factors and Possible Mechanisms in Main Epithelial Cancer Causation and Prevention

Disease	Risk Factors	Mechanism	Protective Elements	Mechanism
Endometrial cancer	Same as above; excessive body weight	Same as above; fat cells generate estrogen, hydroxy radicals	Same as above; weight control/loss	Same as above; lowers excessive nonphysiologic estrogen levels
Pancreatic cancer	Same as endocrine (total dietary fat)	High fat diets increase functional demands, increase cell duplication?	Vegetables, low-fat nutrition	Micronutrients
	Cigarette smoking	Tobacco-specific nitrosamines		
	Fried/broiled meats	HCA	Tryptophan, proline	Prevent formation of HCA
Cervical cancer	Precocious sexual activity; deficient nutrition	Human papillomavirus; low-defense mechanism	Vegetables, fruits	Source of retinoids, folates
	Smoking	Carcinogens		
Skin cancer, melanoma	Sunlight	DNA damage in genetically sensitive with low DNA repair capacity	Avoid exposure; use sun shields	
Esophageal cancer	Salted, pickled food	Specific nitrosamine	Yellow-green vegetables, tea	Role of vegetables unknown if risk factors present in food (β-carotene, protective element); Antioxidants
	Alcohol intake + smoking	Alcohol modifies esophageal metabolism of tobacco-specific carcinogens	Yellow-green vegetables, tea	Antioxidants
	Tobacco chewing	Tobacco-specific carcinogens and promoters	Vegetables?	Same as above
Gastric cancer	Salted, pickled food	Nitrosoindoles, phenolic diazotates	Green-yellow vegetables, tea	Role of vegetables unknown if risk factor present in food; Antioxidants
	Geochemical nitrate and salt	Formation of gastric carcinogens, above, in stomach	Green-yellow vegetables, fruits, vitamins C and E	Prevent formation of carcinogen; increased cellular tissue defenses; Antioxidants
	H pylori	Cell damage, regeneration, hydroxy radicals	Antibiotics	Eliminate *H pylori*
Colon cancer:				
Proximal	Unknown	Unknown	Unknown Soy products?	Unknown ?

Continued

Table 2-8 *Continued.* Factors and Possible Mechanisms in Main Epithelial Cancer Causation and Prevention

Disease	Risk Factors	Mechanism	Protective Elements	Mechanism
Distal	Same as endocrine-related cancers	Biosynthesis of cholesterol, thence bile acids, and colon cancer promotion, including higher cell cycling rates	Cereal fiber	Increases stool bulk; dilutes promoters; lowers intestinal pH
			Calcium/magnesium salts	Bind bile and fatty acids; lower cell cycling
Rectal cancer	Alcoholic beverages; Same as distal colon cancer	Increases cell cycling in rectum?	Cereal fiber?	Dilutes effectors by increasing stool bulk
Liver cancer	Mold-contaminated foods	Mycotoxins	Avoid moldy, pickled foods; improve nutrition; more protein, fruits, and vegetables	Lower carcinogen intake; improved defense systems
	Some plants	Pyrrolizidine alkaloids	Avoid	
	Pickled foods	Nitrosamines	Avoid	
	Chronic virus	Hepatitis B	Vaccination	
	High level of specific alcoholic beverages	Damages liver, risk of of cirrhosis, potentiates carcinogens	Decrease intake of alcohol	Lower cell duplication rates, lower liver damage
	Cigarette smoking; tobacco chewing	Nitrosamines	Stop smoking	
	Occupational	Vinyl chloride	Lower exposure	
	Iatrogenic	Some oral contraceptives (infrequent occurrence)		
Nasopharyngeal cancer	Salted, pickled fish	Contains specific nitrosamine?	Vegetables	Micronutrients
	Viral factors	Can increase cell turnover?	Vaccination?	
	Occupational	Wood and leather workers		Carcinogen-promoters

One of the most frequent gene changes in human tumors is alteration of the p53 tumor suppressor gene.[29] The normal p53 gene functions to arrest cell proliferation and thereby allow cells with DNA damage to undergo repair. When both alleles are inactive due to deletion or mutation, as is required for loss of function of all tumor suppressor genes, the restraint of proliferation is lost. Other notable tumor suppressor genes are the Rb gene, which is defective in retinoblastoma, and the DCC gene, which is missing in colon cancers.

Proto-oncogenes are normal genes involved in cell replication. More than 50 proto-oncogenes are known. Mutation, translocation, or amplification leads to activated oncogenes, which are present in many tumors. A commonly mutated oncogene is the *ras* family: either Ha-*ras* or Ki-*ras*. The *myc* gene is often activated in human tumors by amplification to more than one copy. Also, errors can be introduced into DNA through the lack of fidelity of the DNA polymerase.[30] In general, it appears that tumors attain abnormal growth through alterations in more than one oncogene or alteration of an oncogene and a tumor-suppressor gene.

The rate of cell duplication is important in generating abnormal DNA, with a rapid rate decreasing the chances of successful repair of DNA damage. Thus, growing organisms are often more sensitive to carcinogens.[31] Radiation exposure during the Hiroshima explosion produced a fourfold higher incidence of breast cancer in persons exposed between the ages of

Table 2-9. Estimated Causes of Cancer Mortality in the US, 1994

Agent	Type of Cancer	% of Total
Tobacco related:	Lung, bladder, kidney, renal pelvis, pancreas, cervix	30-35
Tobacco and alcohol related:	Oral cavity, esophagus	3-4
Diet related:	High fat, low fiber, low in vegetables & fruits, broiled or fried foods?— large bowel, breast, pancreas, prostate, ovary, endometrium	30-35
	Pickled, salted foods, low in vegetables & fruits—stomach	2-3
	Alcohol, mycotoxins—liver, esophagus	3-4
Bacterial:	*H pylori*—stomach	?
Sunlight:	Skin (melanoma)	1-2
Occupational:	Various carcinogens—bladder, liver, other organs	1-2
Lifestyle and occupation:	Tobacco and asbestos; tobacco and mining; tobacco and uranium and radium—lung, respiratory tract	3-4
Iatrogenic:	Radiation, drugs—diverse organs, leukemia	0-1
Genetic:	Retinoblastoma, soft-tissue sarcomas	0-1
Viral:	Human T-cell lymphotropic virus type I (HTLV-1), adult T-cell lymphoma; human papillomavirus—cervix, penis, anus	1-5
Cryptogenic:	Lymphomas, leukemias, sarcomas, cervical cancer	3-6

Adapted, classified, and calculated from American Cancer Society Cancer Statistics, 1994.[15]

10 and 15, with mammary gland cells in rapid DNA synthesis and mitosis, than in younger or older groups.[32]

Reactive carcinogens modify not only DNA but also proteins. Both types of interaction can serve as sensitive markers for qualitative and quantitative analysis, especially readily secured hemoglobin adducts.[6,17,34]

The following steps, involving key changes in DNA and specific parts of the cellular genome provoked by reactive forms of chemical carcinogens, by hydroxy radicals, by viruses, or by radiation (including radiation-produced hydroxy radicals), are called neoplastic conversion (Fig 2-1). In the sequence of steps, cells with altered gene structure need to multiply to express the cancer-associated gene structure. Thus, cell duplication determines the rate of expression and essential cancer risk, as noted elsewhere. Neoplastic development is referred to as the segments of the carcinogenic process. This includes promotion, in which nests of preneoplastic cells develop into clinical cancer. Promoters cannot cause cancer without an antecedent cell change.[34] For example, mice with mammary tumor virus (MTV) develop mammary tumors proportional to the level of estrogen administered, but those without MTV do not, no matter what dose of estrogen is used.

Acting on altered cells, promoters facilitate clonal expansion and the development of neoplasms. Promoters can exert their effects through a variety of mechanisms.[35] One cellular event during promotion is an increase in protein kinase C that can be readily measured, even though this enzyme system is complex and may relate to a family of enzymes.[36] Another effect is an inhibition of protein phosphatases, detected through specific inhibitors and distinct from those affecting protein kinase C.[37] Interruption of gap junctions and intercellular communication play key roles in promotion, and promoters can be detected through this characteristic.[38-40] The action of promoters requires their presence at high levels for a long time. These effects are not permanent, and their action is reversible and often tissue specific. For example, bile acids are promoters of colon cancer, and sodium saccharin acts as promoter of cancer of the urinary bladder.

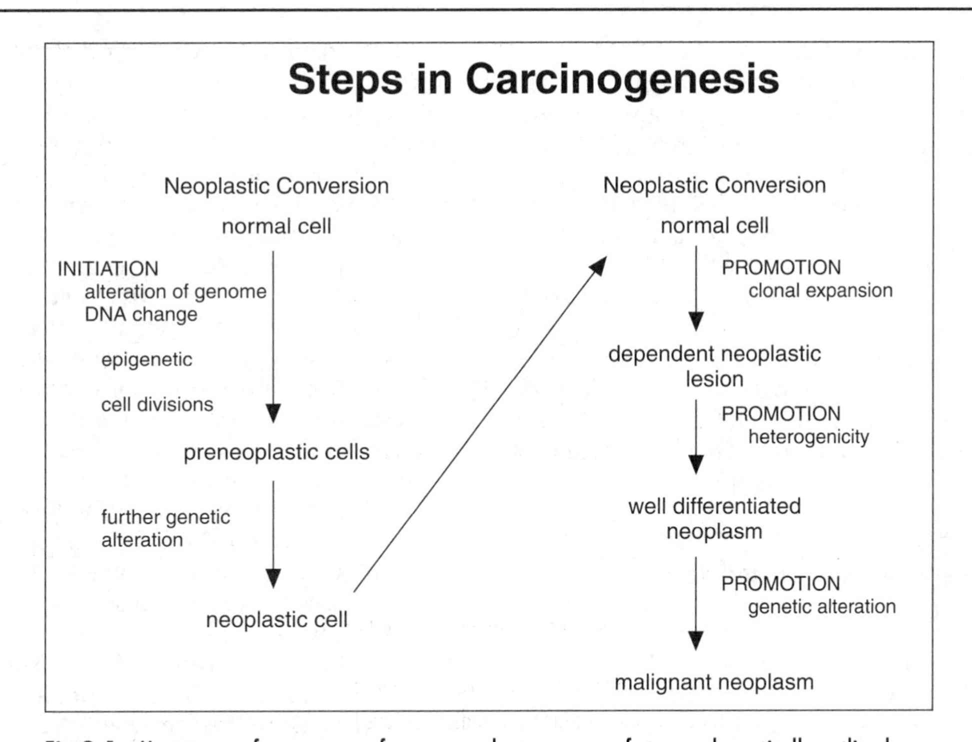

Fig 2-1. Most types of cancer stem from a complex sequence of steps, schematically outlined here. Naturally occurring chemicals related to lifestyle or carcinogens associated with occupational exposure must undergo metabolic activation (or, conversely, are detoxified biochemically). The resulting ultimate carcinogen, a reactive molecule (and also radiation or oncogenic viruses), interacts with cellular macromolecules and specifically with the heritable element, DNA. This altered DNA undergoes further changes during replication, leading to codon (oncogene) rearrangements and amplification. Also involved may be an effect on suppressor genes. This sequence of reactions is the result of "genotoxic" elements. Cells with such abnormal DNA must duplicate and develop, subject to the control of diverse factors at the level of the cell, organ, tissue, whole animal or human being, and external environmental elements. Factors bearing on growth promotion or inhibition may be involved. This sequence of reactions is the result of nongenotoxic, epigenetic events, which are highly dose dependent, with a threshold no-effect dose.

The standard techniques of health risk analysis, involving linear extrapolation of dose-effect experiments, when applied to sodium saccharin have yielded controversial and actually invalid data.[31] The extrapolation methods have yielded uninterpretable results because the techniques generally used for genotoxic carcinogens do not apply to promoters. In fact, new procedures to define the mode of action of epigenetic agents need to be developed for better risk evaluation. A standard S-shaped dose-response threshold is a likely approach.

Thus, chemical carcinogens can be classified into two main groups: (1) carcinogens that are DNA reactive and therefore genotoxic in test systems, and (2) epigenetic agents operating by some other specific biologic effect such as promotion as the basis for their carcinogenicity (Table 2-3). Genotoxic carcinogens alter DNA and are mutagenic.[3,6] Nongenotoxic carcinogens involve other mechanisms such as cytotoxicity, chronic tissue injury, hormonal imbalances, immunologic effects, or promotional activity.[3,34]

Delineating the role of each agent (genotoxic carcinogen, cocarcinogen, promoter) involved in the overall carcinogenic process for each type of cancer by uncovering the mode of action can provide a basis for mechanistic risk assessment. To make further progress in understanding the mechanisms of carcinogenesis, we need to seek information about the nature of the agents—genotoxic or nongenotoxic—associated with the causative factors for a given human cancer (Table 2-4). Reliable information is required on the amount and duration of exposure. Eventually, research on inhibition of the action of carcinogens may provide the basis for effective prevention and should have high priority. Therapy is expensive and, in many instances, only palliative. Prevention is thus the definitive means of cancer control.

Tests for Chemical Carcinogens

Evaluation of human cancer hazards includes the capability to detect and quantitate genotoxic chemicals and, importantly, other agents that act as promoters or enhancers. If the progression from an initiated cell to a neoplasm is susceptible to external influences, procedures will be needed to detect chemicals affecting that part of the process. There are systematic in vitro and in vivo tests to detect and classify chemicals as operating via genotoxic or epigenetic mechanisms. We will briefly review efficient approaches to carcinogen bioassay by the "decision point approach" (Table 2-10). The methods used at each point are described in detail in a monograph by H.A. Milman and E.K. Weisburger.[41]

Table 2-10. Decision-Point Approach to Carcinogen Testing

A. Structure of chemical
B. In vitro short-term tests
  1. Bacterial mutagenesis
  2. Mammalian mutagenesis
  3. Mammalian DNA repair
  4. Chromosome integrity
  5. Cell transformation

Decision point 1: Evaluation of all tests under stages A and B.

C. Tests for promoters
  1. In vitro
  2. In vivo

Decision point 2: Evaluation of results from stages A to C.

D. Limited in vivo bioassays
  1. Altered foci induction in rodent liver
  2. Skin neoplasm induction in mice
  3. Pulmonary neoplasm induction in mice
  4. Breast cancer induction in female Sprague-Dawley rats

Decision point 3: Evaluation from the beginning, plus results from any of the appropriate tests under D.

E. Long-term quantitative bioassay in rodents

Decision point 4: Final evaluation of all available results and application to health risk analysis. This evaluation must include data from stages A to C to provide the basis for mechanistic considerations.

Rapid bioassays have been developed to detect genotoxic (DNA-reactive) carcinogens,[41] which are involved in virtually all human cancers. Any test system has several components: one provides the biochemical activation and detoxification to mimic as closely as possible the situation prevailing in vivo in animals and in humans. A second component is the indicator, or target, DNA and genetic material; a third is the transfer of DNA-reactive metabolite from the site of production to the indicator DNA. A set or battery of select tests provides better evidence than a single test about the potential carcinogenic properties of a chemical, whether synthetic, naturally occurring, or related to human lifestyle activities.

A standard test in any battery is the *Salmonella typhimurium* bacterial mutation assay of Ames.[41] This test uses the S9 fraction of a liver homogenate, which has the required metabolic capability for converting procarcinogens to reactive products, but a low capability of detoxifying phase II conjugation reactions. Thus, one should be aware of false-positive responses. Several flavones, such as quercetin, are positive with the Ames test since they generate hydrogen peroxide, but in the presence of mammalian detoxification systems for these products, and in vivo, such chemicals are negative.[3] Mammalian cell systems are also available for mutagenicity studies.

Another approach is the measurement of DNA damage in cultured cells. Freshly explanted hepatocytes, including human liver cells, have a biochemical competence of activation and detoxification reactions mimicking the in vivo situation.[3] Hepatocytes have the additional advantage of the indicator DNA being in the same cell as the reactive metabolite generated. A procedure has been developed by Williams to detect DNA damage in hepatocytes by carcinogens.[3,41] The hepatocyte test systems can be modified to utilize an in vivo/in vitro scheme, essential when host metabolism, for example by the intestinal bacterial flora, contributes to the production of active compounds.

Other in vitro tests include cell transformation and sister chromatid exchange (SCE). These tests yield information on possible neoplasm-inducing properties in the broadest sense, but are not specific indicators of DNA-reactivity or genotoxicity. SCE can be detected in formed elements from blood; hence the SCE test could be extended to detect possible exposure to harmful chemicals in the workplace, provided results are interpreted in the light of corollary facts and the possible lack of specificity of SCE is kept in mind. Specific biomarkers, immunoassays for specific carcinogen DNA or carcinogen protein adducts, are being developed to estimate populations' exposure.[33] Of interest is a sensitive, widely applicable means of determining the existence of DNA-carcinogen adducts by the ^{32}P-postlabeling technique of Randerath and associates.[20]

A good approach to tests for promoting potential is based on interference with the function of gap junctions and interruption of intercellular communication in cell culture.[3,38-41] Chemicals such as certain halogenated hydrocarbons, the antioxidant butylated hydroxytoluene (BHT), and bile acids are positive for this effect.

The first in vivo tests for promoters used mouse skin. Later studies involved other organs, such as the colon, mammary gland, liver, pancreas, and urinary bladder. The evaluation of recent bioassays for carcinogens has shown that a number of environmental chemicals, pesticides such as DDT and chlordane, and solvents such as trichloroethylene or perchloroethylene, usually led to hepatic neoplasms in the mouse strains used, but not in rats or hamsters. These mouse strains normally display spontaneous liver cancer with a high frequency of activated oncogenes not only in the neoplasms but also in the structure of the DNA of the mouse liver.[24] When these environmental chemicals or their metabolites were tested for genotoxicity, results were overwhelmingly negative. Significantly, however, they were positive in mammalian cell tests for promoters. Thus, the finding of tumors in mouse liver may be due to the promoting potential of chlorinated hydrocarbons, rather than a carcinogenic effect due to genotoxicity. This mechanistic analysis of carcinogenicity tests in rodents is important, as it permits sound, science-based extrapolations of risk to man. Modern, ultrasensitive chemical analyses can detect environmental chemicals and contaminants in water, near waste dumps. This applies, for example, to the family of dioxins, powerful liver enzyme inducers that display a significant dose-response even at low levels, perhaps mediated by specific receptors. Nonetheless, even these chemicals display a threshold. Thus, sound procedures are essential to evaluate human cancer risk and avoid unnecessary "cancer scares." On the other hand, environmental contamination by chemicals should be avoided for ethical and economic reasons.

If in vitro tests have yielded qualitative evidence that a chemical is a genotoxic carcinogen, or a promoter, it is important to secure confirmation in vivo and at the same time generate information on potency. Specific rapid in vivo tests can be applied, based on the probable mechanisms of action, whether genotoxic or promoting.[3]

These diagnostic tests, which usually take <1 year to complete, include the induction of (1) abnormal foci in rodent liver, (2) skin tumors in mice, (3) mammary neoplasms in Sprague-Dawley female rats, and (4) pulmonary tumors in sensitive strains of mice. Tests are conducted at a number of dose levels to provide a dose-response curve, relative to a known positive control carcinogen or promoter.

The tests can be designed to yield potency data for genotoxic initiators, in relation to suitable known control carcinogens, by administering one or a few doses, followed by an appropriate promoter. For tests of promoters, a genotoxic carcinogen for a specific target organ is given, followed by the test substance at four to five dose levels. Use of an appropriate positive control promoter at several dose levels will provide information on relative potency.

Three endpoints can be quantified in these in vivo bioassay systems: (1) proportion of animals with histopathologically validated lesions, (2) the multiplicity and size of neoplasms, and (3) the expression time from exposure to occurrence of tumor. Generally, in vitro tests for genotoxicity or promoting potential, and properly designed, limited in vivo bioassays provide an adequate database for the determination of risk. By applying our current understanding of the mechanisms of cancer causation, and in the light of data from short-term in vitro tests for genotoxicity and for possible promoting substances, the standard long-term bioassay in rodents may no longer be essential in most instances.

Abbreviated procedures of carcinogen bioassay, based on an understanding of the mechanisms of carcinogenesis, can be carried out economically to provide data to forecast potential carcinogenic hazards as well as for health risk analysis. These batteries of rapid tests are deemed no less efficient than the cumbersome, time-consuming, and expensive chronic bioassays.[3,42,43] Advances in molecular biology may provide improvements in diagnosing potential cancer risks. For example, some genotoxic carcinogens lead to activation of cellular proto-oncogenes, which may be an efficient means of determining whether a given chemical causes cancer. Techniques for amplification of segments of DNA, such as the polymerase chain reaction, are being improved continually as specific means to detect abnormal DNA structures typical of neoplasia.[25-28] The method of ^{32}P postlabeling of DNA-carcinogen adducts is a highly sensitive procedure to rapidly generate precise information on such adducts.[20] Application of effective, sensitive methods to problems of food safety inherent in the Delaney clause of the US Food and Drug laws has been proposed.[44] Greater knowledge of the mechanisms involved in promotion may lead to new test systems for the detection of promoters.[39,40]

Lifestyle-Related Cancers

Historic discoveries in the field of cancer causation revealed that chemicals in the workplace were responsible for specific neoplasms. To this day, such discoveries have left the impression that most human cancers are associated with environmental chemical contamination. This opinion has led to public pressure on government to control chemical contamination as a key means of cancer prevention. In most of today's industrialized world, however, work-related cancer is rare, and should remain infrequent by applying the results of tests for carcinogens and promoters. A careful analysis of the causative elements involved in each type of human cancer has shown that locally prevailing lifestyles—in particular, tobacco use, nutritional traditions, and physical activity—account for the cancer incidence.

Tobacco-associated neoplasms and the importance of nutrition are discussed in other chapters, but we will emphasize the relevant mechanisms and how they can be applied to risk reduction and prevention (Table 2-7). We will not comment on leukemias and lymphomas with cryptogenic causes, presumably involving viral elements.[45]

Skin cancer is a high-incidence neoplasm. Its low fatality rate is due mainly to visualization at an early stage and surgical removal by a brief outpatient procedure. The chief cause is sun and other ultraviolet light exposure, causing damage to cellular DNA. People of Celtic descent with poor DNA repair potential are particularly sensitive. An essential preventive measure is avoidance of extensive sun exposure. The allegedly healthy look—tanned skin—can have bad consequences. The view that sun exposure generates vitamin D is now obsolete, as milk and other foods are adequate sources of this vitamin. Furthermore, sun exposure is also the main cause of malignant melanoma—another reason to avoid deliberate tanning.[46,47]

Tobacco

Tobacco has been used for centuries, but commercially manufactured cigarettes were introduced at the beginning of this century. Men in the Western world became heavy users about the time of World War I and women around World War II.[2,18,48] The custom of smoking cigarettes in Japan and some African countries started somewhat later. Female smokers are a recent phenomenon in the Western world. Since about 1986, lung cancer has killed more women per year than breast cancer.[49] Cigarette smoking cessation or, even better, never starting this habit would quickly change these statistics.[50] Chewing tobacco and betel nuts has long been practiced in the Asian subcontinent (India and Pakistan) and in the southern republics of the former Soviet Union. Snuff dipping is common in Scandinavia. These habits are the key causes of oral cavity and head and neck cancer prevalent in users, who often suffer from poor teeth and, thus, malnutrition, especially in regards to protective micronutrients.

Cigarette smoking is directly associated with emphysema and cancer of the lung and has been linked with cancer of the pancreas, cervix, kidney, urinary bladder, and renal pelvis (Table 2-6). It is also a risk factor for fatal myocardial infarction and chronic obstructive lung disease. In the Western world, 40% to 50% of premature mortality occurs in tobacco users, a tragedy with enormous economic impact on lives lost early, on the cost of medical care, and on the economy in general. These losses far outweigh the income of tobacco producers and processors. Chewing or dipping of tobacco with or without other ingredients such as betel nut increases the risk for cancer of the oral cavity and esophagus.

The American Cancer Society, the American Health Foundation, the American Heart Association, the American Medical Association, and the US Public Health Service have warned the public about the risks of tobacco use. An impressive decline in the number of men smoking, especially white men, has been observed in the past 20 years.[49,50] Indeed, in the 1950s, 64% of American men were smokers, while currently only 28% smoke. What would the incidence and mortality of smoking-related diseases be without this reduction in smoking habits? Yet, worldwide tobacco use is increasing, leading to an epidemic rise in disease and deaths.[51,52] The economic impact has been significant, to relatively greater detriment in the developing world.

Carcinogens and Promoters in Tobacco Products

Tobacco smoke contains a number of polycyclic aromatic hydrocarbons, such as benzo(a)pyrene or dibenzo(a,h)anthracene, that are powerful genotoxic carcinogens (Table 2-8).[18] Tobacco smoke and unburned tobacco, used for chewing or snuff dipping, also contain potent nitrosamines, eg, nitrosonornicotine and related compounds, that are derived from nicotine during the curing of tobacco.[6] These compounds are also produced during the combustion process and in vivo from the reaction of nitric oxides with nicotine and related alkaloids. Nitric oxides may play a role in increasing the risk of atherogenesis and heart disease. In addition, burning tobacco leads to certain carcinogenic heterocyclic amines. All of these chemicals are genotoxic carcinogens and mutagens that may be key to the initiation and causation of specific types of cancer. It is important that, overall, the amount of genotoxic carcinogens is small; their impact would be low were it not for the powerful enhancing effect of promoters.

Tobacco and its smoke contain sizable amounts of cocarcinogens and promoters, such as phenolic compounds and terpenes, that are neither carcinogenic nor genotoxic.[18] However, they play major roles in the eventual occurrence of lung cancer through their own specific mechanisms of action, and account for (1) the long latency period usually associated with tobacco smoking; (2) the steep rise in disease risk with increasing consumption, above 20 cigarettes per day (dose-response curve); and (3) the lowered risk of lung cancer on cessation of smoking through elimination of the promoting action. The adverse effects of smoking or other tobacco use are highly dose dependent and are reversible to some extent, because of the mode of action of promoters. This research explains why cessation by addicted smokers or chewers of tobacco yields a progressively lower cancer risk. Similarly, smoking cessation decreases fairly rapidly, in about 2 years, the risk of heart disease. Tobacco smoke also contains chemicals that act as enzyme inducers. Essential endogenous materials like hormones or exogenous products like vitamins are metabolized at different rates or even to different balances of products; as a result, smokers may have higher requirements for vitamins and other essential nutrients. Thus, certain physiologic parameters are distinct in smokers.

Alcohol as a Cocarcinogen

Individuals who smoke cigarettes and consume a considerable amount of alcoholic beverages daily have a high risk of cancer of the oral cavity and esophagus. Alcohol modifies the metabolism of carcinogens in the liver and esophagus.[53] It plays a role in the induction of cancer in select organs by increasing the effectiveness of carcinogens, especially by producing increased amounts of reactive carcinogenic metabolites from procarcinogens in tobacco. In nonsmokers, alcohol can induce cancer of the esophagus through its metabolite acetaldehyde. This risk prevails more in heavy drinkers, especially of hard liquors.

Kidney and Bladder Cancer

These cancers are considered together even though specific agents may have the property of inducing cancer in either kidney or bladder.[25] The main known factor yielding both types of neoplasm is chronic tobacco smoking, through as yet unknown mechanisms. Kidney and bladder cancer are also seen in nonsmokers, and the etiologic elements are unknown. Kidney and bladder are part of the urinary system, excreting metabolic waste products and metabolites in the urine. Clearly, the concentration of such products in urine is a function of water and fluid intake. Low consumption yields a concentrated urine, stored longer in the urinary bladder. This scheme may account for initial damage to the kidney and bladder, giving rise to an increased compensatory cell turnover rate, a situation favoring carcinogenesis. High intake of sodium ion, as with sodium saccharin, leads to such a condition.[31] The group of Kadlubar[33] observed such a sequence in dogs given the bladder carcinogen 4-aminobiphenyl. Dogs consuming less water and having a lower urine volume developed cancer earlier. Thus, regular fluid intake of about 1,200 to 1,500 mL per day can constitute an effective preventive measure in humans. Along those lines, it was noted that tea contains cancer-inhibiting polyphenols, and thus may be beneficial to a healthy lifestyle.[54] In hamsters, estrogen induces kidney cancer. It is not known whether hormonal imbalances and, in particular, estrogen play a role in renal cancer. Obesity, particularly in women, is associated with risk for kidney cancer.[55] Historically, the bladder and renal pelvis were targets of high-level occupational exposure to aromatic amines such as 4-aminobiphenyl or 2-naphthylamine that were intermediates in the production of dyestuffs. In most countries, these hazardous chemicals are no longer produced, or are manufactured in hermetically sealed vessels minimizing human exposure.

Nutrition

Geography determines the incidence of many types of cancer.[2,18,52,56] Pockets of high incidence and other areas of relatively low incidence may occur within the same country. In many, but not all, instances the geographic site of current or longest residence eventually controls the specific risk for different types of neoplasm. In the Western world, diets high in fat, typically representing 40% of calories, are correlated with a higher risk for cancers of the large bowel (Fig 2-2), breast, prostate, ovary, endometrium, and pancreas.[57,58] These neoplasms account for about 35% of premature mortality due to cancer, and for >50% of early deaths from nutritionally linked chronic diseases in the Western world. A high level of dietary fat acts via promoting mechanisms. Genotoxic carcinogens in food may come from various sources, such as broiled or fried meat and fish (in relation to colon, breast, or pancreas cancer), pickled or smoked foods (in relation to gastric or esophageal cancer), or contaminant mycotoxins such as aflatoxins (for liver cancer) (Table 2-7).[52,59] Reactive oxygen may also contribute to the cancer burden in various organs.[6,18,35] The effect can, in great part, be neutralized by antioxidant products in tea, vegetable, and fruits, including some of the antioxidant vitamins.[54,59,60] Oxidative reactions also yield an oxidized LDL-cholesterol, associated with atherosclerosis and heart disease.

Genotoxic Carcinogens

Gastric Cancer

High-risk populations usually consume considerable quantities of dried salted fish, pickled vegetables, and smoked fish; in addition, their intake of fresh fruits and vegetables is low, usually on a seasonal basis, with a concomitant lower intake of vitamins C, E, and A.[59] Descendants of Japanese migrants in Hawaii eat more uncooked vegetables (celery, lettuce, tomatoes), and drink fresh fruit juices; they consequently have a lower gastric cancer risk than native Japanese. The active carcinogenic agent(s) may be nitrosoindoles, diazonium compounds, or as yet unknown chemicals,

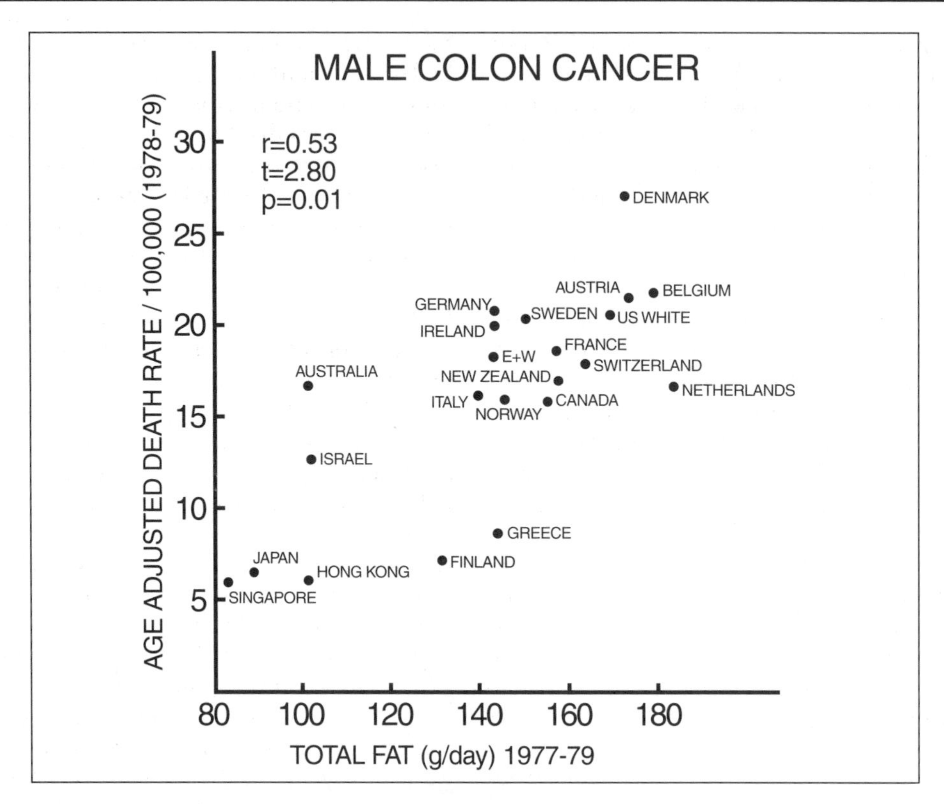

Fig 2-2. Correlation between per capita consumption of dietary fat and age-adjusted mortality from colon cancer (in males). Note the overall relationship of colon cancer risk and total fat, with the important exception of Finland, accounted for by a protective effect from bran cereal fiber intake and a high intake of calcium from dairy products. Greece is another apparent exception, which may be related to consumption of olive oil. Data derived from Kurihara et al[57] and FAO.[58] Similar associations with fat as a function of geography are seen for cancer of the breast in postmenopausal women, prostate, ovary, endometrium, and pancreas.

formed from nitrite and specific substrates. The fact that the formation of such carcinogens may be blocked by vitamin C or E is important. Salt can act as a cocarcinogen in gastric carcinogenesis by increasing lipid peroxidation and cell cycling rates; salt also can lead to atrophic gastritis, a postulated precursor lesion.[5] Salt appears to be the common element in the stroke-stomach cancer mortality relationship, observed as a significant cross-national covariation.[61] Infection with *Helicobacter pylori*, fairly prevalent in many parts of the world, also increases compensatory cell cycling. Eventually, however, it leads to atrophic gastritis and enhances the risk of gastric cancer caused by specific carcinogens.[5,62] A lower intake of salted, pickled, and smoked food would lower the risk of gastric cancer, and also be beneficial in reducing the risk of hypertension and stroke. Reduced consumption of foods preserved by salt, nitrite, or smoking and the improved year-round supply of fresh fruits and vegetables probably account for the large decline in gastric cancer in the US. It is still a numerically important type of cancer worldwide, with declining trends in countries like Japan or Belgium, where public education programs on the need to avoid salted, pickled foods, and to replace them with vegetables and fruits, has begun to be successful.

Esophageal Cancer

Smoking and drinking are major risk factors in the Western world. Alcohol alone, especially in hard liquor, is a risk factor, perhaps through generation of acetaldehyde.[53] There may be a threshold of 8 liters of ethanol per year.[63] Vegetables are protective.[64] The risk factors for esophageal cancer in China and other Asian countries are similar, namely, salted and pickled foods and a low intake of fresh vegetables and fruits.[52] However, the substrates, or fish or vegetables preserved by salt and nitrite treatment, are different from what is used in Japan. In Hong Kong and vicinal areas, esophageal and nasopharyngeal cancer is common.[52,59] This disease has been induced in rats by feeding specific types of fish pickled with salt and nitrite. Some viral agents may also contribute to nasopharyngeal cancer.

In some Near and Middle Eastern countries, one custom associated with esophageal cancer is the frequent intake of boiling hot tea. This habit leads to chronic injury, and thus higher cell repair and turnover, a factor in the increased risk for cancer. These findings suggest food and drink should be at moderate temperatures when consumed.

Colon and Breast Cancers

During the normal process of frying or broiling of fish and meat, certain compounds are formed that are potent mutagens when tested in the Ames assay. These compounds also induce DNA repair in hepatocytes in the Williams test for genotoxicity. These mutagens have been structurally identified as heterocyclic aromatic amines (HCA), such as 2-amino-3-methylimidazo[4,5-*f*]quinoline (IQ), or 2-amino-1-methyl-6-phenylimidazo[4,5-*b*]pyridine (PhIP), and related compounds (MeIQ and MeIQx), which structurally resemble the potent carcinogen 3,2′-dimethyl-4-aminobiphenyl. These heterocyclic amines are potent carcinogens in rats, causing neoplasms in the mammary gland, colon, liver, pancreas, and bladder. PhIP specifically induces cancer in the mammary gland and colon, and is formed in larger amounts than other HCAs. The traditional modes of cooking, frying, and broiling, thus, may be a source of carcinogens for these target organs.[59,65,66] HCAs occur in greatest amounts in well-done meats and gravy, in bacon, and in broiled, dried fish (again, high-temperature cooking).[67] In Sweden, California, and elsewhere, an association with the mode of cooking has been observed.[67] Jägerstad first pinpointed creatinine as the essential ingredient in meats and fish which forms the key aminomethylimidazo part of the HCA molecule.[65,66,67] These molecules are the result of reactions between intermediates formed during Maillard reactions and creatinine. Antioxidants such as propyl gallate or butylated hydroxyanisole (BHA), soy protein, and certain indole-containing amino acids (tryptophan and proline) are effective inhibitors of the formation of these carcinogens during the frying of meat, which may provide a practical means of reducing the formation of this class of carcinogens.[59,65] Brief microwave cooking, under conditions in which fat and juices containing creatinine can escape from the meat, essentially lowers available creatinine and thus the formation of HCAs.[65,67]

Diet may play a carcinogenic role in organs like the breast, endometrium, or prostate, especially when there is fat-associated endogenous production of hydroxy radicals in the absence of adequate antioxidant defenses.

Direct-acting mutagens have been observed in the stools of about 10% to 20% of individuals on a Western (high-fat, low-fiber) diet. Bile acids and anaerobic storage stimulate the formation of these mutagens, called fecapentaenes, which are bacterial products and have some attributes of genotoxicity. Weak carcinogenicity is displayed in some animal models (newborn mice), and questionable carcinogenicity is seen with intrarectal infusion in rats of doses 10 times higher than the mutagenic activity observed in the stools of some humans. The mutagenic activity of fecapentaenes may stem from the production of hydroxy radicals.

Ketosteroids in feces, specifically 4-cholesten-3-one, are not mutagenic but induce nuclear aberrations and sister chromatid exchanges on intrarectal instillation in mice.[68] Such effects are insufficient to classify these cholesterol metabolites as genotoxic, and their role in colon carcinogenesis requires clarification.

Liver Cancer

The overall incidence of primary hepatocellular carcinoma in the US has declined over the past 50 years. In parts of Africa, it is a major neoplasm, affecting men more than women.[18] Presumed etiologic factors include (1) diet, specifically certain genotoxic mycotoxins and liver-specific carcinogens found in certain plants; and (2) high titers of hepatitis B virus; the relative importance of these factors is not known. Current efforts to vaccinate people against the hepatitis virus will serve to delay, if not abolish, primary liver cancer in high-incidence areas such as Africa and China. Mycotoxins are genotoxic carcinogens, and exposure begins in utero and in mother's milk, continuing throughout life; these conditions favor the occurrence of disease. The hepatitis virus can be construed to act as a cocarcinogen, its cytotoxic action leading to liver necrosis and chronic regenerative process. On the other hand, there are data to suggest that the hepatitis virus genome modifies host DNA, leading to neoplastic transformation, so that the risk of hepatocellular carcinoma would stem from the interaction of two genotoxic carcinogens. Also, it may be that chronic hepatitis may generate reactive hydroxy radicals or nitrosating conditions, leading to the formation of hepatocarcinogenic nitrosamines.

Chronic consumption of alcoholic beverages induces cirrhosis, a lesion elevating liver cell turnover and acting as an enhancing factor for primary hepatocellular carcinoma with as yet unknown genotoxic carcinogens (perhaps acetaldehyde, nitrosamines, mycotoxins, or the hepatitis antigen).[53] In Asia, these factors may also play a role; in addition, salting and pickling may generate liver-specific nitrosamines.[52]

High-level occupational exposure of reactor cleaners to vinyl chloride has induced angiosarcoma of the liver. Despite the widespread environmental occurrence of nongenotoxic hepatic carcinogens in rodents (such as carbon tetrachloride, trichloroethylene, and polychlorinated biphenyls in small amounts), the prevailing contamination has not been shown to cause liver cancer in man. Indeed, in the Western world, liver cancer is relatively infrequent, despite the presence of low-level contamination by these chemicals, especially of water as detected by ultrasensitive chemical analysis.

Although few in number, benign liver neoplasms in young women taking oral contraceptives may be fatal because of their hemorrhagic nature. The mechanism of this effect is obscure and must necessarily be attributed to unknown factors, perhaps involving a combination of hydroxy radicals or reactive estrogen metabolites, plus estrogen-mediated promotion. Despite the widespread use of oral contraceptives, the number of cases has been small.

Promoting Epigenetic Phenomena

Clinical Data

Cancers of the breast, prostate, distal colon, pancreas, ovary, and endometrium display similar incidence patterns in most countries.[2,7,9,12,18,56,69] In much of the Western world, the incidence of these cancers is high, but populations in Japan, China, and Arctic areas have or have had low incidence rates. As nutritional customs in those low-risk countries become Westernized, the frequency of these cancers has increased (Fig 2-3).[70] The major lifestyle element associated with disease risk has been total fat intake in each region.[56,70,71] Exceptions to this correlation have been the key to understanding the underlying mechanisms. Thus, in the Mediterranean region, total fat intake is somewhat lower than in other parts of the Western world, and the main fat used is olive oil, a monounsaturated fat, with low promoting attributes.[7,71] Another key exception is the Arctic population (Eskimos), where the total fat intake is as high as in the West—about 40% to 45% of calories—but the fats and oils are derived from fish and eel, and are, therefore, composed mainly of omega-3 fatty acids.[71] These marine oils are protective against cancer and heart disease. Another exception is Finland, particularly the rural areas, where there is a high total fat intake, especially of saturated fats, from dairy foods, but the colon cancer rate is of the same low order of magnitude as in Japan, and the breast cancer rate is lower compared with, for example, Denmark. In this instance, the explanation rests with a substantially higher cereal bran fiber consumption (that increases intestinal bulk and decreases the concentration of bile and fatty acids), and also the enterohepatic circulation of estrogen metabolites.[72]

The question of obesity and body fat distribution as a breast cancer risk has not been resolved. It seems clear that dietary fat and fiber are the prominent factors in the great majority of perimenopausal and postmenopausal disease. In European countries, an association between obesity and breast cancer has been observed,[73] but the waist-to-hip ratio of body fat appears to be irrelevant. In the US, there is not necessarily an association with obesity, but when an association exists, the waist-to-hip ratio ("apple" versus "pear" shape) seems to be relevant.[74] Another risk factor is family history (or perhaps dietary tradition). The latter is more prominent in premenopausal breast cancer, in which micronutrients, but not so much macronutrients, have been found to modulate risk. Soy foods seem to lower the risk of premenopausal breast cancer.[75]

Data from Animal Models

For the past 20 to 30 years, animal models (rats, mice, and hamsters) have been used in the study of etiology of cancer of the breast (mammary gland), colon, and pancreas. When animals are exposed to a carcinogen that induces these cancers and subsequently are fed a nutritional regimen low in fat (10% of total calories), mimicking the traditional diet in Asia, they invariably display a considerably lower incidence of these neoplasms than when the fat level is equivalent to 40% of calories, mimicking the standard Western diet. Although a high total fat level increases tumor yield, exceptions have been noted. When the fat consumed was olive oil or menhaden oil, no significant increase in tumors was noted at any fat level, 10% or 40% of calories. Thus, laboratory models have fairly reproduced the situation found in the Mediterranean countries (regarding olive oil) and in Arctic countries (regarding fish oils).

Mechanisms of Colon Cancer

To evaluate the mechanisms involved in producing cancer in the large bowel or colorectum, we need to consider the three distinct segments of this important digestive organ. No mechanism is known that accounts for cancer in the proximal (or right side of the) colon and cecum. Colon cancer at that site has a fairly uniform distribution worldwide, and where data are available, the incidence of "colorectal cancer" in high-risk regions is only slightly higher than in lower risk areas. Risk factors have not yet been delineated. Inclusion of proximal colon cancer in studies of nutrition and colon cancer has led to confusion, since, among other things, proximal colon cancer does not seem to be affected much by dietary fat.[59,70]

Role of Fat in Distal Colon Cancer

Cancer in the distal (left side of the) colon and the sigmoid junction is common in the Western world, but much less frequent in Japan, the Arctic region, and Finland. A key set of etiologic factors is the type and amount of fat consumed. A high-fat intake pattern

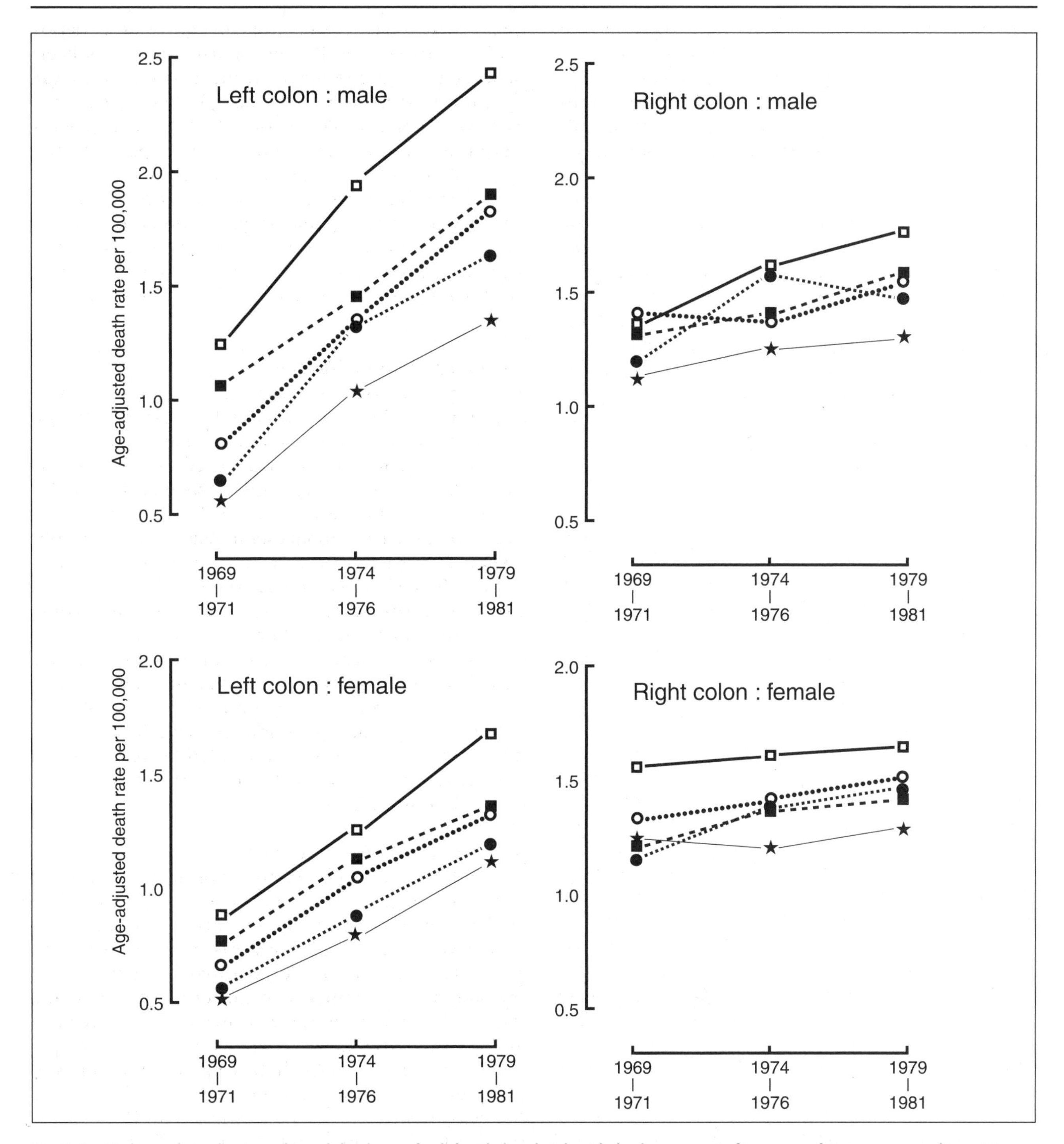

Fig 2-3. Time trends in the age-adjusted death rate for left-sided and right-sided colon cancer in five areas of Japan: metropolitan cities (□); large cities (■); medium-sized cities (○); small cities (•); and counties (*). Considerable increases were found for distal colon cancer and only slight changes for proximal colon cancer, documenting the need to examine time trends separately for proximal and distal colon cancer (and also rectal cancer). The rapid increase in distal colon cancer appears to be associated with the contemporary rise in fat intake. Reprinted with permission from Tajima et al.[70]

controls cholesterol biosynthesis, in turn, related to the total bile acid flow, particularly the secondary bile acid level generated in the intestinal tract by the intestinal bacterial flora. The flora in part controls bile acid activities and intestinal pH, also a function of the amounts and types of fiber and food breakdown products.[76] Laboratory experiments have demonstrated that bile acids are not carcinogens and, despite some claims to the contrary, are not converted to carcinogens; they have been shown to be promoters. In the carcinogenic process, promoters act in a highly dose-dependent manner. Reducing the concentration of bile acids by lowering fat intake to that prevailing in Japan appreciably lowers the risk. The level of bile acids responds rapidly to the amount of total dietary fat, so that a reduction in fat intake can, within days, produce a lower bile acid level in the gut that represents a lower promoting potential (Fig 2-4).[77] This finding has immediate clinical application: on surgical removal of polyps or nonmetastatic tumors, patients would be expected to experience a much lower recurrence rate if they were placed on a low-fat diet.

Role of Fiber

The lower incidence of colon cancer in Finland, particularly in rural areas, may be explained by a higher cereal fiber intake in the form of porridge and rye bread made from whole grains.[59,72] This custom results in a greater stool bulk (about 250 g/day) compared with the daily intake in Denmark or the US (stool, about 80 g/day), where comparative studies have been undertaken. The additional insoluble fiber dilutes the concentration of bile acids in the gut, reducing their promoting potential. Other populations, such as lacto-ovovegetarians or Mormons in Utah, who consume appreciable amounts of fat, but at the same time eat whole-grain cereal foods, also are at lower risk for distal colon cancer. Vegetables and fruits are sources of different types of soluble "fiber" that do not necessarily increase stool bulk, as does wheat or rye bran. Yet, via other mechanisms, they lower the risk for several forms of cancer. Thus, the frequent, regular intake of fruits, vegetables, and bran cereals is desirable.[59,60,78,79] The antioxidants in such foods would significantly assist in neutralizing the generation of reactive oxygen.[71]

Role of Calcium

Wargovich, Newmark, and Bruce first observed the moderating effects of calcium in colon carcinogenesis in animal models.[80] This finding was applied by Lipkin and Newmark in nonpolyposis high-risk families for colon cancer, who displayed a high intestinal cell turnover rate. Increasing the calcium intake of such people dramatically lowered cell turnover rates. An understanding of the mechanisms of carcinogenesis suggests that a proportion of risk can be attributed to cell turnover rates. The lower colon cancer risk seen in Finland may be related to the higher intake of dairy products rich in calcium, in addition to the effect of cereal fiber already described. Optimal intake of calcium and other desirable micronutrients, like magnesium, is obtained through the use of low-fat dairy products, skim milk, certain vegetables, and some types of fish, such as sardines, that are normally consumed with bones.

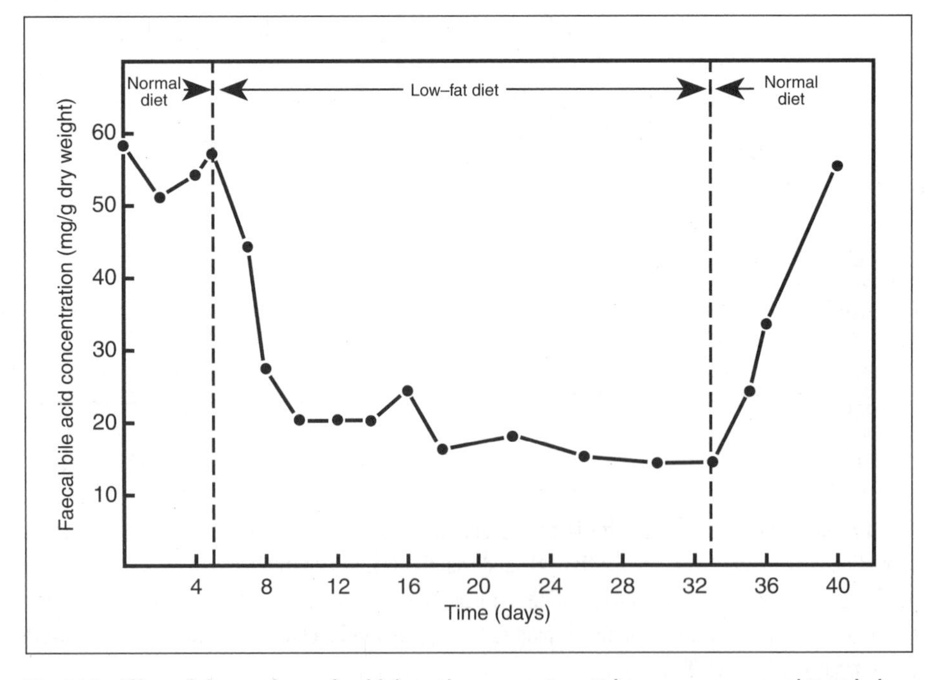

Fig 2-4. Effect of dietary fat on fecal bile acid concentration. Volunteers on a normal British diet of 100-120 g/fat/day were placed on a low-fat diet of <30 g/fat/day. Note the rapid lowering in fecal bile acid concentration, which remained fairly constant and low throughout the low-fat diet. Upon return to the high-fat normal diet, fecal bile acid concentration rapidly rose to the previous level. From Hill.[77]

Rectal Cancer

Incidence and mortality data for rectal cancer need to be reviewed critically on a worldwide basis.[9,11,57] Only in the past 10 to 15 years has there been general agreement on defining the rectum as constituting the tissue 8 cm from the anal verge, in contrast to the rectosigmoid area. Little information exists on etiologic factors. Virtually nothing is known about any genotoxic carcinogens specifically affecting the rectum. There is some parallelism between the occurrence of rectal and distal colon cancers. However, the male:female ratio for rectal cancer in the US is 1.4:1, compared with about 1:1 for colon cancer. The incidence of rectal cancer shows a declining trend, but not the incidence of distal colon cancer (in men). A weak association between distal colon and rectal cancers is noted in international data, perhaps accounted for by a possible promoting element, such as bile acids, common to both neoplasms. This association may be spurious, however, since the rectum is usually not bathed continuously by the intestinal contents as is the distal colon. Some, but not all, epidemiologic studies have correlated the customary consumption of alcoholic beverages with a finding of rectal cancer.[53,81] Laboratory studies attempting to explore the role of alcohol in rectal cancer have, for the most part, produced fruitless results, but Seitz and colleagues have found that alcohol stimulates cell cycling in the rectum of rats.[81] Alcohol would be classified as a cocarcinogen. However, Seitz also identified reactive acetaldehyde in the rectum, perhaps accounting for a direct effect of alcohol. The higher male-to-female ratio for rectal cancer as compared to colon cancer may stem from the greater prevalence of alcohol in men.

Pancreatic Cancer

The worldwide occurrence of this neoplasm generally parallels that of colon cancer.[2,18,56,59] In addition to nutritional elements, cigarette smoking has been pinpointed as a risk factor, which may partially account for the increasing trend in the US from 1950 to 1975, in contrast to a constant incidence rate for colon cancer.[6,18] Two animal models (hamster, rat) have correlated tumor incidence with dietary fat content, although the mechanism for this association has not yet been resolved. In female rats, 2-amino-3-methylimidazo[4,5-*f*]quinoline, an HCA formed during cooking of meats, induced mainly cancer of the mammary gland, but some pancreas adenomas were observed.[59] Dietary fat at 40% of calories would serve to promote neoplasms induced by HAAs. Similarily, fat may enhance the development of pancreatic cancer induced by the tobacco carcinogen 4-[methylnitrosoamino(3-pyridyl)]1-butanone (NNK).

Endocrine-Related Cancers

Cancers of the breast and prostate are prevalent in the Western world, but occur considerably less frequently in Japan and the Arctic countries, and at intermediate rates in Italy, Greece, and Finland.[2,7,12,18,56,59,69] Whereas migrants from a lower-risk area for colon cancer, such as Japan, assume the risk level of the place of residence, such as Hawaii or the US, within the same generation, an increased risk for the endocrine-related cancers is usually found in the offspring of the migrant population.[56] These and other mechanistic analyses of the difference between breast and colon cancer risks suggest that the time of differentiation of the endocrine system is a critical period, and concurrent external influences, such as proper diet, can play a major role in controlling subsequent sensitivity or resistance.[59] In addition to the enhancing effect of fat, cereal bran fiber definitely reduces risk through modification of the enterohepatic cycling and metabolism of estrogen.

Extraordinarily high rates of DNA synthesis and mitosis occur at puberty, rendering the newly forming breast cells extraordinarily sensitive to genotoxic carcinogens. Radiation exposure from the Hiroshima explosion produced a fourfold higher risk of breast cancer in the 10- to 15-year-old age group, compared with older women.[32]

For the study of mechanisms in breast cancers, three different models have been found useful.[65,69] Strains of mice bearing the mammary tumor virus eventually develop mammary gland carcinoma. When female rats of the Sprague-Dawley and derived strains, or Wistar, or Buffalo strains are given the carcinogen 7,12-dimethylbenz(a)anthracene as a single bolus on day 55, during the period of sexual maturation and thus rapid DNA synthesis, mammary adenocarcinoma is induced within 9 months. N-nitrosomethylurea administered intravenously or parenterally likewise leads to tumors of the mammary gland. The carcinogen found in cooked meats, PhIP, is also a useful tool to induce this cancer.[67] In all four models, a low-fat diet is associated with a lower tumor yield than a high-fat diet. These results are obtained with many types of commonly consumed fats. However, exceptions were noted: menhaden and olive oils yielded similar incidence rates whether dietary fat was 10% or 40% of calories. These models, together with appropriate clinical studies, have been useful in investigating relevant mechanisms.[59]

In contrast to colon, breast, or pancreatic cancer, there are at present few reproducible models for prostate cancer[82] for the investigation of dietary factors. However, Bosland has under development such a procedure, based on endocrine modulation of carcinogenic action directed at the prostate.[83] Also, Shirai and colleagues have a model based on the use of an active form of 3,2′-dimethyl-4-aminobiphenyl, originally observed to affect the prostate at the authors' institution.[84]

The development of cancer in endocrine-sensitive tissues (breast, ovary, endometrium, and prostate) is related to hormonal control, with the endocrine balance being especially important. There is a complex, feedback-controlled interaction between hormones of the pituitary gland and hormones of the ovary and testes, adrenals, thyroid, and even liver and kidney concerned with metabolism of steroid hormones.[59,69,85] Nutritional elements, particularly fats, proteins, and fibers, play a significant role in endocrine metabolism and balances. Yet, population studies have been only partially successful in pinpointing the role of different dietary elements in influencing endocrine balances or specific hormone levels. Protein hormones have been analyzed by specific radioimmunoassays with reagents based on specific protein hormone models. The reagents may have been too specific or may not have represented the active bioassayable amount of protein hormone. Investigations of hormone-binding globulins and specific hormone receptors have revealed that the levels of estrogen and androgen unbound by serum globulin may be the element associated with disease risk.[86]

The association of low risk in populations consuming fish oils with specific intracellular effectors (prostaglandin metabolites) has drawn attention to this area as possibly contributing important clues to the underlying mechanisms of dietary effects. Mechanistic studies in appropriate animal models have arrived basically at the same conclusions. Despite the need to pursue more research into the mode of action of diet in influencing carcinogenesis in endocrine-related organs, available information indicates that a low risk for these cancers is associated with (1) a relatively low total fat intake, about 20% of calories; or a monounsaturated fat, such as olive oil, as the main fat component of the diet; or a diet rich in omega-3 polyunsaturated fatty acids, as in fish oils; (2) a low-fat diet during an important time frame: the development of the endocrine system at puberty; and (3) a dietary change from high to low risk status that can occur at any age, because of the reversibility and flexibility associated with endocrine systems.[59,71,86]

Endometrial Cancer

In the Western world, many women are affected by menopausal and postmenopausal symptoms. Physicians used to prescribe pharmacologic replacement with appreciable doses of estrogen or conjugated estrogen. During the late 1960s, women on such estrogen replacement therapy were found to be prone to development of endometrial neoplasia. After discontinuation of the practice of estrogen replacement, the number of women presenting with this condition eventually decreased.[86] This finding attests to the reversibility of promotion by hormones at any age. In addition, dietary modifications would serve to reduce disease risk in endocrine-sensitive tissues. Currently, estrogen replacement therapy involves a considerably lower level of estrogen, with a consequent lower risk of cancer. Furthermore, the previously high estrogen level was not balanced by progesterone, a situation that may have contributed to cancer development. Endocrine preparations that include small amounts of estrogen and progesterone are available, and may serve to ameliorate the postmenstrual syndrome, including the risk for osteoporosis, without increasing cancer risk, although more detailed studies and careful observations are needed.

A major risk factor for endometrial cancer is obesity, explained by the fact that fat cells produce estrogen, itself a key effector in inducing and furthering neoplastic development in this tissue.

Cervical Cancer

Cervical cancer is a major form of neoplasia in developing countries, with an inverse relationship to socioeconomic status in industrialized countries. It may be associated with early sexual intercourse under conditions of poor hygiene, including sex with uncircumcised men. Wider application of circumcision and proper sexual hygiene may help in preventing this disease. The causative elements include the Epstein-Barr, herpes simplex, and human papilloma viruses.[87] Cigarette smoking increases risk, although by unknown mechanisms.[48] Early detection through the widespread use of the Papanicolaou (Pap) smear has improved medical management and lowered mortality appreciably in the past 50 years. Borderline nutritional deficiencies, especially of vitamins A and C and folate, may play a role, especially in lower socioeconomic groups or in the developing world.[69,88]

Causative and Anticancer Prophylaxis

In the preceding sections, our current understanding of the etiology of major human cancers has been described. Clearly, the optimal means of prevention would be to eliminate the relevant causes (or causative prophylaxis). This is possible with occupational cancers, in which specific causes have been pinpointed, and with tobacco-associated cancers. In the Western world, tobacco use accounts for about 40% of premature mortality, mostly due to an increased risk of heart attacks and specific cancer types. Nutritional factors are much more difficult to completely eliminate, although many effective preventive actions can be taken. For the many factors that contribute to the overall cancer burden, there are modulators that can help reduce the risk of specific cancers (or anticancer prophylaxis). Fiber, especially cereal bran fiber, as an effective inhibitor of colon and breast cancer has already been reviewed.

Vegetables, Fruits, and Fibers

Populations that are regular consumers of vegetables and fruits usually have a somewhat lower risk of cancer from various causes, whether they are smoking or nutritionally related.[60,89]

Wattenberg introduced the concept of chemoprevention, or chemoprophylaxis, some 30 years ago.[90,91] He classified chemopreventive agents into three types: One class prevents the formation of carcinogens; for example, fruits containing vitamin C or E eliminate nitrite and, as a result, decrease rate of the formation of carcinogenic nitrosamines or phenolic diazonium compounds. Tryptophan and proline block the formation of carcinogenic heterocyclic amines during cooking of meats. A second class, which Wattenberg calls "blocking agents," reduces the action of carcinogens, by inhibiting the formation of reactive electrophiles or radicals from procarcinogens, or by increasing detoxification of procarcinogens. The last category of inhibitors, called "suppressing agents," operates at steps beyond the reaction of electrophilic carcinogen with cells, preventing the development of clinical neoplasia from transformed cells by a variety of mechanisms.

Vegetables and fruits contain many chemicals belonging to all three classes. Vitamins C and E, noted above, prevent the formation of carcinogens; while vitamin A and carotene may block the expression of carcinogenicity, and carotene, vitamin E, and selenium compounds, together with appropriate enzymes, reduce the development of hydroxy radicals and other active oxygen species.[78] Vegetables, fruits, and tea contain other chemicals and antioxidants with beneficial attributes, including glucaric acid, flavonoids, and enzymes with antioxidant potential.[60,89-92] An important aspect of detoxification of carcinogens is stimulation of epoxide hydrolase, glutathione transferase, and phase II conjugation enzymes, a function not only of chemicals in vegetables, fruits, and tea, but also of certain synthetic antioxidants like BHA or BHT.[93] A whole series of organic selenium compounds are being developed that have anticarcinogenic effects in a variety of situations via several modes of action.[94] Soy and soy products contain a number of chemicals with demonstrated or potential chemopreventive actions, including phytoestrogens, isoflavones, protease inhibitors, saponin, and phytates. Soy protein has high nutritional value, can lower serum cholesterol, and reduce the formation of carcinogens during cooking of meats.[59]

Clearly, therefore, components of vegetables and fruits can exert multiple effects on the activity of genotoxic carcinogens and promoting substances. The benefit associated with chemoprevention, through the broad inhibiting effect of vegetables and fruits in all types of cancer, has already been well documented. Research may lead to isolation of specific components with excellent inhibiting action, for example, isothiocyanates, ellagic acid, and organic sulfur compounds in garlic.[95]

The prominent roles of insoluble and soluble fibers or poorly absorbed starch have been discussed. A health-promoting nutritional scheme would include daily consumption of at least 25 grams of insoluble plus soluble fibers, so as to avoid constipation, and selection of foods that contain such fibers, to prevent intestinal diseases such as appendicitis, diverticulosis, colon cancer, and breast cancer.[96,97] Based on the low risk of breast cancer in Finland, the interactive role of fats and cereal bran fiber was explored in female rats administered a mammary carcinogen.[89] High fat intake was associated with more mammary gland tumors than a low-fat diet. Wheat bran decreased the tumor yield, especially in those consuming more fat (Fig 2-5).[89] Fiber assists in the fecal elimination of lipids (Fig 2-6), but decreases sharply the urinary level of estrogens—evidence of interference with the enterohepatic cycling of estrogen (Fig 2-7).

Excessive sodium salts, as sodium chloride or even the sodium salt of saccharin, can have an "irritating" effect on tissues such as the stomach and urinary blad-

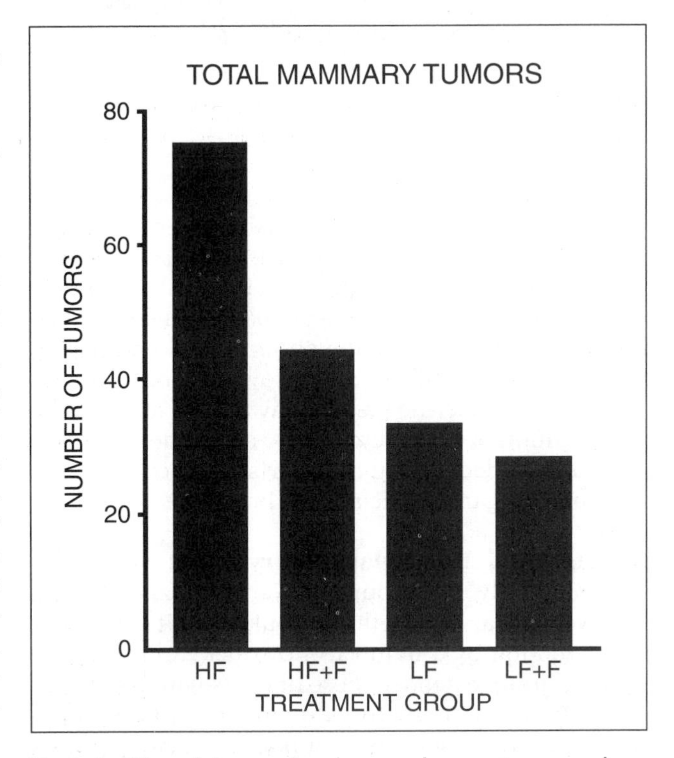

Fig 2-5. Effect of dietary wheat bran supplementation on number of mammary tumors. There were 30 rats in each group. Data are mean ±SE. The four dietary groups were: HF = high fat (23.5% corn oil); HF + F = high fat plus fiber (10% soft white wheat bran); LF = low fat (5% corn oil); and LF + F = low fat plus fiber. From Weisburger et al.[89]

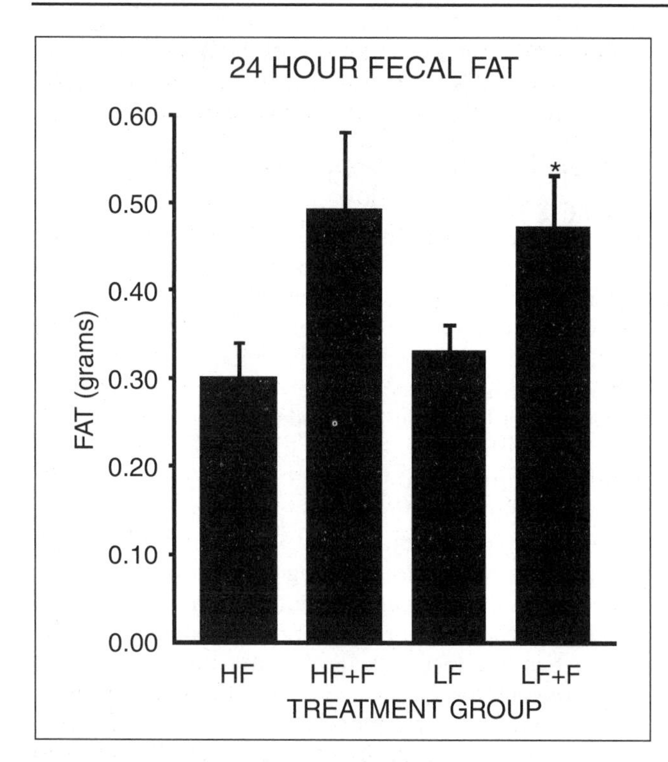

Fig 2-6. Effect of dietary wheat bran supplementation on 24-hr fecal lipid content. Fecal samples (four per group) were obtained in metabolism cages. Assays were performed using standard Soxhlet extraction procedures. Data are mean ±SE. * indicates significance at $p<0.05$ compared with unsupplemented controls. The four dietary groups were as in Fig 2-5.

der, evoking regeneration, increasing cell duplication rates, and thus enhancing the risk of cancer development.[31] The effect of sodium can in part be counteracted by potassium and by calcium or magnesium.[95] In the intestinal tract, calcium and magnesium serve to block the effect of bile acids and lower the risk of colon cancer; the endocrine system may also be affected, by modification of the enterohepatic circulation of estrogens, hence decreasing cancer risk in the hormone-controlled organs, especially the breast.[80]

Nonsteroidal Anti-Inflammatory Drugs

Independently, the groups of Narisawa and Pollard discovered that indomethacin could inhibit colon cancer induction by a number of distinct carcinogens.[98] Reddy's group extended those findings with a series of distinct anti-inflammatory drugs or chemicals modifying specific prostaglandin or polyamine biosynthesis or degradation.[99] Inhibition was apparent throughout the process of colon carcinogenesis while the drugs were administered, but was not maintained when the drug was discontinued. On the other hand, aspirin exerted effects at multiple points in 1,2-dimethylhydrazine-induced colon cancer.[100] Aspirin was most effective in modifying the metabolism of carcinogen to inactive products. In humans, sustained use of nonsteroidal anti-inflammatory drugs, with emphasis on aspirin, appears to have an inhibiting effect on the development of colon cancer.[101] Inasmuch as drug use takes place in the later years of life, this action may depend mainly on the growth inhibition of neoplasms, rather than on carcinogen metabolism. This was also the finding of Narisawa in rats.

Beverages

Not frequently discussed in preventive medicine is the need for adults to consume 1 to 1.5 liters of fluids daily. Adequate fluid intake assists the action of bran fibers to dilute and evacuate products from the intestinal tract in stools. Adequate fluid intake also reduces the concentration of waste products cleared through the kidneys and urinary bladder. It has been demonstrated that dogs given a bladder carcinogen developed cancer earlier if they consumed less water and had more concentrated urine.[33] There have not been many studies on the role of specific beverages. Teas derived from the plant *Camellia sinensis*, as green or black tea, contain antioxidant polyphenols.[102] Tea inhibits the

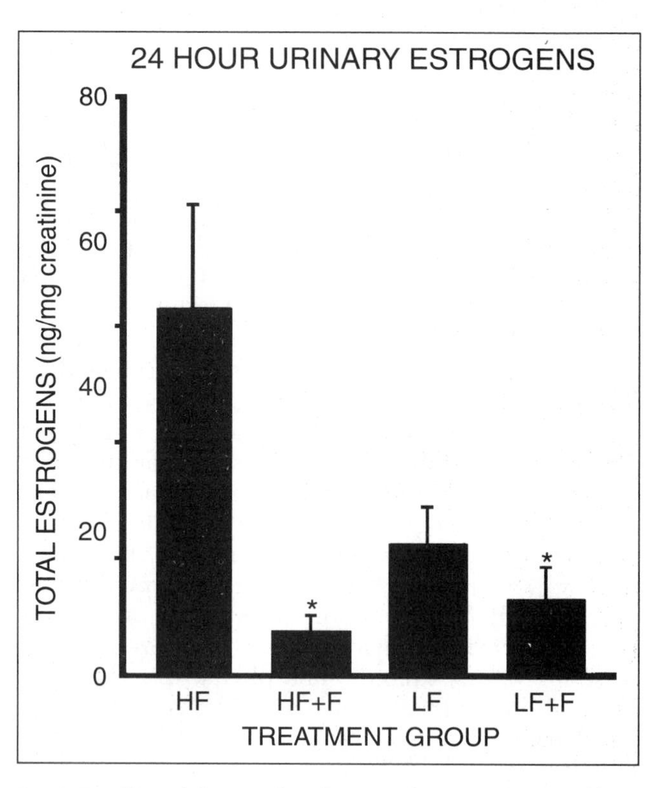

Fig 2-7. Effect of dietary wheat bran supplementation on 24-hr urinary total ($E_1 + E_2$) estrogen levels, analyzed using a kit obtained from ICN/RSL. Urine was obtained in metabolism cages from 4-5 rats per group. Data are mean ±SE. * indicates significance at $p<0.05$ compared with unsupplemented controls. The four dietary groups were as in Fig 2-5.

formation of carcinogens, enhances their detoxification, and inhibits the action of promoting substances. Research is ongoing as to the mechanisms by which green and black tea reduce the risk of cancer and coronary heart disease. The current view is that 4 cups or more of tea at moderate temperature (not boiling hot) would display health-promoting effects.

Exercise

With respect to coronary risk, the beneficial effect of regular, moderate exercise has been demonstrated. Data now reveal that exercise may also benefit cancer of the breast, prostate, and intestinal tract, by mechanisms that are not all known.[103] The database has been obtained through clinical observations of sedentary and active people. Data from animal models indicate that moderate exercise decreases the risk of colon or breast cancer. Clearly, regular exercise can reduce the impact of carcinogens and promoters in humans.

New Developments

Human Cancer Studied in Nude Mice

Nude mice are genetically affected with an immune deficiency stemming from the absence of a thymus. They possess some specific immune functions, but, importantly, will not reject human tumor heterotransplants. Thus, it is possible to devise experiments regarding the growth behavior of human cancers, differentiation, metastasis, and response to therapeutic agents.[104,105] Rose and associates[106,107] have observed that the growth and metastatic potential of a human breast cancer implant responded to the dietary fat level fed to the mice, similar to results in rodent models bearing autochtonous breast cancer, and in women with traditional high or low fat intake. The nude mouse, therefore, permits novel approaches using human tissues or cancers to study underlying mechanisms.

Molecular Mechanisms Studied in Transgenic Mice

Specific exogenous gene segments can be inserted into germ cells of mice to produce transgenic mouse strains bearing the gene integrated in the genetic material. Codons thus introduced can be associated with neoplasia, such as a *myc* segment, or can even carry a human gene, such as for a key enzyme.[108,109] These are important tools, as molecular analysis of the gene structure of human cancer has uncovered select codon changes in a variety of neoplasms. *Ras* and p53 gene mutations, deletions at chromosomes 17p and 18q, and similar translocations, amplification, or losses associated with mutational events were observed in cases of colon cancer.[110] Some changes may be associated with the behavior and aggressiveness of a neoplasm. Related alterations have been noted in cases of pancreatic cancer[111] and mesothelioma.[112] The literature on this topic is expanding rapidly; this technique may supplement and certainly extend histopathologic analysis and provide information of potential prognostic and diagnostic value.

Electromagnetic Fields and Cancer Risk

Epidemiologic observations have suggested that electric power lines generate fields with a risk for childhood malignancies, especially leukemias, and also adult leukemias. However, other research, just as carefully conducted, failed to demonstrate such an association.[113,114] There may be complex confounding elements that need to be unraveled. From the perspective of public health promotion and cancer prevention, even if an association were demonstrated, the number of such cancer cases is small, in contrast to cancers associated with established risk factors, such as tobacco use or improper nutritional habits.

Conclusion

This chapter has outlined our current knowledge of the complex interacting causes of major human cancers. The majority are associated with lifestyle, namely tobacco use and locally prevailing nutritional traditions. In the US, a plan formulated over 10 years ago called for a considerable reduction, originally targeted at 50%, in mortality from cancer by the year 2000.[115,116] Japan also has a national plan to reduce the impact of cancer, through measures such as a low intake of salt and of salted, pickled foods. In Europe, the Code Against Cancer visualizes a sizable decrease in mortality from cancer by the year 2000.[117] Optimistically this worldwide goal could be reasonably met, especially in the Western world, by modifying the known causes of cancer. The effects of tobacco and diet operate mainly through a promoting process, which is highly dependent on the dosage of the promoters, and which can be reversed quickly. Therefore, great efforts by all concerned—government agencies, cancer societies, environmental and public health groups, and especially the powerful influence of the media (television, radio, magazines, newspapers, and books)—are needed to influence the public to change its traditions. Means need to be found to influence the lower socioeconomic groups, which as a rule have greater health problems. The food industries, at least in the US, offer many low-fat, high-fiber products that are being accepted by the public. Such changes in lifestyle would not only serve to decrease sharply the risk of cancer, but also bear on the incidence of hypertension, coronary heart disease, stroke, and adult-onset diabetes mellitus. Therefore, cancer research has provided a strong incentive to encourage the public to make lifestyle changes and remain active and healthy to an older age. Such actions would also be instrumental in sharply reducing the cost of medical care.

These public health recommendations are based on solid research into the mechanisms of carcinogenesis and a mechanistic exploration of the causes of cancer. The oncologic process occurs by a number of successive steps, all of which are needed for the development of clinically invasive cancer. Studies in animal models have reproducibly documented this sequence, and it seems reasonable to suppose that the initiation, development, and progression of human cancers follow such a pattern.

In an occupational setting, fortunately involving few individuals, the early lesions can be the result of neoplastic changes caused by substantial exposure to genotoxic carcinogens. The majority of the cancer burden worldwide stems from certain carcinogens or mixtures associated with lifestyle, specifically tobacco use or nutritional traditions. Genotoxic carcinogens present in tobacco smoke belong to the family of polycyclic aromatic hydrocarbons and the nicotine alkaloid-derived nitrosamines, and are associated with respiratory tract cancers and cancer in the pancreas, kidneys, urinary bladder, and cervix. These nitrosamines, also present in unburned tobacco used for chewing and snuff dipping, account for an effect in the oral cavity and esophagus. Genotoxic carcinogens are formed in salted, pickled, and smoked foods, or in vivo from nitrate and nitrite, and are related to risk for gastric or esophageal cancer, especially when not balanced by the presence of vitamin C, vitamin E, or other antioxidants, and similar means to eliminate nitrite. Instead of salting and pickling, we now refrigerate or freeze foods. Fresh fruits and vegetables are now available year-round instead of seasonally. These combined changes account for the progressive lowering of gastric cancer risk. For other nutritionally linked cancers, research has begun to validate the view that mutagens/carcinogens are formed during the frying or broiling of meat. Their chemical structure involves heterocyclic arylamines (HCAs). HCAs may account for the occurrence of cancer of the colon, breast, or pancreas. Simple, effective means have been developed to decrease the formation of HCAs during cooking, for example by mixing soy protein with ground meat, or applying a mixture of proline and tryptophan before cooking. Brief microwave heating before cooking removes most of the essential creatinine, so that less of the HCAs can form, and incidentally the fat content is also lowered.

Epigenetic agents (or promoters) play a major role in the development of many human cancers; they also operate reproducibly in animal models for these cancers, and their mechanisms of action can be investigated. Fractions of tobacco smoke contain enhancers and promoters that are essential in the development of cancer. The major promoting element for the nutritionally linked cancers is the level of dietary fat, traditionally 40% to 45% of calories in the Western diet. The mechanism by which fat translates to risk has been well outlined for colon cancer, in which there is a relationship between the amount of fat consumed, the quantity of cholesterol biosynthesized in the liver, and the amount of bile acids in the gut. A reduction of the concentration of bile acids, either by a lower intake of dietary fat or by increased luminal bulk produced by cereal fiber, or both, significantly lowers cancer risk. Support for this recommendation comes from the comparison of the high incidence of colon cancer in the Western world, with the low incidence in Japan, where the dietary fat level is 10% to 20% of calories, and the lower incidence in Finland, where the dietary fiber level, and thence stool bulk, is high. In addition, comparative studies of human fecal bile acid concentrations in diverse populations such as the New York area, Finland, Denmark, and Japan provide metabolic evidence correlating percent of dietary fat to fecal bile acid concentrations and thence colon cancer risk. In turn, risk depends on the rate of cell duplication. Similar considerations of a role for dietary fat and fiber intake applies to breast cancer, particularly in postmenopausal women. Fat and fiber modulate estrogen production and metabolism. The endocrine balance, indirectly controlled by these nutritional elements, is also a factor in cancer of the prostate, although the mechanisms by which fat and fiber affect pancreatic cancer development are not clear.

Not all fats exert identical effects. The omega-6 polyunsaturated lipids, effective in lowering serum cholesterol, are better promoters than mostly saturated fats, such as lard or beef fat. It seems probable that the rising incidence of breast and colon cancer in the last 30 years stems from a decreased intake of foods with saturated fats—to avoid heart disease—and an increased compensatory intake of omega-6 polyunsaturated oils. Monounsaturated oils, such as olive oil, have little promoting effect, and omega-3 polyunsaturated oils, found in fish, are protective. All of these fats and oils have identical caloric content and caloric availability. Therefore, the dramatic difference in breast or colon cancer promoting potential cannot be explained by caloric content. Dietary restriction experiments have demonstrated lower incidences in breast and colon cancer even when high-fat diets were fed.[72] It has been known for a long time that dietary restriction depresses cancer development; this association was explained by showing that cell cycling in major organs is reduced by dietary restriction. The importance of cell cycle frequency in (1) controlling the sensitivity of cells to genotoxic carcinogens and (2) furthering growth, development, and progression, needs greater emphasis. This factor is the link to many previously unrelated phenomena, and its relevance in carcinogenesis is the product of recent research. Exposure to a single dose of carcinogenic radiation at the time of the Hiroshima atomic bomb explosion revealed that persons between the ages of 10 and 15 had a four-fold higher breast cancer risk than younger or older age groups. This corresponds precisely to the period of high DNA synthesis and cell duplication rates associated with puberty-linked rapid breast development. Certainly, weight control is an important health-promoting, disease-preventing measure. However, the role of specific lipids in increasing cancer risk is undeniable, and suggests the benefit of limiting intake to about 20% of calories, a demonstrated lower-risk situation irrespective of the type of fat.

Bivalent ions, such as calcium or magnesium, can bind bile acids, decrease cell cycle time, and may play a role in lowering risk for colon and perhaps breast cancer. Calcium ions are also beneficial in controlling the Na^+/K^+ and Ca^{2+} balances bearing on hypertensive disease, and in preventing osteoporosis. Excellent sources of calcium are certain vegetables, low-fat dairy products, skim milk, and, for lactose-intolerant persons, fat-free yogurt.

Physical activity may be protective against cancer development. Because dietary habits and physical activity are often related, controlling for the effect of exercise may provide a truer measure of dietary factors in the etiology of nutritionally linked cancers.

For hormone-related cancers, such as of the breast and prostate, it is not yet known exactly what kind of endocrine balances would favor the growth of neoplastic cells, or indeed would inhibit such growth. It is also unclear precisely how dietary fat affects endocrine balances and specific hormone receptors. It seems probable, however, that the type and amount of fat, endocrine balances, and receptors are related to risk for these cancers. Since these factors all operate through epigenetic mechanisms, their action is dose and time dependent. Thus, a reduction in effective dose by whatever means would be expected to lead to a rapid lowering of risk and hence of incidence.

This concept may apply even to patients with such diseases where dietary intervention promises to be an effective adjuvant therapy. Examples of the reversibility of epigenetic phenomena are the lowering of the risk for lung cancer after cessation of cigarette smoking for a number of years, and the rapid decline in incidence of endometrial cancer when the post-menopausal use of estrogen was discontinued, or the dosage lowered.

In fact, a dietary change to 20% of fat calories from 40% would go a long way to lowering the risk for colon, pancreas, breast, and prostate cancers, and also for ovarian or endometrial cancer if estrogen-generating obesity is avoided. Because caloric restriction and weight loss, along with calcium levels and calcium-phosphate ratios, control cell division, cancer development is decreased. Adequate cereal fiber in the diet, by increasing stool bulk and decreasing promoting elements in the gut, would lower risk for large-bowel cancer. Stool bulk also affects the elimination of conjugated estrogens, in turn benefiting breast and endometrial cancer risk.

For tobacco-linked cancers, promoters and cocarcinogens are present in tobacco and tobacco smoke in much larger quantities than are the genotoxic carcinogens. The presence of promoters probably contributes to the occurrence of cancer after a long latent period, and to the reversibility of lung cancer risk on smoking cessation. Despite the well-documented hazard of smoking, more women have become heavy smokers (from 5% of women in 1950, to about 30% in 1994). The mortality rate in women from lung cancer surpasses that from breast cancer.

In any event, lifestyle is an important controlling element for preventing disease and for patient survival. Physicians should provide guidance along the lines described in Table 2-11.

Table 2-11. Lifestyle Recommendations

1. Don't use tobacco in any form: smoking, chewing, or snuff dipping.
2. Adjust total fat intake to 20% or less of calories, and opt for lipids with less risk for heart disease or cancer, such as monounsaturated oils. Consume fish several times a week.
3. Avoid obesity and adjust overall energy intake to energy needs.
4. Increase intake of cereal bran fiber foods.
5. Consume more vegetables, soy products, and fruits, which are excellent sources of vitamins, antioxidants, anticarcinogens, minerals, and fiber.
6. Avoid salted, pickled, or smoked foods.
7. Limit the intake of fried or broiled foods, or "pretreat" to decrease the formation of carcinogens during cooking.
8. Increase intake of calcium magnesium with low-fat or skim dairy products, milk or yogurt, and certain vegetables.
9. Consume alcoholic beverages in moderation.
10. Drink 1 to 1.5 liters of water or fluids each day; tea contains anticancer antioxidants.
11. Be careful about exposure to sunlight. High-risk individuals, particularly of Celtic ancestry, should use sunscreen creams.
12. Exercise regularly, but only after a health check certifying normal blood pressure and serum cholesterol levels, to ensure cardiovascular patency.

Lifestyle adjustments commensurate with these guidelines, implemented optimally at a young age, are effective in minimizing chronic disease risk. All patients in remission who have had coronary heart disease or cancer of diverse types should be advised of the need to modify lifestyle as part of therapy.

Much has been learned about the causes of the major human cancers in North America and indeed in the world. This chapter has provided factual background and a glimpse of underlying mechanisms leading to the most effective and definitive means of cancer control—prevention.

References

1. International Agency for Research on Cancer: IARC monographs on the evaluation of carcinogenic risks to humans. Lyon, France: 1987;suppl 7.

2. Doll R. Health and the Environment in the 1990s. *Am J Public Health.* 1993;82:933-941.

3. Williams GM, Weisburger JH. Chemical carcinogenesis. In: Amdur MO, Doull J, Klaassen CD, eds. *Casarett and Doull's Toxicology: The Basic Science of Poisons.* 4th ed. New York, NY: Pergamon Press;1991:127-200.

4. Davis DL, Hoel D, eds. Trends in cancer mortality in industrial countries. *Ann NY Acad Sci.* 1990;609:1-347.

5. Correa P. Human gastric carcinogenesis: a multistep and multifactorial process. First American Cancer Society Award lecture on cancer epidemiology and prevention. *Cancer Res.* 1992;52:6735-6740.

6. Brugge J, Curran T, Harlow E, McCormick F, eds. *Origins of Human Cancer: A Comprehensive Review.* Cold Spring Harbor Laboratory Press; 1991.

7. Taioli E, Nicolosi A, Wynder EL. Dietary habits and breast cancer: a comparative study of United States and Italian data. *Nutr Cancer.* 1991;16:259-265.

8. Chlebowski RT, Blackburn GL, Buzzard IM, et al. Adherence to a dietary fat intake reduction program in postmenopausal women receiving therapy for early breast cancer. The Women's Intervention Nutrition Study. *J Clin Oncol.* 1993;11:2072-2080.

9. Kurihara M, Aoki K, Miller RW, Muir CS, eds. *Changing Cancer Patterns and Topics in Cancer Epidemiology.* New York, NY: Plenum Press; 1987:3-219.

10. Howson CP, Hiyama T, Wynder EL. Decline of gastric cancer: epidemiology of an unplanned triumph. *Epidemiol Rev.* 1986;8:1-27.

11. Frey CM, McMillen MM, Cowan CD, Horm JW, Kessler LG. Representativeness of the Surveillance, Epidemiology, and End Results program data: recent trends in cancer mortality rates. *J Natl Cancer Inst.* 1992;84:872-877.

12. La Vecchia C, Lucchini F, Negri E, Boyle P, Maisonneuve P, Levi F. Trends of cancer mortality in Europe, 1955-1989. *Eur J Cancer.* 1992;28:132-235,514-599,927-998,1210-1281,1509-1581; 1993;29:341-470.

13. Baquet CR, Horm JW, Gibbs T, Greenwald P. Socioeconomic factors and cancer incidence among blacks and whites. *J Natl Cancer Inst.* 1991;83:551-557.

14. The Bureau of Vital Statistics, Ministry of Health and Welfare (Japan). Long term trends in cancer mortality rates from 1955 to 1987 in Japan. *Jpn J Clin Oncol.* 1989;19: 305-317.

15. Boring CS, Squires TS, Tong T, Montgomery S. Cancer statistics. *CA Cancer J Clin.* 1994;44:7-26.

16. Byrne J, Kessler LG, Devesa SS. The prevalence of cancer among adults in the United States: 1987. *Cancer.* 1992;69:2154-2159.

17. Weinstein IB, Croce CM, Harris CC. Discoveries and opportunities in cancer research. *Cancer Res.* 1991;51(18, supplement): 5013-5086.

18. Cooper CS, Grover PL, eds. Chemical carcinogenesis and mutagenesis. Berlin: Springer-Verlag; 1990.

19. Weisburger JH, Williams GM. Critical effective methods to detect genotoxic carcinogens and neoplasm-promoting agents. *Environment Health Perspectives.* 1991;90:121-126.

20. Moorthy B, Sriram P, Randerath K. Chemical structure and time-dependent effects of polycyclic aromatic hydrocarbon-type inducers on rat liver cytochrome P450, DNA adducts, and I-compounds. *Fund Appl Toxicol.* 1994;22: 549-560.

21. Feig DI, Loeb LA. Oxygen radical induced mutagenesis is DNA polymerase specific. *Mol Biol.* 1994;235:33-41.

22. Pegg AE, Byers TL. Repair of DNA containing O^6-alkylguanine. *FASEB J.* 1992;6:2302-2310.

23. Grand RJA, Owen D. The biochemistry of *ras* p21. *Biochem J.* 1991;279:609-631.

24. Rumsby PC, Barrass NC, Phillimore HE, Evans JG. Analysis of the Ha-*ras* oncogene in C3H/He mouse liver tumors derived spontaneously or induced with diethylnitrosamine or phenobarbitone. *Carcinogenesis.* 1991; 12:2331-2336.

25. Barrett JC, Huff JE. Cellular and molecular mechanisms of chemically induced renal carcinogenesis. In: Bach PH, Gregg NJ, Wilks MF, Delacruz L, eds. *Nephrotoxicity.* New York, NY: Marcel Dekker Inc; 1991:287-306.

26. Cheng KC, Loeb LA. Genomic instability and tumor progression: mechanistic considerations. *Adv Cancer Res.* 1993;60:121-156.

27 Bloom AD, Deres DA, eds. Genetic susceptibility to cancer. *Mutat Res.* 1991;247:183-292.

28. Ronai Z. *Ras* oncogene detection in pre-neoplastic lesions: possible applications for diagnosis and prevention. *Oncol Res.* 1992;4:120-128.

29. Harris CC. p53: at the crossroads of molecular carcinogenesis and risk assessment. *Science.* 1993;60:477-511.

30. Echols H, Goodman MF. Fidelity mechanisms in DNA replication. *Annu Rev Biochem.* 1991;60:477-511.

31. Cohen SM, Ellwein LB. Risk assessment based on high-dose animal exposure experiments. *Chem Res Toxicol.* 1992;5:742-748.

32. Tokunga M, Land CE, Yamamoto T, et al. Incidence of female breast cancer among atomic bomb survivors. *Radiation Res.* 1987;112:243-272.

33. Kadlubar FF, Dooley KL, Teitel CH, et al. Frequency of urination and its effects on metabolism, pharmacokinetics, blood hemoglobin adduct formation, and liver and urinary bladder DNA adduct levels in beagle dogs given the carcinogen 4-aminobiphenyl. *Cancer Res.* 1991;51:4371-4377.

34. Dragan YP, Pitot HC. The role of the stages of initiation and promotion in phenotypic diversity during hepatocarcinogenesis in the rat. *Carcinogenesis.* 1992;13:739-750.

35. Trosko JE, Jone C, Chang CC. The use of in-vitro assays to study and to detect tumour promoters. In: Borzsonyi M, Day NE, Lapis K, Yamasaki H, eds. *Models, Mechanisms* *and Etiology of Tumour Promotion*. Lyons: International Agency for Research on Cancer;1984:239-252. IARC scientific publications 56.

36. Blumberg PM. Complexities of the protein kinase C pathway. *Mol Carcinog*. 1991;4:339-344.

37. Fujiki H. Is the inhibition of protein phosphatase 1 and 2A activities a general mechanism of tumor promotion in human cancer development? *Mol Carcinog*. 1992;5:91-94.

38. Yamasaki H. Gap junctional intercellular communication and carcinogenesis. *Carcinogenesis*. 1990;11:1051-1058.

39. Ruch RJ, Bonney WJ, Sigler K, et al. Loss of gap junctions from DDT-treated rat liver epithelial cells. *Carcinogenesis*. 1994;15:301-306.

40. Budunova IV, Williams GM. Cell culture assays for chemicals with tumor promoting or inhibiting activity based on the modulation of intercellular communication. *Cell Biol Toxicol*. 1994;10:71-116.

41. Milman HA, Weisburger EK, eds. In: *Handbook of Carcinogen Testing*. Park Ridge, NJ:Noyes Publications;1985.

42. Huff J, Haseman J, Rall D. Scientific concepts, value, and significance of chemical carcinogenesis studies. *Annu Rev Pharmacol Toxicol*. 1991;31:621-652.

43. Swenberg JA, Hoel DG, Magee PN. Mechanistic and statistical insight into the large carcinogenesis bioassays on N-nitrosodiethylamine and N-nitrosodimethylamine. *Cancer Res*. 1991;51:6409-6414.

44. Weisberger JH. Does the Delaney Clause of the US food and drug laws prevent human cancers? *Fund Appl Toxicol*. 1994;22;483-493.

45. Evans AS, Mueller NE. Viruses and cancer: casual associations. *Ann Epidem*. 1990;1:71-92.

46. Dumaz N, Stary A, Soussi T, Daya-Grosjean L, Sarasin A. Can we predict solar ultraviolet radiation as the casual event in human tumours by analyzing the mutation spectra of the p53 gene. *Mutat Res*. 1994;307:375-386.

47. Cascinelli N, ed. Sun exposure, UVA lamps, and risk of skin cancer. *Eur J Cancer*. 1994;30:548-560.

48. Wynder EL. Tobacco and health: a review of the history and suggestions for public health policy. *Public Health Rep*. 1988;103:8-18.

49. Shopland DR, Eyre HJ, Pechacek TF. Smoking-attributable cancer mortality in 1991: is lung cancer now the leading cause of death among smokers in the United States? *J Natl Cancer Inst*. 1991;83:1142-1148.

50. Resnicow K, Kabat G, Wynder E. Progress in decreasing cigarette smoking. *Important Adv Oncol*. 1991;12:205-213.

51. Peto R, Lopez AD, Boreham J, Thun M, Heath C. Mortality from tobacco in developed countries: indirect estimation from national vital statistics. *Lancet*. 1992;339: 1268-1278.

52. Junshi C, Campbell TC, Junyao L, Peto R. Diet, lifestyle and mortality in China. Oxford: Oxford University Press; 1990.

53. Lieber CS. Herman Award Lecture, 1993: a personal perspective on alcohol, nutrition, and the liver. *Am J Clin Nutr*. 1993;58:430-442.

54. Yang CS, Wang ZY. Tea and cancer. *J Natl Cancer Inst*. 1993;38:1049.

55. Mellemgaard A, Møller H, Olsen JH, Jensen OM. Increased risk of renal cell carcinoma among obese women. *J Natl Cancer Inst*. 1991;83:1591-1592.

56. Wynder EL, Fujita Y, Harris RE, Hirayama T, Hiyama T. Comparative epidemiology of cancer between the United States and Japan: a second look. *Cancer*. 1991;67:746-763.

57. Kurihara M, Aoki K, Tominaga S, eds. *Cancer Mortality Statistics in the World*. Nagoya, Japan: University of Nagoya Press;1984.

58. *Food Balance Sheets: 1979-1981 Average*. Rome: Food and Agriculture Organization of the United Nations; 1984.

59. Weisburger JH. Nutritional approach to cancer prevention with emphasis on vitamins, antioxidants, and carotenoids. *Am J Clin Nutr*. 1991;53:226S-237S.

60. Steinmetz KA, Potter JD. Vegetables, fruit, and cancer. *Cancer Causes Control*. 1991;2:325-357, 427-442.

61. Joossens JV, Hill MJ, Geboers J, eds. *Diet and Human Carcinogenesis*. Amsterdam:Excerpta Medica;1985.

62. Talley NJ, Zinsmeister AR, Weaver A, et al. Gastric adenocarcinoma and Helicobacter pylori infection. *J Natl Cancer Inst*. 1991;83:1734-1739.

63. Møller H, Boyle P, Maisonneuve P, La Vecchia C, Jensen OM. Changing mortality from esophageal cancer in males in Denmark and other European countries, in relation to changing levels of alcohol consumption. *Cancer Causes Control*. 1990;1:181-188.

64. Cheng KK, Day NE, Daview TW. Oesophageal cancer mortality in Europe: paradoxical time trend in relation to smoking and drinking. *Br J Cancer*. 1992:613-617.

65. Hayashi Y, Nagao M, Sugimura T, et al, eds. *Diet, Nutrition and Cancer*. Tokyo: Japan Scientific Societies Press; 1986.

66. Aeschbacher H-U. Potential carcinogens in the diet. *Mutat Res*. 1991;259:203-410.

67. Adamson RH, Gustafsson JA, Ito N, et al. Heterocyclic amines in cooked foods. In: *Proceedings of 23rd International Symposium of the Princess Takamatsu Cancer Research Fund*. Princeton, NJ: Princeton Scientific Publications; 1994.

68. Bruce WR, Archer MC, Corpet DE, et al. Diet, aberrant crypt foci, and colorectal cancer. *Mutat Res*. 1993;290: 111-118.

69. The Surgeon General's report on nutrition and health: summary and recommendations. Washington, DC:US Public Health Service; 1988. US Dept of Health and Human Services publication 88-50211.

70. Tajima K, Hirose K, Nakagawa N, Juroshishi T, Tominaga S. Urban-rural difference in the trend of colo-rectal cancer mortality with special reference to the subsites of colon cancer in Japan. *Gann*. 1985;76:717-728.

71. Weisburger JH. Mechanisms of macronutrient carcinogenesis. In: Micozzi MS, Moon TE, eds. *Macronutrients: Investigating Their Role in Cancer*. New York, NY: Marcel Dekker Inc; 1992:3-31.

72. Reddy BS. Dietary fat, calories, and fiber in colon cancer. *Prev Med*. 1993;22:738-749.

73. den Tonkelaar I, Seidell JC, Collette HJA, de Waard F. Obesity and subcutaneous fat patterning in relation to breast cancer in postmenopausal women participating in the diagnostic investigation of mammary cancer project. *Cancer*. 1992;69:2663-2667.

74. Sellers TA, Kushi LH, Potter JD, et al. Effect of family history, body-fat distribution, and reproductive factors on the risk of postmenopausal breast cancer. *N Engl J Med*. 1992;326:1323-1329.

75. Messina MJ, Persky V, Setchell KDR, Barnes S. Soy intake and cancer risk: a review of the in vitro and in vivo data. *Nutr Cancer*. 1994;21:113-131.

76. Macfarlane GT, Cummings JH. The colonic flora, fermentation, and large bowel digestive function. In: Phillips SF, Pemberton JH, Shorter RG, eds. *The Large Intestine: Physiology, Pathophysiology, and Disease.* New York, NY:Raven Press Ltd; 1991:51-91.

77. Hill MJ. Effect of some factors on the faecal concentration of acid steroids, neutral steroids and urobilins. *J Pathol.* 1971;104:239-245.

78. Birt DF, Bresnick E. Chemoprevention by nonnutrient components of vegetables and fruits. In: Alfin-Slater R, Kritchevsky D, eds. *Human Nutrition: A Comprehensive Treatise.* New York, NY: Plenum Press;1991: Vol. 7;221-261.

79. Nixon DW, ed. Nutrition and Cancer. *Hematol Oncol Clin North Am.* 1991;5(1):1-194.

80. Rivlin RS. An update on calcium: applications for the 90's. *Am J Clin Nutr.* 1991;54:177-288.

81. Seitz HK, Simanowski UA. Alcohol and cancer: A critical review. In: Palmer TN, ed. *Alcoholism: A Molecular Perspective.* New York, NY: Plenum Press; 1991:275-296.

82. Nomura A, Kolonel LN. Prostate cancer: a current perspective. *Epidemiol Rev.* 1991;13:200-227.

83. Sukumar S, Armstrong B, Bruyntjes JP, Leav I, Bosland MC. Frequent activation of the Ki-*ras* oncogene at codon 12 in N-methyl-N-nitrosourea-induced rat prostate adenocarcinomas and neurogenic sarcomas. *Mol Carcinog.* 1991;4: 362-368.

84. Shirai T, Iwasaki S, Naito H, Masui T, Kato T, Imaida K. Dose dependence of N-hydroxy-3,2′-dimethyl-4-aminobiphenyl-induced rat prostate carcinogenesis. *Jpn J Cancer Res.* 1992;83:695-698.

85. Welsch CW. Relationship between dietary fat and experimental mammary tumorigenesis: a review and critique. *Cancer Res.* 1992;52:2040s-2048s.

86. Schottenfeld D, Fraumeni JF. *Cancer Epidemiology and Prevention.* 2nd ed. Oxford: Oxford University Press. In press.

87. Griep AE, Lambert PF. Role of papillomavirus oncogenes in human cervical cancer: transgenic animal studies. *Proc Soc Exp Biol Med.* 1994;206:24-34.

88. Van Eenwyk J, Davis FG, Colman N. Folate, vitamin C, and cervical intraepithelial neoplasia. *Cancer Epidemiol Biomarkers Prev.* 1992;1:119-124.

89. Weisburger JH, Reddy BS, Rose DP, Cohen LA, Kendall ME, Wynder EL. Protective mechanisms of dietary fiber in nutritional carcinogenesis. In: Bronzetti G, DeFlora S, Hayatsu H, Walters M, Shankel DM, eds. *Antimutagenesis and Anticarcinogenesis: Mechanisms.* New York, NY: Plenum Press;1992: Vol 3.

90. Visek WJ, ed. Nutrition and cancer. *Cancer Res.* 1992;52:2019-2126.

91. Wattenberg L, Lipkin M, Boone CW, Kelloff G, eds. *Cancer Chemoprevention.* Boca Raton, Fl: CRC Press Inc;1992:1-600.

92. Correa P. Vitamins and cancer prevention. *Cancer Epidemiol Biomarkers Prev.* 1992;1:241-243.

93. Talalay P. Mechanisms of induction of enzymes that protect against chemical carcinogenesis. *Adv Enzyme Regul.* 1989;28:237-250.

94. El-Bayoumy K. The role of selenium in cancer prevention. In: DeVita VT Jr, Hellman S, Rosenberg SA, eds. *Cancer Prevention.* Philadelphia, Pa: JB Lippincott; 1991;1-15.

95. Jacobs MM, ed. *Vitamins and minerals in the prevention and treatment of cancer.* Boca Raton, Fl: CRC Press Inc; 1991:1-298.

96. Burkitt D. An approach to the reduction of the most common Western cancers. *Arch Surg.* 1991;126:345-347.

97. Wynder EL, Weisburger JH, Ng SK. Nutrition: the need to define "optimal" intake as a basis for public policy decisions. *Am J Public Health.* 1992;82:346-350.

98. Rosenberg L, Palmer JR, Zauber AG, Warshauer ME, Stolley PD, Shapiro S. A hypothesis: nonsteroidal anti-inflammatory drugs reduce the incidence of large-bowel cancer. *J Natl Cancer Inst.* 1991;83:355-358.

99. Rao CV, Tokumo K, Rigotty J, Zang E, Kelloff G, Reddy BS. Chemoprevention of colon carcinogenesis by dietary administration of piroxicam, α-difluoromethylornithine, 16α-fluoro-5-androsten-17-one, and ellagic acid individually and in combination. *Cancer Res.* 1991;51:4528-4534.

100. Craven PA, DeRubertis FR. Effects of aspirin on 1,2-dimethylhydrazine-induced colonic carcinogenesis. *Carcinogenesis.* 1992;13:541-546.

101. Gann PH, Manson JE, Glynn RJ, Buring JE, Hennekens CH. Low-dose aspirin and incidence of colorectal tumors in a randomized trial. *J Natl Cancer Inst.* 1993;85;1220-1224.

102. Ho C-T, Lee CY, Huang M-T, eds. *Phenolic Compounds in Food and Health.* Washington, DC:American Chemical Society;1992.

103. Cohen LA. Physical activity and cancer. In: DeVita VT, Hellman S, Rosenberg SA, eds. *Cancer Prevention.* Philadelphia, Pa: JB Lippincott;1991:1-10.

104. Fidler IJ. Rationale and methods for the use of nude mice to study the biology and therapy of human cancer metastasis. *Cancer Metastasis Rev.* 1986;5:29-49.

105. Price JE, Polyzos A, Zhang RD, Daniels LM. Tumorigenicity and metastasis of human breast carcinoma cell lines in nude mice. *Cancer Res.* 1990;50:717-721.

106. Rose DP, Connolly JM, Meschter CL. Effect of dietary fat on human breast cancer growth and lung metastasis in nude mice. *J Natl Cancer Inst.* 1991;83:1491-1495.

107. Rose DP, Connolly JM. Influence of dietary fat intake on local recurrence and progression of metastases arising from MDA-MB-435 human breast cancer cells in nude mice after excision of the primary tumor. *Nutr Cancer.* 1992;18:113-122.

108. Berns A, Breuer M, Verbeek S, van Lohuizen M. Transgenic mice as a means to study synergism between oncogenes. *Int J Cancer.* 1989;4:22-25.

109. Varmus H. Transgenic mice and host cell mutants resistant to transformation as model systems for identifying multiple components in oncogenesis. *Ciba Found Symp.* 1989;142:20-35.

110. Hamilton SR. Molecular genetic alterations as potential prognostic indicators in colorectal carcinoma. *Cancer.* 1992;69:1589-1591.

111. Höhne MW, Halatsch ME, Kahl GF, Weinel RJ. Frequent loss of expression of the potential tumor suppressor gene *DCC* in ductal pancreatic adenocarcinoma. *Cancer Res.* 1992;52:2616-2619.

112. Metcalf RA, Welsh JA, Bennett WP, et al. p53 and Kirsten-*ras* mutations in human mesothelioma cell lines. *Cancer Res.* 1992;52:2610-2615.

113. Boffetta P, Cardis E, Vainio H, et al. Cancer risks related to electricity production. *Eur J Cancer.* 1991;27:1504-1519.

114. Jauchem JR. Epidemiologic studies of electric and magnetic fields and cancer: a case study of distortions by the media. *J Clin Epidemiol.* 1992;45:1137-1142.

115. McGinnis JM, Foege WH. Actual causes of death in the United States. *JAMA.* 1993;270:2207-2212.

116. Gritz ER, Moon TE. The new cancer prevention and control. *Cancer Epidemiol Biomarkers Prev.* 1992;1:163-165.

117. Muir CS, Sasco AJ. Prospects for cancer control in the 1990s. *Annu Rev Public Health.* 1990;11:143-163.

3

CANCER PREVENTION

Dileep G. Bal, MD, MPH, Daniel W. Nixon, MD, Susan B. Foerster, MPH, RD, Ross C. Brownson, PhD

Why Prevention Is A Priority

There are at least three urgent reasons to increase the rather limited attention currently received by cancer prevention. These are trends in incidence and control of the disease itself; the costs to individuals and to society; and the recurrent pattern of lengthy lagtimes between scientific understanding of prevention and control measures and the widespread application of those measures in the community, resulting in tragic numbers of unnecessary deaths.

Cancer Statistics and Disparities Among Population Segments

Cancer is the second leading cause of death, killing more than a half million Americans annually. The total number of new cancer cases grew to about 1.2 million persons in 1994. One in three Americans will experience cancer during his or her lifetime, up from one in four Americans 10 years ago.[1] As described in the first chapter, the incidence rates of several major cancers are rising and, overall, cancer death rates have increased steadily over the past 50 years, primarily due to the impact of lung cancer.

Disparities among population segments are dramatic. While survival rates for various cancers are improving for most patients, there are significant disparities, particularly among the socioeconomically disadvantaged, nonwhite, and other underserved populations. These population segments are growing in size. They are the most likely to develop cancer, to have cancer detected at an advanced stage, and to receive delayed treatment. Statistics related to African-Americans illustrate the point.[2] Black men have cancer incidence and mortality rates well above those for white men, while black women have incidence rates marginally below and mortality rates above those for white women. The current age-adjusted cancer mortality rate is 27% higher for blacks than for the population at large. Over the past three decades, the age-adjusted cancer death rate for black men increased from 21% to 66% above the overall rate, while the rate for black women changed from actually being marginally below the rate for all races to 10% above it.

The causes of these trends are stark and simple. Black men appear to be exposed in greater proportion to the risk factors for cancer, especially the behavioral risks of tobacco use and diet. Moreover, in comparison to nonblacks, cancers in both black men and black women appear to be diagnosed at a later stage, resulting in reduced survival and high case fatality rates.[3]

It is likely that these trends represent myriad social, cultural, economic, behavioral, environmental, and educational factors, rather than a racial or genetic predisposition for cancer. Statistical adjustment for income or education decreases the cancer rates for African-Americans below those for whites.[2] The unfortunate fact remains: being black correlates highly statistically significantly with being poor, less educated, and deprived of a safe, healthy environment to live in. Being black, or in general belonging to certain ethnic groups, becomes a convenient proxy or surrogate measure of these confounding factors and thus seemingly increases one's risk of certain cancers.

The short- and long-range solutions are conceptually easy. For black men, initiate an intensive risk-reduction program, focusing on such risk factors as tobacco use, diet, and worksite exposures to carcinogens. For both black men and women, improve the

---

Dileep G. Bal, MD, MPH, Chief, Cancer Control Branch, California Department of Health Services, Sacramento, California

Daniel W. Nixon, MD, Associate Director, Cancer Prevention and Control, Hollings Oncology Center, Medical University of South Carolina, Charleston, South Carolina

Susan B. Foerster, MPH, RD, Chief, Nutrition and Cancer Prevention Program, California Department of Health Services, Sacramento, California

Ross C. Brownson, PhD, Chairman, Department of Community Health, School of Public Health, St. Louis University, St. Louis, Missouri

availability, accessibility, and range of healthcare services, particularly early detection, treatment, and risk reduction services.[3]

What seems to be a "health" issue is in fact intertwined with larger economic, social, and other concerns. Thus, adequate societal resources must be categorically redirected toward reducing this accelerating difference in the cancer incidence and mortality rates between African-Americans and the rest of the United States population.[3]

Costs of Cancer

Today's exponential rise in healthcare costs has resulted principally from three factors: the displacement of infectious diseases by lifestyle-influenced, chronic diseases such as cancer; the aging of America, which increases the size of the population experiencing the highest rates of chronic disease events; and the high costs of medical technology, especially in the last months of life, when more than one third of Medicare dollars are spent. Lost economic productivity associated with illness, injury, and disability adds further to this fiscal impact. Unchecked, costs will continue to escalate through the year 2000 and beyond.

Cancer accounts for a large share of the nation's healthcare expenditures, totaling $35 billion in direct medical costs, $12 billion in morbidity costs (lost productivity), and $57 billion in mortality costs.[1] The overall cost of cancer is estimated to have reached $104 billion in 1990.

Treatment and rehabilitation are expensive, and the public, employers, and governmental organizations that pay for healthcare all are demanding change. Healthcare reform initiatives, nationwide and in states, are delineating new approaches for greater access to care and more efficient and lower-cost medical services, to keep people well longer and to promote healthy lifestyles. With prevention becoming an increasingly significant strategy for clinicians, patients, and the public at large, funding for prevention activities such as tobacco control and dietary improvement must increase beyond the <4% level of the nation's total healthcare dollars that was allocated in 1989,[4] to a percentage more in keeping with the proven effectiveness of prevention programs in both reducing illness and saving healthcare dollars.

Delays in Cancer Prevention

The history of cancer prevention and control has been characterized by decades of delay between the acquisition of new knowledge, which has led to the development of intervention technologies, or scientific consensus and its widespread application.[5] Three important examples make this point.

First, the Papanicolaou (Pap) test was perfected in 1943, but not widely used until the early 1970s.[5] Second, mammography as a screening procedure became available in the late 1950s, but was not widely promoted until 1985. Third, the Surgeon General first warned about the link between smoking and cancer in 1964, but it was not until the late 1980s that comprehensive population-based interventions to tobacco control were being widely applied.[6] In each case, a delay of 25 to 30 years occurred between the availability of an important new technology and its widespread adoption.

The human cost of these delays is stunning. Between 1943 and the early 1970s, an estimated 7,000 to 10,000 lives were lost annually to cervical cancer.[5] Breast cancer, the second leading cancer killer in women, is estimated to have taken more than 46,000 lives in 1994, and incidence rates are rising about 2% per year.[1,7] Lung cancer has become the number one cancer in both men and women, resulting in an estimated 153,000 deaths in 1994,[1] with the only intervention being the tobacco control programs so belatedly being adopted. In each case, active technology transfer from research and policy decision to medical care and society at large were missing elements.

The same pattern of delay is observed today in other areas of cancer prevention, most notably diet and exercise.[8] It was in 1913 that the first study of a diet-cancer relationship was published. By 1950, associations with alcohol, "protective" foods, obesity, dietary fat, nutritional status, and carcinogens in cooking had been reported. In the 1950s, the literature began to reflect site-specific relationships.[9] There are now hundreds of studies examining diet and cancer risk. Expert panels have called for dietary changes in the general population, and a full array of intervention strategies has been proposed.[10]

The US, like other developed countries in which chronic diseases are rife, is at a healthcare crossroads. The World Health Organization (WHO) calls for massive changes in the type of diet consumed in affluent countries because of associations with the major chronic diseases.[11] The US has led Western countries in developing dietary guidance policy.[12] However, as with the cancer control methods described above, there is as yet no action plan in place to transfer diet-cancer prevention research into practice.

Prevention Science and Policy

Evidence from numerous experimental and clinical population studies suggests that a large proportion of human cancers is associated with what we eat, drink, and smoke.[9,13-16] About one third of the annual 538,000 deaths in the US attributable to cancer, including breast, colon, and prostate cancers, may be attributable to undesirable dietary practices. Another third, principally deaths from lung, other respiratory, and probably bladder and pancreatic cancers, are due to cigarette smoking. A smaller number, including some oral, laryngeal, esophageal, and possibly breast cancers, may be related to the consumption of alcoholic beverages.[17]

The discipline of preventive medicine teaches that the natural history of disease, from onset to death, may be interrupted at three major junctures, thereby "preventing" progressive deterioration to the next, more severe stage. *Primary prevention* refers to health promotion and risk reduction. These first-line efforts promote healthy lifestyles in the general population and reduce exposure to hazards in the environment, thereby avoiding the development of cancer entirely. *Secondary prevention*, as it applies to cancer, includes screening and detection to identify and treat cancer cases early, thus enhancing the prospects of cure. *Tertiary prevention* refers to treatment of cancer patients to avoid clinical complications and recurrence, to promote faster rehabilitation, and to limit disability. In this chapter, the discussion will focus on primary prevention.

National Prevention Policy

National goals for cancer prevention were first set for the US in the mid-1980s. The National Cancer Institute (NCI) has estimated that by applying measures at hand, cancer deaths could be reduced 25% to 50% by the year 2000.[15]

As shown in Table 3-1, mortality reductions projected by NCI from the early 1980s through the year 2000 were dramatic.[15] A total of 8% to 16% of deaths could be avoided by controlling tobacco use (with the higher estimate based on a 15% prevalence rate of tobacco use in adults by the year 1995), 8% by dietary measures (by doubling fiber consumption and reducing the proportion of calories from dietary fat to ≤25%), 3% by screening and early detection (mammograms and Pap smears), and 10% to 26% by applying state-of-the-art treatment more widely.

In 1990, the US Department of Health and Human Services led a consortium of organizations in the establishment of comprehensive national health goals, *Healthy People 2000: National Health Promotion and Disease Prevention Objectives*.[18] Its cancer control goals are significantly less aggressive and therefore more modest in the projected results. These goals, which include specific targets for reducing risk factors and detecting treatable cancers early, would reduce total cancer deaths by only 2% (Table 3-2). Lung cancer deaths would be held to a 6% increase, breast cancer would be reduced 10%, cervical cancer reduced 54%, and colorectal cancer reduced 27%. Risk factor reduction goals included a 48% decline in tobacco use, a 17% decline in consumption of dietary fat, and a 100% increase in consumption of fruits, vegetables, and grain products.

Table 3-1. Estimated Reduction in Cancer Mortality Rate by the Year 2000

Objective	Method	Estimated Reduction (%)
Prevention	Diet	
	Fat reduction to 25% of total calories and fiber increase to 20-30 g/day	8
	Smoking	
	Reduction in adult smoking prevalence rate to 15%	
	If achieved by year 2000	8
	If achieved by year 1990	16
Screening	Achievement of national objectives	3
Treatment	Application of state-of-the-art treatment for specific cancer sites	
	With no future change in therapy	10
	With current trends in survival maintained	14
	With accelerated gains at all sites	26
TOTAL RANGE OF MORTALITY REDUCTION		25-50

From *Cancer Control Objectives for the Nation: 1985-2000*.[15]

Even these modest prevention goals are unlikely to be met. For example, absent large-scale public health interventions, US rates of cigarette smoking in adults arguably show a leveling off at 26%, after several years of decline. Similarly, there have as yet been few discernible improvements in dietary intake.[19,20]

Cancer Risk Factors

Many important risk factors for cancer have been identified through epidemiologic and laboratory studies over the past several decades. The ability to elucidate risk factors has improved mainly due to better methods in chronic disease epidemiology. Epidemiologic concepts have evolved markedly in the areas of quantitative and statistical methods, case-control studies, and clinical epidemiology.[21] While it is beyond the scope of this chapter to describe these methods and concepts, other texts are available for interested readers.[22-27] This section describes the most important and preventable of these risk factors.

Relative risk and *population attributable risk* are epidemiologic measures that underlie the prevention theme of this chapter. *Relative risk* is the risk of disease or death in the exposed population divided by the risk of disease or death in the unexposed popula-

Table 3-2. Healthy People 2000 National Cancer Objectives

Health Status Objectives	
16.1	Reverse the rise in cancer deaths to achieve a rate of no more than 130 per 100,000 people
16.2	Slow the rise in lung cancer deaths to achieve a rate of no more than 42 per 100,000 people
16.3	Reduce breast cancer deaths to no more than 20.6 per 100,000 people
16.4	Reduce deaths from cancer of the uterine cervix to no more than 1.3 per 100,000 women
16.5	Reduce colorectal deaths to no more than 13.2 per 100,000 people
Risk Reduction Objectives	
16.6	Reduce cigarette smoking to a prevalence of no more than 15% among people aged 20 and older
16.7	Reduce dietary fat intake to an average of ≤30% of calories, and average saturated fat intake to <10% of calories among people aged 2 and older
16.8	Increase complex carbohydrate and fiber-containing foods in the diets of adults to ≥5 daily servings for vegetables (including legumes) and fruits, and to ≥6 daily servings for grain products
16.9	Increase to at least 60% the proportion of people of all ages who limit sun exposure, use sunscreens and protective clothing when exposed to sunlight, and avoid artificial sources of ultraviolet light (eg, sun lamps, tanning booths)
Services and Protection Objectives	
16.10	Increase to at least 75% the proportion of primary-care providers who routinely counsel patients about tobacco use, cessation, diet modification, and cancer screening recommendations
16.11	Increase to at least 80% the proportion of women aged 40 and older who have ever received a clinical breast examination and mammogram, and to at least 60% those aged 50 and older who have received these procedures within the preceding 1 to 2 years
16.12	Increase to at least 95% the proportion of women aged 18 and older with uterine cervix who have ever received a Pap test, and to at least 85% those who received a Pap test within the preceding 1 to 3 years
16.13	Increase to at least 50% the proportion of people aged 50 and older who have received fecal occult blood testing within the preceding 1 to 2 years, and to at least 40% those who ever received proctosigmoidoscopy
16.14	Increase to at least 40% the proportion of people aged 50 and older visiting a primary-care provider in the preceding year who have received oral, skin, and digital rectal examinations during one such visit
16.15	Ensure that Pap tests meet quality standards by monitoring and certifying all cytology laboratories
16.16	Ensure that mammograms meet quality standards by monitoring and certifying at least 80% of mammography facilities

From US Department of Health and Human Services, 1991.[18]

tion. For example, the risk of lung cancer is approximately 11 times higher in cigarette smokers than in nonsmokers (ie, relative risk = 11). *Population attributable risk* is a public health benchmark of how much of the disease burden could be eliminated if the exposure were eliminated. For example, the population attributable risk is 0.87 for cigarette smoking and lung cancer.[28] This suggests that 87% of the lung cancer burden in the population is due to cigarette smoking and could be eliminated if this exposure were eliminated.

The great bulk of primary prevention forecasts is based on the elimination of tobacco use and improvement in dietary practices.[29] Tables 3-3 to 3-6 cite two separate data sources to illustrate that there are differences in interpretation of the extent to which different cancer risks contribute to cancer deaths. The 1981 Doll and Peto estimates are the most frequently cited and have recently been corroborated, especially as they relate to diet (Richard Peto, personal communications, September 1992).

Diet and Nutrition

Diet is one of the most important areas in cancer prevention.[9,14,16] As reviewed extensively in Chapter 2, epidemiologic studies from around the world provide evidence that healthier eating will reduce cancer rates dramatically. Experimental studies are delineating the biologic mechanisms that underlie multiple roles played by various dietary constituents in the causa-

Table 3-3. Modifiable Risk Factors for Lung Cancer

Magnitude of Relative Risk	Risk Factor	Best Estimate of Attributable Risk (where available)*†
Strong (relative risk >4)	Cigarette smoking	87%
	Occupation‡	13
Moderate (relative risk 2-4)	Residential radon exposure	10
Weak (relative risk <2)	Environmental tobacco smoke exposure	2
	Diet low in beta-carotene	—
Possible	Dietary fat/low-vegetable diet	5
	Urban air pollution	—

* The population attributable risk percent is the proportion of the rate of a disease that exists in a community, or population, because of a specific exposure.

† Attributable risk percentages exceed 100% due to the overlapping effect of some risk factors (eg, cigarette smoking and occupation).

‡ Includes occupational exposures to asbestos, polycyclic hydrocarbons, arsenic, and radon gas.

Table 3-4. Modifiable Risk Factors for Colorectal Cancer

Magnitude of Relative Risk	Risk Factor	Best Estimate of Attributable Risk (where available)*
Strong (relative risk >4)	None	—
Moderate (relative risk 2-4)	None	—
Weak (relative risk <2)	High-fat/low-vegetable diet	50%
	Physical inactivity†	20
	Occupation‡	—
	Aspirin use§	—
	Obesity	—

* The population attributable risk percent is the proportion of the rate of a disease that exists in a community, or population, because of a specific exposure.

† Includes both occupational and recreational physical activities.

‡ Includes occupational exposures to asbestos, metal and wood dusts, and certain chemicals.

§ Use of aspirin may decrease risk.

tion, promotion, and inhibition of carcinogenesis.

Applying 1994 statistics to the estimated proportion of lives that could be saved through dietary improvement,[15] the impact of diet, by major site, includes: 50% reductions each in colon and rectal cancers, totaling 28,000 lives; 25% reduction in breast cancer, totaling 11,600 lives; and 15% reductions each in cancers of the prostate, endometrium, and gallbladder, totaling 5,700, 885, and 1,600 lives, respectively. In addition, there may be reductions in cancer of the stomach, esophagus, pancreas, ovaries, liver, lung, and bladder. Thus, on the basis of current knowledge alone, more than 47,800 lives, or 9% of all deaths, could realistically be saved in the year 2000. Since everyone eats, exposure to dietary contributors to cancer affects 100% of the population.

Physiologic and behavioral complexity, as well as rapidly changing social forces, makes diet technically very difficult to investigate. Foods contain thousands of chemical components, stimulating an almost infinite number of chemical combinations and possible physiologic interactions. Since food constituents variably inhibit and promote carcinogenesis, it is difficult to isolate clear point-source, cause-effect relationships. Further, with the disappearance of strong local and regional foodways and the emergence of a national rather than local or regional food supply, large natural variations in the types of foods eaten are increasingly rare. At the same time, meal patterns are becoming more varied, and diets are made up of smaller amounts of more different foods.[8]

For these reasons, the study of diet contrasts starkly with the study of smoking, where exposure is fairly clear: who smokes, how much, what brand, and for how long. Long-term dietary behaviors are increasingly difficult to characterize, in contrast to the easier task of counting the number of years of smoking and the number of cigarettes smoked every day. Yet the best evidence available indicates that the contributions of food and tobacco to the occurrence of cancer are quantitatively similar.

Since epidemiologic correlations and animal research are generally viewed as insufficient to conclusively prove causation, traditional programs of human experimental research are designed to fill in the gaps and test different interventions. Long-term research programs generally follow a systematic progression from (1) basic laboratory science, which delineates the biologic mechanisms suggested by epidemiologic observations, to (2) clinical trials, which test specific interventions in defined human population segments, to (3) community trials, which apply interventions in a more natural environment, to culminate in (4) public health approaches involving

Table 3-5. Modifiable Risk Factors for Breast Cancer

Magnitude of Relative Risk	Risk Factor	Best Estimate of Attributable Risk (where available)*
Strong (relative risk >4)	None	—
Moderate (relative risk 2-4)	First full-term pregnancy after age 30	7%
	Oophorectomy†	—
	Large doses of chest radiation	2
Weak (relative risk <2)	Never being married	—
	Never having children	5
	Obesity after menopause	12
	Alcohol consumption	—
Possible	High-fat diet	—
	Low physical activity	—
	Use of diethylstilbestrol	—
	Use of oral contraceptives or estrogen replacements	—

* The population attributable risk percent is the proportion of the rate of a disease that exists in a community, or population, because of a specific exposure.

† Removal of ovaries before menopause reduces risk.

Table 3-6. Modifiable Risk Factors for Cervical Cancer

Magnitude of Relative Risk	Risk Factor	Best Estimate of Attributable Risk (where available)*
Strong (relative risk >4)	None	—
Moderate (relative risk 2-4)	Multiple sex partners	38%
	Early age at first intercourse	25
	History of sexually transmitted diseases†	5
Weak (relative risk <2)	Cigarette smoking	32
	Use of barrier contraceptives‡	—
Possible	Low dietary intake of certain vitamins§	—
	Use of oral contraceptives	—

* The population attributable risk percent is the proportion of the rate of a disease that exists in a community, or population, because of a specific exposure.

† Includes infection with human papillomavirus types 16 and 18.

‡ Use of barrier contraceptive methods (diaphragm and condom) reduces risk.

§ Includes vitamin A, beta-carotene, and folate.

active technology transfer and large-scale application of the interventions in the general population. The research discussed below reflects the fields of study in diet and cancer prevention viewed as most promising by the National Cancer Institute.

Basic laboratory investigations center on the mechanisms by which various dietary constituents contribute to cancer. These food components include dietary fiber; retinoids and carotenoids; and nutritive and nonnutritive constituents of fruits and vegetables (phytochemicals). Micronutrient levels in blood and tissues, dietary surveys, and food intake data are also evaluated. Specific chemopreventive properties are being evaluated in retinoids, phenolic antioxidants, minor dietary components, inhibitors of polyamine biosynthesis, and certain fatty acids.

Prospective clinical trials center on breast cancer, especially the role of dietary fat and calories; on women as a group, especially dietary factors and steroid hormone metabolism; and, for low-income and minority women, on the feasibility and determinants of changing current eating habits to a low-fat pattern.[29]

In the field of *nutritional epidemiology*, active research seeks to disentangle the roles of fat, calories, animal products, and other aspects of a Westernized diet at various cancer sites; to understand how patterns of weight gain, body fat deposition, physical activity, alcohol consumption, and endogenous hormone levels relate to diet and cancer at multiple sites; to assess how dietary exposures at menarche, during early reproductive life, and later in life impact breast cancer; to delineate the protective role of micronutrients, most notably carotenoids, vitamins A and C, folate, and selenium, relative to cervical cancer, as well as the role of nutrient status relative to stage of carcinogenesis; and to examine how fruit and vegetable intake differentially affects rates of lung cancer in women and African-Americans.

Intervention research includes the *Working Well* collaborative study, a large, worksite-based intervention designed to identify effective methods for reducing cancer risk through tobacco control, dietary change, early detection, and reduced occupational exposure to carcinogens. The *National 5 A Day Program*, a unique public-private partnership between the NCI and the nation's produce industry, is a 10-year effort to encourage all Americans to eat five servings or more of fruits and vegetables as part of a low-fat, high-fiber diet. Starting in 1993, NCI funded nine 4-year projects to evaluate defined 5 A Day interventions in schools, workplaces, and other community settings.[30]

Tobacco

Tobacco use is the single best recognized cause of cancer, responsible for fully 30% of all cases. The etiologic agents in tobacco, as well as medical approaches to smoking cessation, are described in Chapters 2 and 8. This section will focus on the emergence of population-based public health approaches as powerful strategies for the prevention and control of tobacco use. Tobacco control may provide insight into measures that can be applied to the equally important fields of dietary improvement and physical activity. This section was extensively adapted from a recent review by one of the authors.[29]

In recent years, the role of environment and policy in influencing individual smoking behavior has become widely appreciated.[6,31] Environmental and policy interventions are based on the premise that individuals are strongly influenced by their social environment, which provides both positive and negative cues to smoke. These interventions are distinguished from individually oriented approaches by their intent to have a sustained "systemic" effect on the population. They seek to alter tobacco use by focusing on factors that precede or establish the context for such use, without specifically focusing on the individual tobacco user.

Changing the environment can involve a combination of forces, including health policies, media coverage, and economic incentives, each of which can be executed through a wide array of specific measures. Health policies can be established at the federal, state, and community levels, or by organizations, through accreditation standards, or at worksites. Media coverage can influence social norms, as demonstrated by the media coverage given to Surgeon General's reports since 1964 and the declines in smoking that have ensued.[32] Similarly, economic incentives such as tobacco taxes have the potential to decrease smoking prevalence.[33]

Environmental and policy approaches to control tobacco use are included in the nation's *Healthy People 2000* goals.[18] (Omitted from these objectives are important measures such as taxation of tobacco and health insurance coverage for tobacco cessation.) The multicomponent strategy outlined for the nation focused primarily on youth smoking.

Examples of effective legislative and regulatory actions include clean indoor air policies in public places and worksites; restricted tobacco advertising and promotion, especially to youth; comprehensive educational curriculum in first through twelfth grades; and restricted youth access to tobacco products. One example of such federal legislation is the Synar Amendment, enacted in June 1992. Effective October 1, 1993, this requires states to enact and enforce a law to prohibit the sale or distribution of tobacco products to youths under the age of 18. The hallmark of the unique carrot-and-stick approach of this legislation is that states failing to comply with these requirements will lose 10% of their prevention and treatment substance abuse block grant funds during the first year, 20% in the second year, 30% in the third year, and 40% in the fourth and subsequent years. This should serve as a powerful incentive for states to comply.

Economic and productivity incentives that work include price policies such as excise taxes, to which youths are especially susceptible; insurance premium differentials, such as nonsmoker discounts; health insurance reimbursement for smoking cessation—an especially important measure for heavy smokers; and differential hiring of nonsmokers by employers, due to the recognition of higher medical costs, sick leave, and accident rates in smokers, as well as concern about the rights and health of nonsmokers.

Media advocacy is the strategic use of mass media to promote public policy initiatives.[16] Media advocacy efforts that frame the smoking issue as being a public health problem rather than a simple matter of personal choice work best. This helps to define public policy initiatives that will change the social environment concerning the use of tobacco.[34] Techniques include placing local spokespersons to gain exposure for the tobacco issue, providing a local angle on national tobacco events, paying for counteradvertising, and using "creative epidemiology" to present scientifically accurate data in a way that catches the media's attention.

Media advocacy conducted by local coalitions is especially effective, as it encompasses a broad-based array of organizations and individuals, helps secure access to media and intervention channels, mobilizes the human resources needed for action, and may include representatives from priority population groups. Other successful techniques include analyzing and publicizing tobacco industry tactics, such as lobbying tactics in state legislatures[35]; product liability and workman's compensation litigation[36,37]; and surveillance related to policy initiatives, such as consumer opinion data about tobacco control. The effectiveness of media advocacy is illustrated by the rapid shift in social acceptability of smoking and the growth of nonsmokers' rights organizations, indicating a shift in the willingness of nonsmokers to speak out and take action.

State initiatives have met with varied levels of success, but each provides lessons for the future. Passed in 1988, California's Proposition 99 has been the model in the growing national and international movements against tobacco use. With an excise tax of 25¢ per pack of cigarettes, designated fractions of the revenue were allocated to fund healthcare services for the indigent, fire prevention and control, statewide anti-tobacco education in schools and communities, and research on tobacco-related disease. The tax sharply accelerated drops in both cigarette sales and smoking, with a 25% decline in adult smoking prevalence in 4 years (from 26.7% to 20%), double the projected decline based on previous trends. In 1992, the per capita rate of cigarette consumption in California was 13.8% lower than it would have been without Proposition 99 activities. Since the campaign began, roughly half of all the smokers in California attempted to quit smoking. The frequency of quit attempts increased with the introduction of local program activities and the quit attempts. By 1992, there were approximately 1 million fewer smokers in California. Included in the effort was an effective 18-month-long, $28 million counter-advertising campaign. More powerful over the long-term is the impact of grassroots efforts stimulated by the funding of anti-tobacco coalitions which focus on clean indoor air ordinances, the removal of cigarette vending machines, prevention and cessation programs for racial/ethnic minorities, increased collaboration among health and education agencies, and technical assistance and evaluation. More than 100 new community ordinances have instituted smoke-free policies, and policies restricting access to cigarettes by minors have been adopted in California since 1990. An interesting twist to state tobacco tax increases is the fact that in these lean fiscal times, this is one of the few sources of revenue still available for health programs not necessarily tobacco related. For instance, in late 1993, the California legislature enacted a bill raising the tobacco tax by 2¢ per pack, with the projected $40 million in annual revenue being equally divided between breast cancer research and breast cancer screening programs.

Other states have made similar efforts. For example, a similar referendum sponsored primarily by the American Cancer Society (ACS) and supported by more than 250 other organizations succeeded in Massachusetts in 1992. In spite of strong legal challenges to its provisions by the tobacco industry, the advocates were able to persevere by using countermeasures such as obtaining twice the required number of signatures and "jawboning" the media to reduce the airtime sold to tobacco proponents.[38]

In Michigan, the legislature created the Michigan Health Initiative Fund, funded in part through a 4¢-per-pack tax on cigarettes, which represented a landmark policy shift toward preventive healthcare in the state and local health departments.[39] In Montana, on the other hand, a 1990 antitobacco initiative failed, succumbing to opponents' themes arguing against new taxes and a larger state bureaucracy, as well as outspending by tobacco proponents by a ratio of 35 to 1.[40]

A case-study methodology was used by the Rand Corporation to analyze the processes by which policies succeeded or failed in becoming law in Florida, Illinois, Minnesota, New York, Texas, and Arizona. It provides insights to states and localities now debating tobacco restrictions in public places.[41] Another review of 15 community intervention trials that used a broad range of education and mass media approaches for cardiovascular disease prevention has shown promising declines in potential morbidity and mortality due to success with smoking cessation and reduced tobacco use, even in the absence of policy and environmental strategies (Rothenberg, unpublished data).

Measures using advertising, promotion, and community empowerment are expected to expand in the future. For example, in 1988 tobacco advertisements were banned in newspapers and magazines published in Canada, as well as point-of-sale advertising and promotion. In Europe, a number of countries have enacted similar restrictions on the use of graphics in tobacco advertising, and it is likely that the European Union will begin to address restrictions that would apply to all member nations.[42]

At the community level, the Uptown Coalition in Philadelphia successfully opposed the introduction by the RJ Reynolds Company of a cigarette specifically targeted to African-Americans, in the first substantive example of an ethnic minority community assuming leadership in a tobacco control initiative. Similarly, the California Healthy Cities Project, which brings tobacco control into the halls of local government and offices of civic organizations, signals an expansion of local ownership and responsibility for tobacco use as a community public health problem.[43]

Throughout these efforts, the ACS has been a strong advocate and leader in the fight against tobacco use.

Physical Activity

The relation of exercise to cancer is a relatively new field of research. An estimated 32% of colon cancers may be related to physical inactivity.[44] This equates to approximately 34,000 new cases and 16,000 deaths from colon cancer each year in the US. Several studies have shown that colon cancer risk is reduced among persons with greater occupational activity, greater adult participation in exercise and other active recreation, and greater levels of total activity.[45,46] In addition, evidence suggests that low physical activity may increase the risk of breast cancer in women[47] and prostate cancer,[48] although these relationships require further study.

Two related physiologic mechanisms have been

proposed. Physical activity appears to stimulate colon peristalsis,[49] as well as prostaglandin production,[50] which also would likely increase peristalsis. Increased colon peristalsis may shorten the transit time of the stool and accompanying exposure of the colon to fecal contents, including carcinogens.

Alcohol

The International Agency for Research on Cancer concluded that there is significant evidence for the carcinogenicity of ethanol and alcoholic beverages in humans.[51] Cancers of the oral cavity, pharynx, larynx, esophagus, and liver are causally related to alcohol consumption.[52,53] Evidence also suggests an association between alcohol consumption and colorectal and breast cancers.[52]

There is also strong evidence that alcohol consumption in combination with cigarette smoking has a synergistic effect on the risk for certain cancers, namely cancers of the oral cavity, pharynx, larynx, and esophagus. It has been suggested that alcohol may act as a solvent, allowing carcinogens in tobacco or in the diet to enter epithelial cells.[54]

Occupational and Environmental Exposure

Many occupations are associated with repeated and prolonged contact with potential carcinogens. Table 3-7 lists a number of industries, industrial carcinogens, and associated cancers.[55,56] In a classic epidemiologic example, Sir Percival Pott recognized an unusual frequency of scrotal cancer among London's chimney sweeps in the late 1700s; the carcinogenic potential of soot was demonstrated more than a century later. During the 1800s skin cancer was commonly noted in workers exposed to coal tar, mineral oil, and arsenic. In the 20th century, lung cancer was identified as an occupational hazard in mineral refining and processing industries. Mining itself may create toxic exposure; radioactivity in mines has been linked to lung cancer.[55]

Exact data are difficult to obtain because of confounding factors (alcohol consumption and tobacco use, for example), but about 20,000 cancer deaths annually may be due to occupational exposure.[56] Observation of tumors (and other diseases) that occur in various occupational groups has led to measures to protect workers' health as well as provide useful background data for experimental research. The Occupational Safety and Health Administration (OSHA), the Environmental Protection Agency, and the National Institute for Occupational Safety and Health (NIOSH) now work together to investigate workplace hazards and to enforce standards for safe exposure levels. Workers must be fully informed about toxic exposure. OSHA and NIOSH require medical surveillance for a total of 23 chemicals or chemical processes used in industry that have carcinogenic potential.[57]

Other Environmental Factors

Despite widespread publicity and concern, the contribution of environmental factors outside the workplace to overall cancer death rates is relatively small compared with tobacco use and diet.

Sunlight

Solar radiation, especially the ultraviolet component, is a major contributor to most skin cancers (basal cell, squamous cell, and melanoma). More than 700,000

Table 3-7. Industries Associated with Exposure to Carcinogens

Industry	Carcinogen	Cancer
Shipbuilding, demolition, insulation	Asbestos	Lung, pleura, peritoneum
Varnish, glue	Benzene	Leukemia
Pesticides, smelting	Arsenic	Lung, skin, liver
Mineral refining and manufacturing	Nickel, chromium	Lung
Furniture manufacturing	Wood dusts	Nasal passages
Petroleum products	Polycyclic hydrocarbons	Lung
Rubber manufacturing/dye workers	Aromatic amines	Bladder
Vinyl chloride	Vinyl chloride	Liver
Radium	Radium	Bone
Petroleum refining/coal hydrogenation	Coal tar products, mineral oils	Skin

basal and squamous cell cancers occur yearly in the US, along with 32,000 cases of melanoma. Fortunately, basal and squamous cancers are rarely fatal, but melanoma accounts for 6,900 deaths per year. For the past two decades, melanoma rates have increased about 4% annually. Reasons for this increase are not well understood, but depletion of the protective atmospheric ozone layer, which absorbs ultraviolet radiation, may be involved. Several by-products of industrialization, including exhausts from high flying aircraft, aerosol propellants, nitrogen-containing fertilizers, and nuclear weapons testing may affect the ozone layer.[58]

Risk factors for skin cancer (that relate to ultraviolet light exposure) include occupations that require outdoor work, having fair skin, living in sunny climates, unprotected recreational sun exposure, and certain inherited diseases that involve defective DNA repair mechanisms and sensitivity to sunlight (albinism, xeroderma pigmentosum).[58] Skin cancer is rare in blacks.

Air and Water Pollution

Clearly, a variety of substances with carcinogenic potential are present as pollutants in our air and drinking water. Low levels of these pollutants, and variations in pollution levels by geography (urban vs rural), by season (eg, coal burning in winter) and over time make any assessment of cancer risk from these sources very difficult. Some common pollutants in air are asbestos, polycyclic aromatic hydrocarbons from fossil fuel (at least 14 different compounds), and various non-aromatic organic compounds. Indoor air pollutants such as formaldehyde from particle board and naturally occurring radon gas also contribute to cancer risk, although to an uncertain extent. In water, many potential human carcinogens have been identified, including viruses, radioactive particles, solid matter such as asbestos, and many inorganic and organic compounds (eg, metals, nitrates, vinyl chloride).[59]

Occupational exposure levels to carcinogens are more likely to be in the hazardous range than incidental exposure outside the workplace. In the latter instance, the concentration of carcinogens is usually lower than the levels known to be carcinogenic in the laboratory.

Efforts to limit or eliminate air and water pollutants are worthwhile. It may not be possible, however, to completely remove all known carcinogens from the air and water supply in an industrialized society. The concentrations of such substances are usually small, and their contribution to overall cancer mortality is undoubtedly minor.

The 1993 Environmental Protection Agency report singles out "second-hand" smoke, or environmental tobacco smoke (ETS), as a hitherto ignored and underemphasized source of indoor air pollution. ETS is now recognized as a significant source of disease and disability among children.

Infections

Many infectious agents have been linked to cancer, by either epidemiologic association or laboratory evidence, or both. Epstein-Barr virus and Burkitt's lymphoma are examples.

Both RNA and DNA viruses cause cancer in animals, and evidence is strong that some human tumors (other than Burkitt's lymphoma) have a viral etiology as well. These include nasopharyngeal carcinoma (also from Epstein-Barr virus), liver cancer (hepatitis B virus) and cervical cancer (human papillomavirus). The human immunodeficiency virus is associated with lymphoma and Kaposi's sarcoma, especially as a component of acquired immunodeficiency syndrome (AIDS).

Several parasitic infections are associated epidemiologically with cancer. Among these are liver flukes (cholangiocarcinoma) and blood flukes (bladder cancer and possibly colorectal cancer).[56,60] Associations between bacterial infections and cancer are uncommon, but a 1991 report linked *Helicobacter pylori* infection of the stomach to stomach cancer.[61] Aflatoxins produced by *Aspergillus* organisms are considered risk factors for liver cancer.

Medications

Drugs in common use that have carcinogenic properties include the sex hormones—estrogens and androgens—and the antiestrogenic agent tamoxifen. Estrogens, widely prescribed for postmenopausal women, have been associated with endometrial and breast cancers. The therapeutic benefits of estrogen use (symptomatic relief, prevention or delay of atherosclerotic disease and osteoporosis) are considered by most to be greater than the remote risk of cancer. Tamoxifen has received considerable attention, because it is being used as a cancer preventive agent in a large NCI study involving healthy women at increased risk for breast cancer. There seems to be a weak causation between use of tamoxifen and the development of liver tumors and endometrial cancers. In the past, diethylstilbesterol has been given to pregnant women to prevent miscarriage, and in 1971 an association was made between such use and adenocarcinoma of the vagina in the female children of exposed women.[62]

Arsenic compounds, also used medicinally in the past, have been associated with squamous cell cancers of the skin, particularly on the palms and soles and in the inguinal area. Alkylating agents, antineoplastics widely used in chemotherapy, have known carcinogenic activity (rarely leukemia and lymphoma occur after solid tumor therapy), as do immunosuppressive agents and radioactive agents. Other commonly used agents with suspected carcinogenic potential include phenacetin (renal pelvic cancer), coal tar ointments (skin cancer), and amphetamines (lymphoma).[56,63] Industrial and pharmacologic carcinogens were reviewed in a 1991 report.[64]

In summary, a succinct description of the state of the science in the primary prevention of cancer is summarized by Henderson, Ross, and Pike[65]:

> *We now have sufficient knowledge to move energetically toward the prevention of a significant proportion of human cancer. The majority of the causes of cancer (such as tobacco, alcohol, dietary fat, obesity, ultra-violet light) are associated with lifestyle; that is, with personal choices and not with the environment in general. The widespread public perception that environmental pollution is a major cancer hazard is incorrect.*

Technologies for Implementing Prevention Programs

Although the primary prevention of cancer in the US is possible through straightforward changes in lifestyle—healthier eating, tobacco cessation, and increased physical activity—the magnitude of exposure to these risk factors in the general population is profound. At least 90% of Americans consume too few fruits, vegetables, and grains and too much fat; 20% to 30% of Americans smoke (and a much larger percent are exposed to environmental tobacco smoke); and over half have sedentary lifestyles.[66] Therefore, interventions must move beyond education and employ more powerful approaches that work for entire populations. To illustrate how prevention science can be transferred from one field to another, we will draw parallels from the well-developed field of tobacco control to demonstrate in practical terms how to apply existing behavioral change theory to another field of cancer prevention, dietary improvement. A similar case could be made for physical activity.

Approaching the Problem

Smoking, eating, and exercising are, first and foremost, social behaviors. They are mediated by societal perceptions and values about health. Tobacco control research shows that a mix of individual, community, and environmental strategies, in tandem with mass media and policy decisions, is extremely powerful. In the case of tobacco, these strategies applied together overcame an addiction as strong as heroin and an industry that spends $4 billion in the US every year promoting, assisting, and encouraging the vulnerable to smoke. The history of tobacco control also clearly indicates that behavioral change occurs fastest once societal norms and values made smoking unfashionable and socially unacceptable.[67]

Behavior Change in Individuals

Many models have been developed to predict how to modify health behavior. The Transtheoretical Model[68,69] blends a number of theories into an intuitively simple approach that has been used successfully in several areas, including smoking. It describes the natural history of behavioral change as individuals going through a series of six stages of change. These are precontemplation, contemplation, preparation, action, maintenance, and termination.

In *precontemplation*, one is not yet considering a behavioral change. The advantages or pleasure of engaging in the risky behavior are still seen as much greater than the benefits of stopping. In *contemplation*, one begins to perceive that the status quo is injurious, to believe that there would be benefits to changing, and to experience dissonance due to the pros and cons being about equal.

In *preparation*, one begins to consider what the costs and benefits of change would be for oneself, and to think about what the changes would entail. One identifies obstacles, begins to see ways to overcome them, and starts testing a new behavior. During this phase, the person replaces arguments against changing with reasons to change, that is, to internalize more "pros" than "cons" for a change. In *action*, one starts to seek out resources and products more consistently, to look and listen for more information and solutions, and to try to form new habits.

In *maintenance*, the person attempts to permanently establish the new behavior, while nonetheless slipping back into long-established and comfortable habits and deflecting social or family pressure to return to the old ways. *Termination* is the stage of zero temptation to engage in the old behavior and 100% self-efficacy in all previous tempting situations. New behaviors such as dietary and exercise change seem to be tougher to deal with than addictive ones such as tobacco use cessation both within and outside Prochaska's model.[69]

Put another way, the staged process involves replacing the number of pros associated with practicing a risky behavior with a larger number of cons, until the pros are essentially removed from a person's belief structure and newly learned skills become habit.

Programming for Health Promotion

Public health education programs are targeted at individuals, their families, and social networks, as well as the institutions and social conditions that impact health behavior.[70] *Health promotion programs* take this further by proactively and assertively combining health education with health advocacy[71] and connecting health education to related organizational, economic, and environmental supports that are conducive to health.[72]

For smoking, decades of applied health education/promotion intervention science have recently been synthesized into easy-to-use principles, guidelines, and protocols through the combined effort of the American Cancer Society and the National Cancer Institute, the two largest cancer and smoking control agencies in the world. Recommendations for planning effective programs are contained in the "gold standard" framework, *Standards for Comprehensive Smoking Prevention and Control.*[73] A second compilation of research findings and recommendations is found in *Strategies to Control Tobacco Use in the United States: A Blueprint for Public Health Action in the 1990s.*[6] Much of the application science base in these expert reports is transferable to other areas of cancer prevention, as discussed below.

To be effective, interventions must be designed to develop synergy from discrete, complementary components. Optimally planned intervention programs involve five steps: (1) clearly identify priority target groups; (2) use multiple, appropriate channels to gain access to the group(s), such as worksites, schools, community networks, the community environment, and/or the health care system; (3) design three types of interventions, namely program services (as in 2, above), media, and policy; (4) deliver the three types of interventions simultaneously; and (5) apply this constellation of interventions at the national, state, and local levels. Fig 3-1 depicts the interrelationships of this planning model using blue-collar workers as an illustration.

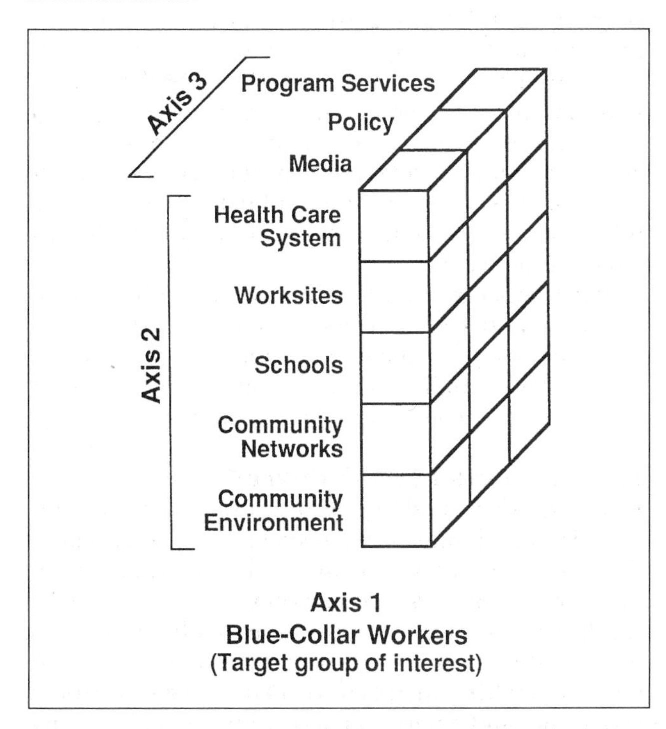

Fig 3-1. Cross-section of planning model for a single target group (blue-collar workers).

For population behavior change, the *mass media* play a critical role in influencing what society knows, believes, and does. For example, tobacco advertising and promotion saturates the environment with messages reinforcing the perception of smoking as a socially approved, accepted, and even desirable behavior.[74,75] Tobacco advertisements reinforce the perception that "smoking must be acceptable, otherwise the government would ban it."[75] Therefore, efforts to control tobacco use must focus on creating a social environment that provides persistent and inescapable cues to counter the advertising messages. Counteracting mass media activities have two goals: to increase the public's exposure to pro-health, anti-tobacco messages, and to reduce the public's exposure to pro-tobacco cues.

Policy and environmental changes strongly influence smoking initiation and cessation. Removal of *environmental stimuli and reinforcement* such as tobacco advertising and promotions and the simultaneous creation of *environmental disincentives* such as worksite policies on smoking markedly alter the personal, psychological, and sociological utility of smoking. This leads to higher rates of smoking cessation and lower rates of smoking initiation.[6] Effective policy and environmental changes include increased tobacco costs, anti-tobacco media campaigns, declining social acceptability of smoking, limitations on where smoking is allowed, and restricted access for youth.[6]

Institutionalizing Behavior Change

Tobacco research also shows that societal positioning of cancer risk factors plays a more powerful role in risk reduction than many health professionals realize. For example, enduring change in health behavior results only when attitudes change about the standards of acceptable behavior in the community.[76] Critical to achieving community behavioral change is acceptance of "ownership" of the problem by the target population and, through community mobilization, empowerment to control the activity. Simply put, the most powerful way to change individual behavior is to affect the social structures in a community that help shape an individual's opinions and attitudes.[77]

Social action and locality development are two practical methods to implement interventions while establishing community ownership. *Social action* involves grassroots organizing of citizen groups that desire change in the social structure, such as the formation of local groups to urge restrictions on public smoking. *Locality development* expands local participation in the intervention by including more than just the most committed groups in the change process. *Coalition building* is a form of locality development. Why does this work?

Because organizations network with each other, change diffuses among them and affects the membership of other organizations, ultimately leading to a change in the community as a whole.[6] Involving organizations in achieving common goals encourages them to divert their resources toward new causes, like tobacco control, which in itself represents a change in policy and in social norms. The changes come full circle when individuals perceive and internalize community norms. They observe opinion and behavior in their immediate environment, which consists of social networks of family, friends, and organizations they belong to; the workplace and other communal facilities such as airports, sports stadiums, and restaurants; and impressions derived from the media.[78] *Denormalization* is a term used in tobacco circles for this broad societal positioning of nonsmoking behavior or depositioning of extended tobacco use behavior.

Leadership for Change

Widely recognized as responsible for the growth of the anti-tobacco movement is the scientific and policy leadership of the Office of the Surgeon General over the past 30 years. In the face of medical skepticism initially, followed by powerful industry opposition to this day, Surgeon General conferences and reports have provided a "steady drumbeat" in support of today's pervasive and highly motivated anti-smoking movement. Such single-minded and principled leadership demonstrates the value of the "bully pulpit" in achieving social changes in the face of massive social and business resistance.

Dietary Recommendations for Cancer Prevention: What Needs To Be Done

While simple in concept, our national dietary goals nonetheless require significant changes for Americans: *a near-doubling of fruits and vegetables; a doubling of dietary fiber; and a reduction by ≥25% of fat intake.* Because dietary habits have changed slowly, if at all, over the last two decades,[16,19] achieving these targets by the year 2000 will require unprecedented acceleration in the rate of dietary change.

Americans have never been better informed or expressed more interest in their diet. However, the food industry is the nation's largest advertiser, spending $8 billion in 1988,[79] the vast majority for foods inconsistent with cancer prevention guidelines. Further, the dominance of incomplete and distorted messages in the media and in food advertising indicates that simple educational strategies are not powerful enough to generate behavioral change of the magnitude needed to reduce cancer risk.[80,81]

Denormalization of a single behavior such as tobacco use is difficult enough, but denormalization of scores of food-related behaviors, some of which are ill-defined and lack scientific consensus, are near impossible. Therefore, the problem needs to be defined more specifically in order for an effective intervention to ensue.

The American Cancer Society has produced research-based dietary guidelines for lowering cancer risk.[19] Similar recommendations are found in multiple consensus documents, including the *National Academy of Sciences Diet and Health,*[16] and the federal government's *Dietary Guidelines for Americans,*[82] and *The Food Guide Pyramid.*[83] The ACS endorses these recommendations. The ACS dietary recommendations and their rationale are described below, together with discussion of the magnitude of exposure of each risk, trends in risk factor reduction, and the progress being made in each goal.

1. Maintain a desirable body weight.

The massive Cancer Prevention Study I, conducted prospectively over a 12-year period (1960 to 1972) by the ACS, showed clearly that obese people are at increased risk of dying from certain cancers.[84] This study found an association between increased deaths from cancers of the uterus, gallbladder, kidney, stomach, colon, and breast and varying degrees of being overweight. Women 40% above desirable weight had up to 55% greater mortality from cancer than did those of normal weight; and similarly, obese men had up to 33% greater mortality. Lesser degrees of being overweight were also associated with increased prevalence of certain cancers.

An estimated 27% of women and 24% of men are overweight.[82] Weight loss and long-term maintenance is one of medicine's most complex physiologic and behavioral challenges, and an estimated $30 billion is spent by Americans annually on weight loss products and programs.[85] While weight loss can be accomplished by combining a reduced intake of total calories with an increase in physical activity, maintaining the new weight is more difficult. In the US, rates of obesity are rising among both adults and youths. There are no population-based interventions in place to reverse this trend.

2. Eat a varied diet.

Variety, balance, and moderation are principles of good nutrition, and they apply as well to risk reduction for cancer. The *Food Guide Pyramid* displayed in Fig 3-2 is the most widely used food guide to help consumers select a healthy mix of foods every day.[83] The system recommends both the number of servings and the variety of foods to eat every day, as well as eating in moderation foods with nutrients that in excess contribute to chronic disease risk. Consistent with cancer recommendations, the *Food Guide Pyramid* calls for an approximate doubling of consumption of fruit, vegetables, and grains with the total amount of animal foods, such as milk and meat, kept at present levels

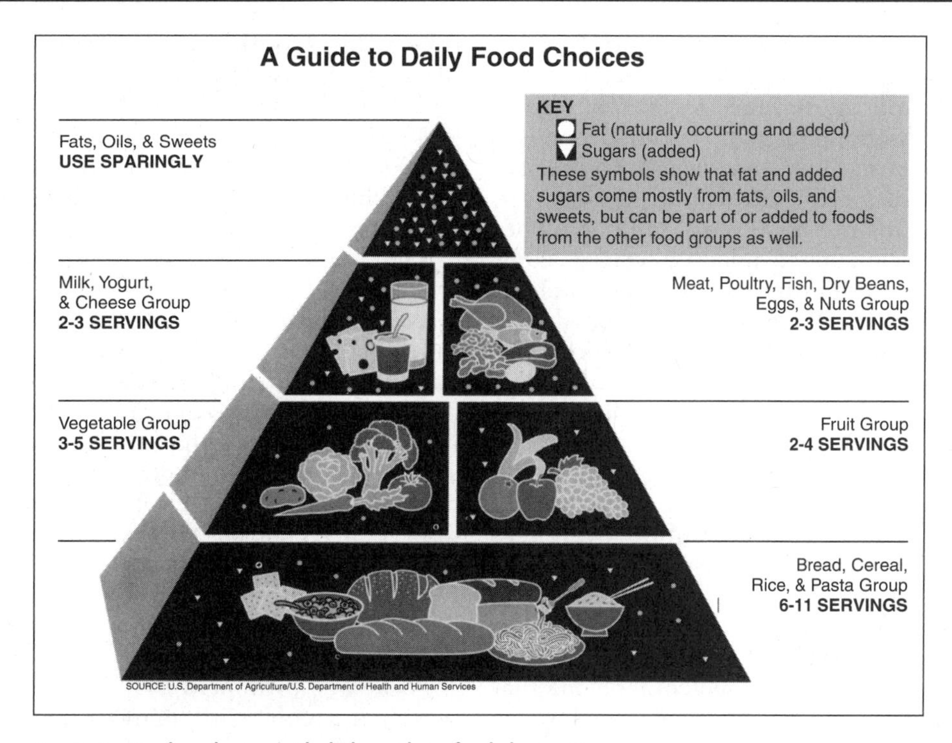

Fig 3-2. Food guide pyramid: daily guide to food choices.[83]

and selected to reduce the fat content. Trends in food consumption indicate that there is little progress toward achieving these goals.

Food and nutrient data for individuals have been available for a relatively short period. As a surrogate, agricultural data on a per capita basis are used to provide some indication of long-term trends. Since 1910, less fruit, vegetable, and grain products have been sold in the marketplace; meat and milk products have increased 23% and 33%, respectively; and supplies of fats, oils, and sugars have increased >60%.[16] Available data suggest that few Americans are achieving the dietary variety, balance, and fat lowering recommended by the *Food Guide Pyramid*.

Historical trends indicate massive shifts in control of the food supply. With industrialization, urbanization, and improved interstate transportation, sources of food entering the kitchen changed early in the 20th century from local farm production and perhaps 300 to 500 foods available for sale in the grocery store to today's huge array of supermarket choices, numbering as high as 60,000 items in a superstore. Control is shifting again, away from the home kitchen to out-of-home preparation.

Other trends are toward fewer sit-down family meals and more "grazing," a larger proportion of food being eaten and/or prepared out-of-home, a high volume of combination dishes such as casseroles, pizzas, frozen dinners, and ethnic dishes containing ingredients that the consumer may not be aware of. As a result, it is more difficult for individuals to monitor how much of each food group they eat every day and to control the content of their meals. This suggests that dietary change interventions must focus on food processors and foodservice operations and not just on individuals.

3. Include a variety of both vegetables and fruits in the daily diet.

A rapidly growing research base shows strong associations between lower cancer rates and patterns of higher fruit and vegetable consumption.[86,87] A recent meta-analysis confirms that eating more vegetables and fruits is associated with a decreased risk of cancers in eleven different sites, including lung, colon, prostate, bladder, esophagus, and stomach.[88] Vegetables and fruits contain vitamins, minerals, fiber, and nonnutritive constituents which, alone or together, may be responsible for the observed reduction in cancer risk. Studies also show lowered risk with many different fruit, vegetable, and legume items, so it is desirable to vary the selection of vegetables and fruits.

The current recommendation is to eat 5 to 9 servings of fruits and vegetables every day. Consumption among American adults is estimated to be between 3 and 4 servings.[20,30] Since the turn of the century, per capita supplies have decreased 20%, with the lowest levels occurring during the 1950s.[16] At present, intake is increasing at a rate of about 1.5% per year, suggesting that the goal for the year 2000 will be met about 2015, or 15 years late.

A model is developing on how to change America's

fruit and vegetable consumption. The *National 5 A Day Program* was launched in 1991 as a major initiative of the NCI and the Produce for Better Health Foundation, representing the nation's produce industry. The program has a simple message: eat 5 or more fruits and vegetables every day as part of a low-fat, high-fiber diet. This initiative seeks to double consumption by the year 2000 to at least 5 servings daily. It has begun by conducting ongoing mass media publicity and involving supermarkets nationwide in voluntarily conducting fruit/vegetable promotions regularly. Additional channels that are or will be involved include produce companies, health departments, schools, community organizations, and foodservice operations, such as restaurants and cafeterias. Coalitions at the state and local levels will be established to organize interventions, conduct public awareness activities, and otherwise encourage policy change.

4. Eat more high-fiber foods, such as whole grain cereals, legumes, vegetables, and fruits.

Dietary fiber consists of plant food components that are not digested in the human intestinal tract. Largely complex carbohydrates of diverse chemical composition, they are abundant in whole grains, fruits, vegetables, and beans. Epidemiologic evidence indicates that colon cancer is low in populations on other continents whose diet includes high amounts of dietary fiber. It is as yet unclear whether these data are applicable to the US. Even if specific types of fiber do not prove to have a direct protective effect against cancer, vegetables, fruits, cereals, and beans can be recommended as nutritious substitutes for higher-calorie or fatty foods. They are also beneficial in the lowering of blood lipids, the control of diabetes, and possibly weight management.

Six to eleven servings of breads, cereals, and grains are recommended daily, several of which should be whole grain. Consumption by women in the mid-1980s averaged about 4 servings. During this century, there has been a 50% per capita reduction in grains in the food supply, and legumes have increased just 12% per capita.

Segments of the food industry have successfully promoted certain grain products. In the late 1980s, a major initiative by the Kellogg's Company and the NCI resulted in a significant percent increase in purchases of targeted cereals, with consumers also buying other brands of high-fiber cereals and breads. Thus, there has been a general gain in awareness about high-fiber eating.[89] More recently, the Wheat Foods Council established the *Check Your 6* initiative which encourages eating at least 6 servings of breads, cereals, and grains daily.

5. Cut down on total fat intake.

Substantial evidence from both clinical and laboratory studies indicates that excessive fat intake increases the risk of developing cancers of the breast, colon, and prostate.

The consensus recommendation endorsed by the American Cancer Society and virtually all major health authorities in the US, including the American Heart Association and the National Cholesterol Education Program, is for all persons older than 2 years to reduce total fat intake by one quarter, so that fat represents no more than 30% of total calorie intake (from the current average of 37%). The ceiling of 30% can be achieved by reducing the use of fats and oils used in food preparation, cooking, and at the table; substituting nutritious foods that are naturally high in fats, such as certain cuts and grades of meat and whole-fat dairy products, with their leaner and lower fat counterparts; and choosing packaged foods with less added fat. (Fat-restricted diets are not recommended for infants or children under the age of two years.)

Between 1971 and 1986, there was no change in average fat consumption in adults aged 19 to 50.[16] In 1986, it was estimated that only 10% of American women ate a diet with no more than 30% of calories from fat.[90] These women ate relatively high proportions of sugar and alcohol with lower levels of vitamins and minerals, raising concern that the single message to lower fat may result in unintended side effects and should therefore be part of a more complete dietary guidance effort.

On a similar note, a phenomenon known as "fat-banking" has been observed in which people reduce fat from certain foods in order to eat more fat in others. This is of particular interest to health professionals because *"precisely those individuals who have been most likely to decrease their consumption of red meat and eggs because of health concerns—educated, middle-aged white women—have at the same time been most likely to increase their consumption of salad oils, cheese, and ice cream. The net effect being that these individuals have not changed the percentage of calories from fat in their diets."*[91]

Clearly, we need a better understanding of fat sources in the food supply and how they are changing. In the late 1970s, prepared animal foods such as milk, meat, poultry, and fish products provided 59% of the fat in the American diet. However, the sources of fat have been shifting to vegetable oils. For example, in 1985, butter and lard were used in only a third of the amount of the early 1900s, with a per capita disappearance of 9 lb annually. During the same period, margarine, shortening, and salad and cooking oils increased >500%, to nearly 60 lb per capita by 1985. (These figures do not represent consumption, as they include fats and oils discarded after use, such as following deep fat frying.) Salad dressings, fried snack foods, and bakery goods now constitute major sources of fat in the diet. This shift, with its accompanying improved ratio of saturated to unsaturated fatty acids, may have had a beneficial effect, namely the recently observed significant reductions in average US blood cholesterol levels.[92]

The meat industry promotes lean and low-fat products to some degree. The *Skinny Six* and *A Change of Plate* are programs of the National Live Stock and Meat Board to promote leaner cuts and smaller portions of meat. The country's largest initiative for low-fat eating was the *National Project LEAN (Low-Fat Eating for America Now)* sponsored by the Kaiser Family Foundation in the late 1980s. This social marketing campaign successfully used mass media to raise public awareness, to promote social norms for low-fat eating, and to help consumers develop new skills in food preparation and eating out.[93,94] *Project LEAN* had counterpart projects in ten states, some of which have continued. The national initiative was transferred to the National Center for Nutrition and Dietetics of the American Dietetic Association in the early 1990s.

A recent policy advance was made with passage of the federal Nutrition Labeling and Education Act (NLEA). More than 20 years in the making, these mandatory food labeling regulations now require disclosure of fat content, standardization of descriptive terms used on foods, such as *low-fat, reduced fat,* and *lean,* and controls on the use of health messages associated with foods, such as for fat and cancer prevention. It is projected that the NLEA will result in many consumers lowering their fat intake, though by how much is as yet unknown.[95] The NLEA is expected to be a powerful factor in stimulating an expanded number of low-fat food items in the marketplace.

6. Limit consumption of alcoholic beverages, if you drink at all.

As cited above, abundant evidence shows that heavy drinkers of all types of alcoholic beverages are at increased risk for cancers of the oral cavity, larynx, and esophagus, with risk being greatly magnified in cigarette smokers. Regular alcohol consumption also may increase breast cancer risk in women.[96] Heavy alcohol intake can result in liver cirrhosis, which may be associated with liver cancer.

The issue of recommendations on alcohol consumption is controversial even though excessive use is associated with adverse consequences besides cancer, including accidents, injuries, homicides, suicide, social disruption, fetal alcohol syndrome, and hypertension. Benefits of light or moderate use have been argued (social enjoyment and lipid lowering). The highly publicized "French paradox" observes that high consumption of red wine is associated with low rates of heart disease in France.

Consensus guidelines from the federal government recommend that if people drink, consumption be limited to two drinks daily for men, one for women, and none for pregnant women. From a nutritional perspective, alcohol provides only calories, and displaces healthful foods in the diet.

Between 1965 and 1985, per capita alcohol availability increased by >25%, from 32 gallons to 41 gallons annually, with beer accounting for most of the rise.[16] In some consumer segments, social norms appear to be shifting toward disapproval of excessive drinking, and nonalcoholic wines and beers are being purchased more widely. Conversely, in some minority communities, the increased sales of beverages such as high alcohol malt liquors are alarming community leaders.

7. Limit consumption of salt-cured, smoked, and nitrite preserved foods.

International data show correlations between stomach and esophageal cancers and the consumption of smoked and pickled foods. In the US, conventionally smoked foods, such as hams, some types of sausage, and fish, absorb tars that arise from incomplete combustion in the smoking process. These substances would also be found in blackened foods and those grilled over charcoal. Tars contain numerous carcinogens similar chemically to the carcinogenic tars in tobacco smoke.

Nitrates and nitrites used in food processing are believed to enhance nitrosamine formation, both in foods and in the digestive tract. Nitrite has been employed traditionally in meat preservation, where it acts as a preventive against botulism and improves the color and flavor of meats. The US Department of Agriculture and the American meat industry have substantially decreased the amount of nitrite used in prepared meats, and many newer methods of meat preservation do not employ these substances. This is an active area of domestic research.

Data are not available about the level of consumption of salt-cured, smoked, and nitrate-preserved foods in the US. Compared to other countries where cured and pickled foods are regularly eaten, domestic consumption is probably substantially lower, except possibly in some traditional cuisines of immigrant groups. There is limited inferential evidence that salt-cured, smoked, pickled, or barbecued foods are a significant concern for cancer prevention.

As a last note, it is ironic that the dietary recommendations of the 1990s are nearly identical to the US Dietary Goals recommended by the US Senate Select Committee on Nutrition and Human Needs in 1978. This is one more example of how decades of delay have occurred between the acquisition of knowledge and its application to cancer control in the community.

Healthy Eating: A New Paradigm for Cancer Prevention

There is as yet no single unifying intervention model of how dietary behavior can be modified in the population at large,[97] and it is not clear what combination of approaches works best.[98] However, the concluding statement of a major National Academy of Sciences report seems to echo what has been learned through years of research in smoking control: media, policy, and program services must be applied to target groups in multiple channels at local, state, and national levels.[16] To change the American diet to prevent chronic diseases:

A concerted effort will be needed to make changes in the food supply and in nutrition policy and programs to increase the availability of [healthier foods] in supermarkets and in public eating facilities such as school cafeterias and restaurants. Consideration may need to be given to the most effective means of achieving such modifications: through technological changes, massive public education efforts, legislative efforts such as food labeling, or a combination of such strategies.

Behavioral Change in Individuals

Returning to the experience of the smoking movement, the stages of change model can be used to segment the American population and plan the type of interventions that would be effective. Many Americans, particularly those who are less educated and otherwise socioeconomically disadvantaged, are either unaware of the significance of healthy eating or unconvinced of the need to change. For these groups, targeted public awareness and educational efforts delivered through the media and channels such as social organizations, worksites, or churches will be needed to move them past the *precontemplation* and *contemplation* stages.

Once in the *preparation* stage, people need to be exposed to new ways of preparing family meals and to new food products, and to see others like themselves (or people they admire) who are successfully changing, either in their immediate environment or through media and popular culture. In the *action, maintenance*, and *termination* stages, reminders and cues to action both through the media and at points of sale in grocery stores, restaurants, and at work help the individual establish and maintain the new habit.

Applied to entire populations and to dietary improvement specifically, interventions tailored appropriately to the stage of change of the individual market segment will accelerate the process by supporting individuals at each stage and by removing or minimizing obstacles. For example, public awareness campaigns and educational efforts by health professionals can increase knowledge of the health benefits of making better food choices, paint an appealing picture of healthy food, and publicize convincing role models. Once people are paying attention and looking for new products to try, there is a greater market for healthier food.

For its part, industry groups will respond to consumer demand by developing more product options, promoting them actively, and competing for market share. The "push-pull" approach uses synergy between the health and industry sectors to develop new social norms and to increase the size of the consumer mar-

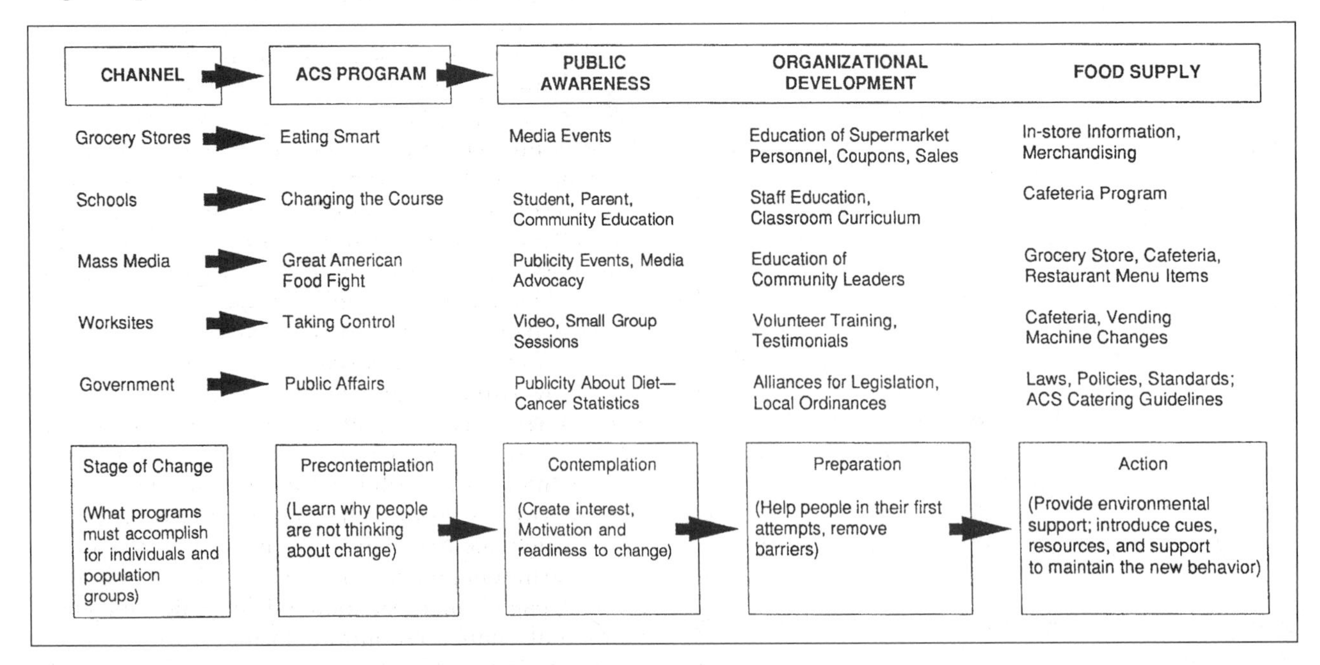

Fig 3-3. A framework for cancer prevention through diet, with existing ACS programs as examples. Adapted from Bal and Foerster.[8]

ket that actively seeks out healthy food. Unlike smoking, with diet and exercise there is the potential for positive, win-win partnerships with large segments of the business community, such as food and physical fitness industries, enlisting them as allies in what otherwise might be an insurmountable public health problem.

Fig 3-3 displays how the stages of change model can be applied to what might at first appear to be unrelated nutrition activities, in this case those of the ACS.[8] This illustrates how, both independently and as part of larger national, state, and local coalitions, ACS activities may be effective in stimulating society-wide dietary improvement to reduce cancer risk.

Programming for Dietary Improvement

Elements in the "gold standard" planning model for smoking control programs also may be transferable to dietary change. In fact, the recently completed *Improving the American Diet: A Strategic Plan* has proposed a three-pronged approach adapted from the ASSIST model (American Stop Smoking Intervention Study) which has been proven effective for smoking control (Fig 3-4).[73,99]

That project calls first for creation of an *infrastructure for action*. It recommends that a public-private foundation be established in order for stakeholder organizations to "partner" and deliver dietary interventions cohesively to the public. Multiple sectors would participate: agricultural organizations and large food companies; voluntary health organizations such as the American Cancer Society and the American Heart Association; local, state, and federal governments and a variety of governmental health, agriculture, education, and aging agencies; professional and consumer organizations, including those representing vulnerable groups; and other sectors with a vested interest in change, such as health insurance companies or large employers.

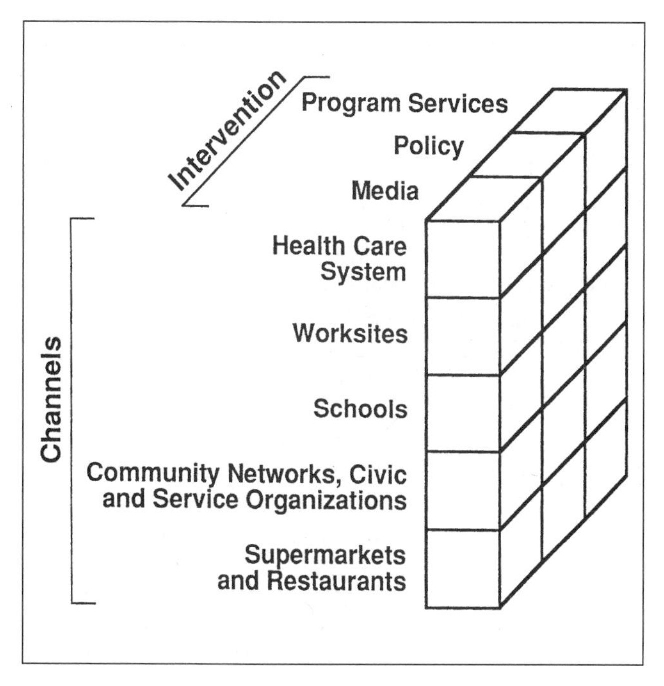

Fig 3-4. Prevention and control model for dietary change, adapted from NCI standards for ASSIST.[73,99]

As with the smoking framework, the second prong outlined in the proposed national plan for dietary improvement involves *media and communications*, and it adds *marketing*. Consumers perceive a great deal of conflict and controversy about what dietary changes to make, in part due to the steady stream of single-issue research studies and corresponding over-interpretation of the dietary implications. Therefore, strong, clear consensus communications are needed to convey convincing, consistent messages about healthy eating. These would be delivered to the public by mass media and reinforced at points of sale.

Cross-promotions are an established effective marketing tool that can be retooled to be more powerful. By executing an authoritative health partner's recommendation about healthy eating with "Madison Avenue" panache (purchased by the industry producers of the food), the healthy eating message cuts through formidable communications barriers. For example, a cross-promotion that demonstrates how to combine foods into a healthy, fast meal (for example, a young working mom stir-frying vegetables and lean meat, served with lots of rice) provides a model for the consumer on how to have fun fixing fast, easy meals in a real-life situation.

Increasing the volume and velocity at which healthy eating messages are delivered is the third prong, akin to *program services* in the tobacco control framework. The plan recommends using multiple channels and a broad array of messengers, not simply the usual list of nutrition advocates. An initial step would be to identify key population segments, and the most effective channels to reach them, then design consumer-driven interventions that also are appealing to the intermediaries in each channel.

The national plan also recognizes the need for *policy* and *environmental* changes, though not necessarily government imposed. A principal vehicle to develop new business and social norms would be a *White House conference on improving the American diet.* Its intent is to mobilize for action organizations and individuals around the nation. Among the outcomes might be the identification of new corporate and government policies to accelerate dietary change. Taking a page from the smoking field, policy and environmental change recommendations could include promoting low-cost healthy eating (as an alternative to taxing low-nutrition luxury foods); large-scale media campaigns; advertising and organizational catering policies that demonstrate the declining acceptability of less healthy foods; limitations on the availability of less healthy foods in noncommercial foodservice operations, like worksites, medical centers, and schools; and restricted advertising to vulnerable groups such as young children.

Institutionalizing Behavior Change

Although dietary improvement will occur fastest when healthy eating becomes the dominant social value surrounding food, it is rarely approached as a fashion issue by health professionals. This is not true in the food industry which is the country's largest advertising sector and spends >$8 billion annually on advertising (and another $16 billion on promotions), almost double the amount spent by the tobacco industry. The great majority of the food ad dollar is directed toward creating a positive social image of high-profit packaged "fun" items, such as snacks, candies, sodas, and fast food. A low proportion of those dollars promotes consumption of foods needed to achieve the nation's health goals. In contrast to tobacco, there are no government programs to counterbalance this powerful medium or to promote good nutrition to the public through mass media. "Normality" on the air waves has been defined by the food industry without any concerted effort to denormalize unhealthy eating or redefine normality by the nutritionally concerned or health advocates.

Because the trends, players, and policies which influence the American food system are largely national in scope, the lack of a national vision and an infrastructure for action was a major barrier to progress. With a national vision now in place, regional, state, and local counterpart partnerships can be established to bring messages, interventions, and decision-making close to the consumer.

Leadership for Change

If diet is to realize its potential in cancer prevention, other major forces acting against it must be understood. In a recent analysis comparing diet with other cancer control measures, four factors that have slowed action on diet as a prevention strategy were identified.[8] The first is the *scientific complexity* of diet in the etiology of cancer, as discussed above, and the demand by many for large clinical trials followed by community intervention trials before implementing dietary interventions widely. In the case of both mammography screening and smoking, similar demands were made. The years of scientific investigation subsequently undertaken did not change what was ultimately done, rather they delayed it. Second is the *lack of any powerful, motivated medical professional specialty* to advocate change, as typically occurs with treatments for specific diseases. Rather, diet as a contributor to or root cause of medical problems crosses many specialties. Its impact is diffuse, and regrettably no one specialty has taken responsibility for solving the problem.

Third is the *profit and loss* factor. Diet as a "treatment" is not medical or technologic in nature, so there also are no pharmaceutical or medical equipment companies motivated by profits to bring the treatment to market. Further, though some segments of the food industry stand to gain, unlike a patented drug or sophisticated piece of medical equipment, food is not a highly differentiated product, market share and profits in the food industry are affected by other consumer and competitive factors, and the history of costly failures in the healthy food sector is well known in the food industry, making companies cautious about undertaking a proven risky strategy. Last is the *diversionary impact of "silver bullet," quick-fix approaches,* which reflect our society's philosophy that technology can fix anything. Examples in the diet area are research programs on cancer preventives for the general population such as nutrient supplements and specially bred vegetables known as "designer foods." Another example is the rapid adoption by physicians of lipid-lowering drugs for cardiovascular disease, instead of the preferred first-line, nonpharmaceutical treatment, dietary modification.

Together, these four factors have contributed to diet being underutilized and inadequately addressed both in biomedical and behavioral research and in medical and public health practice.[8] Understanding them should help to avoid further costly delays, as had occurred with the delayed introduction of other cancer control technologies, namely Pap tests, screening mammography, and tobacco elimination.

The exhaustive reviews of the world's science base contained in the 1988 *Surgeon General's Report on Nutrition and Health* and the 1989 National Academy of Sciences report, *Diet and Health,* show that dietary factors impact multiple diseases and medical specialties. These science-based, consensus policy reports, along with others from abroad,[11] may be convincing enough to by-pass the usual thorough but slow scientific progression from bench to widespread application. Further, today's *Healthy People 2000* dietary objectives and their companion *Food Guide Pyramid* clearly translate the nutrition science into dietary application. Taken together, the US now has a powerful scientific foundation for mobilizing action.

As described above, leaders in the food industry, nonprofit, and government sectors appear to be recognizing their mutual interdependence and to be motivated to work together toward achieving dietary improvement. Reasons for this may include pervasive trends in both the private and public sectors for rethinking how to do business smarter.[100,101] The healthcare reform debates also are focusing attention on stemming long-term demand for health care, encouraging more low-tech approaches, and providing cost-effective preventive services. The proposal for a 6% set-aside in the nation's healthcare budget dedicated to population-based health promotion programs would be a breakthrough, as it would demonstrate understanding of the need for primary prevention programs and, in the case of diet, it would provide funds to jump-start large-scale dietary improvement initiatives designed as described above.

Cancer Prevention Clinical Trials

Cancer prevention can be approached not only through behavioral modification, but also through active intervention with agents designed to interfere with the carcinogenic process. The latter field, broadly designated *chemoprevention*, is one of the most rapidly developing areas of medicine. A large number of clinical trials are now in progress testing nutritional and pharmacologic preventive approaches, and some have been completed.[102]

Dietary prevention trials can be divided into macronutrient and micronutrient interventions. The American Cancer Society is currently conducting two macronutrient trials. The first, piloted by the Virginia Division of the ACS, is an evaluation of a high-fiber cereal supplement (wheat fiber) versus a low-fiber cereal (placebo) in preventing adenomatous polyps of the colon. Subjects with a prior diagnosis of adenomatous polyp are randomized to either the high- or low-fiber cereal and followed by repeat colonoscopy for polyp recurrence. If the study demonstrates the feasibility of this approach, a full-scale project will be implemented. This phase, involving approximately 2,000 subjects, will have an "intermediate marker" endpoint (polyp recurrence) rather than a cancer endpoint (colon cancer), thus permitting a shorter study duration.

The second ACS-sponsored project, the Breast Cancer Dietary Intervention Project (BCDI), is being conducted by the New York State Division and is a prospective, randomized evaluation of two diets (fat constituting 15% versus 30% of total calories) in preventing recurrent breast cancer. Trial participants will have had mastectomy, or lumpectomy with radiation, plus adjuvant chemotherapy or hormonal therapy. As in the colon polyp trial, if feasibility issues are resolved satisfactorily, the project will be expanded to a cancer-endpoint (disease recurrence) phase. The NCI recently funded a similar project called WINS (Women's Intervention Nutrition Study).

Current micronutrient trials involve various vitamins and minerals separately and in combination. Nearly 40 chemoprevention trials are in progress worldwide. Many of these trials involve compounds related to vitamin A (eg, beta-carotene and 13-cis-retinoic acid). A number of cancer sites are being investigated, including breast, colon, lung, skin, cervix, and/or head and neck. Recent studies have demonstrated the effectiveness of 13-cis-retinoic acid in reversing leukoplakia and preventing second primary tumors in previously treated patients with head and neck cancer.[103,104] Oral leukoplakia was found to reverse or stabilize for at least 12 months in 91% of patients on high-dose 13-cis-retinoic acid followed by a lower maintenance dose.[103] After a median follow-up of 42 months, 5% of patients with head and neck cancer receiving this agent for treatment of a primary cancer developed second primary tumors.[104] Furthermore, the combination of beta-carotene, vitamin E, and selenium given for 5 years in 29,000 Chinese at high risk for certain cancers was reported recently to produce a 13% decline in overall cancer mortality (and declines in mortality due to stomach or esophageal cancer of 21% and 4%, respectively).[105] It is not clear whether these results are applicable to other populations.

Other ongoing trials include a cooperative study between the US and Finland evaluating vitamins A and E as preventives for lung cancer in high-risk patients[106]; a large US project evaluating beta-carotene at all cancer sites; and a multicenter trial assessing beta-carotene and retinol in patients at risk for lung cancer.

Nonnutritive hormonal agents are also under clinical investigation. In the US, the National Cancer Institute and the National Surgical Adjuvant Breast & Bowel Project (NSABP) are conducting a randomized placebo-controlled trial of tamoxifen as a chemopreventive in women at increased risk of breast cancer. Tamoxifen is of proven benefit in the treatment of advanced breast cancer and is widely used adjunctively in this neoplasm. As adjuvant therapy, tamoxifen was associated with fewer second primary breast cancers, decreased osteoporotic bone loss, and a favorable effect on circulating lipid levels.[107-109] Possible adverse thrombotic effects and the potential for stimulation of nonbreast neoplasms require close monitoring of subjects in the tamoxifen trial. Randomization of approximately 16,000 subjects will be necessary to determine the efficacy of tamoxifen in this setting.

Another hormonal agent being evaluated by the NCI is finasteride, a 5-alpha reductase inhibitor, for the prevention of prostate cancer. Its potential toxicity has been considered sufficiently limited to justify initiation of a clinical trial. As with the tamoxifen trial, this investigation will be the final determinant of the risk-benefit ratio of this approach.

More than 1,000 natural and synthetic chemicals are known to possess some chemopreventive activity in the laboratory, many with no or extremely limited potential side effects. Garlic alone contains more than 30 such compounds. It is expected that a number of these compounds will be purified and become available for clinical investigation. As we improve our ability to identify high-risk populations for various cancers as a result of progress in molecular biology, clinical prevention trials of these compounds will become more feasible than they are now.

Conclusion

Disease control is defined as a deliberate, discrete, and organized effort, with clearly identified steps, through which research is translated to practice. Real progress is made in reducing the incidence and impact of disease when control efforts are systematically applied in medical practice and in public health. However, in the field of cancer control, there has been a chronically "missing link." For dietary change, as with other areas of prevention, *"the means of control has been discovered before the pathogenic mechanisms or precise etiology has been identified."*[5]

The authors have attempted to demonstrate the high human and economic costs incurred by delays in application of prevention technology and the urgent need for new cancer prevention efforts, especially for diet. The example of smoking, a complex behavioral field in which interventions are well researched, demonstrated that there is a strong theoretical basis on which to design other comprehensive prevention programs. Results from tobacco control indicate that a comprehensive approach is very powerful. A parallel approach could be taken to achieve dietary change in the US.

Achieving the nation's dietary goals would yield benefits of a magnitude similar to those attributable to tobacco control. The one third of all cancers affected by the typical American diet translates into 402,000 fewer new cases of cancer, 180,000 avoided cancer deaths, and $35 billion saved every year.[1] In contrast to tobacco control, though, few comprehensive interventions are in place. Without real resources dedicated to its accomplishment, even the modest goal of 5 fruits and vegetables a day is unlikely to be met on schedule. Significant leadership will be required if cancer control through diet is to realize its potential any time soon.

Regrettably, complex behavioral issues are not amenable to simple solutions. Societal attitudes toward risk factors play a much greater role in cancer prevention than healthcare providers in general and physicians in particular realize. Professional groups have historically overlooked these issues to the extent of not providing leadership in the drafting of public policies, let alone the crafting of the societal solutions. If we are to overcome the barriers to eating healthy in the 21st century and to reduce Americans' risk of cancer, cardiovascular disease, and other diet-related chronic diseases, then physicians, nurses, and other health professionals have to provide leadership in the community. They must be vocal advocates for an entire spectrum of cancer prevention, ranging from healthier societal norms, policy change, and environmental controls through to the design of office- and community-based primary prevention programs with reimbursement mechanisms. In the era of health care reform, we can scarcely do less.

References

1. Boring CC, Squires TS, Tong T, Montgomery S. Cancer Statistics, 1994. *CA Cancer J Clin.* 1994;44:7-26.

2. Boring CC, Squires TS, Heath CW Jr. Cancer statistics for African-Americans. *CA Cancer J Clin.* 1992;42:7-17.

3. Bal DG. Cancer in African-Americans. *CA Cancer J Clin.* 1992;42(1):5-6.

4. Weiner JO. Year 2000 objectives: altering the medical model. *Medicine and Health Perspective.* October 23, 1989.

5. Breslow L, Agran L, Breslow DM, et al. Cancer control: implications from its history. *J Natl Cancer Inst.* 1977;59 (Suppl 2):671-686.

6. National Cancer Institute. *Strategies to control tobacco use in the United States: a blueprint for public health action in the 1990s.* Rockville, Md: US Dept of Health and Human Services, Public Health Service, National Institutes of Health; 1991. Tobacco and smoking control monograph 1. NIH publication no 92-3316.

7. Miller BA, Pies LAG, Hankey BF, Edwards BF. Cancer statistics review, 1973-89. National Cancer Institute, NIH publication no 92-2789.

8. Bal DG, Foerster SB. Dietary strategies for cancer prevention. *Cancer.* 1993;72(Suppl 3):1005-1010.

9. US Public Health Service. Office of the Surgeon General. The Surgeon General's report on nutrition and health. Washington, DC: US Dept of Health and Human Services; 1988. DHHS publication no. PHS 88-50210.

10. Thomas PR, ed. Institute of Medicine (US), Committee on Dietary Guidelines Implementation, Food and Nutrition Board. *Improving America's diet and health: from recommendations to action.* Washington, DC: National Academy Press; 1991.

11. World Health Organization. Diet, nutrition and the prevention of chronic diseases: report of a WHO study group. *World Health Organ Tech Rep Ser.* 1990;797.

12. Truswell AS. Evolution of dietary recommendations, goals, and guidelines. *Am J Clin Nutr.* 1987;45:1060-1072.

13. Doll R, Peto R. The causes of cancer: quantitative estimates of avoidable risk in the United States today. *J Natl Cancer Inst.* 1981;66:1191-1308.

14. National Research Council Committee on Diet, Nutrition, and Cancer. *Diet, Nutrition, and Cancer.* Washington, DC: National Academy Press; 1982.

15. Division of Cancer Prevention and Control, National Cancer Institute. *Cancer Control Objectives for the Nation: 1985-2000.* NCI monograph; 1986:1-93.

16. National Research Council Committee on Diet and Health. *Diet and Health: Implications for Reducing Chronic Disease Risk*. Washington, DC: National Academy Press; 1989.

17. Weinhouse S, Bal DG, Adamson R, et al. American Cancer Society Guidelines on Diet, Nutrition, & Cancer. *CA Cancer J Clin.* 1991;41(6):334-338.

18. *Healthy People 2000: national health promotion and disease prevention objectives.* Washington, DC: US Department of Health and Human Services; 1991. DHHS publication No. PHS 91-50213.

19. Bal DG, Foerster SB. Changing the American diet. *Cancer.* 1991;67:2671-2680.

20. Byers T. Dietary trends in the United States: Relevance to cancer prevention. *Cancer.* 1993;72(3 Suppl):1015-1018.

21. Savitz DA, Harris R, Brownson RC. Methods in chronic disease epidemiology. In: Brownson RC, Remington PW, Davis JR, eds. *Chronic Disease Epidemiology and Control.* Washington, DC: American Public Health Association;1993.

22. Fletcher RH, Fletcher SW, Wagner EH. *Clinical Epidemiology: The Essentials.* 2nd ed. Baltimore, Md: Williams & Wilkins; 1988.

23. Kelsey JL, Thompson WD, Evans AS. *Methods in Observational Epidemiology.* New York, NY: Oxford University Press; 1986.

24. Rothman KJ. *Modern Epidemiology.* Boston, Mass: Little, Brown & Company; 1986.

25. Schesselman JJ. *Case-Control Studies: Design, Conduct, Analysis.* New York, NY: Oxford University Press; 1982.

26. Weiss NS. *Clinical Epidemiology: The Study of the Outcome of Illness.* New York, NY: Oxford University Press; 1986.

27. Kleinbaum DG, Kupper LL, Morgenstern H. *Epidemiologic Research: Principles and Quantitative Methods.* Belmont, Calif: Lifetime Learning Publications; 1982.

28. Centers for Disease Control. Chronic disease reports: deaths from lung cancer, United States, 1986. *MMWR.* 1989;38:501-505.

29. Brownson RC, Reif JS, Alavanja MCR, Bal DG. Cancer. In: Brownson RC, Remington PW, Davis JR, eds. *Chronic Disease Epidemiology and Control.* Washington, DC: American Public Health Association; in press.

30. Havas S, Heimendinger J, Reynolds K, et al. 5 A Day for Better Health: A new research initiative. *J Am Dietet Assn.* 1994:94(1);32-36.

31. McKinlay JB. The promotion of health through planned sociopolitical change: challenges for research and policy. *Soc Sci Med.* 1993;36:109-117.

32. Warner KE. Cigarette advertising and media coverage of smoking and health. *New Engl J Med.* 1985;312:384-388.

33. Flewelling RL, Kenney E, Elder JP, et al. First-year impact of the 1989 California cigarette tax increase on cigarette consumption. *Am J Public Health.* 1992;3:7-9.

34. Erickson AC, McKenna JW, Romano RM. Past lessons and new uses of the mass media in reducing tobacco consumption. *Public Health Rep.* 1990;1:73-77.

35. Doctors Ought to Care. Counter promotion: tennis elbows tobacco company sponsorship at sports. *DOC News and Views.* Summer 1989:4-5.

36. Sweda EL. Summary of legal decisions regarding smoking in the workplace and other places. *Tobacco Products Litigation Reporter.* 1991;6(2):4.11-4.21.

37. Daynard RA. Tobacco liability litigation as a cancer control strategy. *J Natl Cancer Inst.* 1988;80:497-505.

38. American Cancer Society, Massachusetts Division, 1993.

39. Macro Systems. *Obtaining Resources for Prevention: A Michigan Case Study.* Michigan State Department of Health; 1990.

40. Moon RW, Males MA, Nelson DE. The 1990 Montana initiative to increase cigarette taxes: lessons for other states and localities. *J Public Health Policy.* 1993;14:19-33.

41. Jacobson PD, Wasserman J, Raube K. *The Political Evolution of Anti-Smoking Legislation.* Santa Monica, Calif: RAND Publications; 1992.

42. Fielding JE. Smoking control at the workplace. *Annu Rev Public Health.* 1991;12:209-234.

43. Western Consortium for Public Health. *Tobacco Control in California Cities: A Guide for Action.* December 1992.

44. Powell KE, Blair SN. The public health burdens of sedentary living habits: theoretical but realistic estimates. *Med Sci Sports Exerc.* In press.

45. Sternfeld B. Cancer and the protective effect of physical activity: the epidemiological evidence. *Med Sci Sport Exerc.* 1992;24;1195-1209.

46. Shephard RJ. Exercise in the prevention and treatment of cancer: an update. *Sports Med.* 1993;15:258-280.

47. Frisch RE, Wyshak G, Albright NL, et al. Lower lifetime occurrence of breast cancer and cancers of the reproductive system among former college athletes. *Am J Clin Nutr.* 1987;45:328-335.

48. Brownson RC, Chang JC, Davis JR, Smith CA. Physical activity on the job and cancer in Missouri. *Am J Public Health.* 1991;81:639-642.

49. Holdstock DJ, Misiewicz JJ, Smith T, et al. Propulsion (mass movement) in the human colon and its relationship to meals and somatic activity. *Gut.* 1970;11;91-99.

50. Demers LM, Harrison TS, Halbert DR, et al. Effect of prolonged exercise on plasma prostaglandin levels. *Prostaglandins and Med.* 1981;6:413-418.

51. International Agency for Research on Cancer. *IARC Monograph on the Evaluation of Carcinogenic Risks to Humans, Alcohol Drinking.* Volume 44. Lyon, France: International Agency for Research on Cancer; 1988.

52. Blot WJ. Alcohol and cancer. *Cancer Res.* 1992;52:2119S-2123S.

53. Higginson J, Muir CS, Munoz N. *Human Cancer: Epidemiology and Environmental Causes.* New York, NY: Cambridge University Press; 1992.

54. McCoy GD, Wynder EL. Etiologic and preventive implications in alcohol carcinogenesis. *Cancer Res.* 1979;39:2844-2850.

55. Decoufle P. Occupation. In: Schottenfeld D, Fraumeni JF Jr, eds. *Cancer Epidemiology and Prevention.* Philadelphia, Pa: WB Saunders Co; 1982: chap 20.

56. Costanza ME, Li FP, Greene FL, et al. Cancer prevention and detection: strategies for practice. In: *Cancer Manual.* ACS Massachusetts Division; 1990, chap 5.

57. Cone JE, Rosenberg J. Medical surveillance and biomonitoring for occupational cancer endpoints. In: *Occupational Medicine: State of the Art Reviews.* Philadelphia, Pa: Hanley & Belfus Inc; 1990:563-581.

58. Scotto J, Fears TR, Fraumeni JF Jr. Solar radiation. In: Schottenfeld D, Fraumeni JF Jr, eds. *Cancer Epidemiology and Prevention.* Philadelphia, Pa: WB Saunders Co; 1982: chap 14.

59. Shy CM, Struba R. Air and water pollution. In: Schottenfeld D, Fraumeni JF Jr, eds. *Cancer Epidemiology and Prevention.* Philadelphia, Pa: WB Saunders Co; 1982: chap 19.

60. Evans AS. Viruses. In: Schottenfeld D, Fraumeni JF Jr, eds. *Cancer Epidemiology and Prevention.* Philadelphia, Pa: WB Saunders Co; 1982: chap 18.

61. Parsonnet JR, Friedman GO, Vandersteen DP, et al. *Helicobacter pylori* infection and the risk of gastric carcinoma. *N Engl J Med.* 1991;16:1127-1131.

62. Herbst AL, Ulfelder H, Poskanger DC. Adenocarcinoma of the vagina: association of material stilbestrol therapy with tumor appearance in young females. *N Engl J Med.* 1971;284:878-881.

63. Stolley PD, Hibgerd PL. Drugs. In: Schottenfeld D, Fraumeni JF Jr, eds. *Cancer Epidemiology and Prevention.* Philadelphia, Pa: WB Saunders Co; 1982: chap 17.

64. Vainio H. Importance of hazard identification and exposure monitoring in primary prevention of cancer. In: *Recent Results in Cancer Research.* Berlin, Germany: Springer-Verlag; 1991:33-41.

65. Henderson BE, Ross RK, Pike MC. Toward the primary prevention of cancer. *Science.* 1991:254-257.

66. California Morbidity. May 3,1991;17/18.

67. Public Health Service. Reducing the health consequences of smoking: 25 years of progress: a report of the Surgeon General. Rockville, Md: US Department of Health and Human Services, Centers for Disease Control, Office on Smoking and Health: 1989. DHHS publication no CDC 89-8411.

68. Prochaska JO, Velicer WF, DiClemente CC, Fava J. Measuring processes of change: applications to the cessation of smoking. *J Consult Clin Psychol.* 1988;56:520-528.

69. Prochaska JO. A transtheoretical model of behavior change: implications for diet interventions. In: *Proceedings of the conference promoting Dietary Change in Communities: Applying Existing Models of Dietary Change to Population-Based Interventions.* Seattle, Wash: Fred Hutchinson Cancer Research Center; 1992:37-52.

70. Griffiths W. Health education definitions, problems, and philosophies. *Health Education Monographs.* 1972;31:7-11.

71. Minkler M. Health education, health promotion, and the open society: a historical perspective. *Health Educ Q.* 1989;16:17-30.

72. Green LW. Health education models. In: Matarazzo JD, Weiss SH, Herd JA, Miller NE, Weiss SM, eds. *Behavioral Health: A Handbook of Health Enhancement and Disease Prevention.* New York, NY: John Wiley & Sons; 1984:181-198.

73. National Cancer Institute, Standards for Comprehensive Smoking Prevention and Control. December 12, 1989.

74. Davis RM. Current trends in cigarette advertising and marketing. *N Engl J Med.* 1987;316:725-732.

75. Tye J, Warner K, Glantz S. Tobacco advertising and consumption: evidence of a causal relationship. *J Public Health Policy.* 1987;8:492-508.

76. Thompson B, Kinne S. Social change theory: application to community health. In: Bracht N, ed. *Health Promotion at the Community Level.* London, England: Sage Publications; 1990:45-65.

77. Warner KE, et al. Public policy on smoking and health: toward a smoke-free generation by the year 2000. *Circulation.* 1986;73:381a-395a.

78. Novelle-Neuman E. The spiral of silence: a theory of public opinion. *J Communication.* 1974;24:43-51.

79. Economic Research Service. *Food marketing review, 1989-90.* Washington, DC: US Department of Agriculture, 1989-1990. 1990:13-17. Agricultural Economic Report no 639.

80. Wallack L, Dorfman L. Health messages on television commercials. *Am J Health Promotion.* 1992;6:190-196.

81. Story M, Faulkner P. The prime time diet: a content analysis of eating behavior and food messages in television program content and commercials. *Am J Public Health.* 1990;80:738-740.

82. US Department of Agriculture, US Department of Health and Human Services. *Nutrition and your health: dietary guidelines for Americans.* Washington, DC: US Government Printing Office; 1990: Home and Garden bulletin no 232.

83. Human Nutrition Information Service. The food guide pyramid. *Home and Garden Bulletin.* No. 252. US Dept. of Agriculture, 1992.

84. Garfinkel L. Overweight and mortality. *Cancer.* 1986; 58:1826-1829.

85. National Institutes of Health. *Methods for Voluntary Weight Loss and Control.* Technology Assessment Conference Statement. 1992.

86. Block G, Menkes M. Ascorbic acid in cancer prevention. In: Moon TE, Micozzi MS, eds. *Nutrition and Cancer Prevention: Investigating the Role of Micronutrients.* New York, NY: Marcel Dekker Inc; 1989:341-388.

87. Steinmetz KA, Potter JD. Vegetables, fruit, and cancer. *Cancer Causes Control.* 1991;2:325-357,427-441.

88. Block G, Patterson B, Subar A. Fruit, vegetables, and cancer prevention: a review of the epidemiological evidence. *Nutr Cancer.* 1992;18:1-29.

89. Levy AS, Stokes RC. Effects of a health promotion advertising campaign on sales of ready-to-eat cereals. *Public Health Rep.* 1987;102:398-403.

90. Rizek RL, Tippett KS. Diets of American women in 1985. *Food Nutr News.* 1989;61(1):1-4.

91. Levy AS. *Key Findings for Nutrition Education: Quantitative Research at FDA and USDA.* Washington, DC: Center for Food Safety and Education, National Exchange for Food Labeling and Education Conference; 1993.

92. Sempos CT, Cleeman JI, Carroll MD, et al. Prevalence of high blood cholesterol among US adults: an update based on guidelines from the Second Report of the National Cholesterol Education Program Adult Treatment Panel. *JAMA.* 1993;269:3009-3014.

93. Samuels SE. Project LEAN: lessons learned from a national social marketing campaign. *Public Health Rep.* 1993;108:45-53.

94. Samuels SE. Project LEAN: a national campaign to reduce dietary fat consumption. *Am J Health Promot.* 1990; 4:435-440.

95. Zarkin GA, Dean N, Mauskopf JA, Williams R. Potential health benefits of nutrition label changes. *Am J Public Health.* 1993;83;717-724.

96. Willet WC, Stampfer MJ, Colditz GA, Rosner BA, Henneken CH, Speizer FE. Moderate alcohol consumption and the risk of cancer. *N Engl J Med.* 1987;316:1174-1180.

97. Cancer Prevention Research Program. In: *Proceedings of the Conference Promoting Dietary Change in Communities: Applying Existing Models of Dietary Change to Population-Based Interventions.* Seattle, Wash: Fred Hutchinson Cancer Research Center; 1972.

98. McLeroy K. Health education research: theory and practice—future directions. *Health Education Research.* 1992;1-8.

99. *Improving the American Diet: A National Strategic Plan.* Washington, DC: Association of State and Territorial Health Officials, 1993.

100. Hammer M, Champy J. *Reengineering the Corporation: A Manifesto for Business Revolution.* New York, NY: HarperCollins Publishers; 1993.

101. Osborne D, Gaebler T. *Reinventing Government: How the Entrepreneurial Spirit Is Transforming the Public Sector.* New York, NY: Penguin Books USA; 1992.

102. Nixon DE. Status of cancer prevention clinical trials. In: DeVita VT, Hellman S, Rosenbery SA, eds. *Cancer Prevention.* Philadelphia, Pa: JB Lippincott Co; 1992.

103. Hong WK, Endicott J, Itri LM, et al. 13-cis-retinoic acid in the treatment of oral leukoplakia. *N Engl J Med.* 1986; 315:1501-1505.

104. Hong WK, Lippman SM. Hri LM, et al. Prevention of second primary tumors with isotretinoin in squamous-cell carcinoma of the head and neck. *N Engl J Med.* 1990; 323:795-801.

105. Blot WJ, Li JY, Taylor PR, et al. Nutrition intervention trials in Linxian, China. *J Natl Cancer Inst.* 1993;85:1483-1492.

106. The Alpha-Tocopherol, Beta Carotene Cancer Prevention Study Group. The effect of vitamin E and beta carotene on the incidence of lung cancer and other cancers in male smokers. *N Engl J Med.* 1994;330(15):1029-1035.

107. Love RR. Antiestrogen chemoprevention of breast cancer: critical issues and research. *Prev Med.* 1991;20:64-78.

108. Kiang DT. Chemoprevention for breast cancer: are we ready? *J Natl Cancer Inst.* 1991;83:462-463.

109. Love RR, Newcomb PA, Wiebe DA, et al. Effects of tamoxifen therapy on lipid and lipoprotein levels in postmenopausal patients with node-negative breast cancer. *J Natl Cancer Inst.* 1990;82:1327-1332.

4

GENERAL APPROACH TO THE PATIENT

Raymond E. Lenhard, Jr, MD, Walter Lawrence, Jr, MD, Robert J. McKenna, Sr, MD

This chapter will focus on the general principles of cancer management and is meant to serve as an introduction to the disease and organ-specific sections that follow. We will emphasize the philosophy and reasoning that lies behind many of the recommendations for diagnosis, treatment, rehabilitation, and overall management that are discussed in depth in later sections of this book.

The most successful approach to cancer control is the prevention of cancer, the goal of many of our cancer control projects and clinical trials. When we fail to prevent cancer, however, it is important to establish the diagnosis of any cancers that are present at the earliest stage possible. For many primary sites of cancer, early detection is a reasonable goal and, for some, it will yield an improvement in treatment results. In every instance, a well-conceived management plan is critical.

Modern diagnosis, treatment, and rehabilitation of the patient with cancer or suspected cancer relies heavily on the classic principles of the physician-patient relationship. It is as important to understand the patient and his or her family as it is to have detailed information on specific cancer treatments. The latter can be obtained from a variety of current data sources such as the National Cancer Institute's PDQ system and Cancer Information Service, The American Cancer Society's Cancer Response System, textbooks, and meetings and consultations from oncologists. The former requires that you have the discipline to take time to listen to your patients while leading them through this scientifically complex, emotionally daunting experience.

Once the diagnosis of cancer is suspected, there are a number of factors that impact on overall patient management. First, there must be a logical and direct approach to establishing a diagnosis. Evaluation of the patient should include a complete medical history, physical examination, appropriate laboratory tests, radiologic and other noninvasive tests, and an evaluation of the patient's mental and emotional state so that an overall logical plan of action can be developed. After the diagnosis of cancer is established, both local and distant control of the disease are primary objectives, as is maintaining or improving quality of life and extending life, with an emphasis on disease-free survival. A logical and direct evaluation plan leading to an overall strategy for accomplishing all of these objectives also should minimize dollar costs associated with the diagnosis and treatment of the disease process, as well as other less tangible costs to the patient, his or her family, and to society.

Patients with cancer have a disease that is both medical and emotional. Throughout the course of the illness, the diagnosis creates anxiety in the patient, family members, and friends; in the physician who must tell the patient the consequences of the diagnosis; and in the physician's office or hospital staff who see and interact with the patient. The physician must recognize these factors and give the patient a calm, directed, logical evaluation and as optimistic a plan as possible, based on a consideration of all of the treatment modalities available.

Interdisciplinary Evaluation, Planning, and Physician Responsibility

Progress in cancer treatment methods has been relatively slow over the last few decades, but a major advance has been our recent development of a greater

Raymond E. Lenhard, Jr, MD, Professor, Oncology and Medicine, The Johns Hopkins University School of Medicine, Baltimore, Maryland

Walter Lawrence, Jr, MD, Professor of Surgery, Division of Surgical Oncology and Director Emeritus, Massey Cancer Center, Medical College of Virginia, Richmond, Virginia

Robert J. McKenna, Sr, MD, Clinical Professor of Surgery, University of Southern California School of Medicine, Los Angeles, California

appreciation of the value of interdisciplinary activity in patient management. Although the plan for initial evaluation of the patient and for treatment usually requires an interdisciplinary approach to obtain optimal results, leadership in this enterprise still requires a perceptive and knowledgeable coordinating physician who may be a primary physician, internist, or general surgeon. However, once there is a clue that a cancer is actually present, professionals with skills that often cannot be provided by a single individual should be enlisted. The involvement of physicians from several disciplines, nurses, social workers, nutritionists, and other members of the health care team in the early phases of the management of a patient with cancer is the hallmark of modern clinical oncology.

In addition to individual consultations, interdisciplinary considerations may be provided by a tumor board type of conference, where a helpful interchange of ideas may focus on the plan for diagnosis and treatment. Once a treatment plan is formulated for an individual patient, some patients may be treated by a representative of only one of the disciplines initially involved. In many other situations, the ideal treatment program may require a combination of physicians representing the various oncologic specialties.

The physician directing the cancer patient's management should consider how each step in the plan will be evaluated and how the procedures will be carried out to make subsequent treatments easier. For example, at the time of surgery, it may be appropriate for the surgeon to modify the approach to make subsequent radiation therapy more effective or less harmful to normal organs. During the course of a staging laparotomy in a patient with Hodgkin's disease, this might involve moving the ovaries into the mid-line to facilitate delivery of a full dose of radiation to pelvic fields. Placement of radio-opaque clips around the area from which a mass has been resected may provide critical guidance to planning the configuration of radiation therapy fields. The radiation oncologist may plan the treatment area to spare bone marrow for later chemotherapy. The medical oncologist may have to consider the depth or nadir time of aplasia that is planned in a patient who has a partially obstructed intestine that may require surgery in the midst of chemotherapy. These treatment planning decisions are good examples of the multidisciplinary approach and the need for review of the plan at specific decision points following diagnostic or therapeutic interventions.

To assure continuity of care and to provide a consistent source of support and guidance for the patient, a coordinating primary physician is needed during an often prolonged management process. The concepts and considerations discussed in this chapter are directed at that individual.

Communication Between Physician and Patient

One of the most disturbing aspects of the diagnostic situation for the patient—when cancer is suspected—is fear of the unknown. The primary physician involved in and coordinating the diagnostic and evaluation phase cannot afford to delay conferring with the patient until all the facts regarding diagnosis and treatment are known. Compassionate disclosure of information during the diagnostic phase, particularly information regarding the physician's concerns, may be unsettling to the individual who is being evaluated, but not nearly as frightening as having no information. To feel comfortable with the process, patients must understand the reasons for the procedures undertaken during the diagnostic or evaluation phase as well as the treatment options available once a more definitive diagnosis is established. The patient and family often "fear the worst." For this reason, repeated and continued counselling throughout the evaluation and treatment planning process is reassuring to the patient, rather than frightening, and confidence in the physician is established. The patient can then become an effective part of the management team.

Over the years, there has been a healthy and appropriate shift away from a philosophy of hiding the facts of cancer to providing a fuller disclosure. The diagnosis, treatment implications, and survival potential have practical implications for the patient that are beyond any that may be immediately obvious to the physician. What are the patient's plans? Is the patient preparing to assume long-term debt, get married, or become pregnant? The estimated prognosis of survival and the expectation, timing, and severity of symptoms from either the cancer or the treatment are vitally important to the patient but often difficult for the physician to predict.

To discuss treatment planning effectively, the physician, the patient, and the family must have a clear understanding of the clinical situation, an idea of what can be accomplished, and an estimate of the costs involved. The role of the physician is to make a recommendation for action based on an assessment of the clinical goals and the limitations and potential outcomes of various approaches. The physician must allot sufficient time to this process to allow the patient and family to ask all their questions.

The most difficult issue to discuss with a patient is the expectations for survival. Published statistical survival information is based on all patients with a specific diagnosis and stage of disease and may bear little on the expected outcome of a particular patient. Accurate sub-sets of data that relate to clinical stage, distribution of metastases, histologic grade of the cancer, and other newer methods of predicting outcome are important, but are usually not available. In addition, few of the published data take into consideration variations in rate of tumor growth or response to treatment. One needs to assess what factors are important to this patient and how much risk he or she is prepared to take to extend life. How can symptom-free survival be maximized, and can the benefit following intense treatment be translated into a prolonged period of quality life after the treatment has been concluded? The patient may question the value of a few additional months of life if this is accompanied by progressive pain from the cancer or debilitating symptoms resulting from treatment.

The patient will make the ultimate decision regarding treatment options. The physician needs to be prepared to accept the possibility that the patient's decision may not be the one that was proposed. If this decision is seen by the physician as not in the best interests of the patient, the physician should try to persuade without becoming confrontational. Each of us makes different decisions that impact our lives, our careers, and important events in our lives. A slim chance for success may be embraced by one person and rejected by another. This is why a full disclosure is so important. Fear of hospitalization, surgery, irradiation, or chemotherapy may make the patient choose a plan that will result in shorter survival, but less toxicity. The doctor does, however, have a responsibility not to follow through with a program if he thinks that the patient's decision will not result in a good outcome. It may be necessary to assist the patient in finding a replacement physician to direct the patient's care. Establishing the patient's confidence in the treatment team will be absolutely necessary for the days and weeks of treatment that lie ahead once the treatment program has begun.

Assessment of Impact on the Family

In the early phase of evaluation of the patient and, subsequently, as the dynamics of the diagnosis and treatment evolve, the physician, nurse, and other members of the treatment team should assess the patient's occupation and position in the family. What will happen if the patient is admitted to the hospital, becomes ill with either the acute effects of surgery, irradiation, or chemotherapy, or has progression of the disease? Who cares for the family, cooks the meals, and earns the bulk of the family income are important issues requiring assessment at the outset. Answers to these questions may explain why a patient chooses a specific treatment option. A multitude of community and personal support resources exist to serve these needs. These services are accessible and promoted by the American Cancer Society through the Cancer Response System (800-ACS-2345) and through the National Cancer Institute through its Cancer Information Service telephone response program (1-800-4-CANCER).

Concern with Financial Implications

Not the least of the problems facing the patient with cancer is the fact that most of the beneficial services that the physician has to offer the patient are expensive. Although the hospital or other treating facility will collect personal and financial information as part of the process of admission to the facility, the physician should be aware of the current and changing financial status of the patient. What will treatment cost above that provided by insurance? Will the proposed diagnosis and treatment plan change the financial stability of the family and potentially lower their standard of living forever? Understanding the facts and the dynamics of the situation places the physician in a better position to offer strong patient and family support.

Diagnosis and Staging

The primary physician is often in the best position to establish an early diagnosis. There are clues in careful history taking, often of minor symptoms, that should trigger the physician to evaluate the patient for cancer. A number of these clues have been brought to the attention of the public in the form of the American Cancer Society's "Seven Warning Signals." Unfortunately, many of these commonly known signs and symptoms may be evidence of advanced disease, and our efforts to detect cancer in its curative stages must, therefore, focus on screening asymptomatic people. Although the primary focus of the initial physical examination should be to determine the cause of the patient's presenting symptoms, if cancer is suspected, the physician should use the history and physical examination to discover possible sites of metastatic spread of any cancer that may be present. A thorough history and physical examination are still the most effective tools of diagnosis, although specific diagnostic tests have refined our diagnostic capabilities.

Establishing the Diagnosis

The general philosophy of both the diagnosis and staging of various cancers is that these efforts should be both efficient and cost effective. A biopsy of any potential cancer site should be performed early in the process, rather than later, since it establishes the basis for staging and the specific features of the treatment planning process. There are a number of biopsies that can be carried out promptly and with minimal preparation (such as fine needle aspiration biopsy, punch biopsy, or some endoscopic biopsies), while other open incisional or excisional biopsies are usually delayed due to the more extensive nature of the procedure.

Although early biopsy is important, there are specific situations that must be considered appropriate for delaying biopsy, such as when interference in mammographic interpretation would be caused by ecchymosis from a fine needle aspiration biopsy carried out before the mammogram. In addition, there may be areas where it is almost impossible to perform a necessary biopsy due to the location of the tumor, as in the case of retroperitoneal masses. Early biopsy does, however, provide a focus for the continued workup and should be considered as the first diagnostic step whenever feasible and practical.

While biopsy procedures may be appropriate in some cases during the initial history and physical examination, other diagnostic tests should also be considered. Diagnostic testing precision and accuracy have been greatly enhanced in recent years due to radiologic and laboratory advances. However, this refinement of diagnostic tests has been accompanied by an escalation in cost. Therefore, the physician should avoid those tests that have a low likelihood of providing useful information and should avoid duplication by foregoing additional tests that provide similar information. An example of such duplication of diagnostic effort is the use of two slightly different, but expensive, radiologic techniques when the same diagnostic information can be obtained by either approach (eg, abdominal CT and MRI, transhepatic cholangiogram and endoscopic retrograde cholangiopancreatogram [ERCP]). The physician must request the most appropriate test to provide information relevant to both the patient's staging and treatment plan.

An expensive test done early in the diagnostic workup may shorten the process and, in the long run, be the most cost-effective approach. Generally, we recommend doing the least expensive but most revealing test first. All tests must be chosen to further the goal of reaching an informed decision on staging and management. Before ordering complex or expensive diagnostic examinations, the physician should consider how they will affect the overall treatment plan. This applies to tests performed both to establish a diagnosis and to aid in the staging process.

Cancer Staging

Establishing the precise stage of the cancer is important for various reasons (Table 4-1). The primary reason for staging is to help provide optimal treatment selection and planning for the individual patient. Assigning a stage is also a way to determine the eligibility of patients for individual clinical trials. Staging may be used to stratify patients entered in clinical trials, or it may be used as a standardizing tool for making more accurate comparisons of treatment results in patients undergoing two or more treatments that are being compared. Finally, staging is important for prognosis (eg, Dukes' classification of colon and rectal cancer). Prognostic variables are clearly delineated from pathologic findings in surgical specimens removed as part of the treatment process.

There have been many different staging systems employed over the years, but, fortunately, there has been a gradual trend toward the development of a unified staging nomenclature for all primary sites—the TNM system. The TNM system is now accepted worldwide. Size and involvement of the local neoplasm (T) have been defined for each type of cancer. Definitions have also been developed for categorizing regional lymph node involvement (N), since this route is a significant one, prognostically and therapeutically, for a number of cancers. Distant spread (as opposed to local regional involvement) to many anatomic sites is designated by the letter "M." The application of this staging process to each anatomic site is discussed in more detail in other chapters of this book.

Table 4-1. Purpose of Staging

The staging of cancer accomplishes the following objectives:

- Aids the clinician in the planning of treatment for each patient
- Assists in the evaluation of treatment modalities
- Facilitates exchange of information between treatment centers worldwide
- Evaluates the outcome of treatment (ie, patient survival)
- Estimates the prognosis or outcome by stage and treatment

The practice of dividing cancer cases into groups arose from the observation that survival rates were higher if the tumor was localized than if the disease had extended beyond the organ or site of origin. These groups were often referred to as "early cases" and "late cases," implying progression with time. The late cases were divided into "regional" cases if the regional nodes were involved and "distant" if the cancer had spread to distant sites. Until recently, these cases were coded as Localized (L), Regional (R), and Distant (D), in most tumor registries and databases.

Over the past 40 years, the American Joint Committee on Cancer (AJCC) has carried out retrospective studies of outcome on most anatomic sites of cancer and has reviewed staging protocols that were reported in the literature. During the last decade, an international collaboration between the Union Internationale Contre le Cancer (UICC) and the AJCC reached uniform agreement so that one system of staging could be used worldwide. The schema for each site were published in 1992 by the AJCC[1] and by the UICC.[2]

General Rules of the TNM System

The classification of cancer at this time is primarily

anatomic and is based on the assessment of three components:

T The extent of the primary tumor
N The presence or absence and extent of regional lymph node metastasis
M The presence or absence of distant metastasis

The addition of numbers to these three components indicates the clinical extent of the malignant disease, thus showing a progressive increase in tumor size, local involvement, regional lymph node spread, or distant metastasis:

Tumor size	T0	T1	T2	T3	T4
Nodal involvement	N0	N1	N2	N3	
Metastasis	M0	M1			

In effect, the system uses a shorthand notation for describing the clinical extent of a particular malignant tumor in a patient. All cases should also be confirmed histologically. Four staging classifications may be used, but the first two are the most frequently utilized ones.

1. *Clinical classification* (cTNM or TNM) is based on evidence acquired before treatment from physical examination, radiology studies including imaging, endoscopy, and biopsy.

2. *Pathologic classification* (pTNM) is based on information acquired by a surgical procedure that provides additional evidence acquired from surgical exploration and/or pathologic examination of a resected specimen.

3. *Retreatment classification* (rTNM) is used after a disease-free interval and when further definitive treatment is planned. This re-classification is infrequently employed.

4. *Autopsy classification* (aTNM) is done after death and after a complete pathologic study is completed.

After assigning T, N, and M and/or pT, pN, and pM categories, they are grouped into stages and, once established, must remain unchanged in the medical record. If there is doubt concerning the correct T, N, and M category to which a particular case should be allotted, then the lower or less advanced category should be chosen. In the case where multiple simultaneous tumors are present in the same organ, the tumor with the highest T category should be identified and the multiplicity indicated in parenthesis—eg, T2(m). In simultaneous bilateral cancers of paired organs, each tumor should be classified independently.

Staging of cancer is an evolving science. In earlier years this clinical staging process was carried out entirely by physical examination, but various radiologic imaging tests and tumor markers have and will continue to refine clinical staging. Staging schema once requiring only a chest x-ray for detecting metastatic spread now utilize computerized tomography, radionuclide scans, and other diagnostic tools. As new information becomes available about etiology and various methods of diagnosis and treatment, the classifications and the staging system will change. The treating *physician* must be responsible ultimately for appropriate and accurate staging—not the tumor registrar. All residents and fellows should learn and use TNM staging, and all tumor board discussions should specify the stage of the cancer in each patient. Articles prepared for publication in professional journals or books should specify the method of staging employed and the edition of the AJCC *Manual for Staging Cancer* that was used. Most hospitals with cancer programs approved by the Commission on Cancer of the American College of Surgeons utilize staging forms for each case, and this document becomes part of the permanent medical record.

Staging has clear benefits for both physician and patient. In the future, multiple biologic factors such as hormone receptors, genetic markers, cellular proliferation, ploidy, and metastasis potential will probably be used to further classify cancer. All patients who are entered into clinical trials must be accurately staged. As cancer prevention trials are more frequently used, the stage of the cancer diagnosed by early detection and screening tests may become the endpoint rather than disease control or mortality. Finally, the quality of cancer care may be measured in part by the completeness and accuracy of cancer staging.

Therapeutic Goals

Cure

Oncologists are encouraged by the increase in cures for many cancers. The potential for cure is increased if the cancer is sufficiently localized so that it can be eliminated by surgery or irradiation. Cure is also more likely if a histologic cell type is identified for a cancer that can be cured even when the disease is widespread. Information on cancer treatment is changing so rapidly that physicians should take the time necessary to be current. We discussed the important role of staging in treatment planning. All strategies for staging and treatment are based on the premise that patients who can be cured must be found and the appropriate treatments started as promptly as possible.

The first treatment decision is whether the cancer can be cured or if palliation is the only practical goal. Surgery, radiation therapy, chemotherapy, or combinations of these may be used for both palliation and cure of the tumor mass. Reduction of the tumor mass may result in a major relief of symptoms, even if life is not prolonged.

Disease-Free Interval and Survival Time

There are several time intervals that are important to consider as treatment planning proceeds. Increased survival is clearly important, but often equally relevant is the amount of time the patient is free of disease. Many of the issues of quality of life revolve around this point. Cost vs benefit measures include both length of survival and "performance status" quantified by using one of the several measures that rate activity of daily living (eg, Karnofsky scale, Eastern Cooperative Oncology Group standards). Aggressive, highly toxic chemotherapy, radiation therapy, or surgical procedures can be justified if they result in complete regression of the cancer and a prolonged survival time free of disease after treatment. From this group come the patients that remain well for the duration of their life and can be considered cured. Even with later manifestations of recurrence, however, a long disease-free interval contributes to quality of life.

Overall survival data are important and provide a key factor in the selection of treatments. Some treatments remove or diminish the visible cancer but do not change expected survival time. It is important to factor both survival and the expected clinical response to therapy in the development of a treatment strategy. A thorough understanding of oncology is needed as a basis for establishing the chances for prolonged, disease-free survival and overall survival time balanced against cost in terms of physical discomfort, mental distress, family upheaval, and financial loss.

Prevention of Local Recurrence

The optimal extent of surgical resection, the appropriate placement of the radiation therapy fields, and the skilled use of adjuvant irradiation or chemotherapy after surgery all impact on the probability of control of local disease. Although the cancer may recur at a distant site and be the cause of death, control at the original primary site often is a critical factor in the overall success of a treatment plan. Local obstruction (bowel, ureter, airway) and pain arising from locoregional progression of cancer are major medical problems requiring palliation. Initial treatment aimed at preventing these late complications is well worth the extra effort, even if overall survival time is not extended.

Palliation of Symptoms

In many patients, palliation is the only practical goal at the time the diagnosis is initially established. Although, ideally, initial treatment should be potentially curative or life-extending, many patients have advanced disease or a cancer that is poorly responsive to available treatments even at their initial visit. These patients benefit greatly from an intelligent and sensitive approach to both their medical and social problems despite the fact that the disease cannot be cured. The best control of pain associated with cancer may well be achieved by a local surgical procedure or by achieving a limited regression of the cancer with irradiation or chemotherapy. Bypass surgical procedures for various obstructions may provide significant improvement in quality of life. The rate of clinical progression of the cancer and the extent of life-threatening metastases or the presence of other medical problems usually dictate the treatment course to be taken.

Patients who have cancers that are not curable with currently available therapies do not always need to be treated when the cancer is first discovered. However, when the cancer is growing and a decision to treat is made, then the treatment should be vigorous and directed at causing regression of the measured masses. This is generally the best approach for palliation of symptoms and is often associated with a prolongation of disease-free survival.

In the palliative mode, the physician's focus changes from treatment of the cancer to the management of the patient's overall problems. Symptoms may be caused by the cancer or by entirely unrelated medical problems. For example, the patient with an incurable slow-moving cancer may be suffering significant distress from a treatable bladder obstruction secondary to benign prostate enlargement. Not only might this offer an obstacle to future administration of effective pain medication, but surgical relief of this problem may be the one thing that can be done to relieve the patient's most significant symptom. Transurethral resection may be an appropriate step to be taken in this patient's management and should not be overlooked just because the patient has incurable cancer.

It is also important to avoid searching for sites of metastasis or for other diseases for which no effective treatment exists. Diagnostic evaluations that are pursued to prove which of two equally untreatable diagnoses are correct can be counterproductive. The patient and family often focus on the outcome of these tests and will be disappointed to find that considerable time and money has been spent in a futile search that will not directly influence outcome.

Treatment Strategies

Locoregional Treatment

Staging is directed toward finding patients who have localized disease that can be treated with curative intent. If the primary lesion appears localized and suitable for treatment by either surgical resection or radiation therapy, then this should be initiated immediately.

Optimal locoregional treatment implies treatment of the local disease and any regional disease extensions that may be present. Whether the approach is surgical or by irradiation, a margin of safety is usually built into the treatment plan to ensure total eradication of the local disease. For surgical procedures and radiation therapy ports, this usually means a margin of several centimeters of grossly normal tissue that is resected or irradiated in continuity, if this is at all feasible. In the case of a surgical resection, the pathologist can confirm the fact that the margin of resection is clear of microscopic extension of the neoplasm. This is not possible when assessing the adequacy of radiation therapy ports. If the margins around the primary tumor are well designed, however, either irradiation or surgery have a reasonable chance of local control of disease.

When regional lymphatic tissues are involved or there is a suspicion of microscopic involvement, similar therapeutic principles are employed in lymphatic dissections or radiation therapy of the lymphatic bed. Anatomically, this is more easily accomplished for some sites (such as axilla or neck) than others (intra-abdominal). In some instances surgery, followed by irradiation of a wider margin of tissue, offers optimal opportunity for local control or cure.

Strategies for Systemic Treatment

Systemic cancer therapy with chemotherapy and hormonal therapy has curative potential for some neoplastic diseases, particularly childhood leukemia, embryonal carcinoma of the testis, choriocarcinoma, large cell lymphoma, and Hodgkin's disease. In these and other highly responsive cancers, treatment with intent to cure must begin as soon as possible. More commonly, systemic chemotherapy and hormonal therapy have proven to be beneficial in a palliative role, controlling symptoms and extending survival and disease-free survival. Systemic cancer therapy used in the adjuvant situation, combined with either surgery or radiation therapy, has also emerged as an important treatment strategy.

Although oncologists know that carefully quantifying the disease is basic to good clinical research, this process is also critical to the physician's ability to make management decisions at every step along the way. Measurements of the efficacy of treatment are based on knowing the anatomic location of the cancer and its metastases, an observation of the rate of progression or regression of tumor masses, or other biologic measures of the activity of the disease. Quantification of all cancers and their metastases is extremely important. The data must be measured in linear diameters, calculated surface area, or volume and recorded in the patient record. The physician should systematically gather as many correlative measures of tumor size as possible. Number and size of tumor masses, biomarkers, and any other indicators of disease that can be quantified and repeated during the course of the illness are useful. All will help to support the decisions to be made as treatment is begun and periodically evaluated over the days and months of follow-up care. Prognosis in an individual patient is based on changes in these tumor measurements that are recorded in the chart and used to evaluate each step in progression or regression of disease. Calculations of rates of regression and definition of a plateau of growth or regression are useful tools to support clinical decision-making as treatment proceeds.

If a tumor stops regressing or progresses on the same doses of chemotherapy that previously were successful, four possible strategies may be pursued: escalate the doses of these medications, change to another class of agent (other drugs alone or in combination), radiation therapy, or discontinue treatment. The choice of each treatment is initially based on national statistics of predictable response for the histologic tumor type, but the evaluation of the correctness of this selection is based on the individual patient's response to the therapy chosen. Each subsequent treatment will have a lower response rate as predicted by studies of groups of similar patients, but the response of each specific patient is unique. In each patient, assessing the rate of regression and dose-response effect will direct future treatment.

There are numerous common cancers that have a low probability of response to chemotherapy. These patients not only do not benefit from treatment, but suffer toxicities of the treatment added to any symptoms that they may have from the cancer. Important progress is being made in the biologic evaluation of cancer cells. These tests relate to growth rate, metastatic potential, and intrinsic resistance to treatment. As these corollary laboratory tests become more reliable, the definition of sets of patients that can benefit from treatment will become more precise. In the interim, the use of a trial of chemotherapy is still a valid clinical tool.

If the intent is not curative, and anatomic position of metastases are not life threatening or causing local symptoms, then there is time to assess disease progression before treatment begins. Some cancers, without regard to cell type, are indolent and may not progress for long periods of time. Risk of treatment in these tumors includes not only the toxicities of the therapy, but other more subtle changes in host immunity, the relative distribution of populations of tumor cells with differing growth rates, chemotherapy resistance, or metastatic potential. Treatment of a nonprogressive asymptomatic cancer that cannot be cured cannot be recommended for the majority of patients.

When the cancer is no longer regressing or when toxicity, as assessed by the patient and his or her family, exceeds the potential for long-term positive effect, treatment should be stopped. The patient and physician should be in agreement on this point from the outset. Patients should know that beginning a therapy does not commit them to treatment for the duration of their life and that they can decide to stop without jeopardizing their relationship with their physician. There is always a potential to offer the patient an opportunity to participate in clinical research with new drugs in this situation. As alternatives to discontinuing treatment, patients may choose embarking on expensive travel from cancer center to cancer center or seeking treatment from practitioners using unproven methods and quackery. Failure to achieve a regression of the tumor and meaningful palliation is a reason to discontinue treatment, but we owe it to our patients to keep up their morale by not withholding treatment so they don't feel abandoned and lose hope.

Clinical Research

If we are to make significant progress in the diagnosis and treatment of cancer, every patient should be considered a potential candidate for inclusion in a research clinical trial. Much of the progress that has been made in oncology in the last several decades has been based on carefully controlled observations in well-designed clinical trials. Obviously, not all patients either qualify or will choose to be part of a clinical trial, but the option should be offered to all that are eligible.

The clinical trial for cancer management in the 1990s is an improved and more precise clinical investigation compared with many trial efforts in the past. A good definition of a clinical trial is a carefully controlled and highly ethical human experiment that is designed to test a hypothesis relating to possible improvements in patient management. Although such trials may address prevention or diagnostic questions, most clinical trials test questions relating to improved treatment. Phase I trials (preliminary studies of toxicity and definition of appropriate dose and schedule of administration to be used in subsequent tests of therapeutic efficacy) and Phase II trials (studies of effectiveness in specific types of human cancer) are generally employed when patients have failed to respond to current standard treatments. Phase III trials are comparative trials evaluating the relative efficacy of treatment innovations against the most effective treatment now available for a specific histologic cell type and stage. Considerable attention is given to studying comparable groups of patients so that the results of the study can be attributed with confidence to differences in the treatments. This comparison usually requires large numbers of patients participating and a random assignment to treatment choices to determine statistically significant differences between groups.

The selection of a particular treatment by the process of randomization is a particularly difficult idea to convey to the patient, but in many important studies it is the cornerstone of a well-designed study. Selection bias by either patient or physician can influence outcome and lead to the choice of inappropriate treatment for countless patients in the future. One reason given for the limited number of patients entered in clinical trials is the inability of both patient and treating physician to accept the principle of random selection as a method for choosing treatments. Such a concern implies that one of these people knows which treatment arm of a randomized trial is best for that patient. Obviously, if that is the case, it is inappropriate to carry out the study, since the result is already known. If the answer to the question posed by the study is in fact unknown, the clinical trial is the most appropriate choice for treatment, since a "state of the art" therapy is being compared with a potentially superior treatment. The philosophical barrier to research posed by lack of understanding of the value of clinical trials ought to be the subject for education of both patients and physicians.

Information about which specific studies are available is easily found in the National Cancer Institute's PDQ listing of national protocols* or by contacting a National Cancer Institute-sponsored Cancer Center. The National Cancer Institute-sponsored Community Cancer Center (CCOP) program and the outreach research activities of the cooperative clinical trial groups have facilitated access to clinical research being carried out at community hospitals. Practicing physicians should develop a relationship with local research facilities with ties to these national study groups in order to offer their patients this valuable treatment option.

Follow-Up Care of the Cancer Patient

Follow-up may be defined as a planned checkup on a regular basis after cancer therapy has been completed. The benefits of regular checkups are many and include some of the following:

1. The diagnosis and treatment of long-term complications of cancer treatment.

2. The opportunity to institute preventive strategies, eg, diet modification in colon and breast cancer

*PDQ is an on-line computer database product of The National Cancer Institute, International Cancer Information Center, Bethesda, Maryland.

patients or assisting with tobacco cessation in patients who have been treated for a cancer that is tobacco related.

3. The screening for and the early detection of a second cancer, eg, multicentric precancerous lesions that are common in the head and neck, a second cancer in the opposite breast, or a second cancer in the colon.

4. The diagnosis and treatment of recurrent cancer. In some cases therapy may be possible for cure, and in others, for palliation. Examples would be the recurrence of a skin cancer where cure is most likely, a chest wall recurrence of breast cancer where curative therapy is possible in some patients, or in metastatic cancer of the colon to the liver where resection for cure is sometimes possible.

5. The detection of a functional and/or physical disability offers the opportunity to undertake corrective measures; eg, when stomal care is imperfect, offer proper instruction by the enterostomal therapist and/or a visit by another patient with a stoma or a visit to a support group.

In the overall care of the patient with cancer, one must stress the importance of periodic follow-up and continuity of care. In many cases, a patient will receive two or more therapeutic modalities, and multiple physicians will want to follow the patient. To avoid confusion and the potential for the patient's receiving apparently conflicting advice, it is in the patient's best interests to have a single physician assume the central role and coordinate the opinions and management plans of all of those involved in the various aspects of the patient's care. Frequently, this role is assumed by the physician who performed the definitive therapy—the surgeon who did the mastectomy, the radiotherapist or gynecologist who treated the cervical cancer, or the medical oncologist who treated the leukemia. In many cases, the patient may live a significant distance from where the specialized cancer treatment was performed so that the primary care physician assumes primary responsibility for long-term follow-up with oncology specialists consulted as necessary.

The time interval between visits can be variable: the closer to the initial therapy, the more frequent the visit. Knowledge of the biology of each cancer plays a significant role in the selection of the time interval between visits. A reasonable follow-up plan might be: monthly the first year, every 2 months the second year, every 3 months the third year, every 6 months the fourth and fifth year, and yearly thereafter. This schedule should be more frequent if there is a recurrence or if other problems develop. The time intervals may be extended for in-situ and early stage I cases.

Dealing with Relapse

Many patients treated for cancer are not cured. The recurrence rate varies for each site of cancer and is more likely for stage III disease than for stage I disease. There is significant variability in the biology of cancer, and this may be expressed as the probability of recurrence. For example, the majority of patients with lung cancer who are treated for cure will have a recurrence in 6 to 12 months, while the majority of patients with breast cancer will have a recurrence later and less frequently.

Recurrences may be either local/regional, disseminated, or both. The most important predictor of recurrent cancer is the stage at the time of initial therapy. Recurrence may be detected by physical examination or by a variety of tests such as x-rays, CT scans, bone scans, ultrasound, or biologic markers. A workup for recurrent cancer may detect a second cancer in a paired organ or in a residual organ such as the colon.

When a new mass is found in a patient who was treated for cure or in a patient who has had a stable remission and whose clinical status seems to be deteriorating, it is important to establish that the cancer that was originally treated successfully has actually relapsed. Biopsy of a new mass that arises is strongly recommended in the patient being followed for a known cancer. Other more treatable causes of clinical deterioration should be considered. Infection, tumor necrosis, cancer-related metabolic abnormalities, and diseases unrelated to the cancer all can cause symptoms of generalized weakness, pain, disorientation, and other signs that can be misinterpreted as cancer progression. For example, hypercalcemia can mimic progressive brain metastases or bowel obstruction. Anemia arising from a benign duodenal ulcer can mimic progressive bone marrow infiltration. Cancers produce a variety of metabolically active polypeptides that mimic organ dysfunction. A second primary cancer in some cases may be curable or more responsive to treatment than the original diagnosis. This cancer may be incorrectly interpreted as a metastasis. A disciplined search for these new alternatives to the more common diagnosis of recurrent cancer should always be considered.

Rehabilitation

In cancer rehabilitation, the cancer team is concerned with the physical, social, and emotional needs of the patient and family. Modern cancer rehabilitation should be available and offered to all. Rehabilitation is often needed over months or years starting at the time of the diagnosis. It requires a team effort with collaboration among the patient, family, and health professional.

Some patients cope well, others manage poorly or

not at all. The inability to cope may be related to the diagnosis, or its prognosis may result in a failure to comply with treatment or tolerate its side effects. The patient might conceal the diagnosis from the family or significant other or may initiate inappropriate behavior within the family. The patient may sense rejection by fellow employees or management on return to work. A support system is very helpful in getting the patient through this emotional crisis.

Difficulty in coping generates further denial, avoidance of reality, and isolation. Distrust may eventually evolve into depression. An ounce of prevention is said to make a pound of treatment unnecessary. Direct consistent advice and emotional support of the patient by the cancer team will prevent confusion, distrust, and lack of compliance that follow misinformation and unrealistic goals.

The success of helping patients and families in coping with a cancer diagnosis has improved dramatically in the past two decades. Quality of life during and after treatment is now a major concern. Complex social problems may surface and involve diverse issues such as loss of body function, disruption of family and other significant relationships, financial security, employment and insurance, psychologic implications related to cancer and its treatment, as well as additive problems that relate to coexisting medical conditions. Patterns of cancer care are changing rapidly with a shift of treatment away from the hospital to the outpatient setting as well as the home, and the expanded use of support groups and hospice care.

The Beginning of Rehabilitation

The patient may or may not be surprised to learn that he or she has cancer, depending on the symptoms. In either case, there is always a fear that the patient's longevity and ability to carry out the activities of normal living are threatened. The physician who is the first to diagnose cancer has a critical role in communicating to the patient the meaning of cancer, the tests that are indicated, the treatment options, and the possible disabilities. The family is usually involved to varying degrees in this process. Medical personnel in the clinic or office play an important role in educating the patient. Numerous pamphlets are available, and there are telephone hot lines such as those provided by the American Cancer Society or the National Cancer Institute. These hot lines are frequently a lifeline to information.

Age, marital status, cancer site, occupation, emotional stability, and coexisting medical conditions must be taken into consideration at the beginning of the rehabilitation process. The rehabilitation goals should be set to minimize functional, psychologic, and emotional impairments that could result from cancer and its treatment. For example, the patient with a colostomy may retreat from society. However, with a positive and supportive approach, the patient can be trained to cope and care for the stoma and function normally in day-to-day activities. Trained volunteers who have personal experience with colostomy often help on a one-to-one basis. The enterostomal therapist, usually a nurse, provides help in physical and psychologic adjustment. A support group such as provided by the United Ostomy Association allows colostomy patients to share "tricks of the trade" with each other as well as assuring the patient that they are not alone.

The Rehabilitation Care Team

Not every patient will require the services of a rehabilitation team because personal needs, desires, and resources vary. Nonetheless, the physician should be alert to the potential need for services, especially if a cure has not been achieved. Rehabilitative care is still necessary after the patient leaves the hospital. Coordination for continuing care is essential before discharge. The rehabilitation care team's goal is to help each patient readapt and live as normal and full a life as possible.

A physiatrist—a doctor who specializes in rehabilitation techniques—may be required to assist in the strengthening of muscles, the use of artificial limbs, and for retraining for daily activities. A pharmacist may be needed to help with pain management including the use of patient-controlled analgesia (PCA) pumps. The oncology nurse can provide psychosocial support and a variety of educational programs for patients before, during, and after treatment. Nurses also play a major role in at-home care and rehabilitation and in helping patients and family members to deal with the many psychosocial issues of living with cancer.

The physical therapist should be involved in the care of the patient from the outset. For example, the patient with breast cancer always needs some assistance with arm exercises, whether the treatment is primarily surgical or with radiation therapy. This can often be instituted before primary treatment of the cancer has actually begun, with instruction in range-of-motion shoulder exercises to prevent contraction or muscle atrophy. An exception to early application of exercises may be the patient who has immediate breast reconstruction where a delay of 2 or 3 weeks may minimize prosthesis displacement.

The social worker is important in a total rehabilitation effort by helping to plan personal and family activities, introducing the patient to community resources, and in finding appropriate vocational counselors. The social worker also provides emotional support and psychosocial guidance. In addition, a member of the clergy or a lay volunteer also may be helpful in providing assistance and advice in both personal and religious matters. Psychologists and other mental health professionals may be called in to help with the stress and emotional problems that are so common among cancer patients and their families.

Home health care agencies and services are now available in most communities, and their effectiveness is rapidly improving. For patients with advanced cancer that cannot be cured, hospices provide invaluable services. These include continuing care in an institutional setting and in the home, pain management, and supportive care.

Rehabilitation or re-adaption is an essential part of comprehensive cancer care. The goals of rehabilitation, whether preventive, restorative, supportive, or palliative, should be defined before treatment begins. Rehabilitation is best carried out when the primary care physician and the cancer team consider rehabilitation an integral part of the overall treatment. This allows for early recognition of an actual or potential disability so that appropriate referrals can be made. The overall goal of rehabilitation is to return the cancer patient to as nearly normal a life as possible.

Conclusion

This chapter has outlined a philosophy of cancer management from the perspective of the physician who is primarily responsible for the patient. The clinician's approach to the patient who has or is suspected of having cancer should not differ from the organized approach used to analyze other clinical problems. The physician-patient relationship should be established with an honest, but optimistic, discussion of treatment alternatives to assure an environment of confidence and trust.

It is important that a multidisciplinary medical team be involved in planning from the outset. However, a single physician should serve as the patient's primary contact and be available to discuss, explain, and lead. It is also critical that discussions and diagnostic evaluation lead to a coordinated plan. To follow the plan, the physician should gather and record in the chart as much information about the cancer as possible to be able to evaluate treatment progress or progression of the disease and be prepared to shift course as circumstances dictate. The Hospital Tumor Board can facilitate this process, and all hospitals should try to establish approved Commission on Cancer-American College of Surgeons cancer programs.

The primary physician should develop a roster of available consultants and become familiar with the available cancer centers, national databases, and clinical trials.

Finally, modern oncology emphasizes treatment of the whole patient, with the primary goal being rehabilitation and a prompt return to the normal activities of daily living. Although many cancers can be cured, much can be done for all patients with this disease.

References

1. American Joint Committee on Cancer. *Manual for Staging Cancer*. 4th ed. Philadelphia, Pa: JB Lippincott Co; 1992.

2. International Union Against Cancer TNM Atlas. 3rd ed. New York, NY: Springer-Verlag; 1992.

5

THE PATHOLOGIC EVALUATION OF NEOPLASTIC DISEASES

John D. Pfeifer, MD, PhD, Mark R. Wick, MD

Many physicians think of the pathology laboratory only as an unpleasant area of the medical school where they were first exposed to museum specimens of human disease, including neoplasia. Accordingly, they too often forget that abnormalities in these mummified or soggy tissues explained many of the physical findings associated with disorders of living human beings. Indeed, it is advisable to remember the often-quoted statement of Sir William Osler on this topic—"To know Pathology is to know Medicine."

In reality, modern pathology is a dynamic facet of medical practice, in which specialists who are skilled at laboratory analysis actively contribute to the care of patients. Even the autopsy can be included in this statement, because its aim is to serve as a "quality assurance" measure to be used in a prospective educational manner by clinicians. Other areas of laboratory medicine, including surgical pathology, hematopathology, blood banking, clinical chemistry, and microbiology, are regularly involved in the precise definition of disease and in the monitoring of therapeutic results.

The pathologist's understanding of oncologic disorders has progressed far beyond the recognition of abnormal tissues with the microscope, although this activity still retains considerable importance in the diagnosis of cancer. Today, the laboratory specialist plays an integral role in eliminating incorrect differential diagnostic considerations, determining prognostic factors, evaluating treatment outcomes, and otherwise supporting the multidisciplinary care of oncology patients. Recent technologic advances have enlarged the scope of such activities significantly, but they must be utilized prudently with knowledge of their strengths and weaknesses.

This chapter outlines the general activities of pathologists in this context, and presents a practical introduction to the diverse analyses performed by them that have an impact on patients with malignant neoplasms. Because of space constraints, only an abbreviated discussion is possible. For a more complete description of the morphologic analysis of neoplasms, which still plays the central role in diagnosis, the interested reader is referred to the excellent text by Underwood on biopsy interpretation and surgical pathology.[1]

Interactions Between Clinicians and Pathologists

To optimally utilize the services of pathologists, clinicians must be familiar with the strengths and limitations of the technical procedures employed in the laboratory. Oncologists and surgeons are not merely "consumers" of pathologic data; rather, they should be interactive participants in the generation of such information. Much of what the anatomic pathologist is able to say about any given case is dependent on receipt of pertinent clinical facts, prompt and proper submission of specimens, and adequacy of the tissue sample itself. A rapid and confident pathologic diagnosis is assured only when these factors receive proper attention.[1]

Therefore, it is wise for clinicians to consult with the pathology laboratory before scheduling selected invasive diagnostic procedures that will yield pathologic specimens. A discussion may then take place on the best means of obtaining the tissue, the possible need for frozen sections, special processing requirements, and the role, if any, of adjunctive pathologic analyses in diagnosis and prognosis. For example, if lymphoma is suspected in a patient with lymphadenopathy, it is wiser to undertake an excisional lymph node biopsy instead of fine needle aspiration;

John D. Pfeifer, MD, PhD, Assistant Professor of Pathology, Department of Pathology, Washington University School of Medicine, St. Louis, Missouri

Mark R. Wick, MD, Professor of Pathology, Department of Pathology, Washington University School of Medicine, St. Louis, Missouri

conversely, the latter procedure usually yields adequate tissue in cases of probable metastatic carcinoma. In addition, karyotyping, genotypic analyses, and certain immunohistochemical studies can be performed only on fresh tissue, and are precluded if the specimen is placed in fixative solution before dispatch to the pathology laboratory.

With this introduction, an outline will be provided of the conventional and specialized procedures used in the pathologic analysis of malignant tumors. This will include a short discussion of relevant terminology, as well as simplified presentations of macroscopic examination, histopathology, and allied methods.

Definitions of Tumor Types

Current tumor classification systems encompass a multitude of terms that are based on biologic behavior, cellular function, histology, embryonic origin, and anatomic location as well as eponyms (Table 5-1).[2] Although it hardly needs mention, nomenclature is important because it is the means by which pathologists communicate a diagnosis, and because specific tumor designations carry specific clinical implications.

Neoplasms (literally "new growths") may be benign or malignant. They consist of the proliferating tumor cells themselves and a supportive stroma containing connective tissue and blood vessels. An abundant stromal collagenous response to a neoplasm (most often to a malignant one) is called *desmoplasia*.

The most important features used to define a tumor as benign or malignant are the empirically known biologic behavior and the microscopic appearance. Generally, benign neoplasms are innocuous and slow-growing, while malignant lesions often exhibit more rapid proliferation, invade adjacent tissues, and metastasize. Benign neoplasms usually have a bland microscopic appearance, while malignant neoplasms often manifest mitotic activity, abnormal nuclear chromatin, cellular pleomorphism, and areas of necrosis. However, exceptions to these generalizations abound. Benign neoplasms can kill the patient if inopportunely located (eg, an ependymoma blocking the aqueduct of Sylvius, or uterine intravascular leiomyomatosis eventually obstructing the right heart), and some can metastasize (eg, benign giant cell tumor of bone). Malignant neoplasms, on the other hand, may have a bland, mature cellular microscopic appearance, as seen in small lymphocytic lymphoma.

Malignant neoplasms of epithelial origin are called carcinomas. If predominantly glandular or ductal, they are termed *adenocarcinomas*; if derived from a stratified squamous epithelium, *squamous cell carcinomas*. Lesions with hybrid features of glandular and squamous carcinomas are known as *transitional cell carcinomas*. Neoplasms originating in a specific organ may be named accordingly; thus, *hepatocellular* or *adrenocortical* carcinoma. Malignant neoplasms of mesenchymal origin are designated *sarcomas* (if differentiating toward fat cells, liposarcoma; toward fibrous tissue, fibrosarcoma; smooth muscle, leiomyosarcoma; blood vessels, angiosarcoma; and so on). Malignant tumors do not necessarily have benign counterparts, and the converse applies as well.

Modifying adjectives used in diagnosis often reflect prognostic information, as in poorly differentiated adenocarcinoma. Neoplasms with biologically ambiguous names are referred to with a precise modifier, eg, *malignant* versus *benign* schwannoma. Nonspecific anatomic names generally should be avoided; as an illustration of this point, *bronchogenic carcinoma* could refer to squamous cell carcinoma, adenocarcinoma, small-cell neuroendocrine carcinoma, or other tumor types.

Neoplasms of the hematopoietic system usually have no benign analogues. Consequently, the terms *leukemia* and *lymphoma*, together with appropriate adjectives (eg, chronic myelogenous leukemia; follicular, predominantly small cleaved cell lymphoma), always refer to malignant proliferations. Similarly, *melanoma* is always used to describe a malignant melanocytic neoplasm.

Finally, time-honored but idiosyncratic eponyms remain. These are employed in reference to such neoplasms as Ewing's sarcoma (of uncertain histogenesis), Warthin's tumor (a benign lesion of the salivary glands), and Brenner tumor (a neoplasm with both benign and malignant forms derived from the surface epithelium of the ovary).

Macroscopic Examination of Tissue Specimens

As a discipline, pathology had its beginnings in the careful gross examination of diseased tissues at the autopsy table. Even before the microscope had come into general use, several disorders were well recognized at a macroscopic level, including malignant melanoma and various carcinomas. In the current rush to introduce new and ever more molecular techniques to diagnostic medicine, it is tempting to forget about the power of the trained observer's eyes and tactile senses. These simple tools are crucial to good surgical and pathologic practice.

The pathologist grossly examines all resected tumors submitted to the laboratory with several objectives in mind. First, the presence of representative tissue is confirmed, and the suitability of the specimen for further study is judged. Second, margins of excision are labeled with indelible ink, to retain the orientation of the specimen for subsequent histologic analysis. Third, the specimen is opened and sectioned with a scalpel or sharp knife, at which time notes are made on the consistency, color, and extent of the neoplastic growth. By integration of documented macroscopic characteristics with knowledge of the clinical findings, a differential diagnosis may be reached at

Table 5-1. Nomenclature Pertaining to Neoplastic Diseases*

Cell or Tissue of Origin	Benign	Malignant
Tumors of Epithelial Origin		
Squamous cells	Squamous cell papilloma	Squamous cell carcinoma
Basal cells	—	Basal cell carcinoma
Glandular or ductal epithelium	Adenoma	Adenocarcinoma
	Cystadenoma	Cystadenocarcinoma
Transitional cells	Transitional cell papilloma	Transitional cell carcinoma
Bile duct	Bile duct adenoma	Bile duct carcinoma (cholangiocarcinoma)
Liver cells	Hepatocellular adenoma	Hepatocellular carcinoma
Melanocytes	Nevus	Malignant melanoma
Renal epithelium	Renal tubular adenoma	Renal cell carcinoma
Skin adnexal glands		
Sweat glands	Sweat gland adenoma	Sweat gland carcinoma
Sebaceous glands	Sebaceous gland adenoma	Sebaceous gland carcinoma
Germ cells (testis and ovary)	—	Seminoma (dysgerminoma)
		Embryonal carcinoma, yolk sac carcinoma
Tumors of Mesenchymal Origin		
Hematopoietic/lymphoid tissue	—	Leukemia
		Lymphoma
		Hodgkin's disease
		Multiple myeloma
Neural and retinal tissue		
Nerve sheath	Neurilemoma, neurofibroma	Malignant peripheral nerve sheath tumor
Nerve cells	Ganglioneuroma	Neuroblastoma
Retinal cells (cones)	—	Retinoblastoma
Connective tissue		
Fibrous tissue	Fibromatosis (desmoid)	Fibrosarcoma
Fat	Lipoma	Liposarcoma
Bone	Osteoma	Osteogenic sarcoma
Cartilage	Chondroma	Chondrosarcoma
Muscle		
Smooth muscle	Leiomyoma	Leiomyosarcoma
Striated muscle	Rhabdomyoma	Rhabdomyosarcoma
Endothelial and related tissues		
Blood vessels	Hemangioma	Angiosarcoma
		Kaposi's sarcoma
Lymph vessels	Lymphangioma	Lymphangiosarcoma
Synovium	—	Synovial sarcoma
Mesothelium	—	Malignant mesothelioma
Meninges	Meningioma	Malignant meningioma
Tumors of Uncertain Origin		
???	—	Ewing's tumor

Adapted from Lieberman and Lebovitz.[2]

* This list is intended to provide only an introduction to tumor nomenclature. As indicated in the text, the existing terminology has mixed origins.

this stage and appropriate samples taken to resolve it. For example, a soft tissue tumor of the retroperitoneum may have the gross appearance of a leiomyosarcoma; however, to confirm this interpretation definitively, prosected tissues can be placed in special fixative and examined later with the electron microscope. Not uncommonly, macroscopic features alone are sufficient to suggest a final diagnosis. Fig 5-1 shows a renal pelvic tumor from an adult patient, the gross attributes of which are characteristic of transitional cell carcinoma. In Fig 5-2, the darkly colored mandibular mass from a child is macroscopically typical of a pigmented neuroectodermal tumor.

It is imperative that the pathologist examine the *entire* resected tumor before it is subdivided by the surgeon for other purposes (eg, before a portion of a neoplasm is sent directly from the operating room to a research laboratory for investigational purposes). When careful inspection of the lesional borders is important, it is a disservice to patient care to violate the tissue margins before they can be adequately examined pathologically. For example, a malignant rather than benign diagnosis is rendered in cases of follicular thyroid lesions or thymic tumors if they penetrate the capsular boundaries. Obviously, receipt of a "partial" specimen in the gross pathology laboratory prevents proper examination of such lesions.

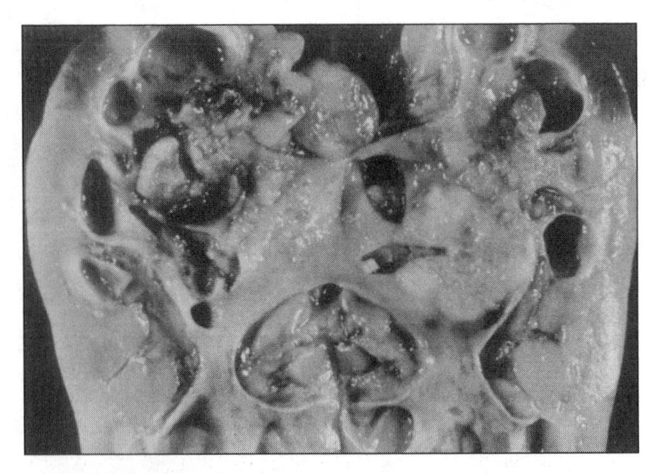

Fig 5-1. Renal pelvic tumor with macroscopic characteristics typical of transitional cell carcinoma. These include a papillary configuration and multifocality.

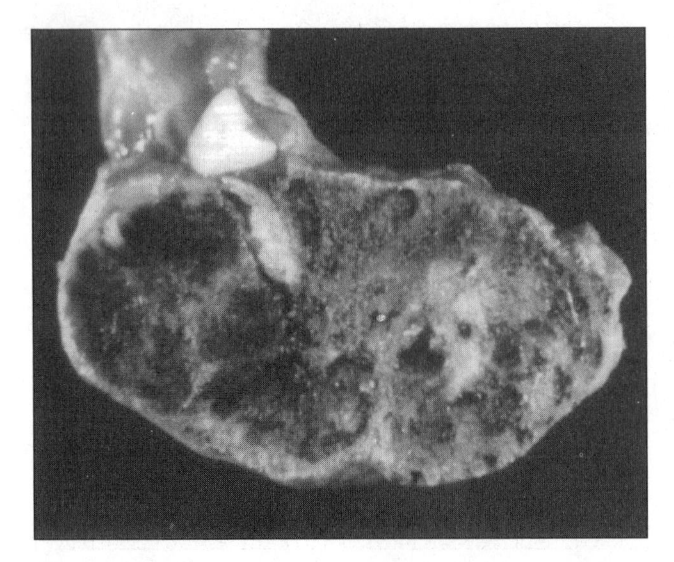

Fig 5-2. Pigmented neuroectodermal tumor of infancy, involving the mandible. The appearance is virtually diagnostic, in light of its known location and the dense pigmentation evident macroscopically.

Anatomic orientation of excised tissues should be a routine part of the information submitted to the pathology department. This allows for the precise localization of a tumor that is present at the margin of resection.

Histologic Study of Human Malignancies

In the hands of individuals well trained in morphologic diagnosis, the light microscope continues to serve as the cornerstone of surgical pathology. With the proviso that the tissue processing requirements outlined above have been met, the simple use of the hematoxylin and eosin staining method on paraffin-embedded tissue sections is sufficient to make the diagnosis with most malignant neoplasms. It should be noted, however, that certain clinical procedures (eg, vigorous compression of tissue specimens during endoscopic biopsy or extensive use of electrical or thermal cautery during resection) have the potential to interfere with diagnosis because they can severely damage microscopic anatomy.

Nevertheless, for the morphologic features of a tissue to be optimally visualized by routine light microscopy, the specimen must undergo proper preparation and processing. First, a minimum period of fixation in formalin (or an alternative mordant) is required; depending on the overall size of the specimen, this interval varies from 1 to 2 hours to more than 12 hours. After fixation, the pathologist completes the gross examination of the specimen and excises slices of the tissue, which are then subjected to automated processing. This additional processing includes further fixation, dehydration of the tissue, and saturation with hot paraffin wax; together, these steps require at least several hours to complete. Finally, the processed tissue slices must be embedded in paraffin, sectioned on a microtome, and stained by histotechnologists in the pathology lab.[3] Routine processing of tissue in practice, therefore, requires at least an overnight time interval. If special studies are warranted for diagnosis (such as routine histochemistry, immunohistochemistry, electron microscopy, or flow cytometry), additional time is obviously required.

This outline of the sequence of events involved in

proper processing of tissue is presented to prevent frustration on the part of clinical physicians, who often wonder why a microscopic interpretation is so long in forthcoming after a specimen has been submitted to the laboratory. Although a quicker method of histologic examination does exist—the frozen section procedure—it is not appropriate in many situations, is technically difficult, and yields microscopic preparations that are vastly inferior to those procured with conventional processing. Consequently, it is used sparingly for the routine evaluation of neoplasia.

Once stained microscopic slides have been obtained, the pathologist employs knowledge of histology and cytology to recognize changes related to neoplasia and other diseases. Tissue growth patterns, the degree of cellular differentiation, and details relating to prognosis, such as adequacy of excision, are assessed. Ideally, a firm diagnosis of cancer would always be possible by brief examination of routinely processed tissue on glass slides. Unfortunately, this is an unrealistic expectation, and often there is no substitute for experience, painstaking analysis, and collegial consultation among laboratory physicians on a difficult case.

There are several potential reasons for uncertainty in the interpretation of biopsy or resection specimens. An important reason relates to the natural history of any given pathologic process. A biopsy may be obtained at a time when a neoplastic lesion is not fully developed and therefore lacks "diagnostic" histologic features. Treatments such as irradiation or chemotherapy often alter the pathologic characteristics of the tissue.[1] Other lesions that cause a great deal of consternation are the so-called borderline or minimal-deviation malignancies. These proliferations, which can be epithelial, mesenchymal, or melanocytic, are characterized by microscopic features that differ minimally from those of benign neoplasms or reactive processes.[4]

In the course of arriving at a diagnosis, the pathologist should *discuss* pertinent findings with the responsible clinician. Ultimately, a written report is issued for all specimens. Documentation is made of the tumor type (and grade, if applicable), as well as information that can be used by oncologists to assign a stage to the lesion in cases of malignant neoplasms. Pathologists may be familiar with the biologic attributes of some tumors that even experienced oncologists have not encountered. Under these circumstances, a comment may be included in the tissue report on the expected behavior of the lesion, and recommendations for therapy may be given in general terms. Previous discussions with clinicians may be distilled into suggestions for the subsequent management of difficult cases, particularly those that fall into the "borderline" category.

Stage and Grade

Determination of tumor stage and grade not only offers important prognostic information but also allows for comparison of therapeutic results using various cooperative treatment protocols. Tumor grading is based primarily on the degree of differentiation of the malignant cells (Figs 5-3 and 5-4), and secon-

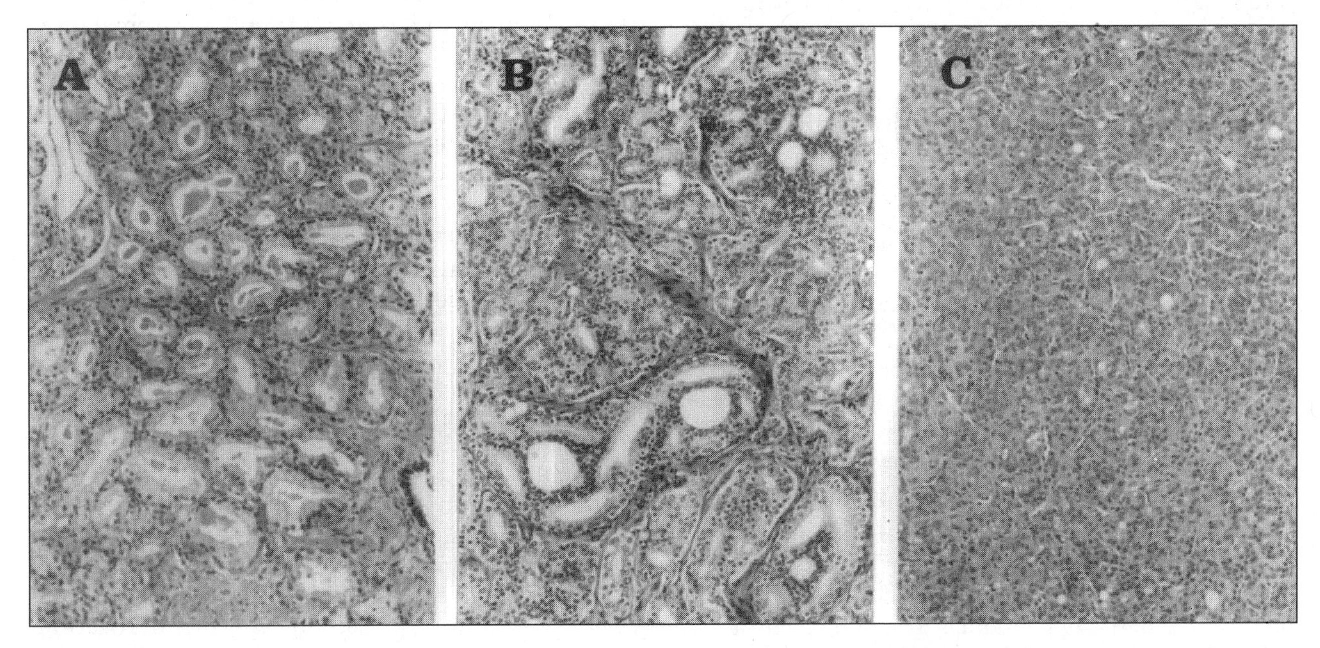

Fig 5-3. Adenocarcinoma of the prostate. ***A:*** Well differentiated (note the single, separate, closely spaced uniform glands). ***B:*** Moderately differentiated (note irregular glands with prominent cribriform epithelium). ***C:*** Poorly differentiated (note fused glandular epithelium and anaplasia of individual cells).

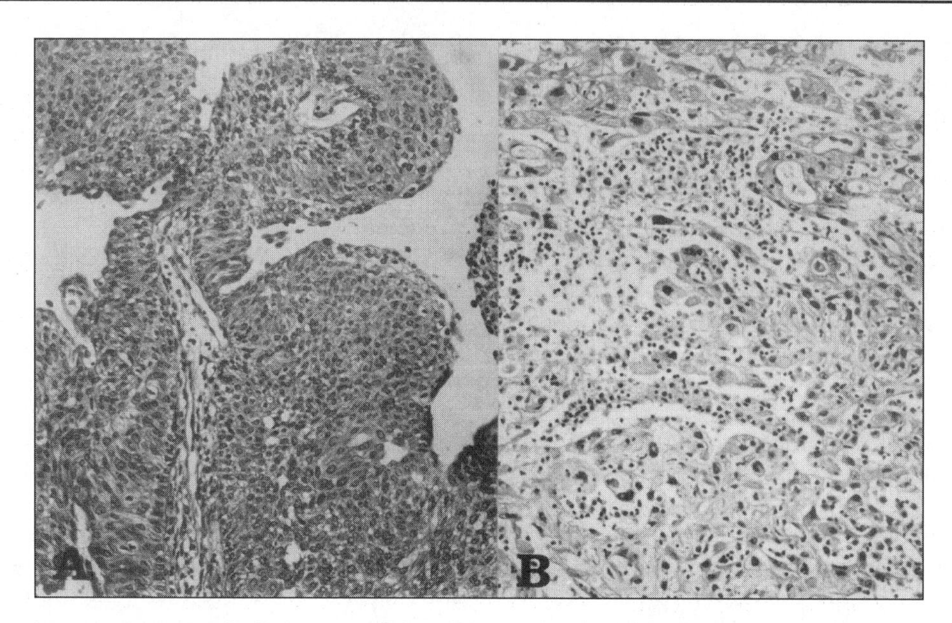

Fig 5-4. Transitional cell carcinoma of the renal pelvis. ***A:*** Grade 2/4; tumor is composed of relatively uniform cells lacking nuclear pleomorphism; papillary growth is demonstrated microscopically. ***B:*** Grade 4/4; neoplasm demonstrates overt nuclear pleomorphism and anisocytosis; it lacks papillary differentiation.

darily on an estimate of the rate of growth as indicated by the mitotic rate. Because the correlation between histologic appearance and biologic behavior is imperfect, grading criteria vary greatly for different neoplasms. Nonetheless, all grading criteria attempt to describe the extent to which the tumor cells resemble their normal tissue counterparts. Accurate grading is complicated by variations in differentiation from area to area in large tumors, as well as by site-related considerations and changes in tumor biology with time.

Tumor stage is based on the size of the primary lesion and the presence of lymph nodal or hematogenous metastasis. The major staging systems in use are the TNM classification (for primary *T*umor size, presence and extent of lymph *N*ode involvement, and distant *M*etastasis) and the AJCC (American Joint Committee on Cancer) system, which divides all tumors into stages 0 to IV.

The details of staging and grading procedures for specific tumors are considered elsewhere in this text. However, a few examples will illustrate the importance of these measures in prognosis and treatment:

1. Although the morphologic subtype of Hodgkin's disease has an effect on prognosis, tumor stage appears to be the most important prognostic variable,[5] given current modalities of therapy. Consequently, the pathologic findings at staging laparotomy (which includes splenectomy and biopsies of the liver, retroperitoneal lymph nodes, and bone marrow) have a far greater influence on the choice of treatment than the determination of a specific histologic subtype.

2. Similarly, the tumor stage of squamous cell carcinoma of the uterine cervix is the most important prognostic variable. The clinical significance of the stage is indicated by studies showing a <1% incidence of pelvic lymph node metastasis in early microinvasive carcinoma that has <3-mm depth of stromal invasion, compared with an 8.1% incidence in tumors that are 3.1 to 5.0 mm deep. Further, the presence of vascular invasion appears to increase the risk of nodal metastasis and vaginal recurrence.[6] Patients with stage Ia (occult invasive) carcinoma have a 5-year survival rate of 96%, while those with stage Ib (frankly invasive) lesions have a survival of 86% at 5 years. For cervical squamous carcinoma, it is noteworthy that histologic grade generally has no influence on survival of patients in any staging group.

3. In contrast, adenocarcinoma of the prostate is an example of a tumor for which microscopic grading is strongly correlated with prognosis and response to treatment. The grading system is based on the degree of glandular differentiation and on the *pattern* of growth, as evaluated by low-power microscopic examination (Fig 5-3). The histologic grade correlates well with clinical stage, as well as with the mortality rate within each stage. A *combination* of microscopic grade and clinical stage provides the best prognostic information.[7]

Histochemical Stains

When hematoxylin and eosin staining of paraffin-embedded tissue sections is insufficient to make a firm diagnosis of a malignant neoplasm, additional histochemical staining often provides sufficient information for definitive diagnosis. Since many of these specialized histochemical stains can be performed on formalin-fixed paraffin-embedded tissue, they often do not require the extra time and expense of many of the more specialized pathologic diagnostic procedures (such as electron microscopy, and flow cytometry). However, because some special stains have specific requirements for uncommon tissue fixation and processing, the pathologist must anticipate the possible need for special stains based on clinical history and the initial gross examination to ensure that adequate tissue samples are appropriately processed. Table 5-2 lists the more common special histochemical stains. The widespread application of immunohistochemical stains (see below) has made many histochemical stains obsolete and limited the usefulness of others.

Table 5-2. Selected Specialized Histochemical Stains of Value in the Pathologic Diagnosis of Neoplasia

Stain	Specificity	Uses and Comments
Alcian blue	Acidic mucosubstances	Demonstration of stromal mucin production by mesotheliomas
Periodic acid-Schiff	Glycogen (with appropriate control); neutral mucosubstances	Demonstration of mucous production
Oil red-O	Neutral lipids	Useful for distinguishing between ovarian fibroma and thecoma, for example; cannot be used on paraffin-embedded tissue
Argentaffin and argyrophilic	Catecholamines or indolamines	Demonstration of neurosecretory differentiation; demonstration of melanin; some modifications require special fixative
Trichrome	Nuclei, cytoplasm, and extracellular collagen	Nonspecific; can often demonstrate immature skeletal muscle cells (myoblasts) in poorly differentiated mesenchymal tumors
Leder	Presence of chloroacetate esterase required	Demonstration of cells of myeloid lineage and mast cells; is actually an enzyme histochemical technique

Frozen Sections

The term *frozen section* is synonymous with an intraoperative microscopic consultation. A sample of fresh tissue obtained during a surgical procedure is frozen by the pathologist; the most widely used method involves rapid cooling in a refrigerated bath of organic liquid. Histologic sections are then prepared using a cryostat (refrigerated microtome), fixed briefly, stained with hematoxylin and eosin, and examined microscopically. The entire procedure, including thorough histologic study, usually can be accomplished in about 10 to 15 minutes. Proper interpretation requires a complete gross examination of the tissue prior to sectioning and a well-trained pathologist with experience. Informative, interactive communication with the surgeon and an adequate clinical history are also essential for optimization of this process.

As with all diagnostic procedures, frozen section consultation has specific indications. In general, these indications include identification of a tissue, demonstration of the presence and nature of a lesion, definition of the adequacy of surgical margins or the extent of disease, and determination that the excised material is sufficient for diagnosis. Frozen sections should not be used merely to satisfy the curiosity of the surgeon, to compensate for inadequate preoperative evaluation, or as a mechanism to communicate information more quickly to the patient or the patient's family. As is well known, some diagnoses are so tenuous in this setting that frozen section interpretation is totally inadvisable. For example, it is often impossible to distinguish benign from malignant follicular thyroid tumors or mammary lesions using this technique.

Although histopathologic interpretation of cryostat sections is technically limited and more difficult than diagnosis using fixed paraffin-embedded tissues, frozen sections are highly regarded as a useful means of intraoperative consultation. The accuracy of frozen section diagnosis is commonly reported to be 94% to 98%, but this figure varies depending on the tissue type and the reason for consultation. It should be obvious that frozen section diagnoses often have a significant influence on the surgical procedure being performed. Hence, they must be utilized wisely by both surgeons and pathologists.

Cytology

Cytology is the science of morphologic examination of individual cells for the purpose of diagnosis. Suitable specimens are collected in one of three basic ways: exfoliation from an epithelial surface (eg, cervical smears obtained with a spatula or brush; bronchial washings or brushings); aspiration of fluid from body cavities; and fine needle suction aspiration of so-called solid lesions of the breast, thyroid, salivary glands, lung, prostate, and other organs. The cytologic preparation is then spread on a glass slide, fixed, and stained by a variety of methods. In most instances, the Papanicolaou's stain yields the greatest clarity of nuclear detail. Special investigations also may be carried out on cytologic specimens (eg, routine histochemistry, immunohistochemistry, and static cytometry), but these must be anticipated before sample procurement and special provisions for such analyses must be implemented.

Although generalizations are difficult, the cytomorphologic evaluation of possible malignancy is predicated on specific features of the cytoplasm and nucleus. The most helpful of these features are anisonucleosis, dyskaryosis, and an abnormal nuclear-to-cytoplasmic ratio. Malignant cells show consistent changes in nuclear structure (dyskaryosis), including coarse or dense granularity, hyperchromasia, abnormal nucleoli, and anisonucleosis (marked variation in shape and size); mitotic abnormalities may also be present (Fig 5-5). Anisocytosis, or pronounced variation in cellular size or shape, is seen in malignancies as well. The volumetric nuclear-to-cytoplasmic ratio is increased; most malignant cells have an oversized nucleus that displaces all but a small peripheral zone of cytoplasm. Intercellular cohesion is likewise aberrant; however, carcinomas do retain enough cell-to-cell adhesion to make their cytologic attributes dissimilar to those of mesenchymal neoplasms. Because reactive cellular changes (due to inflammation, infection, irradiation, or cytotoxic chemotherapy) can easily be confused with malignant proliferations, a complete clinical history is essential for accurate cytologic diagnosis.

Cytology has a high degree of reliability when morphologic interpretations are performed by experienced, well-trained individuals. Nonetheless, an effort should always be made to confirm the diagnosis by conventional biopsy prior to definitive treatment. The reliability of fine needle aspiration, when compared with open surgical biopsy, continues to be a matter of some controversy.

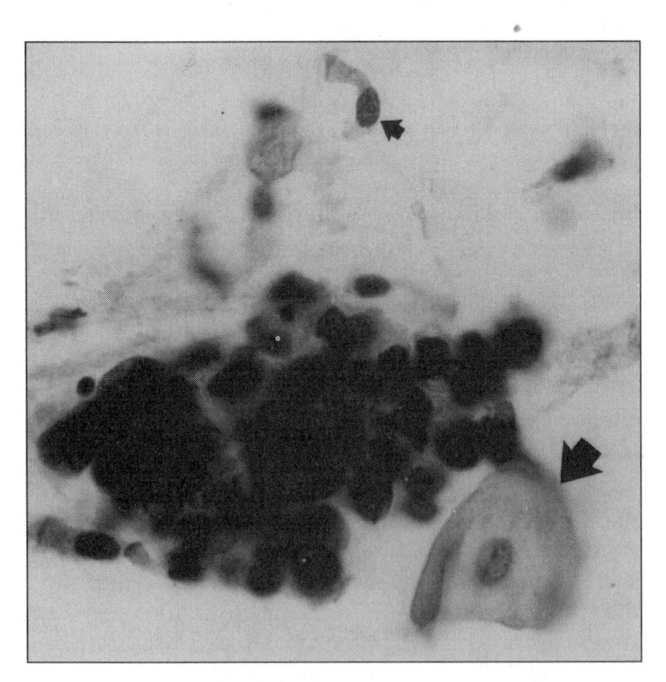

Fig 5-5. Cytologic specimen (bronchial washings) from 60-year-old woman with lung mass. Note the cluster of malignant cells demonstrating pronounced anisocytosis and anisonucleosis. A normal superficial squamous cell is indicated by the large arrow and a normal ciliated columnar cell by the small arrow.

Special Pathologic Procedures

In approximately 10% of all oncology cases, routinely assessed microscopic features of neoplasms may be insufficiently conclusive for a firm diagnosis. For example, malignant melanomas and anaplastic carcinomas are maddeningly similar histologically, often mandating the use of electron microscopy or immunohistochemical studies to distinguish the two through elucidation of submicroscopic, cell lineage-related features (Figs 5-6,A, and 5-7,A). Similarly, spindle cell sarcomas of soft tissue may resemble one another so markedly that adjuvant analyses are necessary for final diagnosis (Fig 5-8).

Of course, such evaluations require additional time for implementation and interpretation. These techniques merit further discussion, as they are used widely and provide extremely useful information.

Electron Microscopy

Electron microscopy is performed after tissue is processed in special fixative, embedded in epoxy resin, sectioned thinly (<1 micron), and impregnated with heavy metals. These heavy metal stains enable differential absorption of a focused electron beam that is passed through the specimen en route to a photographic emulsion plate. The plate provides a pictorial image of intracellular contents, magnified up to 200,000X or more.[8] Based on the presence of certain cytoplasmic organelles and other features, such as

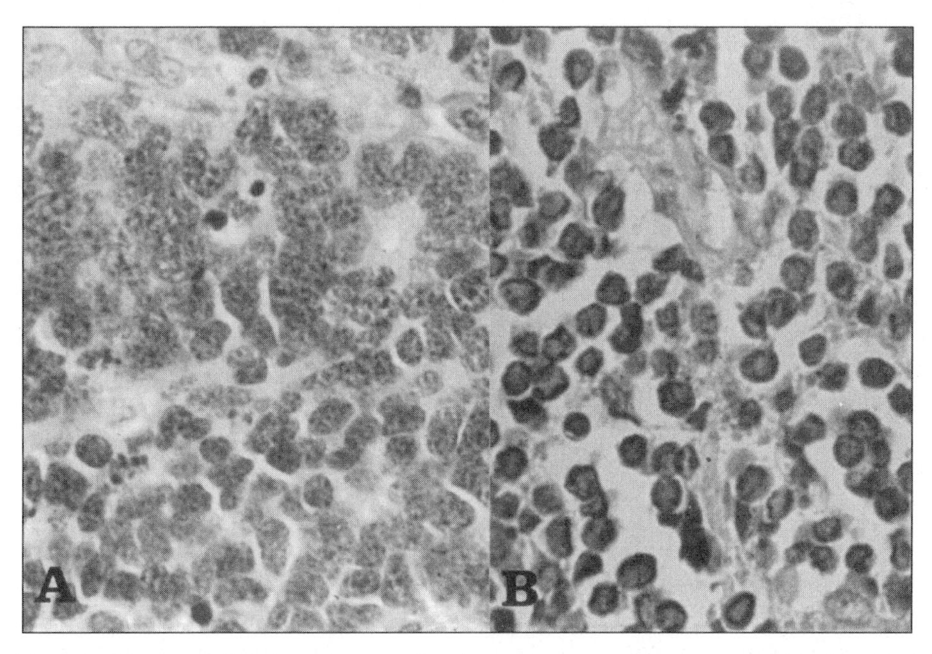

Fig 5-6. Microscopically indeterminate small-cell neoplasm, metastatic to a cervical lymph node, ***A***. This tumor is identified as a carcinoma by immunoreactivity for cytokeratin, an epithelial marker, ***B***.

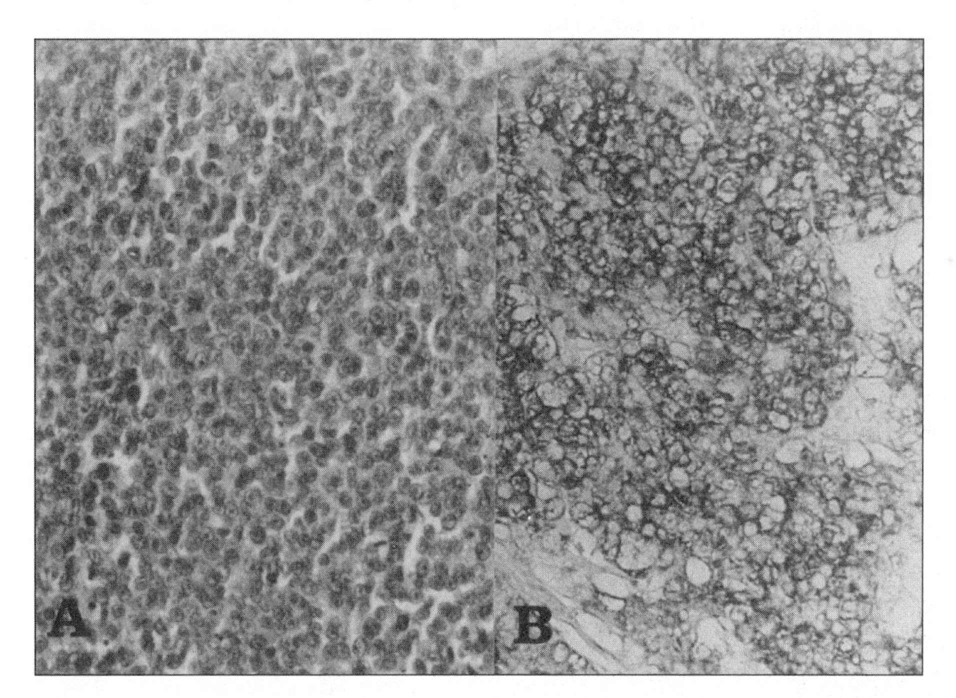

Fig 5-7. Metastatic lymph nodal neoplasm, ***A***, with histologic features virtually identical to those shown in Fig 5-6,A. The two tumors differ in cell lineage, however, as shown by the immunostain for the melanocytic-specific marker HMB-45, ***B***. Hence, the final diagnosis in this case was metastatic malignant melanoma.

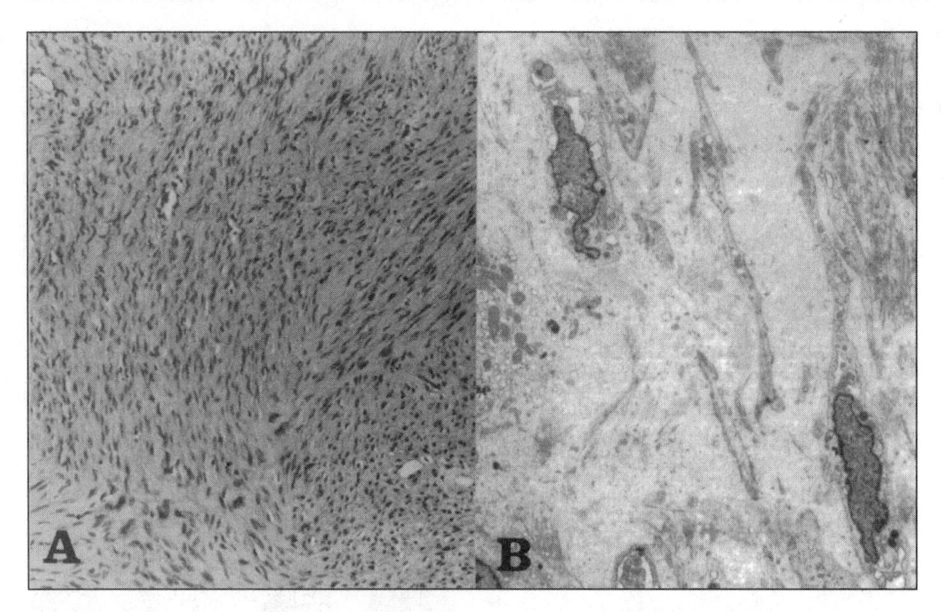

Fig 5-8. Histologically indeterminate malignant spindle cell neoplasm of soft tissue. The differential diagnosis would include leiomyosarcoma, fibrosarcoma, and malignant peripheral nerve sheath tumor based on the light microscopic attributes shown here, ***A***. Electron microscopy in the same case shows attenuated, overlapping cytoplasmic processes, indicating the diagnosis of malignant peripheral nerve sheath tumor, ***B***.

Table 5-3. Selected Electron Microscopic Features of Value in the Pathologic Diagnosis of Neoplasms

Finding	Predominant Distribution	Diagnostic Use
Intercellular junctions	Epithelial cells; selected mesenchymal nonlymphoid tumors	Distinction between lymphoma and carcinoma
External basal lamina (pericellular)	Epithelial cells; selected mesenchymal nonlymphoid tumors	Distinction between lymphoma and carcinoma; aids to identification of some soft tissue sarcomas
Intracellular or intercellular lumina	Glandular epithelia	Identification of adenocarcinomas
Microvillous core rootlets	Glandular epithelium of alimentary tract	Identification of gastrointestinal origin of metastatic carcinomas
Cytoplasmic tonofibrils	Squamous epithelia	Identification of squamous differentiation in epithelial tumors
Premelanosomes	Melanocytic cells	Identification of melanomas
Neurosecretory granules	Neuroendocrine cells	Identification of neuroendocrine neoplasms
Thick and thin filament complexes	Striated muscle cells	Identification of rhabdomyosarcomas
Attenuated cytoplasmic processes	Schwann and neural cells	Identification of peripheral nerve sheath or neuronal neoplasms
Thin filament-dense body complexes	Smooth muscle cells	Identification of leiomyomas and leiomyosarcomas
Birbeck granules	Langerhans cells	Identification of Langerhans cell proliferations (eg, "histiocytosis X")
Cytoplasmic mucin granules	Secretory glandular epithelium	Distinction between malignant mesothelioma and adenocarcinoma; localization of origin for some adenocarcinomas

intercellular junctional complexes, the pathologist may be able to distinguish one malignant cell type from another (such as melanocytic from epithelial).[9] Hence, this technique contributes meaningfully to the differential diagnosis. Examples of salient electron microscopic findings in human malignancies are provided in Table 5-3.

Immunohistochemistry

Practical immunohistochemistry is currently based on an indirect, antibody-enzyme method known in common parlance as the "immunoperoxidase" procedure.[10] In this technique, frozen or rehydrated deparaffinized tissue is overlaid with a specific, well-characterized primary antibody directed at an antigen of diagnostic value. After controlled incubation and subsequent removal of the primary reagent, a second antibody with generic specificity for the first is exposed to the tissue sections. The latter antibody may be labeled with biotin, providing a "bridge" for the subsequent binding of an avidin-biotin-horseradish peroxidase complex that completes the immunochemical assembly (Fig 5-9). The peroxidase enzyme can then be used to catalyze an oxidation-reduction reaction in the presence of a dye that is precipitated at the site of antibody binding. After a counterstaining procedure designed to highlight morphologic details, the presence of the antigen of interest can be visualized at a light microscopic level within the tissue section (Figs 5-6,B, and 5-7,B).

With few exceptions, these antigenic determinants are not absolutely tissue or tumor specific. Therefore, the immunopathologist must employ *panels* of primary antibodies in the study of malignant tumors, building an antigenic "fingerprint" that eventually allows for a final interpretation.[11] A sampling of commonly assessed antigens is listed in Table 5-4. Based on the relative tissue specificities of these antigens, algorithms can be constructed that enable the resolution of differential diagnostic problems with histologically similar neoplasms (Figs 5-10 and 5-11).

Immunohistochemistry is also used to demonstrate components of a neoplasm's phenotype that are not evident on routine light microscopy; these compo-

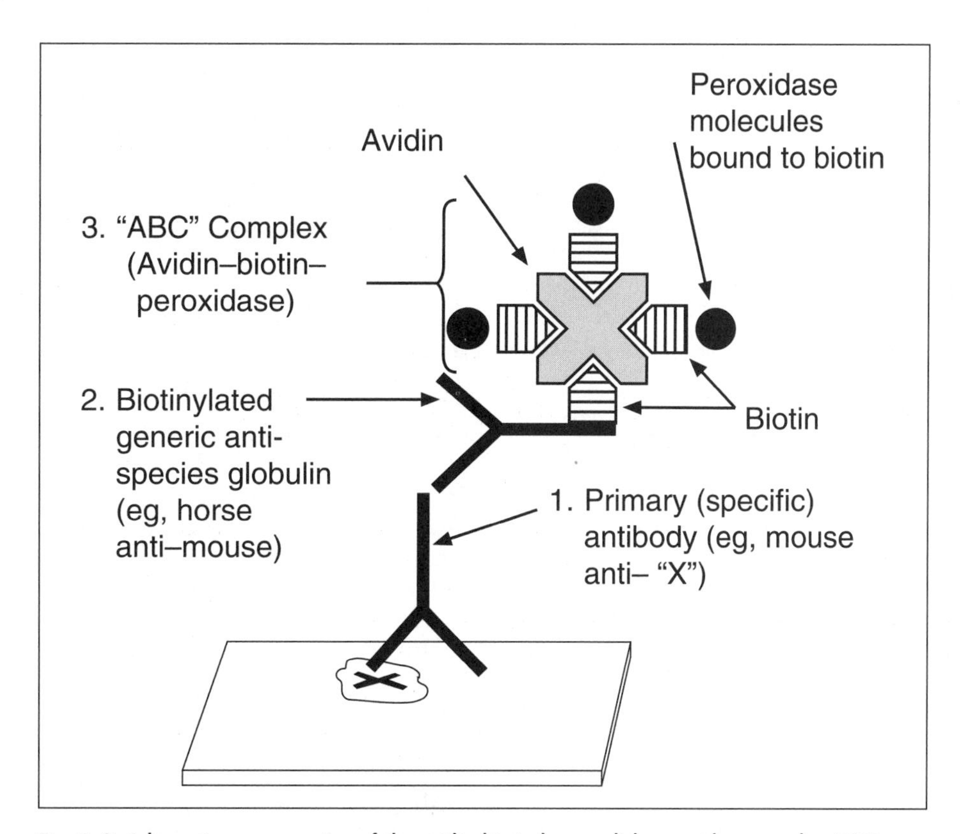

Fig 5-9. Schematic representation of the avidin-biotin-horseradish peroxidase complex (ABC) technique of immunohistochemistry. A primary antibody to an antigen of interest is incubated with test tissue sections, and followed sequentially by biotinylated secondary antibody and ABC complex. If the primary antibody binds (ie, if the antigen is present in tissue), the ensuing sequence of reagent linkages provides the substrate for chromogen localization and light microscopic visibility of the reaction. In this manner, antigens of diagnostic value can be detected in tissue.

Table 5-4. Selected Antigenic Moieties of Diagnostic Value in Practical Immunohistochemistry

Antigen	Predominant Distribution	Diagnostic Use
Cytokeratin	Epithelial cells	Distinction between lymphoma or melanoma and carcinoma
Epithelial membrane antigen	Epithelial cells	Distinction between melanoma and carcinoma
Leukocyte common antigen	Leukocytes	Distinction between lymphoma, carcinoma, and melanoma
Desmin	Myogenous cells	Identification of myogenic sarcomas
Muscle-specific actin	Myogenous cells	Identification of myogenic sarcomas
Thyroglobulin	Thyroid follicular cells	Identification of certain thyroid carcinomas
Prostate-specific antigen	Prostatic epithelium	Identification of metastatic prostatic carcinomas
Calcitonin	Parafollicular thyroid epithelium	Distinction of medullary thyroid carcinoma from other thyroid tumors
Carcinoembryonic antigen	Endodermally derived epithelium	Identification of certain carcinomas; distinction between mesothelioma and adenocarcinoma
Placental alkaline phosphatase	Placental tissue and germ cell tumors	Screening identification of possible germ cell and trophoblastic tumors
Alpha-fetoprotein	Neoplastic hepatic tissue and selected germ cell tumors	Identification of possible hepatocellular carcinoma, embryonal carcinoma, embryonal carcinoma, and endodermal sinus tumor
Beta-human chorionic gonadotropin	Placental tissue; trophoblastic and germ cell tumors	Identification of possible trophoblastic and germ cell tumors
CA-125	Müllerian epithelium	Identification of possible female genital tract carcinomas
CA-19-9	Alimentary tract epithelium	Identification of gastrointestinal and pancreatic carcinomas
Gross cystic disease fluid protein-15	Pathologic mammary epithelium	Identification of metastatic breast carcinomas
HMB-45	Melanocytic cells	Identification of melanomas
Chromogranin-A	Neuroendocrine cells	Identification of neuroendocrine carcinomas
Synaptophysin	Neuroendocrine cells	Identification of neuroendocrine carcinomas and neuroectodermal tumors

nents may affect the prognosis and treatment. As an example, it has recently been suggested that detection of the *neu* oncoprotein is associated with a greater risk of relapse and death in patients with low stage/low nuclear grade breast cancer, a group generally thought to have a rather uniformly good prognosis.[12] An ongoing study suggests that immunohistochemical markers of cell proliferation may represent potential prognostic tools in a wide variety of tumor types.[13]

It must be emphasized that neither electron microscopy nor immunohistochemistry is capable of differentiating benign from malignant tumors. Their purpose is principally to distinguish between microscopic "look-alikes" that have differing prognoses or require dissimilar treatments. Another use for antibody-enzyme staining methods is the localization of clinically important tumor markers within tissue sections, as discussed below.

In Situ Hybridization

Two recent advances have allowed for a wider application of in situ hybridization (ISH) technology to diagnostic pathology: the labeling of DNA probes by nonradioactive methods, and the development of techniques that permit the direct recognition of endogenous nucleic acid sequences in paraffin-embedded tissue sections and cytologic smears. The use of ISH has several diagnostic advantages. Small tissue fragments and archival material can be used with the method, and the reaction product is localized to specific cells (or even subcellular compartments), facilitating simultaneous evaluation of the histology and the ISH result.

Traditionally, nucleic acid probes were labeled by incorporation of a radioisotope of phosphorus. Recently, however, biotin has been linked directly to probes by employing biotinylated derivatives of uridine triphosphate (UTP) or deoxyuridine triphosphate

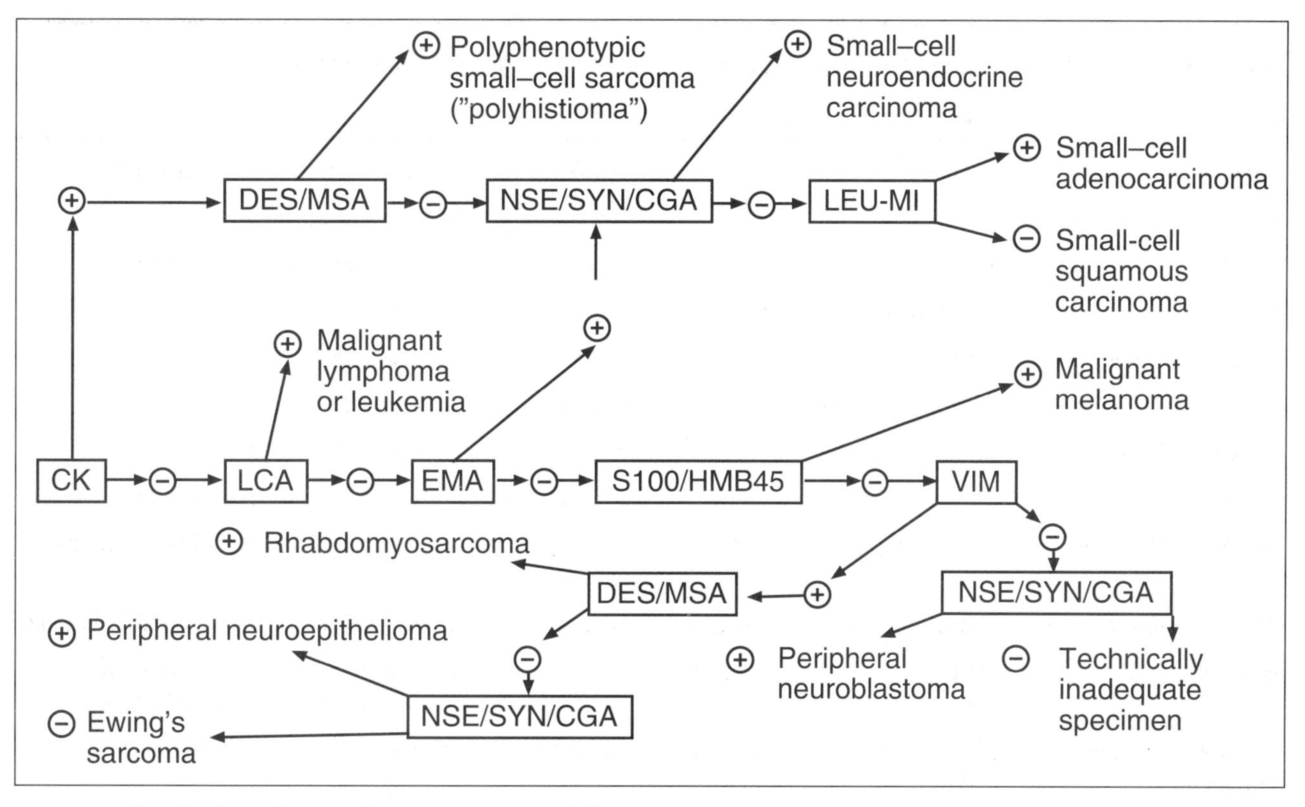

Fig 5-10. Algorithm for application of immunostains to the differential diagnosis of histologically indeterminate small-cell malignancies. (CK = cytokeratin; DES = desmin; MSA = muscle-specific actin; LCA = leukocyte common antigen; EMA = epithelial membrane antigen; NSE = neuron-specific enolase; SYN = synaptophysin; CGA = chromogranin-A; Leu M1=CD15 antigen; S100 = S100 protein; VIM = vimentin).

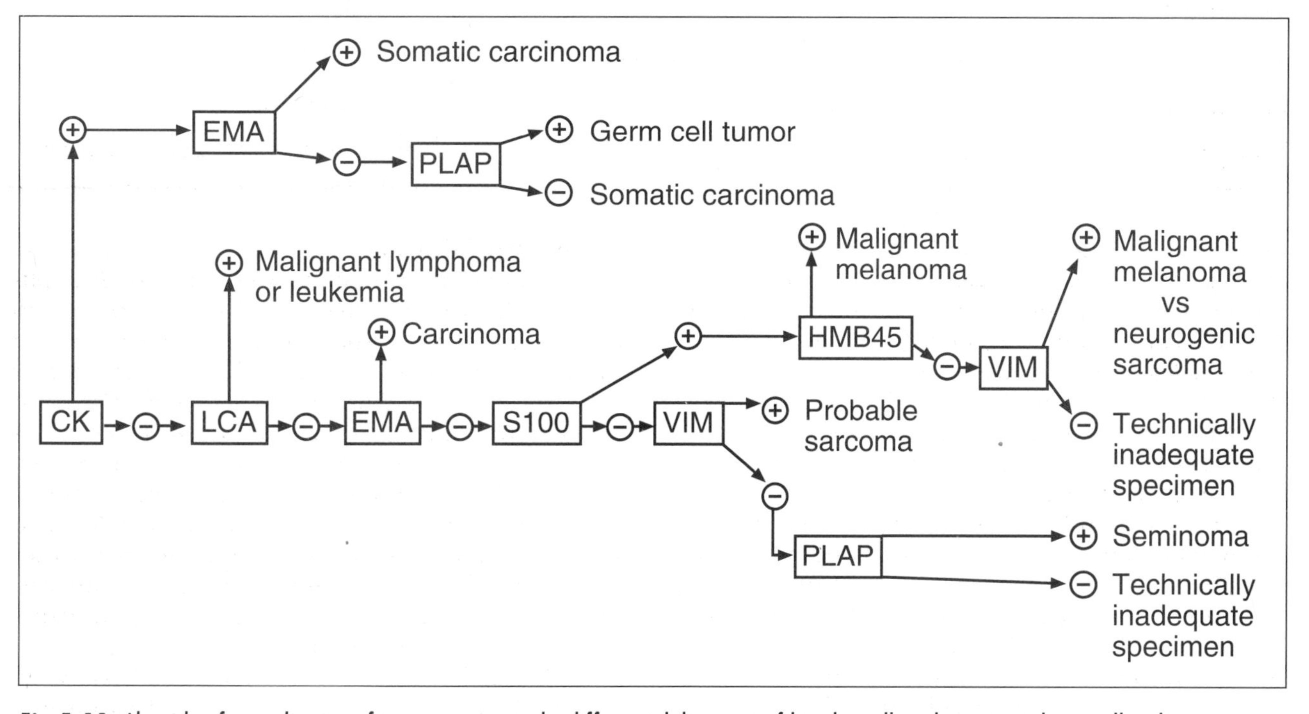

Fig 5-11. Algorithm for application of immunostains to the differential diagnosis of histologically indeterminate large-cell malignancies. (CK = cytokeratin; EMA = epithelial membrane antigen; LCA = leukocyte common antigen; PLAP = placental alkaline phosphatase; S100 = S100 protein; VIM = vimentin).

(dUTP) during probe synthesis. Importantly, the labeled nucleic acid probe exhibits denaturation and renaturation kinetics that are equivalent to those of an unsubstituted template. Through the use of avidin that has been complexed to fluorescent marker molecules (fluorescein), chromogenic enzymes (horseradish peroxidase or alkaline phosphatase), or electron-opaque plastic spheres, the biotinylated probe can be detected after ISH. Other methods for nonradioactive labeling of probes include the direct incorporation of fluorochromes or haptens.[14] ISH has been confirmed as a useful aid for diagnosis, for the identification of patient populations at increased risk of developing malignancies, and for the assessment of prognosis. Some recently described examples of these applications follow:

1. ISH has been widely used in the detection of human papillomaviruses (HPV). Although more than 50 variants of this virus have been identified, certain types (16,18,31,33,35,39,45,51) are correlated with high-grade dysplasias and malignancies of the female genital tract. Because the viral capsid antigen of all types is identical, immunohistochemical techniques are of no value in separating them. However, hybridization with biotinylated or radioactive probes has been used successfully to identify specific HPV types in both cytology specimens and biopsy sections.[15,16] These results show the value of this method for identification of patients with HPV infection who are at risk for progression to uterine cervical carcinoma. In this regard, it is of interest that ISH studies have also identified a predominance of HPV types 6,11,16, and 18 in HPV DNA-positive squamous cell carcinomas of the anus,[17] tongue,[18] penis,[19] and lung.[20]

2. Chronic infection by hepatitis B virus (HBV) is correlated with an increased risk for the development of hepatocellular carcinoma. HBV nucleic acid sequences have been detected by ISH in the liver tissue of some patients who lacked the serologic markers of viral infection.[21] Recently ISH has been suggested to have superior sensitivity in detecting HBV infection when compared with immunohistochemistry.[22]

3. Amplification of the N-*myc* oncogene is a seemingly independent prognostic factor associated with rapid progression of neuroblastomas.[23] DNA probe analysis (in particular, Southern blot analysis as described below) is the standard method by which amplification of N-*myc* is quantified. Recently, the extent of ISH for N-*myc* in neuroblastomas has been shown to correlate well with results of Southern blotting,[24] suggesting the possibility of an alternative method for obtaining this prognostic information.

DNA Probe Analysis

Recombinant DNA technology has been applied increasingly in pathology for tumor diagnosis and classification, as well as for the assessment of prognosis. For Southern blots, DNA is extracted from cells, denatured, electrophoresed in an agarose gel, and transferred to a filter on which it can be hybridized to a complementary DNA probe. Southern blots are used to detect genomic rearrangements, including those of genetic loci that are involved in consistent karyotypic abnormalities of certain tumors. Northern blots (which are completely analogous to Southern blots except that it is RNA that is extracted and so forth) are employed to detect abnormal gene expression in the absence of gross karyotypic abnormalities, or to determine cell lineage on the basis of gene expression.

A powerful advance in recombinant nuclei acid technology that has expanded the use of DNA probe analysis in the pathologic evaluation of neoplasia has been the development of the polymerase chain reaction (PCR). Because PCR provides a means to specifically amplify target nuclei acids, it results in vastly

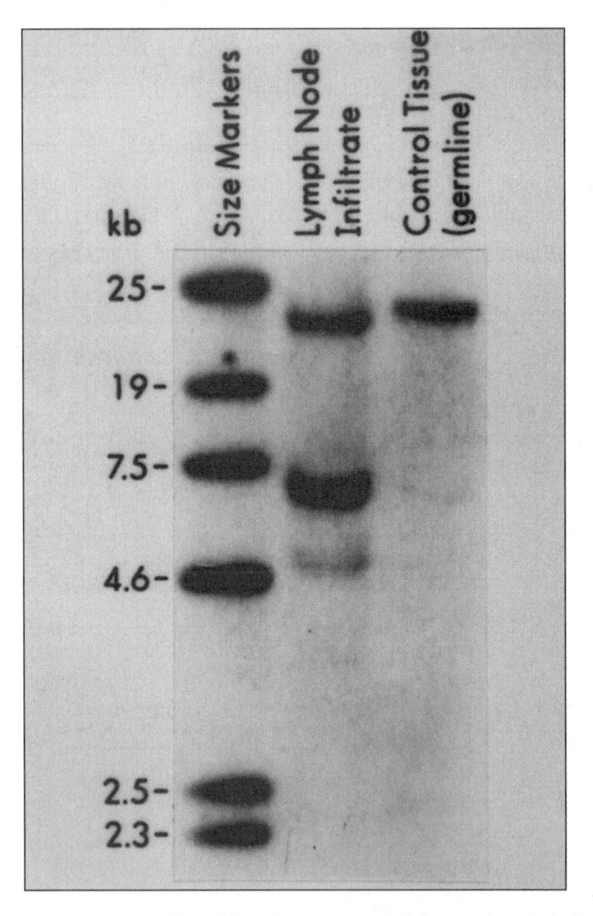

Fig 5-12. Southern blot of DNA extracted from a lymph node that histologically contained an atypical lymphoid infiltrate (DNA digested with the restriction enzyme EcoRI; immunoglobulin heavy chain J-region probe). A discrete set of restriction fragments is detected, indicating that the lymphoid proliferation is monoclonal and suggesting a diagnosis of malignant lymphoma.

increased sensitivity in many diagnostic situations.[25,26] Successful PCR requires only that the nucleotide sequence of at least part of the target DNA is known, to which complementary oligonucleotide primers are synthesized. The oligonucleotide primers flanking the region of interest are added in vast excess to the target sample along with a thermostable DNA polymerase. If the target sequence is present, the primers will hybridize and provide an initiation site for the polymerase to synthesize DNA. After completion of this first polymerization cycle, the reaction mixture is heated to denature the nucleic acid, and then cooled to reanneal the primers and the target DNA. Another cycle of polymerase-catalyzed synthesis then begins. The 20 to 30 cycles of a typical PCR therefore result in exponential amplification of the target DNA. PCR can be performed on fresh or fixed paraffin-embedded tissue. Provided the target DNA is present, the quantity of tissue required is often minute.[27]

Several illustrations of the use of DNA probe analysis in the evaluation of neoplasia follow:

Hematopoietic Malignancies

Molecular analysis is most widely used in the diagnosis and classification of lymphoid neoplasms. The size of DNA restriction fragments (DNA fragments that are obtained after digestion by restriction endonucleases) changes whenever a translocation, inversion, or gene rearrangement occurs in the area detected by a specific probe. This concept has clinical applications in several diagnostic settings in hematopathology (Fig 5-12), including the differentiation of monoclonal from polyclonal lymphoproliferative diseases; detection of rearrangements associated with chromosome translocations in lymphomas and chronic myelogenous leukemias (CML); identification of minimal residual disease during clinical remission; and demonstration of the relationship between a recurrent malignancy and the original clonal population.

A recent study of the diagnostic utility of immunogenotyping lymphoid proliferations demonstrated that Southern blot analysis (with probes to immunoglobulin heavy chain, immunoglobulin light chain, and a T-cell receptor locus) resolved diagnostic problems in more than 50% of cases in which morphology and immunophenotyping yielded indeterminate results.[28] Southern blot analysis itself is quite sensitive, and can detect monoclonality even when the neoplastic proliferation represents only 1% to 5% of the analyzed lymphoid cells.[25]

Detection of rearrangements associated with chromosome translocations is another well-established role for molecular analysis. For example, more than 80% of follicular lymphomas, 20% of diffuse large-cell lymphomas, and approximately 50% of adult "undifferentiated" lymphomas contain a t(14;18) (q32;q21) translocation in which the *bcl*-2 gene from chromosome segment 18q21 moves into the IgH locus of 14q32. The rearrangements are focused on 18q21 and result in a *bcl*-2/immunoglobulin fusion gene with a chimeric transcript. Thus, a translocation-specific rearrangement unique to neoplastic cells can be identified in Southern blots, and used to follow the disease process.[29]

Similarly, 95% of CML and 13% of acute lymphocytic leukemias are associated with a t(9;22) translocation of the c-*abl* oncogene from 9(q34) to 22(q11), known as the Philadelphia (Ph) chromosome. Because the translocation breakpoint on chromosome 22 occurs in a very small region (the breakpoint cluster region, bcr), detection of the fusion gene (*bcr-abl*) transcript or fusion protein is pathognomonic for CML. PCR has been used for diagnosis of the Philadelphia translocation, and exceeds the sensitivity of cytogenetic analysis.[30] In addition, PCR has demonstrated residual chimeric *bcr-abl* transcripts in Ph-positive CML patients who are in clinical remission.[31]

As noted by Lee and coworkers,[31] the sensitivity of PCR has raised several important clinical questions that remain unanswered. For example: Are leukemic patients who are in remission heterogeneous biologically, or do they all have quiescent malignant cells with little proliferative potential? Does the ability to identify the subclinical presence of leukemic cells in patients who are in clinical remission correlate with prognosis? The application of PCR to the evaluation of hematologic malignancies is an example of technology outpacing our ability to apply its benefits in a knowledgeable and practical way.

Human Papillomavirus Infection

As noted above, the correlation of certain types of HPV with high-grade dysplasia and carcinoma suggests the value of PCR for identification of patients at risk for progression to malignancy. PCR has, in fact, been used to detect HPV types 16 and 18 in routinely processed cervical tissue.[32,33] Moreover, PCR has defined differences between individual HPV type 16 isolates. Although type 16b was more prevalent in cervical tissue than 16a in one study, the former subtype was not found in association with carcinoma cases. Instead, subtype 16a was identified in approximately 90% of uterine cervical cancers.[34]

Malignancies with Proto-oncogene Abnormalities

The prognostic value of proto-oncogene abnormalities—specifically, gene amplification as detected by Southern blots—has been demonstrated in both neuroblastoma and breast carcinoma. Amplification of the N-*myc* oncogene is associated with advanced stage and rapid progression of neuroblastoma. The estimated 18-month patient survival is 70%, 30%, and 5% as related to tumors with one, three to ten, and more than ten N-*myc* copies, respectively.[23]

Amplification of the HER-2/*neu* oncogene in breast carcinoma has been correlated with lymph node metastasis. Patients who had tumors with more than five gene copies generally did not survive as long as those with lesions lacking gene amplification. HER-2/*neu* amplification is felt by some to have greater prognostic value than most currently used predictive factors, including hormone-receptor status and size of primary tumor.[35] There is also preliminary evidence that alteration of the c-*myc* gene (amplification or rearrangement) correlates with poor short-term prognosis in breast cancer cases.[36] Studies of malignant tumors of the lung, bladder, pancreas, and colon have demonstrated structural alterations in other proto-oncogenes, including members of the *myc* and *ras* gene families, but the significance of these findings is currently unclear.

Cytogenetics

Specific chromosomal abnormalities are consistently associated with certain malignant neoplasms, and specific aberrations often have diagnostic and prognostic relevance. While application of molecular biology techniques to the detection of such aberrations has defined a new level of cytogenetic analysis, in certain situations routine karyotypic analysis of a tumor is still the only procedure available to probe chromosome structure. Specific abnormalities are best known in leukemias and lymphomas, although characteristic abnormalities have been described in nonhematopoietic tumors as well. For example, it has recently become apparent that virtually all malignant soft tissue tumors contain consistent chromosome aberrations.[37] The most common structural changes are balanced translocations, deletions, and gene amplifications.

The Philadelphia chromosome, present in most CML, is the classic example of a balanced translocation. Because cases lacking the Ph chromosome tend to be resistant to therapy and have a less favorable prognosis,[38] karyotypic analysis can provide clinically relevant information in chronic myeloproliferative disorders. Similarly, Ewing's sarcoma (a tumor of bone and soft tissue) consistently harbors the t(11;22) translocation.[39] This finding has implications for diagnosis and treatment because most neoplasms with a histologic resemblance to Ewing's tumor are not associated with this translocation.

The karyotypic manifestations of gene amplification include homogeneously staining regions (HSR) of single chromosomes and "double minutes" (DM), which are small paired extrachromosomal chromatin fragments. The study of HSR and DM in neuroblastoma resulted in the demonstration of a strong correlation between stage, prognosis, and amplification of the N-*myc* oncogene.

Karyotypic analysis of tumors with chromosomal *deletions* often has little role in diagnosis, often because of a decreased sensitivity compared with other molecular techniques. For example, molecular techniques have revealed a particular deletion (del 13q14) in 95% of patients with hereditary neuroblastoma, while karyotypic analyses have done so in only 5% of cases. However, karyotypic analysis of mesotheliomas has demonstrated that malignant tumors often contain deletions on the short arm of chromosome 1, the short arm of chromosome 3, and monosomy 22; these abnormalities appear to be useful not only in discriminating benign from malignant neoplasms, but also in determining tumor lineage.[37]

Flow Cytometry

Flow cytometry allows for the rapid quantitative measurement of cellular characteristics such as size, surface marker expression, and DNA content. Briefly, the principle of flow cytometry is as follows: A monodispersed cell sample is stained with appropriate fluorochromes and passed through a flow chamber designed to align the stream of cells so that they are individually struck by a focused laser beam. The scattered light and fluorescent emissions are separated according to wavelength by appropriate filters and mirrors, and directed to detectors which convert the emissions into electronic signals that are analyzed and stored for future display by a computer. The data are displayed as a frequency histogram (number of cells versus fluorescent energy) for single-parameter analysis or as a scattergraph for multiparametric evaluation. The principle of "gating" (the placement of electronic windows around areas in the frequency distribution so that the computer analyzes data only on cells falling within the windows) can be used to take full advantage of multiparametric analysis.[40]

The fluorochromes used to stain cells in flow cytometry include compounds that bind stoichiometrically to DNA, that label both DNA and RNA but fluoresce at different wavelengths for each, or that can be attached covalently to antibodies against cell surface antigens. Simultaneous multiparametric analysis is possible using two or more fluorochromes that emit at different wavelengths.

In vivo "single cell suspensions," such as peripheral blood or bone marrow, can be analyzed easily by flow cytometry. Solid tissues, including lymph nodes and solid tumors, require additional preparation (usually gentle enzymatic, detergent, or mechanical treatment) to achieve a monodispersed sample. Methods have been developed for analysis of archival tissue

Table 5-5. Selected Monoclonal Antibodies Used in Flow Cytometry of Hematopoietic Neoplasms (See Fig 5-13)

Antibody (Cluster Designation)	Specificity	% Positive Cells in Gated Regions of Fig 5-13* R1	R3
T-Cell Markers			
CD 3	Pan T cell	58	8
CD 4	Helper/inducer T-cell subset	26	7
CD 8	Cytotoxic/suppressor T-cell subset	26	7
B-Cell Markers			
CD 19	B cells	14	93
HLA-DR	Major histocompatibility complex, class II antigen (B cells, activated T cells)	62	100
Anti-IgM	B-cell subset (immunoglobulin heavy chain isotype M)	2	38
Anti-lambda	B-cell subset (lambda light chain)	13	68

* The staining pattern is diagnostic only for the region of the scattergram containing the atypical lymphocytes (the gated region labeled R3). These cells stain positive for HLA-DR, CD 19, and lambda immunoglobulin light chain, consistent with a monoclonal B-cell population.

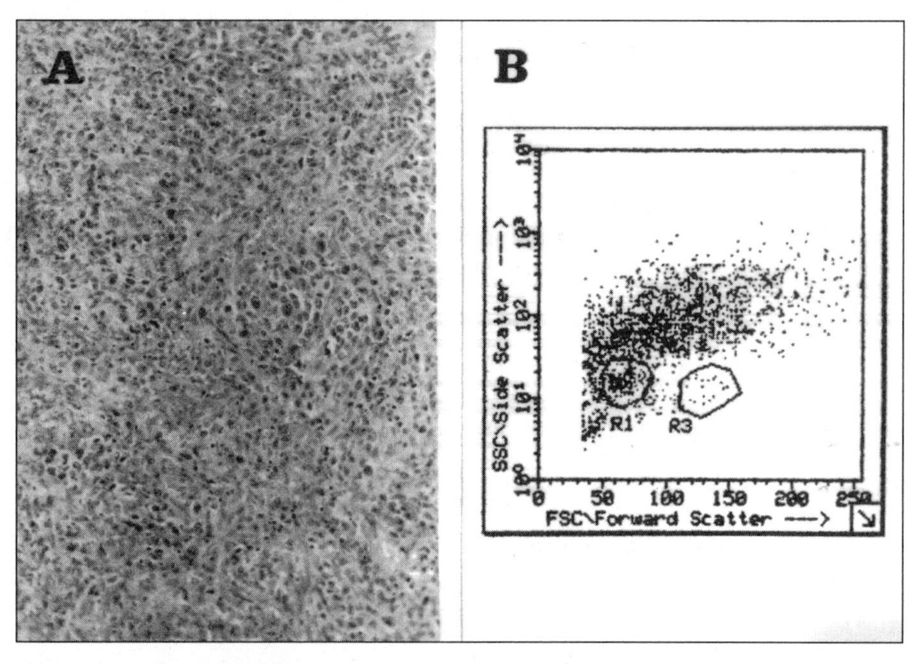

Fig 5-13. Section of spleen from 61-year-old woman; the parenchyma is effaced by large, malignant lymphocytes, ***A***. Scattergram of the malignant infiltrate obtained by flow cytometry, ***B***. Note the presence of two gated regions (arbitrarily labeled R1 and R3); see Table 5-5 for the results of multiparametric analysis of R1 and R3.

that has been formalin fixed and embedded in paraffin. In the pathology laboratory, flow cytometric analysis of tumors is performed to identify cellular subpopulations within a specific histologic tumor type already stratified by stage and grade. These subpopulations are typically not evident on routine histopathologic examination and, to be clinically relevant and therefore useful, their identification must correlate with prognosis or response to treatment.

Surface Marker Analysis

The role of cell surface antigen analysis in the diagnosis of lymphoid and other hematopoietic malignancies is well established. Multiparametric evaluation with a panel of monoclonal antibodies against surface antigens (Fig 5-13 and Table 5-5) facilitates classification of different subtypes of lymphoma and leukemia, and has become a routine facet of diagnosis at many medical centers.

Some progress has been made in extending flow cytometric measurements of surface markers to assessments of solid tumors and to the analysis of intracellular constituents, including oncogene products. However, such procedures remain largely experimental at present.

DNA Measurements

Although many flow cytometric studies have examined DNA ploidy as a prognostic factor, several variables complicate interpretation. For example, very few, if any, malignant tumors have a chromosomal complement normal in number and structure. "Diploid range" malignancies, therefore, actually represent a heterogeneous group of lesions with chro-

Table 5-6. Selected Tumor Markers and Applications in Diagnostic Medicine

Tumor Marker	Exemplary Malignant Neoplasms	Commonly Associated Nonneoplastic Diseases
Hormones		
Human chorionic gonadotropin (hCG)	Gestational trophoblastic disease, gonadal germ cell tumors	Pregnancy
Calcitonin	Medullary cancer of thyroid	—
Catecholamines and metabolites	Pheochromocytoma	—
Oncofetal Antigens		
Alpha-fetoprotein (AFP)	Hepatocellular carcinoma, gonadal germ cell tumors (especially endodermal sinus tumor)	Cirrhosis, toxic liver injury, hepatitis
Carcinoembryonic antigen (CEA)	Adenocarcinomas of colon, pancreas, stomach, lung, breast, ovary	Pancreatitis, inflammatory bowel disease, hepatitis, cirrhosis, tobacco abuse
Isoenzymes		
Prostatic acid phosphatase	Adenocarcinoma of prostate	Prostatitis; nodular prostatic hyperplasia
Neuron-specific enolase	Small-cell carcinoma of lung; neuroblastoma	—
Specific Proteins		
Prostate-specific antigen (PSA)	Adenocarcinoma of prostate	Nodular prostatic hyperplasia, prostatitis
Immunoglobulin (monoclonal)	Multiple myeloma	Monoclonal gammopathy of unknown significance
CA 125	Epithelial ovarian neoplasms	Menstruation, pregnancy, peritonitis
CA-19-9	Adenocarcinoma of pancreas or colon	Pancreatitis; ulcerative colitis

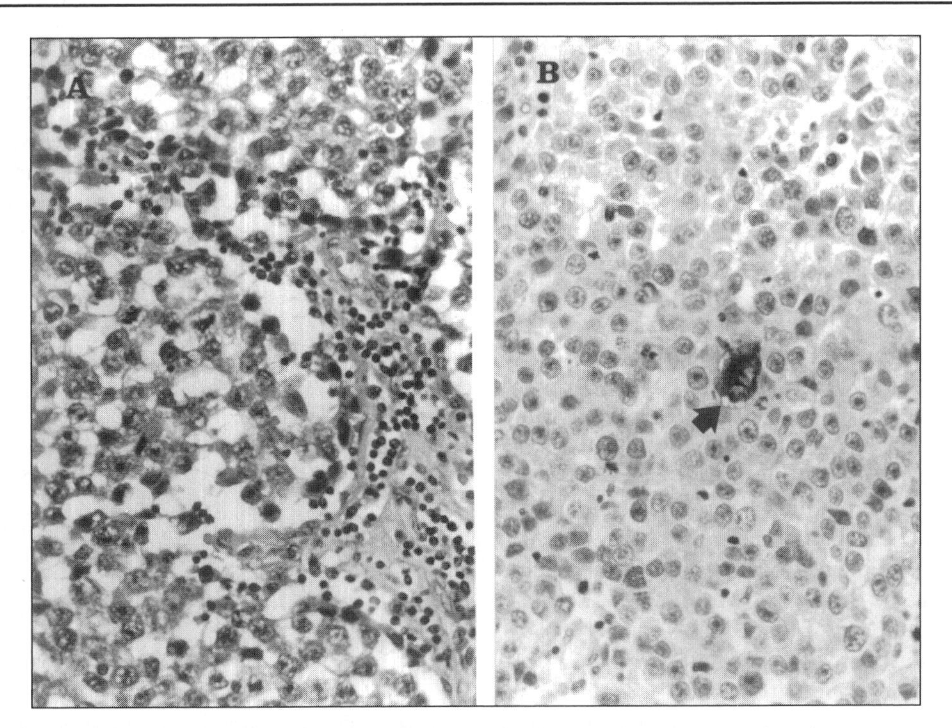

Fig 5-14. Sections of a testicular mass from 57-year-old man. Preoperative workup demonstrated an increased serum beta-hCG level. ***A***: Routine histopathologic examination showed a classic seminoma. Note the uniform malignant cells with abundant clear cytoplasm, arranged in nests divided by fibrous bands; a lymphocytic stromal infiltrate is present. No trophoblastic elements are noted. ***B***: Immunohistochemical stain for hCG, demonstrating isolated, strongly reactive mononuclear cells (arrow), confirming the presence of trophoblastic elements in the tumor.

mosomal abnormalities below the level of resolution of flow cytometry. In addition, a small population of aneuploid cells may not be detected by flow cytometric measurements. Some tissues, such as liver, normally contain tetraploid and even octaploid populations.[41] Aneuploid cellular populations also are observed in several benign neoplastic and reactive soft tissue lesions.

Flow cytometric cell cycle analysis is primarily directed at calculation of the proportion of S-phase cells (the percentage of cells undergoing DNA synthesis) and is used to identify rapidly dividing neoplasms.

It is difficult to arrive at summary statements regarding the correlation of flow cytometric data with prognosis. Published reports suggest that consistent relationships do exist in specific forms of neoplasia.[40,42] A careful prospective study of renal cell carcinoma has documented increased survival in patients with tumors having homogeneously diploid or near-diploid DNA content, as opposed to those with an aneuploid DNA profile.[43] A retrospective study of adenocarcinoma of the prostate demonstrated that only 15% of diploid tumors metastasized or progressed locally, compared with 75% of tumors with an abnormal DNA pattern.[44] A relationship between clinical stage and DNA ploidy in prostate cancer has also been documented.[45]

For many other neoplasms, the correlation between DNA content and prognosis is more uncertain. In carcinoma of the breast, the biologic significance of tumor ploidy and S-phase fractions remains unclear; although aneuploid lesions seem to be associated with a shorter disease-free survival, there is no obvious association between aneuploidy and stage.[46] Similarly, there is no clear pattern with respect to DNA ploidy that can be discerned in cases of colorectal adenocarcinoma. The exact relationship of tumor ploidy to prognosis has not been established for other malignancies, including neoplasms of the lung, uterine cervix, head and neck, soft tissue, thyroid, and stomach. In summary, DNA analysis is still in its infancy and must be approached in a systematic, histologically based fashion.

Tumor Markers

A "tumor marker" is a biochemical indicator of the presence of a neoplastic proliferation. In clinical usage, this term refers to a molecule that can be detected in serum, plasma, or other body fluids. Sensitive methods of measurement—usually radioimmunoassay (RIA) or enzyme-linked immunosorbent assay (ELISA)—are often required for optimal usefulness. No tumor marker is specific; virtually all are present at low levels in the normal physiologic state or in nonneoplastic disease, and any given marker may be seen in conjunction with a variety of neoplasms. Tumor markers can be divided into two broad categories: tumor-derived moieties and tumor-associated (or host-response) markers.

Tumor-derived markers include oncofetal antigens (alpha-fetoprotein [AFP] and carcinoembryonic antigen [CEA]); hormones (human chorionic gonadotropin [hCG], human placental lactogen, antidiuretic hormone, parathyroid hormone, calcitonin, insulin-like growth factors, catecholamine metabolites); tissue-specific proteins (immunoglobulins, prostate-specific antigen [PSA], gross cystic disease fluid protein-15); enzymes (gamma-glutamyl transpeptidase); isoenzymes (prostatic acid phosphatase [PAP], placental alkaline phosphatase [PLAP], neuron-specific enolase [NSE]); oncogene products (src, N-myc, H-ras); various polyamines; sialic acid; and glycolipids.

Tumor-associated (host-response) markers are most often used together with tumor-derived markers. For example, in concert with NSE levels, serum ferritin levels in neuroblastoma have been shown to correlate with stage of disease and response to therapy. Other host-response markers include interleukin-2, tumor necrosis factor, immune complexes, acute phase reactants (C-reactive protein, α_{-2}-macroglobulin), and enzymes (lactic dehydrogenase, creatine kinase BB isoenzyme, glutamate dehydrogenase).

No tumor marker has demonstrated a specificity or sensitivity that is adequate for the screening detection of malignancies in the general population. Because of this limitation, the main utility of tumor markers has been in determining the response to therapy, ie, the detection of residual disease or relapse. Useful tumor markers and associated neoplasms are presented in Table 5-6. As Fig 5-14 demonstrates, the detection of tumor markers may be accomplished by pathologic examination of tumor tissue itself (see the section on "immunohistochemistry"). Excellent general reviews of these topics have been published.[47]

Given the lack of specificity, test *panels* composed of both tumor-derived and tumor-associated markers have been devised. For example, a possible battery of tumor markers for colorectal adenocarcinoma would include CEA, CA-19-9, and PLAP; for small-cell carcinoma of the lung, CEA, NSE, and antidiuretic hormone; and for adenocarcinoma of the prostate, PAP, PSA, and gamma-seminal protein. More experience is needed to determine if such an approach is clinically useful in patients being screened for malignancy.

Summary

This overview has covered a number of conventional and recent techniques available to the pathologist for use in the evaluation of neoplastic diseases. Knowledge of the potential uses and abuses of these procedures is important to the clinician and helps ensure that patient care is not hindered through the omission or misapplication of pertinent studies. We cannot stress too greatly the cooperation required between pathologist and oncologist in the diagnosis of cancer and management of oncology patients.

References

1. Underwood JCE. *Introduction to Biopsy Interpretation and Surgical Pathology*. 2nd ed. New York, NY: Springer-Verlag; 1987.

2. Lieberman MW, Lebovitz RM. Neoplasia. In: Kissane JM, ed. *Anderson's Pathology*. 9th ed. St Louis, Mo: CV Mosby Co; 1990:574.

3. Bancroft JD, Stevens A. *Histopathological Stains and Their Diagnostic Uses*. New York, NY: Churchill-Livingstone; 1975.

4. Grundmann E, Beck L, eds. *Minimal Neoplasia: Diagnosis and Therapy*. Berlin, Germany: Springer-Verlag; 1988.

5. Specht L, Nordentoft AM, Cold S, Clausen NT, Nissen NI. Tumor burden as the most important prognostic factor in early stage Hodgkin's disease: relation to other prognostic factors and implications for choice of therapy. *Cancer*. 1988;61:1719-1727.

6. Ferenczy A, Winkler B. Carcinoma and metastatic tumors of the cervix. In: Kurman RJ, ed. *Blaustein's Pathology of the Female Genital Tract*. 3rd ed. New York, NY: Springer-Verlag; 1987:218-256.

7. Gleason DF, Mellinger GT. Prediction of prognosis for prostatic adenocarcinoma by combined histological grading and clinical staging. *J Urol*. 1974;111:58-64.

8. Peven DR, Gruhn JD. The development of electron microscopy. *Arch Pathol Lab Med*. 1985;109:683-691.

9. Gyorkey F, Min K-W, Krisko I, Gyorkey P. The usefulness of electron microscopy in the diagnosis of human tumors. *Hum Pathol*. 1975;6:421-441.

10. Hsu S-M, Raine L, Fanger H. Use of avidin-biotin-peroxidase complex (ABC) in immunoperoxidase staining techniques: a comparison between ABC and unlabeled antibody (PAP) procedures. *J Histochem Cytochem*. 1981;29:577-580.

11. Wick MR. Immunohistochemistry in the diagnosis of "solid" malignant tumors. In: Jennette JC, ed. *Immunohistology in Diagnostic Pathology*. Boca Raton, Fla: CRC Press, Inc; 1989:161-191.

12. Battifora H, Gaffey M, Esteban J, Mehta P, Faucett C, Niland J. Immunohistochemical assay of neu/c-erbB-2 oncogene product in paraffin-embedded tissues in early breast cancer: retrospective follow-up study of 245 stage I and II cases. *Mod Pathol*. 1991;4:466-474.

13. Linden MD, Torres FX, Kubus J, Zarbo RJ. Clinical application of morphologic and immunocytochemical assessments of cell proliferation. *Am J Clin Pathol*. 1992;97:S4-S13.

14. DeLellis RA, Wolfe HJ. New techniques in gene product analysis. *Arch Pathol Lab Med*. 1987;III:620-627.

15. Crum CP, Nagai N, Levine RU, Silverstein S. *In situ* hybridization analysis of HPV 16 DNA sequences in early cervical neoplasia. *Am J Pathol*. 1986;123:174-182.

16. Pilotti S, Gupta J, Stefanon B, De Palo G, Shah KV, Rilke F. Study of multiple human papillomavirus-related lesions of the lower female genital tract by in situ hybridization. *Hum Pathol.* 1989;20:118-123.

17. Gal AA, Saul SH, Stoler MH. Demonstration of human papillomavirus in anal carcinoma by in situ hybridization. *Lab Invest.* 1988;58:33A. Abstract.

18. de Villiers E-M, Weidauer H, Otto H, zur Hausen H. Papillomavirus DNA in human tongue carcinomas. *Int J Cancer.* 1985;36:575-578.

19. Weaver MG, Abdul-Karim FW, Dale G, Sorensen K, Huang YT. Detection and localization of human papillomavirus in penile condylomas and squamous cell carcinomas using in situ hybridization with biotinylated DNA viral probes. *Mod Pathol.* 1989;2:94-100.

20. Bejui-Thivolet F, Liagre N, Chignol MC, Chardonnet Y, Patricot LM. Detection of human papillomavirus DNA in squamous bronchial metaplasia and squamous cell carcinomas of the lung by in situ hybridization using biotinylated probes in paraffin-embedded specimens. *Hum Pathol.* 1990;21:111-116.

21. Rijntjes PJM, Van Ditzhuijsen TJM, Van Loon AM, Van Haelst UJGM, Bronkhorst FB, Yap SH. Hepatitis B virus DNA detected in formalin-fixed liver specimens and its relation to serologic markers and histopathologic features in chronic liver disease. *Am J Pathol.* 1985;120:411-418.

22. Choi YJ. In situ hybridization using a biotinylated DNA probe on formalin-fixed liver biopsies with hepatitis B virus infections: in situ hybridization superior to immunohistochemistry. *Mod Pathol.* 1990;3:343-347.

23. Seeger RC, Brodeur GM, Sather H, et al. Association of multiple copies of the N-*myc* oncogene with rapid progression of neuroblastomas. *N Engl J Med.* 1985;313:1111-1116.

24. Cohen PS, Seeger RC, Triche TJ, Israel MA. Detection of N-*myc* gene expression in neuroblastoma tumors by *in situ* hybridization. *Am J Pathol.* 1988;131:391-397.

25. Grody WW, Gatti RA, Naeim F. Diagnostic molecular pathology. *Mod Pathol.* 1989;2:553-568.

26. Innis MA, Gelfand DH, Sninsky JJ, White TJ, eds. *PCR protocols: A Guide to Methods and Applications.* San Diego, Calif: Academic Press Inc; 1990.

27. Shibata D, Nichols P, Sherrod A, Rabinowitz A, Bernstein-Singer L, Hu E. Detection of occult CNS involvement of follicular small cleaved lymphoma by the polymerase chain reaction. *Mod Pathol.* 1990;3:71-75.

28. Kamat D, Laszewski MJ, Kemp JD, et al. The diagnostic utility of immunophenotyping and immunogenotyping in the pathologic evaluation of lymphoid proliferations. *Mod Pathol.* 1990;3:105-112.

29. Crescenzi M, Seto M, Herzig GP, Weiss PD, Griffith RC, Korsmeyer SJ. Thermostable DNA polymerase chain amplification of t(14;18) chromosome breakpoints and detection of minimal residual disease. *Proc Natl Acad Sci USA.* 1988; 85:4869-4873.

30. Kawasaki ES, Clark SS, Coyne MY, et al. Diagnosis of chronic myeloid and acute lymphocytic leukemias by detection of leukemia-specific mRNA sequences amplified in vitro. *Proc Natl Acad Sci USA.* 1988;85:5698-5702.

31. Lee M-S, Chang K-S, Freireich EJ, et al. Detection of minimal residual *bcr/abl* transcripts by a modified polymerase chain reaction. *Blood.* 1988;72:893-897.

32. Shibata DK, Arnheim N, Martin WJ. Detection of human papilloma virus in paraffin-embedded tissue using the polymerase chain reaction. *J Exp Med.* 1988;167:225-230.

33. Johnson TL, Kim W, Plieth DA, Sarkar FH. Detection of HPV 16/18 DNA in cervical adenocarcinoma using polymerase chain reaction (PCR) methodology. *Mod Pathol.* 1992;5:35-40.

34. Tidy JA, Vousden KH, Farrell PJ. Relation between infection with a subtype of HPV16 and cervical neoplasia. *Lancet.* 1989;1:1225-1227.

35. Slamon DJ, Clark GM, Wong SG, Levin WJ, Ullrich A, McGuire WL. Human breast cancer: correlation of relapse and survival with amplification of the HER-2/*neu* oncogene. *Science.* 1987;235:177-182.

36. Varley JM, Swallow JE, Brammar WJ, Whittaker JL, Walker RA. Alterations of either c-erbB-2 (neu) or c-myc proto-oncogenes in breast carcinomas correlate with poor short-term prognosis. *Oncogene.* 1987;1:423-430.

37. Fletcher JA. Cytogenetic aberrations in malignant soft tissue tumors. In: Fenoglio-Preiser CM, Willman CL, eds. *Advances in Pathology and Laboratory Medicine.* St Louis, Mo: Mosby Year Book; 1991;4:235-246.

38. Morris CM, Reeve AE, Fitzgerald PH, Hollings PE, Beard MEJ, Heaton DC. Genomic diversity correlates with clinical variation in Ph´-negative chronic myeloid leukaemia. *Nature.* 1986;320:281-283.

39. Whang-Peng J, Triche TJ, Knutsen T, et al. Cytogenetic characterization of selected small round cell tumors of childhood. *Cancer Genet Cytogenet.* 1986;21:185-208.

40. Koss LG, Czerniak B, Herz F, Wersto RP. Flow cytometric measurements of DNA and other cell components in human tumors: a critical appraisal. *Hum Pathol.* 1989; 20:528-548.

41. Mendecki J, Dillmann WH, Wolley RC, Oppenheimer JH, Koss LG. Effect of thyroid hormone on the ploidy of rat liver nuclei as determined by flow cytometry. *Proc Soc Exp Biol Med.* 1978;158:63-67.

42. Auer G, Askensten U, Ahrens O. Cytophotometry. *Hum Pathol.* 1989;20:518-527.

43. Ljungberg B, Stenling R, Roos G. DNA content in renal cell carcinoma with reference to tumor heterogeneity. *Cancer.* 1985;56:503-508.

44. Winkler HZ, Rainwater LM, Myers RP, et al. Stage D1 prostatic adenocarcinoma: significance of nuclear DNA ploidy patterns studied by flow cytometry. *Mayo Clin Proc.* 1988;63:103-112.

45. Stephenson RA, James BC, Gay H, Fair WR, Whitmore WF Jr, Melamed MR. Flow cytometry of prostate cancer: relationship of DNA content to survival. *Cancer Res.* 1987; 47:2504-2509.

46. Visscher DW, Zarbo RJ, Greenawald KA, Crissman JD. Prognostic significance of morphological parameters and flow cytometric DNA analysis in carcinoma of the breast. *Pathol Annu.* 1990;25:171-210.

47. Virji MA, Mercer DW, Herberman RB. Tumor markers in cancer diagnosis and prognosis. *CA Cancer J Clin.* 1988; 38:104-127.

6

BASIS FOR MAJOR CURRENT THERAPIES FOR CANCER

Irvin D. Fleming, MD, (Introduction, Surgical Resection)
Luther W. Brady, MD, Glenn B. Mieszkalski, MD (Radiation Therapy)
M. Robert Cooper, MD, Michael R. Cooper, MD (Systemic Therapy)

Over the past 50 years, a number of primary treatment modalities for cancer have emerged. Surgery, radiation therapy, and chemotherapy have become mainstay approaches, while the effectiveness of other therapies such as hyperthermia, cryotherapy, immunotherapy, and light treatment continues to be evaluated.

Prior to 1940, the primary approach was surgical resection of both local and regional disease, there being little to offer patients with metastatic cancer.

In the 1940s and 1950s, radiation therapy emerged as an alternative option for some primary cancer sites such as the cervix, head, and neck, as well as for lymphomas. Irradiation was also effective as palliative therapy for many forms of metastatic cancer, including metastasis to bone.

With the development of effective agents in the 1950s, cancer chemotherapy began to be used for disseminated cancer, lymphomas, and leukemias.

Since the 1960s, emphasis has focused on the effective combined use of these three methods of cancer treatment to increase the possibility of survival and reduce treatment side effects. Examples of early combined treatment programs include radiation and chemotherapy for Hodgkin's disease; surgery, radiation, and chemotherapy for pediatric Wilms' tumor; and surgery and chemotherapy for choriocarcinoma.

Irvin D. Fleming, MD, Department of Surgery, University of Tennessee, Memphis, Tennessee

Luther W. Brady, MD, Department of Radiation Oncology and Nuclear Medicine, Hahnemann University, Philadelphia, Pennsylvania

Glenn B. Mieszkalski, MD, Department of Radiation Oncology and Nuclear Medicine, Hahnemann University, Philadelphia, Pennsylvania

M. Robert Cooper, MD, Comprehensive Cancer Center of Wake Forest University, Bowman Gray School of Medicine, Winston-Salem, North Carolina

Michael R. Cooper, MD, Health Sciences Center, University of Virginia, Charlottesville, Virginia

More recently, combined therapy has proven to be effective in reducing recurrence of breast cancer (surgery, radiation, and chemotherapy), stage II colon cancer (surgery and chemotherapy), and other neoplasms.

While combination therapy has not remarkably altered the cure rate associated with soft tissue sarcoma in adults, a greater proportion of patients with sarcoma have been spared an amputation by combining complete local excision with radiation therapy and, in some cases, chemotherapy.

In the 1990s, the effort continues to more effectively use combination therapy to obtain the best possible cure rate with the least side effects and toxicity. The three parts of this chapter will present in detail the mechanism of action of the major treatment modalities and explain how each is being used singly and in combination for cancer treatment.

Surgical Resection

Historic Background

Prior to the discovery of anesthesia and antisepsis, the surgical removal of any but superficial malignant tumors was accomplished only with great discomfort and considerable risk to the patient. In 1822, Valpeau made the following comment on mastectomy: "The operation is serious and threatens the patient's life only in those cases in which the cancer is in a very advanced stage, in which it is necessary to penetrate the hollow of the axilla." His reported operative mortality was 32 deaths in 167 operations, and long-term survival was in the range of 5% to 10%. There were serious questions in the 19th century concerning the efficacy of the surgical removal of breast cancer. In 1809, Ephraim McDowell successfully removed a large ovarian tumor at laparotomy—an amazing feat without anesthesia or antisepsis. He performed two additional successful removals of ovarian tumor in 1813 and 1816, publishing his results in 1817. However, no real progress could be made in the surgical management of cancer prior to 1846, at which time general anesthesia was introduced at the Massachusetts General Hospital by Morton, and 1867, when Lister published his results using antisepsis to reduce surgical wound infection.

Gastric and Intestinal Cancers

In 1881, Theodor Billroth in Vienna, using chloroform anesthesia, successfully resected an obstructing carcinoma of the stomach (Fig 6-1), and thus the era of surgical resection of gastric cancer began.

In 1885, Robert Weir reported a resection of colon carcinoma with the proximal bowel brought out as a colostomy.[1] In 1895, Mikulicz-Radceki described a two-staged colon resection, with subsequent colostomy closure reducing the operative mortality to <30%.[2] That same year, Charles H. Mayo reported 14 cases of colon resection with anastomosis using the Murphy button with only two postoperative deaths.[3] With the advent in the 1940s of antibiotics and bowel preparation, routine resection of colon carcinoma and anastomosis became a safe procedure.

In 1826, Jacques Lisfranc of France reported nine cases of resection of rectal cancer. However, in 1907, the English surgeon Ernest Miles first introduced the modern abdominoperineal approach to the resection of rectal carcinoma.[4]

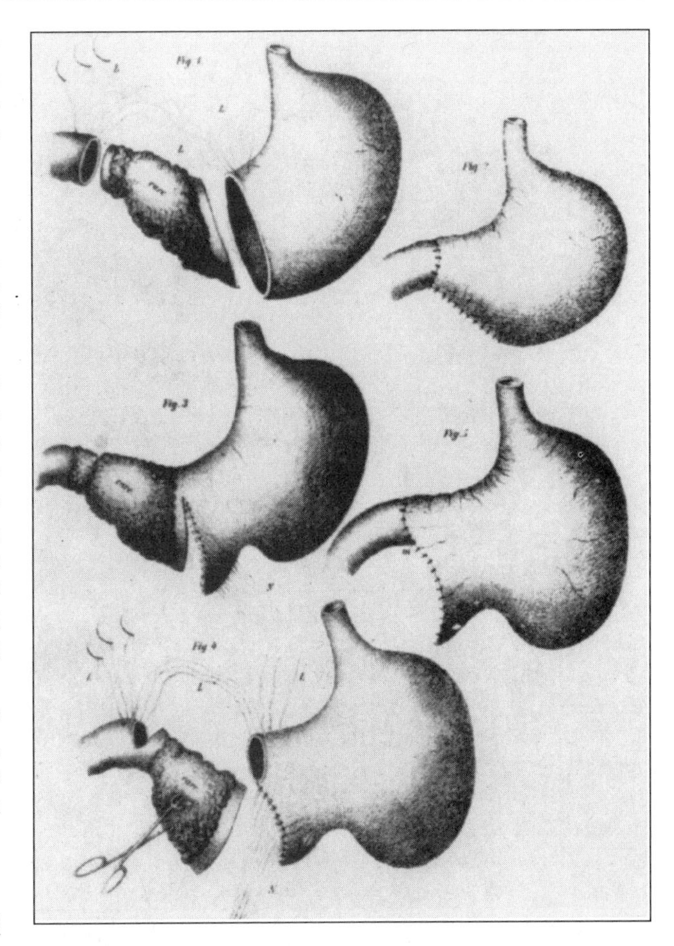

Fig 6-1. Original illustration of gastric resection of cancer by Billroth (1881).

Breast Cancer

C.H. Moore of Middlesex Hospital in London pointed out the importance of "adequate resection" of breast cancer. William Stewart Halsted of Baltimore (Fig 6-2) in 1889 developed a systematic approach to the "radical resection of breast cancer," removing the tumor, breast, overlying skin, and pectoralis muscles and performing axillary dissection. Halsted's method increased the cure rate from 10% to 42.3%, dramatically improving the chance of survival with surgical treatment of breast cancer.[5]

Head and Neck Cancer

Modern thyroid surgery was pioneered by Theodor Kocher of Berne. He developed a technique for safe surgical resection, and in 1883 reported his first 100 thyroidectomies. He subsequently described the effects of thyroid deficiency ("cachexia Strumipriva") following total thyroidectomy.[6] Charles H. Mayo in 1889 reported the first thyroid resection in the United States; by 1918, he described >5,000 cases of thyroid resection.[6]

In the early 1900s, numerous authors developed techniques for successfully resecting carcinomas of the lip, cheek, and tongue. George Crile pointed out that oral carcinoma with cervical node metastasis could be cured by surgical removal of the involved nodes, and in 1906 described a technique for radical neck dissection.[7] Major resections of head and neck tumor in combination with mandibular resection as well as radical neck node dissection were described by Hays Martin of New York in 1948 (Fig 6-3).[8]

Thoracic Cancers

The first successful resection of a cervical esophageal cancer was performed by Vincent Czerny in 1877, and in 1913 Franz Torek reported the resection of a thoracic esophageal cancer.[9]

In 1933, Evarts Graham of St Louis reported the first successful pneumonectomy for cancer,[10] and by 1950 Churchill described the technique for lobectomy in appropriate cases of pulmonary cancer.[11] Alton Ochsner of New Orleans emphasized the importance of cigarette smoking in the etiology of lung cancer.[12]

Role of the Surgeon in Cancer Management

Cancer Prevention and Public Education

The surgeon working in the community should be active in public education, informing patients and the general public about possible cancer risk associated

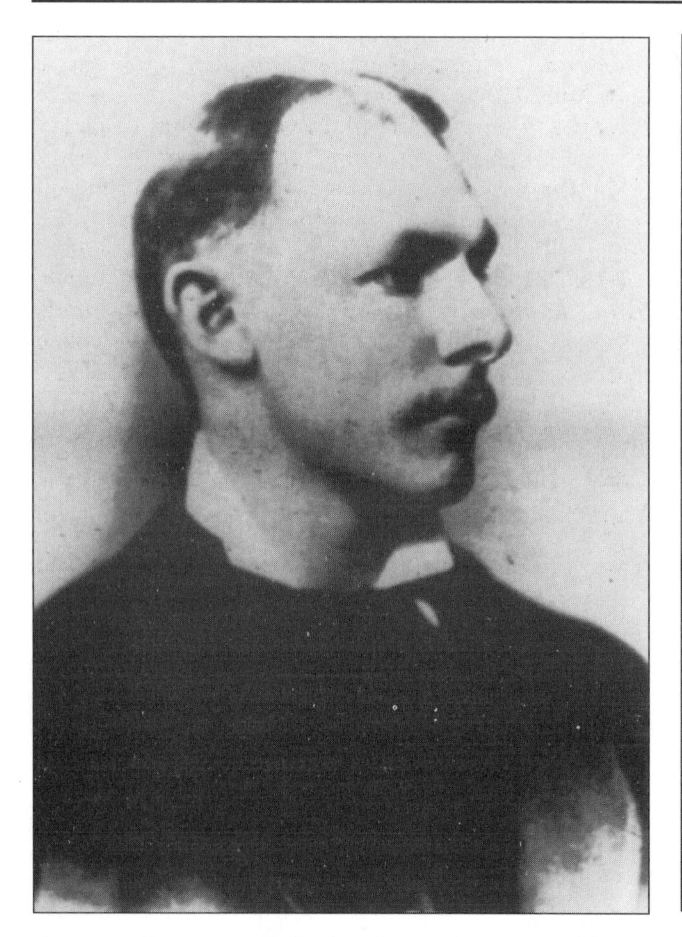

Fig 6-2. William Stewart Halsted, Professor of Surgery at Johns Hopkins University, published results of a radical resection for cure of breast cancer in 1889.

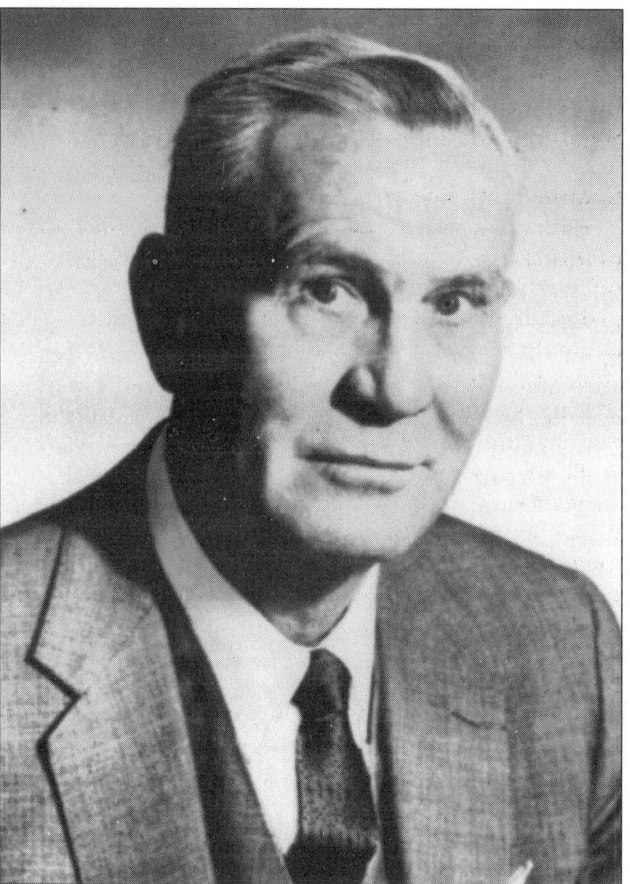

Fig 6-3. Hayes Martin, Chief of Head and Neck Service at Memorial Hospital for Cancer and Allied Diseases, New York, developed techniques for the radical resection of head and neck cancer. From Martin.[8]

with such environmental carcinogens as tobacco, ultraviolet sun exposure, and chemicals. Other factors including family history and lifestyle habits that increase the risk of cancer also should be discussed. In addition, surgeons should participate in community screening activities. Patients seen on routine follow-up should be encouraged to participate in early detection and screening programs such as mammography, Papanicolaou (Pap) smears, and stool blood exam.

Operative Management (Biopsy)

To plan effective treatment, it is essential to establish an accurate histologic diagnosis. In many cases, this can be established by biopsy prior to definitive resection or therapy. Such biopsies are performed routinely for skin cancer, melanoma, and oral cancer. Less accessible cancer sites such as the esophagus, stomach, lung, and rectum are biopsied via endoscopy. Even less accessible tumor sites such as the breast, thyroid, lymph node, soft tissue, and abdomen can be biopsied by fine needle aspiration. Knowing the exact histologic diagnosis enables the multidisciplinary team to plan appropriate staging, evaluation, and definitive treatment. In some situations, it is not practical to establish a histologic diagnosis prior to resection. Thus, in some cases of colon or lung cancer, the diagnosis and stage are established at the time of definitive resection. If the suspected neoplasm is to be treated by any modality other than resection (ie, radiation therapy or chemotherapy), then it is essential for an accurate histologic diagnosis to be established prior to beginning therapy.

Clinical and Pathologic Staging

Following a diagnosis of cancer, effective treatment cannot be done without knowing the extent of tumor spread. Essential elements in the evaluation of the extent of the cancer (stage) are:

(1) size and extent of the primary tumor (T),

(2) extent of regional spread in lymph nodes (N), and

(3) evidence of distant metastatic spread (M).

Using this TNM classification, the American Joint Committee on Cancer has established staging criteria for common cancer sites.[13] This effort has been undertaken in cooperation with the International Union Against Cancer to ensure that a single system of staging is used worldwide. This common international staging system allows scientists, clinicians, and treatment centers to compare end results using varied treatment methods.

Modern cancer treatment often calls for combination therapy, especially for tumors at high risk of not responding to a single treatment modality. Treatment protocols, including surgery, radiation therapy, and chemotherapy, are usually directed by the type and stage of the tumor to be treated. In summary, accurate staging is essential to planning effective therapy, conducting clinical trials, and evaluating end results.

There are two categories of cancer staging. The *clinical stage* is based on clinical evaluation of the tumor supplemented by information from appropriate diagnostic studies (eg, chest x-ray, computed tomographic (CT) scan, blood chemistry tests, and nuclear medicine studies). The *pathologic stage* is based on study of the removed tumor, other removed tissue, or biopsies. A classic example would be the number of positive axillary lymph nodes removed with a modified radical mastectomy for breast cancer. Every treatment facility undertaking the management of patients with malignant neoplasms should evaluate the end results based on the stage of disease at diagnosis. This is accomplished by using a data bank (tumor registry) and follow-up. Evaluation of the end results of cancer treatment can be meaningful only with accurate staging.

Surgical Resection

Currently approximately 90% of cures of solid malignant tumors are achieved by surgical resection alone or in combination with other modalities. The role of the surgeon is to remove the malignant tumor completely with a margin of normal tissue. When there is regional lymphatic spread, the involved area should be resected along with the primary tumor (eg, axillary node dissection for breast carcinoma or mesenteric resection for bowel cancer). This approach is termed therapeutic lymph node removal when there is clinical evidence of tumor involvement and prophylactic or elective removal when there is a high likelihood of microscopic involvement. On some occasions, lymph node dissection is performed in continuity with the primary tumor resection, such as malignant melanoma of the trunk or extremity.

Visceral organs involved with cancer, such as the esophagus, stomach, pancreas, and colon, should be removed so as to ensure complete resection while minimizing changes in the physiologic status of the patient. With the development of improved supportive measures for surgical resection, it was proposed in the sixties and seventies that more extensive surgical resection was feasible and would probably improve cure rates. However, this has not always proved to be true, the chief cause of failure being distant spread of disease. In recent years, the trend has been toward complete, but less radical surgical resection in combination with radiation therapy, systemic chemotherapy, or both. A classic example is the treatment of sarcoma of soft tissue or bone by combined therapy to avoid amputations. Despite the great strides made with combination therapy, few cancers are controlled without removal of the primary tumor (Table 6-1).[14]

Table 6-1. Cancers in Which Surgical Resection Is a Major Factor in Cure

Site	1960-1963 5-Yr Survival		1983-1989 5-Yr Survival	
	Whites	Blacks	Whites	Blacks
Breast	63%	46%	84%	72%
Colon	43	34	60	49
Rectum	38	27	58	45
Melanoma	60	–	84	72
Thyroid	83	–	94	92
Stomach	11	8	17	18
Lung	8	5	13	11

Statistics include all stages of disease. Survival rates are higher if only stages I and II are considered.

Adapted from SEER Program, National Cancer Institute.[14]

Palliative Procedures

On many occasions, patients may present at the time of initial diagnosis with a primary carcinoma that has already metastasized. Such advanced tumors may be associated with obstruction, pain, or a bleeding lesion that must be treated even though the neoplasm cannot be cured. Management by bypass procedure or resection may enhance the patient's quality of life and improve the situation so that other measures of cancer treatment may be applied. Considerable clinical judgment is needed to determine how aggressive the management approach should be.

Surgical Support for Patients Receiving Other Therapies

Aggressive chemotherapy or radiation therapy requires considerable support to manage the complications of malnutrition, neutropenia, infection, sepsis, and opportunistic infections. Many current chemotherapeutic agents cause severe toxicity and local tissue slough if extravasated from intravenous

(IV) injection. The need for frequent blood samples and IV administration warrants a reliable venous access. This is usually accomplished by a longstanding IV line in a central vein like the superior vena cava and brought through the skin by way of a long subcutaneous tunnel to avoid infection (Fig 6-4). The alternative is a central venous catheter attached to a subcutaneous injectable port, which can be used either for administration of chemotherapy or obtaining venous blood. With proper placement and care, the lines and ports can be utilized for months or years if needed. Both chemotherapy and head and neck radiation therapy are associated with oral stomatitis, ulceration, and severe nutritional problems. Supplemental alimentation via the gastrointestinal (GI) tract or total parenteral nutrition is occasionally required in the patient receiving antineoplastic therapy. Other areas of surgical support include removal of pleural fluid or ascites for symptomatic relief or for diagnosis.

Posttreatment Evaluation of Tumor Status

There are occasional clinical settings in which the tumor site must be reevaluated subsequent to treatment to plan further therapy or discontinuation of therapy. Reexploration with appropriate biopsy or other technique may be needed. Results of a diagnostic study such as CT may have to be clarified before subsequent therapy. Some cases of local recurrent tumor can be successfully resected for long-term control or cure.

Long-Term Complications of Cancer Treatment

Now that an increasing number of cancer patients are "cured," delayed complications of the tumor or treatment are being recognized. Irradiation of the abdomen is occasionally associated with bowel strictures, malabsorption, and even fistula formation, which occurs up to 10 years following treatment. New second primary malignant tumors are seen with increasing frequency in patients treated with both radiation and chemotherapy. Thyroid deficiency and thyroid neoplasm have presented in 10% to 30% of patients irradiated in the head and neck. These problems present a challenge to the surgeon and the treatment team with respect to careful surveillance and early detection and treatment of these secondary malignancies.

Rehabilitation and Support

At present, about 50% to 60% of all patients in which cancer is diagnosed either are cured or achieve long-term control of their disease. "Cured" cancer patients have unique problems requiring both physician and community support. Many rehabilitation concerns have been addressed by organizations such as the American Cancer Society (ACS). The ACS has sponsored many programs, including the Reach to Recovery Program for patients treated for breast cancer, the Ostomy Support Programs for colostomy and enterostomy patients, the Lost Cord Program for laryngectomy patients, and self-help programs for cancer patients and their families.

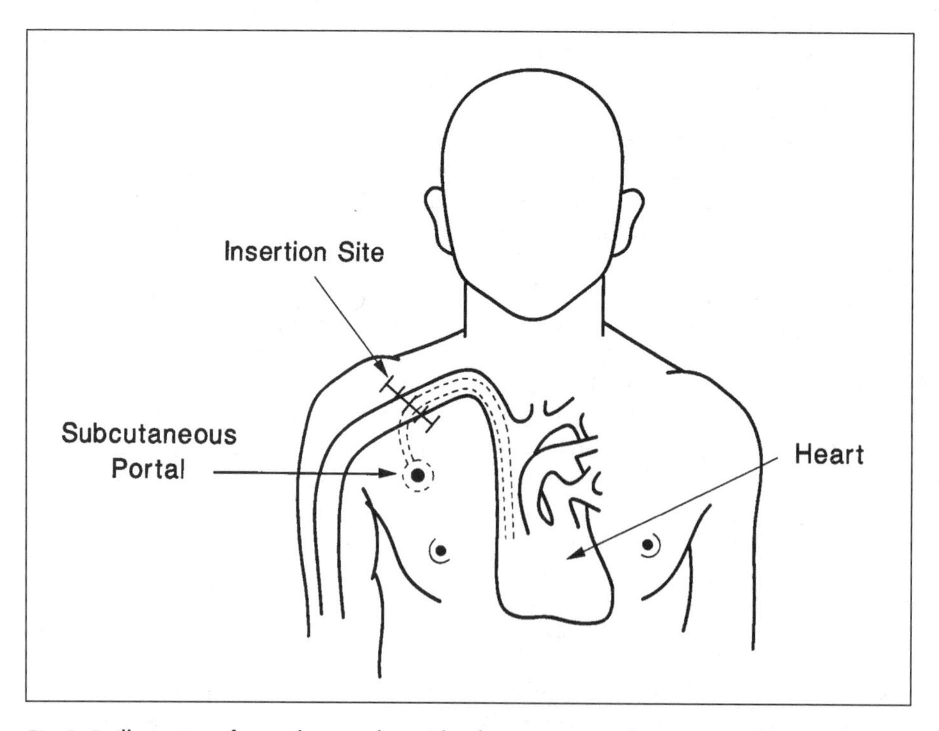

Fig 6-4. Illustration of central venous line with subcutaneous port for venous access in cancer management.

Physicians caring for cancer patients should be aware of such programs and encourage patient participation. Surgeons and others in the treatment team should also play an activerole in the development and maintenance of community rehabilitation programs.

Since about every other cancer patient will have nonoperable, recurrent, or metastatic cancer, the treating physician must be knowledgeable in palliation and symptom relief for advanced cancer. Pain, nausea, anorexia, insomnia, problems of infection, and bleeding are some symptoms associated with advanced cancer; so are depression, anxiety, exhaustion, and frustration on the part of the patient's family. These problems frequently tax the ability of the physician, but when dealt with effectively in a caring and compassionate manner, represent the true "art of medicine" (see Chapter 37 on Supportive Care and Rehabilitation of the Cancer Patient).

Participation in Clinical Trials

New methods of cancer treatment are the outgrowth of basic and clinical research. At some point, new methods must be tested through clinical trials (see Chapter 11 on Clinical Trials). While there are active studies on cancer treatment for virtually all major cancer sites, <4% of adult cancer patients are presently entered in clinical trials.[15] Many of these studies concern surgery and adjuvant therapy.

The surgeon has three clearly defined roles in the area of clinical trials: First, to participate in the development of good clinical research trials that incorporate surgical resection with other modes of therapy. Second, to monitor the surgical aspects of these studies. Poor surgical resection may be more of a factor in a poor outcome than the type of adjuvant therapy. Third and most important, to refer appropriate patients into clinical trials. Coltman has pointed out that approximately one half of clinical research protocols of the Southwest Oncology Cooperative Group are conducted in community hospital oncology programs.[16]

Hospital Cancer Programs

More than 1,300 hospitals in the US have a cancer program in place, which is surveyed and approved by the Commission on Cancer of the American College of Surgeons. These voluntary programs on the part of the hospital are designed to upgrade the care of cancer patients. Hospitals with cancer programs treat >75% of cancer patients in this country. The elements of a hospital cancer program include an active cancer committee and a database (tumor registry) that accesses all cancer patients, stages the cancer, and maintains long-term follow-up to assess the end result of treatment. In addition, these cancer programs have sponsored ongoing educational components, a tumor conference for presentation and discussion of cancer cases, and in-depth patient care evaluations of selected cancer sites. Another aspect of hospital cancer programs is the development of community cancer control activities through public and professional education and community cancer screening activities. Surgeons interested in good cancer care should foster the development of such programs and be active in promoting cancer prevention and early detection.

The Surgical Oncologist

The vast majority of surgical procedures in cancer patients is performed by well-trained general surgeons experienced in treating cancer at the more common sites. The subspecialty of surgical oncology comprises surgeons who on completion of general surgical training have obtained additional training and experience in a university surgical oncology training program or cancer center, and made a career commitment to the surgical treatment of cancer. Surgical oncologists have developed expertise in the management of less common cancers at unusual sites. They usually have expertise in resection of head and neck cancer, pelvic tumors, and unusual bone and soft tissue tumors. The training of surgical oncologists includes an in-depth knowledge of other treatment modalities, and is designed to encourage the most effective combination of treatment. The surgical oncologist is a resource for the community surgeon in dealing with unusual or complicated neoplasms. He is usually active in professional cancer education programs and in the development of cancer treatment protocols and other cancer control activities.

Summary

The role of the surgeon in modern cancer management continues to evolve from heroic and ultraradical operations to remove extensive tumors to an integrated approach combining a variety of modalities—surgery, radiation therapy, and chemotherapy. The best opportunity for care is sought, while reducing associated morbidity and mortality (Table 6-2). The real key to reducing the mortality from cancer lies in prevention and early detection, and the surgeon and treatment

Table 6-2. The Changing Role of Surgery in Cancer Treatment

Before 1850	Early attempts to resect cancer
1850-1950	Development of surgical techniques for resection
1950-1960	Extended radical surgical techniques
1960-1990	Era of combined treatment with surgery, radiation, and chemotherapy

team caring for cancer patients should actively pursue these cancer control efforts.

Radiation Therapy

X-rays were first described in 1895 by Roentgen,[1] and the Curies reported their discovery of radium approximately 3 years later.[2] The biologic effects of these ionizing radiations were soon realized, and they were promptly used to treat a variety of malignant and nonmalignant conditions. During the next decades, technologic advances accumulated rapidly. By 1922, 200 KV x-rays were available for treating patients.

Clinical evidence regarding the effects of ionizing radiations on both normal tissue and malignant tumors also accumulated rapidly. At the International Congress of Oncology in Paris in 1922, Coutard and Hautant presented evidence that advanced laryngeal cancer could be cured by radiation without disastrous, treatment-induced sequelae.[3] This marked the beginning of clinical radiation therapy as a medical discipline.

By 1934, Coutard had developed a protracted, fractionated scheme that remains the foundation of radiation therapy today.[4] The scheme was largely on clinical observations, as basic radiobiologic knowledge was lacking. The science of radiobiology advanced slowly during the first half of this century. It was not until the mid-1950s that in vivo and in vitro assays for mammalian cells, both neoplastic and normal, were developed. This permitted the quantitation of radiation effect by counting surviving cells.[5-7] During the next three decades, radiobiologic science experienced a period of exponential growth. Experiments using cultured mammalian cells led to a wealth of knowledge on the means by which radiation produces biologic injury and the factors that might modify this response. These observations form the basis of modern radiation biology.

Physical Basis of Radiation Therapy

Ionizing radiations used in radiation therapy include both electromagnetic "waves" and particulate radiations. To comprehend the biologic effects of these radiations, it is necessary to have a basic understanding of what these radiations are, how they are produced, and how they react with tissue. Electromagnetic waves are part of a broad spectrum that includes radio waves, microwaves, visible light, x-rays, and gamma rays (Fig 6-5). In radiation therapy, x-rays and gamma rays are used. These types of radiation possess the same general properties, differing only in their source and energy. X-rays are produced when energetic charged particles (usually electrons) impinge on a target and react with either atomic nuclei or orbital electrons. Gamma rays are produced during the decay of an unstable nucleus in a radioactive element. X-rays and gamma rays may be conveniently represented as particles called "photons" using quantum physics. The energy of a photon (E) is determined using the relationship

$$E=hv$$

where h is the constant of proportionality known as Planck's constant, and v is the frequency of the wave.

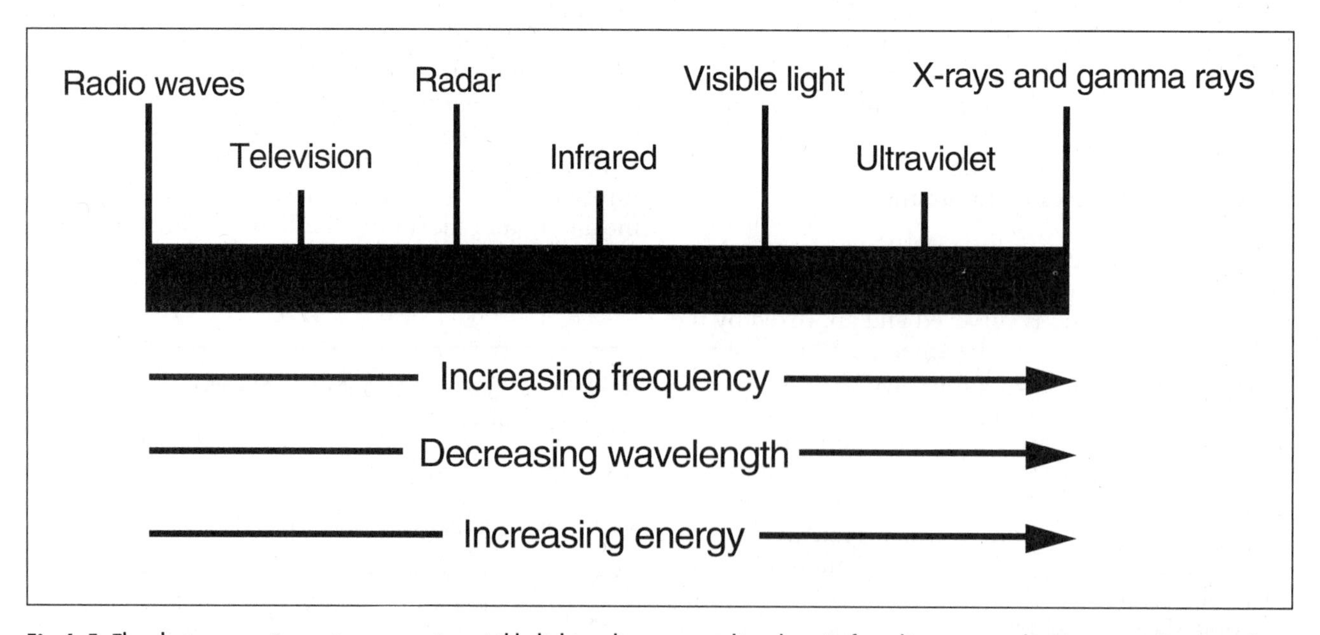

Fig 6-5. The electromagnetic spectrum comprises visible light, radio waves, radiant heat (infrared), x-rays, and gamma rays. X-rays and gamma rays have shorter wavelengths and thus higher energies. This higher energy enables them to break chemical bonds and produce biologic damage.

Substituting for the frequency, this equation becomes

$$E=h\ c/\lambda$$

where c is the speed of light and λ is the wavelength.

Particulate radiation includes electrons, protons, neutrons, alpha particles, negative pi-mesons, and heavy ions. Due to cost and size constraints, heavy particle radiation research is conducted at a limited number of institutions. Currently, only electrons are commonly used in radiation therapy.

Radiation may be directly or indirectly ionizing. Charged particles are directly ionizing. If they have sufficient energy, they may directly disrupt the atomic or molecular structure of the material through which they pass and produce chemical and biologic changes. Electromagnetic radiations and neutrons are indirectly ionizing. When they are absorbed in tissue, they give up their energy to produce fast-moving charged particles which then inflict the damage. In the case of electromagnetic radiations, fast recoil electrons are produced. Neutrons give up their energy to yield fast recoil protons, alpha particles, and heavier nuclear fragments.

In tissue, gamma rays and x-rays may interact in several ways. These include coherent scattering, photoelectric effect, Compton effect, pair production, and photodisintegration. The dominant reaction will vary with the energy of the radiation in use. At the energies commonly used in radiation therapy, the dominant reaction is the Compton effect, in which a photon interacts with a loosely bound orbital electron (Fig 6-6). Part of the energy of the incident photon is transferred to the electron as kinetic energy. This Compton electron may then interact with other electrons in the surrounding tissue. The remaining energy is carried away by another photon, which is less energetic than the original photon. The probability of Compton interactions is essentially independent of the atomic number of the target tissue, depending rather on the electron density of the target tissue. Thus, the amount of radiation absorbed is roughly the same whether the target is bone or soft tissue. In contrast, diagnostic x-rays are of lower energy and react predominantly by the photoelectric effect. The photoelectric effect is highly dependent on atomic number, and therefore bone and soft tissue appear quite different on a diagnostic x-ray film.

Protons, neutrons, and other heavy particles interact with the nucleus of an atom and not with the orbital electrons. Heavy particles dislodge various lower-energy showers of densely ionizing protons, neutrons, and others and deposit a large amount of energy over a short distance. This is the concept of linear energy transfer (LET). Linear energy transfer depends on the type of radiation used. Photons and electrons have a low rate of energy transfer (low LET). Heavy particles tend to deposit their energy in a track over a relatively short distance and are classified as high-LET radiations.

In general, radiation is administered in one of two ways. When the distance between the radiation source and the target is short, the term *brachytherapy* is used.

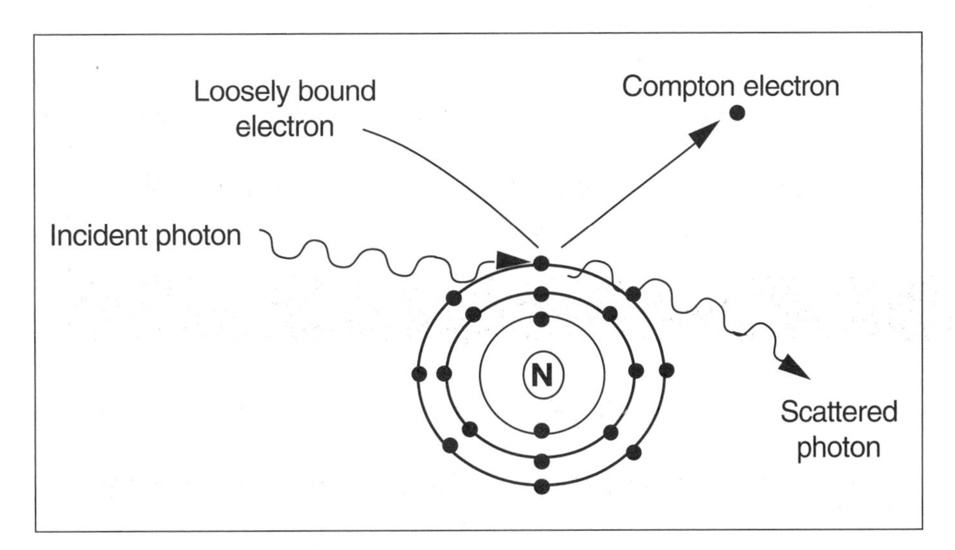

Fig 6-6. The Compton effect is the dominant reaction at the photon energies commonly used in radiation therapy. In this reaction, a loosely bound orbital electron interacts with the incident photon. Part of the photon's energy is transferred to the electron as kinetic energy. This "recoil" electron may then interact with other electrons in the surrounding tissue. The remaining energy is carried away by the scattered photon. N=nucleus.

Brachytherapy allows for a rapid falloff in dose away from the target volume as predicted by the inverse square law

$$I \alpha 1/d^2$$

where I is the intensity and d is the distance from the source. When the radiation source is at a distance from the target (generally 80 to 100 cm), the term *teletherapy* is used. This allows for a more uniform dose across the treatment volume.

Biologic Basis of Radiation Therapy

Radiobiology is the study of the action of ionizing radiations on organisms. The first recorded experiment was conducted in 1901, when Becquerel inadvertently left a container with 200 mg of radium in his pocket for 6 hours. He subsequently described the skin erythema that appeared 2 weeks later and the ulceration that developed and required several weeks to heal. During the early part of this century, radiobiologic experiments were conducted with simple biologic systems. These included measurement of lethal doses in animals, destruction of germination capabilities of seeds, retardation of growth in plants and their roots, and observation of the degree of skin erythema and mucositis.[8] In the 1950s, in vivo and in vitro techniques to culture mammalian cells led to a period of intense investigation.

Despite advances in knowledge, there remains some doubt as to how radiation causes cell death. The energy from radiation is deposited throughout the cell without interference from intracellular structures. It is generally believed that DNA is the critical target for lethal injury.[9] In addition, damage to cell membranes and microtubules may be supplementary mechanisms of cell kill.[10]

Radiation may injure the DNA molecule directly or indirectly. When any form of radiation is absorbed in a cell, it is possible that it will directly interact with a critical intracellular structure and cause biologic damage. This direct action is the dominant process in high-LET radiations, such as neutrons and alpha particles. With x-rays or gamma rays, the dominant process is an indirect action. Approximately one third of the damage may be due to the direct interaction of a recoil electron with a target molecule. The remaining two thirds of the damage will be due to indirect action, in which the recoil electron reacts with water (which constitutes approximately 70% of most cells) to produce hydroxyl radicals, which may then interact with a target molecule. Various substances alter the lifetime and hence the effectiveness of hydroxyl radicals. Electron-affinic molecules such as nitroimidazoles prolong the life of the radicals and increase the radiation effect (radiosensitization). Free radical scavengers such as sulfhydryl molecules shorten the life of the radicals and decrease the radiation effect (radioprotection).

The actual damage to the DNA may take several forms. There may be change or loss of a base, rupture of hydrogen bonds between DNA strands, dimerization, crosslink formation, single strand breaks or double strand breaks. On the chromosomal level, postradiation abnormalities are usually due to chromosome breaks and errors in rejoining postreplication chromosomes. This may lead to chromatid aberrations such as dicentrics, rings, anaphase bridges, and acentric fragments.[11-15] These changes would require two separate damaging events, and they therefore depend on the square of the dose. The improper segregation of DNA with chromosomal damage during mitosis is the most likely cause of radiation-induced mitotic death.

There is a wide disparity in time course for the events involved in biologic injury from radiation. The physical process of radiation absorption is over in roughly 10^{-15} second. Hydroxyl radicals will remain for approximately 10^{-5} second, during which they may inflict damage. The time course between this physical damage and the appearance of biologic damage is variable. If a nonessential area of the cell is damaged, there may be no measurable biologic effect. If the damage is lethal, it may be expressed hours to days later, when the cell attempts to divide. If the damage is oncogenic, its expression may be delayed up to ≥40 years. Finally, if the damage is a mutation, particularly a recessive mutation, it may not be expressed for many generations.

Radiation dose is quantified using the amount of energy absorbed per unit mass. The standard unit for reporting dose is the gray (Gy), which is defined as one joule per kilogram. Older publications may refer to dose in terms of the rad, which is equal to 0.01 Gy or 1 centigray (cGy). Very little energy is actually absorbed from a given dose of radiation. For example, the energy absorbed from a whole-body dose of 4 Gy would be 67 calories. This is roughly the same amount of energy as would be absorbed from drinking a sip of warm coffee. Yet a whole-body dose of 4 Gy will result in bone marrow suppression and death within about a month. The potential for damage from ionizing radiation is due to the way in which the energy is deposited. Energy from x-rays is deposited in discrete packets, each large enough to break a chemical bond and thus cause biologic damage.

Survival Curves

A cell survival curve expresses the relationship between radiation dose and the proportion of cells that survive. Generally, cell death is defined as the loss of reproductive integrity in proliferating cells. In differentiated cells that no longer divide, it may be con-

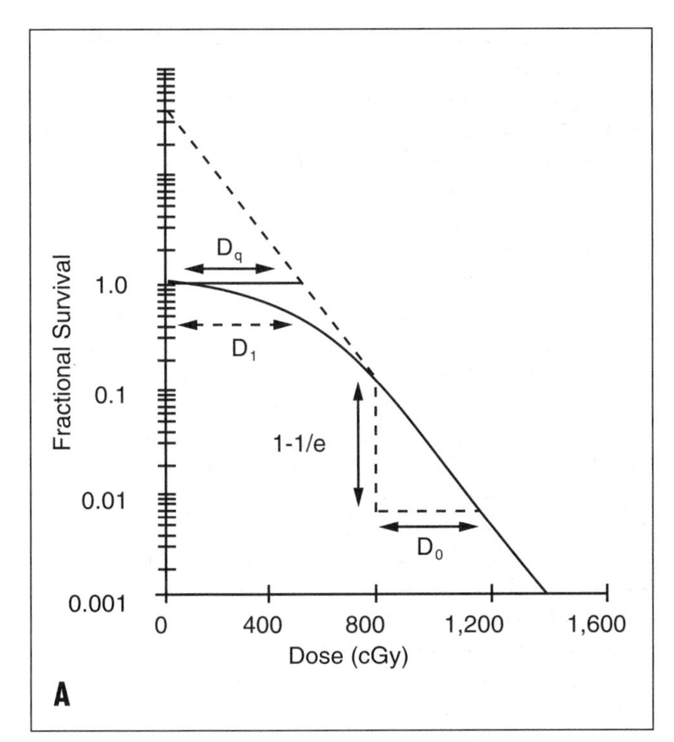

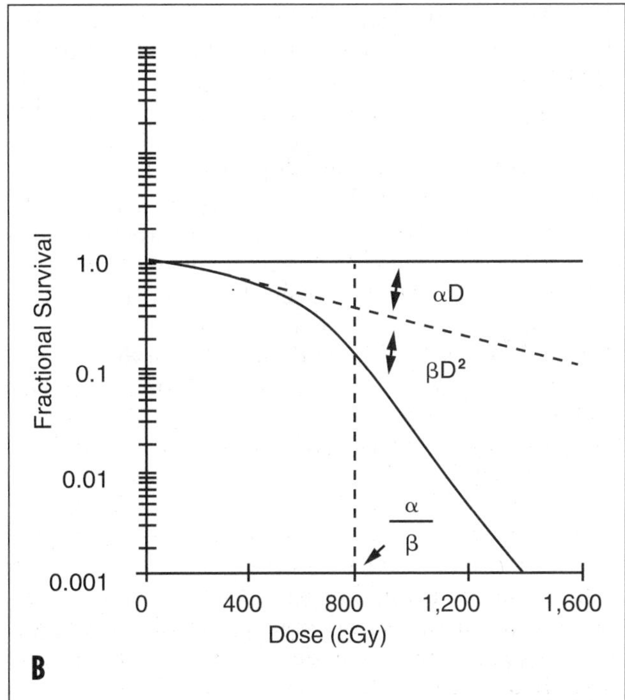

Fig 6-7. ***A*** shows a typical survival curve for mammalian cells exposed to low-LET radiation (x-rays or gamma rays). The curve is described by the initial slope D_1, the final slope D_0, and some expression of the width of the shoulder (either n, the extrapolation number, or D_0, the quasi-threshold dose). ***B*** shows a typical survival curve for mammalian cells exposed to low-LET radiation expressed in terms of the linear-quadratic model. In this model, there are two components to cell killing: one is proportional to dose (αD) and the other proportional to the square of the dose (βD_2). The ratio at which these two components are equal is the ratio of α/β.

sidered to be the loss of a specific function. Cell survival curves are obtained by exposing a population of cells to incremental doses of radiation and counting the number of surviving cells. The data is then plotted using a logarithmic scale for surviving fraction on the ordinate and a linear scale for dose in the abscissa. The overall shape of such curves is nearly the same for all mammalian cells, with some variation in the slope for different cell lines and for different types of radiation. With low-LET radiation, the curve usually begins with a shoulder in the low-dose region before beginning a logarithmic decline. The presence of the shoulder suggests that cells may accumulate some injury without dying. This "sublethal" damage could then be repaired. In contrast, high-LET radiations yield a survival curve that is a straight line from the origin. Survival is essentially an exponential function of dose.

Survival curves may be described using one of two models. First, the curves may be said to have an initial slope D_1 due to single-event killing and a final slope D_0 due to multiple-event killing (Fig 6-7A). The quantities D_1 and D_0 represent the doses that will decrease survival to 37% of the original. On average, this is the dose that will deliver one inactivating event per cell. The shoulder of the curve may be represented by the extrapolation number (n) or the quasi-threshold dose

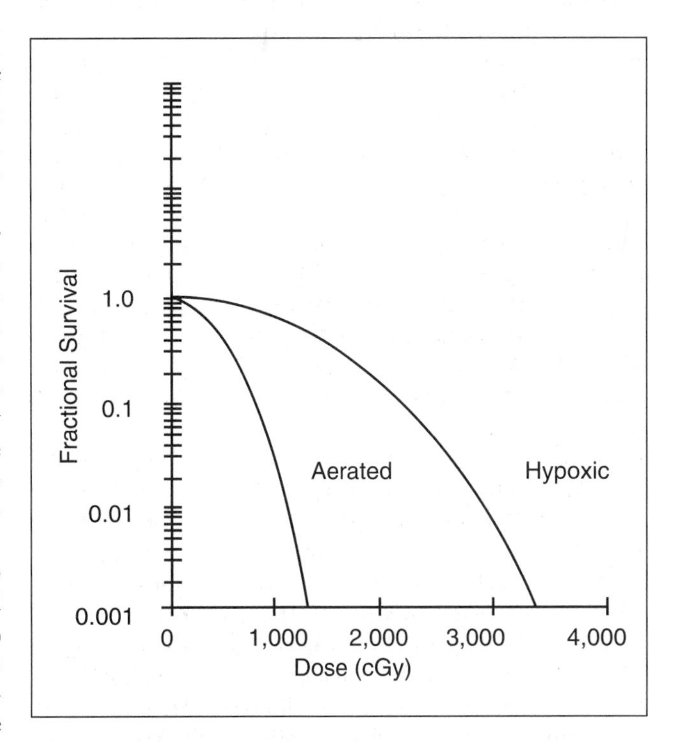

Fig 6-8. Typical survival curves for mammalian cells irradiated during aerobic and hypoxic conditions. Note the smaller shoulder and steeper slope of the cells irradiated under aerobic conditions.

(D_q). The extrapolation number is obtained by extrapolating the straight portion of the curve back through the y axis. In general, curves with a large n will have broad shoulders, and curves with a small n will have narrow shoulders. The quasi-threshold dose is obtained by extrapolating backward from a line extending from the straight portion of the curve to the y axis at a survival fraction of unity. A threshold dose is one below which there is no effect. As there is no radiation dose that produces no effect, the quasi-threshold dose is used instead.

An alternative method of describing survival curves is the linear quadratic model (Fig 6-7B). This model assumes two components to cell killing, one proportional to dose and the other proportional to the dose squared. The survival curve is described by the equation

$$S=e^{-\alpha D-\beta D^2}$$

where S is the fraction of cells surviving a dose D, and α and β are constants. The linear (α) and quadratic (β) portions of cell killing are equal when the dose is equal to the ratio of α to β. This ratio gives an indication of a cell's ability to repair itself. In general, cells from clinically radiosensitive tumors have higher α-to-β ratios than do cells from radioresistant tumors. In addition, tumors with lower α-to-β ratios have a higher dependence on dose per fraction and dose rate than radiosensitive tumors.

Although the general shape of the survival curve is the same for all mammalian cells, there is considerable variation in the inherent radiosensitivity of different cell lines and tumors. These variations are expressed mainly in the width of the initial shoulder and in the slope of the curve. There also may be differences in survival for the same cell lines irradiated under different conditions. In addition, survival is influenced by reoxygenation of hypoxic cells, repair of sublethal damage, repopulation by new cells, and reassortment in the cell cycle. Collectively, these factors are often referred to as the four R's of radiation biology—reoxygenation, repair, reassortment, and repopulation.

Oxygen Effect and Reoxygenation

The effect of oxygen on cells subjected to irradiation has been well documented.[16-18] The ratio of the doses needed to produce the same biologic effect in the presence and absence of oxygen is the oxygen enhancement ratio (OER). In general, the presence of oxygen enhances the effect of ionizing radiation (Fig 6-8). The degree of enhancement varies with the type of radiation. For sparsely ionizing radiations such as x-rays and gamma rays, the OER ranges from 2.5 to 3.0. For densely ionizing radiations such as alpha particles, the OER approaches 1.0 (no oxygen effect). For radiations of intermediate ionizing density such as neutrons, the OER is approximately 1.6.[19] Although it has generally been accepted that the OER is independent of dose, there is evidence that the OER for x-rays and gamma rays may be closer to 2.0 at doses of <200 cGy.[20] There is also evidence that dose rate may affect the OER for x-rays and gamma-rays.[21,22]

The exact nature of the oxygen effect is not known, but it is generally believed that oxygen aids in the production of cell damage via radiation-induced free radicals. This is consistent with the observation that the oxygen effect is much greater with radiations that act via free radicals than for densely ionizing high-LET radiations. The mechanism is believed to involve the combining of the electron-affinic oxygen with an unpaired electron in the outer shell of a free radical to yield a peroxide that is a non-restorable form of the target material.[23] As the lifetime of a free radical is short, oxygen must be present in the nucleus at the time of exposure or within milliseconds of radiation exposure. If bacterial cells are irradiated under anoxic conditions and oxygen is added immediately following the radiation exposure, some sensitization will occur up to approximately 2 milliseconds after irradiation.[24] However, if bacterial cells are exposed to oxygen 5 to 10 milliseconds after irradiation, there will be no biologic injury above that produced under anoxic conditions.[24,25]

Oxygen also must be present in sufficient quantities to have a radiosensitizing effect. Below a partial pressure of 20 mm Hg, cells will have significant protection from radiation damage. Most normal tissues have oxygen concentrations in the range of 40 mm Hg, and therefore are not protected from radiation damage. Tumors, on the other hand, often have areas of poor blood supply and oxygen-deficient cells. There is a decreasing gradient of oxygen with increasing distance from a vascular capillary. Beyond 150 to 200 mm from a capillary, the oxygen tension is essentially zero.[26] Tumor cells farther than approximately 160 mm from a capillary become necrotic and die.[26] Between the regions of well-oxygenated viable cells and hypoxic necrotic cells, one would expect a region in which the oxygen tension was high enough to allow cells to remain clonogenic but low enough to be protected from radiation and thus provide a nidus for regrowth of tumor.

Further evidence for the role of hypoxia in limiting the curability of human tumors is found in reports of improved results with radiation after the correction of anemia[27] or use of hyperbaric oxygen.[28] Despite this evidence, not everyone agrees that hypoxia is a common cause of treatment failure in radiation therapy.[29] This may be due to reoxygenation; tumor cells that are hypoxic one day may be well oxygenated on subsequent days.[30,31]

Repair

Individual cells exposed to a dose of radiation may respond in several ways. First, if no damage occurs at any critical site within the cell, the cell will be unaffected. Second, if sufficient damage occurs at a critical site, the cell will die during one of its subsequent divisions (lethal damage). Finally, cells may experience sublethal damage that may be repaired if the cell is given sufficient time, energy, and nutrients. This repair of sublethal damage is the reason cells can tolerate higher total doses of radiation when the radiation is administered in multiple small fractions. The shoulder of the survival curve reflects the repair of sublethal damage.[32] The capacity for repair varies in different normal tissue and tumors. Slowly responding tissues, such as the spinal cord, tend to repair damage slowly (over 6 to 8 hours), but the repair is essentially complete. In contrast, rapidly responding tissues, such as skin, mucosa, and bone marrow, often have incomplete repair. This may be due to continued stress on the cell to divide, which results in fixation of the injury rather than repair.[33] An important implication is that slowly responding tissues are spared more by using multiple small fractions of radiation than are acutely responding tissues. Clinically, this may be taken advantage of by administering multiple small fractions of radiation daily, with a separation of 6 to 8 hours between fractions to permit repair of normal tissue.[34,35]

Reassortment

Individual cells will vary in their radiosensitivity throughout the cell cycle. After plotting survival curves for Chinese hamster cells irradiated at various stages of the cell cycle, Sinclair found cells to be most sensitive during mitosis (M) and least sensitive during the late phase of nucleic acid synthesis (S).[36] In addition, if the first gap phase (G_1) has an appreciable length, there will be a resistant period in early G_1 followed by a sensitive phase in late G_1. Finally, the second gap phase (G_2) was found to be a sensitive phase, with a sensitivity that may approach that of the M phase.

The reasons for changes in radiosensitivity during the cell cycle are not well understood. It does not appear to be related to oxygen, as studies by Hall and colleagues[37] and Legrys and Hall[38] and have shown no difference in the OER for various stages of the cell cycle. One possible explanation is involvement of sulfhydryl compounds, which are free radical scavengers and therefore natural radioprotectors. Intracellular levels of sulfhydryl compounds tend to be highest during S phase and lowest near mitosis.[39]

Repopulation

Both tumors and normal tissue may undergo cell division during a course of fractionated radiotherapy. Normal tissue may respond to damage by recruiting inactive stem cells and shortening the duration of the cell cycle.[40] This is commonly seen in irradiation of the skin and oral mucosa, during which areas of new tissue can be seen growing within the treatment field. Repopulation is beneficial because it reduces overall injury to the tissue.

In a given tumor, treatment with a cytotoxic agent (such as radiation) may cause cells to divide faster than before treatment. This is known as accelerated repopulation. One of the earliest demonstrations of tumor regeneration during radiation was by Harmans and Barendsen in 1969.[41] They reported a rapid exponential increase in clonogen number in rat rhabdomyosarcoma after a delay of approximately one volume doubling time. There is also evidence that accelerated repopulation may occur in human tumor cells. Withers and associates reviewed the literature on radiotherapy in head and neck tumors and estimated the dose needed to achieve local control in 50% of cases as a function of treatment time.[42] They determined that clonogen repopulation in head and neck cancer accelerates about 28 days after the start of fractionated radiotherapy. To compensate for this accelerated growth, they suggested that an increase of about 60 cGy per day would be required.

It is evident from this data that for head and neck cancer (and most likely for other tumors) radiotherapy should be completed as soon after the initiation of treatment as is feasible. Also, it may be better to delay the start of treatment rather than have a delay during treatment. Finally, with a prolonged course of fractionated radiation, the later dose fractions will be less effective because the surviving clonogens will be undergoing accelerated repopulation.

Dose, Time, and Fractionation

The standard multifraction treatment regimens in common use today were based largely on experiments from France in the 1920s and 1930s.[43] At that time, it was found that it was not possible to sterilize a ram with a single dose of radiation to the testes without producing extensive damage to the skin of the scrotum. However, if the radiation was spread out over a series of daily doses, sterilization was possible without unacceptable skin reactions. By 1934, Coutard had developed a protracted fractionated scheme that is still commonly used today.[4] It is only now, >60 years later, that we can explain the efficacy of fractionated radiation based on well-designed radiobiologic experiments.

Dose-time considerations constitute a complex function that expresses the interdependence of the total dose, time, and number of treatments in the production of a biologic effect in a given tissue volume. This is based on the four R's of radiobiology: repair of sublethal damage, repopulation of cells between fractions, reassortment of cells throughout the cell cycle, and reoxygenation after one or more fractions of radiation. Basically, fractionating a dose spares normal tissue by allowing for repair of sublethal damage and for repopulation of cells between fractions. Also, tumor damage increases due to reoxygenation of hypoxic cells and reassortment of cells into more sensitive phases of the cycle.

Several fractionation schemes are used today. In each, the benefits of sparing acute reactions and allowing reoxygenation of tumors must be weighed against allowing surviving tumor cells to proliferate during treatment. Standard fractionation for radiation therapy consists of five equal fractions weekly. This evolved without solid biologic basis, and was based to a large degree on empiricism and convenience. Hyperfractionation involves giving a larger number of smaller-than-conventional doses (approximately 100 to 120 cGy twice per day). The goal of hyperfractionation is to give a higher total dose, and hopefully a higher probability of tumor control, without increasing the risk of late complications. Accelerated fractionation consists of multiple fractions daily of 150 to 200 cGy per fraction. This decreases the overall treatment time, but because the total dose per day is high, some reduction in overall dose is necessary. Hypofractionation involves a smaller number of larger fractions. Again, the large daily dose necessitates a reduction in overall dose to avoid serious complications. Split-course radiation consists of larger daily fractions (usually >250 cGy daily) with a planned break in the middle of the course to permit acute reactions to subside. Split-course regimens generally are not advisable unless the overall treatment time is decreased.

Clinical Considerations

Many factors enter into treatment planning in radiation therapy. The aim of therapy should be defined prior to the onset of treatment. In curative radiation, it is projected that the patient has a probability of surviving after administration of adequate treatment. In contrast, with palliative treatment there is no hope for cure or extended survival. In curative cases, a certain probability of significant side effects, though undesirable, may be acceptable. In palliative radiation, however, the goal is to improve the patient's quality of life by relieving some symptom or by preventing some tumor-related complication that could impair the patient's self-sufficiency. No major iatrogenic complications should be seen.

In a curative setting, it is extremely important for the radiation oncologist to deliver the highest possible dose to the tumor volume to ensure maximum potential for tumor control while minimizing the incidence of severe sequelae in the normal surrounding tissue. To determine the optimal dose, one must examine the dose-response curves for normal tissue and tumors (Fig 6-9). The farther these two curves diverge, the more favorable is the therapeutic ratio (TR), which can be defined as the percentage of tumor control with therapy A versus therapy B divided by the percentage of major complications with therapy A versus therapy B. Higher therapeutic ratios are found with more efficient radiation technologies.

Improvements in radiation therapy require that the therapeutic ratio be increased. In other words, the

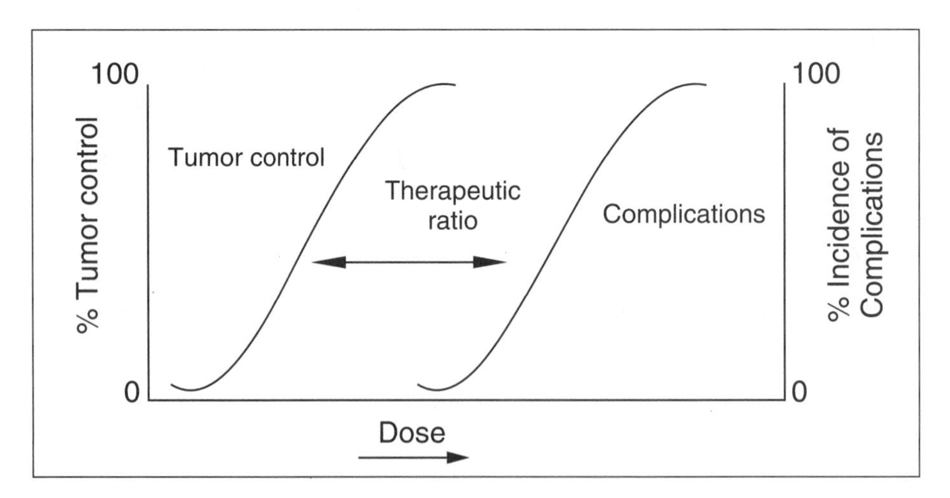

Fig 6-9. The curves for tumor control and normal tissue complications are plotted together. The therapeutic ratio is directly related to the distance between the two curves. Factors that increase the separation between the curves will increase the therapeutic ratio; eg, radiosensitizers shift the tumor control curve to the left, and radioprotectors shift the tissue complications curve to the right.

increase in biologic effectiveness must be greater in the tumor than in normal tissue. This would result in a divergence of the probability curves for tumor control and complications and an increase in the therapeutic ratio. Radiosensitizers increase the therapeutic ratio by making the tumor cells more susceptible to the effects of radiation and thus shift the tumor control curve to the left. Radioprotectors increase the therapeutic ratio by making normal tissue less susceptible to the effects of radiation and thus shift the curve for complications to the right. As the curves for tumor control and complications are sigmoidal, small changes in the midrange of tumor control probability (where the curve is steepest) can provide significant changes in outcome. This has two additional implications. First, if a treatment change produces a modest difference in the percentage of tumor control or complications, that change should not be interpreted as a substantial change in the biologic effectiveness of the dose. Second, it is possible that a small change in a biologically effective dose can translate into a large therapeutic gain or loss.

At incidences of effect approximately <10% or >90%, the curves are relatively flat, and any additional dose is relatively inefficient. For example, if the tumor control probability was already at 90%, there would be no therapeutic gain from dose increases if the incidence of severe complications was already at ≥5%. This is because the probability of complications would increase much faster than the chance of cure. In view of the proximity of the dose-response curves for normal tissue and most human tumors, it is not possible to treat patients with curative intent and produce no complications. In general, radiation oncologists attempt to limit serious complications to ≤5%. The dose that will give a 5% chance of a serious complication at 5 years after treatment is referred to as the $TD_{5/5}$ (Table 6-3).[44]

Tumor control is directly related to total dose. For every increment of radiation dose, a certain fraction of cells will be killed. Thus, the total number of surviving cells will be proportional to the initial number present and the fraction killed with each dose. It is apparent that various levels of irradiation yield a different probability of tumor control, depending on the number of clonogenic cells present. For subclinical disease, which would represent $<10^6$ cells per cubic centimeter, 4,500 to 5,000 cGy is believed to be adequate to control the disease in >90% of patients. This is based on studies of squamous cell carcinoma of the upper respiratory tract[45] and adenocarcinoma of the breast.[46] For microscopically detected disease, which represents $>10^6$ cells per cubic centimeter, doses of 6,000 to 6,500 cGy are required for epithelial tumors. For clinically palpable tumors, doses in the range of 6,000 cGy for T1 tumors up to 7,500 to 8,000 cGy for T4 tumors are required. Again, these doses reflect squamous cell and adenocarcinoma.[47-50]

Table 6-3. Doses for Whole Organ Irradiation That Result in a 5% Incidence ($TD_{5/5}$) and a 50% Incidence ($TD_{50/5}$) of Severe Complications at 5 Years

Organ	Fractionated Dose (cGy)
Testes	100—200
Ovary	600—1,000
Eye (lens)	600—1,200
Lung	2,000—3,000
Kidney	2,000—3,000
Skin	3,000—4,000
Thyroid	3,000—4,000
Liver	3,500—4,000
Heart	4,000—5,000
Bone marrow	4,000—5,000
Gastrointestinal	5,000—6,000
Spinal cord	5,000—6,000
Brain	6,000—7,000
Peripheral nerve	6,500—7,700
Mucosa	6,500—7,700
Bone and cartilage	>7,000
Muscle	>7,000

Modified from Rubin et al.[44]

The "shrinking field" technique makes use of this concept of different doses for different volumes of tumor. In this technique, portals that are progressively reduced in size are used to give progressively higher doses of radiation to the central portion of the tumor, where more clonogenic cells are present. In comparison, the periphery of the tumor, where a lower number of cells is present, receives a lesser dose. This technique minimizes the amount of normal tissue receiving high-dose irradiation.

Tumor Response

Radiocurability refers to the eradication of tumor at the primary or regional site and reflects a direct effect of the irradiation, which may not parallel the patient's ultimate outcome. Radiosensitivity expresses the response of the tumor to irradiation. No significant correlation exists between the responsiveness of a tumor to irradiation and radiocurability. Thus, a tumor may be quite radiosensitive yet incurable. Conversely, a radioresistant tumor may well be curable.

Response of a tumor to irradiation is not necessarily a good measure of radiosensitivity. Most tumors contain a proportion of rapidly proliferating tumor cells and inflammatory cells that show an early response to irradiation. The response of the tumor to irradiation will depend on the programmed lifetime of terminally differentiated cells within the tumor, the proliferation kinetics of the malignant clonogens, and the removal rate of dead cells. In general, local control will be slightly higher for rapidly regressing tumors than for slowly regressing tumors. Despite this observation, reduction in total dose based on tumor response is not warranted.[51]

The interpretation of slow tumor regression is somewhat more complex. Slow regression can be due to slow tumor proliferation and cell loss kinetics. It also may indicate a mass of residual stroma without viable tumor cells, as is commonly seen in Hodgkin's disease, pituitary adenomas, and choroidal melanomas. Finally, slow regression may be due to persistent tumor. The issue is further clouded by the fact that a small proportion of most tumor types will regress slowly even though the majority regress quickly. In view of the heterogeneity of tumor response, it is often unnecessary and sometimes misleading to obtain early postradiation biopsies of a slowly regressing tumor.[51] This is because it is not possible to distinguish tumor cells that are sterilized but still living from tumor cells that have retained their reproductive integrity. As early postradiation biopsies are associated with considerable risk of tissue necrosis, it is usually advisable to avoid them if the tumor continues to regress, and they are not often indicated sooner than 3 months after therapy.

The radiation oncologist is much like the surgeon in that he or she attempts to cure the patient by locally eradicating the tumor. This is the concept of local control, which implies that the tumor will never return to the treated area. By providing local control, one would expect a higher probability of cure.[52] In oncology, we tend to evaluate therapies in terms of response rates. A complete response is defined as the absence of clinically detectable tumor, and a partial response is defined as a >50% reduction in tumor mass. The radiation oncologist tends to place less emphasis on response rates, as a complete response does not necessarily translate into a cure and a partial response will most likely translate into a complete failure.

Summary

There have been many advances in radiation oncology since the discovery of x-rays in 1895. Initially, radiation oncology was based largely on empiricism and clinical observations. Modern radiobiology provides a rationale for both normal tissue and tumor response to radiation. These responses are based largely on the four R's of radiobiology: reoxygenation of hypoxic cells, repair of sublethal damage, repopulation of cells between fractions, and reassortment of cells to more sensitive phases of the cell cycle.

As cell kill is a random process, there is no dose of radiation that will guarantee a cure. The radiation oncologist attempts to provide the highest probability of tumor control while minimizing the risk of serious complications. The radiation oncologist thus is constantly searching for ways to increase the therapeutic ratio and improve patient care. Today, advances in all aspects of oncology have led to cure being a realistic possibility in >50% of newly diagnosed cases.[53,54] Hopefully, future advances will continue to improve radiation oncology and cancer care for all.

Systemic Therapy

Medical oncology has traditionally defined itself as that discipline specializing in the use of systemic forms of treatment for the management of patients with malignancies. It is this focus on systemic therapy that distinguishes medical oncology from surgical and radiation oncology, which are best suited for treating malignancies while they are still localized. Medical oncology had its origins in the 1940s, when nitrogen mustard was first used to obtain a brief remission in a patient with lymphoma.[1] Subsequent advances—notably in the treatment of childhood acute lymphocytic leukemia (ALL), choriocarcinoma, Hodgkin's disease, testicular carcinoma, and diffuse large-cell lymphoma—have generally followed the introduction and combination of other cytotoxic drugs.

Most cytotoxic drugs are effective in destroying cancer cells because they interfere, through various rather direct mechanisms, with the synthesis or function of nucleic acids. Because of this common endpoint, chemotherapeutic agents have gained a certain notoriety for producing undesirable damage to normal tissue, such as hematologic suppression, mucositis, and hair loss. Many patients also fear the use of these drugs because of a tendency to cause nausea and vomiting. Thankfully, major advances have been made in understanding the pharmacokinetics and pharmacodynamics of these agents, enabling less toxicity to normal tissue, and in managing chemotherapy-induced nausea and vomiting.

Furthermore, medical oncology is rapidly changing as new agents with entirely different mechanisms of action are introduced, such as the interferons, interleukins, hematopoietic colony stimulating factors, growth factor antagonists, and agents capable of inducing cellular differentiation. Moreover, medical oncology has begun to make significant contributions to the treatment of localized disease, as witnessed by the combination of 5-fluorouracil (5-FU) and radiation therapy in the curative treatment of rectal carcinoma, a tumor formerly curable only by radical surgical excision.

Although this section will focus primarily on cancer chemotherapy, it should be remembered that the practicing medical oncologist, in collaboration with colleagues in other disciplines, typically spends less time dealing with issues specifically related to the delivery of chemotherapy and more time confronting the fundamental issues of oncology in general: establishment of a tissue diagnosis of malignancy; efficient staging of disease; review of prognosis and treatment options with the patient and family; effective relief of pain; and coordination of auxiliary services to ensure that the patient's emotional and social needs are promptly met.

An understanding of the mechanisms by which nonresectional therapies may thwart the growth of malignant neoplasms—as well as an understanding of why it so often fails to do so—requires an appreciation of the kinetics of tumor growth. Although from a clinical standpoint it is most relevant to describe a tumor's growth as that of a whole tissue, the concepts used to describe tissue growth are built on observations regarding the growth of individual cells; therefore, the kinetics of the cell cycle will be reviewed first.

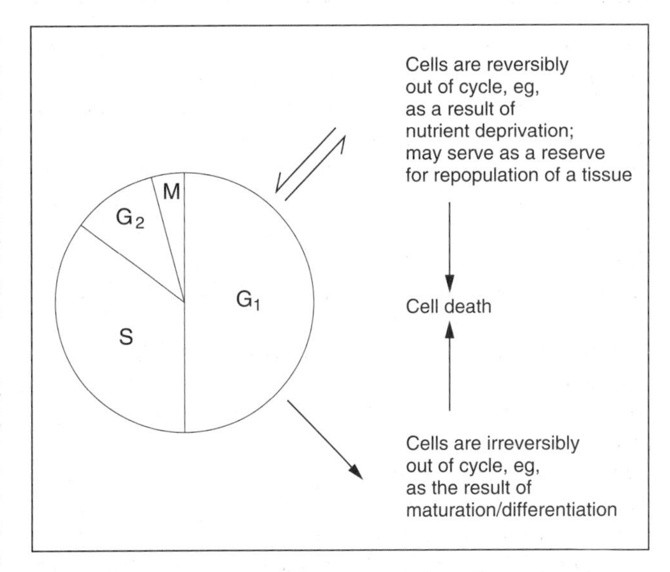

Fig 6-10. Diagrammatic representation of the cell growth cycle, emphasizing the relationships between proliferating and nonproliferating cell populations. M=mitosis, S=DNA synthesis phase.

Cell Cycle Kinetics

The familiar model of cell proliferation, equally applicable to normal and malignant cells, is the result of studies combining tritiated thymidine (^{3}H-TdR) labeling of cells with autoradiography.[2] Thymidine, the nucleoside precursor of the deoxyribonucleic acid (DNA) nucleotide deoxythymidine monophosphate, is essential for the synthesis of DNA; a cell replicating its genome in preparation for mitosis incorporates thymidine into its nucleus. In a typical experiment, ^{3}H-TdR is injected into an animal or a patient and fresh tissue is then obtained by biopsy at serial intervals. The tissue so exposed to the isotope is overlaid with a photographic emulsion; the low-energy β-particles emitted by the tritium have a very short range, so only the silver grains lying directly above labeled nuclei are activated.

Additional techniques are now available to determine the DNA content of cells and the cell cycle characteristics of neoplastic populations. Laser-based flow cytometry is a more rapid and simpler technique of measuring the DNA content of the cell which provides information for ploidy analysis and cell cycle kinetic studies. The use of ^{3}H-TdR requires radioactive materials and fresh tissue and is a tedious process. Flow cytometry is a highly automated procedure that can measure the DNA content of both fresh and frozen tissues in paraffin-embedded specimens. This technique is now widely available for clinical purposes and provides useful prognostic information for patients with breast cancer.[3] Current studies indicate that a high S phase fraction is associated with an increased risk of recurrence and mortality for patients with both node-negative and node-positive invasive breast cancer.

Bromodeoxyuridine (BrdU) labeling of DNA also can provide an assessment of the DNA synthesis of neoplastic tissues. The amount of BrdU incorporated into DNA can be quantitated by either flow cytometry or microscopic techniques. The use of this technique is hampered somewhat by the need for fresh tissue and dual fluorescent staining techniques. Both flow cytometry and BrdU can measure DNA content, but the former is simpler and yields more reproducible results.

The first critical observation to be made from such investigations was that DNA synthesis is not a continuous process from one mitosis to the next, but rather occurs during a discrete period of the intermitotic time, known as S phase.[4] The intermitotic time has been further subdivided into a total of five phases (Fig 6-10). G_1, the time or "gap" between mitosis and S phase, is the portion of the cell cycle dedicated to fulfilling the specialized functions of a given cell type. During G_1, the cell's energy is directed toward the synthesis of ribonucleic acid (RNA) and protein designed to execute these functions. G_2, the gap between the end of S phase and mitosis, represents the usually brief time required to organize the nucleus for the events of mitosis. The onset of mitosis is marked by chromosomal condensation and is followed by chromosomal segregation and cell division, yielding two daughter cells. The fifth phase of the cell cycle, G_0, is often depicted as lying outside the loop connecting one mitosis with the next. This is because cells in G_0 do not respond to the signals that normally prompt initiation of DNA synthesis, in contrast to cells in G_1. However, cells in G_0 are by no means dead: They continue to synthesize RNA and protein and so may carry out some of the differentiative functions of a particular cell type. In addition, they often act as a reserve that given the appropriate cues (eg, increased availability of nutrients), can reenter the pool of proliferating cells and repopulate a tissue.

Measurement of the duration of the various phases of the cell cycle is conceptually simple. Because thymidine is either incorporated into DNA or rapidly metabolized and excreted, only cells that are in S phase at the time of ^{3}H-TdR administration will develop grains over their nuclei on an autoradiograph. A cohort of cells labeled in S phase can be followed by (1) obtaining serial biopsies of tissue for autoradiography following ^{3}H-TdR injection and (2) recording the percentage of mitoses that are labeled in each biopsy.[5] When the percentage of labeled mitoses (PLM) is plotted against the time following ^{3}H-TdR injection, a curve such as the one in Fig 6-11 is obtained. Cells at the very end of S phase during ^{3}H-TdR labeling will be the first to produce labeled mitoses; the elapsed time between exposure to ^{3}H-TdR and the appearance of these first labeled mitotic cells is the length of G_2. Cells poised at the beginning of S phase during labeling are the last to appear in mitosis, so the width of the wave reflects the duration of S phase (T_s). If tissue samples are subsequently examined, waves of labeled mitoses appear as the daughter cells of those originally labeled pass through mitosis. The time separating the beginning of one wave from the beginning of the next yields the total cell cycle time (T_c). When the cell cycle kinetics of mammalian cells are examined in vivo using the PLM method, the durations of S, G_2, and M phases are found to be remarkably similar—about 7, 3, and 1 hour, respectively. Moreover, in most instances, there is no significant difference in the duration of these phases between normal and malignant tissues. The longest and most variable phase is G_1, ranging from 2 to 3 hours to several days. Surprisingly, the intermitotic time (T_c) for most normal human cells is 1 to 2 days, while that of most malignant cells is approximately 2 to 3 days.[6]

It should now be obvious that cell cycle kinetics alone are inadequate for describing the growth of tumors. First, despite rather similar values for T_c, different malignancies have distinctly different growth rates. For example, T_c has been estimated at roughly 2.5 days for acute myelogenous leukemia (AML) and about 2.0 days for squamous cell carcinoma of the skin[6]; yet untreated AML results in death within weeks of diagnosis while squamous cell carcinoma takes a more indolent course, usually measured in years. Second, if tumor growth were determined solely by

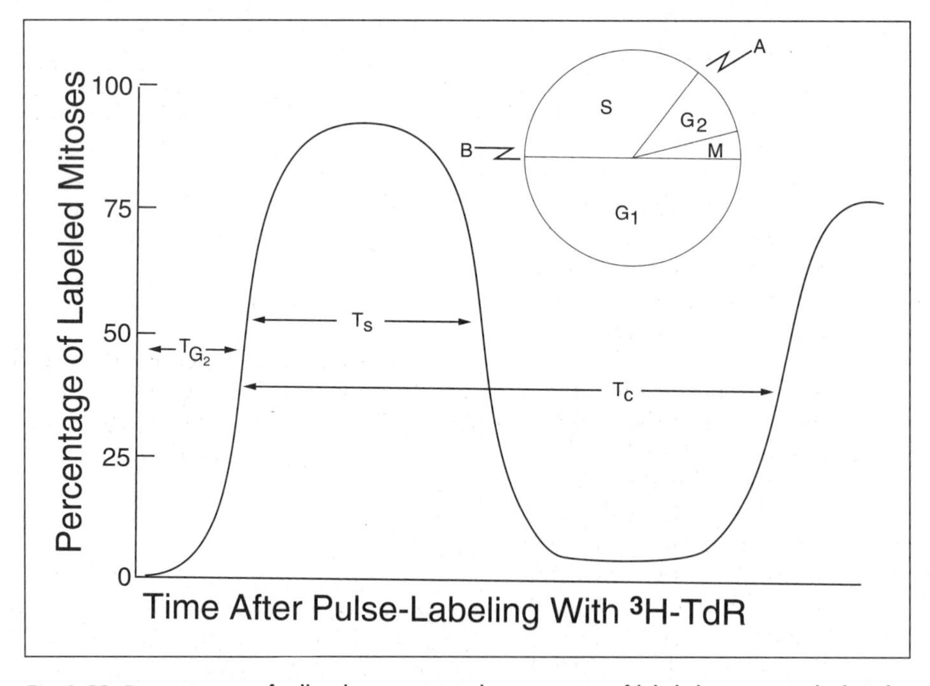

Fig 6-11. Determination of cell cycle times using the percentage of labeled mitoses method. Only cells in S phase become labeled at the time of ^{3}H-thymidine (^{3}H-TdR) administration. Those cells at the very end of S phase (point A) are the first to appear in mitosis, and those just beginning to enter S phase (point B) are the last to do so. The time lag between ^{3}H-TdR pulsing and the appearance of the first labeled mitoses represents the time required for cells to pass through G_2($^TG_2$). The width of the waves of labeled mitoses gives the duration of S phase (T_S), and the time separating one wave from the next yields the total cell cycle time (T_C).

the cell cycle time, then one would anticipate tumors to double in volume every 2 to 3 days. Although Burkitt's lymphoma approximates this rate of growth, clearly it is an exception rather than the rule. To resolve these seeming incongruities, tumor growth must be described in the context of a whole tissue.

Tissue Growth Kinetics

When tumors are examined as whole tissues, it quickly becomes obvious that not all of the cells are proliferating, ie, not all are "in cycle." In fact, only a minority are proliferating, with the bulk in G_0, differentiated to the point that they no longer have the potential to replicate, or simply dead. The fraction of tumor cells that is in cycle can be calculated by ^{3}H-TdR autoradiography. First, one determines the labeling index (LI), the proportion of cells synthesizing DNA at the time of exposure to the isotope (the proportion of cells developing labeled nuclei). Then, if T_s and T_c are known for the cells of that tissue, as might be estimated by the PLM method, the fraction of proliferating cells in the tumor—called the growth fraction (GF)—is determined by:

$$GF = LI \times T_c/T_s \times \lambda$$

By itself the LI does not give the fraction of proliferating cells, since not all cells in cycle will be in S phase at the time of ^{3}H-TdR exposure; hence the term T_c/T_s to make the correction. The constant λ (always close to 1) is necessary to make adjustment for the fact that the distribution of cells in different phases of the cell cycle is not strictly equal (each cell undergoing mitosis yields two daughter cells, so the relative number of cells in each phase of the cell cycle decreases from G_1 to mitosis). When LI has been determined for a variety of solid tumors, it has generally been low, ranging from 1% to 8%.[6] These results should be compared with the LI of the epithelium of the normal gut—roughly 16%.

In addition to a low GF, most tumors suffer from a high rate of cell loss, further limiting their rate of growth.[7] The percentage of newly produced daughter cells that die is high, in part a result of the inherent genetic instability of malignant cells. Moreover, tumors tend to outstrip their vascular supply and so develop large areas of ischemic necrosis. Given this general tendency for low GF and high rates of cell loss, it should be obvious that most tumors are not what on the surface they appear to be—seething masses of rapidly dividing cells. Yet the nature of tumor growth is progressive, so clearly the rate of cell loss ultimately lags behind that of cell production. It is this imbalance between cell production and cell loss—the fact that tumors are not appropriately checked by the homeostatic mechanisms that maintain a predetermined number of cells in normal tissue—that lies at the heart of tumor progression. The importance of this imbalance between cell production and cell loss is well demonstrated by comparing acute with chronic myelogenous leukemia (CML).[6] Acute myelogenous leukemia is rapidly progressive, killing patients within a matter of weeks to months if untreated. On the other hand, CML usually follows an indolent course over several years. Surprisingly, the LI for myeloblasts in AML is about 5% to 11%, while that for myeloblasts of CML is generally up to 43%. The difference is that the myeloblasts of CML, in all but the terminal stages of the disease, are able to differentiate to more mature progeny (eg, neutrophils) with brief life spans. The myeloblasts of AML rarely produce more mature successors and, given their longer life span compared with mature cells, they accumulate rapidly. Even in the terminal phase of CML ("blast crisis"), when the percentage and number of myeloblasts increase rapidly, the LI does not change. The problem at this point in the illness is that the myeloblasts are no longer able to further differentiate and mature, and consequently the clinical course of the disease becomes similar to that of AML.

Gompertzian Growth

The concepts presented thus far describe tumor growth at only one point during its life span. Yet the growth of a tumor changes drastically through time, a fact with important implications for cancer treatment in general and for cancer chemotherapy in particular. During the early phases of a tumor's life span, both the rate at which cells are produced and the rate at which cells are lost from the tumor are proportional to the number of cells in the tumor at a given time. Since cell number (N) and tumor volume (V) are proportional,

$$dv/dt = (K_P - K_L) \times V$$

where K_P equals the rate constant for cell production, and K_L equals the rate constant tor cell loss. The above relationship, on rearrangement and integration, gives the more useful relation

$$V_2 = V_1 e^{(K_P - K_L)(t_2 - t_1)}$$

In short, for a good portion of its life, a tumor grows exponentially. This simple exponential relationship allows one to readily calculate the doubling time of the tumor (T_D):

$$\frac{\ln 2}{K_P - K_L} = T_D$$

By measuring the time required for a tumor to double in size, it should be possible to estimate the time the tumor took to achieve a given size from its beginning as a single cell. When such calculations are made using clinical measurements of T_D, one concludes that the tumor must have started 10 to 20 years prior to its detection!

Such calculations are fundamentally flawed. With occasional exceptions, by the time a tumor becomes clinically detectable it has achieved a mass of approximately 1 g, or 10^9 cells. To reach this size, the tumor has already undergone about 30 doublings and its growth is no longer exponential. The additional 10 doublings required to produce 10^{12} cells, or 1 kg—the burden at which most patients succumb—occur much more slowly than the previous 30 doublings and represent a minority of the tumor's growth.

An English insurance actuary by the name of Gompertz developed a mathematical model to describe the relationship between an individual's age and his expected time of death. The asymmetric sigmoidal curve produced by this model comes close to accurately describing the growth of a tumor over its *entire* life span (Fig 6-12). When the Gompertzian equation is used to calculate the time required for a tumor to reach 10^9 cells, it is estimated that most human malignancies originate <2 years prior to their clinical detection. The exact mechanisms influencing the shape of the Gompertzian curve are not well understood, but the slowing of growth in larger tumors is undoubtedly due in part to (1) hypoxia, as tumors outstrip their fragile vascular supply; (2) decreased availability of nutrients and hormones; (3) accumulation of toxic metabolites; and (4) inhibitory cell-to-cell communication.

As mentioned earlier, most chemotherapeutic agents in clinical use exert their antitumor effects (and the bulk of their toxicities) by interfering directly with the synthesis or function of DNA. It is not surprising, then, that these drugs are in general more toxic to proliferating cells than to those incapable of replication or in G_0, and so are more effective against tumors with high growth fractions.[8] As pointed out above, by the time tumors are clinically detectable, they lie "high on the Gompertzian curve," where their growth fractions are low. However, if this number of cells in a tumor can be reduced, as might occur by surgical debulking or radiation therapy, then the tumor has been brought to a lower point on the Gompertzian curve. Cells previously in G_0 reenter the cell cycle, the GF of the tumor increases, and the growth rate of the tumor may be similar to the rate of a tumor that had just attained the same size from a single cell. If effective chemotherapy is available against the tumor, it would now likely be even more effective. This concept of moving tumors down on the Gompertzian curve prior to the delivery of chemotherapy underlies much of the rationale behind adjuvant chemotherapy[9]—ie, chemotherapy given to patients who have no overt evidence of residual disease after local treatment (eg, surgery or radiation therapy for a primary breast cancer), but for whom past experience with similar patients indicates a high chance of relapse from the presence of undetectable micrometastatic disease.

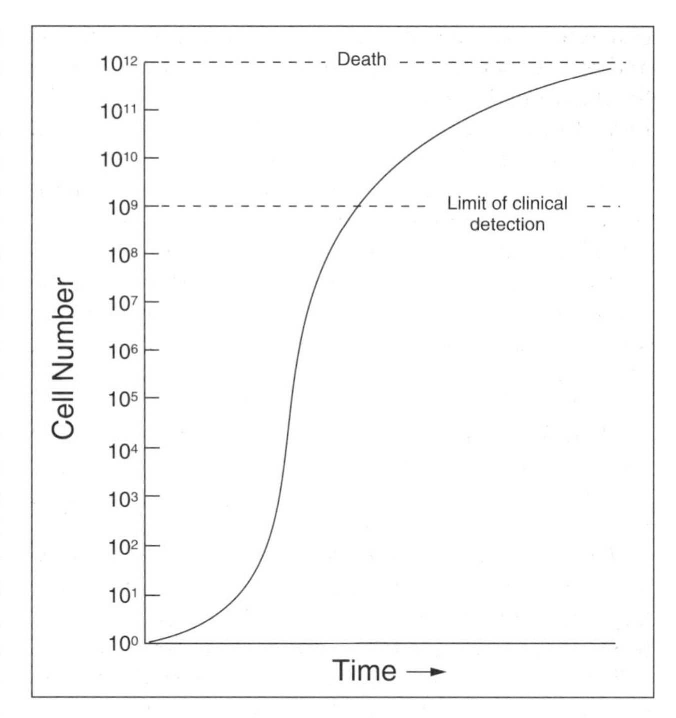

Fig 6-12. The Gompertzian growth curve. During the early stages of development, growth is exponential. As a tumor enlarges, its growth slows. By the time a tumor becomes large enough to cause symptoms and be clinically detectable, most of its growth has already occurred, and the exponential phase is over.

The Stem Cell Model of Tumor Growth

A further impediment to effective chemotherapy is the conclusion that proliferating cells, those that should be most vulnerable to the toxic effects of chemotherapy, are not necessarily the cells that must be eliminated in order to eradicate a tumor. Instead, the critical cell population—the one responsible for the persistence and growth of a tumor—is often largely in G_0. The reasons for this apparent paradox are found in the stem cell model of tissue growth.

This model of tissue growth has been most extensively elaborated for cells of the bone marrow, which are depicted as components of a complex hierarchy. At the top of the hierarchy are relatively undifferentiated cells with an unlimited capacity for self-replication and for replenishing the marrow with all of its elements. Yet these cells are virtually unable to perform the ultimate functions of the marrow, ie, oxygen transport, hemostasis, and defense against infection. At the hierarchic bottom are mature, highly specialized cells (eg, neutrophils, erythrocytes, and platelets) which can execute these tasks but which are unable to divide and renew themselves. Although the proliferative rates for the immediate descendants of stem cells tend to be high (LI for myeloblasts and myelocytes are 40% and 20%, respectively; LI for early erythroid precursors range between 30% and 75%),[6] the stem cells themselves, unless provoked by an appropriate stimulus (eg, blood loss or infection), tend to proliferate slowly.

The sluggish proliferation of marrow stem cells has been inferred by the extent to which their numbers are reduced by the administration of very high doses of ^{3}H-TdR, a technique dubbed "thymidine suicide." As in ^{3}H-TdR autoradiography, only cells synthesizing DNA (those in S phase) will accumulate the isotope in their nuclei. However, in the thymidine suicide experiments, the doses of ^{3}H-TdR are high enough to be lethal to these cells.

The original stem cell assays of bone marrow were performed in mice.[10] If a mouse is given a sufficiently large dose of radiation, it will fail to recover hematopoietic function; both the mature cells and the stem cells of the marrow are irrevocably damaged. If, however, this lethally irradiated mouse is transfused with marrow from a nonirradiated syngeneic mouse, its marrow is repopulated and hematopoiesis resumes. In addition to repopulating the bone marrow, the transfused marrow will establish colonies of hematopoiesis in the spleen, each colony derived from a single stem cell. These spleen cell colonies contain granulocytes, erythrocytes, platelets, and their less mature precursors, so the founding stem cell is referred to as pluripotent, ie, capable of giving rise to cells of all three lineages. When normal bone marrow is exposed to high doses of ^{3}H-TdR and then transfused into a lethally irradiated, syngeneic mouse, the number of spleen colonies formed is reduced only slightly, compared with the number obtained with transfusion of marrow not exposed to the isotope. The conclusion is that the marrow's stem cells are not rapidly proliferating, ie, most are in G_0. Yet if the donor marrow is stimulated to proliferate, as might occur if the donor were rendered anemic by phlebotomy, then exposure of that marrow to ^{3}H-TdR before transplantation results in a more pronounced reduction in the number of spleen colonies formed.[11] The induction of anemia caused the stem cells to move out of G_0 and back into the cell cycle, so that the deficit in erythrocytes might be corrected.

The stem cell model of tissue growth has been extended to describe the growth of nonhematopoietic tissues, including tumors. Several lines of evidence argue for the propriety of applying this model to malignant tissues. First, it is well established that nearly all tumors arise from a single pluripotential, albeit aberrant founding (stem) cell. The monoclonal origin of human tumors was strongly suggested by the unique paraprotein of multiple myeloma and by cytogenetic studies in leukemia (the best example of which is the 9;22 translocation in CML); it was most firmly established by the finding of a single G-6-PD isoenzyme in tumor cells of women heterozygous at the G-6-PD locus. Second, tumors, like bone marrow, contain cells of varying degrees of differentiation. The more differentiated cells have low rates of proliferation and, when transplanted, are incapable of establishing new tumors. The less differentiated cells have higher proliferative rates just as the LI is higher for myeloblasts than for myelocytes) and are more efficient at founding new tumors. Indeed, the more anaplastic tumors tend to have higher growth fractions and follow a more fulminant course if left without effective treatment. The third point in favor of the stem cell model is the response of some human tumors to radiation therapy. Radiation therapy can cure tumors that arise spontaneously in humans at doses that would be incapable of curing experimental tumors of the same size in mice. The increased sensitivity of the spontaneous human tumors appears to reflect a smaller population of stem cells.

Stem cells in tumors have been measured directly through (1) mouse spleen colony assays (eg, injection of lymphoma cells into a mouse with the ensuing appearance of lymphoma colonies in the spleen), (2) the enumeration of metastatic lung colonies following IV injection of tumor cells into mice, and (3) tumor colony formation in vitro.[12] The last method has been applied to human tumors, with somewhat mixed results.[13] The impetus for developing an in vitro assay of human tumor stem cells was the hope that it would enable more rational drug therapy. By noting the effect of varying concentrations of chemotherapeutic agents on stem cell colony formation, one might be able to predict the drugs that would be most likely to have activity in vivo. Unfortunately, although such assays are good at predicting which drugs will not be effective, they fail to accurately predict which drugs will succeed. Nonetheless, the stem cell assay has provided insight into tumor growth. It has demonstrated that only 1/1,000 to 1/10,000 of cells in a tumor is capable of forming colonies of cancer cells in vitro. Although this poor cloning efficiency could be due in part to technical problems related to growing cells in culture, it more likely reflects the fact that most cells in a tumor have a very limited potential, if any, for self-renewal.

Controversy exists over the proliferative status of stem cells in human tumors, some studies indicating that they spend less time in G_0 than do their bone marrow counterparts.[14,15] Nonetheless, it is clear that the proliferating cells of a tumor—perhaps the cells that respond most dramatically to chemotherapy and yield clinical regression of disease (albeit transient)—

are not necessarily the cells that need to be eradicated to effect a cure. Thus, the tumor response to a drug is best assessed by measuring the survival not of all tumor cells but rather only of clonogenic or stem cells.

Relationships Between Tumor Cell Survival and Drug Dose

For most of the commonly employed chemotherapeutic agents, the relationship between tumor cell survival and drug dose is exponential, with the number of cells surviving a given dose of drug being proportional to both (1) the drug dose and (2) the number of cells at risk for exposure to the drug:

$$dN \propto N dD$$

where N = number of cells in the tumor, and D = drug dose, or:

$$dN = -KNdD$$

where the proportionality constant, -K, is introduced with a negative sign since the number of cells decreases with increasing drug dose. Rearranging and integrating the equation above yields the more useful formula

$$N = N_0 e^{-K(D-D_0)}$$

where the subscript *0* indicates the initial dose and cell number.

A simple exponential relationship like this one implies that the death of a tumor cell is the consequence of a simple interaction between the drug molecule and its target in the cell. Of more immediate clinical relevance, exponential cell killing implies that (1) multiple courses of therapy will be needed to eradicate the tumor, since each dose of drug produces the same *proportion* of cells killed, *not* the same number of cells killed; and (2) small changes in the drug dose may translate into large changes in cell survival. Imagine that at the beginning of treatment a tumor contains 10^{10} cells. If each course of treatment results in the death of 99.9% of these cells, and if one log of cell growth occurs between courses of treatment, then five courses of treatment are required to eliminate the last cell (Fig 6-13). Note that this reasoning assumes an ideal situation in which (1) all cells are equally sensitive to the drug and (2) cells resistant to the drug are absent at the outset of therapy and no such cells develop during therapy. These assumptions are not valid, of course, during the treatment of spontaneous human tumors (indeed, nonkinetic forms of drug resistance are the major impediment to the successful treatment of human tumors), but the example makes the point that repeated courses of treatment are necessary. It also demonstrates that complete clinical remission, typically achieved when the number of

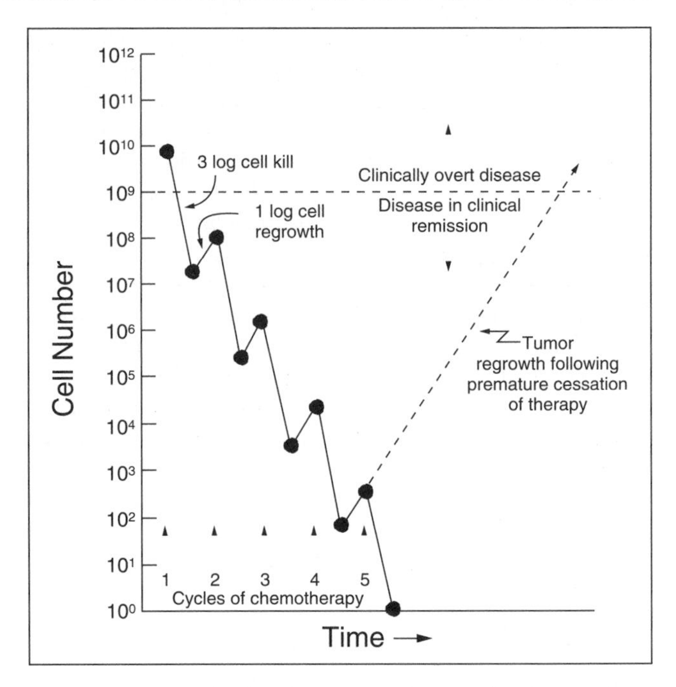

Fig 6-13. Relationship between tumor cell survival and chemotherapy administration. The exponential relationship between drug dose and tumor cell survival dictates that a constant proportion, not number, of tumor cells is killed with each treatment cycle. In this example, each cycle of drug administration results in 99.9% (3 log) cell kill, and 1 log of cell regrowth occurs between cycles. The broken line indicates what would occur if the last cycle of therapy were omitted: despite complete clinical remission of disease, the tumor would ultimately recur.

tumor cells falls below 10^9, does not equal a cure; treatment must be continued despite the absence of an overt tumor. Continued treatment with potentially toxic drugs when no tumor is clinically evident is difficult for both the patient and the oncologist. Only rarely does the oncologist have the benefit of being able to follow a sensitive and specific tumor marker (eg, beta-human chorionic gonadotropin in the management of choriocarcinoma) to monitor the effect of treatment beyond the point of complete remission.

The disproportionate increase in cell survival that results from a decrease in drug dose is readily shown with a simple example. Assume that a tumor before any treatment contains 10^{11} cells. Also assume that the proportionality constant, -K, is -5 for the alkylating agent cyclophosphamide when used in the treatment of this particular tumor. If a dose of 1.5 g of cyclophosphamide is delivered, the tumor will be left with 5.5×10^7 cells:

$$N = N_0 e^{-K(D-D_0)}; N_0 = 10^{11} \text{ when } D_0 = 0$$

$$N = 10^{11} e^{-5(1.5-0)} = 5.5 \times 10^7 \text{ cells.}$$

What happens if the oncologist chooses to administer 0.75 g of cyclophosphamide instead of 1.5 g?

$$N = 10^{11} e^{-5(0.75 - 0)} = 2.4 \times 10^{9} \text{ cells.}$$

The result: a 50% decrease in dose has translated into a 98% increase in cell survival!

A reduction in the drug dose is often unavoidable because of undue toxicity to normal tissue (eg, myelosuppression, mucositis). Nonetheless, it is clear that administering drugs in full dosages (which implies both the amount and frequency with which a drug is given) is an important goal when treating patients. To underscore this point, a retrospective analysis of women receiving adjuvant chemotherapy for stage II, node-positive carcinoma of the breast indicated that women who received the full dose of scheduled drugs were less likely to develop recurrent disease than those receiving lesser doses.[16]

Plots of cell survival as a function of drug dose have rarely been constructed for human tumors under treatment in vivo. Such curves have been constructed, however, for animal tumors using the spleen colony assay or a metastatic lung nodule assay, and for both animal and human tumor cell lines cultured in vitro. It is important to note that these experimental systems measure the survival only of clonogenic tumor cells as a function of drug dose; as emphasized earlier, clonogenic cells are of interest inasmuch as it is *their* elimination that is necessary for a cure.

In the spleen colony assay, tumor cells (eg, from a murine lymphoma) are injected into a lethally irradiated syngeneic mouse following exposure of the tumor cells to varying doses of drug.[17] The number of tumor cell colonies that subsequently appear in the spleen reflects the number of clonogenic cells surviving drug exposure. Some tumors will form metastatic lung nodules following IV injection, and stem cell survival can be assayed in this manner as well. The first conclusion to be drawn from such studies and the analogous in vitro cell culture assays is that the slope of the cell-survival-versus-drug-dose curve is much steeper for rapidly proliferating cells; ie, tumors whose clonogenic cells are more often "in cycle" (not in G_0) are more sensitive to a given drug dose.[18] Only a handful of drugs—specifically cisplatin, the nitrosoureas, nitrogen mustard, and bleomycin—show little increased toxicity for proliferating cells.[19]

The second conclusion to be drawn from these curves is that some chemotherapeutic drugs exhibit a plateau in cell killing as dose is further increased (Fig 6-14). Drugs behaving in this manner have their exclusive or major effect during a single phase of the cell cycle, characteristically during the S phase. To increase cell kill beyond the plateau level, the *duration* of exposure must be prolonged to allow more tumor cells to enter the susceptible phase of the cell cycle. The antimetabolites—drugs structurally similar to normal metabolites that disrupt cell function by competing with these normal precursor molecules in critical metabolic pathways—are the most notable drugs of this type and include cytosine arabinoside, thioguanine, mercaptopurine, methotrexate, 5-FU, and hydroxyurea. Recognition of the plateau in the cell-survival-versus-dose curve for antimetabolites has greatly influenced the manner in which antimetabolites are administered to patients; selected examples are presented later in the section describing individual chemotherapeutic agents.

Mechanisms of Drug Resistance

Given that most chemotherapeutic agents are more toxic to rapidly proliferating tumors, and that the proliferative rate of a tumor increases as its size decreases, it should follow that a tumor, having responded favorably to an initial course of chemotherapy, would become increasingly sensitive to treatment during subsequent courses. Unfortunately, this scenario rarely, if ever, transpires. More typically, tumors regress and may even become clinically undetectable during the initial courses of chemotherapy, but resurge with vigor despite continuation of the same therapy. Tumor growth kinetics clearly fail to explain this sequence of events.

A variety of mechanisms other than a tumor's growth fraction or a cell's location in the cell cycle exist to explain why malignancies are resistant to chemotherapy. First, tumor cells may reside in "sanctuaries" inaccessible to most drugs. The central nervous system (CNS) and testes are often impervious to drugs that distribute freely to other tissues, and represent frequent sites of relapse notwithstanding successful treatment elsewhere. The treatment of childhood ALL advanced with the recognition that the meninges were often a site of recurrent disease and that prophylactic treatment of the CNS, either with radiation or intrathecal methotrexate, could increase the chances for cure in children who had achieved a complete remission with systemic therapy. Second, drug resistance may be more apparent than real, as occurs when a drug is incompletely absorbed, rapidly metabolized and excreted, or incompletely converted to its active form. In many treatment protocols, these forms of what might be called "pseudoresistance" are at least partially circumvented by escalating drug doses until mild normal tissue toxicity occurs. Although these forms of drug resistance are important, by far the most important forms of drug resistance—the most typical explanations for treatment failure—lie in the genetic and biochemical makeup of malignant cells.

The genetic basis of drug resistance in malignant

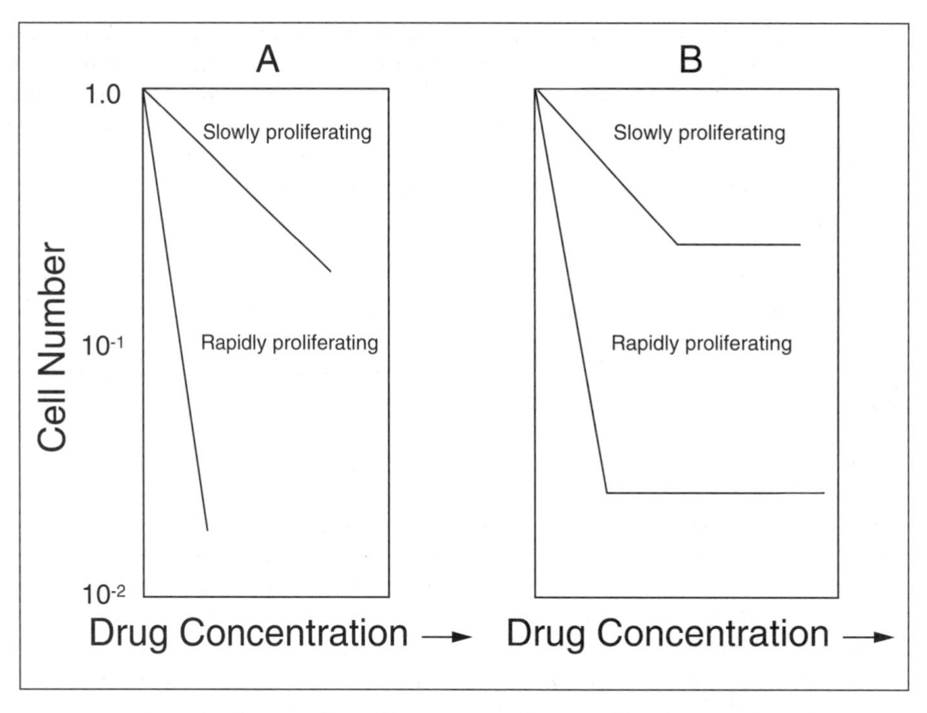

Fig 6-14. Relationship between the proliferative rate of tumor cells and sensitivity to chemotherapy. ***A*** Cell populations are briefly exposed to varying concentrations of drug with subsequent determination of clonogenic cell survival. Rapidly proliferating cells, ie, cell populations with few cells in G_0, are more sensitive to a given drug dose than are slowly proliferating cells. The drugs used in these experiments are without significant specificity for any one phase of the cell cycle. ***B*** These experiments were performed as in A, but with drugs that are specific for one phase of the cell cycle, eg, S phase. Again, rapidly proliferating cells are more sensitive to a given drug dose than are slowly proliferating cells. However, there is now a plateau in survival with increasing drug dose for both types of cell populations. Further decline in cell survival can be achieved only by prolonging the duration of exposure to the drug, allowing more cells to enter the susceptible phase of the cell cycle.

cells is now well established. The same procedures used to prove that bacterial drug resistance results from spontaneous mutation and subsequent selection (the fluctuation test of Luria and Delbruck) have been applied to tumor cells cultured in vivo.[20] If tumor cells are aliquoted in equal amounts onto media containing equivalent concentrations of a given chemotherapeutic agent, the number of tumor colonies appearing on each of those media—the progeny of single resistant cells—is equal. The rate of development of drug resistance calculated from such experiments is consistent with known rates of spontaneous mutation: roughly 1 of 10^6 to 10^7 cells. Moreover, if tumor cells are initially plated onto media without drug and allowed to grow to a given size, and subsequently subplated onto media with drug, then the number of colonies appearing in these subcultures varies significantly from one plate to the next. In the drug-free medium, there is no selection pressure for drug-resistant cells, so their number varies widely, reflecting the random nature of spontaneous mutation. Other evidence for the genetic basis of drug resistance includes (1) the fact that the drug-resistant phenotype may persist despite the absence of drug, and (2) the observation that mutagens may increase the rate at which drug-resistant cells appear. Perhaps most compelling are experiments in which DNA transfer from drug-resistant to drug-sensitive cells confers the drug-resistant phenotype on the formerly vulnerable cells.[21] Although these arguments most readily apply to drug resistance arising from a point mutation, and on the surface appear to exclude the idea that drugs may induce resistance to themselves by means other than simply increasing the rate of spontaneous mutation, it turns out that a Lamarckian view of drug resistance has some validity (see discussion of multidrug resistance below).

Disregarding the complexities of drug resistance for a moment, if the only force causing tumor cells to become resistant were spontaneous mutation, then a tumor containing 10^9 cells, ie, one that has just become clinically detectable, probably already contains 10^2 to 10^3 resistant cells (10^9 cells x $1/10^7$ or $1/10^8$). If the rate of spontaneous mutation is fixed, then the smaller a tumor is, the less likely it is to contain drug-resistant cells. This conclusion makes intuitive sense, but what is not so readily apparent is the exponential relationship between tumor size and the probability of finding drug-resistant cells. Through the use of a mathematical model, Goldie and Coldman have predicted the following relationship:

$$P_0 = 1/e^{\alpha(N-1)}$$

where P_0 equals the probability of finding no drug-resistant cells within a tumor containing N cells and having a spontaneous rate of mutation α.[22] This relationship predicts that the curability of a tumor—here equated with the probability of there being no drug-resistant cells—does not decline gradually as the tumor grows larger, but instead decreases precipitously as the tumor approaches a critical size determined by its rate of spontaneous mutation. A tumor containing 10^6 cells and having a spontaneous mutation rate of 10^{-7} stands only a 10% chance of containing drug-resistant cells, but if the tumor is allowed to grow 1.5 logs (to 5 x 10^7 cells), this chance increases to >99%!

The clinical messages behind the Goldie-Coldman model are that (1) smaller tumors are easier to cure, and (2) the best moment for effective treatment is as soon after detection of the tumor as possible. Delays in treatment, by allowing a modest increase in tumor burden, can result in a greatly increased probability of encountering drug-resistant cells and may thus forfeit the patient's chance for cure or at least meaningful disease regression. The Goldie-Coldman model can be extended to argue that patients should benefit from the use of multiple, noncross-resistant drugs (effectively decreasing the rate of spontaneous mutation) and that equally effective, noncross-resistant regimens should be given alternately rather than sequentially. The use of multiple chemotherapeutic agents in combination has been responsible for much of the success achieved in the treatment of childhood ALL, Hodgkin's disease, and testicular carcinoma; single-agent therapy is clearly inferior in these settings. Admittedly, the superiority of combination regimens is not so evident in some of the more common solid tumors, such as colon cancer. But the failure of multiple agents in the treatment of these tumors is not so much a failure of the Goldie-Coldman model as a reflection of the inherently high levels of resistance of these tumors to all currently available chemotherapeutic agents. And there are, of course, practical limitations on the extent to which the theoretical advantages of combination chemotherapy can be taken. Two or even three drugs may possess activity against a given tumor, but if they all produce similar normal tissue toxicities (eg, if they all are highly myelosuppressive), they will prove difficult to combine in the clinic. Either the combination will result in excessive morbidity and mortality, or the drug doses will be reduced to ineffective levels. Unfortunately, the problem of drug resistance goes well beyond the simple model of random spontaneous mutation to resistance and subsequent selection. The first level of complexity lies in the ability of some drugs to promote resistance against themselves (the Lamarckian view of drug resistance alluded to earlier). Resistance to the antimetabolite methotrexate (MTX) can be effected through several mechanisms.[23] An alteration in the cell surface membrane receptor for folates, as might occur by a point mutation, can decrease intracellular levels of MTX and result in reduced inhibition of the target enzyme, dihydrofolate reductase (DHFR). Once MTX enters the cell, a number of glutamic acid residues are added to the single glutamic acid moiety that forms one end of the MTX molecule. Such polyglutamation, which also occurs with the normal substrate, folic acid, keeps MTX from exiting the cell and yet does not alter its ability to inhibit DHFR. Decreased polyglutamation of the drug is another potential mechanism for resistance. Although uncommon, MTX resistance may be conferred by an alteration in the structure of the DHFR enzyme so that MTX binds to it less avidly.

By far the most common form of MTX resistance (at least in experimental tumors and cell lines) is production by the resistant cell of exceedingly large amounts of DHFR through a process known as gene amplification.[24] In this process, a gene is replicated not once but many times over while the cell is in S phase. Such amplification is promoted by drugs like MTX, which transiently interrupt DNA synthesis in replicating cells. The degree to which the DHFR gene is amplified can be increased by gradually increasing the amount of MTX to which tumor cells are exposed. Moreover, if cells so induced to amplify the DHFR gene are no longer exposed to MTX, they may lose some of their resistance to the drug. This phenomenon is related to the loss of amplified DHFR genes located in relatively unstable, poorly conserved extrachromosomal structures called "double minutes."

Multidrug Resistance

A second level of complexity is found in the observation that the development of resistance to one chemotherapeutic agent often results in the coincident development of resistance to other drugs, albeit structurally unrelated.[25] The appearance of the multidrug-resistant phenotype is associated with the expression of a cell surface glycoprotein, called P-170.[26] Cells expressing P-170 tend to manifest decreased uptake and increased efflux of the drugs to which they are resistant; although not entirely settled, there is evidence implicating P-170 as this "drug pump." The multidrug-resistant phenotype is stable even in the absence of exposure to the drugs to which resistance has developed. Furthermore, the gene encoding the P-170 glycoprotein, called *mdr*1, has been isolated, sequenced, and transferred to a drug-sensitive cell line, thus conferring resistance.[21] Although the phenomenon of multidrug resistance was originally described and subsequently elucidated in vitro, it likely has relevance to the treatment of tumors that arise spontaneously in humans. Indeed, the P-170 glycoprotein has been identified in a resistant human ovarian cell line,[27] and it has been possible to demonstrate expression of the *mdr*1 gene in some human tumors.[28] To date, recognition of this phenomenon of multidrug resistance has borne no obvious fruit in the clinic. In vitro data indicate that compounds inhibiting calcium entry into cells (eg, verapamil) interfere with calcium binding to calmodulin, and other drugs that stabilize cell membranes (eg, quinidine) can partially restore drug sensitivity. An initial clinical trial with verapamil was disappointing; a trial with quinidine should be forthcoming.[29]

Tumor Cell Heterogeneity

A third layer of complexity in the problem of drug resistance emanates from the genetic and phenotypic heterogeneity of human tumors.[30] The origin of all cells in a tumor from a single aberrant stem cell was emphasized earlier. Despite the common ancestry, it is the rule rather than the exception that the cells of a tumor are diversified both genetically and phenotypically. Like their normal tissue counterparts, tumors retain some of the originally programmed ability to mature and differentiate.

In the early stages of growth, a tumor may differ phenotypically only slightly from its tissue of origin, but as it enlarges, a tumor characteristically becomes less differentiated or more anaplastic, and more difficult to treat. The genetic material of malignant cells is more unstable than that of normal cells, a fact most grossly manifested by multiple chromosomal defects (breaks, deletions, translocations, inversions, and the evanescent extrachromosomal double minutes) and expressed by higher mutation rates as measured by clonal selection for drug resistance. Moreover, chemotherapeutic agents may add to this genetic instability by acting as mutagens themselves. Hence, new subclones of malignant cells appear routinely; those with an increased capacity for self-renewal and proliferation gradually replace the more slowly growing, differentiated cells in the tumor, and drug-resistant clones replace sensitive ones in the face of treatment. Classic examples of disease evolution include (1) Richter's syndrome, in which a patient with chronic lymphocytic leukemia (CLL) develops an aggressive diffuse large-cell lymphoma, and (2) the progression of CML, initially an indolent myeloproliferative disorder with a single chromosomal abnormality (the 9;22 translocation), to a more fulminant disease (blast crisis), still accompanied by the 9;22 translocation but heralded by other chromosomal abnormalities.

Standard Chemotherapeutic Agents

It is beyond the scope of this section to describe each standard chemotherapeutic agent in detail and give specific guidelines for its proper clinical use. This critical information is readily available from several sources.[31-33] Rather, the purpose of the current discussion is to introduce the major classes of cytotoxic drugs, emphasizing their mechanisms of action, pharmacology, and unique toxicities. Selected agents will be described in some detail either because they are commonly used or because they are illustrative of the interplay between drug pharmacology and tumor growth kinetics. A classification scheme based on mechanism of action would be ideal, but in many instances a drug kills tumor cells in several ways or is effective for reasons not yet well understood. Therefore a conventional format will be used, categorizing drugs as (1) alkylating agents, (2) antimetabolites, (3) antitumor antibiotics, (4) plant alkaloids, (5) hormonal agents, or (6) miscellaneous compounds. The recently introduced interferons, interleukins, and hematopoietic growth factors, along with other novel approaches to systemic cancer treatment, will be briefly described.

Alkylating Agents

An alkylating agent, mechlorethamine, was the first nonhormonal cytotoxic drug found to be useful in the treatment of malignant disease. Although structurally diverse, all alkylators have or generate via intermediates reactive functional groups that are electron-deficient and that form covalent bonds with electron-rich (nucleophilic) groups in nucleic acids, proteins, and an array of smaller molecules. Despite the wide range of groups with which alkylating agents can form covalent bonds (amino, imidazole, carboxyl, sulfhydryl, and phosphate), the bases in DNA are by far the most important, particularly the electron-rich N-7 position of guanine. DNA alkylation produces a variety of defects (depurination, double-stranded and single-stranded breaks, inter-strand and intrastrand cross-links) that disrupt (sometimes permanently) DNA replication and transcription. This fundamental alteration in the information coded in the DNA molecule, if it cannot be efficiently repaired, may be expressed in cellular death, mutagenesis, or carcinogenesis. The primacy of DNA base alkylation in mediating these effects is underscored by the heightened susceptibility to alkylating agents of cells known to be deficient in DNA repair enzymes. Conversely, an increased ability to repair such damage represents one form of resistance to these drugs. In contrast to the antimetabolites, which interfere with the pathways leading to the synthesis of new DNA (and RNA), alkylating agents react with preformed nucleic acids. Thus, they tend to be active throughout all phases of the cell cycle. Although most alkylating agents are more toxic to proliferating than to nonproliferating cells, the distinction is not as pronounced as it is for the antimetabolites; in fact, for a subset of the alkylating agents, the nitrosoureas, the distinction hardly exists at all.[19] This ability to kill nonproliferating cells makes alkylators attractive drugs to use against tumors with low growth fractions (eg, multiple myeloma). Moreover, alkylating agents have an almost infinite number of potential sites in DNA for disruption and, lacking the cell cycle or cell cycle phase specificity of antimetabolites, they do not typically exhibit a plateau in cell survival with increasing dose. These features make them theoretically attractive drugs to use in testing the notion of drug intensity—ie, the idea that the logarithmic relationship between drug dose and cell survival can be exploited to clinical advantage—as in high-dose chemotherapy followed by bone marrow rescue.

Unfortunately, the same properties that make alkylating agents effective as chemotherapy produce a set of unique long-term toxicities. Their ability to kill the slowly cycling stem cells of tumors also translates into toxicity for the stem cells of the bone marrow. In contrast to the predictable and short-lived myelosuppression of drugs that merely destroy the more mature cells of the marrow (eg, myeloblasts, myelocytes, metamyelocytes, and neutrophils), alkylators are often responsible for producing delayed, prolonged, and even permanent marrow failure. Stem cell toxicity is also manifested by the frequent development of amenorrhea in women and oligospermia or azoospermia in men, often causing irreversible infertility. Finally, the most feared stem cell toxicity of alkylating agents is their mutagenic and ultimately carcinogenic effect on bone marrow stem cells, culminating in a form of AML that is relatively refractory to treatment. The risk of developing AML is directly proportional to the total drug dose a patient receives as well as the length of follow-up; for a group of patients with ovarian carcinoma followed for 10 years after completing alkylator therapy, the risk of AML was as high as 5% to 10%.[34]

The oldest group of alkylating agents, the nitrogen mustards, includes mechlorethamine (the prototype), melphalan, chlorambucil, cyclophosphamide, and ifosfamide. Mechlorethamine is a highly reactive and unstable molecule, liable to cause irritation at the site of injection; its clinical use has become rather limited to the four-drug MOPP regimen used to treat Hodgkin's disease and occasionally other lymphomas. The other nitrogen mustards are derivatives of mechlorethamine; they all contain ring structures that render them more stable and, with the exception of ifosfamide, are available as oral preparations. Chlorambucil has a very narrow spectrum of activity, being restricted to the treatment of slowly growing lymphoid neoplasms such as CLL, Waldenström's macroglobulinemia, and indolent non-Hodgkin's lymphomas. Although in the past melphalan has played a role in the treatment of breast and ovarian carcinomas, it is now used primarily for managing multiple myeloma. Melphalan is notorious for its erratic GI absorption; 20% to 50% of an oral dose can be recovered in the feces. IV administration of melphalan can circumvent this problem, but the usual clinical practice is to titrate the oral dose of melphalan to mild hematologic toxicity.

Cyclophosphamide, the most versatile alkylating agent, is unique among the nitrogen mustards on several accounts. First, cyclophosphamide is itself inactive, requiring hepatic metabolism to 4-hydroxycyclophosphamide before yielding active alkylating metabolites. 4-Hydroxycyclophosphamide (in equilibrium with its acyclic isomer, aldophosphamide) is transported into cells where it spontaneously decomposes into phosphora thought to be responsible for the urothelial toxicity of cyclophosphamide (see below). Second, the metabolites of cyclophosphamide have a more selective toxicity for proliferating cells than do other alkylators: prolonged myelosuppression does not occur, cumulative toxicity to the marrow is unusual, and leukemogenesis appears to be less of a problem than with other alkylating agents.[35] These advantages, coupled with the drug's activity against a very broad spectrum of tumors, have made it the most commonly administered alkylating agent.

The peculiar toxicity of cyclophosphamide and its newer analogue, ifosfamide, is an acute sterile hemorrhagic cystitis, which occurs in up to 10% of patients treated with the former. As mentioned above, the metabolite acrolein is thought to be the culprit. Hemorrhagic cystitis can be largely prevented by simply maintaining a high urine output. However, with high-dose administration of either drug, consideration should be given to the co-administration of either N-acetylcysteine (Mucomyst) or sodium 2-mercaptoethanesulfonate (mesna), thiol compounds that neutralize acrolein.

The pharmacokinetics of cyclophosphamide have not been fully described because some metabolites are difficult to detect in plasma. Nonetheless, it is clear that both the parent compound and its metabolites are excreted by the kidneys. Renal failure results in prolonged blood levels but usually not in increased toxicity, probably because renal clearance of the parent drug is normally low and can be maintained even in patients with marginal renal function. Since cyclophosphamide requires activation by hepatic microsomal enzymes, one would anticipate liver dysfunction to prompt a change in dose. Systematic data on the influence of renal and hepatic dysfunction on the choice of dose is lacking, however. Common sense would suggest attenuated doses of cyclophosphamide in patients with severe renal failure.

There are four other chemical classes of alkylating agents: (1) the nitrosoureas (carmustine, lomustine, semustine, streptozocin); (2) the alkyl sulfonates (busulfan); (3) the triazines (dacarbazine); and (4) the ethylenimines (thiotepa, hexamethylmelamine). The nitrosoureas are distinguished by their lipid solubility, suggesting a potential role in the treatment of intracranial tumors, and by their lack of cross-resistance with other alkylating agents. Their clinical usefulness has been limited, however, by a tendency to cause more delayed, prolonged, and cumulative myelosuppression than other alkylators. Busulfan, the only alkyl sulfonate in clinical use, deserves mention for its longstanding role in CML, which is based on a high degree of selectivity for the myeloid cells of the bone marrow. In some cases, busulfan can produce a period of drug-free clinical remission, albeit always impermanent.

Antimetabolites

Interest in antimetabolite development followed the discovery that folic acid antagonists were effective in the treatment of childhood ALL. Elucidation of the biochemical pathways leading to DNA and RNA synthesis enabled proliferation of a large number of drugs fashioned to be structurally similar to critical intermediates (metabolites) in these pathways. Antimetabolites function by either (1) competing with normal metabolites for the catalytic or regulatory site of a key enzyme or (2) substituting for a metabolite that is normally incorporated into an important molecule, eg, DNA or RNA. Because most antimetabolites interfere with nucleic acid synthesis (rather than with preformed nucleic acids, like the alkylating agents), they have little, if any, effect on cells in G_0 and usually exhibit maximum activity during S phase. The enzymes inhibited by antimetabolites are fewer than the sites potentially available to alkylating agents (ie, the almost innumerable bases of DNA), and complete inhibition of these enzymes may occur at clinically achievable drug levels. Such relatively complete target inhibition, coupled with specificity for cells in a single phase of the cell cycle, explains the plateau in cell survival with increasing drug dose. Also in contrast to the alkylating agents, antimetabolites are not associated with delayed or prolonged myelosuppression, and they appear to present a minimal risk of leukemogenesis or carcinogenesis—all likely reflections of their impotence vis-à-vis slowly proliferating stem cells.

Folic Acid Analogues

A number of folic acid analogues have been produced that inhibit the enzyme DHFR; however, only methotrexate is in current clinical use. DHFR is responsible for the generation of reduced folates, molecules occupying key positions in nucleic acid synthesis. Reduced folates are required for the transfer of methyl groups during the biosynthesis of purines. Moreover, inhibition of DHFR blocks the production of N_5, N_{10}-methylene tetrahydrofolate, a reduced folate coenzyme that participates with thymidylate synthetase in the conversion of 2-deoxyuridylate to thymidylate. DNA synthesis ceases as a result of this lack of dTMP and purines.

Plasma MTX is about 50% bound to plasma proteins and is eliminated primarily by the kidneys without extensive metabolism. Disappearance of MTX from the plasma is essentially biphasic: the initial distribution phase has a $t_{1/2}$ of 2 to 3 hours, while the final phase has a $t_{1/2}$ of 8 to 10 hours. The terminal phase is prolonged with renal dysfunction. A third elimination phase, which occurs very slowly, also has been described and is attributed to enterohepatic circulation of the drug. The renal excretion of MTX can be inhibited by coadministration of weak organic acids, eg, aspirin or penicillin. Aspirin can further compound toxicity by displacing MTX from its binding site on albumin, increasing the concentration of free drug.

The cytotoxicity of MTX depends critically on the duration of exposure of a tissue to the drug above a certain threshold value rather than on the peak level of drug in the tissue.[36] Irrespective of the duration of exposure to MTX, toxicity for many tissues does not occur until the level of drug exceeds 10^{-8} molar. Conversely, exceedingly high levels of MTX may be well tolerated by normal tissues provided exposure is limited to 24 to 36 hours. The availability of a reduced folate "antidote" in the form of 5-formyltetrahydrofolate (leucovorin) allows the duration of methotrexate-induced dTMP and purine depletion to be precisely controlled; the ability to measure serum MTX levels allows one to determine how much leucovorin to give and when leucovorin rescue may be safely discontinued.

An appreciation of these details of pharmacology has allowed MTX to be delivered in doses 10 to 100 times greater than conventional levels. The major impetus to administration of such high doses is the theoretic possibility of overcoming forms of MTX resistance: Defects in active transport of the drug might be overcome by passive diffusion; increased amounts of DHFR from gene amplification might be more completely inhibited; intracellular levels of the drug might remain high despite decreased polyglutamation; and even enzymes with reduced affinity for MTX might be inhibited. Moreover, high-dose MTX followed by leucovorin rescue can achieve tumoricidal drug levels in the CNS and, if properly performed, is without myelosuppression; the latter advantage would permit more frequent drug administration. These theoretic advantages explain the inclusion of high-dose MTX with leucovorin rescue in experimental protocols for diseases such as ALL, lymphomas, and tumors of the head and neck. Yet the only disease for which high-dose MTX with leucovorin rescue has become standard is osteogenic sarcoma. Indeed, it is rare to observe responses to high-dose MTX in patients whose tumors are refractory to conventional doses. One surmises that the resistance of in vivo human tumors to MTX has less to do with the mechanisms of resistance cited above and perhaps more to do with the limited potential of a drug that depends so heavily on DNA synthesis for its toxicity in the treatment of tumors with low growth fractions. The exquisite sensitivity of rapidly proliferating gestational trophoblastic carcinoma to conventional doses of MTX lends additional credence to this argument. Enthusiasm for high-dose regimens is also tempered by (1) the propensity of MTX in high doses to precipitate in the renal tubules (avoided by maintaining a high urine output and by alkalinizing the urine, all of which requires hospitalization); (2) the tendency of MTX in high doses to significantly accumulate within third-space fluid compartments (eg, pleural and peritoneal effusions) and thereafter to slowly diffuse out, producing prolonged exposure to the drug; (3) the need to measure plasma MTX levels; and (4) the enormous cost of leucovorin.

Methotrexate enjoys a wide spectrum of antitumor activity. As cited above, it is usually curative in single-agent therapy for gestational trophoblastic carcinoma. MTX is included in many combination regimens for ALL, lymphomas, carcinoma of the breast, and tumors of the head and neck. It is particularly useful as an intrathecal agent when treating leptomeningeal tumor infiltrates.

Pyrimidine Analogues

5-Fluorouracil resembles both uracil and thymidine. Phosphorylation of 5-FU to 5-fluorouridine triphosphate (5-FUTP) allows the analogue to be incorporated into RNA; nuclear processing of messenger and ribosomal RNA is disrupted, and the fraudulent pyrimidine may cause errors in base pairing during RNA transcription. 5-FU is also converted to 5-fluorouridine monophosphate (5-FdUMP), a compound that irreversibly inhibits thymidylate synthetase; DNA synthesis is brought to a halt because of thymidine depletion. These two mechanisms of cytotoxicity allow 5-FU to be active throughout the cell cycle, not just in S phase. 5-FU is given intravenously because of erratic GI absorption. A single IV bolus of 5-FU has a plasma $t_{1/2}$ of only 10 to 30 minutes, and no drug can be detected in plasma after 3 hours. However, intracellular levels may persist for hours. Although the bulk of 5-FU is catabolized by the liver, the absence of responsible enzymes in some colon carcinomas may explain its usefulness in treating GI carcinomas.

5-FU as a single agent exhibits only modest activity. Recently, the effectiveness of 5-FU appears to have been enhanced by the concomitant administration of leucovorin. When 5-FdUMP binds to thymidylate synthetase, it forms part of a ternary complex that includes N_5, N_{10}-methylenetetrahydrofolate—the normal coenzyme for thymidylate synthetase. Although this ternary complex is covalent, it dissociates with a $t_{1/2}$ of 2 to 3 hours in the absence of excess N_5, N_{10}-methylenetetrahydrofolate. High levels of N_5, N_{10}-methylenetetrahydrofolate, derived from leucovorin, produce optimal conditions for the formation of this complex and deter its subsequent degradation. Clinical trials have yielded evidence to argue that the combination of 5-FU and leucovorin is better than 5-FU alone in the treatment of advanced colon cancer.[37]

Cytosine arabinoside (Ara-C) differs from deoxycytidine only in its sugar moiety, with arabinose replacing deoxyribose. Ara-C penetrates cells via a carrier-mediated process shared with deoxycytidine. Once in the cell, Ara-C, like deoxycytidine, can follow one of two major paths: deamination to the nontoxic compound Ara-U, or sequential phosphorylation to Ara-CTP, the active form of the drug. The toxicity of Ara-CTP arises from its ability to competitively inhibit the binding of the normal substrate, dCTP, to DNA polymerase; DNA synthesis is thereby arrested. Ara-CTP also may be incorporated into DNA and cause defective ligation or incomplete synthesis of DNA fragments. Both effects are consistent with the drug's selective toxicity for cells in S phase.

Following IV injection, Ara-C is rapidly inactivated to Ara-U by cytidine deaminase, an enzyme widely distributed throughout the body. After a single bolus injection, Ara-C has a plasma $t_{1/2}$ of only 7 to 20 minutes. Single bolus injections of Ara-C tend to be nontoxic to normal marrow and are ineffective in treating leukemia as well. However, if the drug is administered in two divided doses separated by 12 hours, a significant number of patients with leukemia respond. The greater effectiveness of the q12h regimen lies in the fact that the S phase of AML blasts lasts approximately 18 to 20 hours. If a leukemia cell is in the cell cycle but not in S phase at the time of a bolus injection of Ara-C, it escapes toxicity (the $t_{1/2}$ of Ara-C being so brief). And if the next bolus of Ara-C is not administered until 24 hours later, the same cell may have already passed through S phase and so evade the drug's effect altogether. Yet when Ara-C is given on a q12h schedule, no cycling cell can pass through a complete S phase without being exposed to the drug. If all leukemia cells were in cycle—ie, if none were in G_0—from a purely kinetic perspective, it would be possible to kill all cells by delivering Ara-C as a bolus every 12 hours or as a continuous infusion over the time required to complete one cell cycle. But many leukemia cells are in G_0, so Ara-C must be administered for a longer period (5 to 7 days) to allow as many of these cells as possible to enter the proliferating pool and pass through S phase.

Most drug combinations in current use have evolved empirically, and the sequence in which the drugs are administered usually reflects little more than an attempt to avoid overlapping toxicities. The sequential use of Ara-C and asparaginase to induce remission in patients with refractory or relapsed AML represents an important exception that shows how the sequence of drug administration can be critical. Asparaginase is an enzyme derived from bacterial sources. When given intravenously, it hydrolyzes serum asparagine and deprives leukemia cells of an amino acid they themselves cannot synthesize; normal cells are spared because they generally have the ability to synthesize their own asparagine. When studied in murine leukemia, pharmacologic antagonism occurred when both drugs were administered concurrently or when the asparaginase preceded delivery of Ara-C.[38] The explanation for this antagonism is that asparaginase depletion shuts down protein synthesis, which inhibits the progression of tumor cells from G_1 to S phase. Since Ara-C is active only in cells in S phase, asparaginase pretreatment is actually protective. However, if asparaginase is given after Ara-C, synergistic killing of leukemia cells is observed, associated with increased formation of Ara-CTP and Ara-CDNA. For unclear reasons, asparaginase treatment lowers the cellular pool of the normal metabolite, dCTP, and thus produces less competition for the target enzyme, DNA polymerase. These laboratory observations led to the design of a clinical trial comparing high-dose Ara-C alone with high-dose Ara-C followed by asparaginase in patients with refractory or relapsed AML.[39] The experimental observations bore fruit: the use of sequential high-dose Ara-C and asparaginase resulted in a 42% complete remission rate, while high-dose Ara-C alone achieved a rate of only 12%.

Purine Analogues

There are two guanine analogues in clinical use: 6-mercaptopurine (6-MP) and 6-thioguanine (6-TG). These two drugs are more alike than different, and resistance to one usually predicts resistance to the other. Both parent compounds are inactive until they undergo metabolic conversion to their respective monophosphate ribonucleotides—a result of the enzyme hypoxanthine—guanine phosphoribosyl transferase (HGPRTase), whose normal function is to salvage purines for nucleic acid synthesis by adding ribose phosphate to them. The monophosphate nucleotides are capable of inhibiting de novo purine synthesis, ie, the formation of adenylic and guanylic acids from inosinic acid. Further phosphorylation gives rise to the respective triphosphate nucleotides; in the case of 6-TG, conversion to the deoxyribonucleotide allows significant amounts of the drug to be incorporated into DNA, the extent of which correlates with the production of strand breaks and cellular cytotoxicity.

In experimental tumors, it has been possible to show that resistance to these two purine analogues can ensue from a deficiency in the activating enzyme, HGPRTase. However, leukemia cells are not typically deficient in this enzyme, and other mechanisms of resistance must be important, eg, rapid dephosphorylation of the active nucleotides by a membrane-bound alkaline phosphatase.

6-MP and 6-TG are used almost exclusively for the treatment of leukemias; they have no significant activity against solid tumors. Because of their use in the treatment of leukemia, it is important to understand the differences in their catabolism. 6-MP is oxidized to 6-thiouric acid by xanthine oxidase. The concomitant administration of allopurinol, an inhibitor of xanthine oxidase used to prevent hyperuricemia and acute uric acid nephropathy during rapid leukemia cell lysis, may increase the toxicity of 6-MP by impairing its degradation. The dose of 6-MP is therefore reduced by 75% if allopurinol is to be coadministered. The catabolism of 6-TG follows a different pathway and no dose reduction is required in the presence of allopurinol.

Several adenosine analogues exist, but their clinical utility is limited. Pentostatin (2-deoxycoformycin) is an adenosine analogue produced by a species of *Streptomyces*. It is a powerful inhibitor of adenosine deaminase (ADA), an enzyme that deaminates adenosine to inosine and deoxyadenosine to deoxyinosine. Accumulation of adenosine and deoxyadenosine is toxic to cells, particularly to those of the lymphoid system, as suggested by the severe lymphopenia of children with congenital ADA deficiency. Pentostatin is probably the most active agent in hairy cell leukemia; it also has activity in cutaneous T-cell lymphoma and in CLL. Fludarabine is a recently tested adenosine analogue that is resistant to deamination by adenosine deaminase; it has been found particularly effective in treating CLL.

Antitumor Antibiotics

The antitumor antibiotics—actinomycin D, the anthracyclines, bleomycin, mitomycin C, and mithramycin—are a structurally diverse group of compounds all derived from species of *Streptomyces*. Their cytotoxicity precludes their use as antibacterial agents, but they have proved to be of great value in treating a broad spectrum of tumors. Only the anthracyclines, chosen because of their widespread use in current clinical oncology, will be discussed below.

The most commonly encountered anthracycline, doxorubicin, consists of a planar 4-ring anthraquinone attached to an amino sugar, daunosamine. The related compound, daunorubicin, differs from doxorubicin only by the substitution of a methoxy for a methyl group in the anthraquinone ring; it is used almost exclusively in the treatment of acute leukemia.

The structure-function relationships of doxorubicin and other anthracyclines have been widely examined because they are among the most effective antitumor agents available, yet produce dose-limiting cardiac toxicity. The clinical benefit of separating the two effects would be substantial. The mechanisms underlying anthracycline cytoxicity are complex. First, the anthraquinone ring can intercalate between base pairs of DNA, the stability of this complex being enhanced by the attraction of the amino group of daunosamine for the phosphate groups of the DNA backbone. DNA intercalation results in disruption of DNA replication and RNA transcription, but it is uncertain just how important intercalation is to anthracycline cytoxicity; DNA is normally organized and folded into chromatin, and perhaps is protected from this type of drug interaction. Second, anthracyclines can produce single-stranded and double-stranded DNA scission and impair DNA repair. The process of DNA scission may be facilitated by intercalation between base pairs or by an interaction with topoisomerase II. A third mechanism for generating DNA breaks as well as other forms of damage is the creation of free radicals. The quinone ring of the anthracyclines can assume a semiquinone form with an unpaired electron; this species reacts with molecular oxygen (O_2) to generate superoxide (O_2^-), which disrupts a wide variety of cellular structures, including DNA. However, doxorubicin retains toxicity under hypoxic conditions when superoxide radicals cannot be formed.[40] Finally, anthracyclines tend to bind to almost everything with which they come into contact, and it is possible that they kill cells through disruption of the cell membrane. In fact, in one experimental system in which doxorubicin was attached to small beads, cell death occurred despite the drug's inability to enter cells,[41] lending credence both to the notion of direct membrane disruption and to the importance of free radical formation. Nonetheless, there exists a large literature to support the idea that anthracycline toxicity is in many systems dependent on the drug's ability to enter cells: witness the phenomenon of multidrug resistance, characterized by either decreased influx or increased efflux of anthracyclines, as well as other natural products, across the cell membrane. As one might anticipate, given their wide-ranging effects, the anthracyclines exhibit activity throughout the cell cycle, although effects are most pronounced for cells in S or G_2 phase.

The ability of anthracyclines to generate free radicals has been implicated in the production of cardiac toxicity. Clinical trials of the free radical scavengers vitamin E and N-acetylcysteine, which lessen the cardiac toxicity of doxorubicin in some animal systems, were unsuccessful. However, initial reports of a randomized clinical trial indicate that the EDTA analogue ICRF-187 can reduce the cardiac toxicity of doxorubicin in man without altering its antitumor activity.[42] ICRF-187 is thought to inhibit free radical formation by chelating iron. Anthracyclines can bind ferric iron which, when reduced to ferrous iron, can react with O_2 to produce O_2^-, H_2O_2, and OH^-.

Doxorubicin is administered intravenously and is widely distributed in the body, with extensive binding to plasma proteins and other tissue. Plasma clearance is triphasic: the half-lives of the three phases are 8 to 25 minutes, 1.5 to 10 hours, and 24 to 48 hours. The second phase is attributed to hepatic metabolism of the drug to yield an active metabolite (doxorubicinol) and a number of metabolites (aglycones) that have no antitumor effect but may contribute to cardiac and other toxicities. The final phase reflects release of drug from tissue binding sites. Because doxorubicin and its metabolites are excreted via the bile, dosage reduction is mandatory for patients with biliary obstruction.

As mentioned above, the unique toxicity of doxorubicin is damage to heart muscle, a problem which increases in incidence with increasing cumulative dose of drug. As the total dose of doxorubicin approaches 550 mg/m_2, the incidence rate of chronic congestive heart failure becomes 1% to 4%; above this cumulative dose, the incidence rises dramatically. Patients who receive significant doses of doxorubicin should be monitored for cardiac toxicity. The gold standard is endomyocardial biopsy. However, while this procedure reflects drug-related myocardial damage in a manner that is linear with dose, it is neither practical nor widely available. Most commonly, the left ventricular ejection fraction (LVEF) is determined by radionuclide cineangiography at serial total doses of the drug, with cessation of doxorubicin therapy if the LVEF drops significantly below the baseline value. It is also important to be aware of the increased risk of anthracycline-induced cardiotoxicity in the presence of other cardiac insults, eg, prior mediastinal irradiation, systemic hypertension, and the coadministration of cyclophosphamide or mitomycin C.

Plant Alkaloids

Vinca Alkaloids

Extracts of the periwinkle plant, long believed in folklore to have medicinal value, were found to cause myelosuppression in rats and led to the isolation of two active alkaloid anticancer compounds, vincristine and vinblastine. These two compounds are complex, multiringed molecules of nearly identical structure. Vinblastine differs from vincristine only by the substitution of a formyl group for a methyl group at one point in a side chain of the parent molecule; nonetheless, this seemingly minor structural variation results in a very different pattern of toxicity and antitumor activity.

Vincristine and vinblastine share a common mechanism of cytotoxicity in that they both bind to tubulin, a dimeric protein. Tubulin normally polymerizes to form the microtubular apparatus along which chromosomes migrate during mitosis, and serves as a conduit for neurotransmitter transport along axons. Binding of the vinca alkaloids to tubulin prevents the protein's polymerization. The results are (1) cytotoxicity, manifested by an arrest of cells in metaphase with subsequent lysis, and (2) neurotoxicity, characterized by depressed deep tendon reflexes and paresthesias if mild and by motor weakness, cranial nerve palsies, and paralytic ileus if severe.

The dose-limiting toxicity of vincristine is neurotoxicity; myelosuppression is infrequently observed with conventional doses. Vinblastine, on the other hand, is decidedly myelotoxic with less neurotoxicity. Vincristine is an important component of regimens used to induce remission in childhood ALL, and it finds its way into a variety of combination chemotherapeutic regimens for other malignancies, especially lymphomas. Vinblastine has made a major contribution to combination chemotherapy for testicular carcinoma.

The two vinca alkaloids are both given by IV injection and display similar pharmacokinetics. Both are extensively bound to proteins, producing rapid biphasic clearance from the plasma as they are distributed into body tissue. The terminal phase of plasma clearance is long (20 to 30 hours), and reflects elimination of the drugs and metabolites via the biliary tract. It is common practice to reduce the dose of vincristine and vinblastine in the presence of obstructive liver disease.

Etoposide (VP-16)

Etoposide is a semisynthetic derivative of podophyllotoxin, a cytotoxic drug isolated from the root of the May apple plant and used for years in the topical treatment of condylomata acuminata. Like podophyllotoxin and the vinca alkaloids, etoposide causes metaphase arrest. Unlike these other alkaloids, etoposide does not inhibit microtubule assembly, apparently the result of a sugar moiety absent in the other compounds. On the other hand, etoposide can induce strand breaks in DNA, an effect that is likely mediated by its interaction with topoisomerase II.

Etoposide is usually given intravenously, its absorption following oral administration being quite variable. However, larger doses by the oral route can achieve equal systemic effects. The pharmacokinetics of etoposide have not been well sorted out, but under normal circumstances some 40% to 60% of a dose appears to be excreted in the urine as unchanged drug and metabolites. Nonetheless, normal clearance of VP-16 has been described in a patient with end-stage renal disease. Similarly, hepatic dysfunction does not seem to alter clearance. The only peculiar toxicity of etoposide is a tendency to produce transient hypotension if given by rapid IV injection; this problem is avoided by infusing the drug over ≥30 minutes.

Etoposide currently enjoys a wide range of clinical use. It is a key component of curative combination chemotherapy for nonseminomatous testicular carcinoma. The drug is also included in several combination regimens directed against aggressive forms of non-Hodgkin's lymphoma. Finally, etoposide is probably the most active single agent in small-cell lung cancer.

Hormones and Hormone Antagonists

Just as hormones influence the growth of many normal tissues, so many malignant cells retain a degree of hormonal sensitivity characteristic of their tissue of origin. This is particularly true of carcinomas of the breast, prostate, and endometrium. To date, the only clinically useful hormonal manipulations have involved, directly or indirectly, the steroid hormones. Steroid hormones mediate their effects by binding to specific intracellular receptors and, as steroid hormone-receptor complexes, interact with nuclear chromatin to stimulate or repress transcription of specific sequences of messenger RNA, ultimately modulating cellular function and growth. Manipulation of this sequence of events has produced important treatment modalities.

Tamoxifen, the most extensively employed and perhaps the most important of the hormonal agents, competes with estradiol for binding to a high-affinity estradiol receptor. The binding of tamoxifen to the estrogen receptor does not result in an estrogenic response in most tissue and renders cells refractory to further estrogen stimulation. A growing body of evidence is accumulating to indicate that the long-term adjuvant (ie, following local treatment) administration of tamoxifen in postmenopausal women with stage II carcinoma of the breast improves their survival.[43] Paradoxically, an older and still effective approach to the palliation of metastatic breast cancer is administration of the synthetic estrogen diethylstilbesterol (DES). The explanation of this paradox probably lies in the fact that DES at pharmacologic doses elicits a different interaction between steroid hormone, receptor, and nuclear chromatin than do the smaller doses of naturally occurring estrogens.

Depletion of steroid hormone in a tumor may be effected indirectly. Prostate carcinoma depends heavily, at least in its early stages, on androgenic stimulation; indeed, the disease does not develop in castrated males. Androgen depletion can be achieved directly with orchiectomy, as well as by administering DES. Although DES may have some slight direct effect on prostate carcinoma, its major effect is to suppress the pituitary's release of luteinizing hormone (LH), which normally stimulates testicular androgen secretion. Neither orchiectomy nor DES is an ideal form of hormonal manipulation: the former approach is emotionally unacceptable for some men, and DES is associated with excessive cardiovascular toxicity. More recently, a group of synthetic gonadotropin-releasing hormone (GnRH) agonists has been developed which offers an important alternative form of hormonal treatment. At first glance, it would seem illogical to use an agent that should elicit increased secretion of LH. However, although the GnRH agonists may initially cause a surge of LH secretion and thus a flare in the disease, they eventually desensitize the pituitary to the effects of GnRH by decreasing the number of GnRH receptors. The end result is the same as in therapy with DES-decreased secretion of LH.

The use of high-dose corticosteroids in the treatment of leukemia and lymphomas appears to be effective for reasons somewhat different from other perturbations of steroid hormone physiology. Lymphoid tumors contain large numbers of cytosolic receptors for corticosteroids, and rather than producing the slow tumor regression typical of other hormonal agents, high dose corticosteroids have a prompt lytic effect on their cells.

At present, no form of hormonal therapy can cure a patient of an established tumor. Hormonal therapy causes tumor regression in approximately 30% of patients with endometrial cancer, 30% to 40% of patients with breast cancer, and 80% of those with prostate cancer. Yet, though tumors regress and on occasion shrink below the limits of clinical detection, and though some tumors may respond to a series of different hormonal treatments, they ultimately become refractory to further hormonal manipulation. In fact, with the exception of tamoxifen for the adjuvant treatment of stage II carcinoma of the breast in postmenopausal women, it has been difficult to show that hormonal therapy even prolongs survival. It is now evident that even hormone-responsive tumors contain from the outset populations of both hormone-dependent and hormone-independent cells. Moreover, the natural history of most tumors is to become increasingly anaplastic (poorly differentiated) and thus less likely to depend on hormonal stimulation for growth. Nonetheless, there is a strong clinical impression that hormonal therapy can be effective, especially when therapy is directed at disease palliation.

Miscellaneous Agents

Of the drugs that fail to fit into a specific category, undoubtedly the most important is cisplatin. The discovery of cisplatin was fortuitous: during experiments on the effect of electrical currents on bacterial growth, growth inhibition was observed in a zone immediately adjacent to platinum electrodes. Of numerous platinum compounds in solution, the active substance was demonstrated to be cisplatin. Subsequent work demonstrated its substantial activity against a variety of tumors.

Cisplatin (cis-diamminedichloroplatinum II) is an inorganic planar coordination complex, the platinum atom coordinated to two amine groups on one side and to two chlorine atoms on the other. Cytotoxicity arises from mechanisms similar to those of classical alkylating agents. The chlorine atoms of the complex behave much like those of mechlorethamine, ie, they function as leaving groups, displaced by nucleophils, such as the bases in DNA. In actuality, the chlorine atoms must first be displaced by water molecules, producing a charged platinum complex, prior to nucleophilic addition. Aquation proceeds slowly in the presence of a high chloride concentration; theoretically, then, formation of the active, aquated, charged complex should occur *intracellularly*, where the chloride concentration is low. As with classic alkylating agents, the preferred site for binding of cisplatin to DNA is the N-7 position of guanine. Being bifunctional (having two leaving groups), cisplatin can form interstrand DNA cross-links, the number of which correlates with the drug's cytotoxicity. The trans-isomer of cisplatin, which is inactive, produces DNA-protein cross-links but cannot form DNA interstrand cross-links at clinically relevant concentrations. Interstrand cross-links form slowly and are opposed by enzymatic mechanisms of excision and repair; resistance to the drug may rise from these processes. Cisplatin is most active in G_1 but behaves predominantly in a phase-nonspecific manner.

Cisplatin may be given intravenously and, in the case of ovarian carcinoma, intraperitoneally as well. In IV injection, about 90% of the drug becomes rapidly bound to proteins and is cleared from the plasma slowly. That proportion of the dose which remains as free drug—the active form of cisplatin—is cleared rapidly; 90% of this free drug is cleared from the plasma during the first 2 hours after injection. Cisplatin is cleared almost exclusively by the kidneys, primarily the result of glomerular filtration. The rate of cisplatin clearance can be accelerated by maneuvers aimed at increasing urinary output, eg, saline or mannitol diuresis, explaining in part the protective effect of diuresis against the drug's toxicities.

The major dose-limiting toxicity of cisplatin is renal damage; it is a direct tubular toxin, preferentially affecting the proximal straight tubule and the distal and collecting tubules. In addition to a decline in glomerular filtration rate, many patients waste magnesium as a result of tubular dysfunction, occasionally to the point of developing tetany. Acute nephrotoxicity attributable to cisplatin therapy is usually reversible; with repeated dosing, however, cumulative damage of a more permanent nature does occur. Ensuring rapid clearance of the free drug by saline or mannitol diuresis is one way of minimizing nephrotoxicity. But an even greater degree of protection is needed when giving very high doses of cisplatin. A simple means of providing additional protection is to administer the drug in 3% (hypertonic) saline; not only is a diuresis established, but the generation of a high urinary chloride concentration slows the formation of the toxic, charged, aquated complex in the lumen of the renal tubule. Other toxicities of cisplatin include ototoxicity (tinnitus, high-frequency hearing loss), peripheral neuropathy (usually in the form of a stocking-glove distribution sensory loss with paresthesias), and relatively severe nausea and vomiting. In contrast to the classical alkylating agents, cisplatin is only mildly myelotoxic, making it an ideal drug for many combination regimens.

Cisplatin is the most active single agent against nonseminomatous testicular cancer; when combined with vinblastine and bleomycin (PVB), it is usually curative. Cisplatin is also the most active single agent in ovarian cancer, often accompanied by doxorubicin or cyclophosphamide, or both. Other important applications include the treatment of squamous cell (head and neck) and transitional cell (bladder) carcinomas and the small-cell lung cancer.

Strategies for Improving Systemic Therapy

Adjuvant Chemotherapy

When an agent produces a high number of palliative responses in overtly metastatic tumors, efforts will be made for its use earlier in the course of the disease, especially in the adjuvant setting. Residual micrometastatic tumor following definitive local therapy should be more susceptible to chemotherapy than the clinically detectable mass for several reasons: a better vascular supply, enabling better drug penetration; a higher proliferative rate; and a decreased likelihood of drug-resistant cells. This rationale has made a significant impact on the treatment of stage II carcinoma of the breast and is being tested in other settings, eg, the adjuvant use of 5-FU and leucovorin in carcinoma of the colon. The more recent notion of neoadjuvant chemotherapy—systemic therapy given prior to definitive local treatment with surgery or radiation—has a slightly different goal: it strives to shrink locally advanced tumors to the point where they are amenable to local therapy, while eradicating or at least controlling distant micrometastatic disease.

Dosage Intensification

The major impediment to exploiting the exponential relationship that exists for many drugs between dose and cell survival is their low therapeutic index, ie, their toxicity in normal tissue. By far the most important dose-limiting toxicity for the bulk of these agents is myelosuppression, which places patients at high risk for infection or bleeding, or both. A successful approach to circumventing the prolonged myelosuppression or permanent marrow ablation that results from high-dose chemotherapy is the technique of bone marrow transplantation. The transplanted bone marrow may be allogeneic (from an antigenically distinct individual), syngeneic (from an identical twin), or autologous (from the patient himself). Allogeneic and syngeneic marrow transplantation following high-dose chemotherapy with or without radiation is currently used in the successful treatment of AML, ALL, and CML.[44] Autologous bone marrow transplantation has been effective in treating some intermediate- and high-grade lymphomas.[45] Efforts are under way to test the potential benefit of high-dose chemotherapy combined with autologous bone marrow rescue in the treatment of more common and typically more resistant solid tumors, such as breast cancer.[46]

Although allogeneic bone marrow transplantation has an established role in treating some individuals with hematologic malignancies, its application is limited by the need for an antigenically suitable donor and by the phenomenon of graft versus host disease, which is more severe in older patients. As a result, a number of techniques are being investigated for purging the bone marrow of malignant cells ex vivo prior to reinfusion, eg, by exposing the marrow to monoclonal antibodies directed against tumor associated antigens or by treatment with cytotoxic drugs.[47,48] Finally, high-dose chemotherapy is toxic not only to bone marrow, but also to other organs. Hepatic, pulmonary, cardiac, and mucosal toxicities create additional barriers to dose escalation that may prove more difficult to surmount than myelosuppression.

The delivery of higher doses of chemotherapeutic agents will also likely be facilitated by the use of hematopoietic growth factors, now available in sufficient quantities for clinical trials as a result of recombinant DNA technology. The hierarchical organization of the bone marrow from progenitor stem cells to mature, highly differentiated end cells was described earlier. Although this organization is fixed, the relative proportions of component in the hierarchy must be flexible to meet the body's ever-changing needs, eg, the need for increased red cell production with blood loss or the need for more neutrophils to combat a bacterial infection. Glycoproteins known as hematopoietic growth factors play major roles in orchestrating such responses. The best described growth factor is erythropoietin, which is secreted by the kidney in response to diminished O_2 delivery. Erythropoietin acts on the marrow in several ways to enhance O_2 delivery: it induces the most primitive erythroid progenitors to undergo differentiation, it increases hemoglobin synthesis, and it stimulates the release of reticulocytes from the marrow. To date, the primary use of erythropoietin is in treating the anemia of end-stage renal disease. However, in high doses it can stimulate platelet formation, suggesting a role in ameliorating thrombocytopenia secondary to cytotoxic drugs.

The myeloid growth factors are highly glycosylated proteins like erythropoietin, but behave in a paracrine fashion, ie, their sites of production are proximal to the target cells on which they act. Myeloid growth factors are produced by cells normally found in the bone marrow: stromal fibroblasts and endothelial cells, lymphocytes, and macrophages. These growth factors are also notable for their occasional ability to act on different progenitor cells and for their somewhat unanticipated ability to alter the function of the end cell of a given myeloid series (eg, by increasing superoxide production of neutrophils or by inhibiting neutrophil migration). Current thinking suggests that when secreted in the bone marrow, these growth factors act primarily to influence the proliferation and differentiation of progenitor cells, and when secreted in local sites of inflammation, they serve to enhance end-cell function. Four myeloid growth factors—IL-3, GM-CSF, G-CSF, and M-CSF (interleukin-3, granulocyte-macrophage colony stimulating factor, granulocyte colony stimulating factor, and macrophage colony stimulating factor)—have been produced in large quantities by recombinant DNA technology. GM-CSF has been used in high-dose chemotherapy followed by autologous bone marrow infusion for the treatment of solid tumors. Infusion of this growth factor shortened the duration of neutropenia from 15 to 12 days.[49] G-CSF has been used in more conventional settings (eg, during aggressive chemotherapy for urothelial transitional-cell carcinoma) and has also shortened the period of significant neutropenia following cytotoxic drug delivery.[50,51]

Interferons

In 1957, the observation was made that it was virtually impossible to infect a mammalian cell with a virus once infection with another virus had been established. The substance responsible for this phenomenon was aptly named *interferon* (IFN). Interferon is now known to be not one but a family of glycoproteins with diverse biologic effects. These molecules are produced normally by leukocytes (IFN-α) or fibroblasts (IFN-β) in response to viral infections, or by lymphoid cells in culture that are stimulated by a mitogen (IFN-γ). The direct antiviral effect of IFNs is unlikely to account for their antitumor activities except in benign cellular proliferative diseases in which viruses have a direct role (eg, juvenile laryngeal papillomatosis and condylomata acuminata). Interferons inhibit cell proliferation and can cause direct cytotoxicity at high concentrations in tissue culture. Lower concentrations have been shown to augment the cytotoxicity of natural killer cells, T cells, and macrophages; to alter antigenic expression on both tumor and effector cells; and to perturb oncogene expression and cellular differentiation. Whether these subtle actions contribute to the antitumor activity of IFNs in vivo is not known. To date, interferon, specifically IFN-α, has made a significant therapeutic impact only in hairy cell leukemia (HCL), a rare B-cell lymphoproliferative malignancy. Objective response to INF-α in HCL is as high as 90%, but complete hematologic remission has been relatively rare.[52] Responses to IFN therapy have also been documented in indolent lymphomas, cutaneous T-cell lymphoma, CML, and multiple myeloma, but the ultimate role of these glycoproteins is less clear. Treatment produces a constellation of symptoms reminiscent of, not surprisingly, viral infection: fever, chills, myalgias, and mild myelosuppression.

Interleukin-2

The idea that a tumor cell can be recognized as foreign by the host's own immune system is supported by scant in vivo evidence. In vitro, at least three subsets of mononuclear leukocytes—cytotoxic T lymphocytes, natural killer cells, and activated macrophages—have been shown to effect tumor rejection. In an attempt to exploit this possible endogenous mechanism of tumor cell killing, peripheral blood lymphoid cells from a patient are induced to proliferate in vitro in a medium containing T-cell growth factor (a lymphokine also known as Interleukin-2); this expanded cell population is subsequently injected back into the same patient, with the simultaneous IV administration of IL-2. Such treatment with IL-2 and IL-2-activated peripheral blood lymphoid cells, or even with IL-2 alone, has produced definite regression in tumors like renal cell carcinoma and melanoma, which are notoriously refractory to all known forms of therapy short of surgery. Unfortunately, the response rate to the combination of IL-2 and autologous IL-2-activated peripheral lymphoid cells has been low. Coupled with the cumbersome, expensive technology required for its use and with its high toxicity, this form of adoptive immunotherapy is not likely to see widespread application.

Directed Drug Delivery

A major limitation of current cytotoxic drugs is the lack of selectivity for malignant cells. The mechanisms of action of these agents (eg, disruption of nucleic acid synthesis and function) fail to discriminate normal from malignant tissues. Given the dearth of truly tumor-specific agents, several approaches have been taken to more precisely target cytotoxic agents for tumor cells. The simplest and, to date, most successful form of directed drug delivery is the instillation of chemotherapeutic agents directly into a body cavity, eg, the pleural or peritoneal space. It is unusual for tumors to be limited to one cavity, but ovarian carcinoma is an important exception. The spread of ovarian carcinoma beyond the ovary's capsule tends to remain confined to the peritoneal surface until the most advanced stages of the disease. Intraperitoneal administration of cisplatin, the single most effective agent for this disease, can induce a substantial number of responses when the disease has become refractory to systemic cisplatin. Encouraged by these results, oncologists have come to use intraperitoneal cisplatin in women with minimal residual disease (lesions <2 mm in diameter) following surgical debulking of tumor.[53] Prospective trials will hopefully validate the approach.

Attempts have also been made to favorably alter drug distribution and uptake by (1) attaching drugs to large molecules, (2) encasing drugs within lipid vesicles, and (3) binding drugs to monoclonal antibodies directed against tumor-associated antigens. Tumor cells often have a high capacity for endocytosis, leading to preferential uptake of, say, a drug-DNA conjugate; once inside the cell, the drug is released from the DNA by enzymatic cleavage of the bonds joining them. This approach is limited by the instability of drug-DNA complexes, by the difficulty such large complexes have in penetrating solid tumors, and by the endocytotic capacity of the tumor. Delivering drugs in liposomes causes a preferential distribution of drug to the reticuloendothelial system (RES)—the lungs, liver, and spleen. However, cloaking drugs in liposomes can change the *relative* availability of a drug to different tissues. For example, when doxorubicin was packaged in liposomes and given to mice, there was decreased drug uptake by the heart and cardiac toxicity with retention of antitumor activity.[54] Substantial obstacles stand in the way of attaching drugs to monoclonal antibodies directed against tumor-associated antigens. First, tumor-associated antigens often are not tumor specific; not only is less drug delivered to the tumor, but the drug may ultimately concentrate in tissues that share the antigen, producing unexpected toxicities. Second, the density of tumor-associated antigens on cancer cells is often low; most tumors cannot be shown to bear *unique* antigenic determinants at all. Finally, the drug-monoclonal antibody complex is usually itself immunogenic, and if successive doses of the complex are given, they will eventually be cleared rapidly by the RES.

Induction of Tumor Differentiation

Since the progressive growth of tumors is a manifestation of their failure to mature and differentiate, attempts are under way to identify agents that might cause malignant cells to "grow up." HL60 cells—an acute promyelocytic leukemia cell line—are susceptible to the induction of differentiation by a number of unrelated compounds: Ara-C, azacytidine, dimethyl sulfoxide, and retinoic acids.[55] Interestingly, maturation is associated with decreased transcription of the c-*myc* oncogene.[56] The mechanisms by which these agents induce differentiation are currently under intensive study; in the case of azacytidine, hypomethylation of DNA may be responsible for altered gene transcription.[57] Efforts are under way to define the potential role of differentiation induction in the clinic. 13-cis-Retinoic acid has met with success in treating oral leukoplakia, a preneoplastic lesion of the oral mucosa,[58] and current trials are evaluating retinoids for other preneoplastic conditions, eg, in metaplasia of the bronchial mucosa and preinvasive cancers, such as recurrent superficial transitional cell carcinoma of the bladder. Although induction of cellular differentiation has yet to become a significant treatment modality, it suggests the possibility of an approach to cancer treatment that is more discriminating for malignant cells than current cytotoxic regimens.

Since the mid-1970s, there has been an explosion in our understanding of the pathogenesis of cancer, specifically through the discovery of oncogenes. It is now well established that oncogenes are derived from normal genes, called proto-oncogenes, which orchestrate cellular growth and differentiate during the early stages of an individual's life. Perturbations of these proto-oncogenes, rarely expressed in the mature individual, allow for their deranged expression as oncogenes, which provoke unbridled and aberrant growth. The protein products of several oncogenes have been identified, and there is hope that they might provide very specific targets for the oncologist. Moreover, the complex pathways of communication that the oncogene product disturbs are just beginning to be unraveled. There is reason to believe that effective interventions based on this understanding will be found as well.

References

Surgical Resection

1. Weir R. Resection of the large intestine for carcinoma. *Am Surg.* 1886;3:469-489.

2. Von Mikulicz-Radceki J. Small contributions to the

surgery of the intestinal tract. *Bost Med Surg J.* 1903;148:608-611.

3. Mayo CH. Gastroenterostomy by means of Murphy button with table of late cases of anastomosis by this method. *Ann Surg.* 1895;21:41-44.

4. Miles WE. A method of performing abdominoperineal excision for carcinoma of the rectum and pelvic colon. *Lancet.* 1908;2:1812-1813.

5. Halsted WS. The results of radical operation for the cure of carcinoma of the breast. *Ann Surg.* 1907;46:1-19.

6. Meade RH. Surgery of the thyroid and parathyroid. In: *An Introduction to the History of General Surgery*. Philadelphia, Pa: WB Saunders Co; 1968.

7. Crile G. Excision of cancer of the head and neck with special attention to the plan of dissection based on 132 operations. *JAMA.* 1906;47:1780-1786.

8. Martin H. Radical surgery in cancer of the head and neck. *Surg Clin of North Am.* 1958;33:329-350.

9. Torek F. The first successful case of resection of the thoracic portion of the esophagus for carcinoma. *Surg Gyneloc Obstet.* 1913;16:614-617.

10. Graham EA. Successful removal of entire lung for carcinoma of the bronchus. *JAMA.* 1933;101:1371-1374.

11. Churchill ED, Sweet RH, Souither L, Scannel JG. The surgical management of carcinoma of the lung. *J Thorac Surg.* 1950;20:329-365.

12. Ochsner A, Debakey M. Primary pulmonary malignancy treatment by total pneumonectomy. *Surg Gynecol Obstet.* 1939;68:435-451.

13. Beahrs OH, Henson DE, Hutter RVP, Kennedy BJ. American Joint Committee on Cancer. *Manual for Staging of Cancer.* 4th ed. Philadelphia, Pa: JB Lippincott Co; 1992.

14. Boring CC, Squirės TS, Tong T, Montgomery S. Cancer Statistics, 1994. *CA Cancer J Clin.* 1994;44:7-26.

15. Friedman MA, Cain DF. National Cancer Institute sponsored cooperative clinical trials. *Cancer.* 1990;65(suppl.):2376-2382.

16. Coltman CA Jr. Southwest Oncology Group. *Cancer.* 1990;65(suppl):2385-2387.

Radiation Therapy

1. Roentgen WC. On a new kind of rays (preliminary communication) translation of a paper read before the Physikalische-medicinischen Gesellschaft of Wurzburg on December 28, 1895. *Br J Radiol.* 1931;4:32.

2. Curie P, Curie Mme P, Bemont G. Sur une nouvelle substance fortement radioactive contenue dans la pechblende (note presented by M Becquerel). *Compt Rend Acad Sci* (Paris). 1898;127:1215-1217.

3. Coutard H. Roentgentherapy of epitheliomas of the tonsillar regional hypopharynx and larynx from 1920 to 1926. *Am J Roentgenol.* 1932;28:313-331.

4. Coutard H. Principles of x-ray therapy of malignant diseases. *Lancet.* 1934;2:1-8.

5. Puck TT, Marcus PI. Action of x-rays on mammalian cells. *J Exp Med.* 1956;103:653-656.

6. McCulloch EA, Till JE. Proliferation of hematopoietic colony-forming cells transplanted into irradiated mice. *Radiat Res.* 1964;22:383-397.

7. Withers HR. The dose-survival relationship for irradiation of epithelial cells of mouse skin. *Br J Radiol.* 1967;40:187-194.

8. Read J. Mode of action of x-ray doses given with different oxygen concentrations. *Br J Radiol.* 1952;25:336-338.

9. Elkind MM, Whitmore GF. *The Radiobiology of Cultured Mammalian Cells.* New York, NY: Gordon and Breach; 1967.

10. Alper T. *Cellular Radiobiology.* Cambridge University Press; 1979.

11. Bender M. Induced aberrations in human chromosomes. *Am J Pathol.* 1963;43:260.

12. Evans HJ. Chromosome aberrations induced by ionizing radiation. *Int Rev Cytol.* 1962;13:221-321.

13. Gerard CR. Effects of radiation on chromosomes. In: Pizzarello D, ed: *Radiation Biology.* Boca Raton, Fla.: CRC Press; 1982:83-110.

14. Ishihara T, Sasaki MS, eds. *Radiation-Induced Chromosome Damage in Man.* New York, NY: Alan R. Liss; 1983.

15. Hall EJ. Radiation-induced chromosome aberrations. In: *Radiobiology for the Radiologist.* Philadelphia, Pa: JB Lippincott Co; 1988.

16. Deschner EE, Gray LH. Influence of oxygen tension on x-ray induced chromosomal damage in Ehrlich ascites tumor cells irradiated in vitro and in vivo. *Radiat Res.* 1959;11:115-146.

17. Elkind MM, Alescio T, Swain RW, et al. Recovery of hypoxic mammalian cells from sublethal x-ray damage. *Nature.* 1964;202:1190-1193.

18. Gray LH, Conger AD, Ebert M, Hornsey S, Scott OCA. The concentration of oxygen dissolved in tissues at the time of irradiation as a factor in radiotherapy. *Br J Radiol.* 1953;26:638-648.

19. Hall EJ. The oxygen effect and reoxygenation. In: *Radiobiology for the Radiologist.* Philadelphia, Pa: JB Lippincott Co; 1988: 137-158.

20. Palcic B, Skarsgard LD. Reduced oxygen enhancement ratio at low doses of ionizing radiation. *Radiat Res.* 1984;100:328-339.

21. Hall EJ, Bedford JS, Oliver R. Extreme hypoxia: its effect on the survival of mammalian cells irradiated at high and low dose-rates. *Br J Radiol.* 1966;39:302-307.

22. Hall EJ. Radiation dose-rate: a factor of importance in radiobiology and radiotherapy. *Br J Radiol.* 1972;45:81-97.

23. Ewing D, Powers EL. Oxygen-dependent sensitization of irradiated cells. In: Meyn RE, Withers HR, eds. *Radiation Biology in Cancer Research.* New York, NY: Raven Press; 1980:143-168.

24. Michael BD, Adams GE, Hewitt HB, Jones WBE, Watts ME. A post effect of oxygen in irradiated bacteria: a submillisecond fast mixing study. *Radiat Res.* 1973;54:239-251.

25. Howard-Flanders P, Moore D. The time interval after pulsed irradiation within which injury to bacteria can be modified by dissolved oxygen, I: a search for an effect of oxygen 0.02 second after pulsed irradiation. *Radiat Res.* 1958;9:422-437.

26. Thomlinson RH, Gray LH. The histologic structure of some human lung cancers and the possible implications for radiotherapy. *Br J Cancer.* 1955;9:539-549.

27. Bush RS, Jenkin RDT, Allt WEC, et al. Definitive evidence for hypoxic cells influencing cure in cancer therapy. *Br J Cancer.* 1978;37:302-306.

28. Cater DB, Silver IA. Quantitative measurement of oxygen tension in normal tissues and in the tumours of patients before and after radiotherapy. *Acta Radiol.* 1960; 53:233.

29. Withers HR, Suite HD. Is oxygen important in the

radiocurability of human tumors? In: Friedman M, ed. *The Biological and Clinical Basis of Radiosensitivity.* Springfield, Ill: Charles C Thomas; 1974: Chap. 23.

30. Thomlinson RH. Reoxygenation as a function of tumor size and histopathological type. In: *Time and Dose Relationship in Radiation Biology as Applied to Radiotherapy.* Brookhaven National Lab Rep. 50203(C-57); 1970: 242-254.

31. Kallman RF. The phenomenon of reoxygenation and its implications for fractionated radiotherapy. *Radiology.* 1972;105:135-142.

32. Elkind MM, Sutton H. X-ray damage and recovery in mammalian cells in culture. *Nature.* 1959;184:1293.

33. Hendrickson FR, Withers HR. Principles of radiation oncology. In: Holleb AI, Fink DJ, Murphy GR, eds. *Textbook of Clinical Oncology.* Atlanta, Ga: American Cancer Society; 1991:39.

34. Suit HD, Howes AE, Hunter N. Dependence of response of a C3H mammary carcinoma to fractionated irradiation on fraction number and intertreatment interval. *Radiat Res.* 1977;72:440-454.

35. Thames HD, Peters LJ, Withers HR, et al. Accelerated fractionation vs hyperfractionation: rationales for several treatments per day. *Int J Radiat Oncol Biol Phys.* 1983;9:127.

36. Sinclair WK. Dependence of radiosensitivity upon cell age. In: *Time and Dose Relationships in Radiation Biology as Applied to Radiotherapy.* Brookhaven National Lab Rep. 50203 (C-57); 1969:97.

37. Legrys GA, Hall EJ. The oxygen effect and x-ray sensitivity in synchronously dividing cultures of Chinese hamster cells. *Radiat Res.* 1969;37:161-172.

38. Hall EJ, Brown JM, Cavanagh J. Radiosensitivity and the oxygen effect measured at different phases of the mitotic cycle using synchronously dividing cells of the root meristem of Vicia faba. *Radiat Res.* 1968;35:622-634.

39. Sinclair WK. Cysteamine: differential x-ray protective effect on Chinese hamster cells during the cell cycle. *Science.* 1968;159:442-444.

40. Ang KK, Landuyt W, Rijnders A, et al. Differences in repopulation kinetics in mouse skin during split-course multiple fractions per day or daily fractionated irradiations. *Int J Radiat Oncol Biol Phys.* 1985;10:95.

41. Hermens AF, Barendsen GW. Changes of cell proliferation characteristics in a rat rhabdomyosarcoma before and after x-irradiation. *Eur J Cancer.* 1969;5:173.

42. Withers HR, Taylor JM, Maciejewski B. The hazard of accelerated tumor clonogen repopulation during radiotherapy. *Acta Radiol.* 1988;27:131-146.

43. Hall E. Time, dose and fractionation in radiotherapy. In: *Radiobiology for the Radiologist.* Philadelphia, Pa: JB Lippincott Co; 1988:240.

44. Rubin P, Constine L, Nelson D. Late effects of cancer treatment: radiation and drug toxicity. In: Perez C, Brady LW, eds. *Principles and Practice of Radiation Oncology.* Philadelphia, Pa: JB Lippincott Co; 1992: chap 5.

45. Mendenhall WM, Million RR, Cassisi NJ. Elective neck irradiation in squamous cell carcinoma of the head and neck. *Head Neck Surg.* 1980;3(1)15-20.

46. Fletcher GH. The scientific basis of the present and future practice of clinical radiotherapy. *Int J Radiat Oncol Biol Phys.* 1983;9:1073-1082.

47. Fletcher GH, ed. *Textbook of Radiotherapy.* 3rd ed. Philadelphia, Pa: Lea & Febiger; 1980.

48. Fletcher GH, Shukovsky LJ. The interplay of radiocurability and tolerance in the irradiation of human cancers. *J Radiol Electrol.* 1975;56:383-400.

49. Meoz-Mendez RT, Fletcher GH, Guillamondequi OM, et al. Analysis of the results of irradiation in the treatment of squamous cell carcinomas of the pharyngeal walls. *Int J Radiat Oncol Biol Phys.* 1978;4:579-585.

50. Shukovsky LJ, Baeza MR, Fletcher GH. Results of irradiation in squamous cell carcinomas of the glossopalatine sulcus. *Radiology.* 1976;120:405-408.

51. Suit H, Lindberg R, Fletcher GH. Prognostic significance of extent of tumor regression at completion of radiation therapy. *Radiology.* 1965;84:1100-1107.

52. Suit HD. Potential for improving survival rates for the cancer patient by increasing the efficacy of treatment of the primary lesion. *Cancer.* 1982;50:1227-1234.

53. DeVita VT Jr. Principles of chemotherapy. In: DeVita VT Jr, Jellman S, Rosenberg SA, eds. *Cancer: Principles and Practice of Oncology.* 2nd ed. Philadelphia, Pa: JB Lippincott Co; 1985:257-285.

54. Rubin P. The emergence of radiation oncology as a distinct medical specialty. *Int J Radiat Oncol Biol Phys.* 1985;11:1247-1270.

Systemic Therapy

1. Gilman A. The initial clinical trial of nitrogen mustard. *Am J Surg.* 1963;105:574-578.

2. Cleaver JE. *Thymidine Metabolism and Cell Kinetics.* Amsterdam: North Holland Publishing Co; 1967.

3. Hedley DW, Clark GM, Cornelisse CJ, Killander D, Kute T, Merkel D. Consensus review of the clinical utility of DNA cytometry in carcinoma of the breast. *Cytometry.* 1993;14:482-485.

4. Howard A, Pele SR. Nuclear incorporation of P^{32} as demonstrated by autoradiographs. *Exp Cell Res.* 1951;2:178-187.

5. Quastler H, Sherman FG. Cell population kinetics in the intestinal epithelium of the mouse. *Exp Cell Res.* 1959;17:420-438.

6. Tannock I. Cell kinetics and chemotherapy: a critical review. *Cancer Treat Rep.* 1978;62:1117-1133.

7. Steel GG. Cell loss as a factor in the growth rate of human tumors. *Eur J Cancer.* 1967;3:381-387.

8. Shackney SE, McCormack GW, Cuchural GJ Jr. Growth rate patterns of solid tumors and their relation to responsiveness to therapy: an analytical review. *Ann Intern Med.* 1978;89:107-121.

9. Weiss RB, DeVita VT Jr. Multimodal primary cancer treatment (adjuvant chemotherapy): current results and future prospects. *Ann Intern Med.* 1979;91:251-260.

10. Till JE, McCullouch EA. Hematopoietic stem cell differentiation. *Biochem Biophys Acta.* 1980;605:431-459.

11. Becker AJ, McCulloch EA, Siminovitch L, Till JE. The effect of differing demands for blood cell production on DNA synthesis by hemopoietic colony-forming cells of mice. *Blood.* 1965;26:296-308.

12. Hamburger AW, Salmon SE. Primary bioassay of human tumor stem cells. *Science.* 1977;197:461-463.

13. Selby P, Buick RN, Tannock I. A critical appraisal of the "human tumor stem-cell assay." *N Engl J Med.* 1983;308:129-134.

14. Shimizu T, Motoji T, Oshimi K, Mizoguchi H. Proliferative state and radiosensitivity of human myeloma stem cells. *Br J Cancer.* 1982;45:679-683.

15. Minden MD, Till JE, McCulloch EA. Proliferative state of blast cell progenitors in acute myeloblastic leukemia (AML). *Blood.* 1978;52:592-600.

16. Hryniuk WM, Levine MN, Levin L. Analysis of dose intensity for chemotherapy in early (stage II) and advanced breast cancer. *NCI Monogr.* 1986;1:87-94.

17. Bruce WR, Meeker BE, Powers WE, Valeriote FA. Comparison of the dose- and time-survival curves for normal hematopoietic and lymphoma colony-forming cells exposed to vinblastine, vincristine, arabinosylcytosine, and amethopterin. *J Natl Cancer Inst.* 1969;42:1015-1023.

18. Van Putten LM, Lelieveld P, Kram-Idsenga LKJ. Cell cycle specificity and therapeutic effectiveness of cytostatic agents. *Cancer Chemother Rep.* 1972;56:691-700.

19. Twentyman PR, Bleehen NM. Changes in sensitivity to cytotoxic agents occurring during the life history of monolayer cultures of a mouse tumor cell line. *Br J Cancer.* 1975;31:417-423.

20. Goldie JH, Coldman AJ. The genetic origin of drug resistance in neoplasms: implications for systemic therapy. *Cancer Res.* 1984;44:3643-3653.

21. Gros P, Ben Neriah Y, Croop JM, Housman DE. Isolation and expression of a complementary DNA that confers multidrug resistance. *Nature.* 1986;323:728-731.

22. Goldie JH, Coldman AJ. A mathematic model for relating the drug sensitivity of tumors to their spontaneous mutation rate. *Cancer Treat Rep.* 1979;63:1727-1733.

23. Bertino JR, Dolnick BJ, Berenson RJ, Scheer DI, Kamen BA. Cellular mechanisms of resistance to methotrexate. In: Sartorelli AC, Lazo JS, Bertino JR, eds. *Molecular Actions and Targets for Cancer Chemotherapeutic Agents.* New York, NY:Academic Press; 1981:385-397.

24. Schimke RT. Gene amplification, drug resistance, and cancer. *Cancer Res.* 1984;44:1735-1742.

25. Biedler JL, Riehm H. Cellular resistance to actinomycin D in Chinese hamster cells in vitro: cross-resistance, radioautographic, and cytogenetic studies. *Cancer Res.* 1970;30:1174-1184.

26. Juliano RL, Ling V. A surface glycoprotein modulating drug permeability in Chinese hamster ovary cell mutants. *Biochem Biophys Acta.* 1976;455:152-162.

27. Bell DR, Gerlach JH, Kartner N, Buick RN, Ling V. Detection of P-glycoprotein in ovarian cancer: a molecular marker associated with multidrug resistance. *J Clin Oncol.* 1985;3:311-315.

28. Fojo AT, Ueda K, Slamon DJ, Poplack DG, Gottesman MM, Pastan I. Expression of a multidrug-resistance gene in human tumors and tissues. *Proc Natl Acad Sci* U S A. 1987;84:265-269.

29. Moscow JA, Cowan KH. Multidrug resistance. *J Natl Cancer Inst.* 1988;80:14-20.

30. Schnipper LE. Clinical implications of tumor-cell heterogeneity. *N Engl J Med.* 1986;314:1423-1431.

31. Dorr RT, Fritz WL. *Cancer Chemotherapy Handbook.* New York, NY:Elsevier North Holland; 1980.

32. Skeel RT. *Handbook of Cancer Chemotherapy.* Boston, Mass:Little, Brown and Co; 1987:1-393

33. Wittes RE. *Manual of Oncologic Therapeutics, 1989/1990.* Philadelphia, Pa:JB Lippincott Co; 1989.

34. Greene MH, Boice JD Jr, Greer BE, Blessing JA, Dembo AJ. Acute nonlymphocytic leukemia after therapy with alkylating agents for ovarian cancer. *N Engl J Med.* 1982;307:1416-1421.

35. Greene MH, Harris EL, Gershenson DM. Melphalan may be a more potent leukemogen than cyclophosphamide. *Ann Intern Med.* 1986;105:360-367.

36. Bleyer WA. The clinical pharmacology of methotrexate. *Cancer.* 1978;41:36-51.

37. Grem JL, Hoth DF, Hamilton JM, King SA, Leyland-Jones B. Overview of current status and future direction of clinical trials with 5-fluorouracil in combination with folinic acid. *Cancer Treat Rep.* 1987;71:1249-1264.

38. Schwartz SA, Morgenstern B, Capizzi RL. Schedule-dependent synergy and antagonism between high-dose 1-β-D-arabinofuranosylcytosine and asparaginase in the L5178Y murine leukemia. *Cancer Res.* 1982;42:2191-2197.

39. Capizzi RL, Davis R, Powell B, et al. Synergy between high-dose cytarabine and asparaginase in the treatment of adults with refractory and relapsed acute myelogenous leukemia: a Cancer and Leukemia Group B study. *J Clin Oncol.* 1988;6:499-508.

40. Tannock I, Guttman P. Response of Chinese hamster ovary cells to anticancer drugs under aerobic and hypoxic conditions. *Br J Cancer.* 1981;43:245-248.

41. Tritton TR, Yee G. The anticancer drug adriamycin can be actively cytotoxic without entering cells. *Science.* 1982;217:248-250.

42. Speyer J, Green M, Ward C, et al. Endomyocardial biopsies provide additional evidence for ICRF-187 protection against Adriamycin induced cardiac toxicity. *Proc Am Soc Clin Oncol.* 1988;7:244.

43. Stewart HJ, et al. Adjuvant tamoxifen in the management of operable breast cancer: the Scottish trial: report from the Breast Cancer Trials Committee. *Lancet.* 1987;2:171-175.

44. O'Reilly RJ. Allogeneic bone marrow transplantation: current status and future directions. *Blood.* 1983;62:941-964.

45. Philip T, Armitage JO, Spitzer G, et al. High-dose therapy and autologous bone marrow transplantation after failure of conventional chemotherapy in adults with intermediate-grade or high-grade non-Hodgkin's lymphoma. *N Engl J Med.* 1987;316:1493-1498.

46. Eder JP, Antman K, Peters W, et al. High-dose combination alkylating agent chemotherapy with autologous bone marrow support for metastatic breast cancer. *J Clin Oncol.* 1986;4:1592-1597.

47. Ramsay N, LeBien T, Nesbit M, et al. Autologous bone marrow transplantation for patients with acute lymphoblastic leukemia in second or subsequent remission: results of bone marrow treated with monoclonal antibodies BA-1, BA-2, and BA-3, plus complement. *Blood.* 1985;66:508-513.

48. Yeager AM, Kaizer H, Santos GW, et al. Autologous bone marrow transplantation in patients with acute nonlymphocytic leukemia, using ex vivo marrow treatment with 4-hydroperoxycyclophosphamide. *N Engl J Med.* 1986; 315:141-147.

49. Brandt SJ, Peters WP, Atwater SK, et al. Effect of recombinant human granulocyte macrophage colony-stimulating factor on hematopoietic reconstitution after high-dose chemotherapy and autologous bone marrow transplantation. *N Engl J Med.* 1988;318:869-876.

50. Morstyn G, Campbell L, Souza LM, et al. Effect of granulocyte colony stimulating factor on neutropenia induced by cytotoxic chemotherapy. *Lancet.* 1988;1:667-671.

51. Gabrilove JL, Jakubowski A, Scher H, et al. Effect of granulocyte colony-stimulating factor on neutropenia and associated morbidity due to chemotherapy for transitional-cell carcinoma of the urothelium. *N Engl J Med.* 1988; 318:1414-1422.

52. Golomb HM. The treatment of hairy cell leukemia. *Blood.* 1987;69:979-983.

53. Myers C. The use of intraperitoneal chemotherapy in the treatment of ovarian cancer. *Semin Oncol.* 1984;11:275-284.

54. Rahman A, Kessler A, More N, et al. Liposomal protection of adriamycin-induced cardiotoxicity in mice. *Cancer Res.* 1980;40:1532-1537.

55. Sporn MB, Roberts AB, Driscoll JS. Principles of cancer biology: growth factor and differentiation. In: DeVita VT Jr, Hellman S, Rosenberg SA, eds. *Cancer: Principles and Practices of Oncology*. 2nd ed. Philadelphia, Pa:JB Lippincott Co; 1985:49-65.

56. Watanabe T, Sariban E, Mitchell T, Kufe D. Human c-*myc* and N-*ras* expression during induction of HL-60 cellular differentiation. *Biochem Biophys Res Commun.* 1985;126:999-1005.

57. Jones PA, Taylor SM. Cellular differentiation, cytidine analogs, and DNA methylation. *Cell.* 1980;20:85-93.

58. Hong WK, Endicott J, Itri L, et al. 13-cis-retinoic acid in the treatment of oral leukoplakia. *N Engl J Med.* 1986;315:1501-1505.

7

PRINCIPLES OF TUMOR IMMUNOLOGY

Ronald B. Herberman, MD

The field of tumor immunology encompasses the wide variety of interactions between the immune system and tumors, emphasizing the immune system's role in resisting the development or progressive growth of cancer and how it can be manipulated to increase such resistance. Tumor immunology also has important applications to the immunodiagnosis of cancer and understanding of altered immunologic competence in tumor-bearing individuals.

The main principles of tumor immunology have emerged from extensive studies performed mainly during the last 30 years.

Immune System Recognition of Tumor Cells

A wide variety of tumor cells express molecular structures that differ from normal cells of the same individual and can be recognized by one or more components of the immune system. Most of the immunologic discrimination of tumor cells from normal cells has been thought to be due to recognition by the host of *tumor antigens* but in addition, tumor cells have been found to have other, nonantigenic differences that may be recognizable by the natural immune system.

Tumor Antigens

Most tumor cells have molecular configurations that can be specifically recognized by immune T cells or by antibodies and hence are termed tumor antigens. The most important tumor antigens, in terms of immunodiagnosis or host resistance, have been termed *tumor associated antigens* (TAAs). They are selectively expressed on tumor cells and are not detectable on normal cells of the same individual. For many years, tumor immunologists sought tumor antigens that would be uniquely present on tumor cells and qualitatively different from antigens on any normal cells, and hence called *tumor specific antigens*. However, most antigens on tumor cells that were initially thought to be tumor specific have been found, by more extensive evaluation of a wider range of normal tissues and the use of highly sensitive immunoassays, to be expressed in some circumstances, at least in low amounts, in some normal cells. Thus, the operational term "TAA" seems more valid. An important subset of TAA is *tumor associated transplantation antigens* (TATAs), which can induce immunologically specific resistance to tumor growth in the autologous host. The immunologic reactions that allow a host to recognize TATAs and to thereby mediate elimination of the tumor cells appear to closely resemble those that mediate rejection of tissue allografts with weak histocompatibility antigenic differences from the host. Tumor cells also contain many normal cellular antigens that are characteristic of the tissue or organ from which the neoplastic cells are derived, or the stage of differentiation of the tumor cells.

Controversy surrounds the issue of whether all or most tumors express TATAs. Although the majority of tumors induced in experimental animals by oncogenic viruses or chemical carcinogens have been shown to have TATAs, some studies of tumors arising spontaneously in aged mice or rats have indicated that most of these spontaneous tumors lacked detectable TATAs. It has thus been argued that most human tumors, which have no known etiology and hence would be considered spontaneous, also lack TATAs.[1] However, as discussed previously in some detail, there are considerable limitations to such arguments.[2] Although there is insufficient evidence about the proportion of human tumors that express TATAs, there is considerable suggestive or circumstantial evidence for the presence of TATAs on many human tumors.[2]

For a TAA to function as a TATA, it must be recognized by the host's immune system and elicit immunologic reactivity that results in destruction or at

---

Ronald B. Herberman, MD, Pittsburgh Cancer Institute, Departments of Medicine and Pathology, University of Pittsburgh School of Medicine, Pittsburgh, Pennsylvania

least growth inhibition of the tumor. During the last several years, there has been a rapid increase in understanding as to how TAAs as well as other antigens are recognized and elicit specific immune reactivity. Small peptide portions of antigens have been shown to physically associate with class II or I major histocompatibility complex (MHC) molecules, and such combined structures interact with helper or cytotoxic T cells, respectively.[3]

In addition to TAAs that evoke cellular immune responses in the host, there are other categories of TAAs, some of which also have considerable practical importance. Any TAA that is recognized by antibodies in the serum of the tumor-bearing host or in the sera of animals immunized against the antigen can potentially be used to discriminate between tumor cells and normal cells, and this may be of value for immunodiagnosis. TAAs that are common to a variety of tumors, at least of the same organ or histological type, are most likely to be useful for diagnostic purposes. Studies in animal model systems have shown that tumors induced by chemical carcinogens and some spontaneous tumors have TATAs that are individually distinct and are not present in other tumors induced by the same agent, even when they arise in the same host. Such antigens would not be helpful diagnostically, since antibodies against one tumor would not be expected to react with any other tumors. Common TAAs have been identified on many tumors, and even those that are not recognized by the immune response of the tumor-bearing individual may be readily detected by antibodies elicited in a different species.

Nonantigenic Differences Between Tumor and Normal Cells

TAAs are the targets for recognition by the components of the classic immune system, immune T cells and/or antibodies. Also, various components of the natural immune system (eg, natural killer cells or macrophages) can selectively recognize and react with tumor cells. Although the basis for such recognition is not well understood, it may be due to the expression on tumor cells of a variety of cell surface molecules in larger quantity or in altered form relative to normal cells. These tumor-associated differences do not seem to be restricted to tumor cells, as virus-infected normal cells or other cells may also be recognized by natural effector cells.[4]

Basis for Differences

The molecular basis for antigenic or other differences between tumor and normal cells is still not completely understood. Several different mechanisms appear to be involved:

1. *Clonally distributed molecules.* Some types of molecules may be highly polymorphic and clonally distributed on normal cells of the population. Because most tumors appear to arise from a single abnormal cell, they may express structurally normal molecules that are characteristic for that clone. The best known example of this type of TAA is the cell surface immunoglobulin on malignant B cells. The immunoglobulin genes of normal as well as malignant B cells undergo recombinations that generate clonal diversity, particularly in the region of the antigen-combining sites. Such idiotypic structures provide individually specific antigens on each malignant clone, and monoclonal antibodies to such idiotypic determinants on human B cell lymphoma have been the focus for some attempts at immunotherapy. More recently, a vaccine trial has been performed to actively immunize lymphoma patients against their idiotypic proteins.[5]

2. *Virus-associated antigens.* Tumors induced by an oncogenic virus, even when they differ in morphologic appearance or arise in different organs, share the same TAAs, some of which may function as TATAs. At least some of these TAAs are determined by new genetic information introduced into the tumor cell by the virus. In other cases, the oncogenic virus may induce or alter the expression of oncogenes that are present within the host genome.

3. *TAAs of carcinogen-induced tumors.* As noted, tumors induced by chemical carcinogens, ultraviolet irradiation, or other physical agents usually express TATAs that are individually tumor specific. The basis for such induction is not clear, but these agents share the ability to cause mutations in DNA, and their TAAs may be due to genetic alterations in normal cellular genes. Recently, detailed molecular studies have been performed on a series of TATAs associated with a murine carcinogen-induced tumor, and each has been attributed to a point mutation in unrelated genes.[6]

4. *Differentiation antigens.* It has been known for some time that antigens present on normal fetal cells may also be expressed on a variety of tumor cells, regardless of etiology. These have been referred to as oncofetal or carcinoembryonic antigens. With more recent and extensive experience, particularly from the extensive analysis of the specificity of antigens detected by various monoclonal antibodies, it appears that a more general categorization of such antigens might be that of differentiation antigens. Tumor cells often are arrested at a particular point in the pathway of differentiation for the normal cell type from which they arose. They express antigens that are characteristic for that stage of differentiation. Antigens of stem cells or of cells at early stages of differentiation may be rare in adults but frequent in fetuses and therefore may appear to be oncofetal in their distribution. Such differentiation antigens may help to classify certain tumors, particularly those derived from hematopoietic cells, where there has been considerable elucidation of the antigens associated with the stages of development in the various hematopoietic lineages.

5. *Tissue antigens.* Large amounts of normal tissue or organ-associated antigens may be expressed in tumor cells derived from that tissue. Especially when the normal cells are relatively infrequent, the tissue antigen may appear to be tumor associated and may only be found to be tissue associated on careful examination of the relevant normal cells.

The Immune System's Role in Resisting Cancer

Many investigators have proposed that the immune system has a general role in preventing or limiting tumor growth. The central concept, known as the *immune surveillance* hypothesis, postulates that the immune system is a key factor in resistance against the development of detectable tumors. The first known suggestion along these lines came from Paul Ehrlich in 1909[7]; the modern formulation of the hypothesis originated from MacFarlane Burnet and Lewis Thomas. When information about thymus-dependent immunity became known, and particularly when T cells were found to play a central role in homograft rejection, Burnet modified the immune surveillance hypothesis to stress the key role of this effector mechanism in antitumor resistance.

The immune surveillance hypothesis has since generated many experimental studies and much discussion and controversy. One of the reasons for the controversy is that the concept leads to a series of predictions; most available evidence relates to tests of one or more of these predictions:

1. Tumor cells have transplantation-type antigens.

2. Resistance against tumors is T-cell dependent and analogous to the homograft reaction.

3. There is a close evolutionary link between malignancy and the development of an immune system with capability for rejection of tumors.

4. Immune depression is associated with, and must precede, development of detectable tumors.

5. A requisite action of carcinogens and/or tumor promoters might be immunosuppression.

The main support for the immune surveillance hypothesis has come from evidence related to prediction No. 4, since naturally occurring or induced immunodepression has been associated with a higher incidence in some types of tumors. In experimental animal systems, this has been most clearly demonstrated with tumors induced by oncogenic viruses. Neonatal thymectomy and other forms of immune suppression have been shown to lead to increased susceptibility to polyoma virus-induced tumors in mice and Marek's disease in chickens.

Considerable clinical evidence shows that immune deficiency diseases are associated with a much higher incidence of lymphoma and leukemia. Allograft recipients receiving immunosuppressive agents, either prednisone and azathioprine or more recently cyclosporine A and/or other immunosuppressive drugs have also been found to have an increased incidence (approximately 100-fold) of lymphoproliferative disease or other tumors.[8] Patients with cancer, arthritis, or other diseases who received chemotherapeutic (mainly alkylating) agents have been subsequently found to develop a relatively high frequency of subsequent primary malignancies, mainly leukemias and lymphomas. The recent observations of a remarkably high incidence of Kaposi's sarcoma or B cell lymphoma in young adults with acquired immune deficiency syndrome (AIDS) are yet another indication of the association of malignancy with immunodepression.

Although such data support immune surveillance, the original hypothesis had several major problems or limitations:

1. The majority of human tumors associated with immunodepression have been leukemias and lymphoproliferative diseases, rather than a complete array of the common types of malignancy. The lymphoproliferative disease occurring in immunosuppressed patients after organ transplantation has been shown to be closely associated with infection by Epstein-Barr virus,[9] derived in at least some cases from the donor organs.

2. There has not been a consistent association between immunodepression and tumors.

3. Neonatally thymectomized mice have been found to have a decreased incidence of mammary tumors, and nude and euthymic mice have similar incidences of spontaneous and carcinogen-induced tumors.

4. Most spontaneous tumors of experimental animals lack detectable tumor-associated transplantation antigens.[1]

5. There appears to be an evolutionary dissociation between the development of tumors and the appearance of a sophisticated immune system and T cells.

These hypotheses have led to the suggestion that immune surveillance may be operative only against tumors induced by oncogenic viruses, which have strong transplantation antigens and for which immune T cells have been shown to be important in resistance.[10] The major exceptions to the central role of immune T cells in resistance to tumor growth have even led Richmond Prehn to formulate a countertheory of immunostimulation, suggesting that the immune system may have mainly enhancing effects on tumor induction and growth.[11,12]

A more likely explanation for many of the discordant results is the involvement of a variety of effector mechanisms in host resistance. In the past several years, it has become apparent that natural immunity, as well as specifically induced immune responses, may contribute to host defenses (see below). When T-cell-mediated immunity is viewed as only one of a series of possible host defense mechanisms, the evidence summarized above need not be viewed in such a negative light. Target-cell structures other than tumor-associated transplantation antigens might be involved in recognition by other types of effector cells; and in T-cell-deficient individuals, natural immunity might still be functional and capable of resisting tumor growth. This is the basis for an updated immune - surveillance hypothesis: transformed cells express surface antigens or other structures that one or more components of the immune system can recognize; one or more components of the natural and/or induced immunological effector mechanisms can eliminate the transformed cells or impede the progression and spread of tumors.

This broader hypothesis leads to a somewhat different set of predictions:

1. Tumor cells have surface structures recognized by one or more effectors.

2. Tumor cells will be susceptible to lysis or growth inhibition by one or more effector mechanisms.

3. One or more of the relevant effector cells should be able to enter the site of tumor growth.

4. Augmentation of relevant effector mechanism(s) will decrease the incidence of tumors or metastases.

5. Depression of relevant effector mechanism(s), either by carcinogen or by immunosuppressive treatment, will increase the incidence of tumors or metastases.

6. Restoration of depressed effector activity will decrease the incidence of tumors or metastases.

In addition to the immune system's postulated role in surveillance against the development of tumors, there is considerable evidence for involvement of both the classic and natural immune responses in host resistance against the progression and metastatic spread of tumors once they arise. In fact, the evidence for an important role of some components of the immune system, eg, natural killer cells, is much more compelling in regard to anti-metastatic effects than for immune surveillance.

The immune system is complex, and there are several different components that may be important effectors of host resistance against tumors.

Role of T Cells in Host Resistance

There is substantial evidence that thymus-dependent immune responses are important in resistance to tumors induced by oncogenic viruses. However, the absence of the thymus has not been associated with increased susceptibility to other types of tumors, suggesting a limited role for T-cell immunity in immune surveillance. Further, the inability to detect tumor-associated transplantation antigens on most spontaneous rodent tumors argues against a major involvement of specific immune responses. Recent evidence indicates, however, the importance of distinguishing between *immunogenicity* and *antigenicity*. Immunogenicity refers to the ability of a TAA to induce an immune response and appears to depend on the degree of expression of the antigen on the tumor cells as well as the expression of major histocompatibility complex (MHC) antigens and the immunologic responsiveness. Ultraviolet light-induced tumors in mice have been found to express strong TATAs but are usually nonimmunogenic in UV-irradiated animals because of a specific form of immune suppression.[13] Some other tumors in mice appear to be nonimmunogenic because they lack expression of MHC antigens. Immunogenicity and MHC antigen expression can be induced by treatment of the tumor cells with a chemical mutagen or ultraviolet irradiation.[14]

The reactivity of specifically immune cytotoxic T lymphocytes (CTL) against TAAs or other cell surface antigens are usually restricted by the MHC, with cytotoxicity only detectable against target cells that share class I MHC determinants with the CTL. Recently, there has been considerable progress in elucidating the basis for the close association between immunogenicity and MHC expression. Some TAA or other exogenous antigens need to be presented to T cells by macrophages or other antigen-presenting cells in physical association with class II MHC molecules. Before presentation, the antigenic molecules are endocytosed and degraded into short peptides, and a physical complex between such peptides and class II molecules is transported to the cell surface. The T cell receptors on helper ($CD4^+$) T cells can specifically bind to and recognize these MHC-peptide complexes. TAAs may also be degraded into short peptides, 8 to 10 amino acids in length, by proteosomes within the tumor cells themselves, which then complex with class I MHC molecules.[3] Such peptide-class I complexes can specifically bind to T cell receptors on $CD8^+$ CTL.

Although most TAAs can only be recognized by T cells when physically associated with MHC molecules, a notable exception has recently been characterized in detail.[15] CTL have been detected in the regional lymph nodes of some patients with pancreatic cancer, which can specifically recognize and lyse not only autologous tumor cells, but also MHC-unrelated pancreatic and breast tumor cells. This lack of MHC restriction has been shown to be due to recognition of repeating peptide subunits on mucin molecules that are preferentially expressed on the tumor cells.

During the past few years, there has been increasing evidence that many tumors, despite their progressive growth and metastasis, contain specifically immune T cells, which are termed tumor-infiltrating lymphocytes (TILs). In studies of human tumors, cultures of TILs from some malignant melanomas or, less frequently, other tumor types have been shown to contain CTL with specific antitumor reactivity. These findings not only provide indications for the immunogenicity of some human tumors but, as discussed below, also provide a basis for specific adoptive therapy with such immune cells.

Antitumor CTL derived from a melanoma patient have also been utilized to identify and characterize the gene (MAGE-1) encoding the recognized TAA.[16] This gene was shown to be selectively expressed on some tumor cells and not in normal cells, and CTL appeared to recognize the encoded antigen in the context of a particular class I molecule, HLA-A1.

The Role of Macrophages in Host Resistance

Macrophages have been suggested as important factors in antitumor defenses and might be primarily responsible for immune surveillance against tumors. This possibility is supported by several lines of evidence:

1. Macrophages can accumulate in considerable numbers in a variety of transplantable tumors and in many primary tumors.

2. Macrophages have natural as well as the rapidly activatable ability to lyse or inhibit the growth in vitro of a wide variety of transformed cells.

3. Several treatments that can depress the function of macrophages (eg, silica or carrageenan) have been associated with an increased incidence of tumors and metastases.

4. Adoptive transfer of in vitro or in vivo activated macrophages was shown to inhibit the metastatic spread of some tumor cell lines.

5. Some carcinogens (eg, methylcholanthrene, acetylaminofluorene) have been shown to depress reticuloendothelial function.

6. Stimulation of macrophage function by various immunomodulators has been associated with decreased tumor growth or a decreased incidence of tumors.

However, there are some major limitations to such evidence:

1. There is remarkably little evidence that macrophages have cytotoxic activity against primary, freshly harvested tumor cells, as opposed to established tumor cell lines.

2. Silica and carrageenan, and virtually all of the other depressive treatments that have been used, may not be entirely selective in their effects. In fact, they may increase some functions, particularly suppressor activity, by macrophages or other cells. The treatment effects on tumor growth are not always in the same direction, even with the same tumor. For example, Mantovani and colleagues found that treatment of mice with silica or carrageenan increased the incidence of pulmonary metastases but inhibited the growth of the primary tumors.[17]

3. The carcinogens shown to depress reticuloendothelial function may also have affected a variety of effector mechanisms, and other carcinogens have had no detectable effects on macrophage or reticuloendothelial function.

4. In experiments with some transplantable tumors in mice, adoptive transfer of macrophages facilitated the development of metastases rather than conferring resistance to metastasis.

As with specific T cell-mediated immunity, some recent evidence suggesting an important antitumor defense role for macrophages has come from therapeutic studies. An immunostimulatory agent, based on the minimal immunomodulatory unit in mycobacteria and shown to be a quite selective activator of macrophages, has had substantial therapeutic efficacy against metastatic tumors in mice and dogs and has also appeared to have activity against lung metastases of patients with osteosarcoma.[18]

The Role of Natural Killer (NK) Cells in Host Resistance

Natural killer (NK) cells are a recently defined subpopulation of natural effector cells. They have the morphologic appearance of large granular lymphocytes and a characteristic cell surface phenotype that distinguishes them from T cells or macrophages.[4] A group of experts in this research area agree that NK cells usually have the morphology of large granular lymphocytes and lack the characteristic cell surface structures of T cells (CD3 and T cell receptors). These cells have spontaneous cytotoxic reactivity against cancer cells and some nonmalignant cells that is not dependent on or restricted by the MHC. In addition to their spontaneous antitumor reactivity, NK cells secrete a variety of cytokines and also have their cytotoxic reactivity augmented substantially by exposure to cytokines, especially interferons or interleukin 2 (IL2), or by various biologic response modifiers

(BRMs).[4] It has recently become clear that most lymphokine-activated killer (LAK) cell activity that is generated on culture of blood or spleen cells with IL2 is attributable to IL2-activated NK cells. LAK cells have very potent cytotoxic activity against most tumor cells, including freshly isolated tumor cells from the autologous or allogeneic solid tumors or leukemias.

There is substantial evidence for the importance of NK cells in in vivo resistance against established tumor cell lines.[19] In addition, some evidence conforms to the predictions of the immune surveillance hypothesis:

1. NK cells are able to accumulate at sites of inflammation and in small primary as well as transplanted tumors.

2. NK cells have a natural and also rapidly activatable ability to lyse a variety of primary autochthonous tumors.

3. NK cells have been shown to have the ability to eliminate metastatic tumor cells and thereby resist tumor spread.

4. An increased tumor incidence (primarily lymphomas) has been found in beige mice with depressed NK activity, patients with Chediak-Higashi syndrome, and immunosuppressed transplant recipients.[8] Some carcinogens (urethane, gamma or x-irradiation, and dimethylbenzanthracene) have been shown to cause early, profound depression of NK activity.

The most convincing data relate to the important function of NK cells in host resistance against metastases.[19] The observation that NK cells appear to be mainly responsible for the rapid elimination of intravenously inoculated tumor cells provided the initial indication that this effector mechanism might be a very effective control of hematogenous spread of tumors. Experimental support for this possibility first came from the finding that cells from the lung metastases of a transplantable tumor in mice were more resistant to NK activity than were locally growing tumor cells. Further support has come from observations that suppression or augmentation of NK activity of mice was associated with parallel alterations in resistance to artificial metastases produced by intravenous inoculation of tumor cells. The patterns of results obtained in these studies suggested that NK cells may primarily influence metastatic spread of tumors by acting during the phase of hematogenous dissemination, presumably by their ability to eliminate rapidly the tumor cells from the circulation of capillary beds. Barlozzari and colleagues further confirmed the association between depressed NK activity and increased metastases by showing that selective restoration of NK activity in rats by adoptive transfer of highly purified large granular lymphocytes was accompanied by increased resistance to pulmonary metastases.[20] Similarly, Warner and Dennert showed that adoptive transfer of a clone of cultured lymphoid cells with NK-like activity protected against development of pulmonary or liver metastases.[21] Immunotherapy studies with transplantable sarcomas in mice by adoptive transfer of LAK cells have indicated appreciable antimetastatic effects even when therapy was initiated after pulmonary metastases had occurred. Highly purified IL2-activated NK cells were shown to have more potent anti-metastatic therapeutic activity than unspecified LAK cells, and this effect has been associated with the selective accumulation of transferred effector cells at the tumor sites.[22]

Direct evidence for the role of NK cells in immune surveillance is limited and relates mainly to two models of carcinogenesis. The first model provides some indicators of NK cells' role in protecting against urethane-induced lung tumors in mice. In studies in highly susceptible A/J mice, a reduction in NK activity by treatment with cyclophosphamide led to a significantly higher tumor incidence. Conversely, adoptive transfer of normal spleen or bone marrow cells, which led to reconstitution of NK activity, inhibited subsequent incidence of lung tumors. In contrast, spleen cells from urethane-treated donors, which had low NK activity and were unable to restore NK activity in the recipients, had no significant ability to transfer resistance to development of lung tumors.

The second carcinogenesis system is the induction of thymic lymphomas by multiple low doses of irradiation of C57BL/6 mice. Tumor development appears to be dependent on a complex series of factors, and it has been difficult to demonstrate a clear contribution of NK cells to the overall process of leukemogenesis. However, NK cells appeared to be involved in protection against the transplantation of preleukemic bone marrow cells from donors that received fractionated doses of irradiation. Warner and Dennert found that adoptive transfer of cloned cells with NK-like activity, during a 4-week period after the last dose of fractionated irradiation, conferred substantial protection against the development of leukemia. Despite such suggestive positive evidence, a series of other experiments have indicated that non-NK-related factors seemed to have a more important influence on the incidence of leukemia than did the NK activity levels.

The Role of Antibodies in Host Resistance

In many tumor-bearing and immunized individuals, specific antitumor antibodies can be demonstrated. Antibodies specific for TAAs have been shown to kill tumor target cells in two ways, and there is some evidence that both mechanisms operate in vivo. The first way is that complement-dependent IgG and IgM antibodies fix to antigenic sites on target cells and activate the complement cascade. Terminal C8 and C9 components bring about lysis by the classic pathway. The second cytocidal pathway is independent of complement and is known as antibody-dependent cellular cytotoxicity (ADCC). Once antitumor IgG antibody fixes to the target cell membrane, various effector cells with receptors for the Fc portion of IgG, particularly NK cells and macrophages, can then bind to the antibody-coated tumor cells and cause their lysis.

Antitumor antibodies may be detrimental to the host. In experimental situations, antibodies administered before transplantation of tumor or infection by oncogenic virus lead to *tumor enhancement* (afferent limb-suppression of response) and thus has been termed *enhancing antibodies*. Other studies suggest that enhancing antibodies attach to the surface of tumor cells, thereby blocking or masking attachment sites for cytotoxic lymphocytes and cytolytic antibodies (efferent enhancement). In some clinical studies, the presence of detectable antibodies or antigen-antibody complexes in the circulation has been associated with the presence of tumor or poor prognosis. However in other clinical studies, high antitumor antibody titers were seen after complete surgical removal of the tumor, and declining titers were associated with recurrence or metastatic spread.

Cancer and the Functioning of the Immune System

The presence of cancer can induce antitumor immune responses, involving T cells and/or antibody-producing B cells. In addition, in many situations, tumor-bearing individuals have more general alterations in their immune system functioning. Usually the direction of modulation of immune function in cancer is negative, with depression of a variety of immunologic activities. This has in part been attributable to the release of immunosuppressive factors by the tumor cells and to the stimulation of suppressor macrophages or T cells.

The various detected deficits in immunologic competence in some tumor-bearing individuals have involved most components of the immune system. These have included decreased cellular immune reactivity, as reflected in vivo by delayed cutaneous hypersensitivity tests and in vitro by lymphoproliferative responses to mitogens or alloantigens, decreased macrophage responsiveness, and decreased NK activity. The literature on depressed immunologic competence in tumor-bearers is particularly extensive at the clinical level. The impairments observed have been most consistent in patients with advanced, metastatic disease, but some studies have detected abnormalities even early in the course of disease or in patients with no detectable tumor. In tests for delayed cutaneous hypersensitivity to dinitrochlorobenzene, which involve sensitization by a large dose of antigen and challenge 2 weeks later with a low dose, the failure of some cancer patients to be sensitized has been a useful prognostic indicator of unresectable disease or early recurrence after surgery. Decreasing the dose used for sensitization would reveal some defects in patients with early Hodgkin's disease, which had previously only been detected in patients with advanced disease.

In vitro assays of cell-mediated immunity have also been used to look for decreased reactivity in cancer patients and, as with the skin tests, the proportion of patients with localized disease who have had evidence of immune depression has varied considerably. Assays designed to detect subtle alterations in lymphoproliferative responses to mitogens and antigens, and standardization of the procedures for testing and data analysis, have yielded substantial evidence for depression in some patients with localized or early disease.[23] In one study of lung cancer patients after surgical removal of their tumors, patients with depressed lymphoproliferative responses to the mitogen concanavalin A or in mixed lymphocyte cultures had a significantly reduced disease-free survival. More recent studies have suggested that poor lymphoproliferative responses in some cancer patients may be attributable to a depressed ability to produce IL2 and for the potential responding T cells to express receptors for IL2. Recently, decreased functional activity of T cells from mice bearing an experimental tumor and from some cancer patients has been attributed to defective signal transduction related to decreased expression of components of the CD3 antigen complex.[24]

Depressed NK activity levels have also been observed in some cancer patients. In some studies, this has been associated with a poor prognosis.[25]

In addition to functional assays, enumeration of the relative proportions and absolute numbers of T and B cells may be useful in immunodiagnosis. In particular, there are indications that many cancer patients, including some with localized disease, have decreased percentages of T cell subpopulations, as assessed by high affinity rosette formation with sheep erythrocytes or by flow cytometry with antibodies to $CD4^+$ T cells.

Practical Applications of the Principles of Tumor Immunology

In addition to the contributions of tumor immunology investigations to the overall understanding of the cancer-host interaction biology, there is a variety of potential ways to apply such information and insights to the detection, diagnosis, classification, prognostic assessment, and therapy of cancer.

Immunodiagnosis

Immunodiagnosis includes several distinct clinical applications (Table 7-1). First, some immunodiagnostic procedures might be useful in the detection of cancer cases by screening of general populations or high-risk groups. Immunologic assays also may aid in distinguishing between patients with cancer and those with benign diseases. Immunodiagnostic procedures can also be used in patients with known cancer to assist in the classification of the tumor cells and assessment of their lineage and stage of differentiation; in in vivo localization of tumor; to determine prognosis; and to monitor patients during the course of disease for early detection of any recurrences or metastases.

Several criteria constitute a useful immunodiagnostic test for cancer (Table 7-2). An obvious point is that the test should be able to detect some consistent difference between cancer and noncancer. It is desirable, but not necessary, that the difference be qualitative, such as expression of a tumor-specific antigen. The presence of a TAA in cancer patients that was absent in nonneoplastic states or the loss of a normal component in cancer patients would provide a strong basis for development of a useful diagnostic test. However, quantitative differences between cancer patients and controls could also be sufficient; carefully determining the normal range would be key. A good diagnostic test should have a high degree of specificity; there should be very few false-positives. Also, the test should be very sensitive and have few false-negative results. In particular, the test should be able to detect cancer in a large proportion of cancer patients, including those with small, localized tumors or with small recurrent or metastatic deposits.

Table 7-1. Potential Applications of Immunodiagnostic Procedures

1. Detection-screening of populations and high-risk groups
2. Aid in differential diagnosis of cancer
3. Aid in classification of tumor cells
4. Localization of tumor
5. Assessment of prognosis
6. Monitoring of course of disease and early detection of recurrences or metastases

A test for initial detection or diagnosis that could localize the tumor mass is needed. One of the main concerns about detection of occult clinically undetectable cancers is the difficulty in determining the type of cancer and its location. Clearly, more information than a diagnosis of "cancer, type and site unknown" would be needed for undertaking rational therapy. Specificity for a particular organ site or histologic type of cancer is important initially, but it is not as essential for monitoring previously diagnosed patients.

Table 7-2. Criteria for Useful Immunodiagnostic Test for Cancer

1. Qualitative or quantitative difference from normal or benign
2. High specificity (low percent of false-positives)
3. High sensitivity (low percent of false-negatives)
4. Organ site specificity for localization

For detection, it is particularly important that the assay be simple and practical enough for testing large numbers of specimens or individuals. The procedures must be sufficiently well developed and standardized so that reproducible results can be obtained in many laboratories. A screening test that would be given to a high proportion of normal individuals should present little or no risk to the recipients. The specificity of a screening test is a particularly important factor because the occurrence of an appreciable number of false-positives in a screened population causes psychologic, logistic, and economic problems. For example, if the frequency of a given type of a cancer in a population is 0.5% and the frequency of positive tests is 10%, most of the individuals with positive results would be needlessly alarmed and subjected to costly, time-consuming diagnostic procedures.

Tests to be used as diagnostic adjuncts must meet different criteria. These tests should be highly accurate in discriminating between cancer and noncancer in an individual, rather than showing significant differences between cancer and noncancer groups. False-positive and false-negative results both have serious implications, but an error rate of 5% to 10% in each direction might be considered acceptable. Also, procedures with some risk might be more acceptable in these patients, since the ratio of potential risk to possible benefit is quite different from that in screening general populations.

For immunologic tests to be useful for prognosis or for monitoring of cancer patients, they must not only discriminate between individuals with cancer and those without, but also reflect the stage of disease and the presence or absence of small amounts of tumor. The monitoring test needs to be acceptable for repeated use by the patients. There may also be special problems of the assays being affected by the therapy, particularly immunosuppressive therapy.

There are several types of approaches to take to the immunodiagnosis of cancer (Table 7-3). The first approach, the detection of antigenic markers in the tumor-bearing individual, has been used the most. Tumor cells may contain antigens that are undetectable or are present in smaller amounts in normal cells. Thus, antibodies in patients' sera, or in the sera of animals immunized against these antigens, can potentially discriminate between tumor cells and normal cells. In order to be useful in immunodiagnosis, the tumor antigens must be common to a variety of tumors, at least of the same histologic type.

Most immunodiagnostic assays have focused on the detection of circulating tumor markers, with the levels generally reflecting the amount of tumor present and the metastatic spread of disease. The expression of TAAs or other markers on the tumor cells has been helpful primarily in classifying tumors and discerning their derivation. This may have therapeutic implications, and the application has been most widely used for the leukemias and lymphomas where the surface phenotype has become a standard aspect of assessment. In addition, the loss of some normal antigens, either organ-specific or not, from tumor cells may be useful in immunodiagnosis. For example, loss of blood group antigens has been correlated with a tendency for metastasis.

Depression in the cancer patient's immune competence might also be useful diagnostically, because deficits in immunologic function or in subpopulations of cells of the immune system have been associated with poor prognosis. Also, there are suggestions that some immunologic assays may be useful in discerning individuals with increased risk of malignancy.

Many tumor-associated antigens can elicit an immune response in a tumor-bearing individual. Antigens present in very small amounts can often be recognized by the host, and it might therefore be expected that immunologic reactions would be detected while tumors were still small and localized. Both humoral antibodies and cell-mediated immune responses can be measured; sufficiently standardized assays might be more sensitive for detection of the tumor-bearing state than the more usual assays of circulating tumor markers.

Table 7-3. Immunologic Approaches to the Diagnosis of Cancer

1. Detection of TAAs or antigens associated with viruses or with certain organs or tissues
   a. On tumor cells
   b. Circulating in plasma or in secretions
2. Immune competence of cancer patients
3. Immune response to TAAs or to virus-associated antigens
   a. Humoral immunity
   b. Cell-mediated immunity

With regard to immunodiagnostic assays currently in clinical use, the value of only a small number of tumor markers has been sufficiently demonstrated. However, a larger array is being actively studied, and the list of useful tests may grow, particularly for assessing prognosis and monitoring therapy. This topic has recently been reviewed.[26] Assays for two circulating markers have given encouraging results, not only for assessing prognosis and the course of disease after diagnosis, but also for initial detection and diagnosis. These markers—prostate-specific antigen for prostate cancer and CA-125 for ovarian cancer—are currently being evaluated for their value in cancer screening in a large, National Cancer Institute-funded multicenter study.

Immunotherapy

The building evidence for the immune system's participation in resistance against the progression and spread of cancer has raised expectations that manipulation of the immune system might also be a valuable treatment. Such optimism has been fostered by the findings that various cytokines and other biologic response modifiers can appreciably stimulate or augment immunologic reactivity against cancer. Some species of genetically engineered interferon have been shown to have had appreciable antitumor effects against experimental tumors and some clinical malignancies. Alpha interferon has already been licensed by the United States Food and Drug Administration (FDA) as effective for treatment of hairy cell leukemia and Kaposi's sarcoma and appears promising for the treatment of several other types of cancer. IL2, particularly in combination with LAK cells (see above), has been shown to have strong antimetastatic effects against some experimental tumors in mice and rats. In some cases it has been able to induce cures. Analogous therapy in some patients with advanced cancer, particularly with malignant melanoma or renal carcinoma, has induced partial or complete regression of detectable metastatic lesions.[27] In detailed studies in an experimental tumor model, it appears that optimal results may be achieved by combining cytoreductive therapy by surgery and chemotherapy with the adoptive immunotherapy with IL2 and LAK cells.

Adoptive therapy with specifically immune T cells and IL2 may even be more potent than LAK cells and IL2, with curative effects induced in some experimental tumor models.[28] Recently, very promising therapeutic results have been obtained by specific in vitro sensitization with irradiated lymphoid tumor cells from mice with growing tumors. Clinically, tumor-infiltrating lymphocytes from patients with malignant melanoma have been expanded in culture with IL2 and have appeared to have specific cytotoxic reactivity against the autologous tumor cells.[29] These IL2-expanded cells, when transferred to the patients, have induced some complete tumor regressions. Considerably more efforts in the overall area of adoptive cellular immunotherapy seem warranted, with a focus on defining and purifying the effector cells responsible for the therapeutic cells, determining the conditions for optimally generating them and stimulating their antitumor reactivity, and maximizing their accumulation in all sites of tumor growth.

In addition to the studies of adoptive transfer of specifically immune T cells, there has been a recent upsurge in the evaluation of active-specific immunotherapy, utilizing "cancer vaccines." Treatment of patients with intact, inactivated tumor cells or with tumor cell extracts has given some encouraging, although still quite preliminary, results, mainly in patients with malignant melanoma, but also with some other tumor types.[30] In recent studies with several animal tumor models, insertion into tumor cells of genes for cytokines such as IL2, interleukin 4, or colony-stimulating factor has resulted in an impressive increase in immunogenicity and antitumor effects. Clinical trials with such genetically altered tumor cells will be initiated in the near future.

Infusion of monoclonal antibodies against TAAs has been another major approach for the treatment of metastatic cancer. The main strategy has been to combine the antibodies with toxic moieties—either radionuclides, toxins, or drugs. The goal is to have the antibodies selectively carry the toxic agents to the tumor site or sites. Although this form of immunotherapy has considerable rationale and should eventually be very useful, many technical problems have limited its therapeutic benefits. In addition to the immunoconjugate approach, some antibodies by themselves appear to have promising therapeutic effects. This might be attributed to such mechanisms as complement-dependent lysis of tumor cells, interactions with effector cells for ADCC, or immunoregulatory effects such as the induction of anti-idiotypic responses. An example of the therapeutic effects of a monoclonal antibody by itself has come from a study with antibodies to the GD3 ganglioside in human malignant melanoma, with partial regression of tumor in several patients with advanced disease.

Other efforts have been directed towards stimulating the host's immune system using a wide variety of immunomodulators. These may be either defined chemical substances or, more frequently, bacterial products such as BCG or OK432. Although the latter group of agents are usually very heterogeneous and ill-defined, they can induce strong stimulation of various components of the immune system, including antitumor effector mechanisms. BCG, which is a low virulence variant of *Mycobacterium tuberculosis*, has been found to be very effective for treatment of superficial recurrent carcinoma of the bladder. OK432, an inactivated form of *Streptococcus pyogenes*, has been used widely in Japan and other countries and appears to be effective for treating malignant effusions and possibly other forms of cancer. A synthetic macrophage activator has also had therapeutic effects against some experimental tumors and is now being evaluated clinically.[18]

Immunotherapy for cancer has had some success to date, but this field is still at a very early stage of development. Most of the promising strategies need to be investigated in considerably greater detail, and the optimal doses and conditions for treatment have to be defined. This will require a methodical approach, with close interaction between the in vivo studies and detailed in vitro evaluation of the effects on the immune system.[31]

References

1. Hewitt HB. Animal tumor models and their relevance to human tumor immunology. *J Biol Response Mod.* 1982;1:107-119.

2. Herberman RB. Counterpoint: animal tumor models and their relevance to human tumor immunology. *J Biol Response Mod.* 1983;2:39-46.

3. Ljunggren H-G, Stam NJ, Öhlen C, et al. Empty MHC class I molecules come out in the cold. *Nature.* 1990; 346:476-480.

4. Ortaldo JR, Herberman RB. Heterogeneity of natural killer cells. In: Paul WE, Fathman CG, Metzger H, eds. *Ann Rev Immunol.* Palo Alto, Calif: Annual Reviews Inc; 1984;2:359-394.

5. Kwak LW, Campbell MJ, Czerwinski DK, Hart S, Miller RA, Levy R. Induction of immune responses in patients with B-cell lymphoma against the surface-immunoglobulin idiotype expressed by their tumors. *N Engl J Med.* 1992; 327:1209-1215.

6. Boon T. Toward a genetic analysis of tumor rejection antigens. *Adv Cancer Res.* 1992;58:177-210.

7. Ehrlich P. Uber den jetzigen Stand der Karzinomforschung. In: Himmelweit F, ed. *The Collected Papers of Paul Ehrlich.* Vol. II. London: Pergamon Press; 1957:550-562.

8. Penn I, Starzl TR. A summary of the status of de novo cancer in transplant recipients. *Transplant Proc.* 1972;4:719-732.

9. Ho M, Jaffe R, Miller G, et al. The frequency of Epstein-Barr virus infection and associated lymphoproliferative syndrome after transplantation and its manifestations in children. *Transplantation.* 1988;45:719-727.

10. Klein G, Klein E. Rejectability of virus induced tumors and nonrejectability of spontaneous tumors—a lesson in contrasts. *Transplant Proc.* 1977;9:1095-1104.

11. Prehn RT, Lappe MA. An Immunostimulation theory of tumor development. *Transplant Rev.* 1971;7:26-54.

12. Prehn RT, Main JM. Immunity to MCA-induced sarcoma. *J Natl Cancer Inst.* 1957;18:769-775.

13. Kripke ML. Immunologic mechanisms in UV radiation carcinogenesis. *Adv Cancer Res.* 1981;34:69-106.

14. Peppoloni S, Herberman RB, Gorelik E. Lewis lung carcinoma (3LL) cells treated in vitro with ultraviolet radiation show reduced metastatic ability due to an augmented immunogenicity. *Clin Exp Metastasis.* 1987;5:43-56.

15. Jerome KR, Barnd DL, Boyer CM, et al. Cytotoxic T-lymphocytes derived from patients with breast adenocarcinoma recognize an epitope present on the protein core of a mucin molecular preferentially expressed by malignant cells. *Cancer Res.* 1991;51:2908-2916.

16. van der Bruggen P, Traversari C, Chomez P, et al. A gene encoding an antigen recognized by cytolytic T lymphocytes on a human melanoma. *Science.* 1991;254:1643-1647.

17. Mantovani A, Giavazzi R, Polentarutti N, Spreafico F, Garattini S. Divergent effects of macrophage toxins on growth of primary tumors and lung metastasis. *Int J Cancer.* 1980;25:617-622.

18. Kleinerman ES, Raymond AK, Bucana CD, et al. Unique histological changes in lung metastases of osteosarcoma patients following therapy with liposomal muramyl tripeptide (CGP 19835A lipid). *Cancer Immunol Immunother.* 1992;34:211-220.

19. Gorelik E, Herberman RB. Role of natural killer (NK) cells in the control of tumor growth and metastatic spread. In: Herberman RB, ed. *Cancer Immunology: Innovative Approaches to Therapy.* Boston, Mass: Martinus Nijhoff; 1986:151-176.

20. Barlozzari T, Reynolds CW, Herberman RB. In vivo role of natural killer cells: involvement of large granular lymphocytes in the clearance of tumor cells in antiasialo GM_1-treated rats. *J Immunol.* 1983;131:1024-1027.

21. Warner JF, Dennert TG. In vivo function of a closed cell line with NK activity: effects on bone marrow transplants, tumor development, and metastases. *Nature.* 1982;31:300.

22. Basse P, Herberman RB, Nannmark V, et al. Accumulation of adoptively transferred adherent lymphokine-activated killer cells in murine metastases. *J Exp Med.* 1991;174:479-488.

23. Dean JH. Application of the microculture lymphocyte proliferation assay to clinical studies. In: Herberman RB, McIntire KR, eds. *Immunodiagnosis of Cancer.* New York, NY: Marcel Dekker, Inc; 1979:738-769.

24. Mizoguchi H, O'Shea J, Longo DL, Loeffler CM, McVicar DW, Ochoa AC. Alterations in signal transduction molecules in T lymphocytes from tumor-bearing mice. *Science.* 1992;258:1795-1798.

25. Schantz SP, Brown BW, Lira E, Taylor DL, Beddingfield N. Evidence for the role of natural immunity in the control of metastatic spread of head and neck cancer. *Cancer Immunol Immunother.* 1987;25:141-145.

26. Virji MA, Mercer DW, Herberman RB. Tumor markers in cancer diagnosis and prognosis. *CA Cancer J Clin.* 1988; 38:104-126.

27. Rosenberg SA, Lotze MT, Muul LM, et al. Observations on the systemic administration of autologous lymphokine activated killer cells and recombinant interleukin-2 to patients with metastatic cancer. *N Engl J Med.* 1985;313:1485-1489.

28. Greenberg PD, Klarnet JP, Kern DE, Cheever MA. Therapy of disseminated tumors by adoptive transfer of specifically immune T cells. *Prog Exp Tumor Res.* 1988;32:104-127.

29. Rosenberg SA, Packard BS, Aebersold PM, et al. Use of tumor-infiltrating lymphocytes and interleukin-2 in the immunotherapy of patients with metastatic melanoma. *N Engl J Med.* 1988;319:1676-1680.

30. Mitchell MS. Active specific immunotherapy of cancer: therapeutic vaccines ("theraccines") for the treatment of disseminated malignancies. In: Mitchell MS, ed. *Biological Approaches to Cancer Treatment.* New York, NY: McGraw-Hill Inc; 1993:326-351.

31. Herberman RB. Design of clinical trials with biological response modifiers. *Cancer Treat Rep.* 1985;69:1161-1164.

8

SMOKING AND CANCER

Ellen R. Gritz, PhD, Michael C. Fiore, MD, MPH, Jack E. Henningfield, PhD

Epidemiology of Smoking and Smoking-Related Cancers

In 1990, almost 30 years after Surgeon General Luther L. Terry first warned the American public that cigarette smoking was the principal cause of lung cancer, 25.5% of all adults in the United States continued to smoke.[1] Since the release of that landmark document, an unequivocal body of scientific evidence has accumulated, further implicating tobacco as a carcinogen for a wide variety of tumor types and sites. Tobacco use is now responsible for 30% of all cancer deaths in the US, resulting in >150,000 cancer deaths each year.[2] Because of this, cigarette smoking has achieved the dubious distinction of being the chief preventable cause of cancer in this country.

The Epidemiology of Cigarette Smoking in the US

In the early 1900s, cigarette smoking was uncommon. A series of events during the first quarter of the twentieth century—the development of the flue-curing process, the first widescale production of machine-made cigarettes and matches, and the outbreak of World War I—combined with the highly addictive nature of nicotine to result in an epidemic of cigarette smoking, particularly among men. This epidemic continued into the 1960s (Fig 8-1) when more than 40% of all adults smoked, including >50% of adult men.[2]

Smoking prevalence rates have declined since the early 1960s, although the rate of decline has varied markedly across different sociodemographic strata. The National Health Interview Surveys (NHIS), collected by the National Center for Health Statistics, have systematically assessed smoking rates among a representative sample of adult Americans since the sixties and provide us with the best source of information on smoking rates.[1,2] Among white men, smoking has declined at an average rate of 0.9 percentage points per year, falling from 51.5% in 1965 to 27.9% by 1990. In contrast, smoking prevalence for white women has fallen from 34.2% in 1965 to 23.5% by 1990, an average of 0.4 percentage points per year. Among black men, the rate of smoking has declined at an average rate of 1.1 percentage points per year, falling from 60.8% in 1965 to 32.6% by 1990. Among black women, smoking has declined from 34.4% in 1965 to 21.2% by 1990, or 0.5 percentage points per year. Among Hispanics, the 1990 NHIS reported smoking prevalence rates of 30.9% in men and 16.3% in women; trend data are unavailable.

Over the past 30 years, there has been a widening gap in smoking rates across socioeconomic parameters, particularly educational status. In the early 1960s, small differences in smoking rates were noted across educational groups. By 1990, this variable was highly associated with risk of smoking: the prevalence rate among high school dropouts remained relatively constant at 31.8%, while the rate among college graduates fell dramatically to 13.5%. Increasingly, the highest rates of smoking are found among the most sociodemographically disadvantaged members of our society—the same individuals who are at increased overall risk for cancer.

The steady decline in smoking rates over the past 30 years allows for cautious predictions into the next century.[3] If current trends continue, the smoking rate among men is projected to fall to 20% by the year 2000, and among women to 22% (Fig 8-2).[2,4] Among whites the prevalence of smoking is projected to fall to

Ellen R. Gritz, PhD, Annie Laurie Howard Research Professorship, Professor and Chair, Department of Behavioral Science, University of Texas MD Anderson Cancer Center, Houston, Texas

Michael C. Fiore, MD, MPH, Director, Center for Tobacco Research and Intervention, Associate Professor, Department of Medicine, University of Wisconsin–Madison Medical School, Madison, Wisconsin

Jack E. Henningfield, PhD, Chief, Clinical Pharmacology Branch, Addiction Research Center, National Institute on Drug Abuse, and Associate Professor, Department of Psychiatry and Behavioral Science, The Johns Hopkins University School of Medicine, Baltimore, Maryland

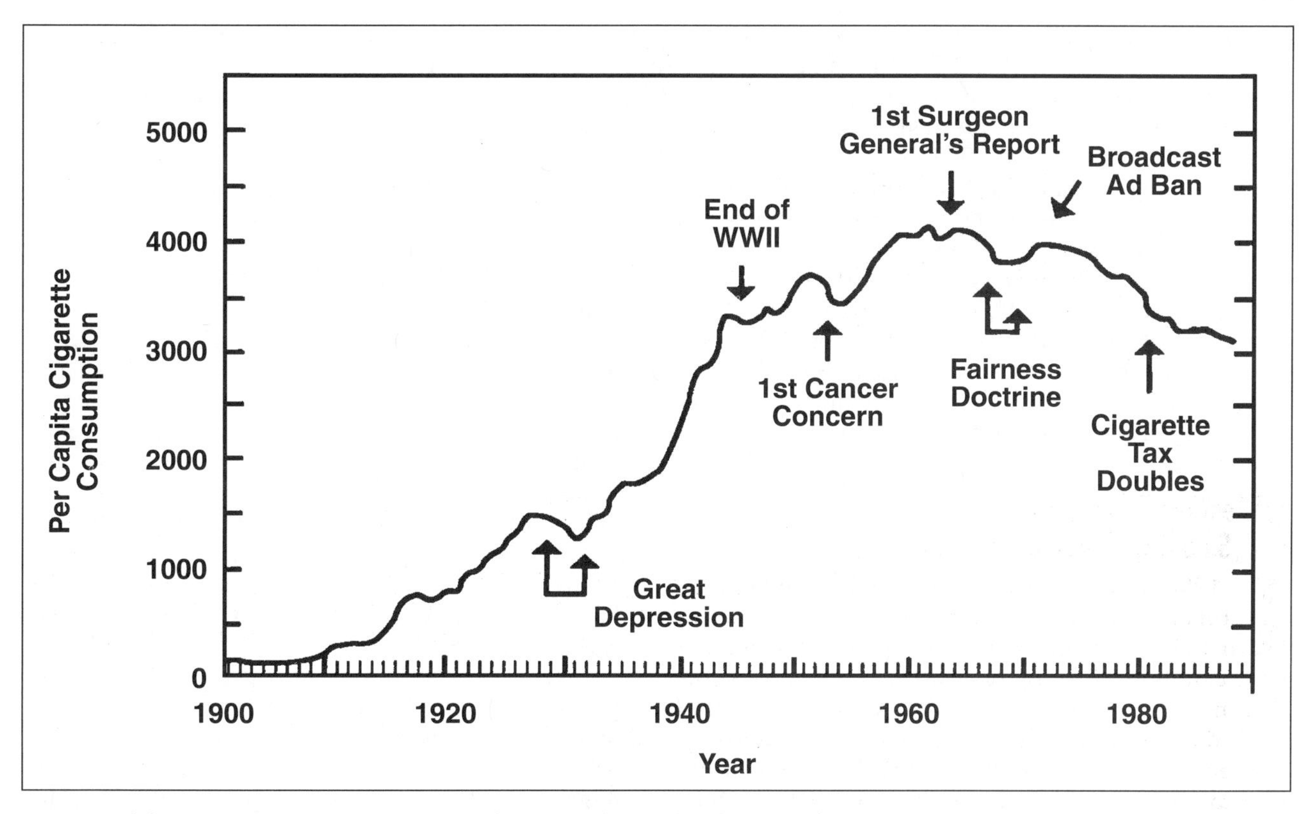

Fig 8-1. Adult per capita cigarette consumption and major smoking and world events (from *Reducing the Health Consequences of Smoking*[2]).

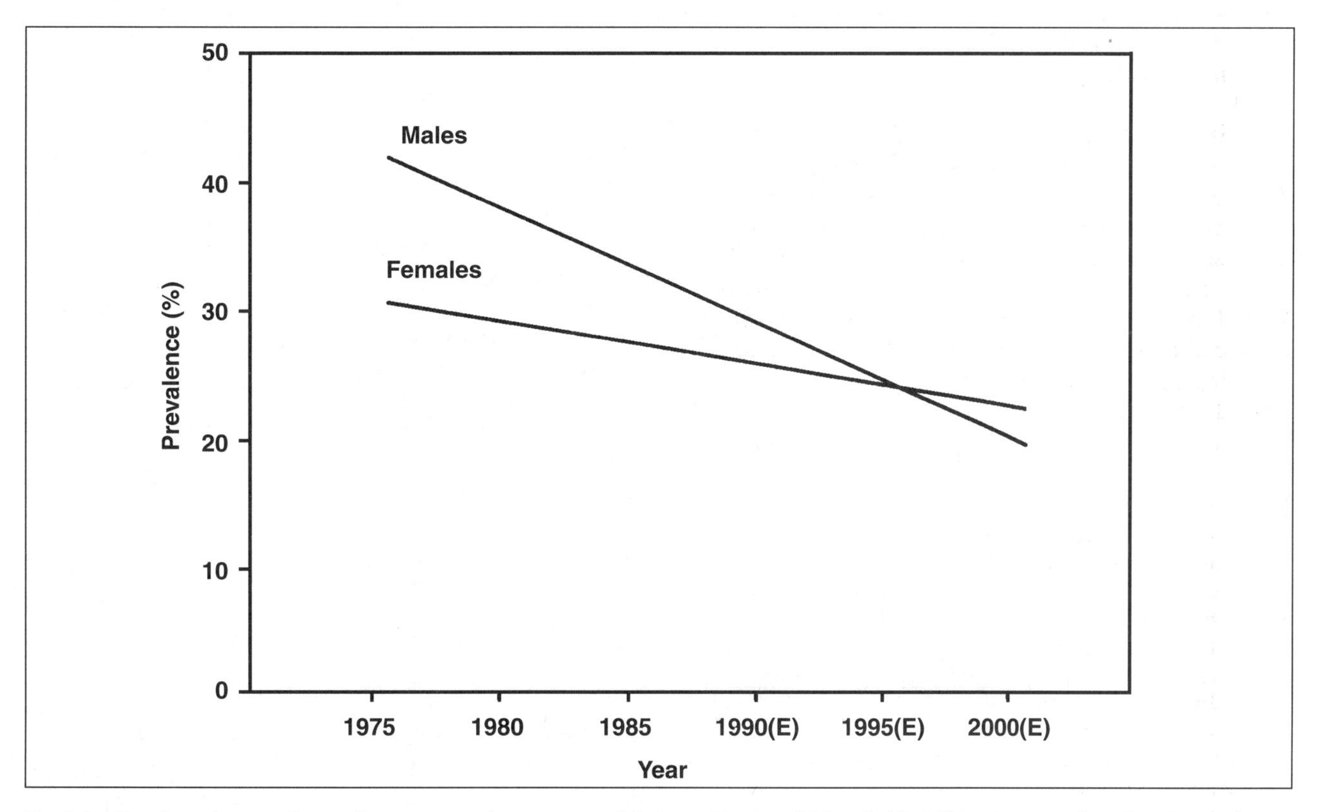

Fig 8-2. Trends in the prevalence of cigarette smoking among adult Americans (aged 20 and older) (from Fiore et al[4] and *Reducing the Health Consequences of Smoking*[2]).

21% by the year 2000, while the rate among blacks is projected to fall to 25% (Fig 8-3).[2,4] Turning to educational status, if current trends continue, smoking rates among high school dropouts will decline only marginally to 30% by the year 2000. In contrast, smoking rates among college graduates are projected to decline to <10% by the turn of the century (Fig 8-4).[2,4]

Overall, approximately 45 million adult Americans (25.5%) currently smoke with 42 million smokers projected for the year 2000.[1] In contrast, one of the objectives of the *Healthy People 2000* program is a reduction in smoking prevalence to 15% by the next century.[5] A significant increase in smoking prevention and cessation activities nationwide will be required to achieve this goal. One example of an effective community-wide intervention is the California Proposition 99 experience. This citizen's ballot initiative, enacted in 1988, mandated a 25 cent per pack increase in cigarette excise tax, with proceeds dedicated to health and tobacco prevention activities. This statewide intervention has resulted in a 17% decline in smoking rates in California in the first 3 years of the program.[6]

In contrast to the success achieved in promoting smoking cessation during the 1980s, rates of smoking initiation have not declined appreciably. The 1991 nationwide, school-based Youth Risk Behavior Survey (YRBS) noted that among 12th grade students, 15.6% reported frequent use of cigarettes over the past month, a proportion essentially unchanged over the past decade.[7] Of students in grades 9 through 12, the prevalence of frequent cigarette use was much higher among whites (15.4%) than Hispanics (6.8%) or blacks (3.1%). The CDC's 1989 Teenage Attitudes and Practices Survey (TAPS) noted that among youths aged 17 to 18, the percentage of high school dropouts who smoked (43.3%) was markedly higher than among those continuing in school or those who had graduated (17.1%).[8]

To achieve the goal of a smoke-free society by the year 2000, significant progress must be achieved in convincing American youngsters to avoid tobacco use. Public health policy changes promoting this goal include establishing tobacco-free schools and including tobacco use prevention programs in school curricula; enacting and enforcing state laws to prohibit the sale and distribution of tobacco products to youths under 19 years of age; eliminating all forms of tobacco product advertising and promotion; and greatly increasing excise taxes on tobacco products.[8]

Cigarette Smoking and Cancer

Cancer accounts for approximately 150,000 of the 434,000 total deaths in the US attributable each year to cigarette smoking.[2] More than 30% of all cancer deaths in this country are directly attributable to tobacco use, as well as approximately 85% of all lung

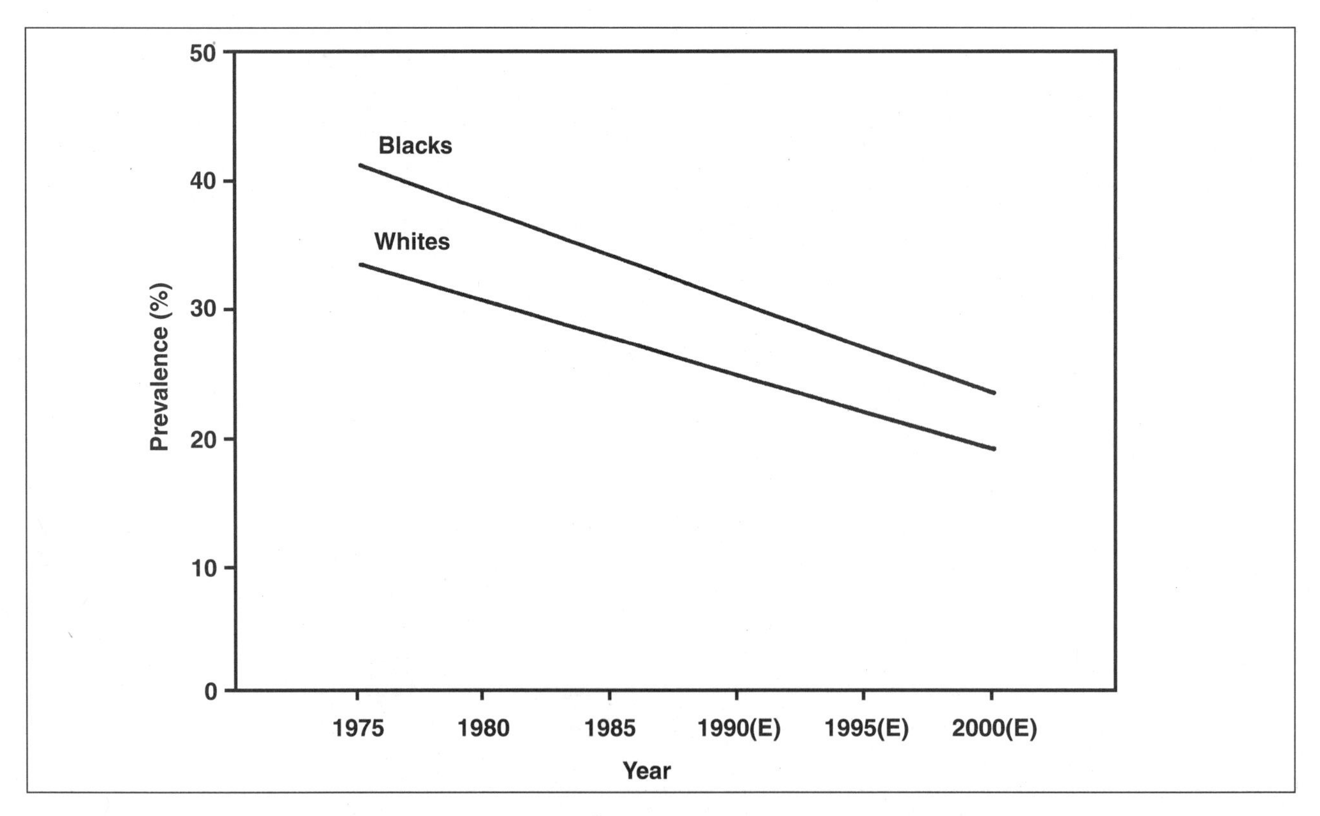

Fig 8-3. Trends in the prevalence of cigarette smoking among black and white adult Americans (aged 20 and older) (from Fiore et al[4] and *Reducing the Health Consequences of Smoking*[2]). E=estimated.

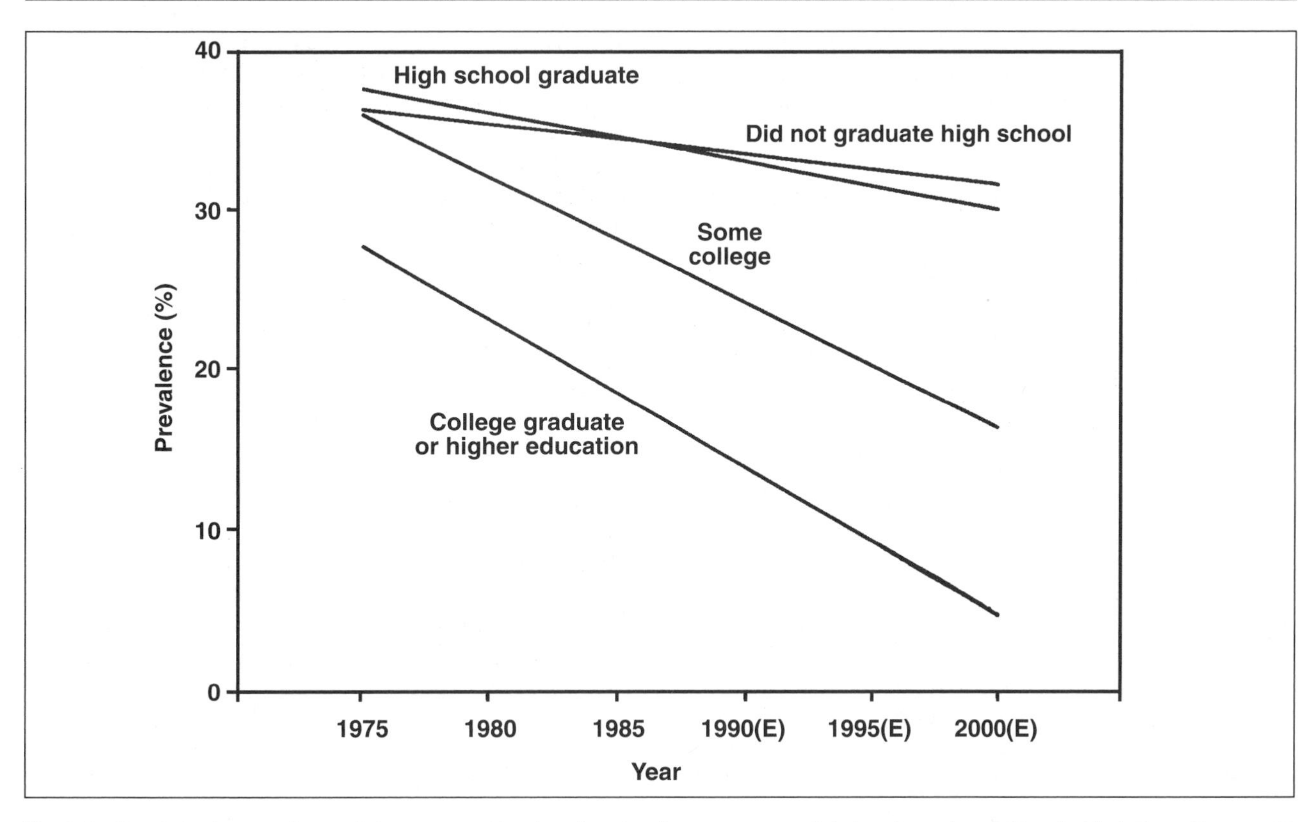

Fig 8-4. Trends in the prevalence of cigarette smoking by educational status among adult Americans (aged 20 and older) (from Fiore et al[4] and *Reducing the Health Consequences of Smoking*[2]). E=estimated.

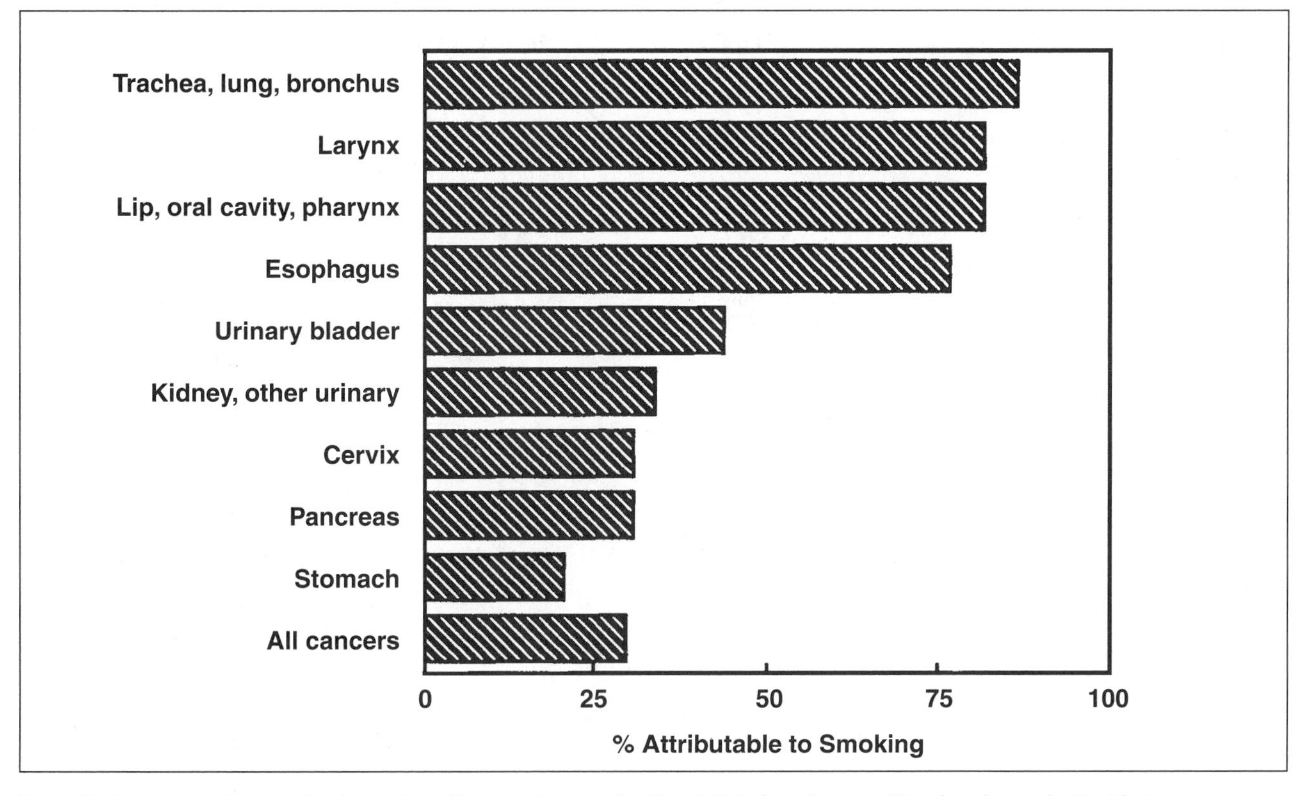

Fig 8-5. Proportion of cancer deaths attributable to smoking in the US in 1985 (from Fiore et al[4] and *Reducing the Health Consequences of Smoking*[2]).

cancer deaths; 80% of larynx, pharynx, oral cavity, and lip cancer deaths; 75% of esophageal cancer deaths; 45% of urinary bladder cancer deaths; 30% of cervical and pancreatic cancer deaths; and 20% of stomach cancer deaths (Fig 8-5).[2,4]

The number of cancer deaths resulting from smoking, particularly the epidemic of lung cancer attributable to smoking, is directly responsible for the steady increase in US cancer mortality over the past 35 years. Overall, cancer death rates for smokers are two times greater than those for nonsmokers; heavier smokers have rates four times greater.[2] Table 8-1 summarizes the relative risks and smoking-attributable mortality for various sites of cancer.[9]

Smoking results in cancer not only at sites in direct contact with tobacco smoke (oral cavity, pharynx, larynx, and lung), but also at distant sites. For example, nearly 50% of all bladder and kidney cancer deaths among men are attributable to smoking, with the risk of bladder and kidney cancers among smokers two to three times greater than among nonsmokers.[9] Aromatic amines found in tobacco smoke are probably important in the development of cancer at these sites.

For cervical cancer, cigarette smoking is believed to account for approximately 30% of the 4,600 deaths each year.[9] The incidence of cervical cancer among smokers is estimated to be about twice that among nonsmokers and appears to be greatest in women who do not have other major risk factors for this neoplasm.[9] With cervical cancer, the effect of smoking cessation appears immediate: former smokers have no increased risk of cervical cancer, suggesting that the effect of cigarette smoking is confined to late-stage or promotional effects.

For a small number of sites, cancer risk is actually less among smokers.[9] For example, there is about a 30% reduction in risk of cancer of the uterine endometrium among smokers, compared with nonsmokers. There may be a decreased risk among smokers for cancer of the breast and large bowel. The public health significance of these relationships, however, is extremely limited. While smoking may confer a modest reduction in risk for certain cancers such as endometrial cancer, the overall annual number of lives lost because of cigarette smoking is 30 times greater.

Table 8-1. Summary of Smoking and Cancer Mortality

		Relative Risk Among Smokers		Mortality Attributable to Smoking	
Type of Cancer		Current	Former	Percent	Number
Lung	Male	22.4	9.4	90	82,800
	Female	11.9	4.7	79	40,300
Larynx	Male	10.5	5.2	81	2,400
	Female	17.8	11.9	87	700
Oral cavity	Male	27.5	8.8	92	4,900
	Female	5.6	2.9	61	1,800
Esophagus	Male	7.6	5.8	78	5,700
	Female	10.3	3.2	75	1,900
Pancreas	Male	2.1	1.1	29	3,500
	Female	2.3	1.8	34	4,500
Bladder	Male	2.9	1.9	47	3,000
	Female	2.6	1.9	37	1,200
Kidney	Male	3.0	2.0	48	3,000
	Female	1.4	1.2	12	500
Stomach	Male	1.5	?	17	1,400
	Female	1.5	?	25	1,300
Leukemia	Male	2.0	?	20	2,000
	Female	2.0	?	20	1,600
Cervix		2.1	1.9	31	1,400
Endometrium		0.7	1.0	–	–

Source: Newcomb and Carbone.[9]

Environmental Tobacco Smoke and Cancer

Recently, environmental tobacco smoke (ETS) has been cited as a cause of cancer in healthy nonsmokers. A number of studies have linked passive smoking with the development of lung cancer, but others have shown no association.[10] On the basis of the conclusions of the former studies, the US Surgeon General concluded that ETS is a cause of lung cancer.[10] The Committee on Passive Smoking from the National Research Council reviewed the existing scientific literature and reached a similar conclusion.[11] Finally, the Environmental Protection Agency's landmark report on environmental tobacco smoke concluded that second-hand smoke has earned the dubious distinction of being classified a group A (known human) carcinogen.[12] This report estimated that approximately 3,000 lung cancer deaths in the US are directly attributable to ETS and that second-hand smoke is particularly harmful to children.

The Role of the Physician in Smoking Cessation

Over the past 10 years, increasing attention has focused on the powerful role of the physician in motivating and assisting patients to stop smoking. This role is appropriate, given that the physician serves as guardian and facilitator of the patient's health, and often that of family members as well. In 1990, a total of 388 million visits were paid to all primary care physicians in the US.[13] Given the estimates that 76% of the US population saw a physician, including 71% of current smokers, and that 24% of all patients were smokers, the potential for physicians to intervene with patients who smoke is great (Centers for Disease Control [CDC], unpublished data from the 1991 NHIS).

Through their own behavior, physicians serve as powerful role models in discouraging tobacco use. They have the lowest smoking prevalence rate of any occupational group in the US. Data collected from 1990 and 1991 showed that only 3.3% of physicians smoked daily.[4] This extraordinary acknowledgment by example of the health-damaging effects of tobacco is unfortunately not true of physicians worldwide, among whom the prevalence is still >40% in many nations.[15]

While most physicians report that they counsel their patients who smoke, this message does not consistently reach patients at risk. In repeated national surveys, only about 50% of patients report ever having been asked by their clinician if they smoke.[16] In contrast, the target set by *Healthy People 2000*, which identifies national health objectives, is for 75% of US physicians to routinely provide antismoking counseling to all their patients.[5] One simple but effective way to promote this goal is to designate smoking status as the *new vital sign*, to be assessed for every patient at every clinic visit.[17]

In controlled trials assessing the effectiveness of clinical intervention, brief advice by primary care physicians to stop smoking yielded 1-year success rates of up to 15% of all patients who smoked.[18] Intervention "quit rates" were as much as six times higher than in control practices. These rates, while statistically significant, may be interpreted as clinically discouraging to physicians, who are oriented toward acute interventions with curative treatments. A more appropriate interpretation of the influence of the physician on lifestyle behavior modification, such as smoking prevention and cessation, is as *one source of influence* in a multifactorial decision matrix that involves the environment as well as individual forces.[19] This requires that clinicians recognize smoking as a chronic disease, with periods of remission and exacerbation for many patients.[17] As with other chronic diseases, such as hypertension or diabetes, physicians must continually intervene with patients throughout the course of the disease, utilizing different interventional strategies and considering a stepped care approach to smoking cessation.[20]

The likelihood that an individual will follow a physician recommendation or regimen has been extensively studied and analyzed in the literature on compliance. The authors prefer to use the term "adherence," which places patient behavior in a systemic context, rather than the more traditional concept of noncompliance, which involves a patient's failure to follow a regimen.[21] For smoking cessation, a preventive health behavior, this distinction becomes even more important since the patient is frequently not seriously ill when advised to stop smoking. A recent formulation of a model for adherence to cancer prevention and control interventions addresses the "art of care"—information and communication, and rapport and trust—which figures prominently among factors influencing intentions to adhere.[21,22] Even if patients decide to follow a regimen or make a lifestyle change, the presence of supports and barriers in their social and physical environments will affect the translation of these intentions into action and the duration of any actions undertaken. Thus, the effect of the physician's recommendation alone can be seen as both time- and place-limited, underscoring the importance of the context in which such messages are delivered.

Stage of change is a concept that has come to have major utility in terms of predicting change in smoking behavior and in planning interventions based on readiness to quit.[23] Individuals move along a continuum from never having smoked through a period of experimentation to regular use, and thence into a cycle of dependent smoking which can eventuate in cessation or relapse (Fig 8-6).[24] It is possible to intervene in the process of smoking uptake, as well as after dependent smoking is established.[19] The major stages in the cessation process are precontemplation (not thinking about stopping), contemplation and preparation (considering cessation), action (within the first 6 months of cessation), and long-term abstinence (more than 6 months). Relapse can interrupt any cessation process; most persons cycle several times before achieving permanent cessation.[19,25]

The physician can influence smoking behavior at many stages in the processes of smoking initiation and cessation (Fig 8-7).[24] Patients advised to quit smoking are both more likely to report being in the contemplation and preparation stages (compared to precontemplation) and to have made a "quit attempt" in the past year.[6] The same message delivered at different times may convey a highly variable impact on the patient's behavior, depending on the complex mix of factors determining decision-making and adherence. For the physician, the "teachable moment" or "window of opportunity" is most often encountered in the context of symptoms or a disease diagnosis, for either the patient or a close friend, family member, or significant other.[19,26,27]

The physician's office and the hospital are the two major settings for offering smoking cessation advice. The National Cancer Institute (NCI) has developed an extensive, state-of-the-art program for the physician, providing a structure for advice and office organization.[18,28] The NCI has also developed guidelines and materials for pediatricians, dealing with prevention and cessation, as well as for allied health professionals, including nurses, respiratory therapists, and pharmacists.

The National Cancer Institute Model

The NCI program, *How to Help Your Patients Stop Smoking*, provides physicians with a brief (3- to 5-minute) but effective intervention strategy to aid smokers to successfully quit.[28] This program is built around the four A's: ASK, ADVISE, ASSIST, and ARRANGE. The first A is to **Ask Every Patient at Every Clinic Visit If They Smoke**. As mentioned earlier, only 50% of patients who smoke report *ever* having been asked by a physician whether they smoke. A much smaller percentage have received specific advice on how to quit successfully. One way to increase the certainty of identifying all patients who smoke is to designate smoking status as the *new vital sign*, assessed for every clinic patient at every visit.[17] A sample vital sign stamp to use on patient history forms is shown in Fig 8-8.

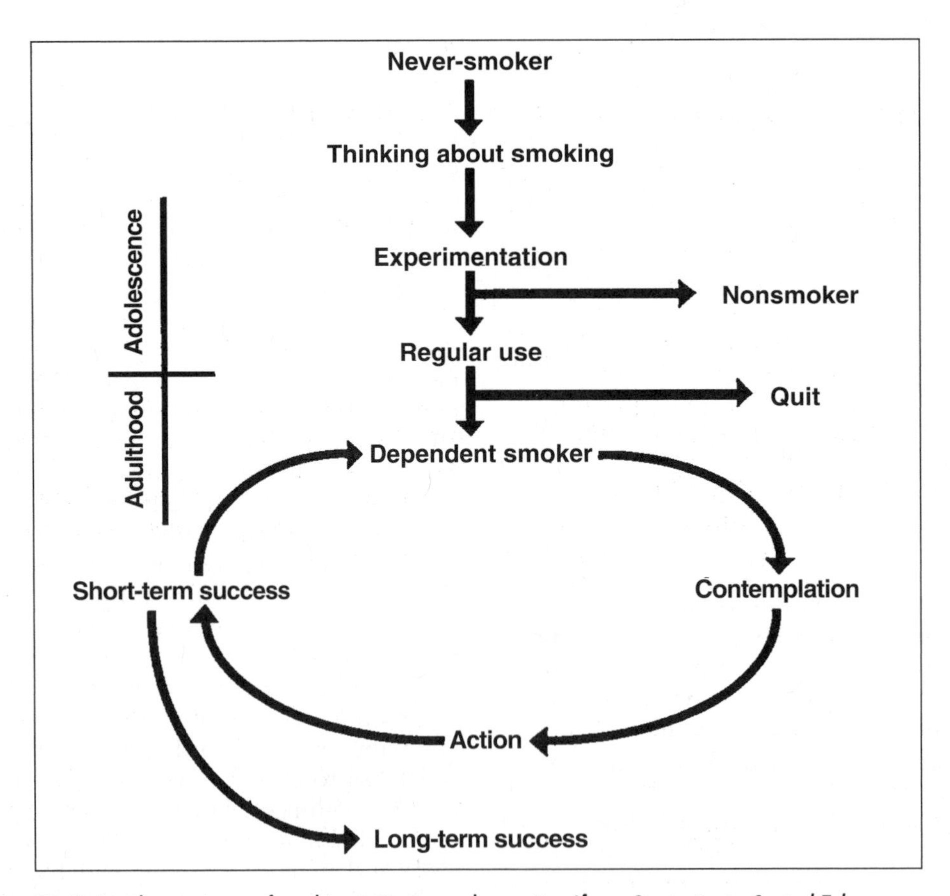

Fig 8-6. The processes of smoking initiation and cessation (from *Strategies to Control Tobacco Use in the US*[24]).

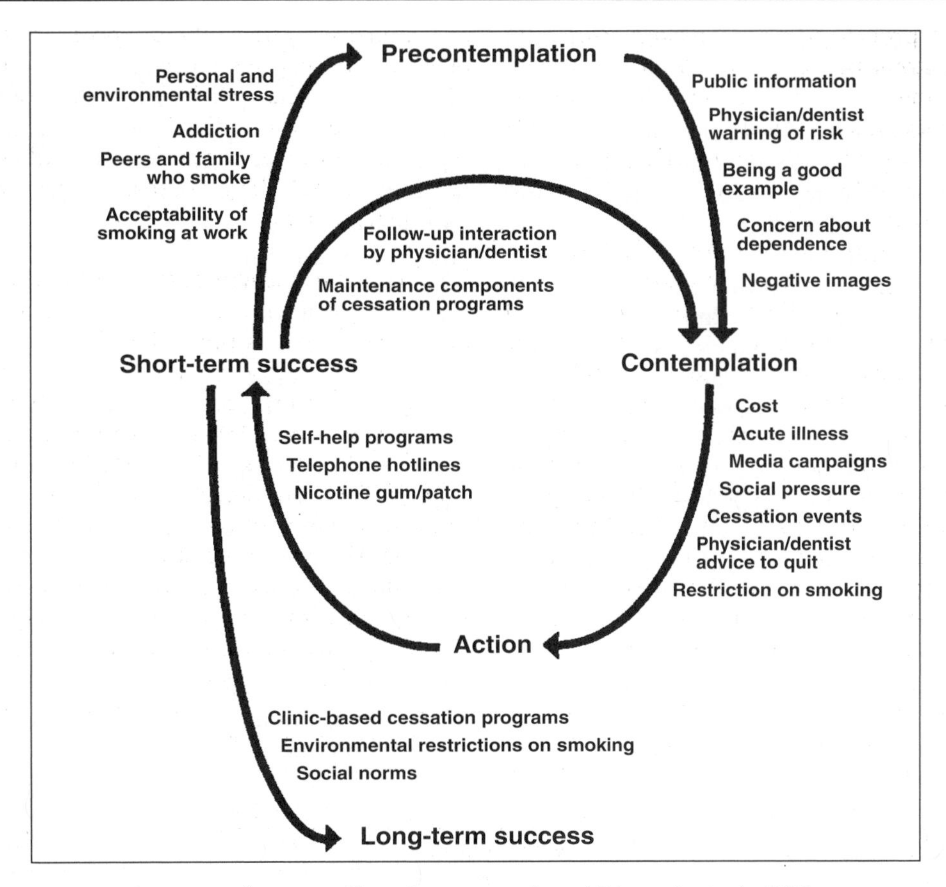

Fig 8-7. The process of cessation (from *Strategies to Control Tobacco Use in the US*[24]).

The second A is to **Advise All Patients Who Smoke to Quit**. This advice should be clear and direct; for example: "As your physician, I must advise you that the most important thing you can do for your current and future health and that of your family is to quit smoking now." It is helpful to personalize the advice—tying it to the patient's social status, to concerns about the dangers of environmental tobacco smoke, and to the illness that precipitated the clinic visit in the first place.

The third A is to **Assist Patients in Quitting Successfully.** This assistance comprises three parts: (1) *set a quit date* usually within 2 weeks of the clinic visit; (2) *provide self-help materials,* such as those available through the American Cancer Society or the NCI; and (3) *consider prescribing nicotine replacement, probably the nicotine patch.* Patients who may benefit from the nicotine patch include motivated individuals who answer yes to any of the following: smoke ≥20 cigarettes per day, have the first cigarette within 30 minutes of awakening; or, during previous quit attempts, reported physical withdrawal symptoms in the first week after quitting.[4]

VITAL SIGNS

Blood Pressure	________
Pulse	________
Temperature	________
Respiratory Rate	________
Smoking Status	Current Former Never (circle)

Fig 8-8. Sample vital signs stamp.

The fourth A is to **Arrange Follow-up.** NCI and other studies have demonstrated that in-person and telephone follow-up visits can double the rates of sustained smoking cessation. The follow-up visits are particularly necessary during the first 2 weeks after the quit date. More than 50% of relapse occurs during this time. At the follow-up visit, it is important to offer reinforcement to those who have achieved abstinence, to evaluate use of nicotine replacement, and to help find solutions for those who are having difficulty.

The NCI program has been effective in markedly increasing the rates of successful smoking cessation. Overall rates of smoking cessation have been shown to increase from a baseline of around 5% to at least 15%. Applying this success rate to all patients who smoke within a practice can have enormous impact over time. *How to Help Your Patients Stop Smoking* is available free of charge by calling 1-800-4CANCER.

Hospital-Based Smoking Cessation Intervention

The concept of hospital-based smoking cessation intervention is not new to clinicians, who regularly advise patients hospitalized for acute cardiovascular and pulmonary problems, as well as for diagnostic workups. Reports of short- and long-term follow-ups in such patient series or trials extend back over 20 years.[29] Only recently, however, have systematic interventions been considered to take advantage of hospitalization as a window of opportunity for smoking cessation intervention, regardless of diagnosis.[30,31] This opportunity becomes even more attractive because of the growing number of hospitals that have smoke-free inpatient and outpatient areas. The Joint Commission on the Accreditation of Healthcare Organizations (JCAHO) has required all hospitals to implement a smoke-free policy (exceptions only by written medical order).

There are multiple advantages to inpatient intervention, as well as notable drawbacks.[30] On the positive side, patients are a "captive audience" focused on a medical problem, and therefore acutely disease oriented. Hospitalization constitutes a generic teachable moment even when the condition is not smoking-related. Furthermore, hospitalization can provide an excellent opportunity to "quit cold turkey," as the beginning of permanent cessation. Behavioral and pharmacologic treatments can be tailored to the patient. Multiple members of the healthcare team (physicians, nurses, respiratory therapists, psychologists, social workers, health educators) can deliver or reinforce the primary advice message. Visiting family and friends can provide social support, and may even benefit personally from advice to the patient. Finally, the opportunities for reimbursement for nicotine addiction may be greater. On the other hand, there are both individual and system barriers to inpatient treatment programs. These include resentment or reactance to enforced smoking restrictions, diffusion of responsibility for nicotine dependence treatment, and lack of continuity of care targeted at smoking behavior after discharge.

The four-step NCI model (ASK, ADVISE, ASSIST, and ARRANGE) described above is readily adaptable to inpatient treatment. The introduction of advice, selection of motivational strategy, implementation of self-help or therapist-assisted cessation treatment, and postdischarge follow-up to ensure sustained abstinence should be tailored to the individual patient, his or her medical condition and readiness to change, and the availability of additional supportive care.[30]

Smoking Cessation in Cancer Patients

In general, cessation rates in medical populations increase according to the severity of disease; long-term quit rates (12 months) in cardiac and oncologic populations range from approximately 25% to 70%, with more recent studies falling at the higher end.[29,32,33] For smoking-related cancers (lung, head and neck), long-term unassisted cessation rates are high (40% to 70%).[34,35] But high initial cessation rates in the preoperative and postoperative periods may be followed by substantial relapse.[34,36]

The benefits of cessation are particularly important for patients with smoking-related tumors in whom early-stage, or curable, disease is diagnosed, although all patients will benefit from cessation in terms of general health and the risk of subsequent smoking-related disease. In the example of head and neck malignancies, smoking cessation following diagnosis has been reported to reduce the rate of second primary cancers, disease recurrence, and radiation-induced morbidity, and to improve overall mortality (see review in Gritz et al[32]). For any cancer patient, quitting also can reduce complications associated with anesthesia, surgery, radiation, and chemotherapy (see review in Gritz et al[32]).

Controlled trials of smoking cessation intervention with cancer patients are just beginning to appear. Gritz and colleagues evaluated a provider-delivered (otolaryngologists and maxillofacial prosthodontists) intervention for current and recent (quit within 1 year) smokers newly diagnosed with a first primary squamous cell carcinoma of the upper aerodigestive tract.[26,37] The intervention was based on the NCI model, and featured strong advice to stop smoking combined with a target quit date and written contract, three tailored self-help and social support booklets, booster advice sessions delivered at the first six regular medical follow-up appointments, and reminder postcards timed to the booster sessions. The control in this study consisted of standardized strong advice to stop smoking, unaccompanied by the additional elements of the special intervention. Initial advice was given to subjects prior to postsurgical hospital discharge or at the beginning of radiation treatment, depending on the primary treatment modality.

The 186 patients enrolled in the study were long-term heavy smokers, averaging 23 cigarettes/day for 40 years.[26] Eighty-eight percent were current smokers; the others had quit within the past year. Health concerns and physician advice were the principal motives for quitting. At 12-month follow-up, 70% of the 116 subjects completing the trial self-reported continuous abstinence from the time of initial advice, with a cotinine validation rate of 90%.[37] Based on multivariate analysis, significant predictors of continuous abstinence included type of medical treatment, stage of change, nicotine dependence, age, and race. Surgical patients (versus primary radiation therapy patients), action stage (versus precontemplators), less (versus more) heavily nicotine-dependent patients, younger, and nonwhite patients were more likely to abstain. The special intervention treatment was not superior to the control advice condition, possibly due to the significant early, as well as sustained, quit rates (a ceiling effect); small sample size; and a confounding effect from the treatment condition.

This trial demonstrates that a "difficult" cancer patient population (those with a history of heavy tobacco and alcohol use) can be successfully enrolled and studied, that surgical and dental specialists are willing and effective providers of smoking cessation advice, and that high, sustained smoking cessation outcomes can be achieved. Additional studies currently under way in cooperative trial groups (Eastern Cooperative Oncology Group [ECOG] and Southwest Oncology Group [SWOG]) involve bladder cancer patients and early-stage cancer patients treated by medical oncologists.

Special issues that arise in counseling the cancer patient to stop smoking include: (1) emphasizing the benefits of cessation as much as the risks of continuing to smoke; (2) avoiding "blaming the victim," especially with smoking-related tumors, by describing long-term smoking as an addictive behavior initiated in youth before the risks were appreciated; (3) featuring quitting as a means of "taking control," of participating actively in the treatment program and facilitating healing; (4) dealing forthrightly with reactance, anger, and feelings of hopelessness voiced by the patient or family member(s), by acknowledging the feelings and then structuring a positive approach, whenever possible; and finally (5) encouraging continuing efforts to stop, even when periods of resumed smoking occur, based on findings that permanent cessation by cancer patients as well as by healthy individuals often occurs only after several efforts.

Smoking Cessation in Other Medical Populations

There are three other special populations of medical patients whose smoking behavior and smoking cessation patterns have been considered at length in the literature—cardiovascular patients, pulmonary patients, and pregnant women (see reviews in references 25, 29, and 32). In each of these populations, smoking exerts a direct damaging effect on the health of the patient (and fetus) in the present and potentially in the future, and cessation will hopefully deter future adverse outcomes. However, each population faces a different configuration of individual and systemic factors concerning smoking cessation.

According to the US Surgeon General, "approximately 30% of women who are cigarette smokers quit after recognition of pregnancy, with greater proportions quitting among married women and especially among women with higher levels of educational attainment."[25] Interventions delivered by healthcare practitioners and via self-help materials can significantly increase further cessation during gestation. Pregnant smokers who quit usually focus on cessation as a benefit to the fetus, parallel to making other lifestyle modifications involving alcohol, diet, and nonprescription medication use. Unfortunately, this approach to cessation often leads to a rapid resumption of smoking in the early postpartum period. Recent emphasis has been placed on relapse prevention efforts during the postpartum period.

Most individuals with cardiovascular disease will stop smoking when hospitalized for a myocardial infarction (MI), although about half will relapse within months of the MI. Over time, the patient's motivation for abstinence may lessen, as contact is reduced with medical providers and rehabilitation programs. Intervention appears to benefit those with more serious cardiovascular disease and those with the strongest desire and motivation for abstinence.[32,33] Relapse prevention efforts are critical for this patient population as part of follow-up medical care, particularly through rehabilitation programs, telephone counseling, and other low-cost adjunctive strategies. Patients with less serious disease appear to require more intensive efforts to promote cessation and abstinence.

Chronic obstructive pulmonary disease (COPD) often takes a slow, progressive course, beginning with shortness of breath and eventually leading to the need for oxygen-assisted respiration. The steady progression of symptoms is usually accompanied by increasing motivation to quit and increasing intensity of advice by the physician. The greatest benefit of cessation comes before development of serious disease or disability; nonetheless, intervention should be a part of comprehensive treatment programs including both inpatient and outpatient respiratory care.[30] Self-blame for the development and progression of COPD is likely, given the clear etiologic connection to smoking and likelihood of past healthcare provider warnings. As in the case of smoking-related malignancies, the provider must make an effort to reframe this counterproductive patient attitude, which is associated with low self-confidence. Supportive advice should acknowledge early addiction to nicotine, the value of past quit efforts, progression through the stages of change (readiness to quit), and the availability of adjunctive pharmacologic aids. Additional motivational tools specific to lung function include spirometry and measurement of alveolar carbon monoxide levels. Intervention at the earliest stages of disease will produce the greatest health benefit.

Nicotine Dependence and Its Treatment

Despite acknowledgment by most smokers that tobacco use is harmful, the desire of most smokers to quit, and the availability of at least some level of aid to cessation offered by many voluntary organizations as well as medical clinics, only about 2.5% of cigarette smokers achieve lasting freedom from smoking each year, as noted by Gary Giovino, PhD (CDC, personal communication, April 1993). Is the difficulty that cigarette smokers are poorly motivated, irrational, or inadequately informed about the dangers of smoking? These and other possibilities are frequently raised and increasingly being addressed in public health programs. But, for most people, the difficulty in quitting remains.

The powerful hold of tobacco involves the pathophysiologic effects of rapid nicotine exposure, which induces changes in physiology and behavior, termed dependence. From this perspective, the difficulty of many smokers to even bring themselves to make a quitting attempt, let alone enjoy long-term remission from their dependence, is no less physically based than the many diseases that result from continued tobacco exposure. Health professionals who understand the pathophysiologic basis of tobacco dependence will be better armed to assist their tobacco-dependent patients to achieve and sustain remission from tobacco use.

Nomenclature

Drug addiction is widely used to describe medical and social disorders related to the compulsive ingestion of psychoactive chemicals. In 1983, the US Public Health Service recognized nicotine itself as an "addicting" and "dependence-producing" drug; in 1988, the US Surgeon General came to the following three major conclusions[38]:

1. Cigarettes and other forms of tobacco are addicting.

2. Nicotine is the drug in tobacco that causes addiction.

3. The pharmacologic and behavioral processes that determine tobacco addiction are similar to those that determine addiction to drugs such as heroin and cocaine.

Perhaps more useful from a clinical perspective is delineation of two medical disorders pertaining to nicotine addiction by the American Psychiatric Association:

(1) *Nicotine dependence,* which is a type of psychoactive substance use disorder. The essential feature of this type of disorder is "a cluster of cognitive, behavioral, and physiologic symptoms that indicate that the person has impaired control of psychoactive substance use and continues use of the substance despite adverse consequences."[39]

(2) *Nicotine withdrawal,* which is a type of psychoactive substance-induced organic mental disorder. The essential feature is "a characteristic withdrawal syndrome due to the abrupt cessation of or reduction in the use of nicotine-containing substances (eg, cigarettes, cigars, and pipes, chewing tobacco, or nicotine gum) that...includes craving for nicotine; irritability, frustration, or anger; anxiety; difficulty concentrating; restlessness; decreased heart rate; and increased appetite or weight gain."[39]

Two other commonly used terms are *tolerance* and *physical dependence*. *Tolerance* refers to the decreased responsiveness to the same dose of the drug as drug exposure increases. This is often accompanied by increased drug taking over time, as is the case with tobacco. A toxicologic consequence of tolerance to nicotine is that cigarette smokers expose themselves to much higher levels of tobacco-borne toxins than they would if they had not become tolerant and able to ingest many cigarettes per day. The cellular and neurologic adaptations that result in tolerance also result in the body coming to need continued drug intake to function relatively normally. At this point, the person is said to be physically dependent; acute drug deprivation will result in many responses, including some that are opposite to those produced by drug administration. Depending on the individual, and the duration and amount of drug intake, it may take several days to many months for complete recovery to a state in which the person feels normal in the absence of the drug.

The Addicting Chemical

Many substances are present in trace amounts in tobacco (eg, carbon monoxide) that could theoretically be involved in the establishment of highly controlled behavior; however, only nicotine is delivered by all commonly used forms of tobacco in amounts sufficient to produce such effects on brain function and behavior. Nicotine is a naturally occurring alkyloid present in the many strains of tobacco leaf cultivated to produce cigarettes. Because nicotine is a small molecule that is both lipid and water soluble, it is rapidly absorbed through the skin or lining of the mouth and nose.

The Drug Delivery System

Tobacco is not necessary for the delivery of nicotine. Nicotine can also be taken orally, nasally, or intravenously, in chewing gum form, inhaled from nontobacco aerosol generators, or absorbed through the skin. However, as vehicles for the delivery of nicotine, tobacco products are convenient to use and provide readily controllable means of regulating dose level. Moreover, tobacco-based vehicles appear to optimize the addictive potential of nicotine, much as the addictive potential of coca is optimized when converted to formulations such as injectable cocaine hydrochloride or smokable free base ("crack").

Most cigarettes on the American market contain about 8 to 9 mg of nicotine, of which the smoker usually obtains about 1 to 2 mg per cigarette. In general, the type of cigarette or the nicotine delivery rating reported by tobacco manufacturers bears almost no relation to the amount of nicotine obtained per cigarette by the typical smoker.[38] Exceptions are the so-called ultra low nicotine-delivering cigarettes, which are highly ventilated and deliver such a high volume of air along with the smoke that it may be more difficult for smokers to obtain a milligram or more of nicotine per cigarette unless they cover the ventilation holes with their lips.

The tobacco cigarette would appear to be the most highly addictive and toxic form of nicotine delivery that has ever been widely used. The low pH of the smoke delivered and the small doses delivered per puff require users to engage in large amounts of repetitive behavior to maintain their addiction. Toxins in the tobacco, as well as new toxins produced in the nearly 2,000° microblast furnace at the burning tip of the cigarette, are inhaled deeply into the lungs approximately 300 times each day by a person smoking a pack and a half per day. Such repetition occurs because the acute effects of smoke-delivered nicotine, which are desired by the smoker, last only a few minutes.

Smokeless tobacco products are also highly addictive and toxic, but these toxins are not inhaled into the lungs and do not include carbon monoxide and other products of tobacco pyrolysis. It may be easier for young people to become addicted to smokeless tobacco, however, because the products that tend to be marketed to young people (termed "starter products" by the tobacco industry) deliver nicotine in doses that are lower and more slowly delivered than those from maintenance smokeless products or cigarettes; starter tobacco products are also heavily sweetened and flavored.[40]

There are distinct advantages to the replacement of tobacco-based nicotine delivery systems with non-tobacco-based systems. For example, nicotine polacrilex (gum) and transdermal delivery systems (patch) do not deliver the multitude of highly toxic chemicals present in tobacco or produced during tobacco pyrolysis. Furthermore, for most patients, total daily nicotine delivery will be lower from nicotine replacement medications than with tobacco use. Finally, the advent of nicotine replacement medications with controlled delivery and limited total dose enables the clinician to determine, to a considerable degree, the nicotine exposure of the patient. In contrast, gradual reduction of nicotine intake is difficult with tobacco-based systems because of the ready ability of patients to defeat the effort by measures as simple as taking a few extra puffs per cigarette.

Kinetics

Nicotine is a lipid- and water-soluble molecule that is rapidly absorbed through the skin and buccal mucosa and via inhalation in the lungs. Following oral smokeless tobacco use, nicotine levels peak within approximately 15 minutes.[41] Time to peak may take 30 minutes or longer following administration of nicotine gum[41] and several hours for any of the four commercially available transdermal nicotine delivery systems.[42] Fig 8-9 compares nicotine absorption curves from several types of delivery systems.[40,41,43]

The rate of absorption of nicotine is enhanced in a mildly alkaline environment and severely reduced in an acidic environment. Thus, the nicotine in starter smokeless tobacco products, with a low pH, is absorbed more slowly than maintenance smokeless tobacco products.[40] Similarly, nicotine polacrilex gum is buffered to enhance delivery, but absorption is compromised if the patient consumed acidic foods or beverages immediately before taking the medication.[44] Cigar and pipe smoke is sufficiently alkaline to be well absorbed if held in the mouth, but cigarette smoke must be inhaled into the lungs, where efficient absorption is not pH dependent.[38]

Because of the massive area for gaseous exchange in the alveoli of the lungs, nicotine delivered by smoke inhalation is almost immediately extracted from the smoke and funneled from the alveoli into the pulmonary veins. It is then pumped through the left ventricle of the heart into the arterial circulation where this highly concentrated wave of nicotine-laden blood reaches organs such as the brain in less than 10 seconds, as well as to the fetus of a pregnant woman via the umbilical artery. Arterial nicotine boluses may be 10 times or more concentrated than the levels produced by use of nicotine polacrilex gum or nicotine transdermal patches.[45]

The terminal half-life of nicotine is approximately 2 hours, following an initial redistribution "half-life" phase of about 20 minutes.[46] The half-life of nicotine administered by transdermal patch appears to be approximately 4 hours,[42] probably reflecting the continued release of some nicotine absorbed by the dermal tissues at the site of application.

Changes in Brain Structure and Function Due to Nicotine Exposure

Even prenatal exposure to nicotine stimulates the growth of excess nicotine receptors.[38] Postmortem studies of smokers have revealed elevated concentrations of nicotine receptors, as well as other changes in brain tissue due to cigarette smoking.[47] Such morphologic changes in the nervous system are being investigated for their possible contribution to the development of nicotine tolerance and physical dependence.[38] Nicotine also produces a wide range of changes in the function of the central nervous system, including alterations in brain metabolism and energy utilization in various regions similar to those produced by other addictive drugs, changes in spontaneous electroencephalographic (EEG) patterns, and changes in evoked electrocortical potentials.[38]

Development of Dependence

Although the distinction between physiologic and psychologic dependence is useful heuristically, as well as in the development of treatment protocols, the dichotomy is blunted on closer analysis. For example, the subjective pleasure reported in studies and advertised by tobacco manufacturers is due, in part, to the actions of nicotine in the brain. These actions are related to the dose of nicotine administered, and the time since the last dose, and can be blocked by chemicals that inhibit the actions of nicotine in the brain, such as mecamylamine. Conversely, nicotine withdrawal symptoms include anxiety, irritability, and impaired cognition; these psychologic symptoms can be prevented or reversed by administration of nicotine. The severity of the syndrome depends on the time since the last nicotine dose and the level of nicotine that the person had become accustomed to until the point of abstinence. Most people who smoke regularly have become dependent, both physiologically and psychologically. The time course of addiction has not been well studied, but it is assumed that physical dependence on nicotine takes at least several weeks to develop.[39]

Reinforcing Effects

Cigarette smoking is a complex behavior that becomes powerfully conditioned by several entrenched mechanisms. Let us briefly review the ways in which the behavior of the smoker becomes controlled. First, sensory stimuli associated with the effects of nicotine become immediately and powerfully reinforcing to the user in their own right. These include the sight, feel, and taste of cigarettes, as well as the effects of various smoke constituents, including nicotine, in the mouth, nose, and throat.[38,48] Second, environmental stimuli may come to signal the occasion for smoking, such as friends who smoke, the ringing of the telephone, tobacco advertisements, or a cup of coffee. For some people, such stimuli do more than set the occasion; they elicit powerful urges that occur throughout the day even in the person who has been smoking periodically. The effects of environmental stimuli have also been documented as important factors in addictions to heroin, cocaine, and alcohol.[38]

Finally, nicotine itself directly reinforces the behavior of tobacco smoking; because such reinforcements

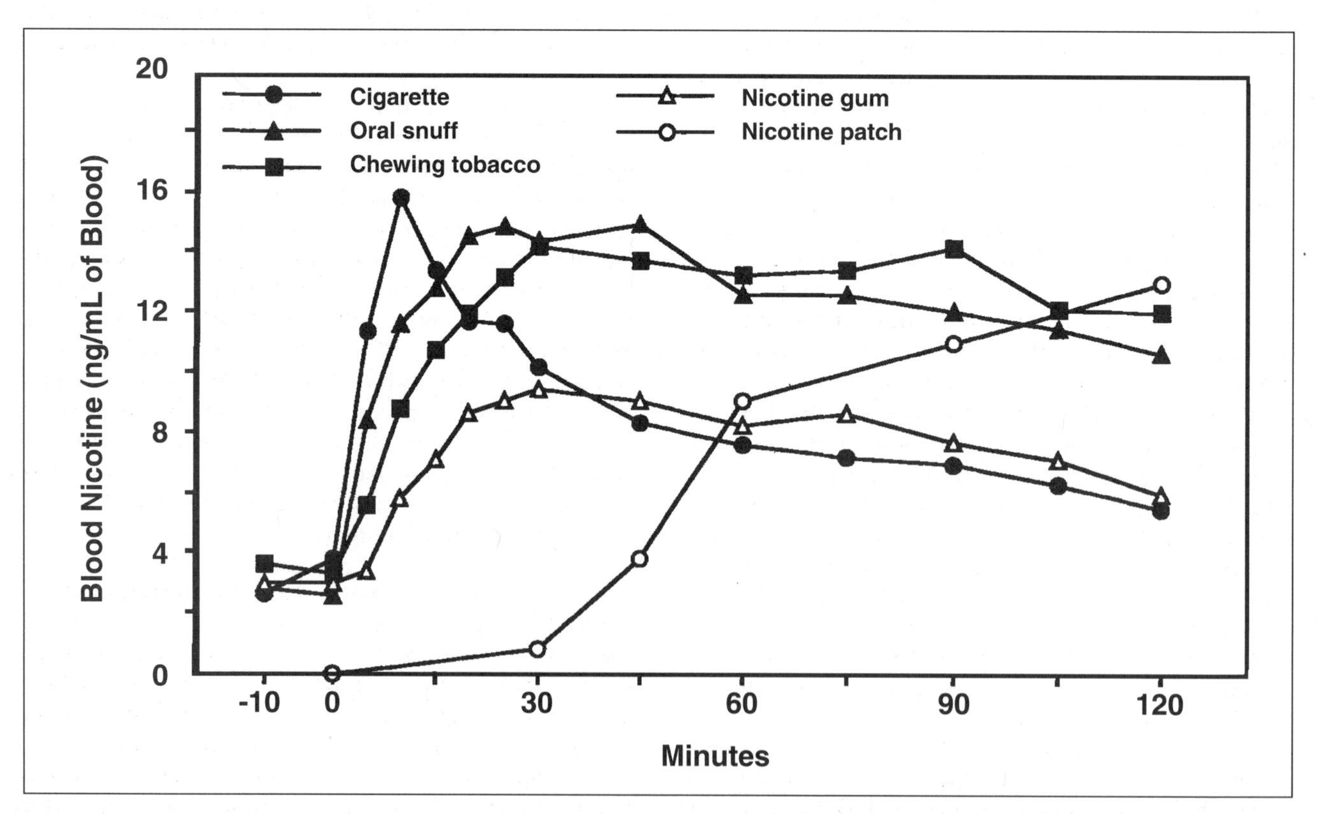

Fig 8-9. Venous blood nicotine concentrations over time for each of five nicotine delivery systems. (The transdermal [patch] nicotine data are from Benowitz et al[43]; other data are from Benowitz et al.[41] This figure is used with permission from Henningfield and Keenan.[40])

occur hundreds of times per day and hundreds of thousands per time per year in people smoking a pack or more per day, the behavior of seeking, lighting, and self-administering cigarettes becomes exceedingly entrenched. Such reinforcements "stamp in" nicotine self-administration in both humans and animals.[38]

Nicotine administration also provides relief of negative symptoms of withdrawal, which begin to emerge within a few hours of the last cigarette. It is plausible that cigarette smoke inhalation optimizes these reinforcing effects of nicotine since the arterial bolus of nicotine would maximize the effects at brain nicotine receptors, as well as on hormone release.[38] Nicotine gum and the transdermal patch systems also reduce withdrawal symptoms, but with apparently much less pleasure than is provided by smoke inhalation. Thus, the cigarette smoker may get with nicotine gum or patch what he or she needs to avoid withdrawal, but not a pleasurable euphoria.

Physical Dependence

As discussed earlier, repeated exposure to nicotine leads to the development of tolerance and physical dependence. However, some degree of tolerance is lost overnight, so that the first cigarettes of the day are reported as the strongest or the best. Over the course of the day, tolerance increases and the effects diminish. These observations indicate that with nicotine, as with other addicting drugs, the development of tolerance is only partial. For example, the first few cigarettes of the day may produce a substantial increase in heart rate, lasting only a few minutes beyond the duration of the cigarette; thereafter, heart rate follows the same diurnal rhythm of nonsmokers and is elevated about seven beats per minute.

As with morphine and alcohol, the chronic administration of nicotine leads to physiologic or physical dependence; abrupt abstinence is accompanied by signs and symptoms that can be unpleasant and debilitating.[37] The clinical course has been described in detail.[38] In brief, the syndrome includes increased craving, anxiety, irritability, and appetite, and decreased cognitive capabilities and heart rate. Onset is within approximately 8 hours of smoking the last cigarette; symptoms peak in the first few days, then subside over the next few weeks. In some individuals, symptoms may persist for months or more. Cognitive deficits described by many smokers who quit are correlated with disruption in various measures of brain function; these effects occur within a few hours of the last cigarette, and appear to subside over the next few weeks for most people.[38]

The withdrawal syndrome varies somewhat with each tobacco user, although certain symptoms are pervasive (eg, cognitive impairment). Other symptoms are not part of the generally recognized syndrome of withdrawal, but may be related to psychiatric comorbidities; eg, people with a history of major depression may develop serious depression. Most symptoms of nicotine withdrawal do not return to pre-abstinence levels until 2 to 4 weeks after cessation, and increased hunger and craving for tobacco may persist 6 months or longer.[25]

The magnitude of the withdrawal syndrome is directly related to the level of nicotine dependence, as measured by cotinine or Fagerstrom tolerance questionnaire score, although there is considerable variability within and across individuals.[38] Rates of relapse are also related to the level of dependence, with the majority of people who quit smoking relapsing within approximately 1 week.[38]

The tobacco withdrawal syndrome is pharmacologically mediated by nicotine deprivation. In addition, behavioral conditioning factors are at least as important for this addiction as they are for other drug addictions for both the strength of the dependence and the magnitude of withdrawal symptoms.[38] Thus, the sight, smell, and feel of a cigarette and the ritual of handling, lighting, and smoking become an important source of pleasure for the smoker. Nicotine gum and patch do not replace these aspects of tobacco.

That cigarette withdrawal effects are largely specific to nicotine, and can be alleviated by nicotine in the absence of tobacco, is illustrated in Fig 8-10.[49,50] Fig 8-10 also shows that nicotine replacement can alleviate both the physiologic and cognitive aspects of the withdrawal syndrome.

A clinically important, but poorly understood, feature of the nicotine withdrawal syndrome is "craving for tobacco." Cravings and urges to smoke cigarettes or use smokeless tobacco have been described, both clinically and theoretically, as major obstacles confronting tobacco users attempting to quit, and have been identified as one of the most prominent symptoms of nicotine withdrawal.[38] Unfortunately, there is little evidence that suppressing cravings with medications, for any type of drug addiction, enhances quitting success.[38] Nicotine gum and patch only weakly reduce cravings; fortunately, they are efficacious in reducing the overall severity of the withdrawal syndrome as well as in helping people to enter and sustain remission from tobacco use.

Treatment Guidelines for Nicotine Replacement Therapy

While historically most smokers have quit on their own (without the assistance of a formal smoking cessation program), the advent of effective pharmacologic aids, coupled with the increasing sociodemographic marginalization of smokers in the US, has increased the importance of clinical intervention with patients who smoke. The characteristics of

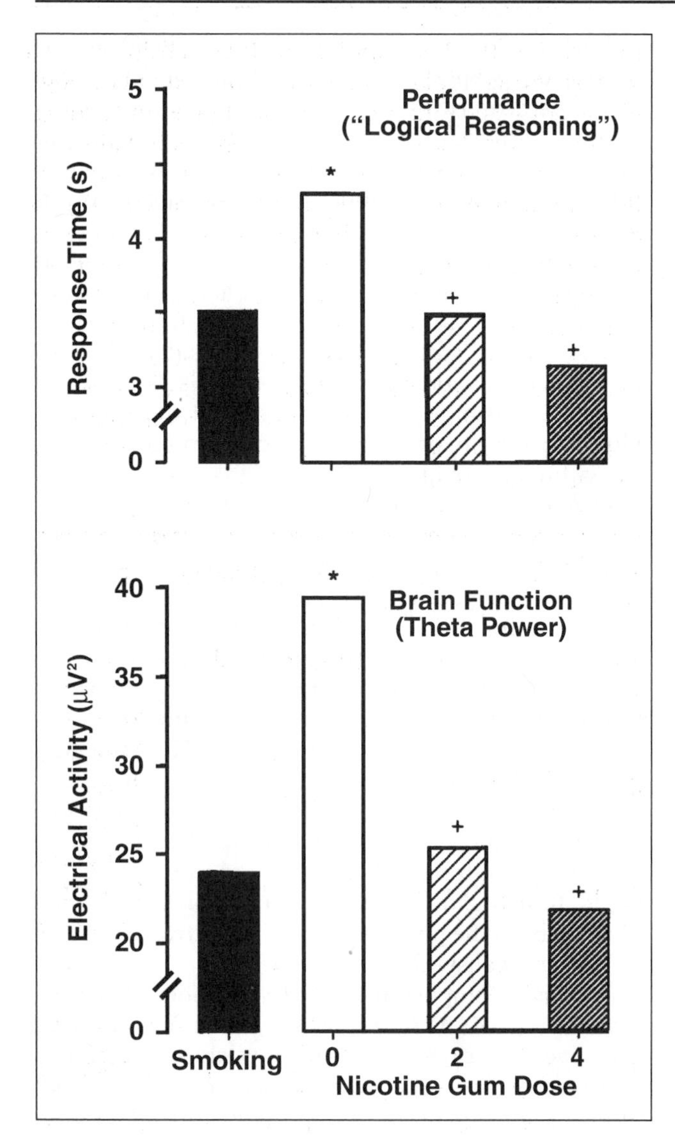

Fig 8-10. Cognitive performance and electrophysiologic measures of brain function in human volunteers during smoking or in the absence of tobacco (after treatment with placebo or nicotine-delivering polacrilex gum). Nicotine gum or placebo were given after either 12 hours (performance study) or 29 hours (EEG study) of nicotine deprivation. Adapted from Snyder et al[49] and Pickworth et al.[50]
* = Significantly different from libitum smoking;
+ = Significantly different from placebo.

tobacco dependence and nicotine addiction suggest that the most effective way to treat smokers clinically may require the use of nicotine replacement therapy paired with counseling and advice.

This paired approach requires that clinicians take a more active role in the identification of smokers for effective intervention. As described previously, <50% of smokers report ever being asked by a clinician whether they smoke and <5% report that a clinician has ever offered specific advice on how to quit. The NCI model described above, *How to Help Your Patients Stop Smoking,* provides clinicians with a brief but effective advice and counseling message for their patients who smoke. A necessary second step is to develop skills to identify patients who will benefit from nicotine replacement therapy and to use these pharmaceutical aids effectively.

By 1993, >90% of new prescriptions for nicotine replacement therapy were for the nicotine patch, a product approved by the US Food and Drug Administration (FDA) in November 1991. The popularity of the patch as the first-line nicotine replacement therapy can be attributed to increased compliance and markedly improved ease of use when compared with the only other available nicotine replacement product, nicotine gum. Because of current prescribing patterns, guidelines on the use of nicotine replacement products will focus primarily on the nicotine patch.

Four different brands of the nicotine patch are now available in the US. These products all deliver a selected amount of nicotine transdermally over either a 24-hour (Habitrol, Nicoderm, Prostep) or a 16-hour (Nicotrol) period. No clinical trial has directly compared the four brands, and there is no evidence to suggest that any one brand is associated with a higher rate of smoking cessation.

A recent review demonstrated that the nicotine patch is a highly effective aid to smoking cessation, with an overall doubling of the rate of smoking cessation.[4] Results have been markedly variable, however, with cessation rates at 6 months ranging from 22% to 42% for nicotine patch use; overall, more intense adjuvant counseling was associated with higher success rates with the nicotine patch. Community-based trial results with the nicotine patch have not been reported to date.

An important clinical challenge is to identify patients appropriate for nicotine patch use. Unfortunately, no *a priori* characteristics have yet been identified in clinical trials to predict those patients most likely to benefit from nicotine patch use. The Center for Tobacco Research and Intervention at the University of Wisconsin has developed empiric criteria to identify patients who may benefit from nicotine patch use (Table 8-2).[4]

Patients should be informed to begin patch use as soon as they awaken on the morning of their quit day.

Table 8-2. Empiric Criteria for Identifying Patients for the Nicotine Patch

Patient MUST be motivated to make a quit attempt and report at least one of the following:

- Smokes at least 20 cigarettes per day, or
- Smokes first cigarette within 30 minutes of awakening, or
- Has experienced a strong craving for cigarettes during the first week following previous quit attempts

Source: Fiore et al.[4]

At that time, all smoking should stop, with continued abstinence maintained throughout patch use. Patients should place the patch on a hairless part of the body between the neck and the waist, changing the patch every morning and not reusing the same patch site within the same week. About 30% of patients develop a local, erythematous, sometimes pruritic skin reaction at the patch site. This rarely leads to termination of therapy and can be treated locally with 5% hydrocortisone cream or 0.1% triamcinolone cream (3 times daily for 3 days after removing the patch). The only other clinically significant side effect is sleep disruption. Because sleep disruption is a hallmark of the tobacco withdrawal syndrome, it is sometimes difficult to discern whether this is a result of tobacco withdrawal or nicotine replacement therapy. There are ongoing trials to determine the effects of smoking cessation and nicotine replacement on sleep.

Dose and length of treatment are also important factors in the clinical use of the nicotine patch. The four patches vary greatly in the recommended for length of treatment, ranging from 6 to 16 weeks. No published trials have documented a benefit of longer therapy with the nicotine patch. Because of this, a recent review of the nicotine patch recommended a 6- to 8-week course of therapy for most patients (Table 8-3).[4] Clinicians are urged to individualize treatment when appropriate.

Use of the nicotine patch is recommended with caution in patients with cardiovascular disease, although there has *not* been a documented association between nicotine patch and acute MI. The patch is classified as Class D, for use with pregnant patients. It should be used with particular caution in this population, according to FDA guidelines, and only after the patient has failed to successfully quit using a nonpharmacologic intervention.

Conclusion

The physician has the opportunity to become the gatekeeper for smoking cessation interventions for the majority of the US population. Intervention begins with querying smoking status, and can extend through giving advice to quit, providing assistance, and arranging follow-up. The stepped care approach delineates the degree of intervention and availability of supportive care, including ancillary personnel on the healthcare team, nicotine replacement therapy, printed materials, and referrals to formal group and individual treatment programs. Given the extraordinary quantity and strength of the evidence supporting the causal relationships between tobacco use and numerous forms of cancer, as well as other diseases, physicians must adopt a primary sense of responsibility for intervening in patient smoking behavior. The health of the nation is at stake.

Table 8-3. Recommendations for Nicotine Patch Therapy for Tobacco Dependence

Brand	Duration (weeks)	Dose
Prostep (Lederle Labs)	3-5	22 mg/24 h
	3	11 mg/24 h
Habitrol (Ciba-Geigy)	2-4	21 mg/24 h
	2	14 mg/24 h
	2	7 mg/24 h
Nicoderm (Marion Merrell Dow)	2-4	21 mg/24 h
	2	14 mg/24 h
	2	7 mg/24 h
Nicotrol (Parke-Davis)	2-4	15 mg/16 h
	2	10 mg/16 h
	2	5 mg/16 h

Source: Fiore et al.[4] Derived from available data. Manufacturers' recommendations vary and in most cases exceed the above recommendations. Patch therapy needs to be used in the context of a smoking cessation counseling program.

References

1. Centers for Disease Control. Cigarette smoking among adults—United States, 1990. *MMWR.* 1992; 41:354-355, 361-362.

2. *Reducing the Health Consequences of Smoking: 25 Years of Progress: A Report of the Surgeon General, 1989.* Rockville, Md: Public Health Service, Centers for Disease Control, Center for Chronic Disease Prevention and Health Promotion, Office on Smoking and Health; 1989. US Dept of Health and Human Services publication CDC 89-8411.

3. Pierce JP, Fiore MC, Novotny TE, Hatziandreu EJ, Davis RM. Trends in cigarette smoking in the United States: projections to the year 2000. *JAMA.* 1989; 261:61-65.

4. Fiore MC, Jorenby DE, Baker TB, Kenford SL. Tobacco dependence and the nicotine patch: clinical guidelines for effective use. *JAMA.* 1992; 268:2687-2694.

5. *Healthy People 2000: National Health Promotion and Disease Prevention Objectives: Full Report With Commentary.* Washington, DC: Public Health Service; 1991. US Dept of Health and Human Services publication PHS 91-50212.

6. Burns D, Pierce JP. *Tobacco Use in California, 1990-1991.* Sacramento, Calif: California Dept of Health Services; 1992.

7. Centers for Disease Control. Selected tobacco-use behaviors and dietary patterns among high school students—United States, 1991; *MMWR.* 1992; 41:417-421.

8. Centers for Disease Control. Cigarette smoking among youth—United States, 1989. *MMWR.* 1991; 40:712-715.

9. Newcomb PA, Carbone PP. The health consequences of smoking: cancer. In: Fiore MC, ed. *Cigarette Smoking: A Clinical Guide to Assessment and Treatment.* Philadelphia, Pa: WB Saunders Co; 1992: 305-331, *Medical Clinics of North America.*

10. *The Health Consequences of Involuntary Smoking: A Report of the Surgeon General, 1986.* Rockville, Md: Public Health Service, Centers for Disease Control, Center for Health Promotion and Education, Office on Smoking and Health; 1986. US Dept of Health and Human Services publication CDC 87-8398.

11. National Research Council, Committee on Passive Smoking. *Environmental Tobacco Smoke: Measuring Exposures and Assessing Health Effects.* Washington, DC: National Academy Press; 1986:336.

12. *Respiratory Health Effects of Passive Smoking: Lung Cancer and Other Disorders.* Washington, DC: US Environmental Protection Agency, Office of Research and Development, Office of Health and Environmental Assessment; 1992. Publication EPA/600/6-90/006F.

13. Schappert SM. National ambulatory medical care survey: 1990 summary: advance data from Vital and Health Statistics. No. 213. Hyattsville, Md: National Center for Health Statistics; 1992. US Dept of Health and Human Services publication PHS 92-1250.

14. Nelson DE, Giovino GA, Emont SL, et al. Trends in cigarette smoking among US physicians and nurses. *JAMA.* 1994;271:1273-1275.

15. Adriaanse H, Van Reek J. Physicians' smoking and its exemplary effect. *Scand J Prim Health Care.* 1989;7:193-196.

16. Gilpin E, Pierce J, Goodman J, et al. Trends in physicians' giving advice to stop smoking, United States, 1974-1987. *Tobacco Control.* 1992; 1:31-36.

17. Fiore MC. The new vital sign: assessing and documenting smoking status. *JAMA.* 1991; 266:3183-3184.

18. Manley M, Epps RP, Husten C, Glynn T, Shopland D. Clinical interventions in tobacco control: a National Cancer Institute training program for physicians. *JAMA.* 1991; 266:3172-3173.

19. Burns DM, Cohen S, Gritz ER, Kottke TE, Shopland D, eds. *Tobacco and the Clinician: Interventions for Medical and Dental Practice.* Rockville, Md: US Department of Health and Human Services, Public Health Service, National Institutes of Health, National Cancer Institute; 1994. Smoking and Tobacco Control Monograph 5. NIH Publication 94-3693.

20. Fiore MC, Jorenby DE. Optimizing nicotine-dependence treatment: a role for inpatient programs. *Mayo Clin Proc.* 1992; 67:901-902.

21. DiMatteo MR, DiNicola DD. *Achieving Patient Compliance: the Psychology of the Medical Practitioner's Role.* New York, NY: Pergamon Press; 1982.

22. Gritz ER, Bastani R. Cancer prevention—behavior changes: the short and the long of it. *Prev Med.* 1993;22: 676-688.

23. Prochaska JO, DiClemente CC, Norcross JC. In search of how people change: applications to addictive behaviors. *Am Psychol.* 1992; 47:1102-1114.

24. Shopland DR, Burns DM, Samet JM, Gritz ER, eds. *Strategies to Control Tobacco Use in the United States: A Blueprint for Public Health Action in the 1990s.* Rockville, Md: US Department of Health and Human Services, Public Health Service, National Institutes of Health, National Cancer Institute; 1991. Smoking and Tobacco Control Monograph 1. NIH Publication 92-3316.

25. *The Health Benefits of Smoking Cessation. A Report of the Surgeon General, 1990.* Rockville, Md: Public Health Service, Centers for Disease Control, Center for Chronic Disease Prevention and Health Promotion, Office on Smoking and Health; 1990. US Dept of Health and Human Services publication CDC 90-8416.

26. Gritz ER, Carr CR, Rapkin DA, Chang C, Beumer J, Ward PH. A smoking cessation intervention for head and neck cancer patients: trial design, patient accrual and characteristics. *Cancer Epidemiol Biomarkers Prev.* 1991; 1:67-73.

27. Orleans CT, Slade J, eds. *Nicotine Addiction: Principles and Management.* New York, NY: Oxford University Press; 1993.

28. Glynn TJ, Manley M. *How to Help Your Patients Stop Smoking: A National Cancer Institute Manual for Physicians.* Washington, DC: National Cancer Institute; 1991. US Dept of Health, Education, and Welfare publication 90-3064.

29. *The Health Consequences of Smoking: Chronic Obstructive Lung Disease: A Report of the Surgeon General, 1984.* Rockville, Md: Public Health Service, Centers for Disease Control, Center for Health Promotion and Education, Office on Smoking and Health; 1984. US Dept of Health and Human Services publication PHS 84-50205.

30. Orleans CT, Kristeller JL, Gritz ER. Helping hospitalized smokers quit: new directions for treatment and research. *J Consult Clin Psychol.* 1993;61(5):778-789.

31. Stevens VJ, Glasgow RE, Hollis JF, Lichtenstein E, Vogt TM. A smoking-cessation intervention for hospital patients. *Med Care.* 1993; 31:65-72.

32. Gritz ER, Kristeller J, Burns DM. High-risk groups and patients with medical co-morbidity. In: Orleans CT, Slade J, eds. *Nicotine Addiction: Principles and Management.* New York, NY: Oxford University Press. 1993:279-309.

33. Ockene J, Kristeller JL, Goldberg R, et al. Smoking cessation and severity of disease: the coronary artery smoking intervention study. *Health Psychol.* 1992; 11(2):119-126.

34. Gritz ER, Nisenbaum R, Elashoff R, Holmes EC. Smoking behavior following diagnosis in patients with stage I non-small cell lung cancer. *Cancer Causes Control.* 1991; 2(2):105-112.

35. Spitz MR, Fueger JJ, Chamberlain RM, Goepfert H, Newell GR. Cigarette smoking patterns in patients after treatment of upper aerodigestive tract cancers. *J Cancer Educ.* 1990; 5:109-113.

36. Davison G, Duffy M. Smoking habits of long-term survivors of surgery for lung cancer. *Thorax.* 1982; 37:331-333.

37. Gritz ER, Carr CR, Rapkin D, et al. Predictors of long-term smoking cessation in head and neck cancer patients. *Cancer Epidemiol Biomarkers Prev.* 1993; 2:261-269.

38. *The Health Consequences of Smoking: Nicotine Addiction: A Report of the Surgeon General, 1988.* Rockville, Md:

Public Health Service, Centers for Disease Control, Center for Health Promotion and Education, Office on Smoking and Health. US Dept of Health and Human Services publication CDC 88-8406.

39. *Diagnostic and Statistical Manual of Mental Disorders.* 3rd ed (DSM-IV) Washington, DC: American Psychiatric Association; 1994:166,180.

40. Henningfield JE, Keenan RM. Nicotine delivery kinetics and abuse liability. *J Consult Clin Psychol.* 1993;61(5);743-750.

41. Benowitz NL, Porchet H, Sheiner L, Jacob P III. Nicotine absorption and cardiovascular effects with smokeless tobacco use: comparison with cigarettes and nicotine gum. *Clin Pharmacol Ther.* 1988; 44:23-28.

42. Palmer KJ, Buckley MM, Faulds D. Transdermal nicotine: a review of its pharmacodynamic and pharmacokinetic properties, and therapeutic efficacy as an aid to smoking cessation. *Drugs.* 1992; 44:498-529.

43. Benowitz NL, Chan K, Denaro CP, Jacob P III. Stable isotope method for studying transdermal drug absorption: the nicotine patch. *Clin Pharmacol Ther.* 1991; 50:286-293.

44. Henningfield JE, Radzius A, Cooper TM, Clayton RR. Drinking coffee and carbonated beverages blocks absorption of nicotine from nicotine polacrilex gum. *JAMA.* 1990; 264:1560-1564.

45. Henningfield JE, London ED, Benowitz NL. Arterial-venous differences in plasma concentrations of nicotine after cigarette smoking. *JAMA.* 1990; 263:2049-2050.

46. Benowitz NL. Pharmacologic aspects of cigarette smoking and nicotine addiction. *N Engl J Med.* 1988; 319:1318-1330.

47. Balfour DJ. The influence of stress on psychopharmacological responses to nicotine. *Br J Addict.* 1991; 86:489-493.

48. Rose JE. The role of upper airway stimulation in smoking. In: Pomerleau OF, Pomerleau CS, eds. *Nicotine Replacement: A Critical Evaluation.* New York, NY: Alan R Liss Inc; 1988: 95-106.

49. Snyder FR, Davis FC, Henningfield JE. The tobacco withdrawal syndrome: performance decrements assessed on a computerized test battery. *Drug Alcohol Depend.* 1989; 23:259-266.

50. Pickworth WB, Herning RI, Henningfield JE. Spontaneous EEG changes during tobacco abstinence and nicotine substitution in human volunteers. *J Pharmacol Exp Ther.* 1989; 251:976-982.

9

PRINCIPLES OF CANCER BIOLOGY

Dennis J. Templeton, MD, PhD, Robert A. Weinberg, PhD

Study of Tumor Cells Grown in Culture

The biological traits of cancer cells are known largely from experiments in which these cells are grown in vitro under a variety of culture conditions. This permits the study of a number of cancer cell traits that are not readily observed when cells are growing in the midst of a tumor mass in vivo. Since the 1950s, when routine in vitro culturing of mammalian cells was first achieved, a large number of tumor cells have been adapted to grow in culture as permanent cell lines.

Although culturing techniques have created a number of distinct tumor cell lines, cells derived from recent biopsies do not always grow well on initial introduction into cultures. Instead, the explanted tumor cell population must undergo extensive adaptation during which variant tumor cell clones grow out and show traits beyond those exhibited by their recently explanted progenitors. Accordingly, knowledge of the biology of human tumor cells is often distorted by studying the traits of variants that may deviate substantially from tumor cells growing in vivo.

An alternative to studying cultured cells derived from spontaneous human tumors arises from experiments designed to transform normal cultured cells into tumor cells during their growth in vitro. Such experiments utilize several types of oncogenic agents, notably carcinogenic chemicals and oncogenes. By inducing malignant conversion with precisely defined reagents, researchers have hoped to clearly delineate the changes that accompany the conversion of a normal cell into a tumor cell.

With rare exceptions, attempts at transforming normal human cells in vitro have been notably unsuccessful. For reasons that remain unclear, human cells are refractory to agents that are able to readily induce the neoplastic conversion of rodent cells; thus, the great bulk of what is understood about the mechanisms of neoplastic transformation is derived from rodent models. Implicit in the following discussion of rodent cells is the assumption that they represent good models of the processes that intervene to create human cancer.

Rodent models of cancer offer additional advantages, perhaps most importantly the ability to grow rodent tumor cells in culture and introduce these into fully syngeneic (ie, genetically compatible), immunocompetent hosts at will. The ensuing tumor-host interactions presumably mirror many of the interactions that occur in a human bearing a tumor of endogenous origin. Most studies of in vitro transformation have utilized fibroblasts or closely related mesenchymal cells, which can be readily grown in vitro. Mesenchymal cells have some, but hardly all, of the attributes of the epithelial cells that are the precursors to the common human tumors, the carcinomas.

The Pleiotropic Nature of Malignant Conversion

A comparison of normal cells and their transformed, tumorigenic derivatives reveals a large number of distinct shifts in cell phenotype. These encompass traits as diverse as morphology, energy metabolism, and response to growth-stimulatory factors; a thorough cataloguing of these differences might include changes in hundreds of cell parameters. A central problem in tumor biology over the past century has been to explain how cancer cells can acquire so many distinctive, novel phenotypes.

A partial answer to this quandary is provided by the notion of the multistep progression of tumor cells.[1] This model states that cells pass through a

Dennis J. Templeton, MD, PhD, Department of Pathology, Case Western Reserve University School of Medicine, Cleveland, Ohio

Robert A. Weinberg, PhD, Professor of Biology, Massachusetts Institute of Technology, Cambridge, Massachusetts, Member, Whitehead Institute for Biomedical Research, Cambridge, Massachusetts

number of distinct intermediate stages during their evolution from normalcy to full malignancy. The notion of ongoing evolution is central to this model, which depicts tumors as large, heterogeneous populations of cells from which rare variants emerge with selective growth advantage; subpopulations of these favored cells then expand and ultimately dominate the tumor cell population. This process is repeated in successive cycles to yield the end stage—highly evolved tumor cells that differ substantially from their normal ancestors.

The kinetics of tumor formation in experimental animals and humans suggest a rather small number of distinct stages occurring during tumor progression. The estimates range from three to six, but the small number of stages is dwarfed by the large number of cellular changes associated with malignant transformation. This gives rise to the concept of *pleiotropy*, in which changes in a relatively small number of central regulators are able to elicit a large number of distinct changes in cell phenotype.

Tumor Cells Have an Altered Cell Structure

Tumor cells usually can be distinguished from their normal counterparts by an examination of their morphology in microscopic sections. In many cases, the diagnosis of malignant cells can be made by examining the appearance of isolated tumor cells; diagnostic cytologists use the features of increased nuclear size, increased nuclear-to-cytoplasmic ratio, irregular chromatin distribution, and prominent nucleoli to formulate a diagnosis. When isolated tumor cells are examined on cytologic smears, they retain most of the features of tumor cells growing within a tumor mass.

When studied in culture, normal untransformed cells growing in monolayers make many contacts with the substratum, often displaying a flattened "fried egg" appearance. Tumor cells make fewer contacts, frequently in the form of long processes that extend from the cell body and cross over the extended processes of adjacent cells.

Cells in culture are usually observed on phase-contrast microscopy. The tumor cell body is often seen to be round, having either a spheroid or a spindle shape. The round shape causes tumor cell bodies to refract light, producing a bright highlight at the round edge. In contrast, the edges of the flattened normal cells refract little light.

The cell's overall shape is dictated by its internal architecture in the form of its cytoskeleton. A major component of the cytoskeleton is the protein actin, which is present in normal fibroblasts as linear polymers called actin cables or microfilaments. Actin cables can be visualized in intact cells by using fluorescent antibodies directed against the protein. In normal cells, this process demonstrates actin cables spanning nearly the entire length of the cell. The actin cables are believed to be anchored to the inner surface of the cell membrane at sites which are in turn connected through the plasma membrane to cell surface receptors responsible for tethering the cell to a substrate such as the bottom of a culture dish.

Transformed cells also contain actin, but immunofluorescence staining fails to reveal the organized cables found in normal cells.[2] This observed disruption of the actin cytoskeleton results in significant changes in the cell's external morphology. The mechanisms leading to this disruption are unclear. Thus, the actin cable disruption may be a consequence of overall metabolic alterations in the tumor cell. Alternatively, the architectural changes may effect the metabolic changes found in tumor cells. The cytoskeletal alterations may be a very early event in the sequence of changes that lead to a transformed cell. Furthermore, the cytoskeletal protein vinculin, which serves to anchor the termini of actin cables to the cell surface, has been shown to be modified directly by the transforming protein encoded by the *src* oncogene.[3]

Tumor Cells Display Altered Interactions with Neighboring Cells

Cells growing in normal tissues have an ordered growth pattern, characterized by regular, predictable relationships with their neighbors. The structural order characteristic of each tissue depends on each component cell conforming to a precise growth pattern. The predominant growth pattern in body tissues is a two-dimensional sheet of cells (albeit often rolled or convoluted) that is one or several cell layers thick. This is true at both the macroscopic and microscopic levels, as evidenced by the orderly sheets of cells that make up the skin or intestinal mucosa and the single layer of cells that line the tiny follicles found in the thyroid gland. Even a bulky organ like the liver is organized at the microscopic level as cells joined to their neighbors at their sides, forming a single-layer sheet; in the liver, this sheet is rolled into a convoluted tube called an acinus.

Cells explanted from the body and grown in culture mimic the tendency of their progenitors to form a single layer (monolayer) of cells. For example, cells taken from chicken or mouse embryos (largely fibroblasts and other mesenchymal cells) will adhere to glass or some plastic surfaces and will divide until each cell is touching neighbors on all sides. These cells then will stop dividing.[4] Within such a confluent cell monolayer, each cell maintains contact with the substratum (the culture dish) and will not grow over adjacent cells. Further cell division is inhibited by contacts made with other cells; this is the phenomenon of *contact inhibition*.

Tumor cells have escaped the controls that normally regulate orderly tissue growth. In the organism, this is evidenced by the formation of tumor masses that displace adjacent normal tissue. When grown in culture, tumor cells also display a disordered growth pattern. They will continue to divide after contact is made with their neighbors, forming jumbled piles of cells growing on cells. Unless they are divided into subcultures and placed in fresh medium, the tumor cells will continue to divide until they have exhausted the culture medium and die.

This loss of contact inhibition can be exploited to identify cancer cells growing amid normal cells, and in turn yields a sensitive assay for agents that induce cell transformation in culture. Thus, a population of normal cells can be grown in culture dishes and treated with chemical carcinogens or cancer-causing viruses. When one or another cell becomes transformed, it will acquire the altered growth behavior that allows it to continue to divide long after the cell monolayer has grown to confluence; its progeny will pile up to form a thick clump of cells that can be distinguished from the normal monolayer by staining.[5] These piles of transformed cells are termed *foci*. Formation of foci in vitro usually serves as a good predictor of in vivo behavior. Thus, cells taken from a focus of transformed cells growing in a culture dish usually exhibit the attributes of spontaneously arising tumor cells, such as the ability to form tumors and metastases in appropriate host animals. This suggests that the changes exhibited by a transformed cell growing in vitro are tightly linked to its altered growth properties seen in vivo.

The mechanism that maintains contact inhibition is uncertain, but it clearly involves the transfer of signals between adjacent cells. At least two kinds of contacts are made between normal cells in culture: (1) tight junctions, visualized as *desmosomes* by the electron microscopist, and (2) gap junctions, which allow passage of small molecules between the cytoplasm of two adjoining cells. Passage of small molecules between cells may explain how a cell is able to announce its presence to its neighbors, thus preventing growth once the confluent monolayer is formed. Tumor cells grown in culture (and tumors observed microscopically) usually retain the tight junctions found in nontransformed cells. Gap junctions, however, are frequently reduced or absent, suggesting again that intercellular communication may be important for maintenance of normal growth patterns.[6,7]

With the exception of cells from hematopoietic lineages, normal cells grown in culture must have a solid substrate on which to grow. The presence of a basement membrane, which underlies epithelial cell layers, may represent an analogous phenomenon in the intact tissue. If normal cells are prevented from adhering to a substrate by being suspended in a viscous medium or a semisolid medium containing agar, they stop dividing and, as a consequence, are said to exhibit anchorage-dependent growth. The reason for this dependence on substrate is unclear, but it is possible that cells require contact with extracellular proteins or glycoproteins (often mimicked by serum proteins coating the tissue culture plate surface) to organize their growth pattern and to continue dividing. Transformed cells grown in culture frequently grow even when they are deprived of association with substrate by being suspended in a semisolid medium.[8] This *anchorage independence* displayed by many tumor cells indicates that transformed cells do not require the same level of external stimulation as normal cells in order to maintain a state of active growth.

In addition to growth in a semisolid medium, many tumor cells can grow in a fluid medium without attachment to a substrate. These cells grow singly or in small clumps; in the laboratory they are usually agitated gently to keep them from settling to the bottom of the culture vessel. This phenomenon has a counterpart to the behavior of tumor cells in the cancer patient; many types of tumors tend to grow along the pleural surfaces of the thorax or abdomen, producing a suspension of tumor cells in a protein-rich fluid that may seriously compromise the patient's respiratory or circulatory function.

Normal cells produce proteins that are exported to the outer cell surface and are used to coat the cells and their immediate surroundings. The best studied of these proteins is *fibronectin*, which, by itself, is sufficient to promote the adhesion of cells to the surface of a culture dish. Signals from extracellular proteins are not required for the growth of many types of tumor cells in culture, so it may not be surprising that tumor cells usually make significantly less fibronectin and other extracellular matrix proteins than normal cells.[9]

Tumor Cells Have Reduced Requirements for Growth Factors

Growing body tissues are bathed in a complex mixture of nutrients, including amino acids, minerals, and vitamins, and a still undetermined number of growth-stimulatory and growth-inhibitory substances. When in vitro culture methods were being formulated, nutrient mixtures (cell culture media) of defined chemical composition were devised to provide many of the compounds necessary for cell growth. Nevertheless, it was always necessary to supplement the mixtures with sera (usually from calves or fetal calves) to optimize growth rate and cell survival. These sera contain a complex and still poorly defined mixture of growth-stimulatory factors. Recently, rodent cells have been found to grow in a chemically defined medium supplemented with three growth-stimulatory peptide growth factors: insulin, transferrin, and epidermal growth factor.

Normal human cells typically require fetal calf

serum for growth, presumably because some essential factor is present in fetal calf serum and absent or reduced in calf serum. Significantly, the growth of human cancer cells is usually much less dependent on serum factors; tumor cells frequently can be grown in greatly reduced concentrations of fetal calf or calf serum. When normal cells are placed in medium containing reduced levels (<1%) of serum, they become arrested in the G_0 phase of the cell growth cycle and stop dividing. Tumor cells often will continue to grow even under conditions of reduced serum levels.

The reduced dependence of tumor cells on serum growth factors may be explained, in part, by the discovery of biochemical alterations within cancer cells resulting from some genetic alterations. These biochemical alterations mimic the changes experienced by a normal cell on exposure to polypeptide growth factors. As a consequence, direct exposure of the tumor cell to these growth-stimulatory factors is obviated, and this cell no longer shows substantial dependence on them for its proliferation.

Cancer Cells Are "Immortal"

When populations of normal rodent cells are explanted from an animal and grown in culture, they will divide for a limited number of generations and then experience a so-called senescent crisis, in which most cells stop dividing and die. A small number of these cells may emerge from this crisis, having undergone a poorly defined change that enables them to continue to divide without limitation. The descendants of these cells can then be cultured through an unlimited number of passages. Such *immortalized* cultures, established to grow indefinitely in culture, are termed *cell lines*.[10]

Normal human cells undergo a crisis similar to rodent cells, but for unknown reasons no cells survive to establish permanent cell lines. Explanted human tumor cells (though they are frequently difficult to adapt to tissue culture in the first place) do not exhibit this phenomenon; they usually have an unlimited potential for growth and are thus immortalized. Similarly, human tumors transplanted experimentally into immunodeficient mice exhibit an apparently unlimited potential to regenerate tumors after repeated rounds of transplantation.

Although established rodent cell lines share the phenotype of immortality with tumor cells, they exhibit few other characteristics associated with malignant cells. Established cell lines retain contact inhibition and are anchorage dependent. Most will not form tumors when injected into appropriate host animals. Consequently, the phenotype of immortality in culture is only one of several phenotypes of tumorigenic cells. Immortalization may be an essential prerequisite for tumorigenesis, but it is hardly sufficient. This conclusion is corroborated by studies of the genes carried by some oncogenic viruses and used by them to transform infected cells. Some of the genes carried by these tumor viruses are known to promote the establishment of immortal cell lines at high frequency. In nearly all cases, these immortalizing genes are not capable of converting an infected cell to the fully tumorigenic state; yet other cellular changes are clearly required to reach this state.

Tumor Cells Must Escape Immune Surveillance

Experimental tumors arising from treatment of animals or cultured cells with carcinogenic chemicals or oncogenic viruses frequently express on their surfaces novel antigens that are not present on the surfaces of their untransformed progenitors. One type of novel antigen may be common to many kinds of tumor cells and may be recognized by a class of lymphocytes called natural killer (NK) cells.[11] NK cells can recognize some tumor cell antigens even without specific prior immunization, and may be able to destroy tumor cells bearing this type of antigen.

In other instances, novel antigens specific to a particular type of tumor may be displayed. When animals are immunized with killed tumor cells bearing such an antigen, they subsequently may be protected from the growth of injected viable cells bearing the same antigen. These antigens are referred to as tumor-specific transplantation antigens (TSTAs). The molecules constituting TSTAs are usually not involved causally in cell transformation, but are best regarded as markers or consequences of the central transforming event or events.[12]

According to one model for the development of tumors in humans, all individuals develop numerous transformed cells over the course of their lives, but most of these cells are recognized as foreign and are killed by one or another component of the host's immune system. Proponents of this model of immune surveillance point to the fact that some tumors evoke a lymphocytic response (as evidenced by the lymphocytic infiltrates seen in microscopic sections of some testicular seminomas and medullary carcinomas of the breast), and that the clinical severity of these tumors is inversely correlated with the degree of lymphocytic involvement. The increased frequency of B-cell neoplasms and the otherwise rare Kaposi's sarcoma in patients with the acquired immune deficiency syndrome (AIDS) is often explained by a lowered efficiency of immune surveillance in these immunocompromised hosts.[13] Immunocompromised individuals experience almost 200-fold more malignancies than the population as a whole.[9]

One mechanism by which the tumor cell may escape the host immune response is to down-regulate the expression of HLA antigens, which normally serve to assist lymphocyte recognition of the target cell. Among the many effects produced by oncogenic adenoviruses, one is a reduction in the expression of HLA antigens in the transformed cell. In certain types of spontaneously arising human tumors, such as neuroblastomas, cells from advanced tumor stages often have reduced levels of HLA antigens.

Tumor Cells Exhibit Some Features of Cell Differentiation

Many tumor cells display some characteristic features of the normal cells found in their tissue of origin. Thus, cells from breast tumors may make duct-like tubules; those from thyroid tumors, tiny colloid-filled follicles; and cells of rhabdomyosarcomas, cross-striations similar to those found in skeletal muscle. The distinction between the common adenocarcinoma and squamous or epidermoid carcinoma depends on the features of glandular mucosa (mucus secretion and tubule formation) in the former and squamous mucosa (keratin production) in the latter. In general, tumors that express more of the features of the mature tissue (so-called well-differentiated tumors) have a less malignant clinical course than their poorly differentiated counterparts. Some tumors, notably the neuroblastomas of infancy, spontaneously differentiate into a more benign tumor type and may actually regress without treatment.

This partially differentiated state of most tumor cells requires explanation. It is thought that the initial transforming event leading to the tumor often occurs in a dividing and still-undifferentiated stem cell, the precursor of the differentiated cells within a tissue. One mechanism of the transformation process may involve the establishment of a partial or complete block in the normal developmental pathway toward full differentiation. As a consequence, the resulting transformed cell may be trapped in a relatively undifferentiated, highly proliferative cell compartment.

These concepts offer some explanations for the origin of tumors. Growth of tissues is normally limited by the fact that as cells differentiate, they lose the proliferative ability of their stem-cell precursors. Tumor cells become blocked in this differentiation pathway and retain the potential for unlimited growth. As an example, cells of the epidermal layer of the skin originate from stem cells in the basal layer and begin to express keratin. These cells are displaced outwardly by the newer cells which follow them, and as their cytoplasm fills with keratin, the cells elongate and become metabolically inactive until they are eventually sloughed from the surface. Tumor cells arising from the epidermis do not exhibit the features of mature skin cells (eg, they may make little keratin) and retain the proliferative activity which, in the normal skin, is restricted to the stem cells in the basal layer. With this model in mind, recent attempts have been made to induce tumor-cell differentiation, circumventing the block to differentiation by treating patients with chemicals (eg, retinoic acid, a relative of vitamin A) known to induce differentiation in culture.[14] To date, however, no conclusive evidence of long-term therapeutic value has been shown.

In addition, many tumor cells express proteins that are not found in the mature tissue, but are part of the normal pattern of protein expression from the corresponding embryonic tissue. For example, the embryonic liver produces and secretes alpha-fetoprotein (AFP), which is analogous to serum albumin produced by the adult liver. Alpha-fetoprotein is not found in mature liver tissue, except under conditions in which the organ is injured and is actively regenerating. Hepatocellular carcinomas, the common cancers of liver cell origin, frequently express large quantities of AFP, which is found both in the tumor cells and in the circulation of patients bearing hepatocellular tumors.[15] Similarly, an embryonic protein termed carcinoembryonic antigen (CEA) is secreted by many tumors of lung and gastrointestinal tract origin; the circulating level of CEA is a rough indicator of the tumor burden carried by the patient.[16]

Tumor cells frequently release biologically potent polypeptides that may announce the tumor's presence long before it becomes evident on the basis of its size. One example is the insulinoma, an insulin-secreting pancreatic islet cell tumor. Patients with these tumors will usually present with symptoms of hypoglycemia resulting from insulin excess. Another tumor that produces an active hormone is choriocarcinoma, which arises from the placenta and is retained by the uterus after delivery. This tumor releases into the circulation large quantities of the hormone hCG (human chorionic gonadotropin), which is a normal product of the placenta. Fortunately, choriocarcinoma is quite sensitive to the chemotherapeutic agent methotrexate. Patients who have undergone chemotherapy for this tumor are regularly monitored for the appearance of hCG in their serum as a sensitive and thus early indicator of recurrence. Tumors may also express products not typical of their tissue of origin. Such inappropriate, or "ectopic," hormone production is exemplified by certain lung carcinomas that produce parathyroid hormone and renal cell carcinomas that elaborate erythropoietin.

Tumor Cells Have an Altered Metabolism

Tumor cells exhibit a vast array of metabolic differences distinguishing them from their untransformed counterparts. The overall trend is toward simplified metabolic activities and an increased synthesis of material necessary for cell division. This generalization is understandable in light of the process of selection that has taken place over the tumor's lifetime. Tumor cells have no need to express proteins relevant to the specialized functions of the original tissue, and their growth is favored when they divert much of their resources to the purposes of cell division.

One very apparent metabolic change in culture-grown tumor cells is the production of large amounts of acid, which is due, at least in part, to utilization of anaerobic pathways of glycolysis even in the presence of oxygen. This was observed decades ago by Warburg,[17] but has since been shown to occur as well in rapidly growing untransformed cells. An increased rate of glucose transport is another striking feature of tumor cells.

The increased metabolic rate and rapid rate of cell growth cause an increased demand for blood-borne nutrients in the expanding tumor. Since the diffusion of solutes and oxygen is limited to a few millimeters, many rapidly growing, poorly vascularized neoplasms suffer necrosis of their central portions. This is seen in tissue sections as poorly defined cell bodies with degenerated nuclear material and infiltrating granulocytes, surrounded by a ring of viable tumor tissue. Most tumors larger than several millimeters in diameter manage to stimulate the ingrowth of nonneoplastic blood vessels from the surrounding normal tissue into the expanding tumor. The resulting infiltration of the tumor mass by blood vessels—the process of *neovascularization*—is achieved through the release by the tumor cells of polypeptide angiogenic growth factors. The capillary beds generated through neovascularization also provide the tumor cell populations with a direct access to avenues for metastasizing to distant sites. Indeed, the future ability of a still-localized breast carcinoma to metastasize is correlated to its degree of neovascularization.[18]

Tumor Cells Are Capable of Invasion and Metastasis

Invasion of adjacent tissue and metastasis to distant organs are the most ominous features of a malignant tumor. Without these features, surgical resection could control most cancers. A tumor's ability to metastasize is a complex phenomenon, which requires at the minimum the following steps: (1) invasion by tumor cells through adjacent structures such as underlying basement membranes; (2) entrance into blood or lymphatic vessels with release of tumor cells into the circulation (intravasation); (3) survival of tumor cells within the circulation and evasion of immune surveillance; (4) escape from the circulation (extravasation); and (5) implantation in a foreign tissue with establishment of a new tumor locus.

Invasion is a feature common to nearly all types of malignant tumors. Microscopically, this is apparent when tumor cells are seen to be admixed with nonmalignant cells in the adjacent tissue. In some tumors, malignant cells mingle with or replace adjacent normal cells, but remain confined to the original plane of cells from which the tumor cells originated. For example, tumor cells arising in breast ducts may fill the lumen of the duct and replace the normal duct cells for several millimeters without penetrating through the basement membrane into the adjacent tissue. These tumors are referred to as in situ ductal carcinomas, and they metastasize infrequently. Invasive breast carcinomas include those that have penetrated the wall of the duct and are found growing in the adjacent stromal tissue. These tumors are thought to arise from earlier in situ carcinomas, although their pattern of invasiveness may have developed very early in the course of tumor progression.

Another example is provided by the highly malignant skin cancer, melanoma. The superficially spreading form of melanoma initially grows in a radial pattern; ie, it spreads laterally through the skin but remains confined to the epidermal cell layer. The vertical growth phase is a later stage in which the tumor invades the dermis and develops a propensity to metastasize.

Most carcinomas arise in epithelial cell layers that are underlain by a basement membrane composed of dense proteoglycans; the basement membrane represents a barrier to early tumor cell spread. Invasive tumor cells frequently secrete enzymes, including several types of collagenase, heparanase, and stromelysin, that are capable of degrading this type of physical barrier.[19] Expression of these enzymes may be a critical step in the invasion by tumor cells through adjacent structures and cell layers and thence into the circulation.

Once a tumor has eroded through the wall of the blood or lymphatic vessel, individual tumor cells or a small clump may detach and circulate through the body as an embolus. These cells can become encased in fibrin or in aggregates of platelets, which may protect them from destruction by the cell's immune system. The presence of tumor cells in the circulation does not guarantee the establishment of metastatic tumor loci, since the survival of tumor cells in the circulation appears to be quite low. Only about 0.1% of tumor cells injected intravenously into rats survive for more than 24 hours.[20]

Cells of many tumor types demonstrate the ability to "home" to a specific target organ. Clinically, this is demonstrated by the tendency of certain tumors to preferentially metastasize to specific organs. Sometimes the pattern of metastasis may reflect the pattern of the blood circulation; thus, the major site of blood-borne metastasis from the colon is the liver, which is the recipient of blood flow from the colon through the portal vein. However, most patterns of metastasis are not readily explainable on the basis of anatomic blood flow patterns; examples of this are the frequent metastasis of gastric carcinoma to the ovary and of lung carcinoma to the adrenal gland. These target organs receive <1% of the total blood circulation, but the frequency of metastasis is much higher than to the kidneys, which receive about 10% of the circulation. The ability of some tumors to develop a mechanism for homing to specific target organs has been demonstrated experimentally with B16 murine melanoma cells. Mice injected with these tumor cells develop tumor metastases in several organs. However, when tumor cells are recovered from metastases to the lung and then regrown in culture, these cells have a much higher tendency subsequently to form metastases in the lungs on reinjection into mice.[21] Thus, the tumor cells are capable of expressing a certain pattern of metastasis which, at least in these cases, is apparently genetically determined. It is not clear how these patterns of metastasis arise, but some evidence suggests that tumor cells can respond to specific chemotactic signals released by certain organs. A tumor cell may therefore pass through the circulation or lymphatic system until it receives an appropriate signal, and then be stimulated to attach to a vessel wall and extravasate into the tissue bed. Recently, specific receptors have been identified on the surfaces of metastasizing tumor cells that appear to play important roles in enabling these cells to adhere to complementary structures displayed by endothelial cells in certain organs.[22]

Genetic Mutation as a Basis of Neoplastic Transformation

Experimental data accumulated over more than half a century have suggested that neoplastic changes in cell phenotype occur as a direct consequence of alterations to the cell genome. The derived genetic theories of cancer contrast with an alternative theory, that cancer results because of changes in nongenetic (epigenetic) regulatory circuits that occur without alteration of the cellular genome.

The strongest support for the genetic origins of cancer comes from observations that agents known to damage DNA (mutagens) are often found to act as carcinogens. This association was first observed in work with x-rays. Early experimenters succumbed to cancer at high rates. Several decades later, it was realized that x-rays could act as potent agents for inducing genetic damage. In the 1970s, the work of Bruce Ames focused attention on a wide variety of chemicals that exhibit both mutagenic and carcinogenic properties. The correlation between their relative mutagenic and carcinogenic potencies suggested that these agents induce cancer through their ability to damage DNA.[23]

A corollary to these findings was the notion that the progenitors of tumor cells sustain a number of genetic alterations that create mutant genes, the expression of which then dictates the cell's malignant phenotype. These genetic changes occur in cells of the target organs in which tumors eventually appear and are called *somatic mutations* to distinguish them from the mutations that occur in germ cells and are transmitted from one individual to his or her offspring.

The search for the hypothesized mutant cancer-causing genes proceeded slowly. Their number and mode of action were initially totally obscure. Initial progress in understanding such cancer genes came from work with several tumor viruses, among them the small DNA-containing viruses SV40 and polyomavirus. In the early 1960s, these viruses were found to be able to infect and transform cultured rodent cells into a tumorigenic state. This showed that the process of neoplastic conversion of a cell, hitherto thought to occur only within the complex tissues of an animal, could be induced as well in vitro. Moreover, such transformation was achieved by small, relatively simple biological agents.[24] The resulting transformed cells were found to retain several viral genes in their DNA, and the continued presence of these genes was found to be essential for the cells' continued display of cancer traits. It was clear that the viral oncogenes were orchestrating the malignant properties of these cells: they initiated the process of transformation and their continued presence was required for maintenance of the transformed state.

The viral oncogenes retained in these cells were relatively simple and small in size. This led to the realization that a small number of genes, in this case viral oncogenes, can induce a large number of concordant shifts in cell phenotype. Thus, oncogenes could act pleiotropically to elicit multiple changes, apparently through an ability to trigger a small number of central regulatory controls within the cell. Some speculated that this logic could be transferred to human tumor cells in which no viral oncogenes were apparent; perhaps a small number of mutant cellular genes could also act as oncogenes to induce the many behavioral aberrancies associated with malignant cells. Indeed, the existence of such cellular genes was indicated by work on RNA-containing tumor viruses (retroviruses), such as the Rous sarcoma virus of chickens. The oncogene used by this virus to transform cells was found to originate from one of the normal genes of the chicken cell. This led in turn to the realization that the chicken genome must contain a normal gene which can be converted into an active, transformation-inducing oncogene by a retrovirus. By extension, the mammalian genome might also contain such a gene, if not a number of such genes, each of which could become activated into a potent oncogene.[25]

The Search for Cellular Oncogenes

Substantial progress was made in the late 1970s in the search for oncogenes within cancer cells prepared from human tumors or from chemically induced rodent tumors. The cancerous state of these particular cells did not appear to be derived from infection by oncogene-bearing tumor viruses.

One strategy to detect oncogenes within the nonviral tumors was to extract DNA from cancer cells and introduce it into normal nontransformed recipient cells via the procedure known variously as gene transfer or transfection. The transfected recipient cells were then studied to detect any changes in their phenotype. In a number of cases, the recipients took on some of the neoplastic traits that had been exhibited by the donor cells from which the DNA had been prepared.[26] This yielded a simple yet important conclusion: the information encoding cancerous behavior could be passed from cell to cell via DNA molecules. This meant that among the transfected DNA molecules, there must be several carrying cancer-inducing genes: oncogenes. As oncogenes were not detectable in the DNA of normal cells, it was clear that they appeared in cancer cells as part of the processes that led to the malignant state.

With the advent of gene cloning technologies, it was possible to isolate these cellular oncogenes in the early 1980s. One well-studied example stemmed from a human bladder carcinoma cell line termed EJ/T24.[27] This oncogene was relatively small, encompassing only 6,000 base pairs of DNA; the cell nucleus by contrast contains about 6 billion base pairs of human DNA. Nonetheless, this small oncogene could exert profound effects on a cell by inducing concomitant changes in cell shape, secretion of growth factors, loss of contact inhibition, anchorage independence, increased glucose transport, and a host of other changes, including, in many cell types, tumorigenicity and metastasis.

This bladder carcinoma oncogene was found to arise from a normal cellular gene of very similar structure. Such a normal antecedent is often termed a *proto-oncogene*, a term that implies the ability of a normal gene to acquire oncogenic powers following appropriate mutations in its DNA sequence. Proto-oncogenes are present in a wide variety of organisms.[28] Their ubiquitous presence in many distantly related life forms is a testimonial to the essential role they play in normal cellular and organismic physiology. Such an essential role has ensured conservation over vast evolutionary distances in relatively unchanged form. The involvement of proto-oncogenes in cancer occurs only as a consequence of rare genetic accidents that cause a deregulation of their function and, with this, a resulting deregulation in the complex apparatus responsible for governing cell growth.

Many of the oncogenes detected in human tumors were known from earlier work on RNA tumor viruses (retroviruses), among them the Rous sarcoma virus. As described earlier, many tumor viruses carry oncogenes in their genomes, using them to transform cells that they infect. The retroviral oncogenes, in particular, were found to be derived ultimately from normal cellular proto-oncogenes. It is now realized that during their infectious passage through cells, retroviruses are capable of picking up and mobilizing proto-oncogenes residing in the genomes of infected host cells. These acquired genes, carried now in the viral genome, assume the role of oncogenes and are responsible for the tumorigenic properties of these hybrid viruses.

Many of the oncogenes originally detected by virtue of their association with various retroviruses were then found to be activated through nonviral mutational mechanisms in human tumors (Table 9-1). The Ha-*ras* oncogene, associated initially with a rat sarcoma retrovirus, was seen to be closely related to the EJ/T24 bladder carcinoma oncogene.[29,30] The *myc* oncogene, discovered in the context of the avian myelocytomatosis virus genome, was seen in activated form in many Burkitt's lymphomas.[31] The *abl* oncogene of mouse Abelson leukemia virus was discovered as an activated oncogene in many, if not all, chronic myelogenous leukemias.[32]

Mechanism of Oncogene Activation

A variety of somatic mutational mechanisms are responsible for creating activated cellular oncogenes. The mutation responsible for the bladder carcinoma oncogene was surprisingly subtle: a single base change out of the 6,000 bases constituting the original proto-oncogene. This *point mutation* affected, in turn, the amino acid sequence of the protein specified by the gene.[33] The structurally altered protein is the molecule that ultimately affects cell metabolism, thereby inducing malignancy.

Yet other oncogenes arise through mutations that affect the structure of their encoded proteins. In chronic myelogenous leukemia, the oncogenicity of the *abl* gene is derived from the fact that this gene undergoes fusion with a fully unrelated gene, *bcr*.[34] The bcr-abl hybrid protein encoded by these fused genes differs substantially in structure and function from the normal abl proto-oncogene protein.

Oncogenes like *myc* or the related N-*myc* acquire their malignant properties through mechanisms that affect the level of expression of their encoded proteins but leave their protein structures intact. These deregulations of protein quantity are achieved through several distinct mechanisms. In childhood neuroblastomas, the copy number of the N-*myc* gene frequently is amplified from its usual diploid number to many dozens per cell.[35] Because this amplified state is

Table 9-1. Cell Oncogenes Involved in Human Tumors

Oncogene	Retrovirus Association	Example of Human Tumor Involvement	Subcellular Localization of Protein	Name of Protein
abl	Abelson murine leukemia virus	Myelogenous leukemia	Myelogenous plasma membrane	Tyrosine kinase receptor
erb-B	Avian erythroblastosis virus	Mammary carcinoma, glioblastoma	Plasma membrane	Tyrosine kinase receptor
erb B-2 HER-2/*neu*		Mammary, ovarian, and stomach carcinoma	Plasma membrane	Tyrosine kinase receptor
Ha-*ras*	Harvey murine sarcoma virus	Wide variety	Cytoplasmic membranes	GDP/GTP binding
Ki-*ras*	Kirsten murine sarcoma virus	Wide variety	Cytoplasmic membranes	GDP/GTP binding
N-*ras*		Wide variety	Cytoplasmic membranes	GDP/GTP binding
myc	MC-29 avian myelocytomatosis virus	Lymphoma	Nucleus	Transcription factor
N-*myc*		Neuroblastoma	Nucleus	Possible transcription factor
L-*myc*		Small-cell lung carcinoma	Nucleus	Possible transcription factor
hst		Stomach carcinoma	Secreted	Related to fibroblast growth factor
bcl-2		Follicular lymphoma	Cytoplasmic membranes	Not known
GSP		Pituitary adenoma	Cytoplasmic membranes	G-protein
Ret		Thyroid carcinoma	Plasma membrane	Tyrosine kinase
Trk		Thyroid carcinoma	Plasma membrane	Tyrosine kinase

GDP = guanosine diphosphate; GTP = guanosine triphosphate.

often correlated with poor prognosis, it is thought that N-*myc* amplification is an important cause of the aggressiveness of such tumors. In mammary carcinomas, the HER-2/*neu* oncogene is often amplified in tumors having a high metastatic potency.[36] This amplification may provide a useful diagnostic index and a possible explanation for the metastatic aggressiveness of the tumor cells.

In Burkitt's lymphomas, the deregulation of *myc* gene expression is due to chromosomal translocations that fuse the *myc* proto-oncogene with immunoglobulin genes. This unusual juxtaposition places the *myc* gene under the control of regulatory elements of the immunoglobulin gene. Expression of the *myc* gene is normally modulated by a complex array of physiological stimuli. When its expression is placed under the control of elements of the immunoglobulin gene, a steady expression results that is uncoupled from normal regulatory circuits.

Oncogenes and Tumor Progression

As oncogene action was explored in detail, it became clear that single oncogenes were unable to induce transformation of fully normal cells into fully malignant cells. Instead, the actions of a single oncogene usually induce only partial conversion to malignancy. This point is made most graphically by introducing single oncogenes into normal cells recently explanted from a normal tissue or embryo. For example, when a *ras* oncogene originating from a human tumor is introduced into rat embryo fibroblasts growing in monolayer culture, the recipient cells may show anchorage independence but are unable to form tumors when inoculated in host animals. Moreover, these cells soon die after several passages in culture, unlike well-established tumor cells. A *myc* oncogene has quite different effects on the cellular phenotype. Cells bearing *myc* may be able to grow indefinitely in culture, but they too are nontumorigenic. Full tumorigenicity ensues only when the *myc* and *ras* oncogenes are introduced concomitantly into these embryo cells.[37] Analogous results have been reported with other oncogene pairs acting in other cell types.

While human tumors bearing both a *myc* and a *ras* oncogene have been observed only rarely, this experimental model teaches a number of lessons that appear to be widely applicable to cancer cell biology. Growth regulation of the mammalian cell appears to be organized in such a way that single oncogenes are unable to induce full conversion to malignancy. This serves as a protective mechanism operating in normal cells by acting to prevent the outgrowth of tumors whenever single oncogenes arise through isolated genetic accidents.

The observed oncogene cooperation also shows that different oncogenes act in distinct ways on cell metabolism. Each oncogene may induce only a subset of the changes associated with full malignancy; several acting in concert can achieve the end result of creating a highly malignant cell. In the case of the *ras*-*myc* pair, the *ras* oncogene can induce anchorage independence and growth factor secretion while the *myc* oncogene can immortalize cells. Together, these responses encompass many of the important aspects of the growth deregulation observed with cancer cells.

Yet a third point has arisen from attempts to relate the phenomenon of multistep carcinogenesis with the observed complementary effects of various oncogenes. It would appear that each step through which cells pass in the progression from normalcy to malignancy is demarcated by a distinct genetic change, often one that creates an oncogene like *myc* or *ras*. The precise number of distinct steps is poorly documented in human tumorigenesis, and in most cases the precise nature of the gene mutations involved in delineating these steps is also unknown. One exception is provided by human colon carcinomas, in which the histopathologic changes occurring as normal colonic epithelial cells progress to malignant carcinomas have been correlated with distinct genetic lesions in the genomes of these various cell types. Early adenomatous polyps carry lesions in the APC (adenomatous polyposis coli) gene; larger polyps show additional mutation of their K-*ras* genes; carcinomas acquire lesions in their DCC (deleted in colon carcinoma) and p53 genes.[38] These associations are not absolute, and alternative genetic paths to full malignancy may be taken by some colonic tumors. Nonetheless, this work does provide the beginnings of a precise road-map of the genetic changes undergone by most developing colonic tumors and represents a model for the genetic description of multistep tumorigenesis that will be developed for a number of other tissues in the future. Significantly, of these four target genes, only one is an oncogene; the remaining three genes are tumor suppressor genes, as described below.

Tumor Suppressor Genes and Tumor Progression

Oncogenes represent only one of several classes of genetic elements that play critical roles in tumorigenesis. Another group of genes, known variously as tumor suppressors or anti-oncogenes, appears to be equally important. Unlike oncogenes and antecedent proto-oncogenes, all of which function as growth-promoting elements in the cell, tumor suppressor genes appear to function in the normal cell to restrict or repress cellular proliferation.[39]

Proto-oncogenes participate in cancer through their hyperactive or deregulated alleles. In contrast, tumor suppressor genes are involved in tumorigenesis when they suffer genetic inactivation. Loss-of-function mutations affecting the two redundant copies of these genes serve to remove a normally existing barrier to cell growth, unleashing in turn the clonal proliferation that leads to a tumor mass. Such inactivating mutations occur much more readily than the precisely targeted mutations that activate proto-oncogenes, increasing the likelihood that tumor suppressor genes are frequently involved in cancer pathogenesis.

Inactive alleles of tumor suppressor genes can be acquired in two ways: they may be created through somatic mutation occurring in a target organ, or they may be passed through the germ line, being present in the conceptus and consequently in all body tissues. The latter situation may create a congenital predisposition to cancer because one of the two required mutational events needed to knock out both homologous copies of the gene has already occurred in all cells of the target organ.[40] This nicely describes the origins of retinoblastoma. When a defective allele of the retinoblastoma (Rb) gene is acquired congenitally, a familial retinoblastoma ensues, involving multiple independent tumor foci in both eyes of the afflicted child. In the founding cells of each of these tumor foci, the loss of one Rb gene copy through germ line mutation is compounded by the loss of the surviving, intact copy through somatic mutation. In the sporadic form of the disease, both alleles are inactivated somatically in a single cell—a rare constellation of events that leads to only a single tumor-cell focus.

The easiest mechanism for inactivation of both copies of a tumor suppressor gene like Rb involves an initial inactivation of one allele and the subsequent replacement of the surviving wild-type allele with a duplicated copy of the mutant allele. The processes creating homozygosity—two identical versions—of this gene may also lead to homozygosity of other closely linked genes on the chromosome. Accordingly, workers have searched the genomes of tumor cells for regions that were initially heterozygous for different genetic markers prior to tumorigenesis and have been reduced to a homozygous condition during the course of tumor progression.[41] Indeed, homozygous regions have been found in a number of distinct tumor types; in each case, changes in a specific chromosomal region are associated with a specific form of cancer (Table 9-2). Although largely unproven, it is assumed that these reductions to homozygosity reflect loss of function of specific tumor suppressor genes, which in turn triggers cancer. Oncogenes and tumor suppressor genes together appear to represent the two most important groups of genetic elements participating in cancer formation.

Tumor Cells and Growth Factors

As described earlier, a hallmark of tumor cells is their reduced dependence on mitogenic growth factors. For example, while normal cells will often require the addition of 10% serum to their culture medium, tumor cells will often grow well in only 1% serum. Because the serum functions as a source of factors, these observations indicate that tumor cells have acquired a measure of growth factor autonomy.

This autonomy has important implications for understanding the essential nature of cancer. The disease is best characterized as a breakdown of communication and interdependence between cells within a tissue. Since much of the cell-to-cell communication is mediated by transmission of growth factors, a loss of growth factor dependence represents an important breakdown in the regulatory network maintaining normal tissue architecture.

Oncogenes represent important means by which tumor cells acquire growth factor independence. They confer such autonomy in at least four different ways. The first mechanism depends on the observation that tumor cells often secrete mitogenic growth factors. Sporn and Todaro postulated that these secreted growth factors may stimulate growth of the same cell that has just released them, resulting in an autostimulatory or *autocrine* positive feedback loop.[42] Stated differently, the endogenous production of growth factor renders their importation from elsewhere in the tissue unnecessary. Oncogenes may participate in autocrine stimulation in two ways. Some oncogenes, like *ras* and *src*, may induce the expression of normally tightly regulated growth factor genes. Alternatively, growth factor genes may themselves suffer alterations that cause their uncontrolled expression.[43] A growth factor gene so altered takes on the role of an oncogene.

Table 9-2. Identified or Suspected Tumor Suppressor Genes

Name	Tumor Involvement	Chromosomal Site
	Neuroblastoma	1p 36
	Small-cell lung carcinoma*	3p 21
	Kidney carcinoma	3p 12-14
APC	Colon carcinoma	5q 21
WT-1	Wilms' tumor	11p 13
	Bladder carcinoma	11p
MEN-1	Parathyroid, pancreas, pituitary	11q 13
RB	Retinoblastoma, osteosarcoma	13q 14
	Small-cell lung carcinoma	
	Liver carcinoma	16q 22
NF-1	Neurofibromatosis type 1	17q 11
p53	Many tumor types	17q 12
DCC	Colon carcinoma	18q 21
	Meningioma, acoustic neuroma	22q

Tumor cells have been found to secrete a great variety of growth factors. Among these are tumor growth factor-α (TGF-α), which acts as a surrogate of epidermal growth factor (EGF); platelet-derived growth factor (PDGF); and TGF-β. If the factor-secreting cell also displays cell surface receptors that bind the secreted product, then these released factors may succeed in driving autocrine growth.

A second mechanism of growth factor autonomy stems from the growth factor receptors displayed on the surface of normal cells. These receptors release growth-stimulatory signals into the cell when they bind their cognate ligands. Recent work suggests that alterations in receptor number or structure can result in the release of gratuitous mitogenic signals into the cell, even in the absence of any encountered growth factor ligands.[44] These aberrantly expressed or structured receptors then operate as oncogene proteins. Aggressively growing mammary carcinomas often display enormous numbers of the receptor protein encoded by the HER-2/*neu* proto-oncogene.[36] Cells of the human epidermoid carcinoma-cell line A431 display versions of the EGF receptor that are both truncated and present in several hundred-fold increased amounts.[45] In both cases, these aberrantly expressed receptors appear to drive cell growth independently of binding exogenous growth factor ligands.

A third mechanism of growth factor autonomy pertains to components of the cytoplasmic signaling pathway responsible for picking up signals from cell surface receptors and transducing them to central growth-regulatory switches within the cell. Although the details of these pathways are still poorly understood, it appears that proteins of genes like *ras* and *src* participate in signal-transducing events in these pathways. When these proteins undergo certain structural alterations, they may release signals constitutively, even in the absence of prior prompting by upstream components in their signaling pathway. Growth factors are rendered unnecessary because mitogenic signals now originate through an alternative mechanism—the misfiring of cytoplasmic signal transducers downstream in the signaling cascade.

A final route to growth factor autonomy stems from the behavior of nuclear proto-oncogenes that are normally regulated through a wide range of expression. For example, genes like *fos* and *myc* may be virtually silent in nongrowing cells and increase their expression 20- to 50-fold when the cell encounters appropriate growth factors such as PDGF. The mutations that convert these genes into active oncogenes often cause their constitutive expression in a way that no longer depends on growth factor stimulation. One striking example of this is the translocation seen in Burkitt's lymphomas that removes the *myc* gene from its normal regulatory sequences and places it under the control of regulatory elements of the immunoglobulin gene. Similar end results may be obtained in childhood neuroblastomas, in which amplification of the N-*myc* proto-oncogene results in its vast overexpression.

The Metabolic Basis of Oncogene Action

While oncogenes have been found to induce many of the distinctive traits of neoplastic cells, a fundamental puzzle remains: How do the oncogene proteins succeed in altering the cell in such profound ways? This question must ultimately be reduced to the biochemical mechanisms of action of these proteins. Progress in understanding this has been slow, but it is now clear that a number of oncogene proteins, exemplified by the pp60 protein of the *src* oncogene, act as tyrosine kinases and, as such, serve to phosphorylate tyrosine residues on target proteins.[46] Other oncogene proteins, such as those of the *fos, myc,* and *jun* oncogenes, act as transcription regulators.[47,48]

Even these insights leave the major questions unanswered. In the case of the tyrosine kinases, a decade of work has provided little insight into how protein phosphorylation can induce cancer-specific phenotypes. The nuclear oncogene proteins acting as transcriptional regulators may well modulate the expression of banks of important responder genes, but the identities of these genes are elusive.

A further aspect of cancer biochemistry addresses the small molecules, known as second messengers, that function as intracellular hormones by conveying mitogenic signals from one part of the cell to another. A number of second messengers have been found within cells, including elements as diverse as calcium ions and cyclic AMP. Perhaps the most critical of these are the breakdown products of the phosphatidylinositol (PI) phosphates, compounds that act as pharmacologically potent intracellular growth agonists.[49] Some suspect that many oncogene proteins act through their ability to deregulate the PI pathway.

An understanding of the biochemical basis of oncogene action remains incomplete and, in many respects, highly speculative. This will change rapidly; within a decade, many of these puzzles will have been worked out in great detail. With this progress will come insight into how oncogenes act pleiotropically to induce a multitude of cancer cell phenotypes. Such insights may be applicable to the causal mechanisms of many types of cancer. In addition, an understanding of the biochemistry of the cancer cell may lead to the first perception of molecular targets within the cancer cell that can be attacked by totally new types of therapeutics. In the end, this faith drives much of contemporary cancer research: By understanding the cause, we can create the cure.

References

1. Foulds L. *Neoplastic Development.* London: Academic Press; 1969; 2.

2. Verderame M, Alcorta D, Egnor M, Smith K, Pollack R. Cytoskeletal F-actin patterns quantitated with fluorescein isothiocyanate-phalloidin in normal and transformed cells. *Proc Natl Acad Sci USA.* 1980;77:6624-6628.

3. Sefton BM, Hunter T, Ball EH, Singer SJ. Vinculin: a cytoskeletal target of the transforming protein of Rous sarcoma virus. *Cell.* 1981;24:165-174.

4. Abercrombie M, Heaysman JEM. Observations on the

social behaviour of cells in the tissue culture, II: "monolayering" of fibroblasts. *Exp Cell Res.* 1954;6:293-306.

5. Temin HM, Rubin H. Characteristics of an assay for Rous sarcoma virus and Rous sarcoma cells in tissue culture. *Virology.* 1958;6:669-688.

6. Weinstein RS, Merk FB, Alroy J. The structure and function of intercellular junctions in cancer. *Adv Cancer Res.* 1976;23:23-89.

7. Loewenstein WR. Junctional intercellular communication and the control of growth. *Biochim Biophys Acta.* 1979;560:1-65.

8. Macpherson I, Montagnier L. Agar suspension culture for the selective assay of cells transformed by polyoma virus. *Virology.* 1964;23:291-294.

9. Vaheri A, Mosher DF. High molecular weight cell surface-associated glycoprotein (fibronectin) lost in malignant transformation. *Biochim Biophys Acta.* 1978;516:1-25.

10. Todaro GJ, Green H. Quantitative studies of the growth of mouse embryo cells in culture and their development into established lines. *J Cell Biol.* 1963;17:299-213.

11. Herberman RB, Ortaldo JR. Natural killer cells: their role in defenses against disease. *Science.* 1981;214:24-30.

12. Old LJ. Cancer immunology: the search for specificity. GHA Clowes memorial lecture. *Cancer Res.* 1981;41:361-375.

13. Ziegler JL, Drew WL, Miner RC, et al. Outbreak of Burkitt's-like lymphoma in homosexual men. *Lancet.* 1982;11:631-633.

14. Gouveia J, Hercend T, Lemaigre G, et al. Degree of bronchial metaplasia in heavy smokers and its regression after treatment with a retinoid. *Lancet.* 1982;1:710-712.

15. Abelev GI. Alpha-fetoprotein in oncogenesis and its association with malignant tumors. *Adv Cancer Res.* 1971;14:295-358.

16. Concannon JP, Dalbow MH, Liebler GA, Blake KE, Weil CS, Cooper JW. The carcinoembryonic antigen assay in bronchogenic carcinoma. *Cancer.* 1974;34:184-192.

17. Warburg OH. *The Metabolism of Tumors: Investigations From the Kaiser Wilhelm Institute for Biology.* London: Constable; 1930.

18. Weidner N, Semple JP, Welch WR, Folkman J. Tumor angiogenesis and metastasis: correlation in invasive breast carcinoma. *N Engl J Med.* 1991;324:1-8.

19. Recklies AD, Tiltman KJ, Stoker TAM, Poole AR. Secretion of proteinases from malignant and nonmalignant human breast tissue. *Cancer Res.* 1980;40:550-556.

20. Fisher ER, Fisher B. Experimental studies of factors influencing hepatic metastases, I: the effect of number of tumor cells injected and time of growth. *Cancer.* 1959; 12:926-941.

21. Brunson KW, et al. Selection and altered tumor cell properties of brain-colonizing metastatic melanoma cells selected from B16 melanoma. *Int J Cancer.* 1979;23:854.

22. Günthert U, Hofmann M, Rudy W, et al. A new variant of glycoprotein CD44 confers metastatic potential to rat carcinoma cells. *Cell.* 1991;65:13-24.

23. McCann J, Ames BN. Detection of carcinogens as mutagens in the salmonella/microsome test: assay of 300 chemicals: discussion. *Proc Natl Acad Sci USA.* 1976;73:950-954.

24. Dulbecco R. Cell transformation by viruses. *Science.* 1969;166:962-968.

25. Stehelin D, Varmus HE, Bishop JM, Vogt PK. DNA related to the transforming gene(s) of avian sarcoma viruses is present in normal avian DNA. *Nature.* 1976;260:170-173.

26. Shih C, Shilo BZ, Goldfarb MP, Dannenberg A, Weinberg RA. Passage of phenotypes of chemically transformed cells via transfection of DNA and chromatin. *Proc Natl Acad Sci USA.* 1979;76:5714-5718.

27. Krontiris TG, Cooper GM. Transforming activity of human tumor DNAs. *Proc Natl Acad Sci USA.* 1981;78:1181-1184.

28. Shilo BZ, Weinberg RA. DNA sequences homologous to vertebrate oncogenes are conserved in *Drosophila melanogaster. Proc Natl Acad Sci USA.* 1981;78:6789-6792.

29. Der CJ, Krontiris TG, Cooper GM. Transforming genes of human bladder and lung carcinoma cell lines are homologous to the *ras* genes of Harvey and Kirsten sarcoma viruses. *Proc Natl Acad Sci USA.* 1982;79:3637-3640.

30. Parada LF, Tabin CJ, Shih C, Weinberg RA. Human EJ bladder carcinoma oncogene is homologue of Harvey sarcoma virus *ras* gene. *Nature.* 1982;297:474-478.

31. Taub R, Kirsch I, Morton C, et al. Translocation of the c-*myc* gene into the immunoglobulin heavy chain locus in human Burkitt lymphoma and murine plasmacytoma cells. *Proc Natl Acad Sci USA.* 1982;79:7837-7841.

32. de Klein A, van Kessel AG, Grosveld G, et al. A cellular oncogene is translocated to the Philadelphia chromosome in chronic myelocytic leukaemia. *Nature.* 1982;300:765-767.

33. Tabin CJ, Bradley SM, Bargmann CI, et al. Mechanism of activation of a human oncogene. *Nature.* 1982;300:143-149.

34. Groffen J, Stephenson JR, Heisterkamp N, de Klein A, Bartram CR, Grosveld G. Philadelphia chromosomal breakpoints are clustered within a limited region, *bcr*, on chromosome 22. *Cell.* 1984;36:93-99.

35. Seeger RC, Brodeur GM, Sather H, et al. Association of multiple copies of the N-*myc* oncogene with rapid progression of neuroblastomas. *N Engl J Med.* 1985;313:1111-1116.

36. Slamon DJ, Clark GM, Wong SG, Levin WJ, Ullrich A, McGuire WL. Human breast cancer: correlation of relapse and survival with amplification of the HER-2/*neu* oncogene. *Science.* 1987;235:177-182.

37. Land H, Parada LF, Weinberg RA. Cellular oncogenes and multistep carcinogenesis. *Science.* 1983;222:771-778.

38. Bos JL, Fearon ER, Hamilton SR, et al. Prevalence of *ras* gene mutations in human colorectal cancers. *Nature.* 1987;327:293-297.

39. Klein G. The approaching era of the tumor suppressor genes. *Science.* 1987;238:1539-1545.

40. Knudson AG Jr. Mutation and cancer: statistical study of retinoblastoma. *Proc Natl Acad Sci USA.* 1971;68:820-823.

41. Cavenee WK, Hansen MF, Nordenskjold M, et al. Genetic origin of mutations predisposing to retinoblastoma. *Science.* 1985;228:501-503.

42. Sporn MB, Todaro GJ. Autocrine secretion and malignant transformation of cells. *N Engl J Med.* 1980;303:878-880.

43. Doolittle RF, Hunkapiller MW, Hood LE, et al. Simian sarcoma virus *onc* gene, v-*sis*, is derived from the gene (or genes) encoding a platelet-derived growth factor. *Science.* 1983;221:275-277.

44. Downward J, Yarden Y, Mayes E, et al. Close similarity of epidermal growth factor receptor and v-*erb-B* oncogene protein sequences. *Nature.* 1984;307:521-527.

45. Ullrich A, Coussens L, Hayflick JS, et al. Human epidermal growth factor receptor cDNA sequence and aberrant expression of the amplified gene in A431 epidermoid carcinoma cells. *Nature.* 1984;309:418-425.

46. Collett MS, Purchio AF, Erikson RL. Avian sarcoma virus-transforming protein, $pp60_{src}$, shows protein kinase activity specific for tyrosine. *Nature.* 1980;285:167-169.

47. Franza BR Jr, Rauscher FJ III, Josephs SF, Curran T. The Fos complex and Fos-related antigens recognize sequence elements that contain AP-1 binding sites. *Science.* 1988;239:1150-1153.

48. Vogt PK, Bos TJ, Doolittle RF. Homology between the DNA-binding domain of the GCN4 regulatory protein of yeast and the carboxyl-terminal region of a protein coded for the oncogene *jun*. *Proc Natl Acad Sci USA.* 1987;84:3316-3319.

49. Kaplan DR, Whitman M, Schaffhausen B, et al. Common elements in growth factor stimulation and oncogenic transformation: 85 kd phosphoprotein and phosphatidylinositol kinase activity. *Cell.* 1987;50:1021-1029.

10

CANCER DETECTION: THE CANCER-RELATED CHECKUP GUIDELINES

Diane J. Fink, MD, Curtis J. Mettlin, PhD

In 1980 the American Cancer Society (ACS) published its Guidelines for the Cancer-Related Checkup to assist physicians and their patients in making better decisions concerning examinations for the early detection of cancer.[1] When these guidelines first appeared, the specific recommendations, as well as the very concept of guidelines, provoked substantial comment and controversy. In the ensuing years, the ACS has monitored the impact of the guidelines and modified them as new data and new technologies have become available.[2] This chapter examines the criteria and methods used to evaluate early detection interventions and reviews the current Guidelines for the Cancer-Related Checkup. Particular emphasis is given to the recommended early detection protocols for breast, colorectal, prostate, lung, and uterine cancers.

Criteria for Evaluation of Early Detection Procedures

Screening is the search for disease in asymptomatic people. An asymptomatic person is someone who does not have symptoms or who does not recognize the symptoms as being related to disease. Once an individual has a positive screening test, or signs or symptoms have been identified, further tests are considered diagnostic, not screening. It is important to distinguish interventions for asymptomatic persons from those used for persons presenting with signs or symptoms of disease. The risks versus benefits of a medical intervention when used in persons not previously suspected of having cancer necessarily differ from the risk versus benefits when the intervention is used for a specific indication. Similarly, the costs of medical procedures directed to large numbers of well persons must be weighed differently from the costs of medical care to the smaller numbers of persons suffering the acute effects of known disease.

Because of the unique nature of early detection interventions, special criteria have been developed to evaluate them. When the ACS guidelines were first developed, four concerns were stressed: There had to be evidence that the test was effective in detecting cancer early enough to influence cancer morbidity or mortality, or both. Medical benefits had to outweigh the risks. The cost had to be reasonable relative to the expected result, and the recommendation had to be practical and feasible.

These four criteria may be most appropriate in advanced healthcare systems, but in some developing nations, resources for diagnosis, treatment, and follow-up may be limiting factors. The World Health Organization (WHO) has identified ten criteria by which the value of screening in all settings may be evaluated.[3] Those criteria are:

1. The disease under study should be an important health problem.

2. There must be an effective treatment for patients suffering from localized disease.

3. Facilities for further diagnosis and treatment must be available.

4. There must be an identifiable latent or early symptomatic stage of the disease.

5. The technique to be used for screening must be effective.

6. The test must be acceptable to the screened population.

7. The natural history of the disease, including the development of the latent phase to clinical disease, must be sufficiently known.

8. There must be a generally accepted strategy

Diane J. Fink, MD, Group Vice President for Cancer Control, American Cancer Society, California Division, Inc., Oakland, California

Curtis J. Mettlin, PhD, Chief of Epidemiologic Research, Roswell Park Cancer Institute, Buffalo, New York

enabling determination of patients who should be treated and those who should remain untreated.

9. The expenses of the screening must be acceptable.

10. Case-finding should be a continuous process and not a "once and for all" project.

Outcome Measures of Screening Effectiveness

Ideally, all early detection recommendations are supported by rigorous randomized controlled trials (RCTs) that show reduced mortality for persons who receive early detection interventions. Beyond that, there should be controlled comparisons of its costs, risks, and benefits when used in different combinations, in different age and risk groups, and at different frequencies. These ideal data are seldom available, however, when decisions about the use of a detection procedure must be made. RCTs are expensive to conduct and require many years to complete. RCT results are available now only for demonstrating the benefit of breast cancer screening and the absence of benefit of lung cancer screening. With only limited RCT data available, it often is necessary to make decisions on the basis of measures other than death rate reduction. The following sections describe several such measures of early detection effectiveness.

Sensitivity, Specificity, and Predictive Value

The most commonly used criteria to evaluate early detection methods are sensitivity, specificity and predictive value. The sensitivity of a test is its ability to detect cancer when it is present. Specificity is the accuracy of a test to demonstrate the absence of cancer when it is not present. Both are important. A test with low sensitivity will provide false reassurance and waste the resources expended to detect cancer. A test with low specificity has the opposite result of causing alarm when there is no threat, leading to potentially costly and unnecessary further diagnostic evaluation. Often it is not possible to directly measure sensitivity because persons who test negative in a screening do not receive further evaluation and there is no independent evidence to confirm the absence of disease. Data are more often available concerning the positive predictive value of a test. The positive predictive value is the likelihood that a result indicative of the presence of cancer will prove correct on further evaluation.

Yield

The yield of an early detection program is the proportion of persons discovered by the test to have the disease in question. It is a function of the prevalence of detectable disease in an asymptomatic population, which in turn is determined by the incidence rate of the disease and the duration of its preclinical stage. Although yield often is interpreted as a measure of cost-effectiveness, yield alone tells little about whether an early detection effort is effective. For example, a disease might be common and early detection might have a high yield, but if the disease is not detected at an earlier stage or if there is no effective treatment for the disease, no benefit will result. On the other hand, screening for low-yield, rare conditions may be justified when there is a large benefit to the fewer patients detected with early cancer.

Stage of Disease at Diagnosis

The benefit of early detection mainly derives from the opportunity to treat disease before it has spread, when cure or control is most achievable. Therefore, earlier stage of disease at diagnosis is an important measure of the usefulness of a screening test. If a test fails to detect cancer at any earlier stage than when patients present with symptoms, it is unlikely to have benefit. It does not follow, however, that earlier stage of disease at detection alone demonstrates the success of the intervention. If treatments applied at an earlier stage are no more effective than when used later in the natural history of the disease, the early stage at diagnosis may be clinically irrelevant.

Case-Survival Rates

One goal of early detection is to provide greater opportunity to survive cancer. This can be assessed by measuring cancer survival rates in screened and unscreened populations. If the screened group has no better survival following detection by screening than persons who present with symptomatic disease, it suggests an absence of benefit. On the other hand, better case-survival in the screened population is not proof of benefit because of some of the biases that can affect interpretation of survival rates. These include lead time and length bias, which will be discussed later.

Cost, Cost-Effectiveness, Cost-Benefit

Many screening procedures are inexpensive, but price alone is a poor indicator of cost. An inexpensive test that is not sensitive can prove much more costly than the more sensitive, albeit more expensive, method. An alternative measure that takes into account differences in test performance is cost per cancer detected. While this measure combines information about the yield with the program cost, it also can lead to some obviously incorrect recommendations. For example, the lowest cost per case detected is achieved by not screening at all. Any cancers not detected will eventually be found by the patients themselves at zero cost per cancer detected.

It also is possible to analyze early detection interventions relative to their effects or benefits. Cost benefit can be expressed in such terms as the dollar cost of achieving an additional interval of life expectancy in the screened population. While providing a common basis on which to compare alternative interventions, this measure alone will not necessarily determine the best strategy. For example, which is better: a $1,000 program that delivers 30 days of life expectancy or a $4,000 program that delivers 50 days of life expectancy? The answer will depend on the value a person assigns to an additional day of life expectancy. In addition, there is no good way to assign dollar value to other outcomes such as reduction of pain or alleviation of anxiety.

Experimental Biases in Early Detection Programs

That a test can detect a condition before it is detectable by other means, that it appears to detect cancers at earlier stages, and that it delivers higher case-survival rates do not necessarily mean that it will increase the chances for a cure or that it will prolong a patient's life. Lead-time bias, length bias, selection factors, and overdiagnosis all are factors that can result in misleading interpretations of screening effectiveness.

Lead-Time Bias

The interval between the moment a condition can be detected and the moment that condition would have been brought to attention by patient awareness of signs or symptoms is known as lead time. Unless lead time is accounted for, comparisons of survival rates in screened and unscreened populations will be misleading. There always is a bias toward better survival rates in the screened group because the point at which survival begins to be measured is moved forward by the length of the lead time. It is possible that earlier detection only moves forward the time of a patient's diagnosis, without moving back the time of death.

Length Bias

The period in the natural history of a cancer during which the tumor may be detected before symptoms appear is the detectable preclinical phase. The detectable preclinical phase is the practitioner's "window of opportunity" to advance the point of detection. Different types of cancer offer "windows" of different length because of variations in tumor growth rates and other biologic characteristics. It is also possible that the same disease in different persons will demonstrate different lengths of detectable preclinical phase. Because of the greater opportunity for detection, more of the cancers with a long preclinical phase will be detected when a population is screened. A tumor with a longer preclinical phase probably also has a longer clinical phase and will be a more indolent and less threatening lesion. This bias toward detection of less threatening cancers is length bias. This will complicate the interpretation of outcome differences between cancers detected by screening and those found outside the screening program because the cancers most likely to escape detection may be the very cancers that have the greatest likelihood of causing death.

Patient Self-Selection Bias

Persons who elect to receive early detection tests may be different from those who do not in ways that could affect their survival or recovery from disease. For example, users of early detection services may be more health conscious, more likely to control risk factors such as smoking or diet, more alert to the signs and symptoms of disease, more adherent to treatment, or generally healthier. Any of these factors could produce a longer survival from cancer that is independent of early detection, and the better survival observed in screened patients compared with the general population could be due more to the selection of patients than to the effect of early detection.

Overdiagnosis

The purpose of early detection examinations is to find cancers at an early stage. It is possible, however, to detect some tumors at so early a stage that their biological propensity to progress and cause death is uncertain. Because early detection intervention is more likely than symptom recognition to yield lesions that might never become clinically significant cancers, survival statistics for screening detected cancers may be inflated. Comparison of overall death rates in screened and unscreened populations is one means of controlling for this bias.

Summary of ACS Recommendations

The ACS Guidelines for the Cancer-Related Checkup are designed for application in asymptomatic persons on an individual basis. In addition to the guidance they offer to the patient and practitioner, the guidelines can provide information to public health policymakers. They are not intended for the evaluation of individuals with signs or symptoms of cancer. Such individuals require a careful diagnostic workup to determine the cause of their complaint.

For each cancer site, the Cancer-Related Checkup Guidelines list recommended tests and/or procedures, sometimes by age and sex. In general, the same guidelines apply to average-risk and high-risk persons, an exception being the protocol for colorectal cancer. Table 10-1 reviews the Cancer-Related Checkup. Tables 10-2 and 10-3 summarize the recommendations by sex.

The American Cancer Society recommends a cancer-related checkup every three years for asymptomatic men and women 20 to 39 years of age, and every year for asymptomatic men and women aged 40 and older. This checkup should include examination for cancers of the oral cavity, thyroid, skin, lymph nodes, testes, prostate, and ovaries. Specific protocols designed to detect asymptomatic cancers of the breast, colon and rectum, prostate, and uterus are also recommended.

In addition to these procedures, the healthcare provider is encouraged to offer counseling on personal risk factors, such as tobacco use, exposure to ultraviolet rays, sexual practices, and other environmental or occupational exposures; on the role of diet and nutrition in tumorigenesis; and on the advantages of

Table 10-1. ACS Recommendations for the Early Detection of Cancer in Asymptomatic People

Test or Procedure	Population: Sex	Population: Age	Frequency
Sigmoidoscopy, preferably flexible	Male & female	50 and over	Every 3-5 years, based on advice of physician
Fecal occult blood test	Male & female	50 and over	Every year
Digital rectal examination	Male & female	40 and over	Every year
Prostate examination*	Male	50 and over	Every year
Pap test	Female	All women who are, or have been, sexually active, or have reached age 18, should have an annual Pap test and pelvic examination. After a woman has had >3 consecutive satisfactory normal annual examinations, the Pap test may be performed less frequently at the discretion of her physician	
Pelvic examination	Female	18-40 Over 40	Every 1-3 years with Pap test Every year
Endometrial tissue sample	Female	At menopause, women at high risk+	At menopause and thereafter at the discretion of the physician
Breast self-examination	Female	20 and over	Every month
Breast clinical examination	Female	20-40 Over 40	Every 3 years Every year
Mammography++	Female	40-49 50 and over	Every 1-2 years Every year
Health counseling and cancer checkup§	Male & female	Over 20	Every 3 years
	Male & female	Over 40	Every year

* Annual digital rectal examination and prostate-specific antigen should be performed in men 50 years and older. If either is abnormal, further evaluation should be considered.

+ History of infertility, obesity, failure to ovulate, abnormal uterine bleeding, or unopposed estrogen therapy or tamoxifen therapy.

++Screening mammography should begin by age 40

§ To include examination for cancers of the thyroid, testicles, ovaries, lymph nodes, oral region, and skin self-examination of the breasts, testes, and skin.

Self-examination should be encouraged in asymptomatic, healthy adults, but it is not a substitute for the recommended early detection procedures. Benefit has not been confirmed by research, but self-examination may be helpful for individuals who cannot obtain medical care easily, such as the elderly, economically disadvantaged, and those residing in remote locations.

Breast Cancer

Breast cancer is the most common cancer in American women and the second most common cause of cancer-related deaths, after lung cancer. In 1994, an estimated 183,000 new breast cancer cases were diagnosed and 46,300 deaths occurred.[4] Based on data from the Surveillance, Epidemiology, and End Results Program (SEER), the incidence rates for in situ and localized invasive tumors increased sharply between 1982 and 1986, while the rates for regional and distant tumors remained stable.[5] In women aged 50 and older, the incidence rates of small, localized tumors (diameters of <1.0, 1.0 to 1.9, and 2.0 to 2.9 cm) rose more rapidly than those of tumors ≥3.0 cm. Although other factors cannot be ruled out, these data suggest a role for early detection with mammography in the increase in breast cancer incidence.

Table 10-2. Recommended Guidelines for Early Detection of Cancer in Asymptomatic Women at Average Risk

Age	Recommendation
20-39	Cancer-related checkup every 3 years, to include counseling and examination of the oral cavity, thyroid, skin, lymph nodes, and ovaries, plus: • breast self-examination monthly, • clinical breast examination every 3 years, • Pap test and pelvic examination every year (after 3 or more consecutive satisfactory normal annual examinations, the Pap test may be performed less frequently at the discretion of the physician); for women who are or have been sexually active or are 18 years of age or older
40-49	Cancer-related checkup yearly, to include all the above plus: • digital rectal examination yearly, • breast self-examination monthly, • clinical breast examination yearly, • mammography every 1 to 2 years, • at menopause, endometrial tissue sample in high-risk women, • pelvic examination yearly
50 and older	Cancer-related checkup yearly, to include all the above, plus: • stool blood test yearly, • sigmoidoscopy every 3 to 5 years, • mammography yearly

Table 10-3. Recommended Guidelines for Early Detection of Cancer in Asymptomatic Men at Average Risk

Age	Recommendation
20-39	Cancer-related checkup every 3 years, to include health counseling and examination of the oral cavity, thyroid, skin, lymph nodes, testes, and prostate
40-49	Cancer-related checkup yearly, to include all the above, plus: • digital rectal examination with palpation of the prostate, yearly
50 and older	Cancer-related checkup yearly, to include all the above, plus: • digital rectal exam with palpation of the prostate yearly, • fecal occult blood test yearly, • sigmoidoscopy every 3 to 5 years, • prostate-specific antigen yearly

In patients with localized breast cancer, the 5-year survival rate has increased from 78% in the 1940s to 93% today. If breast cancer is not invasive or is in situ, the survival rate reaches 100%. In the presence of regional spread, however, survival falls to 72%, and distant metastasis is associated with an 18% survival. At the time of diagnosis of breast cancer, the proportion of patients without lymph node involvement is usually 53%. When breast cancer detection includes mammography, nodal involvement is absent in >75% of cases, suggesting again the value of the screening test in detecting early disease.[5]

Screening Recommendations

The American Cancer Society recommends three interventions for early detection of breast cancer: breast self-examination (BSE), clinical breast examination (CBE), and screening mammography (Table 10-4). These recommendations are for asymptomatic women of appropriate age regardless of the presence or absence of risk factors. Women with symptoms of breast cancer (a persistent lump or thickening, dimpling, skin irritation, nipple retraction, nipple scaling, discharge, bleeding,

Table 10-4. Breast Cancer Detection Protocol in Asymptomatic Women at Average Risk

Age	Recommendation
20-39	Breast self-examination monthly Clinical breast examination every 3 years
40-49	Breast self-examination monthly Clinical breast examination yearly Mammography every 1 to 2 years
50 and older	Breast self-examination monthly Clinical breast examination yearly Mammography yearly

or breast pain) should undergo complete diagnostic evaluation. In symptomatic women, mammography may be indicated as a diagnostic tool before biopsy, but not as a screening technique. Even if the mammogram is normal, a biopsy is indicated in persons with positive findings on physical examination, such as a localized mass.

The Cancer-Related Checkup Guidelines recommend screening mammography for women aged 40 to 49. Unlike in women age ≥50, screening mammography in this younger age group has not been convincingly demonstrated by an RCT to reduce mortality. On the basis of the totality of evidence, however, the American Cancer Society has concluded that mammography can save lives in this age group.

Evidence of Effectiveness

A number of studies have evaluated the effectiveness of mammography and CBE as screening procedures. The most widely cited is the RCT initiated in 1964 in New York City by the Health Insurance Plan (HIP), which assessed screening by annual CBE and mammography in 62,000 women aged 40 to 65.[6] Participants in the study group were offered an annual detection examination, including an initial exam. About 67% accepted the invitation for an initial screening, and a large proportion returned for reexaminations. During the first 10 years of follow-up, mortality from breast cancer for women aged ≥50 in the study group was reduced about 30%. At 18 years' follow-up, the reduction was 25%. In women aged 40 to 49, a favorable effect appeared later, at 10 years' follow-up. By 18 years' follow-up, similar effects were seen in the two age groups.

A Swedish RCT evaluated 160,000 women assigned either to a study group, in which a single-view mammogram was offered approximately every other year, or to a control group.[7] Over a 7-year follow-up, breast cancer mortality was one third lower in the study group, primarily among women 50 years of age and older.

A large cancer screening program, conducted by the ACS and the National Cancer Institute (NCI) and called the Breast Cancer Detection Demonstration Project (BCDDP), was initiated in 1973 to promote the results of the HIP study to physicians and women.[8] By 1975, twenty nine community projects were organized across the country, with an enrollment of 280,000. Each woman was screened by history, physical examination, and mammography annually for 5 years. Breast self-examination was taught and encouraged throughout the project.

One third of the 3,500 cancers diagnosed in the BCDDP were minimal, ie, noninfiltrating and <1 cm in diameter. More than 75% of detected cancers showed no lymph node involvement. CBE and mammography detected neoplasms not found on BSE, but the role of mammography in detection was greater. Mammography alone detected 40% of all cases, compared with 10% for CBE. Higher survival rates were found in cases detected by mammography alone in the BCCDP, compared with rates in women registered in the SEER system. This benefit was seen in women aged 40 to 49 as well as in older women.

Shapiro has summarized the experience with breast cancer screening programs in the US (the HIP and BCDDP trials), Canada, Netherlands (case-control studies in Nijmegen and Utrecht), Sweden (the two-county and Malmo trials), and the United Kingdom (the eight-district and Edinburgh trials).[9] He concluded that these studies showed a consistent pattern of benefit from screening at age ≥50, but less conclusive evidence for benefit in women aged 40 to 49.

A Canadian RCT completed in 1992 evaluated more than 50,000 women aged 40 to 49 who received either annual screening mammography plus CBE or a simple CBE plus an annual self-administered questionnaire.[10,11] In addition, more than 39,000 women aged 50 to 59 were randomly assigned to receive an annual screening mammography plus CBE or an annual CBE. All participants were taught BSE. At 7 years' follow-up, screening with annual mammography and CBE had no effect on the rate of breast cancer in either age group. The publication of these results attracted considerable public and scientific interest, and the adequacy of randomization, as well as the quality of the mammography, follow-up, and management of breast cancer in the study, has been debated.

International conferences have been conducted to review all available data on the efficacy of screening mammography. A meeting convened by the American Cancer Society and the International Union Against Cancer (UICC) concluded that the existing data clearly demonstrate the benefits of mammography and CBE in women aged 50 and older and were supportive of their use in individuals aged 40 to 49.[12] Based on this review of the evidence, the ACS elected not to modify its guideline recommendations. After similar review, the NCI changed its guidelines for average-risk asymptomatic women aged 40 to 49 and no longer recommends mammography on a regular basis to detect early breast cancer.

The interval for optimal screening in women aged 40 to 49 remains an unresolved issue. It may be that the lower incidence of breast cancer in women younger than 50 makes annual screening too costly for its yield. On the other hand, it is possible that breast cancer in younger women progresses more rapidly and more frequent screening in younger compared with older women is necessary. No trial has yet examined the influence of different screening frequencies, and the ACS recommendations provide latitude for patient and physician discretion in choosing a frequency of breast cancer screening in the fifth decade.

Early Detection in Women Aged 65 and Older

Women aged 65 and older are particularly vulnerable to the development of breast cancer, the risk for which increases with age. On average, these women have an appreciable number of years of remaining life, ie, close to 20 years for women aged 65 and 13 years for those aged 75.

In the Swedish two-county study, which is the sole source of data on screening in older women, the relative risks for breast cancer mortality (study versus control) were 0.60 among women aged 60 to 69, and 0.84 among 70- to 74-year-olds.[7] Although the latter figure was not statistically significant because of the small number of women in the older age groups, it does suggest a reduced risk of death associated with mammographic screening. A physician must evaluate each woman to determine whether screening would be beneficial, taking into account comorbid conditions and the woman's health status. The ACS guidelines should be heeded in this age group, unless comorbidity mitigates against screening. Some investigators recommend a 2-year mammography screening interval for women aged ≥65. As with screening in younger women, there are insufficient data to determine an exact early detection interval.

Risk of Mammography and Quality Assurance

The radiation exposure from modern mammographic technology is extremely low, making the risk of radiation-induced cancer extremely low.[13] Although studies have linked radiation exposure to breast cancer in atomic bomb survivors, in women irradiated for acute mastitis, and in tuberculosis patients who were repeatedly given chest fluoroscopies, the doses involved were significantly higher than those used in screening mammography. Modern technology provides a favorable benefit-risk ratio in women aged 40 and older when image quality is maintained using a two-view examination of each breast with a dose of ≤0.08 cGy.

A high-quality, low-dose mammogram is critical for breast cancer detection. Quality assurance involves improving the ability of radiologists and technologists to provide mammography, as well as enhancing the quality of the mammographic image. In the past, mammography was not part of the board examinations in diagnostic radiology. The American College of Radiology (ACR) now provides a large number of educational courses. An accreditation program for facilities offering mammography reviews radiation levels and image quality, and provides advice for modifications when needed. With the support of an ACS grant, the ACR has developed a home study course. Practicing radiologists can request these programs from the ACR.

New federal laws mandate that facilities offering mammography meet requirements similar to ACR or state standards for mammography quality assurance. It will take some time for these standards to be met. In the interim, a woman can locate an ACR-accredited facility by calling her local American Cancer Society office.

Other Imaging Techniques

The role of other breast cancer imaging techniques, including thermography, diaphanography, and ultrasound, has been reviewed by the ACS, which concluded that there was insufficient proven value to justify their routine use in screening in asymptomatic women. None should be considered a substitute for physical examination or mammography, or a preliminary screen to identify asymptomatic women suitable for mammography. Their use does not eliminate the need for biopsy or breast aspiration when indicated by physical examination; thus, the cost of breast cancer detection may rise without an increase in benefit. Magnetic resonance imaging (MRI), computed tomography (CT), and other newer imaging techniques have not been evaluated adequately to determine their role in breast cancer detection.

Breast Self-Examination

Women are encouraged to do breast self-examinations, to be aware of their breasts so they can recognize changes as early as possible. Historically, most women detect their own breast cancers. For persons unable to receive medical examinations (CBE and mammography) due to lack of access or economic factors, BSE is an available and inexpensive option. The American Cancer Society recommends that BSE be done monthly, but surveys show that a minority of women perform BSE that frequently.

Retrospective studies of BSE have reported a variable effectiveness in detecting early breast cancer. One study showed fewer deaths among breast cancer patients who practiced BSE. According to one review, there is accumulating evidence that BSE can be helpful despite the lack of prospective RCT data.[14] Even though many issues are unresolved, it appears prudent to continue to recommend BSE as a cancer detection technique, while not detracting from the importance of screening mammography and CBE.

A woman must know how to perform BSE properly. The optimal content and extent of instruction are not known. Approaches have ranged from handing a woman a pamphlet and offering verbal encouragement, to one-on-one training using films and models, to demonstrations before large groups. Pamphlets containing simple instructions on how to perform BSE are available at all local ACS offices.

Barriers to Breast Cancer Screening

Two important factors have been identified in women who have not had mammography: they were not aware they needed a mammogram, and they were not informed by their physician that they should have one. Reminder systems to the individual and the physician may help to increase utilization. The challenge is to foster heightened media awareness and develop special educational programs for women who are not participating in screening, especially older women and women of low income. In addition, physicians should be encouraged to follow guidelines and recommend mammograms to their patients.

A 1990 survey of breast cancer practices showed about two thirds of women aged ≥40 have ever had mammography, but only about 50% have had more than one mammogram.[15] Women who have had mammograms tend to be white and have higher educational status. African-Americans, Hispanics, and women older than 75 tend to have lower rates of mammography screening. Women are more likely to have screening with Papanicolaou (Pap) smears and mammograms if they see a female physician, particularly if the physician is an internist or family practitioner.[16] In an ACS survey of physician attitudes, obstetricians and gynecologists tended to follow ACS guidelines more often than do other primary care providers. Thus, women in child-rearing years may have a greater chance of access to breast cancer early detection. However, as women pass menopause and age, their healthcare providers must be diligent in recommending breast cancer early detection, especially mammography. It is in this age group that the data are the most conclusive.

Use of Resources

The introduction of breast cancer early detection into a physician's practice or into a community screening program is likely to require the use of significant resources. An important determinant of workload is the ratio of the number of biopsies taken to the number of cancers found. The peak in workload occurs with the first screening and then levels off. Surgical workload may increase, with very small lesions requiring special techniques for localization.

Compared with other screening programs, the costs associated with breast cancer early detection are relatively high. While the direct cost of a mammogram can be as low as $27, this is achieved only in well-organized screening programs. Mammograms performed by private physicians and radiologists can cost the individual $50 to $100, or more. If 25% of women aged 40 to 70 were screened annually with mammography and physical examination, the cost would total approximately $1.3 billion.[17] At present, there are insufficient facilities and personnel to accomplish this task. Methods to lower the costs of screening mammography have been described in an ACS workshop report.[18]

The cost of a CBE also varies tremendously, depending on whether the individual is in a well-organized program with cost-containment incentives. The charge to the individual for an office visit to do a CBE could be $10 to $25, or more.

Swedish investigators sought to determine the cost of screening and follow-up examinations, including diagnostic mammography, clinical examinations, aspiration cytology, and screening.[19] Their estimate was $49 for current (prevalence) cases and $37 for future (incidence) cases. In terms of prevalence, the cost per cancer detected was $7,040; in terms of incidence, $12,000. The authors pointed out that costs will change based on the screening intervals selected and the populations targeted for screening. In Sweden, there are 1,594,000 women aged 40 to 74 and 1,132,000 women aged 50 to 74. If all women from 40 to 74 years of age were screened annually with a two-view mammography, the total cost would be $71 million for a screening program, including follow-up investigation. If screening were limited to women aged 50 to 74, with 90% receiving annual single-view mammography, the cost would decline to $30.5 million.

A modeling study by Eddy and associates analyzed the economic consequences of adding annual mammography to annual CBE in asymptomatic women aged 40 to 49. In this analysis, if 25% of women in this age group were screened annually, the breast cancer mortality would decrease by about 373 deaths.[20] In 1984 dollars, the cost of screening, workups, continuing care, and treatment was calculated at $402 million. The authors did not suggest a blanket recommendation for all asymptomatic women aged 40 to 49, but indicated that a flexible policy of "see your physician" might be advisable.

Summary

Despite controversies, the ACS guidelines for breast cancer early detection appear to be sound advice for women and healthcare providers. Based on the results of clinical trials in women aged 50 to 74, regular breast cancer detection examinations can be life saving. Less conclusive evidence of benefit in women aged 40 to 49 should not preclude a recommendation for early detection examination, including screening mammography, in these women. Our goal must be to ensure access to information and advice about the ACS guidelines. Healthcare providers must recommend screening to women in a proactive manner.

Cancer of the Colon and Rectum

Colorectal cancer is a major public health problem for American men and women. In 1994, a total of 149,000 new cases are expected, as well as 56,000 deaths from this cancer.[4] Colorectal cancer is highly curable if found at its earliest stage. Five-year survival rates for early, localized cancers are 91% in the colon and 85% in the rectum. Once the cancer is no longer localized, survival declines to 60% and 51%, respectively.

Persons with possible cancer of the colon and rectum are good candidates for early detection. It appears that most colorectal cancers arise from adenomatous polyps and slowly progress, after 10 years, to an invasive, more lethal malignant stage. Thus, the detection and removal of colorectal polyps can reduce the risk for subsequent development of colorectal cancer. Furthermore, 94% of colorectal cancers occur in persons older than 50, so targeting early detection by age is important.

Screening Recommendations

A triad of early detection tests is recommended by the American Cancer Society for persons at average risk: digital rectal examination (DRE), fecal occult blood test, and sigmoidoscopy (Table 10-5). The NCI has adopted identical guidelines for early detection of colorectal cancer in persons at average risk. Studies indicate that early detection tests in asymptomatic individuals can reduce mortality.

Persons at high risk for colorectal cancer may require additional testing beginning at an earlier age. Risk factors and recommended cancer detection protocols for these high-risk individuals are discussed in a subsequent section.

Table 10-5. Colorectal Cancer Detection Protocol for Asymptomatic Men and Women at Average Risk

Age	Recommendation
40-49	Digital rectal examination yearly
50 and older	Digital rectal examination yearly Stool blood test yearly Sigmoidoscopy every 3 to 5 years

Digital Rectal Examination

Inspection of the anal region and palpation of the perineal and sacrococcygeal areas are integral to the detection of colorectal cancer. In men, it is also important to palpate the prostate.

DRE has been in clinical use for so long that formal studies of efficacy have been considered unnecessary. Its usefulness is supported by results of a multiphasic health examination study conducted by the Kaiser Health Foundation.[21] Study participants were randomly assigned to a screened or control group. Those in the screened group were urged to have an annual health checkup, which included DRE and sigmoidoscopy; controls were not given such encouragement, but could arrange for a health examination on their own. After 16 years of follow-up, subjects in the screened group had a lower cumulative mortality from colorectal cancer (2.3 deaths per 1,000 versus 5.2 in controls).[22] Although this study was not designed to assess the specific effects of various detection techniques, digital rectal examination may have contributed to the decline in mortality.

DRE is safe, and its cost, as part of a general examination, is relatively low. Therefore, it is recommended annually in patients older than 40. The use of DRE may be limited by an individual's emotional reaction, by the cost of follow-up tests after a false-positive result, and by the potential for a false sense of security with a false-negative result.

Fecal Occult Blood Test

The testing of stool for occult blood was popularized by Greegor, who used a guaiac-impregnated slide in asymptomatic individuals.[23] The methodology for occult blood testing has been refined, and controversies surrounding its use have been reviewed.[26]

The presence of fecal occult blood is not specific for colorectal cancer. Any condition, benign or malignant, that leads to gastrointestinal bleeding can result in a positive test. Evidence suggests that stool blood testing in asymptomatic individuals can detect cancer polyps. There has been a shift in incidence of colon cancer favoring the right colon; such cancers, which may constitute about 50% of colon cases, lie beyond the reach of standard sigmoidoscopes. Thus, there is great interest in using the fecal occult blood test to detect cancer throughout the colon.

Studies of fecal occult blood testing have tended to show an earlier stage at diagnosis for persons receiving early detection.[25-27] The results of the Minnesota study, a prospective RCT, are reviewed. This study randomized more than 46,000 individuals aged 50 to 80 to annual screening for colorectal cancer, to screening every two years, or to no screening (the control group).[28] Participants in either screening group submitted six guaiac-impregnated paper slides, with two smears from each of three consecutive stools. Those who tested positive received a diagnostic evaluation that included colonoscopy. The 13-year cumulative mortality rates from colorectal cancer were 5.88 per 1,000 in those screened annually, 8.33 in those screened biennially, and 8.83 in controls. Thus, annual screening reduced the 13-year cumulative mortality by 33%. There was a significantly higher incidence of Dukes stage D cancers in the control group. Only 2.4% of patients with Dukes stage D cancer survived 5 years, while 5-year survival ranged from 94% for stage A to 57% for Stage C.

The limitations of fecal occult blood testing include high false-negative and high false-positive rates.[24,29,30] In one study, the test missed 70% of cancers and 90% of precancerous conditions. About 92% of people testing positive did not have cancer. In addition, colorectal cancers and polyps may bleed intermittently, and a negative stool blood test does not rule out colorectal cancer. The procedure should not be used as a prescreening test for DRE or sigmoidoscopy.

Patient Preparation

Preparation for the stool blood test must include guidance concerning pretest dietary intake. A positive test depends on the phenolic oxidation of guaiac in the presence of hemoglobin. Compounds with peroxidase-like activity that are found in vegetables such as broccoli, turnip, cauliflower, radish, horseradish, and parsnip, and in meat can cause false-positive results. The test reaction also may be inhibited by foods or supplements containing iron or vitamin. Aspirin or nonsteroidal anti-inflammatory drugs should be avoided, but aspirin substitutes such as acetaminophen may be used.

Follow-Up

For the fecal occult blood test to be an effective screening procedure, persons with a positive result must be followed up appropriately. Cancers may bleed intermittently; therefore, a positive test result should lead to examination of the entire large bowel, either by barium enema with sigmoidoscopy or by total colonoscopy.

A high-quality barium enema, which is an x-ray examination of the entire colon, is effective in identifying polyps and cancer. Contrast material can be used in one of two ways: by filling the entire colon (single-contrast barium enema) or by using the contrast material to form a thin coating over the inner bowel surface and then filling the entire colon with air (double-contrast barium enema). Most investigators prefer a double-contrast to a single-contrast barium enema.

Double-contrast barium enema plus sigmoidoscopy is about as accurate as, but may be less expensive than, colonoscopy. The value of colonoscopy depends on the extent to which the entire colon can be examined. With colonoscopy, suspicious lesions can be biopsied and polyps removed. Preparation of the subject, consisting of adequate cleaning of the colon, is similar for both approaches.

If the barium enema or colonoscopy is negative in an asymptomatic person with positive fecal occult blood test, evaluation for upper gastrointestinal tract disease may be considered, depending on other clinical findings and the clinical judgment of the physician. Neither barium enema nor colonoscopy is cost-effective for screening asymptomatic persons at average risk for colorectal cancer.

Sigmoidoscopy

Rigid sigmoidoscopy has been in use since the 1920s. Because about 50% of colorectal polyps and cancers are within the range of the sigmoidoscope, this procedure is a major diagnostic test for colorectal disease. However, there has been controversy about its value as a screening procedure.

A number of studies have suggested benefits from screening sigmoidoscopy. In 1960, the Strang Clinic in New York City evaluated more than 26,000 people older than 45, about 10% of whom had minimal symptoms.[31] Sixty percent (n=58) of cancers were found by periodic rigid sigmoidoscopy, and another 17% by barium enema after a sigmoidoscopic finding of polyp or blood in the bowel lumen. Eighty-one percent of detected cancers were localized (Dukes stage A or B). In 50 patients followed for ≥15 years, survival was almost 90%, or double the expected 10-year rate. This study was uncontrolled and subject to several biases.

In the Kaiser Health Foundation multiphasic health examination study, participants who were urged to undertake a battery of tests, including sigmoidoscopy, had a lower cumulative mortality rate from colorectal cancer (2.3 versus 5.2 deaths per 1,000) over a 16-year period.[22] An 18-year follow-up study examined cancers arising in the distal 20 cm of the large bowel wall, which was within reach of the rigid sigmoidoscope.[32] The screened group had a 50% lower cumulative incidence of colorectal cancer and a higher proportion of localized tumors.

In a case-control study, data from 261 members of the Kaiser Permanente Medical Care Program who died of colorectal cancer were examined to determine the use of rigid sigmoidoscopy screening in the 10 years before diagnosis.[33] The use of screening was compared in 868 control subjects matched for age and sex. Patients with one or more screening sigmoidoscopic examinations in the preceding 10 years had a 60% to 70% decrease in the risk of death from colon or rectal cancer within reach of the sigmoidoscope. The risk of death was markedly reduced for 10 years after a single examination.

At the University of Minnesota, more than 18,000 patients older than 45 were followed for up to 25 years using rigid sigmoidoscopy.[34] All adenomatous polyps were removed. At the end of the surveillance period, only 15% of the anticipated number of cancers occurred, suggesting benefit by discovery and removal of polyps. In addition, all cancers detected were localized, and after 21 years of follow-up, no patient had died of colorectal cancer.

The long-term risk of colorectal cancer after rigid sigmoidoscopy and polypectomy has been assessed in 1,618 persons with colorectal symptoms.[35] The risk of cancer in the proximal colon was related to the size and extent of villous change in the adenomas found in the rectosigmoid area. Low-risk patients had small (<1 cm in diameter) tubular adenomas. High-risk patients had relatively large adenomas or adenomas with tubulovillous or villous features. The number of polyps found in the rectosigmoid colon did not influence risk group status.

Compliance

The value of rigid sigmoidoscopy has been diminished by poor patient acceptance combined with a relatively low rate of physician use. According to ACS surveys, most people are unwilling to undergo the discomfort of the procedure and few return for follow-up. The more comfortable flexible scopes, available in 60- and 35-cm lengths, may increase patient and physician acceptance. The 60-cm flexible scope requires more training and examination time. Proficiency with the 35-cm scope is easier to achieve, and there is less patient discomfort than with the longer flexible scope. Perforation rates have been estimated by Eddy to be 0.0125% for the rigid scope, 0.02% for the 35-cm flexible scope, and 0.045% for the 60-cm flexible scope.[36] The training of physicians in flexible sigmoidoscopy is critical so that it can replace the rigid sigmoidoscopic examination.

Screening sigmoidoscopy is controversial. Its use has been advocated by the American Cancer Society, the National Cancer Institute, the American Gastroenterological Association, and the World Health Organization. In contrast, the United States Preventive Services Task Force has concluded that there was insufficient evidence to recommend sigmoidoscopy for asymptomatic persons.[32]

Evaluation and Follow-Up of High-Risk Persons

Certain conditions place individuals at high risk for colorectal cancer: a family history of polyps or colorectal cancer; inflammatory bowel (ulcerative colitis or Crohn's disease) lesions; familial polyposis syndromes; a history of adenomas; and a history of breast, ovarian, or endometrial cancer. The American Cancer Society considers surveillance necessary for most of these high-risk groups.

A family history of colorectal cancer is often overlooked in the evaluation of an asymptomatic person. If the family member is a first-degree relative (parent, sibling, or blood relative) and if the cancer occurred at age ≤55, examination of the entire colon and rectum by barium enema or colonoscopy is advised beginning at age 35 to 40 and repeated every 5 years.

Members of families with familial polyposis syndromes require earlier and more intensive surveillance with colonoscopy. Persons with inflammatory bowel lesions are at exceptionally high risk for colorectal cancer and require individual management. Persons with a history of breast, ovarian, or endometrial cancer are at some increased risk, but the risk is lower than those of the groups just mentioned. These individuals should follow guidelines for average-risk asymptomatic persons.

A history of colorectal adenoma places individuals at higher risk for colorectal cancer. All polyps should be removed for histologic evaluation. Individuals with adenomatous polyps detected by flexible sigmoidoscopy or barium enema need to have the entire large bowel cleared of all polyps. Individuals with one or more adenomas should have a follow-up program to identify subsequent (metachronous) adenomatous polyps. Most individuals can be followed every 3 to 5 years after polypectomy, provided the entire large bowel has been cleared. It may be possible to increase the interval between follow-ups to 5 years for individuals with very small tubular adenomas. Surveillance should be individualized in persons with numerous adenomas or a malignant or large sessile adenoma. In the elderly, individual considerations such as general health and comorbid conditions determine when follow-up can be discontinued.

Cost of Colorectal Cancer Detection

The cost of colorectal cancer detection is becoming increasingly important, as healthcare financing becomes a national agenda. Several investigators have provided cost estimates of early detection.[37-42] The workup of a patient with a positive fecal occult blood test can take several days and cost more than $1,000, depending on the protocol followed. Even if the bleeding is not caused by cancer, the workup can have significant benefit. For example, a study of 81 patients with a positive test revealed cancer in 12%, polyps in 55%, and diverticulosis in 19%.[43]

Direct and indirect costs need to be considered. The former includes the cost of the screening tests as well as follow-up examinations. Indirect costs can be incurred, especially when the detection examination is part of a community-based program: rental of facilities, personnel, materials, and public education activities are contributing expenditures.

Investigators from the Congressional Office of Technology Assessment in Washington, DC, developed a model to evaluate four colorectal screening strategies in the elderly.[42] They determined that annual fecal occult blood testing cost $35,000 per year of life saved, while screening schedules with periodic sigmoidoscopy could cost $43,000 to $47,000 per year of life gained. The cost per year of life gained from use of both tests did not exceed $61,000. It was concluded that although colorectal cancer screening is costly in the aggregate, the potential medical benefits make it a reasonably cost-effective preventive intervention in the elderly.

Prostate Cancer

Prostate cancer is the most common neoplasm and the second leading cause of death in men in the US. In 1994 about 200,000 new cases and 38,000 deaths from prostate cancer were projected.[4] The incidence of prostate cancer is increasing at an unprecedented rate. Among African-American males, the incidence is one-and-a-half times the rate in the general population.

The early detection of prostate cancer is an important public health issue facing medicine during the 1900s and beyond. The survival rate of patients with prostate cancer has improved steadily over the past 30 years, from 50% to 77%. When prostate cancer is detected at its earliest stages, the 5-year survival rate is 92%.

Screening Recommendations

For many years, DRE alone was recommended for the detection of colorectal and prostate cancer as part of the Cancer-Related Checkup Guidelines. In 1992, the American Cancer Society added a second annual screening procedure for prostate cancer in asymptomatic men aged >50: serum prostate-specific antigen (Table 10-6).

DRE and PSA

When DRE alone is used to evaluate men with signs and symptoms of prostate disease, approximately 65% of cancers detected are thought to be clinically localized, but only half of these are confirmed on surgical staging to be confined to the prostate.[44] Screening with DRE alone fails to increase the proportion of pathologically organ-confined cancers detected.[45,46]

Table 10-6. Prostate Cancer Detection Protocol for Asymptomatic Men

Age	Recommendation
40-49	Digital rectal examination yearly
50 and older	Digital rectal examination yearly Prostate-specific antigen yearly

Prostate-specific antigen (PSA) is a glycoprotein that lyses the seminal-vesicle coagulum and is essential for normal male fertility. While PSA is organ specific, it is not cancer specific. Normal as well as hyperplastic prostate cells manufacture and release PSA.[47,48] Elevated PSA levels are associated with acute prostatitis, prostatic infarction, benign prostatic hypertrophy, prostate cancer, and prostate needle biopsy.[49] Up to one quarter of patients with prostate cancer may have normal PSA levels. DRE does not appear to raise serum levels above normal.

While PSA has proved useful in the evaluation and management of prostate cancer, it is still being evaluated as an examination for early detection. In a 1991 study of 1,653 men aged 50 and older, 137 individuals with elevated PSA levels (>4 ng/mL) were evaluated by DRE and transrectal ultrasound (TRUS).[50] A total of 37 cancers were detected; DRE and TRUS would have missed 12 and 16, respectively, if used alone. In a comparison group of 300 consecutive men who were evaluated by biopsy because of symptoms or an abnormal DRE, normal PSA levels were detected in 13 men with a diagnosis of prostate cancer. The authors concluded that the combination of DRE and PSA was the best means of detecting early prostate cancer.

In another study, 263 cancers were detected in 1,807 men between 50 and 89 years of age.[51] Abnormal findings on DRE were reported in 203 patients with a positive biopsy and elevated PSA levels in 211. These tests appear to have the same predictive power, but may not detect the same tumors. Again, the combination of DRE and PSA seems reasonable. In a study of 10,251 men followed by PSA and a comparison group of 266 men referred because of an abnormality on DRE, twice the number of organ-confined prostate cancers were detected by serial PSA screening as compared to DRE.[52]

In the multicenter American Cancer Society National Prostate Cancer Detection Project, the coordinated use of DRE, TRUS, and PSA was shown to be effective in detecting early prostate cancer.[53] In a cost-benefit analysis of this study, DRE was the least costly approach when performed by highly skilled clinicians.[54] However, it became one of the most costly when a minor decrease in performance was assumed. The authors suggested that the pivotal factor in lowering cost would be pricing PSA below $30. It was concluded that the combination of PSA and DRE seemed to be an economical and ethical choice for individual patients in consultation with their physicians. TRUS is not recommended as a screening procedure for asymptomatic males, but should be used to evaluate persons with abnormal DRE or PSA findings.

While data are accumulating that PSA is useful in detecting early prostate cancer, there is no evidence that testing with PSA and DRE reduces the mortality from prostate cancer. Perhaps the NCI early detection trial, which includes prostate cancer screening, will provide an answer. The decision on whether to recommend screening is complicated by the low disease-specific mortality rate, especially in patients with highly and moderately well-differentiated tumors who do not receive early tumor-directed treatment.[55] In the interim, until the results of RTCs are in, the American Cancer Society has elected to recommend PSA testing as part of its checkup guidelines for prostate cancer.

Lung Cancer

Lung cancer screening with chest x-ray examination and sputum cytology has not been demonstrated by studies to be beneficial in reducing mortality.[56] Clearly, the risks, resources, and cost of chest x-rays and sputum cytology must be evaluated when considering screening in asymptomatic individuals. According to available data, lung cancer mortality is unaffected by these techniques when normal-risk persons are screened. The physician and the asymptomatic person must decide in each case whether screening is warranted based on the possible benefits and risks. In the individual at high risk for lung cancer, it may not be prudent to withhold these tests if the physician judges them to be useful.

At present, efforts aimed at primary prevention are the best hope for reducing the impact of lung cancer. The ACS thus urges physicians and all health professionals to advise their patients, especially those at high risk, not to smoke. Other national and international experts in disease control have reached similar conclusions. The Canadian Task Force on the Periodic Health Examination, the UICC, the NCI, and other organizations agree with the ACS lung cancer detection recommendations.

Uterine and Cervical Cancers

The Pap test is one of the most important examinations for asymptomatic women. The effectiveness of regularly scheduled Pap tests in detecting early cervical cancer has been documented by worldwide epidemiologic trials, which show dramatic reductions in the incidence and mortality of invasive cervical cancer in screened populations. Coupled with a pelvic examination, the Pap test is a life-saving procedure.

A review of existing data, including evidence of changing sexual patterns, suggests that all women who have had vaginal intercourse are at risk for cervical cancer. Vaginal intercourse started at an early age and intercourse with multiple partners are factors that place women at high risk for the disease. Human papillomavirus has been implicated as the venereal factor associated with the development of cervical cancer.

The exact interval between screenings remains under debate. The ACS does not advocate an upper age limit for termination of cervical cancer checkups (Table 10-7); such decisions must be made by each individual and her physician. Although data for the early detection of endometrial cancer are still evolving, it now appears prudent to provide endometrial tissue sampling for high-risk women beginning at menopause.

After deliberations with leading health professional groups, the ACS Board of Directors adopted the following recommendation for cervical cancer detection:

> That all women who are or have been sexually active, or have reached age 18 years, have an annual Pap test and pelvic examination. After a woman has had three or more satisfactory normal annual examinations, the Pap test may be performed less frequently at the discretion of her physician.

To provide the best national strategy for cervical

Table 10-7. Uterine Cancer Detection Protocols for Asymptomatic Women

Population	Recommendation
Cervical Cancer	
Women who are or have been sexually active or are age 18 or older	Annual Pap test and pelvic examination. After 3 or more consecutive satisfactory annual normal examinations, the Pap test may be performed less frequently at the discretion of the physician.
Endometrial Cancer	
High-risk women at menopause	Pelvic examination Endometrial tissue sample

cancer detection, every effort must be made to institute screening at a regular basis in unscreened women to decrease the remaining burden of this disease, especially in underserved women.

Endometrial Cancer

Cancer arising in the uterine endometrium is the most frequent malignancy in the female pelvis. Tissue sampling of the endometrium, an office procedure, should be considered in all women at increased risk. High-risk status is defined by infertility, obesity, failure to ovulate, abnormal uterine bleeding, estrogen therapy unopposed by progestin intake, and tamoxifen therapy (which acts as a weak estrogen). These risk factors indicate the importance of unopposed estrogenic stimulation of the endometrium in the development of endometrial cancer and its precursor, adenomatous hyperplasia.

Research has shown that so-called hormone-dependent tumors are generally low in virulence and mostly curable. The detection of all endometrial cancers in asymptomatic postmenopausal women, including the 30% at low risk who develop virulent tumors, would require universal screening, which is currently not feasible.

Sampling of asymptomatic women should begin at menopause and may be indicated depending on the degree of risk and other factors as determined by the physician. It should be emphasized that the Pap test alone is insufficient to exclude early endometrial cancer or its precursor.

Discussion

Major changes in health practice and public behavior have occurred since the ACS Cancer-Related Checkup Guidelines were first promulgated. In a 1989 survey, 80% of 1,029 primary care physicians reported giving greater attention to early cancer detection in asymptomatic patients than they did 5 years earlier.[57] In 1984, 11% of primary care physicians had reported following the ACS guidelines for screening mammography; by 1989, the number rose to 37%. There also has been greater public adherence to breast cancer early detection guidelines. Between 1983 and 1987, the proportion of women older than 40 who reported having had a mammogram increased from 41% to 64%.[2] In the same survey, the proportion of women who reported having had a mammogram every 1 to 3 years increased from 18% to 40%.

Progress in promoting early detection interventions has resulted partly from the consensus on early detection guidelines that has been achieved among several health-related organizations. The American Cancer Society has sponsored conferences on cancer detection that have been attended by experts in the field, representatives of major health organizations, legislators, and health insurance industry officials.[58] Following these meetings, many organizations, including the National Cancer Institute,[59] developed their own guidelines for early detection that were very similar to the ACS recommendations.

Complete agreement among different organizations is difficult to achieve, however, given the different professional perspectives that shape views of the topic. For example, the United States Preventive Services Task Force, the American College of Physicians, and the Canadian Task Force on the Periodic Health Examination have adopted different recommendations for some examinations.[60-62] An important challenge for the future is to continue the process of research and evaluation that leads to the greatest degree of cancer control achievable within the limits of available resources.

References

1. American Cancer Society Guidelines for the Cancer-Related Checkup: recommendations and rationale. *CA Cancer J Clin.* 1980;30:4-50.
2. Mettlin C, Dodd GD. The American Cancer Society Guidelines for the Cancer-Related Checkup: an update. *CA Cancer J Clin.* 1991;41:279-282.
3. Wilson JMG, Jungner G. *Principles and Practice of Screening for Disease.* Geneva: World Health Organization; 1968. Public health papers #34.
4. *Cancer Facts and Figures, 1994.* Atlanta, Ga: American Cancer Society; 1994.
5. Miller BA, Feuer EJ, Hankey BF. Recent incidence trends for breast cancer in women and the relevance of early detection: an update. *Cancer Causes Control.* 1991;2:67-74.
6. Shapiro S, Venet W, Strax P, Venet L. *Periodic Screening for Breast Cancer: The Health Insurance Plan Project and Its Sequelae, 1963-1986.* Baltimore, Md: John Hopkins University Press; 1988.
7. Tabar L, Fagerberg G, Duffy SW, Day NE, Gad A, Grontoft O. Update of the Swedish two-county program of mammographic screening for breast cancer. *Radiol Clin North Am.* 1992;30:187-210.
8. Baker L. Breast Cancer Detection Demonstration Project: 5-year summary report. *CA Cancer J Clin.* 1982;32:194-225.
9. Shapiro S. Periodic breast cancer screening in seven foreign countries. *Cancer.* 1992;69:1919-1924.
10. Miller AB, Baines CJ, To T, Wall C. Canadian National Breast Screening Study, I: breast cancer detection and death rates among women aged 40 to 49 years. *Can Med Assoc J.* 1992;147:1459-1476.
11. Miller AB, Baines CJ, To T, Wall C. Canadian National Breast Screening Study, II: breast cancer detection and death rates among women aged 50 to 59 years. *Can Med Assoc J.* 1992;147:1477-1488.
12. Murphy GP, Odartchenko N. Report on the UICC workshops on breast cancer screening in premenopausal women in developed countries. *CA Cancer J Clin.* 1993;43:372-373.
13. *Mammography: A User's Guide.* Bethesda, Md: National Council on Radiation Protection and Measurements; 1986.
14. Baines CJ. Breast self-examination. *Cancer.* 1992; 69:1942-1946.

15. Smith RA, Haynes S. Barriers to screening for breast cancer. *Cancer.* 1992;69:1968-1978.

16. Lurie N, Slater J, McGovern P, Ekstrum J, Quam L, Margolis K. Preventive care for women: does the sex of the physician matter? *N Engl J Med.* 1993;329:478-482.

17. Eddy DM. Screening for breast cancer. *Ann Intern Med.* 1989;111:389-399.

18. Dodd GD, Fink DJ, Bertram DA. Proceedings of an American Cancer Society workshop on strategies to lower the costs of screening mammography. *Cancer.* 1987;60(7, suppl):1669-1701.

19. Jonsson E, Hakansson S, Tabar L. Cost of mammography screening for breast cancer screening: experiences from Sweden. In: Day NE, Miller AB, eds. *Screening for Breast Cancer.* Toronto: Hans Huber Publisher; 1988: 113-115.

20. Eddy DM, Hasselblad V, McGivney W, Hendee W. The value of mammography screening in women under age 50 years. *JAMA.* 1988;259:1512-1519.

21. Dales LG, Friedman GD, Collen MF. Evaluating periodic multiphasic health checkups: a controlled trial. *J Chronic Dis.* 1979;32:385-404.

22. Friedman GD, Collen MF, Friedman BH. Multiphasic health checkup evaluation: a 16-year follow-up. *J Chronic Dis.* 1986;39:453-463.

23. Greegor DH. Diagnosis of large-bowel cancer in the asymptomatic patient. *JAMA.* 1967;201:943-945.

24. Simon JB. Occult blood screening for colorectal cancer: a critical view. *Gastroenterology.* 1985;88:820-837.

25. Winawer SJ, Andrews M, Flehinger B, Sherlock P, Schottenfeld D, Miller DG. Progress report on controlled trial of fecal occult blood testing for the detection of colorectal neoplasia. *Cancer.* 1980;45:2959-2964.

26. Hardcastle JD, Armitage NC, Chamberlain J, Amar SS, James PD, Balfour TW. Fecal occult blood screening for colorectal cancer in the general population. *Cancer.* 1986; 58:397-403.

27. Ekiland G, Carlson V, Jonzon L. The feasibility of large-scale population screening. *Br J Surg.* 1985;72:571-590.

28. Mandel JS, Bond JH, Church TR, et al. Reducing mortality from colorectal cancer by screening for fecal occult blood. *N Engl J Med.* 1993;328:1365-1371.

29. Gnauck R, Macrae FA, Fleisher M. How to perform the fecal occult blood test. *CA Cancer J Clin.* 1984;34:134-147.

30. Ahlquist DA, Wieand HS, Moertel G, et al. Accuracy of fecal occult blood screening for colorectal neoplasia: a prospective study using Hemoccult and Hemo-Quant tests. *JAMA.* 1993;269:1262-1267.

31. Hertz RL, Deddish MR, Day E. Value of periodic examinations in detecting cancer of the rectum and colon. *Postgrad Med.* 1960;27:290-294.

32. Selby JV, Friedman GD, US Preventive Services Task Force. Sigmoidoscopy in the periodic health examination of asymptomatic adults. *JAMA.* 1989;261:594-601.

33. Selby JV, Friedman GD, Quesenberry CP Jr, Weiss NS. A case-control study of screening sigmoidoscopy and mortality from colorectal cancer. *N Engl J Med.* 1992; 326:653-657.

34. Gilbertsen VA. Proctosigmoidoscopy and polypectomy in reducing the incidence of colorectal cancer. *Cancer.* 1974;34:936-939.

35. Atkin WS, Morson BC, Cuzick J. Long-term risk of colorectal cancer after excision of rectosigmoid adenomas. *N Engl J Med.* 1992;326:658-662.

36. Eddy DM. Screening for colorectal cancer. *Ann Intern Med.* 1990;113:373-384.

37. Levin B. Screening sigmoidoscopy for colorectal cancer. *N Engl J Med.* 1992;326:700-701.

38. Winawer SJ, O'Brien MJ, Waye JD, et al. Risk and surveillance of individuals with colorectal polyps. *Bull World Health Organ.* 1990;68:789-795.

39. Ransohoff DF, Lang CA, Kuo HS. Colonoscopic surveillance after polypectomy: consideration of cost effectiveness. *Ann Intern Med.* 1991;114:177-182.

40. Eddy DM, Nugent FW, Eddy JF, et al. Screening for colorectal cancer in a high risk population: results of a mathematical model. *Gastroenterology.* 1987;92:682-692.

41. Barry MJ, Mulley AG, Richter JM. Effect of working strategy on the cost-effectiveness of fecal occult blood screening for colorectal cancer. *Gastroenterology.* 1987; 93:301-310.

42. Wagner JL, Herdman RC, Wadhwa S. Cost effectiveness of colorectal cancer screening in the elderly. *Ann Intern Med.* 1991;115:807-817.

43. Winawer SJ, Leidner SD, Miller DG, et al. Results of a screening program for the detection of early colon cancer and polyps using fecal occult blood testing. *Gastroenterology.* 1977;72(5 pt 2):A-127/1150.

44. Catalona WJ, Bigg SW. Nerve-sparing radical prostatectomy: evaluation of results after 250 patients. *J Urol.* 1990;143:538-543.

45. Chodak GW, Keller P, Schoenberg HW. Assessment of screening for prostate cancer using the digital rectal examination. *J Urol.* 1989;141:1136-1138.

46. Gerber GS, Thompson IM, Thisted R, Chodak GW. Disease-specific survival following routine prostate cancer screening by digital rectal examination. *JAMA.* 1993; 269:61-64.

47. Oesterling JE. Prostate specific antigen: a critical assessment of the most useful tumor marker for adenocarcinoma of the prostate. *J Urol.* 1991;145:907-913.

48. Hara M, Inorre T, Fukugama T. Some physiochemical characteristics of gamma-seminoprotein. *Jpn J Legal Med.* 1971;25:322-335.

49. Stamey TA, Yang N, Hay AR, McNeal JE, Freiha FS, Redwine E. Prostate-specific antigen as a serum marker for adenocarcinoma of the prostate. *N Engl J Med.* 1987; 317:909-916.

50. Catalona WJ, Smith DS, Ratliff TL, et al. Measurement of the prostate-specific antigen in serum as a screening test for prostate cancer. *N Engl J Med.* 1991;324:1156-1161.

51. Cooner WH, Mosley BR, Rutherford CL Jr, et al. Prostate cancer detection in a clinical urological practice by ultrasonography, digital rectal examination, and prostate specific antigen. *J Urol.* 1990;143:1146-1154.

52. Catalona WJ, Smith DS, Ratcliff TL, Basler JW. Detection of organ-confined prostate cancer is increased through PSA screening. *JAMA.* 1993;270:948-954.

53. Mettlin C, Lee F, Drago J, Murphy GP. The American Cancer Society National Prostate Cancer Detection Project: findings on the detection of early prostate cancer in 2425 men. *Cancer.* 1991;67:2949-2958.

54. Littrup PJ, Goodman AC, Mettlin CJ. The benefit and

cost of prostate cancer early detection. *CA Cancer J Clin.* 1993;43:134-149.

55. Johansson JE, Adami HO, Andersson SO, Bergstrom R, Holmberg L, Krusemo UB. High 10-year survival rate in patients with early, untreated prostatic cancer. *JAMA.* 1992;267:2191-2196.

56. Eddy DM. Screening for lung cancer. *Ann Intern Med.* 1989;111:232-237.

57. 1989 Survey of physicians' attitudes and practices in early cancer detection. *CA Cancer J Clin.* 1990;40:77-101.

58. McKenna RJ, Fink DJ. Proceedings of an American Cancer Society workshop on the community and cancer prevention and detection. *Cancer.* 1988;61(11 suppl):2363-2406.

59. *National Cancer Institute PDQ Cancer Information: Cancer Screening Guidelines.* Bethesda, Md: National Cancer Institute; 1992.

60. Canadian Task Force Report on the Periodic Health Examination. The periodic health examination. *Can Med Assoc J.* 1979;121:1193-1254.

61. US Preventive Services Task Force. *Guide to Clinical Preventive Services: An Assessment of the Effectiveness of 169 Interventions.* Baltimore, Md: Williams and Wilkins; 1989.

62. Eddy DM, ed. *Common Screening Tests.* Philadelphia, Pa: American College of Physicians; 1991.

11

CLINICAL TRIALS

Michael A. Friedman, MD

While results of well-designed clinical trials are important to all physicians, they are absolutely essential to oncologists. Everything we know about oncology was learned from clinical trials. Since we are far from having adequate clinical treatments and preventive measures against cancer, clinical research should be viewed as the essential foundation for tomorrow's therapy.

Despite the fact that most researchers, health care deliverers, and even patients support the concept of clinical trials, only a tiny fraction of all cancer patients are enrolled in formal studies. While there are about 1,250,000 newly diagnosed cancer patients in the United States each year, fewer than 50,000 patients participate in federally sponsored therapeutic clinical studies. Perhaps an equal number of individuals participate in clinical studies focusing on prevention or diagnosis. For rarer forms of cancer (especially pediatric malignancies), there is a somewhat greater efficiency in clinical research. More than 50% of children with Wilm's tumor, neuroblastoma, acute lymphocytic leukemia, and Ewing's sarcoma enter clinical trials. For adult patients with common epithelial cancers (such as lung, breast, or colon), less than 5% are enrolled in studies annually. This is unfortunate, as the clinical challenges are immense.

As the population ages, and as competing causes of death (ie, cardiovascular disease) diminish, the importance of finding better cancer prevention and therapy grows. Enormous public and private resources are devoted to cancer care, and there is both an economic and a compassionate imperative to increase our clinical skills.

Moreover, the intellectual challenges of oncology are compelling—there have never been so many legitimate scientific hypotheses to pursue. Currently, clinical trials are being conducted in all conceivable aspects of oncology. These topics include (but are not limited to) such investigative disciplines as biology (eg, prognostic factor studies of immunogenetics), diagnosis, epidemiology, prevention, rehabilitation, cancer control, and therapy.

One of the most active areas of research is in therapy. Therapy includes surgery, radiation, hyperthermia, chemotherapy, biologic therapy (eg, monoclonal antibodies or immune augmentation), hematopoietic cell transplantation, and genetic therapy.

The National Cancer Institute sponsors research on more than 250 investigational agents at this time. Researchers are investigating new agents alone or in various combinations with standard therapies. In addition, both pharmaceutical companies and universities are independently studying their own agents. There are literally thousands of interesting and potentially important lines of investigation. Hence, for humanitarian as well as scientific reasons clinical trials will remain central to oncology. Studies must be promoted and fostered.

Clinical Trial Requisites

Clinical studies must be carefully and responsibly designed, carried out, analyzed, and reported. Patient safety and welfare must be assured. These studies may only be conducted with the freely granted permission of the patient (informed consent). The informed consent process requires that the patient have an understanding of the treatment protocol to be used during the clinical trial, including potential risks and benefits, as well as alternative treatments. After patients have been recruited to the clinical trial, the investigator is obligated to modify care based on new information. In a randomized trial, if one treatment is proven to be superior to another, the best treatment can be offered to patients not originally assigned to that therapy.

The Department of Health and Human Services'

Michael A. Friedman, MD, Cancer Therapy Evaluation Program, Division of Cancer Treatment, National Cancer Institute, National Institutes of Health, Bethesda, Maryland

policy for federally sponsored research requires that patients be recruited from both genders and from a broad range of racial and ethnic groups. This policy allows for equal access to new therapies while at the same time providing important comparative research for possible genetic differences across these groups.

Unfortunately, lack of health care coverage for the indigent and those with limited resources discourage patients, especially racial minorities, from participating in clinical trials. Clinical trials in the areas of cancer prevention and early detection are very important for this population, since this approach has the potential for being exceedingly cost effective.

In summary, properly designed clinical trials may focus on any discipline or goal. Studies of cancer treatment, prevention, diagnosis, etiology, and rehabilitation are currently being conducted. The best studies are those that provide definitive scientific information without regard to clinical outcome. Correlative laboratory investigations can be linked to clinical research to provide additional insights. Well-designed studies provide answers to multiple hypotheses.

General Aspects of Clinical Trials

Formal clinical trials (those which are properly designed and conducted) attempt to arrive at answers by studying relatively small populations and extrapolating the findings over similar individuals. In designing the study, attention should be given to identifying the research objectives and the study population. These subjects should be homogenous in all critical parameters (eg, they must all have the same disease, stage of condition, co-morbid conditions, or other prognostic features). The essential statistical considerations should include the recruitment of an adequate number of study subjects to ensure confidence in the conclusions. The study's endpoint(s) should be clear and achievable. Ideally, a study should yield valuable information whether or not a "positive" clinical result is achieved.[1]

With respect to research conduct, an attempt should be made to statistically account for all subjects entered in a study with few, if any, patients excluded, ineligible, or lost to follow-up. Data should be collected in a timely, complete, and accurate manner. Moreover, quality assurance is essential—whether it is a chemoprevention trial (such as insuring adherence to the prevention program), a diagnosis trial (such as spot-checking the quality of diagnostic tests or their interpretation), or a therapeutic study (such as checking the thoroughness of a surgical intervention)—attention to accuracy is the only means of assuring credibility.

Analysis of clinical trials should be conducted with equal care. Proper statistical methodology should be employed and inappropriate comparisons or conclusions avoided.[2] Premature analysis, too frequent analysis, and so-called "data dredging" (utilizing inappropriate techniques to reach fake conclusions) can be avoided by establishing formal analysis plans in the protocol document itself. Indeed, such statistical considerations are necessary at the very inception of the study protocol document.

Types of Clinical Trials

For convenience, therapeutic cancer trials have usually been divided into distinct phases.

Phase I Trials

Although all clinical trials seek to benefit patients, the main goal of Phase I studies is to determine the qualitative and quantitative aspects of treatment-associated toxicity. Therapeutic trials usually involve patients with refractory, incurable cancer, since there is no assurance of direct personal benefit. Healthy individuals may be the subject of Phase I trials for prevention studies. Often pharmacokinetic and pharmacodynamic studies are performed; but other biologic studies are now being performed more often. For biologic response modifiers, so-called Phase IB studies may attempt to evaluate relevant immunologic endpoints (such as specific T-cell population dynamics or activation or production of a specific cytokine of interest). The endpoints of Phase I studies are either the achievement of some biologic goal (eg, targeted reduction of glutathione [GSH] or inhibition of topoisomerase I) or detection of significant, but acceptable, toxicity judged to be dose-limiting or maximally tolerable. The number of subjects required should be the smallest number compatible with demonstration of reproducible and reversible toxicity.

Many types of Phase I trials are currently being sponsored by the National Cancer Institute. These studies include (1) evaluations of adults with relatively normal organ function, (2) those with abnormal function, (3) young children, and (4) the elderly. If hematologic toxicity is thought to be the dose-limiting factor, attempts are made to escalate doses of the agent, along with hematopoietic growth factors. For agents with marrow ablative potential (and little other toxicity even at high doses), evaluation with marrow or peripheral stem cell transplantation is appropriate.

Phase II Trials

Phase II trials are designed to employ the dose, schedule, and route of administration determined in the Phase I study.[3] However, the study population is usually better defined and more homogenous with respect to type of cancer, physiologic state, and prior therapy. Efficacy is usually judged based on a convenient surrogate endpoint, such as objective partial or complete antitumor response. Further data on toxicity is obtained, but the principal goal of a Phase II study is the detection of antitumor effect. The requisite sample size of such a study depends on a minimal threshold of activity. Identifying a minimum response rate of 20% usually requires the accrual of 25 to 40 eligible patients. If no response is noted in the first 14 patients studied, there is a less than 5% chance of an actual response probability of 20%.[4]

There are many possible designs for Phase II studies that are worth consideration.[5] The goal of a Phase II study is to provide the best chance of identifying an active drug with the minimal number of patients so that patients are not unnecessarily exposed to an ineffective therapy.

Combination trials of multiple agents also must undergo testing to assure tolerability. However, the value of Phase II combination studies of agents of recognized activity is questionable. The vagaries of patient selection make it nearly impossible to determine whether a new combination is better or worse than a standard approach. Selecting fit, good-risk patients makes it more likely that a positive benefit will be observed. It is unlikely that dramatic synergism or antagonism will be detected; more likely a moderate (more intermediate) effect will be observed. A formal Phase III study is usually required in order to confidently draw efficacy conclusions.

Phase III Trials

Phase III trials are perhaps the most crucial type of study for influencing clinical practice. One or more investigational therapy is compared to one or more standard approach. The presence of a concurrently randomized comparison group is a highly attractive feature, since it avoids the need for a historical control group. No matter how carefully selected, a historically derived group of patients previously studied is never as satisfactory as a contemporaneous group. The chance of unexpected or unpredictable introduction of bias or the inclusion of biologically dissimilar groups is thus minimized. Requiring larger numbers of patients, these studies can define the state-of-the-art therapies for each type of cancer. However, it should be noted that a Phase III trial is only necessary if a dramatic effect is not observed in a Phase II trial. A curative therapy for advanced pancreatic cancer patients would be easily demonstrated in a Phase II study. However, for common adult tumors, modest benefits (on the order of 5 to 15 percentage point increases in 5-year survivals) are well worth identifying. For adjuvant populations of breast, large bowel, or ovarian cancer patients, hundreds to thousands of patients may be needed to demonstrate an improvement of this magnitude. In addition, these large, precise trials provide an outstanding opportunity to evaluate laboratory tests of prognostic value or to characterize biologically diverse patient groups that deserve different clinical interventions.

For all their advantages, Phase III studies are also the most complicated and demanding for everyone. These studies must be carefully designed. Proper randomization, data monitoring, and analysis are required. For the research sponsor, the investigator, and the patient, Phase III studies require commitment and discipline.

All of these studies are valuable and necessary. No one type is complete in itself. Phase I and II trials are prerequisites for Phase III, but each is a specialized research instrument.

Obstacles to the Conduct of Clinical Trials

The Patient

It is obvious from the small number of participants in clinical trials that enrolling patients is a challenge. There are many reasons why patients are reluctant to be a study participant. Patients with a serious disease like cancer are not comforted by their physician's frankly admitting that the single best form of treatment is not obvious or uniformly accepted. The concept of "research" may be foreign to some or anathema to others. The patient may fear that his or her individual interest will be subservient to the research (ie, they will be utilized as "guinea pigs"). Entering a clinical trial may require extra visits to the physician or additional tests that result in time lost from home or work or heightened anxiety.

An important impediment is the threat that insurance coverage may be denied if the patient's care is within the context of a clinical trial. Many of these agencies (both for profit and not-for-profit) refuse coverage for what they define as investigational therapies of unproven worth.

Another reason patients give for not entering a study is that they have already decided on a course of therapy, whether it be the new or traditional approach.

The Health Care Professional

From the health care professional's perspective, there are also many reasons not to join. Every aspect of a clinical trial requires extra time, effort, and expense—petitioning the local Institutional Review Board for permission to perform the trial, explaining the study to the patient, obtaining informed consent, filling out forms, as well as other tedious tasks. Some physicians are not comfortable with clinical trials because the trials interfere with their ability to manage their patient's therapy. The physician may be biased against the treatment under study or may simply wish to customize each patient's treatment.

Encouraging Participation

How can the concerns of patients and health care professionals be addressed? The best answer is that the extra effort, discomfort, and financial and emotional costs have the potential to directly benefit the patient as well as others. Participating in a clinical trial is an important investment in the welfare of the individual and society.

Recruiters can stress that patients who participate in peer-reviewed, scrupulously monitored clinical trials have access to the best treatment available. Designers of the trials have carefully considered issues of science, clinical medicine, and ethics. Of course, excellent clinical care is available without participation in a study. However, some of the very best care is found as part of a clinical trial.

Clinical trials are not a societal right but rather a precious privilege. In the United States tax revenues or charitable donations are devoted to supporting research. All physicians who administer clinical trials have duties, rights, and obligations. What we know today is a result of the devotion, courage, and industry of those who precede us. Future generations of patients will hold us accountable for our successes and failures in doing the most ingenious, efficient, and valid clinical trials possible. Good clinical research requires some effort, but so does good clinical care.

References

1. Simon R, Friedman M. *The Chemotherapy Source Book.* Baltimore, Md: Williams & Wilkins; 1991.

2. Simon RS. *Cancer: Principles and Practice of Oncology.* Philadelphia, Pa: JB Lippincott Co; 1989.

3. Wittes RE, Marsoni S, Simon R, et al. The phase II trial. *Cancer Treat Rep.* 1985;69:1235-1239.

4. Gehan EA. The determination of the number of patients required in a preliminary and follow-up trial of a new chemotherapeutic agent. *J Chron Dis.* 1961;123:346-353.

5. Fleming TR. One sample multiple testing procedure for phase II clinical trials. *Biometric.* 1982;38:143-151.

Selected Readings

1. Fleming TR, Green SJ, Harrington DP. Considerations for monitoring and evaluating treatment effects in clinical trials. *Controlled Clin Trials.* 1984;5:55-66.

2. Peto R, Pike MC, Armitage P, et al. Design and analysis of randomized clinical trials requiring prolonged observation of each patient, I: Introduction and design. *Br J Cancer.* 1976;34:585-612.

3. Peto R, Pike MC, Armitage P, et al. Design and analysis of randomized clinical trials requiring prolonged observation of each patient, II: analysis and examples. *Br J Cancer.* 1977;35:1-39.

4. Fleming TR, Green SJ, Harrington DP. Designs for group sequential tests. *Controlled Clin Trials.* 1984;5:348-361.

5. Fleming TR, Watelet L. Approaches to monitoring clinical trials. *J Natl Cancer Inst.* 1989;81:188-193.

6. Yusuf S, Simon R, Ellenberg S, eds. Symposium on methodology for overviews of randomized clinical trials. *Stat Med.* 1987;6:217-410.

12

BREAST CANCER

I. Craig Henderson, MD

No single statistic describes the status of breast cancer relative to other cancers. On the one hand, it is the most common cancer among women. It is estimated that breast cancer will be diagnosed in 183,000 American women in 1994, and the incidence has been increasing at an annual rate of 1.2% since 1940. Between 1982 and 1986, the rate of increase was 4% per year. Since 1940, breast cancer mortality has also increased, but more slowly. In fact, breast cancer mortality has been stable since 1950, but this overall figure masks a 15% increase among women 55 years of age and older and a concomitant 15% decrease among those younger than 55.[1] An estimated 46,300 American women will die of breast cancer in 1994, and it is the leading cause of death among American women aged 40 to 55. However, lung cancer is now a greater contributor to cancer mortality among women of all ages.

This disparity between a rapid rise in incidence and a modest increase in mortality is not easily explained. Part of the reason may be increased registration of the disease and widespread use of mammography in recent years. Prior to the 1980s, <15% of women had regular screening. Many of the cancers now being diagnosed might never become clinical problems if left undetected. As many as 12% (ACS estimate) of cancers diagnosed in 1994 may be of the in situ variety, and it is not known for certain that these tumors all would have gone on to become invasive if not diagnosed. Another reason for the disparity may be the apparently less aggressive character of many of the newer invasive tumors. For example, a higher percentage of recently diagnosed cancers are estrogen receptor positive.[1] Finally, with improvements in treatment, especially during the past 30 years, a real increase in cancer incidence may have been partly counterbalanced by an increase in the percentage of breast cancers that are cured.

Breast cancer incidence rates greatly underestimate the number of women who will be affected by this disease in one way or another, since for every woman with a diagnosis of breast cancer, another five or ten will have a biopsy that shows benign disease. It is plausible that for every woman biopsied, another 10 go to their physician because they either have a breast symptom or are worried that they may be in a high-risk group. Overall, it is likely that nearly 20 million American women will see their physician this year about a potential breast cancer.

Risk Factors for Developing Breast Cancer

A proper interpretation of relative risk requires an understanding of the baseline risk for all women. These risks are determined by actuarial methods and reported as cumulative probabilities from birth to some age between 85 and 110. Currently, the cumulative baseline risk for any American woman developing breast cancer is 12%, but the cumulative risk of dying from breast cancer is only 3.6%.

It is common practice (and technically correct) to multiply an individual woman's relative risk of developing or dying of breast cancer by the underlying risks for the entire population. However, such figures may overestimate a woman's real risk for two reasons. First, there may be attenuation of risk with time. In other words, the increased risk associated with the risk factor may not be constant throughout a woman's life, and the risk of developing breast cancer may be much higher during the first decade following identification of the factor than in subsequent decades (see below). Second, much of the increased risk is expressed in old age, and this may be of less importance to a woman than her immediate risk. Thus, in explaining and counseling a woman about her relative risk of breast cancer, 10- and 20-year intervals

I. Craig Henderson, MD, Professor of Medicine, Chief, Medical Oncology, Director, Clinical Oncology Programs, University of California, San Francisco, Cancer Center, Mt. Zion, San Francisco, California

Table 12-1. Cumulative Probability of Eventually Developing and Dying of Breast Cancer, Based on 1985 Estimates of Overall Risk*

Age Interval	Risk of developing any breast cancer %	Risk of developing invasive breast cancer %	Risk of dying of breast cancer %
Birth to 110	10.2	9.8	3.6
20 to 30	0.04	0.04	0.00
20 to 40	0.49	0.42	0.09
20 to 110	10.34	9.94	3.05
35 to 45	0.88	0.83	0.14
35 to 55	2.53	2.37	0.56
35 to 110	10.27	9.82	3.56
50 to 60	1.95	1.86	0.33
50 to 70	4.67	4.48	1.04
50 to 110	8.96	8.66	2.75
65 to 75	3.17	3.08	0.43
65 to 85	5.48	5.29	1.01
65 to 110	6.53	6.29	1.53

*Data from Surveillance, Epidemiology, and End Results (SEER) Program, white females.

From Seidman et al.[2]

may be more meaningful. For example, the risk that a 35-year-old woman will develop breast cancer by the age of 55 is about 2.5% and the risk that she will die of breast cancer during this interval is 0.56% (Table 12-1).[2] If her relative risk were calculated to be 3, her cumulative risk of developing breast cancer during this interval would be 7.5% and her risk of dying of breast cancer would be 1.7%. A patient's perception of her risk may substantially affect her behavior and quality of life. In some cases, the perception that her risk is excessively high may lead her to avoid routine mammography.[3]

The list of factors that have been shown in one study or another to be associated with an increased risk of developing breast cancer is almost endless. The factors demonstrated in multiple epidemiologic studies to be important are more manageable (Table 12-2). The single most important factor is age, especially in Western countries. The probability that a 60-year-old white American woman will develop breast cancer in a single year (1 in 420) is fourteen times that of a 30-year-old (1 in 5,900). At least two hereditary patterns can be ascertained, one a familial aggregation associated with a modest increase in risk and the other a truly genetic pattern with high penetrance and linkage to a specific gene. Familial aggregations are very common. Truly genetic breast cancers have been estimated to account for only 5% of the incidence rate.

Table 12-2. Risk Factors for Developing Breast Cancer

- Age
- Hereditary factors
  - Familial
  - Genetic
- Prior history of breast cancer
  - In situ
  - Invasive
- Benign breast disease
  - Atypical hyperplasia
- Endogenous endocrine factors
  - Age at menarche
  - Age at menopause
  - Age at first pregnancy
- Exogenous endocrine factors
  - Postmenopausal estrogen replacement
  - Oral contraceptives
- Environmental factors
  - Region of birth
  - Diet
  - Alcohol

Although any family history of breast cancer is associated with an increase in risk, only a history of breast cancer in a first-degree relative (parent, sibling, or child) is associated with more than a trivial increase. Familial patterns based on the number of first-degree relatives with cancer and the age of onset and bilaterality of cancers in the affected relatives are associated with relative risks varying from 1.1 to more than ninefold. For example, a woman's relative risk of developing breast cancer is 1.8 if only her mother had breast cancer, 2.5 if one sister had breast cancer, and 5.6 if both her mother and one sister had breast cancer.[4] Expressed as cumulative probabilities, the likelihood that a 30-year-old woman will develop breast cancer by age 70 is 8% if either her mother or sister had breast cancer, 18% if two first-degree relatives had breast cancer, and 28% if two first-degree relatives had bilateral breast cancer.[5,6]

Genetic breast cancers occur at a younger age, are more likely to be bilateral, and appear in multiple family members over three or more generations. Specific genes linked to these cancers have now been identified on chromosome 17. One of these is p53, a tumor suppressor gene that appears in both carriers and patients in Li-Fraumeni families.[7] The BRCA1 gene, on 17q, is associated with families who have the breast ovarian syndrome.[8] The discovery of these genetic links opens up new possibilities for identifying women at high risk of developing breast cancer, but at present genetic screening is inappropriate unless a woman has a pedigree highly suggestive of genetic breast cancer.

A woman with a history of either invasive or in situ cancer in one breast has an increased lifelong risk of developing a new breast cancer in any remaining breast tissue. This risk is approximately 0.5% to 1% per year. The reduction in risk is not entirely proportional to the amount of tissue removed, and breast cancers have been reported to occur in the very small remnant of tissue remaining after subcutaneous mastectomy in women with a history of in situ or micro-invasive breast cancer. Fortunately, two breast cancers, whether concomitant or sequential, do not impart a worse prognosis than one breast cancer. The risk is determined by the tumor with the worst prognostic features, and this provides incentive for careful follow-up examinations and periodic screening mammography in all women with a diagnosis of breast cancer.

Some types of benign breast disease carry an increased risk of breast cancer. Approximately half of all patients who are biopsied and found not to have breast cancer will have evidence of ductal or lobular hyperplasia, which is associated with a relative risk of breast cancer of 1.6.[9] Only about 7% of such patients will carry a diagnosis of atypical hyperplasia, but the relative risk in this group is 4.4. There is evidence of an interaction between family history and atypical hyperplasia, and the very small group (1.2% of biopsied women) with both these risk factors has a relative risk of 8.9. This translates into a slightly less than 40% probability of developing breast cancer over 25 years. The risk of these women dying of breast cancer is the same as, or even slightly less than, that of women who have a diagnosis of breast cancer but are not in such a high-risk group. The relative risk of developing breast cancer after a diagnosis of benign breast disease is not constant throughout a woman's life. Women with biopsy-proven atypical hyperplasia will have a relative risk of 9.8 during the first 10 years, but only 3.6 in the subsequent two decades.[10]

Endogenous endocrine factors appear to promote the development of breast cancer and may even be involved in etiology. Longer intervals from menarche to the first full-term pregnancy and from menarche to cessation of menses are associated with significantly higher risks of breast cancer. Women whose menarche begins at age 12 or earlier have twice the risk of developing breast cancer as those whose menarche begins after age 13. The time when regular ovulatory cycles are established may be even more important, since women who have onset of regular menses at or before age 12 have a 3.7-fold greater risk of developing breast cancer than women who have menarche after age 13 and take >5 years to establish regular menstrual cycles.[11] Women who have a natural menopause after age 55 are at twice the risk of developing breast cancer as those with a natural menopause prior to age 44. Therapeutic oophorectomies performed between ages 50 to 54 are associated with a 1.34 relative risk, compared with oophorectomies performed between ages 45 to 49. The number of full-term pregnancies is important, but only if the first pregnancy occurs before age 30. A woman whose first full-term pregnancy occurs prior to age 19 has 50% of the risk of a nulliparous woman. If the first full-term pregnancy is between ages 30 to 34, the relative risk equals that of a nulliparous woman; if the first full-term pregnancy is after age 35, the relative risk is actually greater than that of a nulliparous woman. Presumably this is due to a transient increase in risk associated with pregnancy compounded by other risk factors associated with aging. The increase in risk persists approximately one decade after the first pregnancy, and as a woman grows older, this higher risk associated with pregnancy likely becomes more important.

The increased risk associated with the use of estrogen replacement therapy (ERT) in postmenopausal women or oral contraceptives in premenopausal women is either very small or nonexistent. However, prolonged use of these therapies may result in a modest increase. In a meta-analysis of ERT studies, the relative risk of developing breast cancer was 1.3 (95% confidence interval, 1.2 to 1.6) among women taking ERT for >15 years.[12] The risk seems to be somewhat greater if estradiol, rather than conjugated estrogens, is used and if ERT is begun during the menopausal years. There may be some interaction with family history. The use of progestins with ERT does not decrease, and may even augment, the risk of developing breast cancer. The effect of oral contraceptive use on the subsequent development of breast cancer may be related to the time and duration of administration. A meta-analysis of oral contraceptive studies failed to demonstrate any association between oral contraceptive use and overall risk of developing breast cancer, but prolonged use, especially prior to the first full-term pregnancy, was associated with an increased risk of developing breast cancer before age 45.[13] The relative risk from oral contraceptive use for >10 years was 1.46 (P=.001), and the relative risk from oral contraceptive use for 4 years prior to the first full-term pregnancy was 1.72.

There are large regional differences in the incidence of breast cancer. In the San Francisco bay area, the annual incidence among whites is 87 per 100,000, in contrast to only 18.6 per 100,000 population in rural Japan. Incidence studies among migrants who move from low- to high-incidence areas have demonstrated that the risk of developing breast cancer in the migrant population will gradually rise to the level of the population in the new locale. In the case of the Japanese, this rise in incidence does not occur until the second generation following migration. This pattern of change in risk suggests that environmental factors are important in the development of breast cancer, and the fact that the increase in risk primarily occurs in second generations suggests that environmental factors may be operative in a woman's youth rather than in later life. Among the environmental factors studied thus far, a region's total production of dietary fat is most closely associated with breast cancer risk.[14] The results from case control studies of fat intake have been contradictory, but a meta-analysis of 12 such studies suggests that 24% of breast cancers in postmenopausal women and 16% of those in premenopausal women might be attributable to dietary factors.[15] Large cohort studies lead to exactly the opposite conclusion. In the largest of these, women with a *high* fat content in their diet had a 15% lower risk of developing breast cancer than those in the lowest quintile (a difference that was not significant);[16] in a second, somewhat smaller cohort study, the group with the highest fat content had a 61% lower incidence of breast cancer than those on a low-fat diet![17]

The dietary factor most consistently shown to be associated with an increased risk of breast cancer is alcohol intake. A meta-analysis of epidemiologic studies demonstrated that an alcohol intake of 6 g/day (about 1/2 drink) may be associated with a relative risk of 1.3; an intake of 36 g/day was associated with a relative risk of 2.[18] One study suggests that alcohol intake prior to age 30 is more closely correlated with breast cancer risk than alcohol consumed later in life.

Attributable Risk

In the development of public health policies on the use of screening mammography or in the design of chemoprevention trials, it would be desirable to focus on high-risk groups because of the substantial savings from evaluating or treating smaller numbers of women. However, the increased risk associated with most risk factors or constellation of risk factors is relatively modest. In the Nurses' Health Study, breast cancer incidence among women who had a menarche before age 11, their first child after age 35, and either benign breast disease or a family history of breast cancer in a first-degree relative, was only 54% higher than in the remainder of the population.[1] In an American Cancer Society (ACS) survey conducted several decades ago, only 21% of cancers in women aged 30 to 54 and 29% of those in women aged 55 to 84 were attributable to one or more risk factors.[19] Most breast cancers occur in patients not at high risk. For this reason, it is inadvisable to use any factor other than age in determining diagnostic vigilance for detecting breast cancer.

Prevention

Increasing attention is being paid to the development of breast cancer prevention strategies. Trials are ongoing to determine whether 5 years of tamoxifen or a reduction in dietary fat intake to levels <20% will reduce breast cancer incidence, and studies to evaluate retinoids (vitamin A derivatives) are being developed. Although promising, none of these strategies has been shown to reduce breast cancer mortality among women who do not already have the disease.

Natural History and Biology of Breast Cancer

Two of the most striking features of breast cancer biology are variable behavior in different patients and a relatively slow growth rate compared with other tumor types. The median survival of patients who decline all forms of treatment for breast cancer is about 2.8 years, but the tail of these survival curves is very long, with some patients living 15 to 20 years. Studies of untreated patients were done in the 19th and early 20th century, and it is likely that these studies underestimate the median survival today of untreated patients with a diagnosis. Using conventional forms of treatment, the median survival of patients with metastatic breast cancer is >2 years.[20] The tail of this curve is also quite prolonged, and in one recent series 10% of patients with metastatic or locally inoperable breast cancer lived more than one decade following diagnosis of metastases.[21] There are anecdotal reports of patients living >30 years with recurrent disease.

Some breast cancers will double in size within a few days, while others will take >2,000 days. The average doubling time for human breast cancers is estimated at about 100 days. Cancers can be readily palpated in the breast when they reach a diameter of approximately 1 cm. A "sphere" of this size contains approximately one billion cells, which is the result of 30 doublings of a single cell. Assuming that a preclinical breast mass grows logarithmically with a doubling time of 100 days, it would require 10 years to reach a point where it could be diagnosed. Although it is unlikely that metastases occur during the first 20 doublings, some breast cancers metastasize soon after that point, and the probability of metastases increases steadily the longer the breast cancer grows before detection. Most patients with a diagnosis of breast cancer have likely had the disease for 5 to 10 years prior to diagnosis, and a substantial percentage will have had well-established metastases for several years even if these cannot be detected on physical examination, x-rays, bone scans, or magnetic resonance imaging (MRI). (Very few of these methods, with the notable exception of mammography, will detect a lesion <1 cm in diameter.)

For a cancer to be curable using surgery and radiotherapy, it must be diagnosed prior to the development of metastases. Just because a cancer is diagnosed earlier does not mean that it will be more readily cured. Fortunately, because the preclinical period for most breast cancers is very long, enabling earlier detection, and because mammography is a sensitive means of detecting early breast cancer, we have been able to increase the breast cancer cure rate with routine screening evaluations of asymptomatic women.

Even patients whose tumors cannot be detected prior to the development of metastases may benefit from early detection, since subsequent metastases will still be very small and less resistant to drugs and hormones than if additional doublings had occurred. Larger tumors are less sensitive to these therapies for a number of reasons: less favorable kinetics with larger metastatic deposits, inadequate vasculature for drug delivery, and mutant clones that are either estrogen receptor negative or drug resistant. For this reason, early treatment with endocrine and chemotherapy (ie, adjuvant systemic therapy) may substantially reduce or even eradicate the undetectable micrometastases. Since breast cancer is more sensitive to systemic treatment than most other tumor types, this strategy has proven successful in prolonging survival.

Studies dealing with prognosis provide further evidence of the heterogeneity of breast cancer. About two thirds of patients have tumors with estrogen receptors (ER) on the cell surface, but the percentage of ER-positive cells varies enormously among tumors that are labeled "ER positive." Tumors with a larger percentage of receptor-positive cells will grow more slowly, are more likely to respond to endocrine therapy, and are more likely to have a durable response if it occurs.[22] Recently, a number of oncogenes have been identified in patients with breast cancer. Approximately 25% to 30% of tumors will have overexpression of the *erb*B-2 oncogene. Such patients have a greater probability of developing distant metastases, have a more rapid-growing form of the disease, and may have greater resistance to some forms of chemotherapy while being more responsive to others.

The heterogeneity and natural history of breast cancer confound the interpretation of clinical studies. If a small cohort of patients is selected for the evaluation of a new treatment strategy and these patients have a long survival, this may be due to the superiority of the treatment under evaluation or to the fortuitous selection of patients with a slower-growing form of the disease. These problems are particularly prominent in the evaluation of various methods for early diagnosis, such as breast self-examination (BSE) and mammography. A breast cancer might be detected several years earlier because of BSE or mammography and yet not be curable because metastases have already begun to grow. In such cases, the patient would die at the same time she might have died without early detection, but the period in which she was observed to have the cancer would be prolonged. This is called lead-time bias. Patients with more slow-growing tumors have a longer preclinical phase and are more likely to be detected at a screening evaluation. This, too, will give the false impression that screening has resulted in a better outcome. This is called length bias. These problems are not limited to evaluations of screening strategies, and will occur if a cohort of patients with particularly slow-growing disease is selected for the evaluation of a new therapy for metastatic breast cancer. Both these problems can be circumvented relatively easily if a new diagnostic or treatment modality is evaluated in a randomized trial involving large numbers of patients, since a larger trial is more likely to include a cross-section of all types of breast cancer patients.

Symptoms and Diagnosis

Despite increasing use of mammography, >80% of cancers are diagnosed as a result of symptoms, and in the vast majority of cases the important symptom is a painless mass. However, the presence of pain should not lead to a false reassurance of the patient, since as many as 10% of patients may present with breast pain and no mass. Less common symptoms leading to a diagnosis are nipple discharge, nipple erosion or ulceration, diffuse erythema of the breast, axillary adenopathy, and symptoms associated with distant metastases. Most conditions associated with nipple discharge are benign, whether the discharge is serous or bloody. However, a clear nipple discharge that is also Hemeoccult negative will almost never be associated with cancer.[23] Paget's disease of the nipple may present as an innocent pimple, scaling, erosion, or ulceration, and these are often treated inappropriately with a steroid cream. Persistent lesion of the nipple should be biopsied. A substantial percentage of these patients will have a palpable mass on physical examination or an abnormality on mammogram deep within the breast. Enlargement of the breast with or without a distinct mass, erythema, and peau d'orange are the hallmarks of an inflammatory breast cancer. The physical findings of this type of cancer suggest a mastitis, but infections of the breast are rare in non-lactating women. Inflammatory breast cancer carries a particularly poor prognosis, and the diagnosis should be confirmed by skin biopsy.

Physical examination of the breast should begin with an inspection of the patient in the sitting position. Any evidence of nipple inversion, skin dimpling, or architectural distortion may provide clues of a breast cancer deeper within the breast. These signs may be brought out if the patient contracts her pectoralis muscles, pressing her palms together above her head. While the patient is in the sitting position, it is convenient to examine the supraclavicular, infraclavicular, and axillary areas for evidence of lymphadenopathy. Finally, the breast should be gently palpated while the patient is still sitting. The area beneath the nipple should be specifically evaluated by bringing two opposing fingers together, compressing this area. More extensive palpation of the breast should be performed with the patient in a supine position with a pillow under the ipsilateral breast and the ipsilateral arm raised above the head. In this position, the breast is relatively evenly distributed over the chest wall and the deeper regions of the breast are more accessible to the examining fingers. The breast should be systematically evaluated using the palmar surfaces of the second, third, and fourth fingers rather than the fingertips. The hand should move in a circular motion, systematically traversing the breast from the nipple to the outer edges in a pattern suggestive of wheel spokes. It is particularly important to evaluate the tail of the breast, which extends high into the axilla.

Breast self-examination is performed by the patient using techniques very similar to those employed by the physician or nurse (Fig 12-1).[24] At the time of the physician examination, patients should be instructed in performing BSE. The use of a model is sometimes helpful. The patient should always have ready access to the physician or a trained nurse in the months following her first attempts at BSE, since many normal areas of the breast may seem abnormal to the inexperienced examiner, and this may produce considerable anxiety. The patient should be informed that lumpiness of the breast is not, in itself, abnormal or the sign of a woman at high risk of developing breast cancer.

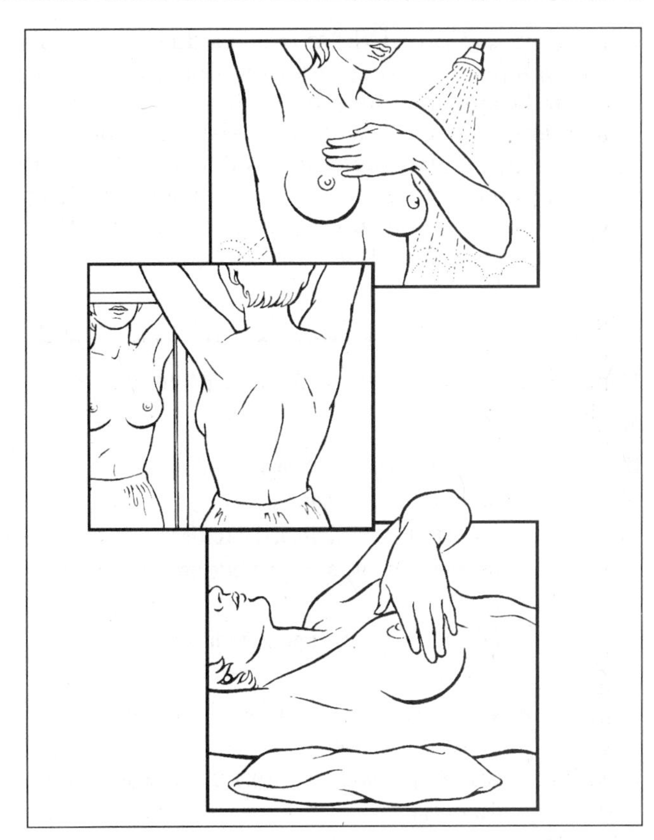

Fig 12-1. American Cancer Society's recommended procedure for breast self-examination. Courtesy of American Cancer Society.[24]

The characteristics of a breast cancer cannot be precisely defined. In general, however, breast cancers have a much firmer character than the surrounding tissues and have somewhat indistinct edges.[25] A suspicious area is usually described as "a dominant mass," because it is so distinctly different from the remaining breast tissue. Solid masses often confused with breast cancers include fibroadenomas, fat necrosis, and sclerosing adenosis. Fibroadenomas are usually very well defined and freely movable; they occur more frequently in younger women. None of these lesions can be distinguished definitively from the others without a biopsy. Cysts or a large area that includes small cysts and reactive fibrosis are also difficult to distinguish from breast cancer. In general, cystic areas are somewhat more diffuse and less firm. A well-defined cyst can be confirmed by either aspiration of clear fluid or demonstration of a fluid-filled cavity on ultrasound. While extremely rare, a cancer growing in the wall of a cyst should be suspected if the cyst recurs rapidly, if there is a residual defect on mammography following cyst aspiration, or if there is blood in the cyst aspirate.[25] Following cyst aspiration, the patient should return for at least one follow-up visit to confirm that the cyst has disappeared completely. Lobular carcinomas are particularly difficult to diagnose on physical examination because they usually present as a diffuse thickening rather than a discrete mass.

Table 12-3. TNM Staging for Breast Carcinoma

Primary Tumor (T)

TX		Primary tumor cannot be assessed
T0		No evidence of primary tumor
Tis		Carcinoma in situ: Intraductal carcinoma, lobular carcinoma in situ, or Paget's disease of the nipple with no tumor
T1		Tumor 2 cm or less in greatest dimension
	T1a	0.5 cm or less in greatest dimension
	T1b	More than 0.5 cm, but not more than 1 cm in greatest dimension
	T1c	More than 1 cm, but not more than 2 cm in greatest dimension
T2		Tumor more than 2 cm, but not more than 5 cm in greatest dimension
T3		Tumor more than 5 cm in greatest dimension
T4		Tumor of any size with direct extension to chest wall or skin
	T4a	Extension to chest wall
	T4b	Edema (including peau d'orange) or ulceration of the skin of breast or satellite skin nodules confined to same breast
	T4c	Both T4a and T4b
	T4d	Inflammatory carcinoma

Regional Lymph Nodes (N)

NX		Regional lymph nodes cannot be assessed (e.g., previously removed or not removed for pathologic study)
N0		No regional lymph node metastasis
N1		Metastasis to movable ipsilateral axillary lymph node(s)
	N1a	Only micrometastasis (none larger than 0.2 cm)
	N1b	Metastasis to lymph node(s), any larger than 0.2 cm
	N1bi	Metastasis in 1 to 3 lymph nodes, any more than 0.2 cm and all less than 2 cm in greatest dimension
	N1bii	Metastasis to 4 or more lymph nodes, any more than 0.2 cm and all less than 2 cm in greatest dimension
	N1biii	Extension of tumor beyond the capsule of a lymph node metastasis less than 2 cm in greatest dimension
	N1biv	Metastasis to a lymph node 2 cm or more in greatest dimension
N2		Metastasis to ipsilateral axillary lymph nodes that are fixed to one another or to other structures
N3		Metastasis to ipsilateral internal mammary lymph node(s)

Table 12-3 *Continued.* TNM Staging for Breast Carcinoma

Distant Metastasis (M)

MX	Presence of distant metastasis cannot be assessed
M0	No distant metastasis
M1	Distant metastasis (includes metastasis to ipsilateral supraclavicular lymph node(s))

Stage Grouping

Stage 0	Tis	N0	M0
Stage I	T1	N0	M0
Stage IIA	T0	N1	M0
	T1	N1	M0
	T2	N0	M0
Stage IIB	T2	N1	M0
	T3	N0	M0
Stage IIIA	T0	N2	M0
	T1	N2	M0
	T2	N2	M0
	T3	N1	M0
	T3	N2	M0
Stage IIIB	T4	Any N	M0
	Any T	N3	M0
Stage IV	Any T	Any N	M1

From American Joint Committee on Cancer.[26]

Following examination of the patient, a physician should determine his/her level of suspicion regarding breast cancer and carefully note the size and character of the lesion, as well as the presence or absence of lymphadenopathy. Together, these characteristics can be used to determine the patient's clinical stage (Table 12-3).[26] When information is available from the pathology report, the stage is usually further refined. The patient's clinical stage will frequently determine which primary and adjuvant therapy is appropriate. Prior to biopsy of a suspicious lesion, a patient should have a mammogram both to define the extent of the areas thought on examination to be suspicious and to identify other suspicious areas. Mammographic abnormalities characteristic of breast cancer include spiculated, "crablike," or "puckering" lesions; microcalcifications; and an architectural distortion of the breast without an obvious mass (Fig 12-2, A). Less commonly, a breast cancer may appear as a perfectly round coinlike lesion. Microcalcifications may occur within a mass lesion or independently. Suspicious microcalcifications occur in clusters with at least three separate flecks of calcium, and the calcium deposits are usually much smaller in cancerous than in benign lesions (Fig 12-2, B).[27] Approximately 15% of cancers will not be apparent on mammograms; this is true of both small and large lesions. Therefore, a negative mammogram should never dissuade a physician from performing a biopsy if a dominant mass has been found on physical examination. If both physical examination and mammogram are negative, the probability of a cancer being undetected has been reported to be 3.7%. If both are positive, the probability of not finding a cancer is only 3.6%.[28]

An ultrasound may be of value as a supplement to, but never as a substitution for, mammography. Ultrasounds are particularly valuable in distinguishing cystic from solid lesions. Microcalcifications and other very early signs of breast cancer cannot be detected on ultrasound. Thermography and diaphanography are both associated with unacceptably high false-positive and false-negative rates and have no role in the routine management or early detection of breast cancer. Breast cancers can be identified on computed tomography (CT), but this modality has not been shown to be superior to mammography and is associated with much greater radiation exposure. MRI does not involve radiation exposure, but is no more accurate and considerably more expensive than mammography.

Fine needle aspiration (FNA) biopsy is increasingly being used because of the ease of performance and the rapidity with which a diagnosis can be made. However, cytologic evaluation from an FNA cannot distinguish in situ from invasive cancers and does not provide clues that a cancer might be multicentric. When used as an adjunct to physical examination and mammography, it may be quite reliable. In one study, only 0.6% of patients were later found to have cancer on biopsy when the physical examination, mammogram, and FNA were all negative.[28] When all three evaluations were positive, 99.4% of patients were found to have cancer. However, when the physical examination and mammogram suggested a cancer but the FNA was negative, 36% were found subsequently to have cancer. When the physical examination was positive but both the mammogram and FNA were negative, 7% were found to have cancer. The use of FNA requires experience on the part of the individual

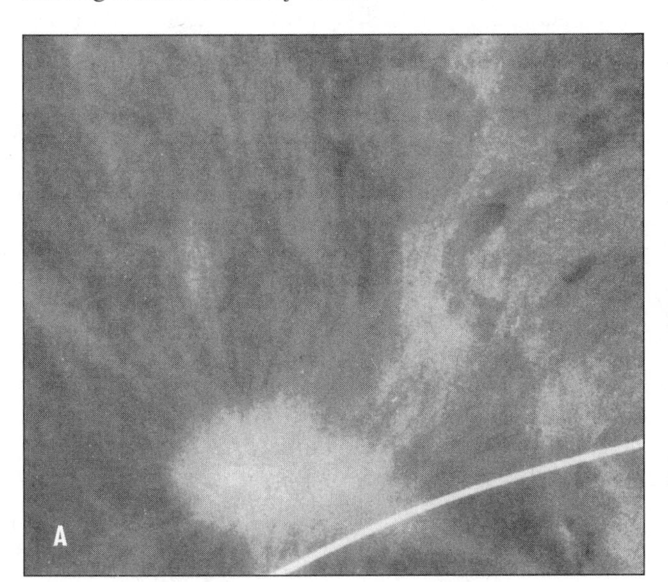

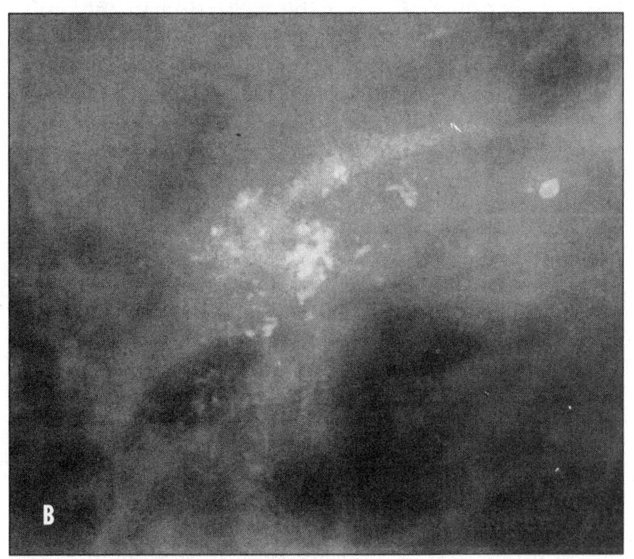

Fig 12-2. ***A***, mammogram of surgical specimen from a patient with breast cancer, showing the tumor as a dense (white) mass in the center with "crablike" extensions. ***B***, mammogram showing microcalcifications, which appear as a cluster of small, white specks in the center of the image. Courtesy of Edward Sickles, MD, University of California, San Francisco.

performing the test, an experienced cytologist, and good clinical judgment.

The ultimate proof that a patient has breast cancer must, as in years past, come from a biopsy. In most cases, this can be done under local anesthetic. It may be a needle core, an incisional, or an excisional biopsy. It is rare that a patient will have a biopsy and definitive therapy at the same time unless she has previously had at least an FNA biopsy. If a lesion is seen on mammography but cannot be palpated, needle localization is performed. The tips of two needles are placed in the center of the lesion under mammographic guidance. The removed specimen is then x-rayed to determine that the abnormality originally seen on mammography has been totally excised. In addition, the patient should have a follow-up mammogram in 6 to 12 weeks to confirm complete excision. If there is any suspicion of inflammatory breast cancer, a skin biopsy should be obtained at the time of breast biopsy. If there is reason to suspect Paget's disease of the nipple, a separate biopsy of the nipple should be performed at the time a mass deeper in the breast is biopsied.

Early Diagnosis and Screening

Routine screening mammography will reduce breast cancer mortality by at least 30%. No strategy has been shown to have a larger impact on breast cancer mortality, and the use of a screening modality has not been as well established for any other disease. Since these estimates of benefit were derived from randomized clinical trials, lead-time and length biases do not confound the results. Since many of the patients randomized to the screened groups in these studies may have been noncompliant, the reduction in mortality among women older than 50 who actually obtain regular screening may be as high as 39%.[29] This translates into a reduction in all-cause mortality of 1.5% to 2% for women older than 50. Although mammography *may* pick up some cancers that would never cause symptoms or lead to death if undetected, there is very little evidence of this in the studies conducted thus far.

Major controversies surrounding the use of mammography center on the benefits for women aged 40 to 49 and on the optimal frequency for obtaining mammograms. Without exception, randomized and case control studies of mammography have demonstrated a benefit in women aged 50 and older (Fig 12-3, A).[29-32] In contrast, the results of studies among younger women are contradictory: some demonstrate a benefit, while others show an increase in breast cancer mortality among younger women randomized to the screened group (Fig 12-3, B).[29-32] Most of these trials, especially the earlier ones, were not designed to evaluate the efficacy of mammography in younger women independently of assessment in older women. Since the incidence of breast cancer is smaller among younger women, a substantially larger trial is needed to reliably demonstrate a 30% reduction in mortality. Thus, the results shown in Fig 12-3, B may be due to the play of chance in a series of inadequate studies. In the earliest studies, mammography was clearly less capable of detecting breast cancer in the younger, more dense breast. However, the percentage of cancers detected by mammography alone (ie, not detectable on physical examination) appears to be approximately the same in younger and older women when modern mammographic techniques are used. One study has demonstrated a statistically significant reduction in mortality from screening women aged 40 to 49. In this study, the Health Insurance Plan (HIP) of New York study, no survival benefit emerged during the first decade of follow-up, but at year 9 the survival curves of the screened and control groups began to separate.[33] By the 18th year, a 23% reduction in mortality was apparent for women aged 40 to 49. No other trial has a similar duration of follow-up. These data suggest that a cohort of younger women with a more indolent form of the disease benefit from screening. This possibility has been given credence by other studies that demonstrate a longer sojourn time for breast cancer among older women.[29] Practically, this means that there may be a longer interval for older women during which breast cancer has not metastasized to distant organs but still can be detected by mammography. It is plausible that the ideal frequency for mammograms in younger women may be higher than in older women. However, it is difficult to recommend more frequent mammograms for younger women not only because of the lack of properly controlled trials evaluating this hypothesis but also because of the substantial increase in cost. Since breast cancer is substantially less common among younger women, the cost of screening will be proportionally much greater, relative to any benefit.[34] For this reason, various professional groups evaluating this information have reached different conclusions about the appropriate public health policy for screening women aged 40 to 49.

The optimal frequency for screening older women also has not been established by randomized trials. The original HIP trial and the American Breast Cancer Detection Demonstration Project (BCDDP) used a 1-year interval. In other countries, 2- and 3-year frequencies have been used. All these intervals have been shown to reduce breast cancer mortality in women aged 50 and older. It seems plausible that the maximum benefit is achieved when a yearly interval is used, but it is plausible that a substantial portion of the benefit is achieved with less frequent intervals. These questions could and may be addressed by future randomized controlled studies. Routine mammogra-

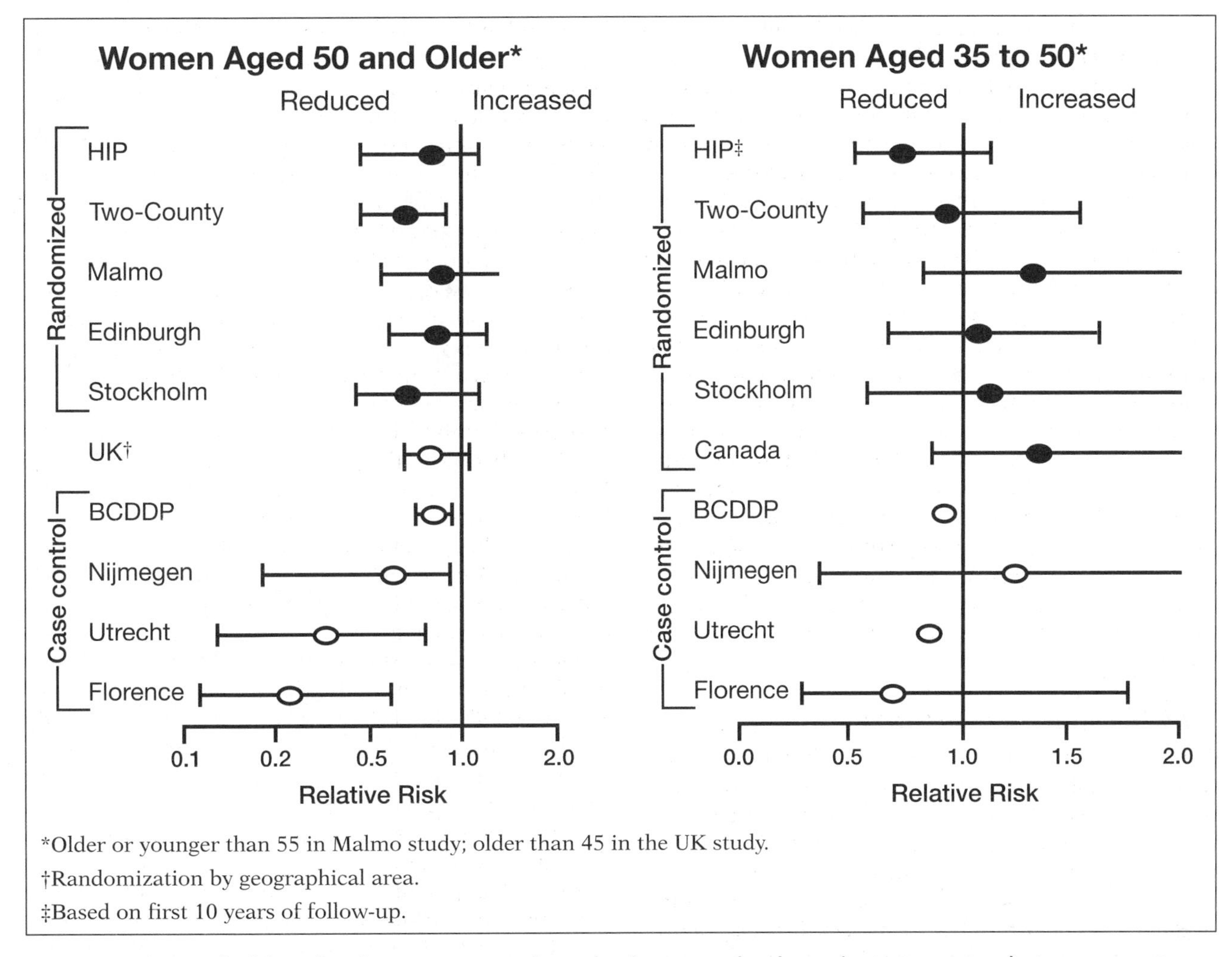

Fig 12-3. Relative risk of dying from breast cancer in randomized and case control studies evaluating mammography in asymptomatic women. A solid dot to the left of the vertical line at 1.0 indicates that patients screened at regular intervals by mammography had a lower mortality rate than unscreened patients. If the dot is to the right of the solid line, the mortality rate in screened patients was higher than that of controls. The horizontal lines extending from each dot represent the 95% confidence interval (CI) for that study. If the CI crosses the vertical line, then the effect of mammography on breast cancer mortality did not reach a level of conventional statistical significance ($P \leq .05$). In some studies, such as the HIP trial, the reduction in mortality was statistically significant when women in both age groups were analyzed together. For example, the overall reduction of breast cancer mortality was 29% (95% CI, 11-44) in the HIP study, 31% (95% CI, 17-43) in the two-county study. BCDDP=Breast Cancer Detection Demonstration Project; HIP=Health Insurance Plan (of New York). Adapted from Cancer Research Campaign,[30] Day,[29] Miller et al,[31] and Morrison et al.[32]

phy will reduce breast cancer mortality in women in their 70s or 80s, just as it does for younger women. However, there are no data on which to base recommendations for stopping mammograms if a woman has had 15 or 20 sequential yearly evaluations. At least one study suggests that there may be a time beyond which continual mammograms have only a marginal benefit. At the other end of the scale, there are no data on which to base recommendations for obtaining a so-called baseline mammogram, and this recommendation has recently been dropped by the ACS.

Patients who perform routine BSE present with smaller lesions. It is well established that women with early-stage breast cancer have a better survival. For example, using a staging system similar to that outlined in Table 12-3, the 5-year relative survival rates for patients with stage I, II, III, and IV breast cancer have been reported to be 86%, 58%, 46%, and 12%, respectively.[29] Unfortunately, most of the studies of BSE are subject to length and lead-time biases. Randomized trials in St Petersburg, Russia, and the United Kingdom have not demonstrated a survival benefit for BSE. However, these studies do not rule out a benefit as large as half of that seen with mammography. In light of the very low costs associated with the performance of BSE, the cost-to-benefit ratio of this method of early detection favors its use despite potentially smaller benefits. For this reason, the lack of data from randomized trials need not be used as a rationale for abandoning BSE altogether.

There is no role for thermography, diaphanography, ultrasound, or other methods of routine screening.

Recommendations for Screening

In the United States, the most widely used recommendations for screening mammography are those of the ACS (Table 12-4),[35,36] which represent the considered opinions of experts in radiology, cancer treatment, and epidemiology throughout the US and are based on a consideration of all the facts summarized above.

Table 12-4. American Cancer Society Recommendations for Screening

Age	Examination	Frequency
20-39	Breast self-examination	Monthly
	Clinical examination*	Every 3 years
40-49	Breast self-examination	Monthly
	Clinical examination*	Yearly
	Mammography*	Every 1-2 years
≥50	Breast self-examination	Monthly
	Clinical examination*	Yearly
	Mammography*	Yearly

*Recommendations agreed on by the American Cancer Society, American Academy of Family Physicians, the American Association of Women Radiologists, the American College of Radiology, the American Medical Association, the American Osteopathic College of Radiology, the American Society of Therapeutic Radiology and Oncology, the American Society of Clinical Oncology, the American Society of Internal Medicine, the College of American Pathologists, the National Cancer Institute, and the National Medical Association.[35] For recommendations by other American groups and by public health agencies in other countries, see Stomper and Gelman.[36]

Histology and Prognostic Factors

Almost all cancers arising in the breast will be adenocarcinomas. About 80% of these will be infiltrating ductal carcinomas and 10% lobular (or small-cell) carcinomas. The prognoses of these two major histologic types are identical. Their behavior differs primarily in the slightly greater tendency for lobular tumors to present in both breasts and to metastasize to meningeal and serosal surfaces. A number of different histologic patterns constitute the remaining 10% of breast cancers, but most have a slightly to somewhat better prognosis than infiltrating ductal or lobular breast cancer. The largest of these, accounting for about 5% of all breast cancers, is the medullary type. Medullary carcinomas less frequently metastasize to regional lymph nodes and are characterized by a mononuclear cell infiltrate surrounding the tumor. However, medullary carcinomas with nodal metastases have about the same prognosis as node-positive ductal carcinomas. Pure tubular carcinomas have an extremely good prognosis, but this is not necessarily true of cancers with "tubular elements."

The rare nonadenocarcinomas include squamous cell carcinoma, which has a worse prognosis than adenocarcinoma; cystosarcoma phyllodes; and angiosarcoma, which should be treated in a manner similar to sarcomas in other parts of the body.

Staging

Clinical staging systems for breast cancer were first developed in the 1930s to identify patients most likely to be cured by radical mastectomy. Since a mastectomy was performed immediately after biopsy and during the same general anesthesia, staging was completed before any surgery was undertaken and, of necessity, was based on physical findings. The most important of these findings were tumor size, the presence of palpable lymphadenopathy, and the appearance of "grave" signs, such as skin ulceration, satellite nodules, fixation to the chest wall, matted lymph nodes, or supraclavicular lymphadenopathy. This staging system was eminently rational, since patients with the higher clinical stages were more likely to have distant metastases, and patients with distant metastases were unlikely to be cured with local therapies such as surgery and radiotherapy. In subsequent years, greater emphasis was placed on surgical staging, using the pathologist's measurement of tumor size and lymph node involvement. Since surgery will already have been performed, the value of this staging is primarily academic, and it has been used to match cohorts of patients in an effort to compare the efficacy of various forms of treatment.

Many as yet undetermined factors are at least as important prognostically as histologic node involvement and tumor size, with the result that randomized clinical trials have largely supplanted this method of evaluating treatment effects. In more recent years, patients perceived to have a worse prognosis have been subjected to early systemic therapy (eg, adjuvant chemotherapy or high-dose chemotherapy and bone marrow transplant) because of the limited value of local treatment alone in this group of patients, but it has not been shown that patients in the worst prognostic categories are more likely to benefit from systemic treatment.

Despite the widespread search for better prognostic factors, no single factor is as predictive as the number of involved lymph nodes or tumor size. The 10-year survival rate in patients without histologically involved nodes is about 65% to 70%. Each involved node worsens the patient's prognosis, but by convention patients have been divided into three groups: those with 1 to 3 involved nodes (10-year survival rate, 48% to 63%), 4 to 9 nodes (10-year survival rate, 28%), and ≥10 positive lymph nodes (10-year survival rate, 18%). Patients with larger tumor size are more likely to have histologically involved nodes, but within any nodal category, tumor size is an independent prognostic factor. Thus, in one series, the 10-year recurrence and mortality rates were 9% and 7%, respectively, among patients with node-negative tumors ≤1 cm, and 17% and 14%, respectively, for patients with node-negative tumors ≤2 cm.[37]

Newer Prognostic Factors

Since most patients with histologically involved lymph nodes are now treated with some form of early systemic (adjuvant) therapy, considerable emphasis is placed on identifying the node-negative patients who need (or do not need) this therapy because the breast cancer is likely to recur despite adequate local treatment.

The earliest staging systems were based on the assumption that stage was related to the length of time the cancer had been growing prior to diagnosis. For this reason, lower stage numbers were referred to as "early." However, the great variability in survival among patients within each stage suggests that intrinsic biologic factors are as important as the length of time the tumor has been growing. For example, the tumor's histologic differentiation (ie, the degree to which it forms glands and the extent to which individual cells have cytoplasmic and nuclear characteristics similar to those of normal breast cells) reflects the tumor's invasive and metastatic potential. Undifferentiated tumors are more likely to recur than well-differentiated tumors, even when they are small and node negative. Although several grading systems score the degree of differentiation, the Scarf-Bloom-Richardson (SBR) system is most commonly used. A low number reflects a well-differentiated and "good prognostic" tumor; a SBR score of 9 is at the other end of the scale.[38] A major drawback of histologic grading is the lack of reproducibility from one pathologist to another. In some studies, tumors graded at one end of the scale by one pathologist may be at the opposite end according to another.

It has long been known that patients who respond to endocrine therapy have more slowly growing tumors. Tumors with an estrogen receptor (ER) or a progesterone receptor (PR), or both, are more likely to respond to endocrine therapy; thus, it is not surprising that they are more likely to relapse later than tumors without a receptor. Determining ER or PR values is an important part of the initial evaluation of a tumor, because it is helpful in selecting between adjuvant endocrine and chemotherapy as well as in providing prognostic information. It is more helpful in node-positive than node-negative patients, since the survival of node-negative patients with a receptor-positive tumor will be only 4% to 8% better than the survival of those with receptor-negative tumors at the end of 5 years.

Tumors with multiple mitotic figures have a worse prognosis. Thus, it is not surprising that other measures of increased DNA synthetic activity are also associated with a worse prognosis. These include thymidine-labeling indices (TLI); S-phase fraction (SPF), determined by flow cytometry; and increased Ki-67, as measured by immunocytochemistry. Although all these tests are used frequently today, there are no generally agreed-on values that define a "bad prognostic" or a "good prognostic" tumor. Frequently all values above the median are treated as "bad," but this obscures the fact that these tests all measure a continuous variable. The prognosis differs little in patients with a tumor just above and just below the median value. The difference is likely to be much less than the difference in prognosis between a patient with four positive lymph nodes and one with three positive nodes.

Ploidy, or the DNA index, is determined by flow cytometry, and, like histologic grading, is a measure of the tumor differentiation. Although some studies demonstrate a good correlation between aneuploidy and poor prognosis, others fail to confirm this, especially for node-negative patients, and this test is used less frequently than the others. Tumors capable of generating new blood vessels are more likely to grow rapidly and to metastasize, and it has been shown that tumors that stain with monoclonal antibodies directed at blood vessels have a worse prognosis than those without evidence of increased blood vessel development (angiogenesis). The value of this test relative to other prognostic factors and the reproducibility of scoring from one pathologist to another have not yet been fully established.

Before a prognostic factor is used routinely, the relationship between cutoff values and recurrence or survival should be well established in independent studies, and its importance relative to other, readily available factors should have been demonstrated in a multivariate analysis.[39] A large number of factors have been reported to have prognostic value in one or even several studies, but none meets all the criteria necessary to justify its use outside of the study environment. These include cathepsin D, p53, HER-2/*neu* (*erb*B-2), epidermal growth factor receptor (EGF-R), transforming growth factor alpha (TGF-α), PCNA, heat-shock proteins, pS2, haptoglobin-related protein, urokinase plasminogen activator, *nm*23, tissue ferritin concentrations, laminin receptor expression, cyclic adenosine monophosphate (AMP)-binding protein, and the monoclonal antibody NCRC11.

Thus far, none of the factors described in this section, except the estrogen and progesterone receptors, has been shown to reproducibly predict a patient's response to therapy. Therefore, the primary use of prognostic factors is to define a group of patients whose prognosis is so good after local treatment, without adjuvant systemic therapy, that any degree of toxicity is unacceptable. Many oncologists would define this point as a 10-year recurrence-free survival >90%. The critical question, then, is whether any of these prognostic factors or a constellation of factors can define such a group with certainty. The answer is no. None of the newer prognostic factors, including receptor status, levels of DNA synthetic activity, or ploidy, adds substantially to the information gained from measurement of tumor size and careful measurement of the number of histologically involved lymph nodes.[40]

Evaluation for Metastases

Breast cancer may metastasize to almost any organ in the body. The most common sites are skin, especially around a lumpectomy or mastectomy scar and on the scalp; regional and distant lymph nodes; bone; lung parenchyma; pleura; and liver. The initial evaluation of the patient should include a careful physical examination of these areas. In a patient with stage I or II breast cancer, the yield from performing radiologic studies is small, and for some tests, such as liver and brain scans, the odds of a false-positive exceed the true-positive rate in asymptomatic patients. Patients with metastatic breast cancer have elevations of carcinoembryonic antigen (CEA) and CA15-3, and abnormalities of these tests or abnormal white blood count, platelet count, hematocrit, or liver function studies may provide clues to the presence of occult metastases at relatively low cost. However, as with radiologic tests, these blood tests are infrequently positive in patients with operable breast cancer. If any radiologic tests are to be performed for routine staging, a chest x-ray and bone scan should suffice.

Following the completion of primary therapy, including any adjuvant systemic therapy, patients may find it reassuring to return with some regularity for follow-up. These follow-up evaluations should include a careful physical examination of remaining breast tissue and a mammogram at least once yearly, since the patient is at high risk of developing a second breast cancer. (A second neoplasm will not appreciably alter her overall prognosis if found at an earlier stage than the first breast cancer.) Most tests, such as bone scans, will not become abnormal more than 3 to 6 months prior to the onset of symptoms, and there is no evidence that treatment of metastases while the patient is asymptomatic will substantially improve survival. For this reason, no specific blood test or radiologic evaluation is mandatory, and those selected by the physician to provide some warning of impending problems should be simple, such as a periodic chest x-ray and a limited number of blood tests.

Primary Treatment: Invasive Cancer

Less than one third of all patients with a diagnosis of breast cancer will die of this disease, and the majority of those cured will have benefited from local treatment alone. While no studies have ever been performed in which patients were randomized to receive mastectomy or no local treatment at all, randomized screening trials provide proof that early mastectomy cures more patients than late mastectomy.

While it is clear that some form of local treatment is beneficial, there is almost no evidence that any particular type is superior. More extensive surgery, such as the Halsted radical mastectomy, provides better local control of the disease than lesser operations such as a simple mastectomy or a lumpectomy alone. The addition of radiotherapy to any form of surgery improves local control. However, there is a very poor association between improved local control and long-term survival.[41] This is presumably due to the fact that recurrences in the skin and subcutaneous tissues around the mastectomy or lumpectomy site are blood borne and not a result of inadequate local therapy. Such metastases are harbingers of spread to distant organs that are outside the scope of the local treatment.

Multiple randomized trials have now demonstrated that the 10- to 20-year survival of patients treated with lumpectomy and radiotherapy is equivalent to that achieved with mastectomy or mastectomy plus adjuvant radiotherapy.[42] For example, more than 1,800 women were randomized in the National Surgical Adjuvant Breast Project (NSABP) trial B-06 to treatment with total mastectomy, lumpectomy, or lumpectomy plus radiotherapy. All three groups had node dissection as well. At the end of 8 years, there were significant differences in local failure rates and, to a lesser extent, distant failure, but there were no differences in overall survival (Table 12-5).[43] Because of these results, either a modified radical mastectomy or lumpectomy plus radiotherapy is currently considered optimal local treatment of patients with stage I or II breast cancer.

It is reasonable to ask whether any subset of patients is better treated with one or another of these forms of treatment. If only the effects of treatment on

Table 12-5. Effects of Mastectomy, Lumpectomy, and Lumpectomy Plus Radiotherapy on Eight-Year Survival*

	Node Negative	Node Positive†
	Disease-Free Survival‡	
Total Mastectomy	66	45
Lumpectomy	61§‡	42
Lumpectomy + Radiotherapy	66	47
	Distant-Disease-Free Survival	
Total Mastectomy	74	51
Lumpectomy	70**	49
Lumpectomy + Radiotherapy	71	53
	Overall Survival	
Total Mastectomy	79	60
Lumpectomy	77	60
Lumpectomy + Radiotherapy	83	68

*Results from the National Surgical Adjuvant Breast Project (NSABP) trial B-06; all patients also had axillary node dissection.

†All node-positive patients received adjuvant chemotherapy.

‡An initial local failure within the breast is not counted as an event if patient is free of recurrence in skin and distant sites at end of follow-up period.

§P =.05 vs mastectomy

**P =.03 vs mastectomy (other differences not statistically significant)

From Fisher et al.[43]

survival are considered, the answer is no. However, the only advantage of lumpectomy plus radiotherapy over mastectomy is "cosmetic," with all that this implies regarding quality of life and the patient's sense of body integrity. If inadequate long-term local control is achieved with lumpectomy and radiotherapy, the patient may require a delayed mastectomy. This clearly obviates any advantage of lumpectomy plus radiotherapy. Tumors that cannot be fully excised, including multicentric tumors and very large tumors, are likely to fall into this category. In such cases, the cosmetic defect left by complete excision may approach that of mastectomy. Tumors characterized by multiple, suspicious clusters of microcalcifications scattered throughout the breast are often treated preferentially with mastectomy, especially if several of these lesions have been shown to be cancerous on biopsy. In addition, there is a higher probability of local recurrence following lumpectomy and radiotherapy in patients with a histologic pattern termed extensive intraductal component (EIC).[42] To meet the diagnostic criteria for EIC, ≥25% of the primary cancer focus must be composed of in situ carcinoma; *in addition*, one or more independent foci of in situ carcinoma must be found in otherwise normal breast tissue separate from the primary focus. At a very minimum, these patients should be re-excised, especially if the in situ component extends to the original excision margin, to evaluate the extent of the multicentricity before making a final choice between mastectomy and lumpectomy plus radiotherapy.

For patients electing mastectomy, the breast may be reconstructed at the same time the mastectomy is performed or months, or even years, later. Reconstruction may be performed with a saline or silicone implant, or the patient's own tissue may be used by moving a flap of skin and fat with either the latissimus dorsi or the rectus abdominis (TRAM flap) muscles. Rarely, a free flap is created from gluteus maximus muscles. If the skin over the mastectomy site is inadequate, a tissue expander may be implanted at the time of mastectomy and slowly inflated postmastectomy to stretch the skin before placement of a permanent implant. Not infrequently, a combination of synthetic implant and tissue flap is employed. The patient should review the pros and cons of each procedure with her plastic surgeon before proceeding, since the time required to perform the surgery, the postsurgical recovery time, the complications, and the cosmetic effects of each procedure are distinct.[44]

Primary Treatment: In Situ Cancer

In an American College of Surgeons survey, the incidence of carcinoma in situ prior to 1972 was found to be 1.4%. In the BCDDP screening study conducted between 1973 and 1981, 22% of cancers were of the in situ variety. It is estimated today that approximately 12% of all cancers are in situ. Much of our knowledge regarding the natural history of in situ carcinoma is based on lesions that were palpable or found incidentally before 1972, and it is not clear that this knowledge is entirely applicable to the disease so prevalent today.

The two types of in situ carcinoma—lobular and ductal (or intraductal)—differ in a number of ways. Lobular carcinoma never forms a palpable mass, is rarely the cause of an abnormality on mammography, and is usually found accidentally when some other lesion is biopsied. Ductal carcinoma in situ may form a mass, but is most often diagnosed today as a result of biopsy for microcalcifications seen on mammography. Lobular carcinoma occurs primarily in the premenopausal years, while ductal carcinoma in situ may occur at any age. The single most important distinction between these two types of in situ carcinoma is location. Lobular carcinoma occurs diffusely throughout both breasts, while ductal carcinoma in situ is usually unilateral and frequently found in only one quadrant of one breast. Both forms of in situ carcinoma are associated with a subsequent risk of invasive breast cancer. The latency period between diagnosis and the appearance of invasive cancer may be measured in decades, and risk persists throughout the patient's life. However, subsequent cancers following a diagnosis of lobular carcinoma in situ are equally distributed between both breasts, while a subsequent cancer following a diagnosis of ductal carcinoma in situ will usually be in the ipsilateral breast. Practically, intraductal carcinoma can be fully excised with a lumpectomy, quadrantectomy, or unilateral mastectomy. A unilateral mastectomy for lobular carcinoma in situ decreases the subsequent risk of breast cancer by only 50%. For this reason, lobular carcinoma is increasingly viewed as a risk factor for subsequent breast cancer and more closely related to atypical hyperplasia than to ductal carcinoma in situ.[45] Increasingly, patients with lobular carcinoma in situ are given one of two options: observation with very careful follow-up or bilateral mastectomy.

Conventional therapy for ductal carcinoma in situ has been simple mastectomy without lymph node dissection, since lymph node involvement is rare, especially in patients with small lesions of the noncomedo type. With this procedure, mortality and distant recurrences are usually <2% and have never been reported to exceed 5%. However, it is difficult for patients to understand why mastectomy and lumpectomy plus radiotherapy are considered equivalent options if they have an invasive tumor, while mastectomy is recommended for an in situ lesion. For this reason, it has been impossible to perform randomized trials comparing mastectomy and breast-conserving surgery. Currently, there are six ongoing studies comparing lumpectomy alone with lumpectomy plus radiotherapy in patients with ductal carcinoma in situ. In the most mature of these trials, patients have been followed for an average of 43 months, at which time in situ recurrences within the breast had developed in 10.4% of patients treated with lumpectomy alone and 7.5% of those treated with lumpectomy plus radiotherapy (P=.055); invasive recurrences were seen in 10.5% and 2.9% of the lumpectomy alone and lumpectomy plus radiotherapy patients (P<.001), respectively.[46] Three patients have died, all in the group randomized to lumpectomy and radiotherapy. Based on the early results of this study, lumpectomy plus radiotherapy appears to be a reasonable alternative to mastectomy and provides better short-term control within the breast than lumpectomy alone. It remains to be seen whether long-term survival is as good with either of these treatments as with mastectomy or whether there are some patients who can be treated with lumpectomy only.

Ductal carcinoma in situ should be fully excised in all patients. When a mastectomy is chosen, it should be a simple rather than subcutaneous or modified radical mastectomy. Tylectomy, or lumpectomy, may be a reasonable option if the tumor size is <25 mm in a single focus, the histologic type is noncomedo, all microcalcifications seen on mammography have been removed, and the patient understands the importance of regular follow-up. Tylectomy plus radiotherapy is a reasonable option for all other patients if the tumor can be fully excised, but the patient should understand that the addition of radiotherapy is likely to decrease the chances of a local recurrence even if the tumor is small and noncomedo.

Adjuvant Systemic Therapy

Patients die from breast cancer because of metastases to distant organs that occur years or months prior to the diagnosis. Since these metastases cannot be detected by physical examination or radiologic evaluation, they are referred to as "micrometastases." Their growth will be largely unaffected by surgery or radiotherapy directed at the breast and regional lymph nodes. However, adjuvant systemic therapy (chemotherapy or endocrine therapy given immediately after local treatment) will substantially reduce the number of cancer cells in these metastatic foci. This adjuvant therapy may actually eradicate all of these micrometastases in some cases, but it is not known whether this ever happens. It certainly does not happen frequently. Since a single focus of micrometastasis may consist of almost one billion cells and still be undetectable, adjuvant therapy may substantially reduce the number of cancer cells in these foci without eradicating the micrometastases altogether. When this happens, the woman's life will be prolonged even if she is not cured. This is likely the most common effect of adjuvant systemic therapy.

Several hundred adjuvant therapy trials have, together, enrolled more than 100,000 women. As often happens when so many studies have been performed, results are somewhat contradictory. To circumvent this problem, a meta-analysis, or overview, of these trials has been done that provides the most accurate summary of our current knowledge regarding adjuvant treatment.[47] Adjuvant chemotherapy or ovarian ablation given to premenopausal women or adjuvant tamoxifen given to postmenopausal women will reduce the odds of death by approximately 25% annually. At the end of 10 years, the survival of patients with positive lymph nodes who are given adjuvant systemic therapy will be about 10% better than that of patients not given this therapy. This does not mean that only 10% of the patients have benefited, or that 10% of the patients have been cured. The improvement arises from the fact that most patients have had some prolongation of survival, even though most have not been cured of their disease. It is impossible to calculate the average prolongation of survival for these women, but a rough estimate might be derived from comparing median survival in recipients and nonrecipients of adjuvant therapy. The difference in median survival is approximately 2 years. Of course, some patients may have derived a much shorter prolongation of survival, while others may have had their lives prolonged by a decade or more.

Adjuvant chemotherapy will reduce the odds of death for women with negative lymph nodes by 25% per year, just as it does for patients with positive lymph nodes. However, since many fewer women are at risk of recurrence among the negative-node group, the absolute difference in survival at the end of 10 years will be much smaller. For those with a low to average risk of recurrence, the 10-year survival difference might be only 2%. For a group considered to be at high risk of recurrence because of poor tumor differentiation, high S-phase fraction, or other factors (see above), the 10-year survival advantage from receiving adjuvant systemic therapy might be as high as 6%. Because the absolute survival advantage for treating node-negative patients (2% to 6%) is smaller than for treating node-positive patients (10%), a physician must carefully weigh the benefits of therapy against the toxicities the patient will experience before recommending treatment, especially adjuvant chemotherapy, for node-negative patients.[48]

Adjuvant chemotherapy is about half as effective as adjuvant tamoxifen in postmenopausal women.[47] Adjuvant tamoxifen has not been adequately studied in premenopausal women, but the available evidence suggests that it may be somewhat less effective than adjuvant chemotherapy or ovarian ablation. If chemotherapy plus tamoxifen is administered to postmenopausal women, there may be some added benefit compared with using tamoxifen alone, but many studies have failed to demonstrate any added benefit. Many postmenopausal women and their physicians are likely to conclude that the benefit is too small or too uncertain to justify the additional toxicity that occurs when chemotherapy is added to tamoxifen. Among premenopausal women, it has not been shown that tamoxifen provides additional benefit once chemotherapy has been given, but studies are under way to evaluate this question more carefully in premenopausal women with receptor-positive tumors.

A second generation of adjuvant therapy trials has been undertaken to determine the best chemotherapy regimen and the ideal duration of treatment.[49] These studies have established that a combination of cytotoxic drugs is better than a single agent. However, no regimen has been shown to be better than cyclophosphamide, methotrexate, and 5-fluorouracil (CMF), which was described in one of the earliest trials.[50] A combination of cyclophosphamide plus doxorubicin (or Adriamycin) (CA) is often used, and randomized trials have demonstrated that this is at least equivalent to CMF. Both regimens cause nausea, vomiting, myelosuppression, and thrombocytopenia. Adjuvant chemotherapy may also increase the risk of secondary leukemia, but the benefits clearly outweigh this risk in node-positive patients.[40] More visits to the physician's office and intravenous injections are required with CMF. CA is associated with more rapid and total hair loss and may cause heart damage. Adjuvant chemotherapy should be administered for longer than 1 month, but there is no evidence that a treatment period in excess of 4 months imparts additional benefit. Presumably the optimal treatment duration is either 3 or 4 months, but available evidence is inadequate to choose between these. Tamoxifen should be administered for at least 2 years. It has been given safely to many women for up to 5 years, but as yet there is no evidence of additional benefit from treatment periods in excess of 5 years. For women over age 50, the optimal duration of treatment may be somewhere between 2 and 5 years.[47] Although tamoxifen has very few short-term side effects, some patients experience mild nausea, hot flashes if postmenopausal, or menstrual irregularities if premenopausal. An increased incidence of endometrial cancer has also been seen, and this risk may be greater with more prolonged administration.[51]

Many questions are currently being addressed in ongoing studies. Because it is not clear that chemotherapy and ovarian ablation produce equivalent results in premenopausal women, the former is the preferred adjuvant systemic treatment for premenopausal women until such trials have been completed. Adjuvant therapy is usually begun within the first month of completion of surgery or surgery plus radiotherapy, but there is no evidence that a somewhat longer delay is harmful, nor is there evidence that beginning chemotherapy before surgery or radiotherapy ("neoadjuvant therapy") is more effective than postoperative systemic therapy. It is common practice in many centers to excise the tumor fully and administer chemotherapy for 4 to 6 months before administering radiotherapy. There is no evidence that this delay in radiotherapy compromises local control of the disease, nor is there evidence from properly controlled trials that this approach improves survival. The reduction in chemotherapeutic dose will compromise the survival benefit achieved with more conventional chemotherapeutic doses, but there is no evidence that escalation of chemotherapy dose, including the use of very-high-dose chemotherapy with autologous bone marrow transplant, imparts any survival advantage over that achieved with conventional chemotherapy, even in patients with many positive lymph nodes.

Because the field of adjuvant systemic therapy is evolving so rapidly, it is difficult to make firm recommendations regarding use. There are several situations in which agreement is nearly universal that treatment is indicated. These include the use of chemotherapy for premenopausal women with histologically involved nodes and the use of tamoxifen for postmenopausal women with an ER-positive tumor, whether node positive or node negative (Table 12-6). A consensus conference held in 1991 concluded that the prognosis of patients with tumors <1 cm in diameter was so good that adjuvant systemic therapy should not be used. No data have emerged since to reverse that recommendation. For other groups of patients, there is controversy regarding the optimal treatment, and physician judgment coupled with a thorough and current knowledge of the medical literature is required. For postmenopausal, node-positive patients with ER-negative tumors, adjuvant tamoxifen has been shown to have as much benefit as adjuvant chemotherapy.[47] However, since the benefit from either of these therapies is very small in these patients, some physicians will opt for no adjuvant treatment at all. In other clinical situations shown in Table 12-6 as requiring "physician judgment," the benefits may be considered too small to justify the toxicity of chemotherapy (eg, in premenopausal, node-negative, ER-negative patients) or are still somewhat uncertain (eg, premenopausal, node-negative, ER-positive patients or postmenopausal, node-negative, ER-negative patients).

Treatment of Metastatic Breast Cancer

Once breast cancer has metastasized to distant organs, it is not curable. However, this does not mean that death is imminent, since half the patients will live >2 years and as many as 10% will live more than a decade. Most of these patients will require several types of therapy, and each therapeutic decision should be made with an eye to its impact on subsequent decisions. When properly used, treatment will substantially improve the patient's quality of life, even when the treatment has many side effects. Despite its toxicities, chemotherapy is often more effective than pain medications and supportive treatment alone in relieving pain from bone metastases. Although the primary goal in treating patients with metastatic breast cancer is relief of symptoms, these therapies do prolong survival as well. It is possible that when all therapies are considered together, the median survival may be prolonged as much as 6 months to a year.[52] However, there is no evidence that treating an asymptomatic patient with metastatic breast cancer will have a greater impact on survival than waiting until the patient's first symptoms appear. For this reason, some physicians will elect to use a new or innovative therapy when a patient is asymptomatic and desires treatment, saving therapies with proven palliative value until the patient is symptomatic.

Surgery, radiotherapy, chemotherapy, and endocrine therapy all have a role in the management of metastatic breast cancer. This disease never metastasizes to a single focus, and for this reason systemic therapies are used more often than surgery and radiotherapy. However, there are some situations in which surgery or radiotherapy will be clearly more effective, and there are others in which the pace of the disease may justify delaying the initiation of systemic treatment.

- About 10% of patients with metastatic breast cancer will eventually have symptoms from metastases to the central nervous system. Patients with headache, seizure, localized neurologic deficits, or personality change should have a CT scan or MRI and lumbar puncture. The treatment of choice for brain metastases or metastases to the choroid, which usually can be seen on funduscopic examination, is dexamethasone followed immediately by radiotherapy.
- Most patients with metastases to bone will have multiple involved sites, but if a lytic lesion has eroded >50% of the cortex of a weight-bearing bone, a combination of surgery and radiotherapy should be considered. Although systemic treatment and radiotherapy, alone or in combination, will relieve pain and may result in healing of this lytic area, it will be many months, or even years, before normal tensile strength is regained, if it is regained at all.
- A local recurrence on the chest wall is always a harbinger of distant disease, but if it is the only site of metastasis after a long disease-free interval (eg, 5 to 10 years from mastectomy to recurrence), it may be many months or years before another local recurrence or distant recurrence is identified. Under these circumstances, surgery alone, radiotherapy alone, or a combination of these without systemic therapy may be reasonable treatment.
- Malignant pleural effusions are frequently a manifestation of metastatic breast cancer, and these often persist even when disease at other sites responds to systemic therapy. The optimal management of symptomatic effusions may require chest tube drainage and sclerosis.
- When there are multiple metastatic sites, systemic therapy should be used. About one third of patients will respond to endocrine treatment and about two thirds will respond to chemotherapy. The characteristics of patients likely to benefit from endocrine treatment are well established and include an ER-positive and/or PR-positive tumor, a disease-free interval >2 years, disease limited to soft tissue and bone, late premenopausal or postmenopausal status, and prior response to endocrine treatment.[22] Approximately two thirds of patients who have one or several of these characteristics will respond to endocrine treatment. The factors predictive of a response to chemotherapy are not nearly as well defined. In general, however, chemotherapy candi-

Table 12-6. Minimum Recommendations for Using Adjuvant Therapy

	Premenopausal Patients	Postmenopausal Patients
Node Positive		
ERP* Negative	CMF x 6 mos or CA x 4 mos	PHYSICIAN JUDGMENT†: *No Adjuvant or TAM x 2-5 Yrs or Chemotherapy**
ERP Positive	CMF x 6 mos or CA x 4 mos	TAM x 2-5 yrs
Node Negative, T>1 cm		
ERP Negative	PHYSICIAN JUDGMENT†: *No Adjuvant or CMF x 6 Mos* *CA x 4 mos*	PHYSICIAN JUDGMENT†: *No Adjuvant or TAM x 2-5 yrs*
ERP Positive	PHYSICIAN JUDGMENT†: *No Adjuvant or Tam x 2-5 yrs*	TAM x 2-5 yrs
Node Negative, T≤1cm	NO TREATMENT	NO TREATMENT

*Estrogen receptor protein.

†Areas of controversy; read text carefully.

CMF = cyclophosphamide orally and methotrexate plus 5-fluorouracil intravenously, monthly for 6 cycles.

CA = cyclophosphamide and doxorubicin (Adriamycin) intravenously, every 3 weeks for 5 cycles.

TAM = tamoxifen, 10 mg orally twice daily

dates are those who have either failed to respond to endocrine therapy or who do not have any of the characteristics described above. A 65-year-old woman with an ER-negative tumor that recurs on the chest wall and in several bony sites 5 years after mastectomy might reasonably be treated with endocrine therapy, since she has many, even if not all, of the characteristics of a patient who will respond to endocrine therapy. A 35-year-old woman with an ER-positive tumor that recurs in the liver and brain 6 months after mastectomy might be better treated with immediate chemotherapy despite her positive receptor status. The median duration of response to endocrine therapy is usually about 12 months; median duration of response to chemotherapy is closer to 9 months, reflecting the fact that endocrine therapy patients are more likely to have an indolent form of breast cancer. However, responses of several years, or even a decade, may be seen following treatment with either modality. There is no evidence that patients will respond more rapidly to chemotherapy than to endocrine treatment.

Endocrine Therapy

Since patients who respond to one form of endocrine therapy have a better than average chance of responding to a second at the time of disease progression, endocrine therapies are usually administered in sequence. There is very little evidence that one endocrine treatment is better than another. Therefore, the least toxic treatment is used first. In postmenopausal women, this is generally considered to be tamoxifen. When patients progress, they are then treated with progestins (megestrol acetate or medroxyprogesterone) or aminoglutethimide. The rare patient who responds sequentially to all three of these could then be treated with estrogens; androgens are usually left as a last form of endocrine treatment because they are slightly less effective than estrogens. For premenopausal women, either tamoxifen or ovarian ablation (oophorectomy, radiation therapy to the ovary, or a luteinizing hormone-releasing hormone [LHRH] agonist) is roughly equivalent in efficacy and toxicity. If the premenopausal woman has responded to both these therapies, then progestins or aminoglutethimide might be used. Aminoglutethimide is not effective in women who have not had ovarian ablation, but progestins may be considered as an alternative to either first-line treatment. When a patient progresses after responding to endocrine therapy, merely discontinuing the therapy may result in a further response. This is especially true after estrogen therapy, but also has been observed after tamoxifen treatment. There is no evidence that combinations of endocrine therapy are more effective than a single agent, nor are alternating regimens of endocrine treatment superior. Combinations of chemotherapy plus endocrine treatment will result in a higher response rate than endocrine therapy alone, but such combinations do not result in better survival and will deny some patients the opportunity of a response with minimal toxicity. There is no evidence that higher doses of any hormone therapy have an advantage over conventional dosages.

In general, endocrine therapies are less toxic than chemotherapy. However, approximately 10% of patients with breast cancer will develop hypercalcemia during the course of their disease, and oftentimes this occurs as part of a "flare" after the initiation of endocrine therapy.[22] Although the mechanism of flare is not well understood, it is characterized by diffuse aching, increased pain at sites of known disease, erythema around the sites of skin metastases, and hypercalcemia that can be life threatening. These symptoms usually occur within a few days to a few weeks of the start of treatment, but the course will be self-limited in most cases, even if endocrine treatment is continued. If calcium values exceed 14 mg/dL, it is prudent to discontinue the endocrine therapy. If the calcium values are below this level, continuation of the endocrine treatment with intravenously administered fluids, diuretics, bisphosphonates, and careful observation is reasonable. Flare also can be seen following endocrine ablation (oophorectomy, adrenalectomy, hypophysectomy) or, rarely, chemotherapy. Patients who respond to endocrine or chemotherapy may also have a transient elevation of tumor markers, such as CEA or CA15-3, and increased intensity of abnormal areas on bone scans. For these reasons, evaluation of response to therapy may be difficult and, whenever possible, the patient should be kept on therapy for at least 3 months unless there is unequivocal evidence of disease progression.

Chemotherapy

A wide array of cytotoxic drugs has been shown to induce response in patients with breast cancer, but only a handful have established roles in the treatment of early or advanced disease.[53] These include cyclophosphamide (C), doxorubicin (A), methotrexate (M), and 5-fluorouracil (F), the drugs most commonly used in combinations as "first line" for patients who have failed or who are not good candidates for endocrine treatment. Mitomycin C is frequently used alone or with vinblastine in patients who have failed these first-line regimens. Recently, taxol has been shown to be very effective in the treatment of metastatic breast cancer, including tumors that have proven resistant to doxorubicin. Taxol combinations have not been fully developed, and the value of taxol relative to the more established treatments is not yet clear. Mitoxantrone and epirubicin are active agents with somewhat less toxicity than doxorubicin; each is available in some countries. Ifosfamide, cisplatin, carboplatin, and etoposide all have shown some activity in patients without prior chemotherapy, but they have no role in patients resistant to cyclophosphamide or doxorubicin.

When chemotherapy is begun for the first time after the diagnosis of metastasis, a combination of drugs is usually employed. The most popular combination regimens are similar to those used in the adjuvant setting: CMF, CA, or CAF. The optimal duration of chemotherapy for women with metastatic breast cancer is clearly >3 months and likely >6 months, but there is no evidence that continuous treatment beyond a year or so will result in a much better quality of life or longer survival than shorter courses. There is also no evidence that crossover to a new combination of drugs or that alternating chemotherapy combinations has any advantage over the use of a single regimen until disease progression. Thus, all treatment might reasonably be stopped after a year in patients who have had a response and who are asymptomatic. About 20% to 30% of patients will respond to second-line regimens when the disease has become resistant to the initial regimen, but there is no evidence that these second-line regimens prolong survival, that a combination of drugs is better than a single agent in this setting, or that net quality of life is substantially improved by chemotherapy in the end stages of the disease. A variety of high-dose chemotherapy combinations with autologous bone marrow transplant are being tested in patients with metastatic disease, but there is no evidence that this treatment prolongs life to a greater extent than conventional doses.[53]

Special Problems

Stage III Breast Cancer

Patients with stage III breast cancer fall into three broad categories: those who have technically operable breast cancer and are classified as stage III by virtue of tumor size, those who have inoperable breast cancer because of extensive skin involvement or attachment to the chest wall, and those with inflammatory breast cancer.

Patients with operable breast cancer may reasonably be treated with mastectomy and adjuvant therapy following the same principles as in the management of patients with stage II disease. Some of these patients can even be treated with lumpectomy and radiotherapy if sufficient breast tissue remains after the tumor has been fully excised. Many physicians prefer to use radiotherapy or chemotherapy first. Although this is a reasonable option, there is very little or no evidence that it provides better long-term local control or survival.

Patients with inoperable stage III breast cancer may live for long periods despite poor prognostic features. In one series, the 5-year survival of patients treated with radiotherapy alone was 38%.[54] More commonly, these patients are treated with chemotherapy or endocrine therapy before or after radiotherapy, and randomized trials have shown that this imparts a survival benefit.[55]

Inflammatory breast cancer has a much worse prognosis than either of the other two forms of stage III disease. This is true whether the disease is diagnosed on the basis of symptoms or because of dermal lymphatic invasion found only on biopsy of the skin. Following mastectomy alone, inflammatory breast cancer recurs frequently and rapidly on the chest wall. The use of chemotherapy as a primary modality substantially and significantly improves the survival of these patients.[56] Radiotherapy is invariably added, and the use of mastectomy in addition to radiotherapy will improve local control. However, it is not clear that this will improve overall survival.

Pregnancy

Breast cancer is particularly difficult to diagnose in the engorged breast during pregnancy and lactation. However, the most recent studies suggest that these patients do as well as nonpregnant patients who receive a diagnosis at a similar stage, and treatment is nearly the same. There is no evidence that survival will be prolonged if the fetus is aborted. The tumor can usually be fully excised and mastectomy can be performed during pregnancy. Radiotherapy is usually avoided until after delivery. There is no evidence that chemotherapy administered in the third trimester is teratogenic, but there is also no evidence that delaying chemotherapy until after delivery will substantially compromise the value of adjuvant chemotherapy. For this reason, many physicians and patients prefer to wait.

Most case control studies have failed to demonstrate a harmful effect from pregnancy begun after completion of primary treatment for breast cancer. Very few women choose to become pregnant within 2 years of diagnosis, possibly because of the desire to recover from the emotional trauma associated with breast cancer before undertaking a pregnancy. However, when these patients are matched with women of a similar age and stage who did not become pregnant, their survival is about the same, or possibly even slightly better.

Male Breast Cancer

Male breast cancer occurs at a frequency of about 1/100th that of female breast cancer. The ratio of male to female breast cancer is strikingly similar to the ratio of breast glandular tissue in the two sexes. The natural history of the disease and its treatment are nearly identical. Men who present with a freely movable mass are usually treated with mastectomy and node dissection, since few are concerned about the cosmetic result. Positive lymph nodes have the same prognostic importance in men as they do in women. However, the number of men with breast cancer is too small to evaluate adjuvant treatment in randomized clinical trials. In node-positive patients, an argument can be made for using either chemotherapy or tamoxifen, since male breast cancers may be receptor positive and respond to hormone therapy with about the same frequency as female breast cancers. When metastatic, male breast cancer can be treated with tamoxifen, orchidectomy, progestins, aminoglutethimide, and possibly other endocrine maneuvers. If the cancer is unresponsive to endocrine therapy, the same drugs and drug combinations proven effective in women can be used to palliate male breast cancer.

References

1. Harris JR, Lippman ME, Veronesi U, Willett W. Breast cancer. *N Eng J Med.* 1992; 327:319-328,390-398,473-480.
2. Seidman H, Mushinski MH, Gelb SK, et al. Probabilities of eventually developing or dying of cancer: United States, 1985. *CA Cancer J Clin.* 1985; 35:36-56.
3. Kash KM, Holland JC, Halper MS, Miller DG. Psychological distress and surveillance behaviors of women with a family history of breast cancer. *J Natl Cancer Inst.* 1992; 84:24-30.
4. Bain C, Speizer FE, Rosner B, et al. Family history of breast cancer as a risk indicator for the disease. *Am J Epidemiol.* 1980; 111:301-308.
5. Anderson DE, Badzioch MD. Risk of familial breast cancer. *Cancer.* 1985; 56:383-387.
6. Ottman R, King MC, Pike MC, Henderson BE. Practical guide for estimating risk for familial breast cancer. *Lancet.* 1983; 2:556-558.
7. Malkin D, Li FP, Strong LC, et al. Germ line p53 mutations in a familial syndrome of breast cancer, sarcomas, and other neoplasms. *Science.* 1990; 250:1233-1238.
8. Hall JM, Lee MK, Newman B, et al. Linkage of early-onset familial breast cancer to chromosome 17q21. *Science.* 1990; 250:1684-1689.
9. Dupont WD, Page DL. Risk factors for breast cancer in women with proliferative breast disease. *N Engl J Med.* 1985;312:146-151.
10. Dupont WD, Page DL. Relative risk of breast cancer varies with time since diagnosis of atypical hyperplasia. *Hum Pathol.* 1989;20:723-725.
11. Henderson BE. Endogenous and exogenous endocrine factors. In: Henderson IC, ed. *Endogenous and Exogenous Endocrine Factors.* Philadelphia, Pa: WB Saunders Co; 1989:577-598.

12. Steinberg KK, Thacker SB, Smith SJ, et al. A meta-analysis of the effect of estrogen replacement therapy on the risk of breast cancer. *JAMA.* 1991; 265:1985-1990.

13. Romieu I, Berlin JA, Colditz G. Oral contraceptives and breast cancer: review and meta-analysis. *Cancer.* 1990; 66:2253-2263.

14. Prentice RL, Kakar F, Hursting S, Sheppard L, Klein R, Kushi LH. Aspects of the rationale for the Women's Health Trial. *J Natl Cancer Inst.* 1988; 80:802-814.

15. Howe GR, Hirohata T, Hislop TG, et al. Dietary factors and risk of breast cancer: combined analysis of 12 case-control studies. *J Natl Cancer Inst.* 1990; 82:561-569.

16. Willett WC, Stampfer MJ, Colditz GA, Rosner BA, Hennekens CH, Speizer FE. Dietary fat and the risk of breast cancer. *N Engl J Med.* 1987; 316:22-28.

17. Jones DY, Schatzkin A, Green SB, et al. Dietary fat and breast cancer in the National Health and Nutrition Examination Survey, I: epidemiologic follow-up study. *J Natl Cancer Inst.* 1987; 79:465-471.

18. Longnecker MP, Berlin JA, Orza MJ, Chalmers TC. A meta-analysis of alcohol consumption in relation to risk of breast cancer. *JAMA.* 1988; 260:652-656.

19. Seidman H, Stellman SD, Mushinski MH. A different perspective on breast cancer risk factors: some implications of the nonattributable risk. *CA Cancer J Clin.* 1982; 32: 301-313.

20. Clark GM, Sledge GW Jr, Osborne CK, McGuire WL. Survival from first recurrence: relative importance of prognostic factors in 1,015 breast cancer patients. *J Clin Oncol.* 1987; 5:55-61.

21. Henderson IC. Window of opportunity. *J Natl Cancer Inst.* 1991; 83:894-896.

22. Henderson IC. Endocrine therapy of metastatic breast cancer. In: Harris JR, Hellman S, Henderson IC, Kinne DW, eds. *Breast Diseases.* 2nd ed. Philadelphia, Pa: JB Lippincott Co; 1991:559-603.

23. Chaudary MA, Millis RR, Davies GC, Hayward JL. Nipple discharge: the diagnostic value of testing for occult blood. *Ann Surg.* 1982;196: 651-655.

24. Diagram on BSE special touch: participant's guide. American Cancer Society: 1987.

25. Donegan WL. Evaluation of a palpable breast mass. *N Engl J Med.* 1992; 327:937-942.

26. Beahrs OH, Henson DE, Hutter RVP, Kennedy BJ, eds. *American Joint Committee on Cancer Manual for Staging of Cancer.* 4th ed. Philadelphia, Pa: JB Lippincott Co; 1992:149-154.

27. Kinne DW, Kopans DB. Physical examination and mammography in the diagnosis of breast disease. In: Harris JR, Hellman S, Henderson IC, Kinne DW, eds. *Breast Diseases.* 2nd ed. Philadelphia, Pa: JB Lippincott Co; 1991: 81-106.

28. Layfield LJ, Glasgow BJ, Cramer H. Fine-needle aspiration in the management of breast masses. In: Rosen PP, Fechner RE, eds. *Pathology Annual,* part 2 (volume 24). Norwalk, Conn: Appleton & Lange; 1989: 23-62.

29. Day NE. Screening for breast cancer. *Br Med Bull.* 1991; 47:400-415.

30. Austoker J. Breast cancer screening. *Cancer Research Campaign.* 1991: Factsheet 7.5.

31. Miller AB, Baines CJ, To T, Wall C. Canadian National Breast Screening Study, 1: breast cancer detection and death rates among women aged 40 to 49 years. *Can Med Assoc J.* 1992; 147:1459-1476.

32. Morrison AS, Brisson J, Khalid N. Breast cancer incidence and mortality in the Breast Cancer Detection Demonstration Project. *J Natl Cancer Inst.* 1988; 80:1540-1547.

33. Shapiro S. Determining the efficacy of breast cancer screening. *Cancer.* 1989; 63:1873-1880.

34. Eddy DM, Hasselblad V, McGivney W, Hendee W. The value of mammography screening in women under age 50 years. *JAMA.* 1988; 259:1512-1519.

35. Dodd GD. American Cancer Society guidelines on screening for breast cancer: an overview. *CA Cancer J Clin.* 1992;42:177-180.

36. Stomper PC, Gelman RS. Mammography in symptomatic and asymptomatic patients. In: Henderson IC, ed. *Hematology/Oncology Clinics of North America: Diagnosis and Therapy of Breast Cancer.* Philadelphia, Pa: WB Saunders Co; 1989:611-640.

37. Rosen PP, Groshen S, Saigo PE, Kinne DW, Hellman S. A long-term follow-up study of survival in stage I ($T_1N_0M_0$) and stage II ($T_1N_1M_0$) breast carcinoma. *J Clin Oncol.* 1989; 7:355-366.

38. Elston CW, Ellis IO. Pathological prognostic factors in breast cancer, I: the value of histological grade in breast cancer: experience from a large study with long-term follow-up. *Histopathology.* 1991; 19:403-410.

39. McGuire WL, Clark GM. Prognostic factors and treatment decisions in axillary-node—negative breast cancer. *N Engl J Med.* 1992; 326:1756-1761.

40. Henderson IC. Breast cancer therapy: the price of success. *N Eng J Med.* 1992;326:1774-1775.

41. Fisher B, Anderson S, Fisher ER, et al. Significance of ipsilateral breast tumour recurrence after lumpectomy. *Lancet.* 1991; 338:327-331.

42. Harris JR, Recht A. Conservative surgery and radiotherapy. In: Harris JR, Hellman S, Henderson IC, Kinne DW, eds. *Breast Diseases.* 2nd ed. Philadelphia, Pa: JB Lippincott Co; 1991: 388-419.

43. Fisher B, Redmond C, Poisson R, et al. Eight-year results of a randomized clinical trial comparing total mastectomy and lumpectomy with or without irradiation in the treatment of breast cancer. *N Engl J Med.* 1989;320:822-828.

44. Bostwick J III. Breast reconstruction after mastectomy. In: Harris JR, Hellman S, Henderson IC, Kinne DW, eds. *Breast Diseases.* Philadelphia, Pa: JB Lippincott Co; 1987:668-683.

45. Haagensen CD, Lane N, Lattes R, Bodian C. Lobular neoplasia (so-called lobular carcinoma in situ) of the breast. *Cancer.* 1978; 42:737-769.

46. Fisher B, Costantino J, Redmond C, et al. Lumpectomy compared with lumpectomy and radiation therapy for the treatment of intraductal breast cancer. *N Eng J Med.* 1993; 328:1581-1586.

47. Early Breast Cancer Trialists' Collaborative Group. Systemic treatment of early breast cancer by hormonal, cytotoxic, or immune therapy: 133 randomised trials involving 31,000 recurrences and 24,000 deaths among 75,000 women. *Lancet.* 1992; 339:1-15,71-85.

48. Henderson IC. The nature of the benefit. In: Henderson IC, ed. *Adjuvant Therapy of Breast Cancer.* Boston, Mass: Kluwer Academic Publications; 1992:57-68.

49. Tripathy D, Henderson IC. Systemic adjuvant therapy

of breast cancer. *Curr Opin Oncol.* 1992; 4:1041-1049.

50. Bonadonna G, Brusamolino E, Valagussa P, et al. Combination chemotherapy as an adjuvant treatment in operable breast cancer. *N Engl J Med.* 1976;294:405-410.

51. Fornander T, Cedermark B, Mattsson A, et al. Adjuvant tamoxifen in early breast cancer: occurrence of new primary cancers. *Lancet.* 1989; 1:117-120.

52. Henderson IC, Harris JR. Principles in the management of metastatic disease: integration of local and systemic therapies. In: Harris JR, Hellman S, Henderson IC, Kinne DW, eds. *Breast Diseases.* 2nd ed. Philadelphia, Pa: JB Lippincott Co; 1991:547-558.

53. Henderson IC. Chemotherapy for metastatic disease. In: Harris JR, Hellman S, Henderson IC, Kinne DW, eds. *Breast Diseases.* 2nd ed. Philadelphia, Pa: JB Lippincott Co; 1991:604-665.

54. Sheldon T, Hayes DF, Cady B, et al. Primary radiation therapy for locally advanced breast cancer. *Cancer.* 1987; 60:1219-1225.

55. Rubens RD, Bartelink H, Englesman E, et al. Locally advanced breast cancer: the contribution of cytotoxic and endocrine treatment to radiotherapy. An EORTC breast cancer co-operative group trial (10792). *Eur J Cancer Clin Oncol.* 1989; 25:667-678.

56. Jaiyesimi IA, Buzdar AU, Hortobagyi G. Inflammatory breast cancer: a review. *J Clin Oncol.* 1992; 10:1014-1024.

13

LUNG CANCER

Edward W. Humphrey, MD, Herbert B. Ward, MD, Robert T. Perri, MD

At present, cancer of the lung is the leading cause of death from cancer in both men and women. It is estimated that in 1994 some 28% of all cancer deaths, or 153,000 deaths per year, in the United States were due to lung cancer.[1] Based on estimates for 1993 in *SEER Cancer Statistics Review* using Surveillance, Epidemiology, and End Results program data, 61% of deaths from lung cancer occurred in men and 39% in women.[2] Fig 13-1 illustrates the continuing change in the male-to-female ratio observed for this disease, a change due to the increasing number of women developing cancer of the lung. For people younger than 40 years of age, 55% of lung cancers are in men and 45% in women, whereas in the eighth decade of life, 64.3% are in men and 35.7% in women. While the death rate from cancer of the lung in black women is similar to that in white women, the death rate in black men is 44% greater than in white men. A substantial portion of the increased death rate is associated with increased smoking.[3]

Anatomy

Carcinomas originating in the lung commonly invade adjacent structures, including other thoracic viscera, the chest wall, and the diaphragm. After first traversing the parietal pleura and endothoracic fascia, peripheral carcinomas on the lateral surfaces of the lung may invade the ribs, intercostal nerves, and intercostal muscles. Peripheral carcinomas at the apex of the lung, termed superior sulcus carcinomas, may invade the first rib and the brachial plexus, which is adjacent to the posterior portion of this rib. At particular risk from tumors in this location are the eighth cervical nerve, just above the first rib, and the first thoracic nerve, just below the first rib, which together supply fibers to the ulnar nerve through the medial cord of the brachial plexus. Also at risk for invasion from these tumors is the stellate ganglion, which lies on the upper part of the body of the first thoracic vertebra.

On the right side, the superior vena cava, the inferior vena cava, and the right and left atria are adjacent to the medial side of the lung and may be invaded by central carcinomas or peripheral carcinomas on that side. The phrenic nerve, which runs anterior to the pulmonary hilus on the right surface of the superior vena cava, the pericardium, and inferior vena cava, is also at risk of invasion and paralysis. Posterior to the hilus, the esophagus and the vertebral bodies may be invaded.

On the left side, the arch of the aorta, the left subclavian artery, and the left common carotid artery are adjacent to the medial surface of the lung above the anterior end of the second interspace. The left recurrent laryngeal nerve branches off from the vagus nerve on the lateral surface of the aortic arch and

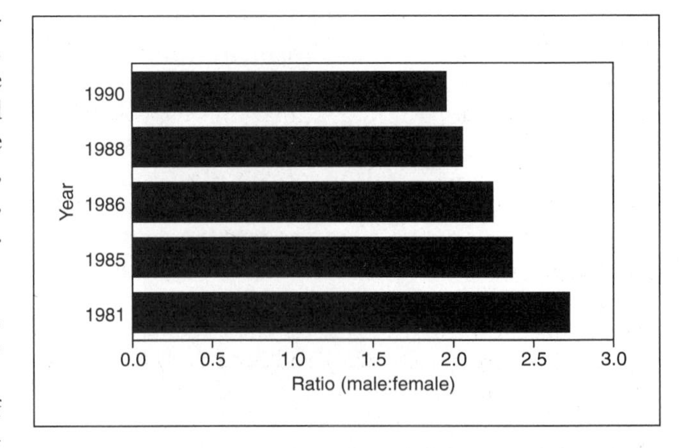

Fig 13-1. Time trends in the male-to-female ratio of lung cancer cases.

Edward W. Humphrey, MD, Professor and Interim Chairman, Department of Surgery, University of Minnesota, Minneapolis, Minnesota

Herbert B. Ward, MD, Assistant Professor, Department of Surgery, University of Minnesota, Minneapolis, Minnesota

Robert T. Perri, MD, Associate Professor, Department of Medicine, University of Minnesota, Minneapolis, Minnesota

encircles the arch. This nerve is frequently paralyzed by carcinoma invading from lymph nodes under the arch of the aorta or from a central carcinoma of or near the left main bronchus. The left atrium and distal portion of the pulmonary artery trunk lie on the left side of the mediastinum, and may also be invaded by a central carcinoma of the lung. As on the right side, the left phrenic nerve may be invaded by carcinoma where it runs on the surface of the pericardium anterior to the hilus of the lung. Posterior to the hilus, the medial surface of the lung is in contact with the descending aorta and vertebral bodies.

The anatomy of the lymph drainage from the lung is described in the section on the natural history of lung cancer.

Risk Factors

Tobacco

Cigarette smoking is by far the most important risk factor for the development of carcinoma of the lung. A woman smoking 1 to 20 cigarettes per day has a 10.3-fold greater risk of developing lung cancer than a woman who has never smoked, while a woman smoking >20 cigarettes per day has a 21.2-fold greater risk. After ≥16 years of cessation, the risk to the first group falls to 1.6 times and to the second to 4.0 times that of a woman who has never smoked.[3] The rate of cancer of the lung in nonsmokers has remained relatively constant over the past 26 years: 12 per 100,000 women and 15 per 100,000 men. Although the prevalences of most histologic types of cancer of the lung have increased with smoking, the most striking rises have been seen in squamous cell carcinoma and small-cell carcinoma. Histologic characteristics of smoking-related carcinoma of the lung, however, are a function of age and sex. Squamous cell carcinoma increases in frequency with age and is more common in men than in women.

Tuberculosis

Carcinoma of the lung can develop in regions of scar, particularly in scars from tuberculosis. In one study, the risk of developing lung cancer in persons with a previous diagnosis of tuberculosis was five times greater in men and ten times greater in women than in the general population.[4] The most common histologic diagnosis of such lesions is adenocarcinoma. The diagnosis of carcinoma in a lung scar is often difficult to make. It is one source of error in percutaneous needle biopsies, and is the reason why any growth in a previously observed lung nodule necessitates an excisional biopsy of that nodule.

Asbestos

The relationship between carcinoma of the lung and asbestos inhalation was first noted in the US in 1935.[5] More recently the magnitude of this risk has been compiled by Selikoff.[6] Men who were asbestos workers have a 6- to 7-fold greater risk of death from cancer than the general population.[6] Indeed, exposure to asbestos for as short as 1 month is associated with an increased risk of cancer after 25 years. Asbestos exposure and cigarette smoking together act synergistically to produce a 53-fold increase in the risk of lung cancer.[7]

Low-Level Radiation

Radon and its decay products are thought by the National Radiological Protection Board to cause 5% of the lung cancer in the United Kingdom after a survey of radon levels in homes. The International Commission on Radiological Protection has estimated that 10% to 30% of lung cancer in the general population can be attributed to radon exposure. For the most part, these estimates are based on extrapolations from risk estimates for uranium and other types of mining. At present there is no direct evidence to incriminate radon or its decay products at the levels found in most homes. More and better data are needed to resolve this question.

Air Pollution

The air pollutant most widely accepted as increasing the risk of lung cancer is passive tobacco smoke. Other air pollutants postulated to increase this risk are diesel exhaust, pitch and tar, dioxin, arsenic, chromium, cadmium, and nickel compounds.

Natural History

As a rule, carcinoma of the lung originates in the cells lining the bronchi. It is probably an oversimplification to think that cigarette smokers have one abnormal cell that becomes malignant, and its progeny then determines the course of the patient's disease. In one study of male cigarette smokers who died of a cause other than carcinoma of the lung, the entire tracheobronchial tree was sectioned.[8] Of those who smoked 1 to 2 packs per day, areas of carcinoma in situ were found in 48%, with an average of 4.3 areas per patient. Of those who smoked 2 packs per day, areas of carcinoma in situ were found in 75%, with an average of 11.4 areas per patient. In another study, patients with lung cancer who had undergone a resection with curative intent were followed up for 14 years. Even after that period, the annual mortality rate was still 2.3 times greater than expected, and the greatest cause of death was carcinoma of the lung, probably from a second or third primary tumor.[9]

Most carcinomas of the lung have an aneuploid DNA content and exhibit striking chromosomal abnormalities, such as a deletion of the short arm of chromosome 3 and trisomy of chromosome 7. Genetic abnormalities have been identified in several oncogene families. *Ras* gene mutations and *myc* family overexpression can be found frequently in human lung cancer. Mutant p53 genes are common.[10] Thisis an exciting field of study for the future control of lung cancer.

Carcinoma of the lung, especially small-cell carcinoma, has the ability to metastasize early and widely. Common sites are the brain, bone (including the bone marrow), lung, liver, adrenals, and skin. Initial spread, however, is usually to the regional lymph nodes. It is therefore important to understand the lymphatic drainage of the lungs. The first sites of cancer deposits are hilar lymph nodes. These nodes surround the origin of lobar or segmental bronchi from the main bronchus within the lung. The lymph nodes are adherent to both bronchi and pulmonary arteries in the depth of the interlobar fissures. These lymph nodes are not accessible by mediastinoscopy.

The second level of spread is to the mediastinal lymph nodes. From the right lung, the mediastinal nodes first involved are the tracheobronchial nodes around the origin of the right main bronchus from the trachea. These are identified in Fig 13-2,A, as the anterior subcarinal, the azygos, and the anterior tracheal nodes. Later, the paratracheal nodes at or just below the level of the innominate artery become colonized. All these nodes are accessible by cervical mediastinoscopy and all may be identified by computed tomography (CT).

From the left lung, cancer usually spreads to the nodes identified in Fig 13-2,B, as aortic pulmonary or para-aortic nodes, but metastasis may also occur to the left anterior mediastinal lymph nodes. These are not accessible by cervical mediastinoscopy, but may be reached by left anterior mediastinotomy or by thoracoscopy. Left lower lobe carcinoma may on occasion spread up the right side of the mediastinum by way of the subcarinal nodes, and the spread from both lower lobes may involve lymph nodes in the pulmonary ligament, just inferior to the inferior pulmonary vein.

The third level of lymph node spread is to nodes located in the fat pad overlying the scalenus anterior muscle just above the clavicle. From the scalene nodes, cancer may spread to the supraclavicular nodes. The levels of lymph node spread described are the commonly experienced order of metastasis. But when the usual lymph drainage channels become plugged with tumor, spread may occur to nodes on the contralateral side of the mediastinum or even retrograde into the abdomen.

Clinical Presentation

The most frequent signs and symptoms of carcinoma of the lung are listed in Table 13-1. Early symptoms are not characteristic of a malignancy, but rather are common to many respiratory disorders. In *asymptomatic* patients, the diagnosis is usually made from a chest x-ray done for some other medical condition. A *cough* is the most common symptom of lung cancer. However, it is also common to other diseases, and since most patients with lung cancer are cigarette smokers, many will have had a cough for the greater part of their lives. Frequently it becomes more severe following the development of lung cancer. *Hemoptysis* is a nonspecific symptom that may occur with bronchitis, broncholithiasis, tuberculosis, paragonimiasis, aspergillosis, and other pathologic conditions. It is very common in carcinoma of the lung. A patient with even one episode of hemoptysis should be examined by bronchoscopy in addition to a chest x-ray. *Dyspnea*, like coughing, is associated with cigarette smoking and emphysema. It frequently becomes more severe with the development of bronchial obstruction from a carcinoma. *Wheezing* occurs with partial bronchial

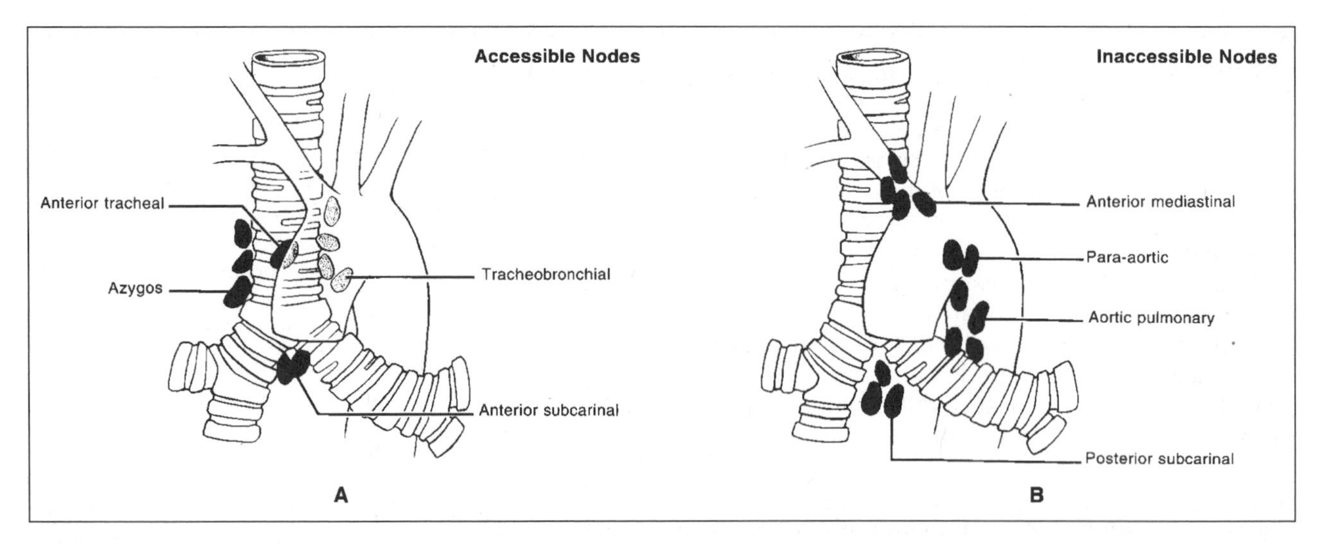

Fig 13-2. Mediastinal lymph nodes accessible ***A*** and inaccessible ***B*** for biopsy by mediastinoscopy.

Table 13-1. Symptoms of Carcinoma of the Lung

- Cough
- Hemoptysis
- Dyspnea
- Pneumonia
- Chest, shoulder, or arm pain
- Weight loss
- Bone pain
- Hoarseness
- Headaches or seizures
- Swelling of the face or neck

obstruction. *Pneumonia* may occur distal to bronchial obstruction. Any patient with an unresolved pneumonia for ≥2 months should have a bronchoscopic examination. *Chest or shoulder pain* usually occurs from invasion of the chest wall, although it seems to present in some patients with cancer of the lung who have no such involvement. A common physician error is to assume that patients with shoulder and arm pain have a herniated cervical disk or cervical osteoarthritis when they may have a carcinoma of the lung in the superior sulcus of the chest that is invading the brachial plexus. As the cancer progresses, it invades the first and second thoracic vertebrae and ribs as well as the stellate ganglion. The finding of pain along the distribution of C-7 or T-1 nerves, a tumor in the apex of the chest, and Horner's syndrome is termed Pancoast's syndrome.

Weight loss, a late symptom, is associated with a poor prognosis. *Bone pain* usually is a sign of distant metastasis, although fairly severe pain, particularly of the lower legs, may occur secondary to osteoarthropathy without metastasis. *Hoarseness*, when caused by carcinoma of the lung, is usually due to paralysis of the left recurrent laryngeal nerve by invasion of the tumor at the point at which it loops around the arch of the aorta. *Headaches or seizures* usually indicate metastasis to the central nervous system. *Swelling of the face*, along with dilatation of cutaneous venules of the upper chest, is caused by compression and invasion of the superior vena cava (termed superior vena cava syndrome). A *pleural effusion* may occur either from dissemination of carcinoma onto the parietal and visceral pleurae or from pneumonia secondary to a hilar carcinoma. It is mandatory that a diagnostic thoracentesis be performed on such a patient, since the finding of malignant cells in the pleural fluid is a contraindication for a surgical resection.

In addition to the signs, symptoms, and findings caused by the physical presence of the carcinoma, there are some rare syndromes—termed paraneoplastic—caused by substances elaborated by the different types of carcinoma of the lung. These are listed in Table 13-2 by histologic type.

Diagnosis

The workup of a patient with a problem that could be caused by carcinoma of the lung has three goals: (1) to determine whether the patient's problem has a high or low probability of being caused by carcinoma of the lung; (2) to determine whether the patient might have a protracted survival from any therapy; and (3) to determine whether the patient can survive the necessary therapy.

Probability of a Diagnosis of Lung Cancer

History and Physical Examination

The diagnostic workup should include a thorough history and physical examination. An easily recognizable feature, clubbing of the digits can be found with any

Table 13-2. Incidence of Histologic Diagnoses in Patients with Paraneoplastic Syndromes

Cell Type	Carcinoid Syndrome	Clubbing of Digits	Cushing's Syndrome	Hypercalcemia	Hypertrophic Pulmonary Osteoarthropathy	Antidiuretic Hormone Secretion	Peripheral Neuropathy
Squamous cell	.09	5	.08	3.3	.6	.8	1
Adenocarcinoma	.1	4.4	.09	.9	1.2	.8	.9
Small cell	.2	3.4	.6	1.6	.4	5.4	1.6
Large cell	.07	5.2	.07	2.1	1.1	1	1.3
Carcinoid	5.7		1.3	.4			

In addition to the syndromes listed above, subacute cerebellar degeneration, a myasthenia-like syndrome, acanthosis nigricans, dermatomyositis, and an intravascular coagulopathy may also occur.

type of primary lung tumor. The facies of Cushing's syndrome is also readily apparent and may be indicative of a small-cell carcinoma, while Horner's syndrome can result from a superior sulcus tumor. Tenderness of the thorax to palpation may be associated with tumor invasion of the chest wall, and tenderness of the tibia is associated with hypertrophic pulmonary osteoarthropathy. An enlarged, nodular liver may be indicative of hepatic metastasis. Auscultation and percussion of the lung may reveal unilateral wheezing or evidence of a pleural effusion.

Radiographic Examination

The plain chest x-ray remains the single most important test in the diagnosis of lung cancer. Many lung tumors are asymptomatic and are discovered as a mass on a screening chest x-ray. A careful review of previous chest x-rays, while viewing the current roentgenogram, provides invaluable information on the presence of a lung opacity on old x-ray films, the rate of growth of the lesion, and evidence of mediastinal involvement. The importance of reviewing old films cannot be overemphasized, as the decision to operate is not uncommonly based on this comparison alone. It is important, therefore, that chest x-rays (not just reports or microfilm) be retained for at least 10 years.

The appearance of the lesion on chest x-ray may be diagnostic and is described as malignant, benign, or indeterminate. Large, spiculated masses with rib erosion and mediastinal widening are considered to be malignant. Small, smooth, concentrically calcified lesions are considered to be benign and no further diagnostic workup is needed. A significant percentage of lung lesions found on chest x-ray fall into the indeterminate category, however, requiring further diagnostic workup.

A CT scan of the chest and upper abdomen with lung and mediastinal windows (attenuation) provides the most detailed anatomic assessment of the lung currently available. This examination clearly demonstrates the location, size, and shape of the lung mass. In addition, previously unsuspected lesions may be identified. Evidence of invasion into adjacent structures may also be found. Masses located in the lung hilum are better defined by CT scanning than by chest x-ray, and endobronchial lesions can be better visualized. CT scanning is an excellent means of evaluating mediastinal lymph nodes for size.

The therapeutic decision when a solitary pulmonary nodule (SPN), or coin lesion, is found constitutes a special case. One third to one half of SPNs are malignant, and efforts are directed toward differentiating benign from malignant disease. An SPN that has been stable for at least 2 years, has smooth round borders, is <3 cm in diameter, or contains concentric calcification on chest x-ray can be safely diagnosed as benign. When previous x-ray films are unavailable for comparison and the lesion is not obviously malignant on chest x-ray or CT scan, special radiographic tests may be helpful.

In the past, tomographic examination of an SPN has been the standard technique for identifying calcification not apparent on the plain chest x-ray. Tomography is relatively insensitive, however, and involves a relatively high dose of radiation to the patient.

A far more sensitive test is the phantom CT scan. The scientific basis for this examination is its ability to determine the density of a given SPN and to compare this density number (Hounsfield unit) with the density of a known standard (phantom) nodule. Multiple thin-section (1 mm thick) CT cuts are obtained through the area of the SPN and the Hounsfield number determined. An epoxy resin model of the chest, which approximates the patient's body habitus, is then substituted for the patient in the CT scanner. A calcium carbonate phantom nodule of similar size and configuration to the patient's nodule is positioned in the model chest, and a repeat scan is obtained. By comparing the Hounsfield units of the actual and phantom nodules, the likelihood of the nodule being benign or malignant can be predicted based on calcification. The false-negative rate of this technique is almost zero (1 in 345 patients), but 60% to 70% of nodules will not show calcification and are labeled indeterminate. Therefore, while the phantom CT study will decrease the number of needless thoracotomies by 25% to 33%, invasive procedures are still required for diagnosis in a large percentage of patients.[11]

New radiographic techniques are being developed to distinguish benign from malignant disease. Monoclonal antibodies with an affinity for certain cancer proteins can be tagged with technetium (^{99m}Tc) and injected into the patient.[12] The ^{99m}Tc-antibody complex will concentrate in the malignant SPN and in metastatic mediastinal lymph nodes and appear as a bright spot on the single photon emission computed tomographic (SPECT) image. Positron emission tomography (PET) scanning is being used in a similar fashion and may hold promise for the future.

Magnetic resonance imaging (MRI) of the chest also can provide high-quality images of the lung and mediastinum. It is most useful for examining areas perfused by blood such as the heart, aorta, and venae cavae. Images can be obtained in the coronal and sagittal planes, leading to greater versatility than CT imaging. MRI may prove superior to CT scanning in determining when a lung cancer has invaded adjacent structures, such as the brachial plexus by a superior sulcus tumor. It offers advantages over CT scanning for the assessment of the mediastinum in that it can image organs containing blood flow without contrast enhancement. Therefore, MRI may prove to be the test of choice for patients who are at risk for allergic reactions or renal failure from contrast administration. The disadvantages of MRI include the amount of time required to obtain an image, the claustrophobic environment in the scanner, and the as yet unproven nature of its results. Magnetic resonance spectroscopy (MRS) is an old technique that is currently being investigated as a means of distinguishing benign from malignant disease.

Cytology

Cytologic characteristics of sputum can be used to diagnose malignant disease in patients in whom a lung mass is visible on chest x-ray. This test is not helpful for evaluation of peripheral SPNs and cannot be used to rule out cancer in any instance. Technique is very important in obtaining an adequate sample, and the accuracy of the test can also be improved by using induced and pooled sputum. Positive cytologic results in patients with negative chest x-rays can be a dilemma for the clinician. Panendoscopy of the oropharynx, larynx, and tracheobronchial tree is required, and if no lesion is found, the examinations should be repeated at frequent intervals.

Invasive Procedures

Bronchoscopic examination of the trachea and bronchi should be performed in all patients with centrally located lung masses and in selected patients with peripheral lesions. Because of the ease of use, the flexible fiberoptic bronchoscope has replaced the rigid scope for most diagnostic studies. The procedure can be performed on an awake, mildly sedated patient in an office setting with excellent results. A combination of washings, brushings, and direct biopsies from centrally located lesions provides a definitive diagnosis in >85% of these patients. The usefulness of bronchoscopy in patients with a peripheral SPN is only fair. These lesions are investigated using fluoroscopically directed brushing and transbronchial biopsies. Positive results are obtained in about two thirds of lesions that eventually prove to be malignant, and the yield is directly related to the size of the mass.[13] The number of false-negative results using this technique is unacceptably high, however, and limits its potential as a decision-making tool.

CT-guided transthoracic needle aspiration (TNA) of a suspicious lung mass is a simple, effective technique for obtaining a definitive diagnosis in a high percentage of appropriately selected patients. The technique is most successful in peripheral lesions that are not located under a rib or next to a large vascular structure. The specificity of TNA is excellent (approaching 100%), and when malignant cells are seen, the lesion is assumed to be cancer. When no malignant cells are encountered, however, benignity cannot be ensured, as the false-negative rate of this test is unacceptably high (approximately 15%). TNA is recommended, therefore, in patients with marginal lung function, in those who refuse a suggested thoracotomy, and in those who require a definitive diagnosis prior to the initiation of radiation or chemotherapy. Pneumothorax occurs in approximately one fifth of patients treated in this manner and usually can be managed conservatively. Other complications include hemoptysis and air embolism.

Open thoracotomy has been the definitive diagnostic maneuver in many patients. The technique of video-assisted thoracoscopic surgery (VATS), while still invasive, may supplant open thoracotomy in this regard. VATS involves three or four small (1 to 2 cm) incisions in the chest wall. A thoracoscope fitted with a miniature video camera is inserted into the chest through one incision, and the other incisions are used as working ports for instrumentation. VATS provides an excellent view of the chest wall, diaphragm, lung parenchyma, and mediastinal structures, enabling biopsy of visible lesions. The drawbacks of VATS are a need for general anesthesia with one-lung ventilation and the difficulty of sampling nonvisible lesions located deep within the parenchyma of the lung (because they cannot be readily palpated). Wire-guided localization techniques used in the diagnosis of breast cancer may solve this problem and allow for accurate diagnosis of microscopic lesions.

Likelihood of Protracted Survival from Therapy: Staging

In current use is the TNM classification for carcinoma of the lung, devised at a 1986 international meeting for unification of staging and reported by Mountain.[14] The *T* refers to the size and extent of the primary tumor, *N* represents the involvement of the hilar and mediastinal lymph nodes, and *M* refers to metastatic disease. This staging method is described in Table 13-3 and illustrated in Figs 13-3 through 13-6.

Lung cancer should be staged at the time of diagnosis (clinical staging) and again postoperatively (pathologic staging) when the final pathology report is available. The initial therapy is determined by the clinical stage and the histologic diagnosis of the cancer. The prognosis is a function of the pathologic stage.

One half of all patients found to have non-small-cell lung cancer (NSCLC) will be inoperable at the time of diagnosis. The reasons for inoperability are given in Table 13-4. Profound weight loss often indicates metastatic disease. Vocal cord paralysis or superior vena cava syndrome is apparent from observation of the patient. Malignant cells found on thoracentesis indicate stage IIIB disease, and these tumors are considered to be nonresectable for cure. Parane-

Table 13-3. TNM Staging for Lung Carcinoma

Primary Tumor (T)

TX	Primary tumor cannot be assessed, or tumor proven by the presence of malignant cells in sputum or bronchial washings but not visualized by imaging or bronchoscopy
T0	No evidence of primary tumor
Tis	Carcinoma in situ
T1	Tumor 3 cm or less in greatest dimension, surrounded by lung or visceral pleura, without bronchoscopic evidence of invasion more proximal than the lobar bronchus (ie, not in the main bronchus)*
T2	Tumor with any of the following features of size or extent: More than 3 cm in greatest dimension; Involving main bronchus, 2 cm or more distal to the carina; Invading the visceral pleura; Associated with atelectasis or obstructive pneumonitis that extends to the hilar region but does not involve the entire lung
T3	Tumor of any size that directly invades any of the following: chest wall (including superior sulcus tumors), diaphragm, mediastinal pleura, or parietal pericardium; or tumor in the main bronchus less than 2 cm distal to the carina but without involvement of the carina; or associated atelectasis or obstructive pneumonitis of the entire lung
T4	Tumor of any size that invades any of the following: mediastinum, heart, great vessels, trachea, esophagus, vertebral body, carina; or tumor with a malignant pleural effusion**

*Note: The uncommon superficial tumor of any size with its invasive component limited to the bronchial wall, which may extend proximal to the main bronchus, is also classified as T1.

**Note: Most pleural effusions associated with lung cancer are due to tumor. However, there are a few patients in whom multiple cytopathologic examinations of pleural fluid are negative for tumor. In these cases, fluid is non-bloody and is not an exudate. When these elements and clinical judgment dictate that the effusion is not related to the tumor, the effusion should be excluded as a staging element and the patient should be staged T1, T2 or T3.

Table 13-3 *Continued.* TNM Staging for Lung Carcinoma

Regional Lymph Nodes (N)

The regional lymph nodes are the intrathoracic, scalene, and supraclavicular nodes.

NX	Regional lymph nodes cannot be assessed
N0	No regional lymph node metastasis
N1	Metastasis in ipsilateral peribronchial and/or ipsilateral hilar lymph nodes, including direct extension
N2	Metastasis in ipsilateral mediastinal and/or subcarinal lymph node(s)
N3	Metastasis in contralateral mediastinal, contralateral hilar, ipsilateral, or contralateral scalene or supraclavicular lymph node(s)

Distant Metastases (M)

MX	Presence of distant metastasis cannot be assessed
M0	No distant metastasis
M1	Distant metastasis

Stage Grouping

Occult	TX	N0	M0
Stage 0	Tis	N0	M0
Stage I	T1	N0	M0
	T2	N0	M0
Stage II	T1	N1	M0
	T2	N1	M0
Stage IIIA	T1	N2	M0
	T2	N2	M0
	T3	N0	M0
	T3	N1	M0
	T3	N2	M0
Stage IIIB	Any T	N3	M0
	T4	Any N	M0
Stage IV	Any T	Any N	M1

Source: Beahrs OH, Henson DE, Hutter RVP, Kennedy BJ, eds. *American Joint Committee on Cancer Manual for Staging of Cancer.* 4th ed. Philadelphia, Pa: JB Lippincott Co; 1992.

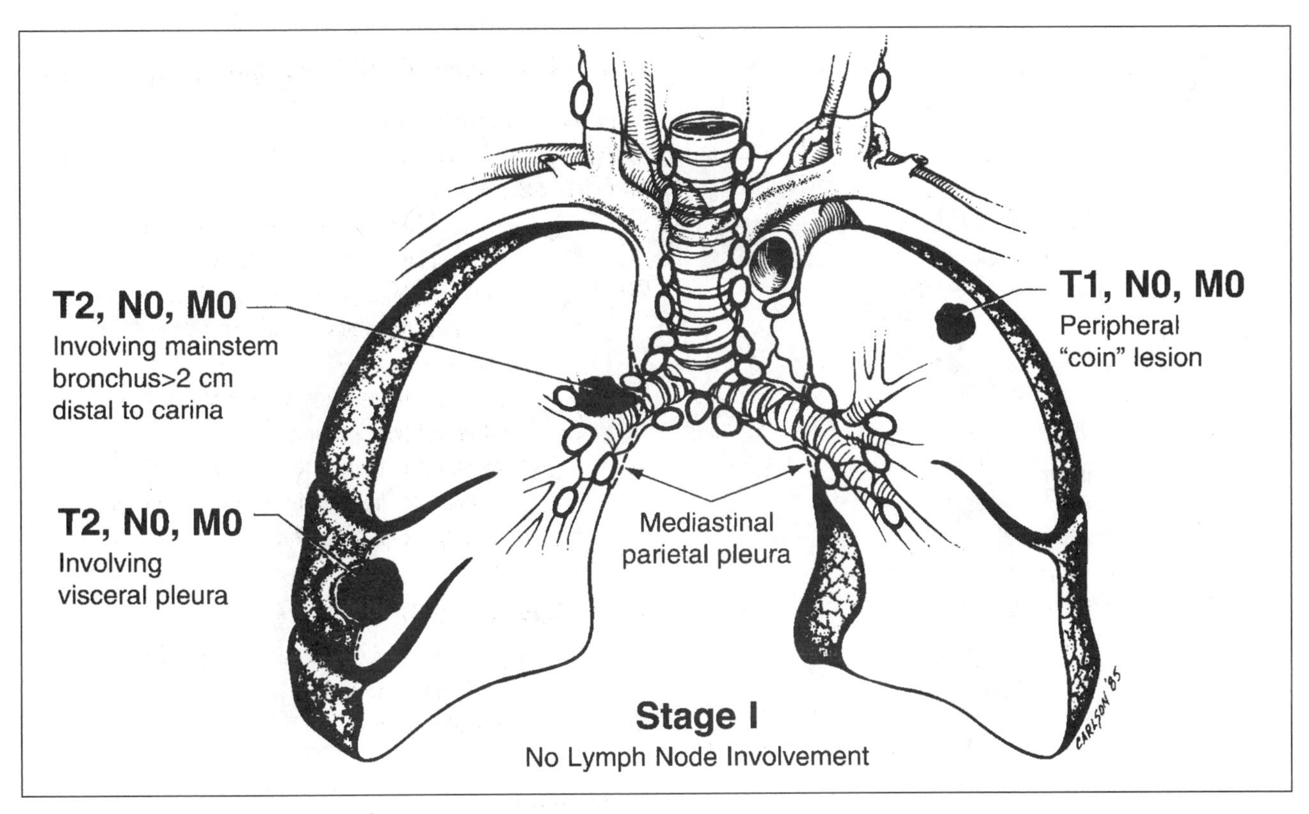

Fig 13-3. Stage I disease. Adapted from Mountain.[14]

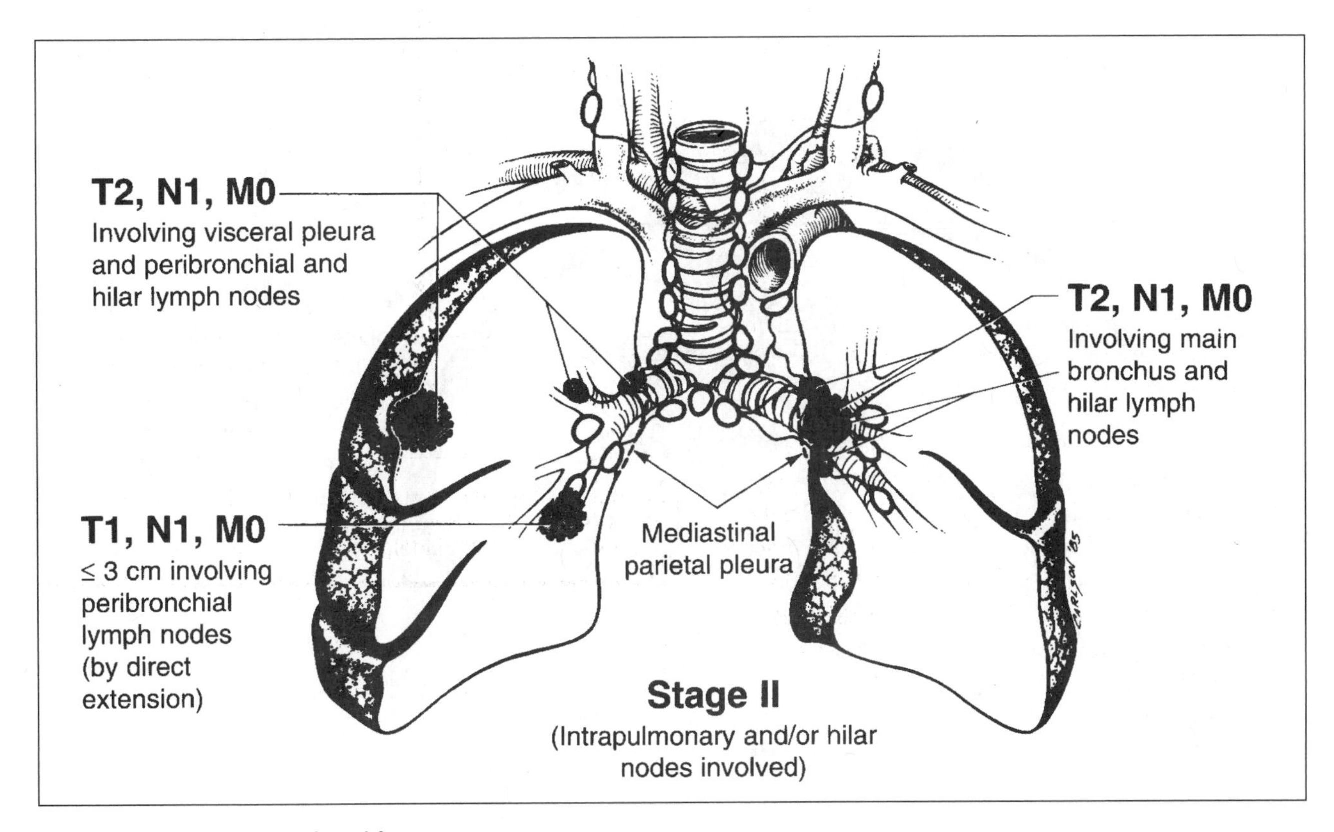

Fig 13-4. Stage II disease. Adapted from Mountain.[14]

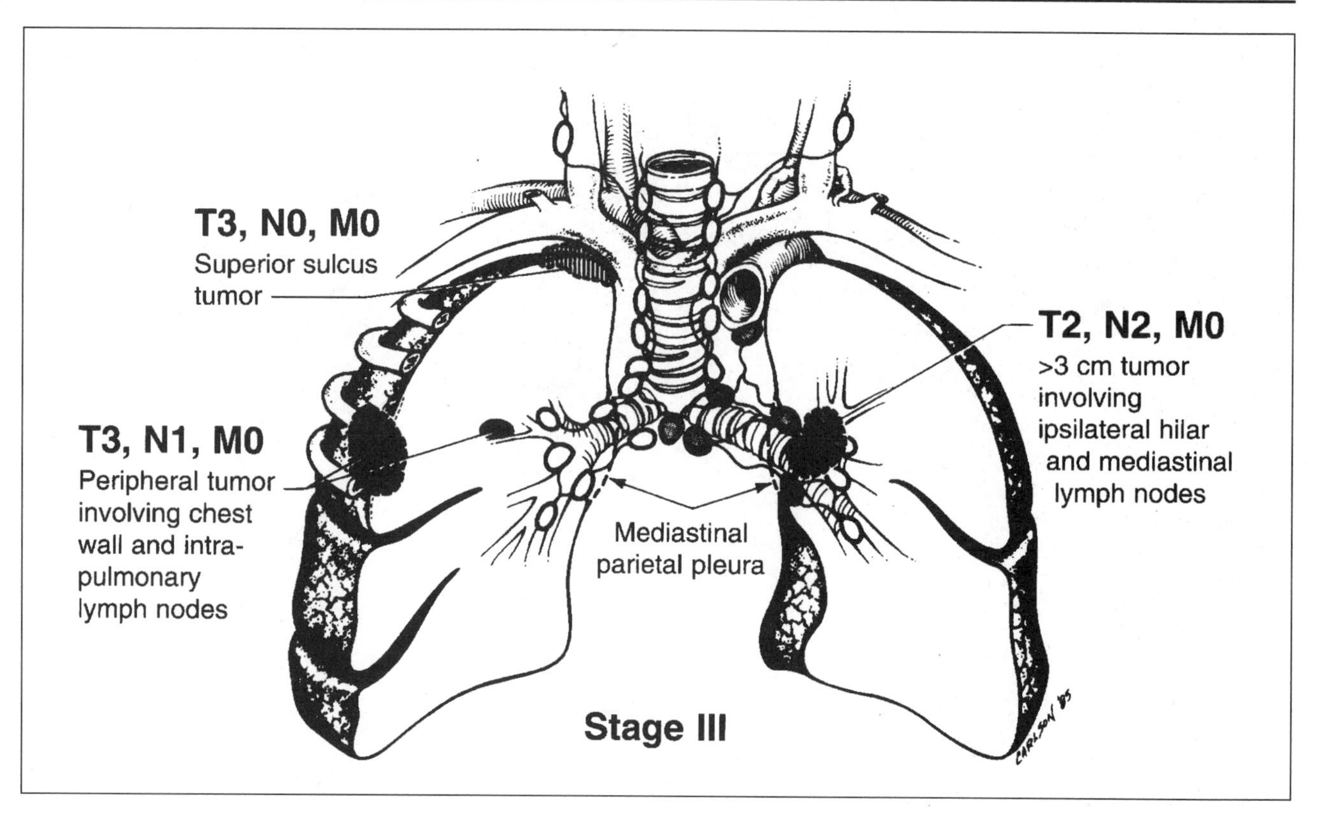

Fig 13-5. Stage IIIA disease. Adapted from Mountain.[14]

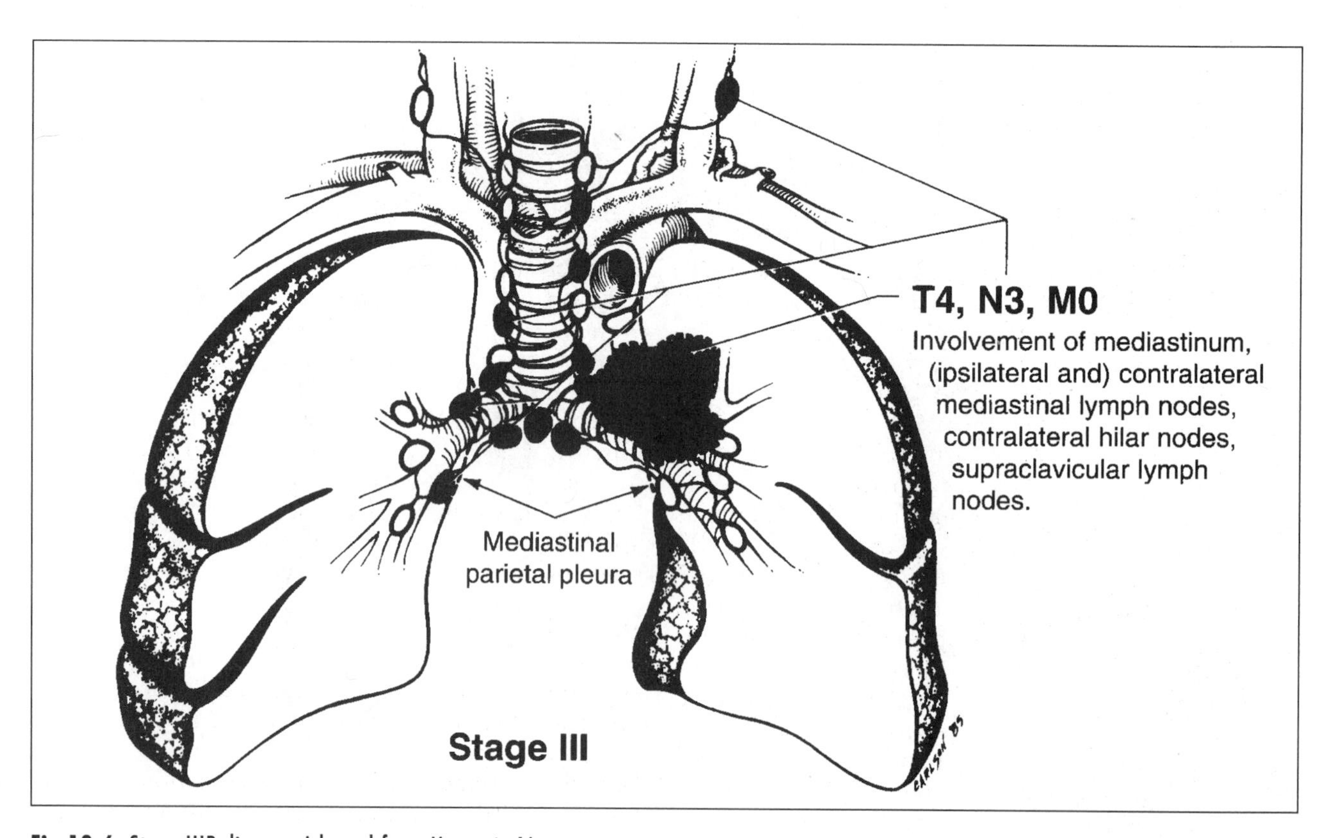

Fig 13-6. Stage IIIB disease. Adapted from Mountain.[14]

oplastic syndromes are not necessarily associated with metastatic disease, and the symptoms will often disappear on resection of the tumor.

Staging of NSCLC allows the clinician to recommend a therapy that may extend the life of the patient. When the disease has become systemic (stage IV), surgical resection has not been shown to prolong life. Surgical resection, therefore, is the treatment of choice for patients with stage I and stage II NSCLC and for selected patients with stage IIIA disease. While life expectancy is less in patients with stage II disease than in those with stage I disease, prolonged survival has been achieved with surgical therapy. Patients with tumors that invade nonvital structures (stage IIIA), such as the chest wall, and patients with ipsilateral hilar lymph node metastasis are also best treated by surgical therapy.

Table 13-4. Reasons for Inoperability in Patients with Lung Cancer

1. Distant metastasis
2. Involvement of trachea or contralateral main bronchus with carcinoma
3. Mediastinal lymph node metastasis
4. Superior vena cava obstruction
5. Malignant cells in pleural effusion
6. Recurrent laryngeal nerve paralysis from carcinoma
7. Histologic diagnosis of small-cell carcinoma

Bone, brain, and liver-spleen scans have been used in the past to rule out metastatic disease. Without preexisting evidence of disease in these organs, however, the specificity of a positive test is extremely low, and the cost of these examinations is not justified.

The CT scan of the chest and upper abdomen has a much higher yield for staging than radionuclide scanning and should be used on a routine basis. Mediastinal windows provide pertinent information on tumor invasion into adjacent structures such as the chest wall and spinal column. The mediastinum is assessed for tumor metastasis by administering oral and intravenous contrast material in an effort to differentiate vascular and esophageal structures from lymph nodes. Metastatic spread to these nodes markedly diminishes the likelihood of long-term survival. Lymph nodes <1 cm in diameter are considered to be benign as they are rarely occupied by tumor (13%), while nodes >2 cm in diameter are much more likely to contain tumor cells (>60%).[15] The finding of enlarged mediastinal lymph nodes on CT scan is almost never used as the final determinant of operability, as postobstructive pneumonia can create an inflammatory reaction resulting in benign nodal hyperplasia. Therefore, the size of the lymph nodes is used to decide only whether mediastinoscopy or mediastinotomy should be performed prior to surgical exploration. Finally, CT examination of the upper abdomen may show possible tumor involvement of the liver or adrenal glands; confirmation can be obtained with a CT-guided needle aspiration.

Invasive Staging

Mediastinoscopy is commonly used in combination with the CT scan to determine whether the cancer has metastasized to ipsilateral, contralateral, or superior mediastinal lymph nodes in the paratracheal, subcarinal, or right tracheobronchial regions. Under direct vision, the nodes are isolated and biopsied. On the left side, when the enlarged lymph nodes are located in the aortopulmonary window area on CT or MRI scan, a mediastinotomy rather than a mediastinoscopy is performed. This involves a small incision in the left second or third intercostal space and direct visualization of the aortopulmonary window.

The paraesophageal area of the mediastinum is not accessible by mediastinotomy or mediastinoscopy and previously was assessed by open thoracotomy. VATS may prove to be the procedure of choice for the staging of disease in this area. Transbronchial needle aspiration (TBNA) may be useful in sampling subcarinal and paratracheal lymph nodes for evidence of metastatic disease. The technique uses a sheathed needle passed through a flexible fiberoptic bronchoscope. The sensitivity and specificity of this test are highly dependent on the skill and experience of the bronchoscopist. As with TNA, a positive result is accurate, but a negative result will not rule out metastatic spread.

Probability of Surviving Therapy

A surgical resection is the mainstay of therapy with curative intent for non-small-cell carcinoma of the lung. The type of operation performed should depend on the extent and location of the cancer, as well as the patient's pulmonary and cardiac reserve. The surgeon must decide whether the patient will tolerate the necessary resection or whether he or she would be better served with a less effective, but less dangerous approach to treatment. This subjective decision is made using the following data:

History

A history from the patient and family members should elicit the patient's recent ability to perform physical exercise such as climbing stairs and walking at a reasonable pace. A recent history of smoking becomes extremely important, as cessation of smoking for as little as 2 weeks prior to surgery reduces the incidence of postoperative complications. On physical examination, the patient's overall appearance and ability to perform physical tasks, such as the climbing of two flights of stairs and counting to 20 in two or three breaths, correlate with his ability to withstand a major lung resection. A patient with a substantial recent weight loss who appears weak and is unable to climb stairs without stopping is likely to have an unacceptably high surgical risk.

Laboratory Data

Spirometric testing of lung function plays an integral role in determining which patients will tolerate a major pulmonary resection. The single most consistent predictor of outcome is the forced expiratory volume in 1 second (FEV_1). If the preoperative FEV_1 is sufficient to allow a postoperative FEV_1 of >800 mL/s, the patient should be able to clear his or her own secretions and not become a pulmonary "cripple." Predicting the postoperative FEV_1 relates directly to the amount of functioning lung tissue to be removed as a percent of the total functioning lung mass. A split-function radionuclide scan may offer useful information on pulmonary function in an otherwise marginal patient.

Analysis of arterial blood gases also provides strong predictors of outcome in patients undergoing lung resection. A Pao_2 of <50 torr on room air generally precludes surgery until the ventilation-perfusion mismatch can be corrected. Similarly, a $Paco_2$ of >46 torr is associated with an increased risk of postoperative respiratory failure and ventilator dependence.

Serum biochemical tests may correlate with the ability to perform the necessary ventilatory work after a lung resection. Serum albumin and transferrin levels provide an indication of the patient's nutritional status. Studies have reported improved survival in debilitated general surgical patients who receive preoperative nutritional repletion.

Pathologic Classification

Table 13-5 lists the 1977 World Health Organization (WHO) classification of malignant lung tumors. Although other schemas have been published, most are variations of the WHO classification.[16]

The various histologic types of carcinoma of the lung have a predilection for different parts of the lung. The lung, as seen on a radiogram, may be divided into central and peripheral zones. The former is occupied by the main, lobar, segmental, and first-order subsegmental bronchi, all available to inspection with a fiberoptic bronchoscope. The rest of the lung parenchyma is in the peripheral zone. Of squamous cell carcinomas, 65% occur in the central zone. Of the one third that occur in the peripheral zone, approximately 30% will have cavitated when discovered. Of small-cell undifferentiated carcinomas, 90% to 95% occur in the central zone. Often, however, they cause only narrowing of the involved bronchus by submucosal infiltration and have no intraluminal mass. Thus, bronchoscopic biopsy of these tumors may be difficult. Of adenocarcinomas, 75% occur in the peripheral zone. The large-cell undifferentiated group comprises poorly differentiated squamous cell carcinoma, poorly differentiated adenocarcinoma, and a truly undifferentiated set. They occur more frequently in the peripheral zone.

The prognoses of squamous cell carcinoma and adenocarcinoma are essentially the same. In addition, both are relatively insensitive to current cancer chemotherapeutic drugs. Small-cell carcinoma car-

Table 13-5. World Health Organization Histologic Classification of Malignant Lung Tumors

I. Malignant epithelial tumors
- A. Squamous cell carcinoma (epidermoid carcinoma)
  - Variant:
    1. Spindle cell carcinoma
- B. Small-cell carcinoma
  1. Oat cell carcinoma
  2. Intermediate cell type
  3. Combined oat cell carcinomas
- C. Adenocarcinoma
  1. Acinar adenocarcinoma
  2. Papillary adenocarcinoma
  3. Bronchiolo-alveolar carcinoma
  4. Solid carcinoma with mucus formation
- D. Large-cell carcinoma
  - Variants:
    1. Giant cell carcinoma
    2. Clear cell carcinoma
- E. Adenosquamous carcinoma
- F. Carcinoid tumor
- G. Bronchial gland carcinomas
  1. Adenoid cystic carcinoma
  2. Mucoepidermoid carcinoma
- H. Others

II. Malignant mesothelial tumors
- A. Malignant mesothelioma
  1. Epithelial
  2. Fibrous (spindle cell)
  3. Biphasic

III. Miscellaneous malignant tumors
- A. Carcinosarcoma
- B. Pulmonary blastoma
- C. Malignant melanoma
- D. Malignant lymphoma
- E. Others

From Yesner et al.[16]

ries a poorer prognosis. It has long been thought that surgery is not indicated for these tumors. They are quite sensitive, however, to chemotherapy. Recently several centers have reported relatively good 5-year survival rates from T1, N0 small-cell carcinomas treated by surgical resection and chemotherapy.

Management

Operative Management

The operative treatment of lung cancer is complete extirpation of the tumor and its regional lymphatic drainage. This generally means an anatomic lobectomy for disease confined to one lobe (most stage I and stage II lung cancers) or a pneumonectomy for disease extending into the mainstem bronchus or the main pulmonary artery. Lung-sparing procedures, such as a sleeve resection of the right upper lobe in continuity with the right mainstem bronchus, are excellent means of preserving functioning lung tissue without compromising the integrity of the operation. Resections that remove a smaller amount of lung tissue, such as a segmentectomy or a wedge resection, are reported to give poorer results with a 2.7-fold increased local recurrence rate. They should be used only in patients who cannot tolerate a more extensive lung resection.[17]

The 30-day operative mortality for a wedge resection is about 0.4%. For a pulmonary lobectomy, this rate has been reported to be <3%.[18] In the majority of patients with stage I and stage II lung cancer, the latter operation is sufficient and results in adequate postoperative pulmonary function. A pneumonectomy involves a far greater alteration of pulmonary and cardiac function. Right ventricular failure is not an uncommon long-term sequela in these patients due to an increase in pulmonary artery resistance. The operative mortality is also higher (6%) with this procedure than with a lobectomy, and complications such as a bronchial stump leak, while rare, can be devastating. Because long-term survival with a lobectomy is equal to that following a pneumonectomy, lobectomy should be the procedure of choice when it is technically feasible.

VATS is currently being evaluated in several large trials to determine its role in the diagnosis and treatment of lung cancer. While it is technically feasible to perform wedge resections, lobectomies, and even pneumonectomies using VATS, the results of carefully controlled trials should be available before these procedures are used as definitive therapy. Under no circumstance should a simple procedure such as a wedge resection be substituted for a conventional lobectomy in order to experiment with this new technique.

Management of Recurrent Lung Cancer

Repeat chest x-ray is the most cost-effective means of follow-up after a lung resection. Postoperative films provide a baseline that includes changes induced by the surgical procedure itself. Repeat examinations are then performed at 6-month intervals for the next 2 years and on an annual basis thereafter. Comparison with the immediate postoperative film will provide an excellent means of follow-up and early detection of recurrent disease. If recurrent disease is suspected, the CT scan and other diagnostic tests are repeated and a workup for metastasis initiated.

Elevation of carcinoembryonic antigen (CEA) after a return to normal following lung resection may be a predictor of recurrent disease. While there is no evidence that this knowledge will improve survival, a recent publication has reported that completion pneumonectomy is safe and effective for recurrent disease.[19] Combined with neoadjuvant chemotherapy and radiotherapy, this modality may improve the otherwise dismal survival statistics for patients with recurrent lung cancer.

Table 13-6. Actuarial Survival Estimates by Stage in Patients Who Underwent a Resection in 1981

	Squamous Cell		Adenocarcinoma		Bronchoalveolar		Large Cell	
Pathologic AJC Stage	No. of Patients	5-Year Survival (%)	No. of Patients	5-Year Survival (%)	No. of Patients	5-Year Survival (%)	No. of Patients	5-Year Survival (%)
Stage I	848	51.9	757	53.7	287	61.7	155	44.3
Stage II	290	32.2	176	21.9	43	21.9	46	16.4
Stage III	548	13.6	394	14.1	70	15.8	128	4.6

AJC = American Joint Committee for Cancer Staging and End-Results Reporting.

Adapted from Humphrey et al.[20]

Prognosis

Based on a survey by the Commission on Cancer of the American College of Surgeons of more than 15,000 patients in whom carcinoma of the lung was diagnosed in 1981, the overall 5-year survival was 14.4%. The survival rate from the time of initial treatment for non-small-cell carcinoma, however, depends on the stage of the carcinoma. Table 13-6 gives the actuarial survival by stage for patients who underwent a resection in 1981.[20] The staging, since it was done in 1981, is based on the 1979 system, not the system described in this chapter, but the two classifications have many similarities. Notice that little difference in survival exists between patients with squamous cell carcinoma and those with adenocarcinoma. However, other data show that the survival of women with adenocarcinoma exceeds that for women with squamous cell carcinoma.[21] The 5-year survival rate varies from >50% for patients with stage I carcinoma to about 14% for those with stage III disease.

The survival rate also varies with the patient's sex and the type of operation performed, as shown in Table 13-7, but since the type of operation should be a function of the stage, one might think that Tables 13-6 and 13-7 represent a tautology. This is not completely true. The survival of patients who underwent a lobectomy exceeded that of patients who had only a wedge or segmental resection despite the fact that wedge resections are recommended only for carcinomas ≤3 cm in diameter while lobectomies are often performed for considerably larger tumors. This finding is in agreement with another report of increased local recurrence after limited resections.[17] Survival, at present, is also a function of race. In addition to an increased incidence of carcinoma of the lung, black patients have a poorer survival from the time of diagnosis than whites. This is true for each histologic category and for both localized disease and overall.[21]

Alternative Forms of Therapy and Clinical Trials

Non-Small-Cell Lung Cancer

Approximately one third of patients with NSCLC will have clinically resectable disease based on initial staging evaluation. Even patients with completely resectable disease are at significant risk for tumor recurrence. The Lung Cancer Study Group (LCSG) found that 65% to 75% of initial recurrences in stage I and stage II patients involve distant sites. These high rates of disease recurrence emphasize the systemic nature of most NSCLCs.[22]

For patients with surgically resected stages II and IIIA disease, the poor survival associated with resection has led to considerable interest in adjuvant therapy as a means to improve survival. Unfortunately, despite the attractiveness of postoperative radiotherapy in reducing local recurrence, there is no evidence that survival is improved compared with surgery alone. The LCSG investigated the use of adjuvant chemotherapy in patients with completely resected stage II or stage III adenocarcinoma and large-cell undifferentiated carcinoma of the lung.[23] Patients received adjuvant chemotherapy consisting of cyclophosphamide, doxorubicin, and cisplatin (CAP) or immunotherapy consisting of bacillus Calmette-Guerin (BCG) (by chest tube or thoracentesis) and levamisole. The median survival of patients receiving CAP was 22.5 months versus 15.5 months for patients on immunotherapy. Unfortunately, two-thirds of relapses still occurred outside the thorax.

The LCSG also compared postoperative radiotherapy alone with the combination of postoperative chemotherapy plus radiotherapy in patients with incompletely resected NSCLC. Incomplete resection was defined as microscopic residual disease following surgical resection or tumor involvement of the most proximal lymph node. Chemotherapy again was CAP. Patients who received CAP plus radiotherapy

Table 13-7. Three-Year Relative Survival of Lung Cancer Patients Undergoing a Resection by Histologic Diagnosis, Sex, and Type of Surgery

	Adenocarcinoma		Squamous Cell		Large Cell	
	Male	Female	Male	Female	Male	Female
	(% of patients)					
Wedge-segmental	41	54	47	52	30	31
Lobe-bilobectomy	59	70	58	59	47	45
Pneumonectomy	32	36	46	49	52	*

*Fewer than 10 observations.

Adapted from Humphrey et al.[20]

had a median survival of 20 months versus 13 months for those receiving only radiotherapy. An analysis based on cell type indicated that chemotherapy had a greater impact in patients with a histologic diagnosis of non-squamous cell carcinoma than in those with squamous cell carcinoma.[24] These LCSG studies were initiated in the late 1970s. Today it is generally accepted that CAP is not "state of the art" treatment, and higher dosages of cisplatin are necessary for optimal tumoricidal results.

Approximately one-third of NSCLC patients present with locally advanced but inoperable tumor. For these patients, thoracic irradiation is often recommended with a resultant median survival of only 9 to 11 months; survival at 2 years is 10% to 20% and at 3 years, 5% to 10%. In theory, "systemic" therapy in locally advanced NSCLC patients might control extrathoracic micrometastases, thus rendering such patients "more curable" with a local treatment modality (ie, radiotherapy, surgery, or both). Chemotherapy administered before definitive local-regional treatment is referred to as "neoadjuvant" therapy. The Cancer and Leukemia Group B (CALGB) recently reported that in patients with stage III NSCLC, two courses of cisplatin plus weekly doses of vinblastine for 5 weeks followed by thoracic radiotherapy resulted in a significant survival advantage compared with radiotherapy alone.[25] The median survival was 13.8 months versus 9.7 months in favor of the combined-modality approach. Rates of survival at 1 year (55% versus 40%), 2 years (26% versus 13%), and 3 years (23% versus 11%) all favored the combined-modality approach. Thus, in stage III patients, combined treatment improved the median survival and doubled the number of long-term survivors as compared with radiotherapy alone.

Treatment of metastatic NSCLC remains disappointing. Few studies have demonstrated a survival advantage resulting from chemotherapy in NSCLC. The median survival of such patients is 5 to 6 months. It is generally accepted that there is no "standard" regimen or treatment plan for NSCLC. To date, no single chemotherapeutic agent has demonstrated improved survival. Of >50 agents evaluated in the past two decades, only 6 have demonstrated significant antitumor activity in >15% of tested patients: cisplatin, ifosfamide, mitomycin C, vindesine, vinblastine, and etoposide. Adding to the confusion of how to identify agents active against NSCLC is the observation by the Eastern Cooperative Oncology Group (ECOG) that carboplatin, which as a single agent had a response rate of only 9%, resulted in a longer survival than three separate cisplatin-based combination chemotherapy programs.[26] In general, however, response rates are higher for combination chemotherapeutic regimens.

There have now been some prospective randomized trials comparing combination treatment with no treatment. In the National Cancer Institute of Canada (NCIC) study, patients were randomized to either cisplatin plus vindesine, CAP, or best supportive care. Patients given either combination regimen survived longer than patients given best supportive care (32.6, 24.7, and 17 weeks, respectively).[27] In contrast, a study in Australia and the UK compared cisplatin plus vindesine versus best supportive care. Median survivals were not significantly different for either approach (23 versus 16 weeks).[28] Thus, it remains unclear whether combination chemotherapy in metastatic NSCLC confers a survival advantage over best supportive care. In addition, the clinical significance of the noted survival differences is small, and the true benefit of administering combination chemotherapy in this group of patients remains open to question.

Principal factors predicting a response to chemotherapy and survival in NSCLC include performance status, tumor bulk, site of metastases, sex (females do better than males), and age. Histologic subtype does not appear to play a significant role in prognosis. In an ECOG study, it was demonstrated that treatment factors associated with a survival of at least 1 year included ECOG performance status 0; no bone, liver, or subcutaneous metastasis; female sex; a histologic diagnosis other than large-cell carcinoma; no weight loss; and no symptoms of shoulder or arm pain.[29]

Future therapeutic approaches in NSCLC will include the use of agents such as the retinoids in chemoprophylaxis. The risk of dying from a second tumor persists for many years after lung resection and may exceed 25% in patients observed for 5 to 10 years. Preliminary reports from Italian investigators suggest that high-dose retinol palmitate reduced the number of cancer failures in patients curatively resected for stage I NSCLC. Only 33% of patients receiving chemopreventive therapy developed either recurrent or new primary tumors, compared with 44% of patients receiving placebo. A similar approach using 13-cis-retinoic acid in cancers of the head and neck has been reported to reduce the occurrence of second primary tumors.

Small-Cell Lung Cancer

Small-cell lung cancer (SCLC) is one of the most biologically aggressive neoplasms and leads rapidly to death in the untreated patient. Results of clinical trials have demonstrated that long-term survival can be improved with intensive combination chemotherapy. As a result, chemotherapy is the cornerstone in the management of SCLC. Active chemotherapeutic agents include cisplatin, etoposide, cyclophosphamide, vincristine, vinblastine, doxorubicin, and carboplatin.

The most effective chemotherapy programs require simultaneous administration of chemotherapeutic agents at relatively intensive doses at frequent intervals (eg, every 3 to 4 weeks) to achieve optimal results. Using these combination chemotherapeutic programs, one can achieve an overall tumor response rate of 70% to 90%. Complete responses are achieved in one-half of patients with limited disease and 20% of patients with extensive disease. This results in a median survival of 14 months in patients with limited disease and 7 to 9 months in patients with extensive disease. A small subset of patients with limited disease (10% to 15%) are long-term survivors following treatment. Few formal trials have addressed the optimal duration of therapy, but it appears that first-line treatment programs administered for only 4 to 6 months achieve results similar to 12- to 24-month programs. There appears to be no role for maintenance chemotherapy.

Despite the high response rate to first-line chemotherapy, up to 90% of patients will eventually relapse and die of SCLC, even if a complete remission had been achieved. Because most patients with SCLC ultimately relapse with drug-resistant tumors, treatment approaches that attempt to address the problem of drug resistance have been explored. This has consisted of the use of so-called non-cross-resistant chemotherapeutic regimens. The rationale for this approach comes from the Goldie-Coldman hypothesis that maximally effective therapy results from the simultaneous use of as many active agents as possible early in treatment. The results of randomized trials testing non-cross-resistant chemotherapy in SCLC have not been encouraging. No study has yielded a major benefit in median or long-term patient survival. These studies have been criticized, since sufficiently non-cross-resistant regimens have not yet been identified.

Critical analysis of failure patterns in SCLC patients treated with chemotherapy alone, especially those with limited disease, indicates that a substantial percentage will relapse solely within the chest, usually at the site of the primary lesion. It seems logical that some limited-stage patients might benefit from chest radiotherapy designed to control local recurrence. Results of several randomized studies using combined-modality therapy (ie, chemotherapy plus radiotherapy) are mixed. Variations in scheduling and in dose of radiation and chemotherapy complicate inter-trial comparisons. Approaches including radiotherapy administered concomitantly with the start of chemotherapy, after chemotherapy is completed, or as a split course between cycles of chemotherapy have all been advocated.

Brain metastases are detected in 10% of SCLC patients at diagnosis. Actuarial analysis indicates a 50% to 80% probability of brain metastases in 2-year survivors of SCLC, without prior central nervous system therapy. Therefore, those patients who achieve complete remission of SCLC should receive prophylactic cranial irradiation. For SCLC patients who fail to achieve a complete remission, prophylactic cranial irradiation is not recommended.

An occasional SCLC patient presents with a peripheral stage I lesion (ie, T1, N0 or T2, N0). These lesions should be surgically resected and combination chemotherapy given postoperatively as adjuvant therapy. When chemotherapy is given postoperatively to this subset of patients with stage I SCLC, a 5-year survival rate of 50% has been reported.[30]

References

1. Boring CC, Squires TS, Tong T, Montgomery S. Cancer Statistics, 1994. *CA Cancer J Clin.* 1994;44:7-26.

2. Miller BA, Ries LAG, Hankey BF, Kosary CL, Harris A, Devesa SS, Edwards BK, eds. *SEER Cancer Statistics Review: 1973-1990.* (NIH Pub. No. 93-2789) Bethesda, Md: National Cancer Institute, 1993.

3. Garfinkel L, Silverberg E. Lung cancer and smoking trends in the United States over the past 25 years. *CA Cancer J Clin.* 1991;41:137-145.

4. Steinitz R. Pulmonary tuberculosis and carcinoma of the lung: a survey from two population-based disease registers. *Am Rev Respir Dis.* 1965;92:758-766.

5. Lynch KM, Smith WA. Pulmonary asbestosis: carcinoma of the lung in asbesto-silicosis. *Am J Cancer.* 1935;24:56-64.

6. Selikoff IJ, Hammond EC, Seidman H. Mortality experience of insulation workers in the United States and Canada, 1943-1976. *Ann N Y Acad Sci.* 1979;330:91-116.

7. Hammond EC, Selikoff IJ, Seidman H. Asbestos exposure, cigarette smoking and death rates. *Ann NY Acad Sci.* 1979;330:473-490.

8. Auerbach O, Stout AP, Hammond EC, Garfinkel L. Changes in bronchial epithelium in relation to cigarette smoking and in relation to lung cancer. *N Engl J Med.* 1961;265:253-267.

9. Humphrey EW, Keehn RJ, Higgins GA Jr, Shields TW. The long term survival of patients with visceral carcinoma. *Surg Gynecol Obstet.* 1979;149:385-394.

10. Viallet J, Minna JD. Dominant oncogenes and tumor suppressor genes in the pathogenesis of lung cancer. *Am J Respir Cell Mol Biol.* 1990;2:225-232.

11. Ward HB, Pliego M, Diefenthal HC, Humphrey EW. The impact of phantom CT scanning on surgery for the solitary pulmonary nodule. *Surgery.* 1989;106:734-739.

12. Rusch VW, Macapinlac H, Heelan R, et al. NR-LU-10 monoclonal antibody scanning: a helpful new adjunct to CT in evaluating non-small cell lung cancer. *J Thorac Cardiovasc Surg.* In press.

13. Radke JR, Conway WA, Eyler WR, Kvale PA. Diagnostic accuracy in peripheral lung lesions: factors predicting success with flexible fiberoptic bronchoscopy. *Chest.* 1979;76:176-179.

14. Mountain CF. A new international staging system for lung cancer. *Chest.* 1986;89(suppl 4):225S-233S.

15. McLoud TC, Bourgouin PM, Greenberg RW, et al. Bronchogenic carcinoma: analysis of staging in the mediastinum

with CT by correlative lymph node mapping and sampling. *Radiology.* 1992;182:319-323.

16. Yesner R, Sobin L, et al. *Histologic Typing of Lung Tumors, Revised.* Geneva: World Health Organization; 1977.

17. Ginsberg RJ, Rubenstein L. Lung Cancer Study Group: randomized comparative trial of lobectomy vs. limited resection for patients with T1, N0 non-small cell lung cancer. *Lung Cancer.* 1991;7(suppl):83.

18. Ginsberg RJ, Hill LD, Eagan RT, et al. Modern thirty-day operative mortality for surgical resections in lung cancer. *J Thorac Cardiovasc Surg.* 1983;86:654-658.

19. Gregoire J, DesLauriers J, Guojin L, Rouleau J. Indications, risks and results of completion pneumonectomy. *J Thorac Cardiovasc Surg.* In press.

20. Humphrey EW, Smart CR, Winchester DP, et al. National survey of the pattern of care for carcinoma of the lung. *J Thorac Cardiovasc Surg.* 1990;100:837-843.

21. Humphrey EW. Lung cancer. In: *National Cancer Data Base. Annual Review of Patient Care 1992.* Atlanta, Ga: American Cancer Society and Commission on Cancer of American College of Surgeons; 1992.

22. Feld R, Rubinstein LV, Weisenberger TH. Sites of recurrence in resected stage I non-small-cell lung cancer: a guide for future studies. *J Clin Oncol.* 1984;2:1352-1358.

23. Holmes EC, Gail M. Surgical adjuvant therapy for stage II and stage III adenocarcinoma and large-cell undifferentiated carcinoma. *J Clin Oncol.* 1986;4:710-715.

24. The Lung Cancer Study Group. The benefit of adjuvant treatment for resected locally advanced non-small-cell lung cancer. *J Clin Oncol.* 1988;6:9-17.

25. Dillman RO, Seagren SL, Propert KJ, et al. A randomized trial of induction chemotherapy plus high-dose radiation versus radiation alone in stage III non-small-cell lung cancer. *N Engl J Med.* 1990;323:940-945.

26. Finkelstein DM, Ettinger DS, Ruckdeschel JC. Long-term survivors in metastatic non-small-cell lung cancer: an Eastern Cooperative Oncology Group study. *J Clin Oncol.* 1986;4:702-709.

27. Rapp E, Pater JL, Willan A, et al. Chemotherapy can prolong survival in patients with advanced non-small-cell-lung cancer: report of a Canadian multicenter randomized trial. *J Clin Oncol.* 1988;6:633-641.

28. Williams CJ, Woods R, Levi J, Page J. Chemotherapy for non-small-cell lung cancer: a randomized trial of cisplatin/vindesine v no chemotherapy. *Semin Oncol.* 1988;15(6, suppl 7):58-61.

29. O'Connell JP, Kris MG, Gralla RJ, et al. Frequency and prognostic importance of pretreatment clinical characteristics in patients with advanced non-small-cell lung cancer treated with combination chemotherapy. *J Clin Oncol.* 1986;4:1604-1614.

30. Shepherd FA, Ginsberg RJ, Evans WK, et al. Reduction in local recurrence and improved survival in surgically treated patients with small cell lung cancers. *J Thorac Cardiovasc Surg.* 1983;86:498-506.

14

COLORECTAL CANCER

Glenn Steele, Jr, MD

Approximately 149,000 new cases of colon and rectal cancer will have been diagnosed in the United States in 1994.[1] The 5-year survival rate remains at approximately 45%. The death rate for colon and rectal cancer in the US remains second to that for cancer of the lung, with an expected 56,000 deaths from the former cause in 1994.[1] This mortality rate has been unchanged for at least three decades. However, major advances in multimodality therapy for stage III colon adenocarcinoma and stages II and III rectal adenocarcinoma are expected to improve survival during the next decade.[2]

Epidemiology and Pathology

Recent data from national patterns-of-care surveys, such as the Patient Care Evaluation Study and the National Cancer Data Base of the Commission on Cancer, have shown no dramatic changes in either sex or age distribution for the diagnosis of "sporadic" colon and rectal cancer (Table 14-1).[3] However, these surveys do confirm earlier databases showing a trend toward more proximal bowel tumors (Table 14-2).[3] The reason for this apparent change is unclear, but probably is not simply a function of access to the proximal bowel by increasing application of colonoscopy.

The pathologic variations of colon and rectal cancer are relatively limited. Morphologic interpretation of the most common histologic type, adenocarcinoma, is relatively unrewarding in predicting outcome. Only in patients with poorly differentiated or highly mucin-producing tumors is there any secure correlation with biologic aggressiveness. The biologic behavior pattern is quite unpredictable in patients with moderate to well-differentiated adenocarcinomas

Table 14-1. Age Distribution for Diagnosis of Colon and Rectal Cancer (Patient Care Evaluation Study, 1992)

Age	1983 Colon (% of total)	1983 Rectum (% of total)	1988 Colon (% of total)	1988 Rectum (% of total)
<20	0.1	0.1	<0.1	<0.1
20-39	1.6	1.5	1.4	1.8
40-59	16.8	21.3	15.1	20.1
60-79	61.2	62.1	61.8	62.6
80-99	20.2	15.0	21.5	15.5
100-119	0.1	<0.1	0.1	<0.1
Mean Age	75.4	71.5	73.4	71.5
Median Age	70.8	68.7	71.6	68.8

From Beart et al.[3]

Table 14-2. Distribution of Colon and Rectal Cancer by Site (Patient Care Evaluation Study, 1992)

	1983 (% of total)	1988 (% of total)
Ascending–cecum	25.2	26.8
Trans-Hep-Spleen	12.8	13.5
Descending	6.3	5.7
Sigmoid	26.9	26.1
Multiple sites	0.5	0.5
Colons NOS	1.6	1.5
Rectum	17.1	16.0
Rectosigmoid	9.5	9.7

From Beart et al.[3]

Glenn Steele, Jr, MD, William V. McDermott Professor of Surgery, Harvard Medical School and Chairman, Department of Surgery, New England Deaconess Hospital, Boston, Massachusetts

(90% to 95% of cases). Carcinoid tumors of the large bowel are most often found in the appendix and rectum. These tumors have little propensity to metastasize, even to regional lymph nodes, unless they have progressed through the entire bowel wall and are >2 cm. The determination of carcinoid tumor metastasis (in the absence of liver spread and carcinoid syndrome) is relatively unhelpful since there is no way to preempt or, in fact, treat most regionally or distantly aggressive carcinoid tumors, other than with complete initial resection. In the anal canal, most carcinomas are epidermoid or cloacogenic in type, with some rare anal adenocarcinomas.[4] The treatment of anal cancers is quite distinct from that of colorectal cancer, and their biologic pattern of spread is unique. Other than noting simply that Nigro and colleagues[5] and their successors have led the way in sphincter preservation using combination chemotherapy and radiotherapy as primary treatment, the application of sphincter preservation in the treatment of adenocarcinoma will not be optimal until more effective nonsurgical staging and therapeautic modalities are available for adenocarcinomas in the most distal segment of the rectum.

Etiology

Predisposing Conditions

Known predisposing conditions for colorectal cancer include familial polyposis; inflammatory bowel disease, including both chronic ulcerative colitis (UC) and Crohn's disease; family cancer syndromes, identified in several pedigrees by Lynch and coworkers[6]; and adenomatous polyps (sessile or tubular). In addition, a subset of patients have the propensity to develop flat polyps in the large bowel, particularly in the ascending colon.

The biologic and treatment focus on familial adenomatous polyposis (FAP) has extended recently from a set of relatively pragmatic and clinically effective rules for screening and surgical preemption to dramatic technical improvements (sphincter preservation and a variety of neo-reservoirs) for patients who would like to retain their sexual and sphincter function but at the same time minimize the risk of dying from colorectal cancer. Screening for FAP is based on its inheritance as an autosomal dominant trait. Adenomatous polyps will generally not develop until puberty, and transformation of these polyps in patients who carry the gene generally occurs 10 to 15 years after onset of polyposis. Typically then, relatives of patients with FAP should have colonoscopic screening at or shortly after age 15 and should give consideration to a preemptive surgical approach before the age of 25 to 30. Patients who do not have their large-bowel mucosa removed will ultimately undergo transformation in one of their multiple polyps. The ability to remove the colon and the rectal mucosa with reconstruction using either a Parks procedure or some modification has been a remarkable technical advance in preserving function as well as in preventing bowel cancer. In the near future, use of the recently defined gene product from 5q should result in a blood or tissue typing test to screen for the FAP phenotype.[7]

Similarly, patients with chronic ulcerative colitis who have an individually indeterminate but definite predisposition to transformation may also now have less resistance to the move to preemption of possible colon cancer, after about 10 years of UC diagnosis. The ability to remove diseased mucosa without sacrificing sphincter function is based, as in the FAP patient group, on a modification of the Parks procedure and does allow the "best of both worlds." One or, quite frequently, several surgeries may be subsequently warranted for obstruction or pouch problems, but there is not the previous high probability of permanent sexual or sphincter dysfunction.

The cancer risk for each individual patient with ulcerative colitis or Crohn's disease is difficult to establish. For populations of patients with UC, more recent investigations have tended to challenge the dogma of colon cancer incidence being approximately 1% annually 10 years after the diagnosis of UC is made and increasing with each subsequent year. Such individually difficult clinical dilemmas have led to a series of investigations into the molecular biology of large-bowel mucosa predisposed to either familial or sporadic adenocarcinomas.

A number of potentially interesting markers now exist to qualitatively determine the degree of dysplasia and may, in fact, allow more precise quantitation of individual patient risk for mucosal transformation in inflammatory bowel disease.[8] Such molecular markers might also be valuable in defining other areas of the gastrointestinal (GI) tract known to be at risk for transformation. At present, however, the risk for transformation cannot be adequately quantitated in the individual patient, such as the patient with gastric dysplasia, gastroesophageal reflux, Barrett's esophagus, or dysplasia of the mucosa at the gastroesophageal junction. The use of sucrase-isomaltase has just begun to be discussed in the clinicopathologic literature, in place of simple morphologic monitoring of the qualitative aspects of progress dysplasia in such groups.[9]

However, the major clinical yield from recent breakthroughs in the molecular biology of colon and rectal adenocarcinoma will depend on application not simply to known predisposing conditions but to the majority of patients who develop so-called sporadic large-bowel carcinoma. The watershed work of Vogelstein[10] and others[11,12] has translated clinical access to known premalignant colon phenotypes—ie, patients with polypoid disease—to model systems in which the genetics of initiated and promoted GI mucosa can be linked (Fig 14-1).[13] Within a few years, tests of stool samples, in patients with no known predisposition to colorectal cancer, and perhaps even blood tests will allow us to define candidates for screening with either double-contrast roentgenography or colonoscopy. If this "high risk" group for sporadic colorectal cancer is relatively limited, then colonoscopy will become cost-effective in terms of both screening and preempting at a polyp stage the progression that occurs at a low frequency but is accepted as a precursor in most sporadic bowel cancers.

Screening

Individuals who are not at known increased risk for large-bowel cancer and who are asymptomatic should be screened annually with a digital rectal exam beginning at age 40. In patients who are aged 50 or over, additional screening should include not only an occult blood test at the time of the annual digital examination but also sigmoidoscopy at 3- to 5-year intervals.[14] Screening in large asymptomatic populations with a variety of occult blood testing of stool samples has not been uniformly productive for polyp or carcinoma diagnoses.[15] The American Cancer Society has recently updated its screening recommendations for the early detection of colorectal cancer. These have been published by Levin and Murphy in a 1992 issue of *CA—A Cancer Journal for Clinicians.*[16]

It is important to note that new screening recommendations have been developed over the past several years for first-degree relatives of patients with sentinel sporadic large-bowel carcinomas. Thus, the relative risk for such individuals depends on the age of the "proband" with the cancer but definitely is increased compared with nonrelated, age-matched controls.[17] Thus, the use of colonoscopic or double-contrast screening may be justified in most first-degree relatives at age 40. In addition, patients with colonic polyps or colon cancer remain at increased risk for metachronous malignancy or premalignancy of the large bowel and should undergo interval screening as defined in a number of studies, with at least an annual survey followed every 2 to 3 years by complete mucosal surveillance if metachronous polyps are not found in the first follow-up study.

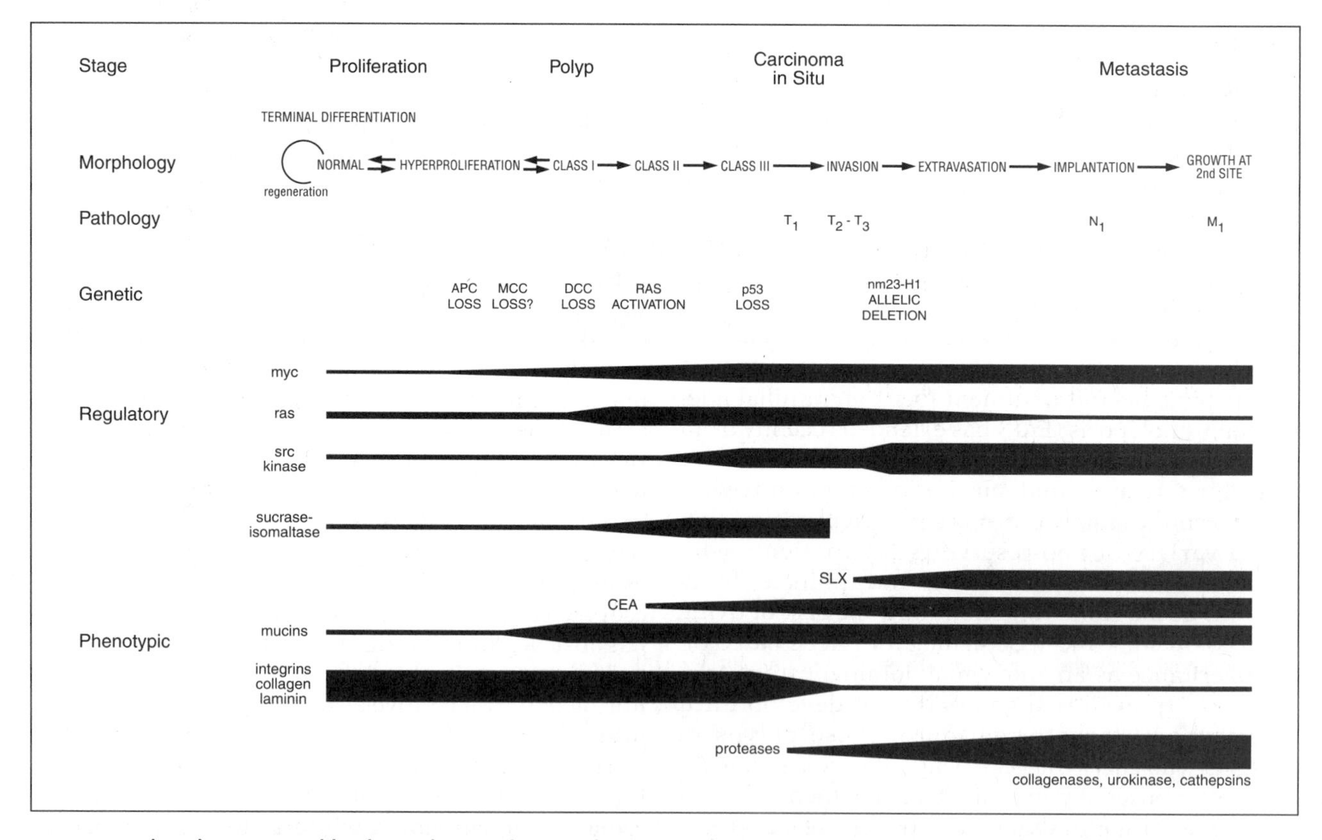

Fig 14-1. Clinical, genetic, and biochemical events during malignant transformation and progression to metastasis of colonic and rectal epithelial cells. Depicted are the various stages of colon cancer development and, below, the approximate time at which molecular changes occur. Genetic changes are depicted at the time they become frequent. Regulatory and biochemical changes are illustrated by increasing and decreasing levels of activity. From Jessup and Gallick.[13]

Staging

At present, staging criteria still depend on the pathologic examination of a completely resected colon or rectal cancer and the surrounding mesenteric tissue. The TNM (primary tumor, nodal involvement, and distant metastases) classification is used to stage colorectal cancers (Table 14-3).[18]

The TNM classification has largely replaced the Dukes system described in 1932 and modified innumerable times. Although the more recent modifications of Dukes have attempted to focus on improved prognostic information, particularly valuable as "tailored" adjuvant and neoadjuvant therapy is addressed, the proliferation of Dukes terminology has accentuated the need for a uniform terminology for staging. This remains the major rationale for TNM. Evaluation of diagnostic and treatment standards, for both practitioner and hospital, in caring for tumor patients will soon be inferred by the frequency of correct staging (ie, TNM) applied to all appropriate patients, as monitored by national survey techniques.[19]

Staging is based on the natural history of a tumor. For adenocarcinomas of the large bowel, spread occurs sequentially from the primary tumor through the bowel wall into pericolonic or perirectal mesentery, into adjacent lymph nodes, and then through the mesenteric lymph node chain and mesenteric venous channels into regional and distant target organs. The most distal rectal adenocarcinomas and anal cancers spread laterally to perineal nodes and may appear in

Table 14-3. Carcinoma of the Colorectum: Stage Classification and Stage Grouping

AJCC 1992 (4th ed)	UICC 1978 (3rd ed)	Dukes (1932, 1935)*	Astler-Coller†
Stage 0	Stage 0		Stage 0
Carcinoma in situ			
Tis, N0, M0	Tis, N0, M0		0
Stage I	Stage I	A	Stage I
Tumor invades submucosa	1A		
T1, N0, M0	T1, N0, M0	A	A
Tumor invades muscularis propria	1B		
T2, N0, M0	T2, N0, M0	A	B1
Stage II	Stage II	B	Stage II
Tumor invades through muscularis propia into the subserosa, or into nonperitonealized pericolic or perirectal tissues	T3, T4, N0, M0 (T3a with fistula) (T3b without fistula)		B2
T3, N0, M0			
Tumor directly invades other organs or structures and/or perforates the visceral peritoneum			
T4, N0, M0			
Stage III	Stage III	C (1932)	Stage III
Any degree of bowel wall invasion with regional node metastasis but without distant metastasis	Any T, N1, M0	C1 (1935) C2 (1935)	C1 C2
Any T, N1-3, M0			
Stage IV	Stage IV	Type 4	Stage IV
Any degree of bowel wall invasion with or without regional lymph node metastasis but with evidence of distant metastasis	Any T, any N, M1	(so-called D)	D
Any T, any N, M1			

*Dukes: A = limited to bowel wall; B = spread to extramural tissue; C = involvement of regional nodes (C1: near primary lesion, C2: proximal node involved at point of ligation); Type 4 (so-called D) = distant metastasis

† Astler-Coller: A = limited to mucosa; B1 = same as AJCC Stage I (T2); B2 = same as AJCC Stage II (T3); C1 = limited to wall with involved nodes; C2 = through all layers of wall with involved nodes

From American Joint Committee on Cancer.[18]

both inguinal as well as hypogastric and periaortic node basins. Target organs for distant dissemination most often include the liver and lung. Less often, but still frequent, sites of spread include the brain and bone. The overall distribution of regional versus distant recurrence remains approximately 50/50.

The concept of distant metastatic tumor spread has changed with the current realization that target-specific metastatic spread is not based simply on the probability of tumor cells entering either lymphatic or vascular circulation. Recent data have shown a surprisingly high number of patients with insidious epithelial marker positivity in marrow samples, without clinically apparent advanced-stage disease at the time of primary colon and rectal cancer surgery. Thus, a predisposition to either regional recurrence or distant recurrence, to the liver, lung, bone, or brain, may depend more on specific biologic factors such as interactions between transmembrane molecules on predestined metastatic tumor clones and specific receptors on endothelium or perhaps Kupffer's cells in the liver or fixed alveolar macrophages in the lung.[20] The marrow may be either a marker of systemic disease proclivity or a reservoir of disseminated tumor cells that are temporarily clinically latent.[21,22] A number of investigators (including our group) have been asking if carcinoembryonic antigen (CEA), a known tumor marker used in the serologic follow-up of many patients with colon and rectal cancer, is functionally equivalent to an adhesion molecule, with particular relevance to target-specific metastatic ability in the liver and lung.[23]

At present, the major clinical rationale for determining metastatic spread is to place in perspective the role of primary surgical extirpation of large-bowel cancer. Almost all patients will need surgery for their primary disease, at least to prevent obstruction or bleeding, even if they are known preoperatively to have stage IV disease. Thus, the preoperative evaluation should be limited to the least number of studies necessary to define co-morbid disease and, if appropriate, to define regional spread. Unless there is a specific need, patients should not undergo computed tomography (CT) or intravenous pyelography (IVP) before surgery for a primary tumor. However, surveillance of the entire large-bowel mucosa is mandatory prior to definitive tumor resection (if the tumor is not distally obstructing) or within several months of removal of the distally obstructing tumor because of the high frequency of synchronous malignant or premalignant lesions in other segments of the large bowel.

Clinical Symptoms

The presenting symptoms in patients who have large-bowel cancer depend on the site of the tumor. Circumferential adenocarcinomas of the descending colon, the sigmoid colon, and the mid to upper rectum are the most frequent causes of perturbation in bowel habits, changes in the caliber of the stool, and occasionally—in the more advanced lesions that are close to complete obstruction—paradoxical diarrhea. Tenesmus is often a sign of adenocarcinomas infiltrating into and around the perisphincteric lymphatics. The more proximal bowel lesions are those associated with iron deficiency anemias of unknown origin. Table 14-4 presents a summary of the symptoms and their association with the probability of site of large-bowel cancer.[24] Diagnostic tests and staging studies should be appropriate to each of the symptom complexes seen by the physician.

Principles of Surgical Treatment

The primary therapy for colon and rectal adenocarcinoma remains surgical. Principles of cancer surgery include: (1) removal of the entire cancer or precancerous lesion; (2) analysis of the depth of invasion of the cancer into or through the bowel wall or, in the case of a polyp, into the base of the polyp or its stalk; (3) removal and histologic review of the pericolonic or

Table 14-4. Variation in Symptoms of Right Colon, Left Colon, and Rectal Cancer

Symptom	Right Colon	Left Colon	Rectum
Pain	Ill defined	Colicky*	Steady, gnawing
Obstruction	Infrequent†	Common	Infrequent
Bleeding	Brick red	Red, mixed with stool	Bright red, coating stool
Weakness§	Common	Infrequent	Infrequent

* Made worse by the ingestion of food.

† If obstruction occurs, tumor often is located at ileocecal valve region.

§ Weakness secondary to anemia.

From Sugarbaker.[24]

perirectal soft tissues; (4) analysis of the pericolonic or perirectal lymphatic tissues; (5) surgical visualization, palpation, and, now, intraoperative ultrasonographic evaluation of adjacent and noncontiguous target organs for distant spread; (6) minimization of the functional consequences of surgery without sacrifice of any of the above precepts for staging or treatment. Adherence to the above-mentioned "design parameters" for cancer therapy has supported the rationale for conventional surgical techniques to remove right, transverse, and left colon cancers. Thus, right hemicolectomy, transverse colectomy, or left hemicolectomy continues to be founded on clearly definable anatomic structures, specifically the ileocolic, the middle colic, and the right colic vessels. These structures also conveniently encompass the boundaries for regional lymphatic staging and curative resection as defined in Figs 14-2 to 14-5.[25-29]

More extensive lymphatic or colonic resection, "no touch" techniques, and various regional radiation therapy techniques have largely been touted using anecdotal information or nonformally designed or casually performed studies. With the exception of surgical changes that are presently being investigated for mid and distal rectal adenocarcinomas, standard surgical procedures offer the best assurance of cure and adequate staging. Moves to "sleeve" bowel resection or laparoscopic-assisted colon resections hopefully will remain limited to patients with either far-advanced distant disease or significant co-morbid illnesses, or in highly formalized, controlled, ideally multi-institutional trial settings.

For patients with mid and distal rectal adenocarcinomas, sphincter preservation approaches have been evaluated (without sacrifice of the curative surgical principles listed above) in institutional and now multi-institutional trials in which perianal, transanal, transcoccygeal, or transsacral approaches, as well as low anterior approaches with colo-anal reanastomoses, have been addressed.[30] The application of colonic J pouches and additional physiologic modifications in order to obtain the best functional results early have also recently occurred.[31] The gist of all this, although still experimental, may be that in patients with T1, T2, and perhaps even T3 adenocarcinomas, abdominoperineal resection as described by Miles[32] will not be nec-

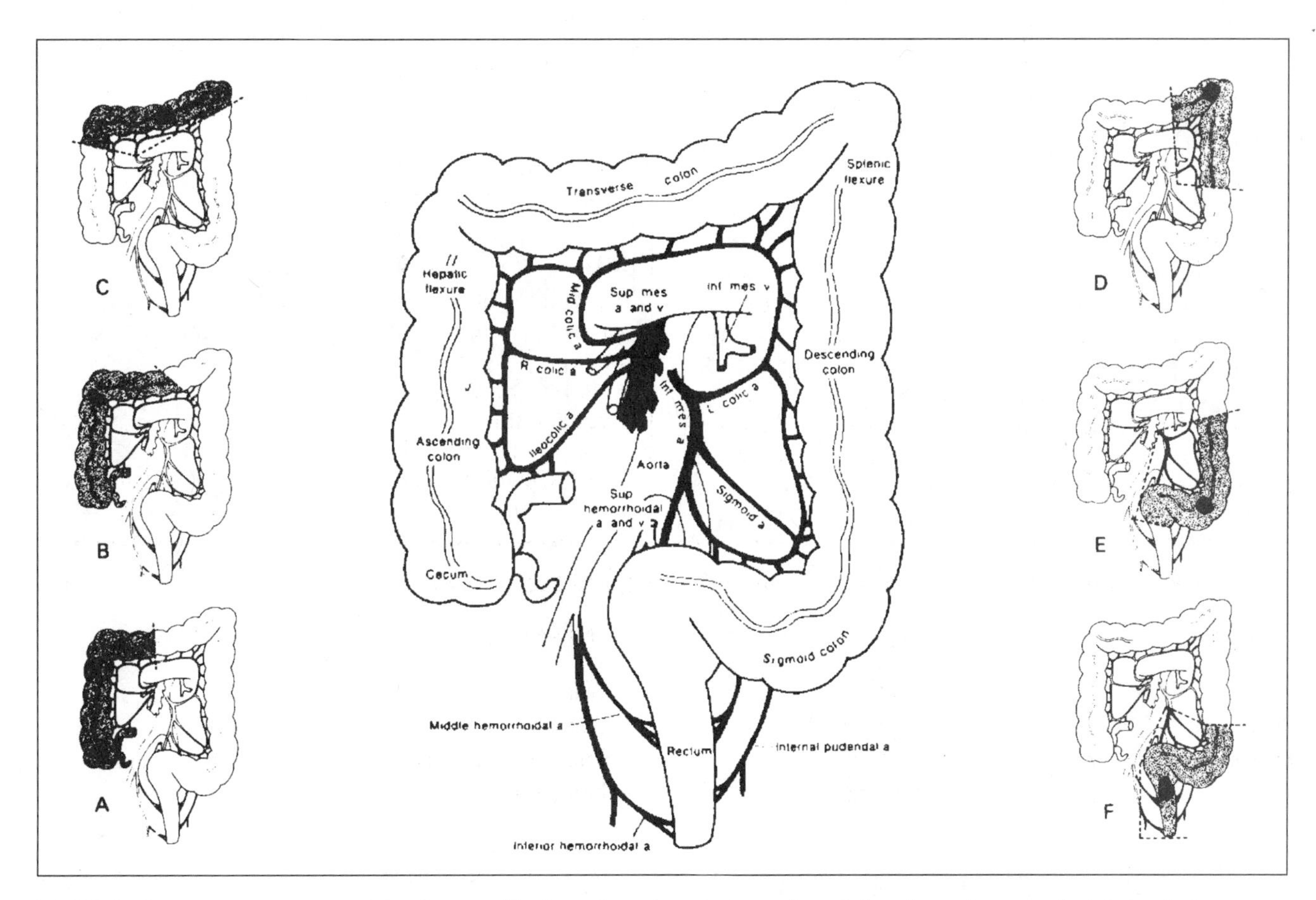

Fig 14-2. Anatomic segments, arterial and venous blood supply, and surgical resections of the colon and rectum. ***A***: right hemicolectomy; ***B***: extended right hemicolectomy; ***C***: transverse colectomy; ***D***: left hemicolectomy; ***E***: sigmoid resection; ***F***: rectosigmoid resection. From Steele and Osteen;[25] adapted from Coller[26] and Jones and Shepard.[27]

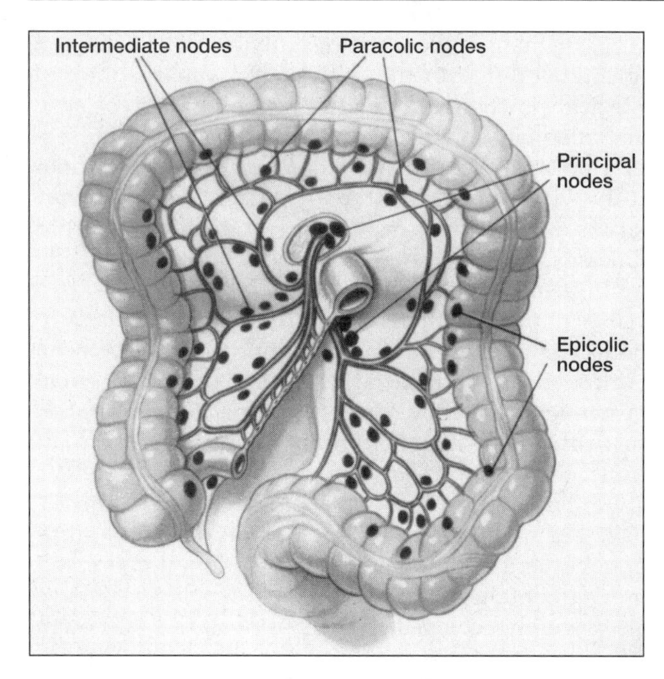

Fig 14-3. The epicolic, paracolic, intermediate, and principal lymph node groups accompanying the vessels of the colon. From Grinnell.[28]

essary to achieve cure, except those with tenesmus or actual physical evidence of tumor extending into the perisphincteric lymphatics. For patients with T2 and T3 lesions, and even some with T1 lesions that show poor morphologic differentiation or lymphatic or vascular infiltration,[33] the addition of concurrent chemotherapy and radiation will be necessary to obviate insidious or microscopic lymphatic spread.

Optimal application of precisely tailored therapy will await more appropriate preoperative staging capacities. Thus, although endoscopic rectal and colonic ultrasound has increased our ability to preoperatively assess the depth of penetration of bowel tumors, the ability to define microscopic pericolonic, perirectal, or mesenteric nodal disease (in nodes of <1 to 1.5 cm in diameter) is negligible. Only with more adequate preoperative staging can neoadjuvant approaches be more intelligently pursued.

Outcome

The best monitor of outcome is examination of the surgery-only control arms of the most recent multi-institutional, multimodality trials with adjuvant therapy. Since the mid 1970s, numerous such trials have involved major referral institutions throughout North

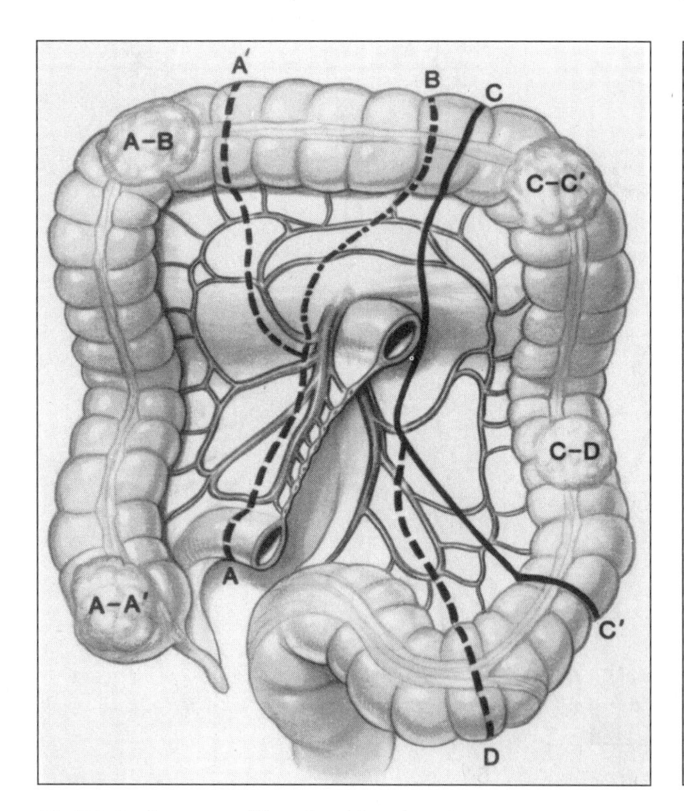

Fig 14-4. Segments of bowel and lymph node containing mesentery to be removed for carcinoma of the cecum (A-A′), hepatic flexure (A-B), splenic flexure (C-C′), and descending colon (C-D). From Steele and Osteen;[25] adapted from McKittrick.[29]

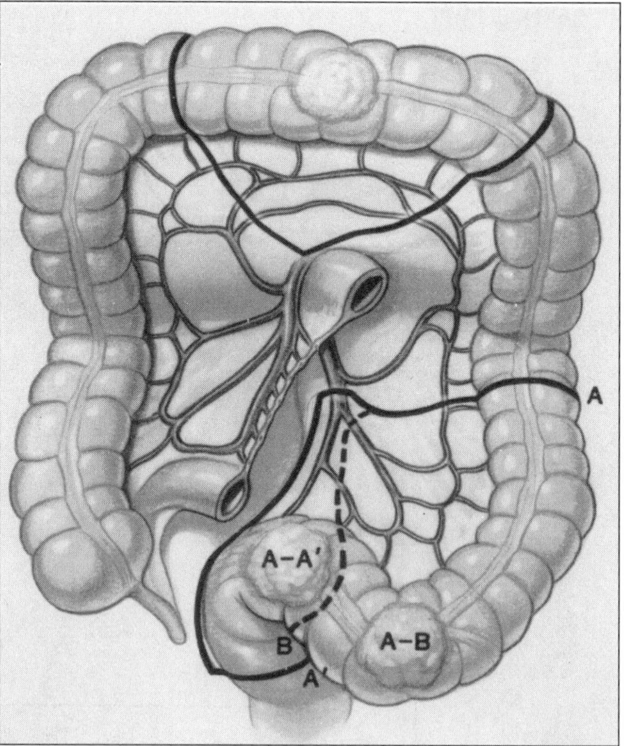

Fig 14-5. Segments of bowel and lymph node containing mesentery to be removed for carcinoma of the transverse colon, the apex of the sigmoid (A-B), and the lower sigmoid or rectosigmoid (A-A′). From Steele and Osteen;[25] adapted from McKittrick.[29]

America; it became obvious that standardized surgery and standardized pathologic staging produced better than expected outcome. Thus, survival for patients even with positive nodes was considerably better than had been expected at the time of the trial design (Figs 14-6 and 14-7).[34,35] This apparent improvement is undoubtedly based on stage shifting and not necessarily on any intrinsic change in the biology of colon and rectal cancer or in any particular surgical treatment. Nevertheless, it has accentuated the need for appropriate control arms in any multimodality treatment plan such as the initial and subsequent adjuvant therapy trials.

For rectal cancer, the same apparent (but not real) improvement in outcome stage for stage was defined in the multi-institutional trial settings. Again, this emphasizes the need for appropriate concurrent control arms prior to concluding any multimodality therapy benefit.

Clinical Trials

The National Consensus Panel on Adjuvant Therapy for Colon and Rectum Cancer, convened in 1990, examined all the appropriately designed multi-institutional trials initiated in the early 1970s or later that addressed adjuvant therapy in stages II and III colon and rectal cancer.[2] For colon cancer, the surprising positive result reported by Laurie and colleagues from the North Central Cancer Treatment Group study (Fig 14-8) implied that stage III colon cancer patients benefited in terms of both disease-free as well as overall survival if they received 5-fluorouracil (5-FU) and levamisole compared with surgery alone.[36] Although this conclusion was based on a retrospective subset analysis of stage III patients (in other words, the effect was not seen in stage II patients), a subsequent intergroup study published in 1990 by Moertel and associates reproduced in part the Laurie result. Specifically, the 1990 report confirmed the benefit in terms of both survival and disease-free survival among stage III colon cancer patients if they received concurrent 5-FU and levamisole after surgery (Figs 14-9 and 14-10).[37]

For rectal cancer, the earliest Gastrointestinal Tumor Study Group (GITSG) trial clearly foreshadowed the benefit of combination chemotherapy and radiation therapy after either low anterior resection or abdominoperineal resection for patients with stages II and III rectal carcinoma (Fig 14-11).[38] However, because of numerous methodologic problems in that early trial, it was not until 1991, when Krook and associates published an important, somewhat similar,

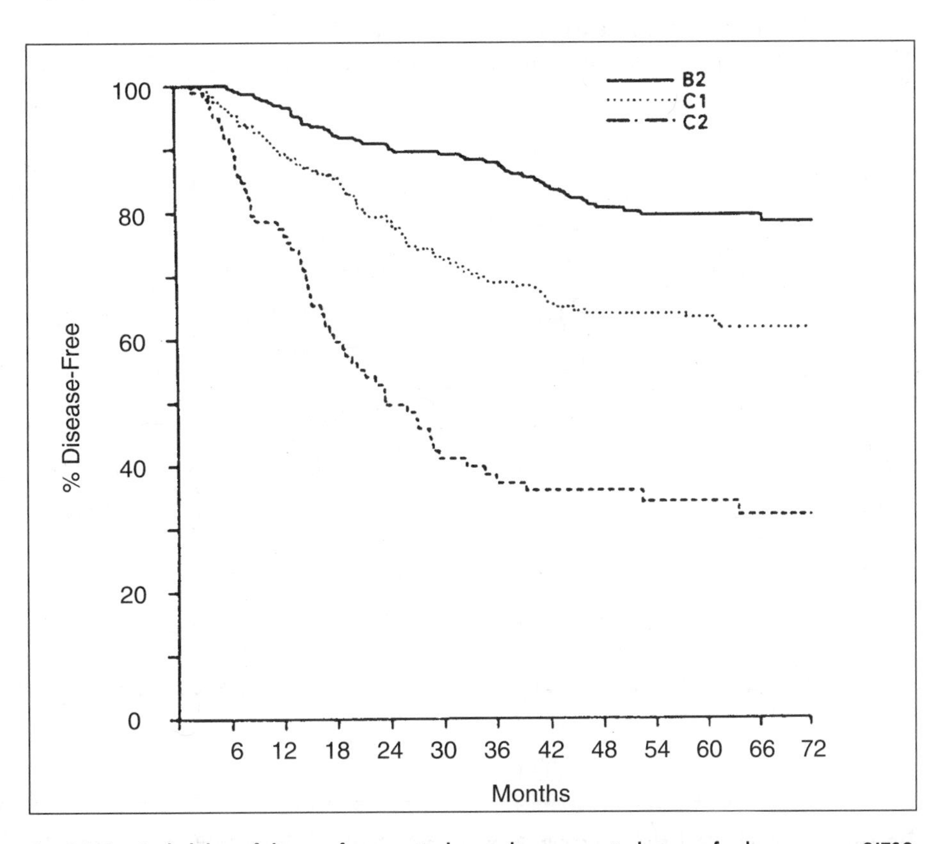

Fig 14-6. Probability of disease-free survival according to surgical stage of colon cancer—GITSG modification of Astler-Coller classification. From Gastrointestinal Tumor Study Group.[34]

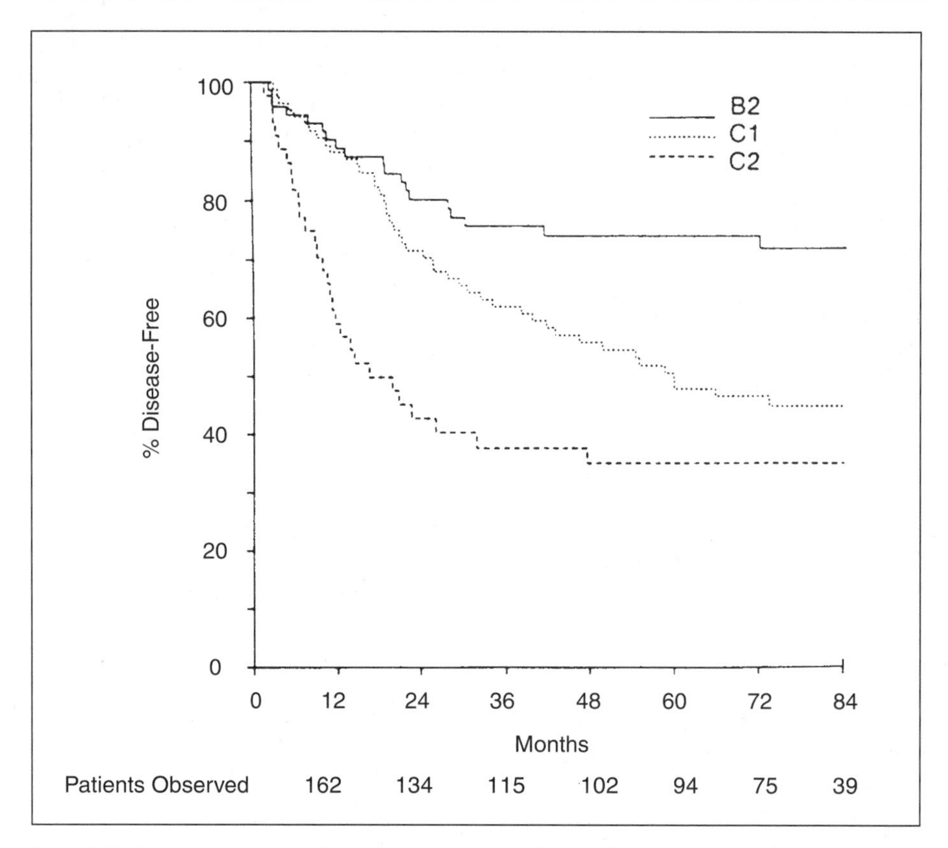

Fig 14-7. Time to recurrence of rectal carcinoma according to disease stage of colon cancer—GITSG modification of Astler-Coller classification. From Gastrointestinal Tumor Study Group.[35]

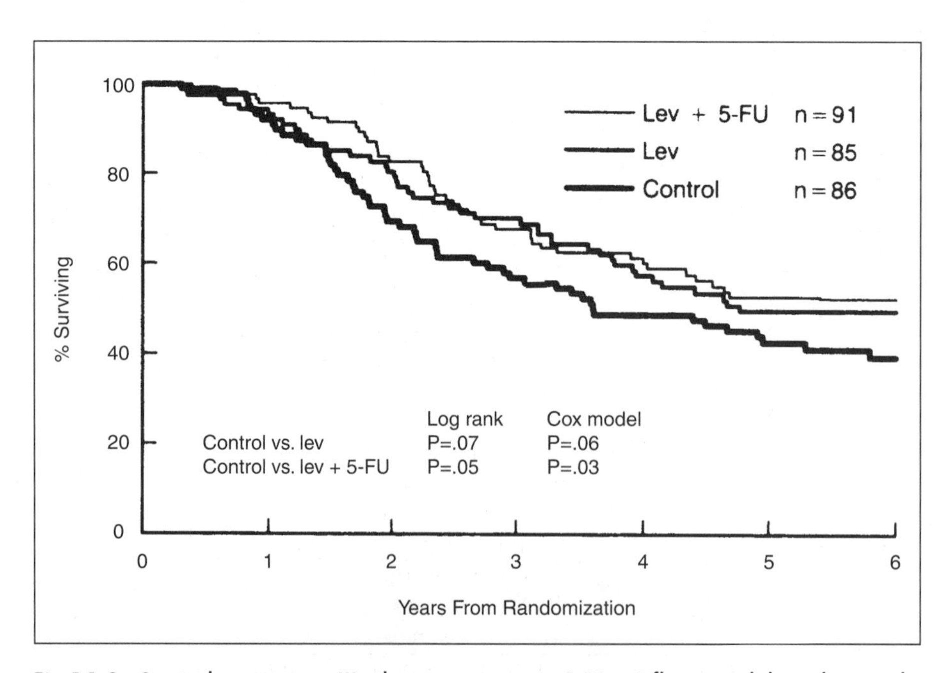

Fig 14-8. Survival rate in stage III colon cancer patients. 5-FU = 5-fluorouracil; lev = levamisole. From Laurie et al.[36]

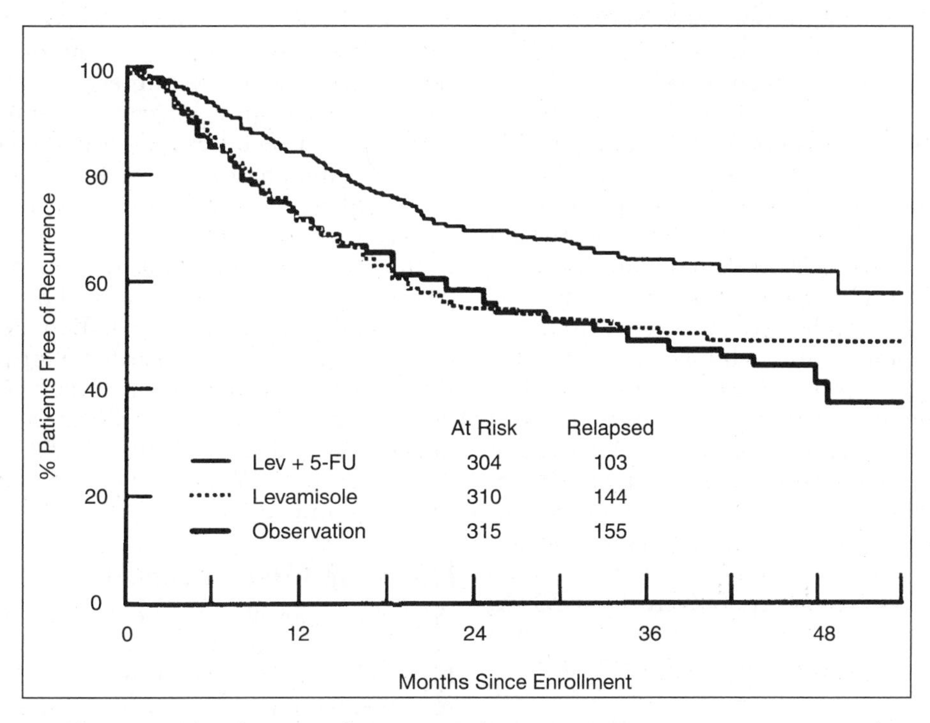

Fig 14-9. Recurrence-free interval in stage III colon cancer patients. LEV + 5-FU = Levamisole plus 5-fluorouracil combination therapy. From Moertel et al.[37]

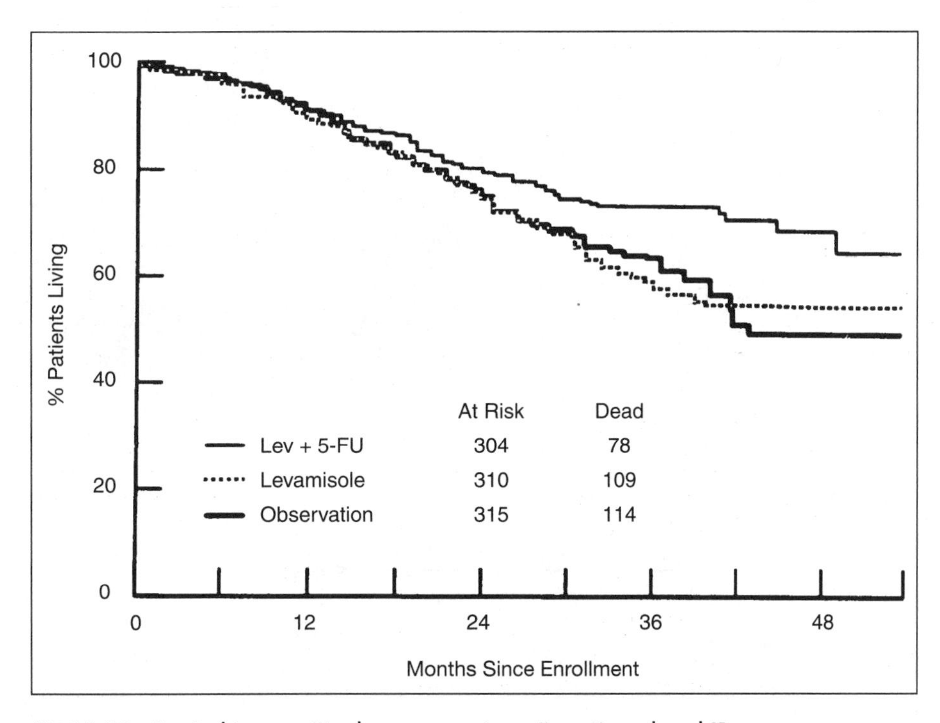

Fig 14-10. Survival in stage III colon cancer patients. From Moertel et al.[37]

data set from a well-executed adjuvant study, that the benefit of concurrent radiation and chemotherapy after conventional surgery for stages II and III rectal adenocarcinoma was confirmed.[39]

Subsequent studies, again in multi-institutional national trial settings, have confirmed that lomustine (methylCCNU) should not be a part of the chemo/radiation therapy combination. Interesting trials by other groups, including the National Surgical Adjuvant Breast and Bowel Project, have implied that combination chemotherapy may be as beneficial as concurrent radiochemotherapy, particularly in males with rectal carcinoma. Although interesting intellectually, the use of preoperative therapy—most frequently radiation therapy alone—has repeatedly been shown to improve freedom from regional disease in patients with T4 colon cancer or stages II and III rectal cancer, but have no significant benefit on patient survival.[40] In addition, the radiation-alone adjuvant studies in rectal cancer patients, whether administered preoperatively or postoperatively, have shown only one half of the regional disease protection when compared with concurrent 5-FU and external beam radiation therapy.[35,39]

New questions concerning adjuvant therapy are based, to a large extent, on the most effective systemic regimens that have recently been evaluated in patients with advanced disease (Table 14-5).[41] The remarkable consistency in results with 5-FU and folinic acid for advanced colorectal cancer makes this particular 5-FU modulation plus concurrent radiotherapy adjuvant study of extreme interest. In addition, results with levamisole for colon cancer can be evaluated for patients with rectal cancer. Whether leucovorin, in fact, is better than levamisole in high-risk primary colon and rectal cancer patients is being evaluated in present adjuvant protocols.

In summary, almost all patients presenting with proven colon or rectal cancer will be operable, if not for cure, then at least for palliation. Fewer than 10% will be unresectable or resectable for palliation only. Fewer than 5% will die from surgery. About 20% will die from associated causes within 5 years. Approximately 50% will survive without evidence of disease 5 years after their cancer diagnosis. These statistics continue to improve.

Follow-Up After Treatment

When large-bowel cancer resection is thought to have been curative, follow-up is based on two precepts. First, the patient needs to be colonoscoped or screened with double-contrast roentgenography on a regular basis. Initial complete surveillance is based on the need to define any synchronous malignant or premalignant lesions. Timing of subsequent studies will be based on whether or not concurrent polyps are

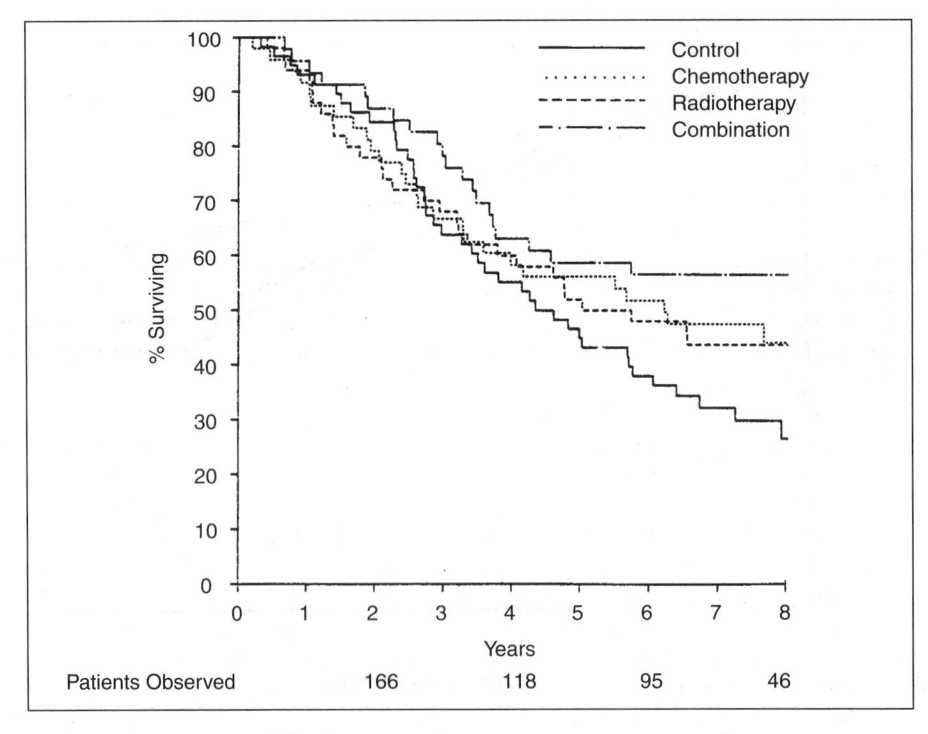

Fig 14-11. GITSG survival distribution according to treatment in patients with stage II or III rectal carcinoma. From Douglass et al.[38]

Table 14-5. Controlled Trials of 5-FU/Folinic Acid Chemotherapy in Advanced Colorectal Cancer

Institution	5-FU Schedule	Folinic Acid Duration	Folinic Acid Dose (mg/m^2)	Tumor Response*
Roswell Park	weekly	2 hr	500	yes
GITSG	weekly	2 hr	500	yes
Italian	weekly	2 hr	500	yes
City of Hope	loading	24 hr	500	yes
Princess Margaret	loading	push	200	yes†
Mayo/North Central	loading	push	200	yes†
Northern California Oncology Group	loading	push	200	no

* Yes = indicates statistically significant improvement in response rate for 5-FU/folinic acid compared with 5-FU alone.
† Statistically significant prolongation of patient survival compared with 5-FU alone.
From Mayer et al.[41]

found at the initial screen. If none are found, the first endoscopic or double-contrast roentgenographic surveillance should occur in a year. If polyps are found, then the initial study should be at 3- to 6-month intervals until complete clearance of the colonic mucosa is achieved. If, at 1 year, endoscopic or double-contrast roentgenographic clearance is documented, the subsequent study probably need not occur for another 2 to 3 years. Obviously, if symptoms arise prior to this interval, appropriate diagnostic studies should be pursued. The rationale for mucosal surveillance in these patients is not to define early evidence of suture line recurrence. Suture line recurrence as an isolated phenomenon is extraordinarily rare and almost always foreshadows regional recurrence with tumor that has grown from the outside of the bowel in through the anastomosis. Thus, anastomotic recurrence is almost always regional. Although the recurrence may necessitate surgery, the procedure is by definition palliative, with cure being limited to regional therapy approaches if any are applicable.

The other major reason for follow-up is based on several data points. First is the kinetics of recurrence: 80% to 90% of recurrences of colon and rectal adenocarcinoma take place in the first 2 to 3 years. Thus, interval follow-up should be more frequent early on. Next, specific target organs are at risk, including the liver, lung, and, to a lesser degree, bone and brain. Finally, only in a very few cases will asymptomatic recurrence be curable. At present, these include the liver and lung and encompass only those patients with isolated, removable asymptomatic recurrences. Thus, in the absence of protocols in which disease-free as well as overall survival is assessed or in the absence of environments where there are experimental therapies for a variety of asymptomatic recurrences, minimal "asymptomatic" follow-up should be undertaken.

In the setting of isolated liver or lung metastasis, patients who have no significant co-morbid disease can be expected to have a probability of 20% to 25% cure if all metastatic disease can be removed or ablated surgically (Figs 14-12 and 14-13).[42,43] All other patients, including those with regional recurrence, are probably not going to be cured. Therefore, the rationale for follow-up should be attentiveness to symptoms and need for palliation once those symptoms occur.

CEA remains an extraordinarily effective marker for patients who have CEA-producing adenocarcinomas. However, its limitation is the absence of curative approaches (for most patients) once recurrence is defined by serial CEA elevation. Thus, CEA follow-up, particularly during the first 2 to 3 years of highest-probability recurrence, is appropriate if the primary tumors in these patients have been proven to produce CEA by immunohistologic staining techniques or by elevated serum CEA levels preoperatively sampled. However, it should be understood that such CEA follow-up studies have a curative potential in a limited number of patients with isolated distant disease in two specific target organs (liver and lung).

The decision to initiate therapy for advanced, noncurable colorectal cancer should depend on availability of formalized treatment protocols in which new techniques are being applied, new combinations of treatment modalities are being compared with old approaches, or conventional systemic therapies are used for patients with symptomatic disease. It should be remembered that in most settings, there is little evidence that systemic disease in patients with

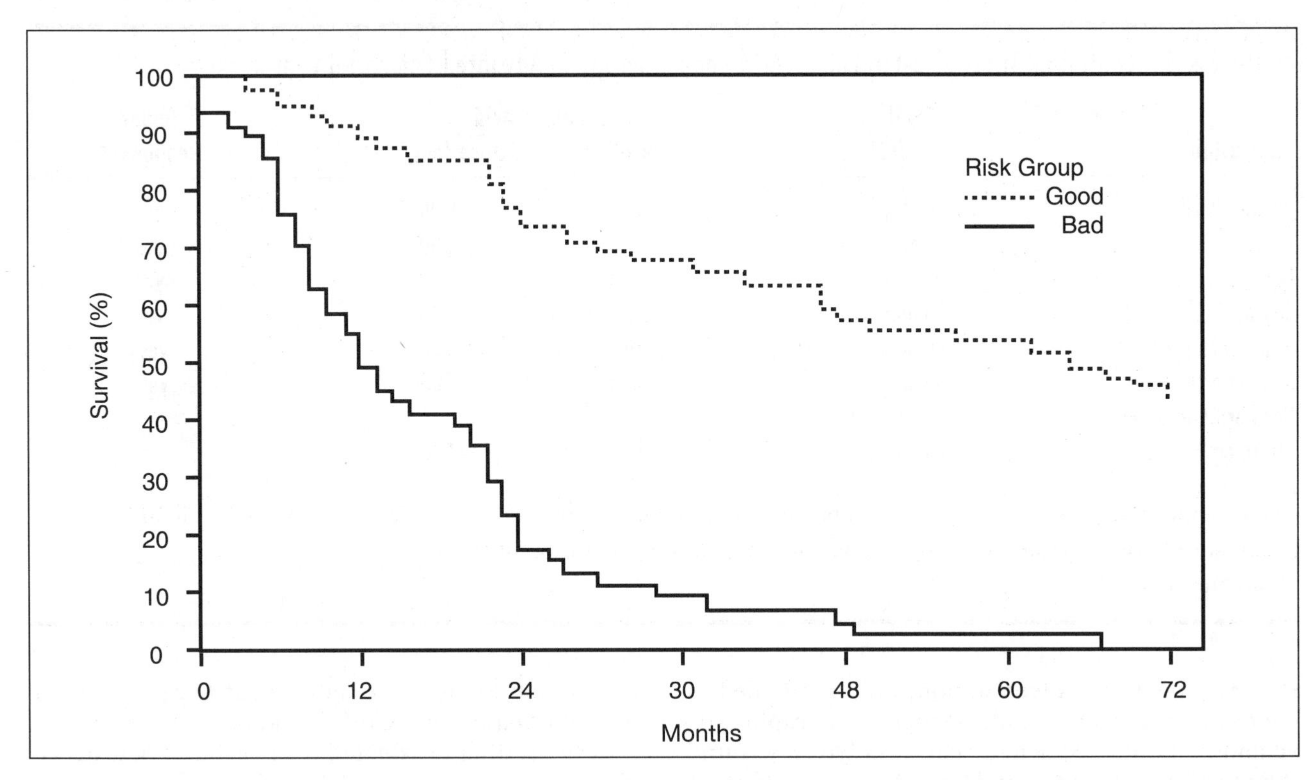

Fig 14-12. Projected disease-free survival for good- and bad-risk groups. Risk group based on margin, disease-free interval (DFI), and number of nodules. Good = all factors favorable; Bad = all unfavorable. Modified from Cady.[42]

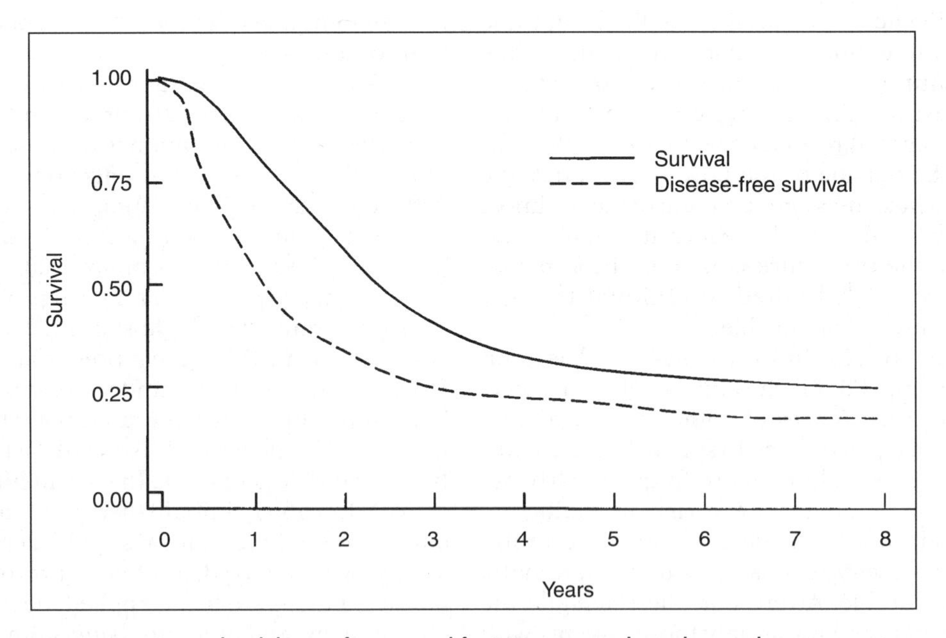

Fig 14-13. Survival and disease-free survival for 859 patients who underwent hepatic resection for metastases of colorectal carcinoma to the liver. From Hughes et al.[43]

advanced colorectal carcinoma can be treated effectively with any significant lengthening of life. This is true of a variety of regional as well as systemic disease treatment options available currently and should moderate enthusiasm for conventional systemic therapy unless there are compelling circumstances—such as symptoms to palliate.

References

1. Boring CC, Squires TS, Tong T, Montgomery S. Cancer Statistics, 1994. *CA Cancer J Clin.* 1994;44:7-26.

2. Steele GD Jr, Augenlicht LH, Begg CB, et al. National Institutes of Health Consensus Development Conference: Adjuvant Therapy for Patients with Colon and Rectal Cancer. *JAMA.* 1990;264:1444-1450.

3. Beart R, Doggett S, Steele G Jr. *Patient Care and Evaluation Study—Colorectal Cancer.* In press.

4. Beart RW Jr. Rectal and anal cancer. In: Steele G Jr, Osteen RT, eds. *Colorectal Cancer: Current Concepts in Diagnosis and Treatment.* New York, NY: Marcel Dekker Inc; 1986:163-185.

5. Nigro ND, Vaitkevicius VK, Buroker T, Bradley GT, Considine B. Combined therapy for cancer of the anal canal. *Dis Colon Rectum.* 1981;24:73-75.

6. Lynch HT, Watson P, Lanspa S, et al. Clinical nuances of Lynch Syndromes I and II. In: Steele G Jr, Burt RW, Winawer SJ, Karr JP, eds. *Basic and Clinical Perspectives of Colorectal Polyps and Cancer.* New York, NY: Alan R Liss Inc; 1988: 177-188.

7. Kinzler KW, Nilbert MC, Vogelstein B, et al. Identification of a gene located at chromosome 5q21 that is mutated in colorectal cancers. *Science.* 1991;251:1366-1370.

8. Wiltz O, O'Hara CJ, Steele GD Jr, Mercurio AM. Expression of enzymatically active sucrase-isomaltase is a ubiquitous property of colon adenocarcinomas. *Gastroenterology.* 1991;100:1266-1278.

9. Andrews CW Jr, O'Hara CJ, Goldman H, et al. Sucrase-isomaltase expression in chronic ulcerative colitis and dysplasia. *Hum Pathol.* In press.

10. Vogelstein B, Fearon ER, Hamilton SR, et al. Genetic alterations during colorectal-tumor development. *N Engl J Med.* 1988;319:525-532.

11. Bodmer WF, Bailey CJ, Bodmer J, et al. Localization of the gene for familial adenomatous polyposis on chromosome 5. *Nature.* 1987;328:614-616.

12. Weinberg RA. Tumor suppressor genes. *Science.* 1991; 254:1138-1146.

13. Jessup JM, Gallick GE. The biology of colorectal carcinoma. In: Steele G Jr, ed. *Current Problems in Cancer.* St Louis, Mo: Mosby-Year Book Inc; in press.

14. Steele G Jr. Colorectal cancer. In: McKenna RJ Sr, Murphy GL, eds. *Cancer Surgery.* Philadelphia, Pa: JB Lippincott Co; in press.

15. Winawer J, Schottenfeld D, Flehinger BJ. Colorectal cancer screening. *J Natl Cancer Inst.* 1991;83:243-253.

16. Levin B, Murphy GP. Revision in American Cancer Society recommendations for the early detection of colorectal cancer. *CA Cancer J Clin.* 1992;42:296-299.

17. Levin B. Screening sigmoidoscopy for colorectal cancer. *N Engl J Med.* 1992;326:700-702.

18. Beahrs OH, Henson DE, Hutter RVP, Kennedy BJ, eds. *American Joint Committee on Cancer Manual for Staging of Cancer.* 4th ed. Philadelphia, Pa: JB Lippincott Co; 1992; 75-82.

19. Steele GD Jr, Winchester DP, Menck HR, Murphy GP. National Cancer Data Base. Annual Review of Patient Care. Atlanta, Ga: American Cancer Society/American College of Surgeons Commission on Cancer; 1992.

20. Thomas P, Toth CA, Steele G Jr. Carcinoembryonic antigen binding proteins from Kupffer cells. In: Wisse EW, Knook DL, McCuskey RS, eds. *Cells of the Hepatic Sinusoid, III.* Leiden, The Netherlands: Kupffer Cell Foundation; 1991;506-509.

21. Cote RJ, Rosen PP, Lesser ML, et al. Prediction of early relapse in patients with operable breast cancer by detection of occult bone marrow micrometastases. *J Clin Oncol.* 1991;9:1749-1756.

22. Schlimok G, Funke I, Bock B, Schweiberer B, Witte J, Riethmuller G. Epithelial tumor cells in bone marrow of patients with colorectal cancer: immunocytochemical detection, phenotypic characterization, and prognostic significance. *J Clin Oncol.* 1990;8:831-837.

23. Meterissian S, Ford R, Toth CA, et al. Carcinoembryonic antigen is an adhesion molecule for colorectal carcinoma. *Proc Am Assoc Cancer Res.* 1991;32:A432.

24. Sugarbaker PH. Clinical evaluation of symptomatic patients. In: Steele G Jr, Osteen RT, eds. *Colorectal Cancer: Current Concepts in Diagnosis and Treatment.* New York, NY: Marcel Dekker Inc; 1986;59-98.

25. Steele G Jr, Osteen RT. Surgical treatment of colon cancer. In: Steele G Jr, Osteen RT, eds. *Colorectal Cancer: Current Concepts in Diagnosis and Treatment.* New York, NY: Marcel Dekker Inc; 1986;127-162.

26. Coller JA. *Cancer of the Colon and Rectum.* New York, NY: American Cancer Society Inc; 1956.

27. Jones T, Shepard WC. *A Manual of Surgical Anatomy.* Philadelphia, Pa: WB Saunders Co; 1945.

28. Grinnell RS. Lymphatic metastases of carcinoma of the colon and rectum. *Ann Surg.* 1950;131:494-506.

29. McKittrick LS. Principles old and new of resection of colon for carcinoma. *Surg Gynecol Obstet.* 1948;87:14-25.

30. Steele G Jr, Busse P, Huberman MS, et al. A pilot study of sphincter-sparing management of adenocarcinoma of the rectum. *Arch Surg.* 1991;126:696-702.

31. Berger A, Tiret E, Parc R, et al. Excision of the rectum with colonic J pouch-anal anastomosis for adenocarcinoma of the low and mid rectum. *World J Surg.* 1992;16:470-477.

32. Miles WE. A method of performing abdomino-perineal excision for carcinoma of the rectum and of the terminal portion of the pelvic colon. *Lancet.* 1908;2:1812-1813.

33. Brodsky JT, Richard GK, Cohen AM, Minsky BD. Variables correlated with the risk of lymph node metastasis in early rectal cancer. *Cancer.* 1992;69:322-326.

34. Gastrointestinal Tumor Study Group. Adjuvant therapy of colon cancer: results of a prospectively randomized trial. *N Engl J Med.* 1984;310:737-743.

35. Gastrointestinal Tumor Study Group. Prolongation of the disease-free interval in surgically treated rectal carcinoma. *N Engl J Med.* 1985;312:1465-1472.

36. Laurie JA, Moertel CG, Fleming TR, et al. Surgical adjuvant therapy of large-bowel carcinoma: an evaluation of levamisole and the combination of levamisole and fluorouracil. *J Clin Oncol.* 1989;7:1447-1456.

37. Moertel CG, Fleming TR, MacDonald JS, et al. Levamisole and fluorouracil for adjuvant therapy of resected colon carcinoma. *N Engl J Med.* 1990;322:352-358.

38. Douglass HO Jr, Moertel CG, Mayer RJ, et al. Survival after postoperative combination treatment of rectal cancer. *N Engl J Med.* 1986;315:1294-1295. Letter.

39. Krook JE, Moertel CG, Gunderson LL, et al. Effective surgical adjuvant therapy for high-risk rectal carcinoma. *N Engl J Med.* 1991;324:709-715.

40. Gerard A, Buyse M, Nordlinger B, et al. Preoperative radiotherapy as adjuvant treatment in rectal cancer: final results of a randomized study of the European Organization for Research and Treatment of Cancer. *Ann Surg.* 1988;208:600-614.

41. Mayer RJ, O'Connell MJ, Tepper JE, Wolmark N. Status of adjuvant therapy for colorectal cancer. *J Natl Cancer Inst.* 1989;81:1359-1364.

42. Cady B, Stone MD, McDermott WV Jr, et al. Technical and biologic factors in disease-free survival after hepatic resection in colorectal metastases. *Arch Surg.* 1992;127:561-569.

43. Hughes KS, Simon R, Songhorabodi S, et al. Resection of the liver for colorectal carcinoma metastases: a multi-institutional study of indications for resection. *Surgery.* 1988;103:278-288.

15

TUMORS OF THE PANCREAS, GALLBLADDER, AND EXTRAHEPATIC BILE DUCTS

Robert M. Beazley, MD, Isidore Cohn, Jr, MD

Tumors of the Pancreas

Pancreatic exocrine cancer is the second most common visceral malignancy as well as the fifth leading cause of cancer mortality in the United States, accounting for one fifth of all gastrointestinal (GI) cancer deaths. According to the American Cancer Society, about 27,000 new cases of pancreatic cancer were diagnosed in 1994 and 25,900 deaths will be recorded.[1] The retroperitoneal location of the pancreas is considered a major obstacle to early treatment. Nevertheless, recent developments have influenced the diagnosis and clinical management of this difficult disease and are reviewed in this chapter.

Epidemiology and Risk Factors

The incidence of pancreatic cancer in the US rose sharply until the mid 1970s, when the rate stabilized at 9 per 100,000. Pancreatic cancer is a disease of the industrialized world, with a tenfold difference between the highest incidence rate, in American black males (15.2 per 100,000), and the lowest rates, in Hungary, Nigeria, and India (1.5 per 100,000).[2] High risk has also been observed in Polynesian males, including native Hawaiians and New Zealand Maoris. The incidence in Japan has risen from 1.8 per 100,000 in 1960 to 5.2 per 100,000 in 1985.

Whittemore and colleagues studied cancer precursors in 50,000 graduates of Harvard and the University of Pennsylvania, using results of college physical examinations and subsequent alumni questionnaires. Nonsmoking classmates were used as age- and sex-matched controls. An increased relative risk of 2.6 was observed for males who were smokers during college.[3] Additional studies have confirmed an increased risk for cigarette smokers, which may be directly proportional to total cigarette consumption.[4] The risk for ex-smokers approaches that of lifetime nonsmokers 10 to 15 years after cessation of smoking. Consumption of cigars, cigarillos, and pipe tobacco as well as chewing tobacco does not appear to be associated with increased risk.

The geographic distribution of pancreatic exocrine cancer as well as migrant studies strongly suggests a causative role for environmental factors such as diet. Diets high in fat have been associated with the development of pancreatic cancer, a correlation supported by experimental animal studies. Other factors include ingestion of meat and total caloric intake, especially that derived from carbohydrates, dairy products, and seafood. Burney and associates found low serum levels of both lycopene (a carotenoid structurally similar to beta carotene but with no retinoid or preretinoid activity) and the trace element selenium in individuals with pancreatic cancer.[5] An inverse association has been demonstrated with the consumption of a high-fiber diet, fruits, and fresh vegetables. An increased risk was thought to be associated with coffee drinking and alcohol intake; however, studies have failed to confirm these observations.

Similarly, many studies have failed to show an association between diabetes and pancreatic cancer, although several prospective studies have demonstrated up to a fourfold risk. The onset of diabetes in the months prior to the diagnosis of pancreatic cancer has been recognized for years. This finding may alert a clinician to the possible presence of an early pancreatic carcinoma, particularly in the middle-aged patient without a family history of diabetes.

Previous studies have suggested that certain occupations such as chemists and metal workers may have an increased risk of pancreatic cancer mortality. Mancuso and El Attar have shown an associated risk in men employed in the manufacture of betanaphthylamine and benzidine.[6]

Robert M. Beazley, MD, Professor of Surgery, Boston University School of Medicine and Chief, Section of Surgical Oncology, University Hospital, Boston, Massachussetts

Isidore Cohn, Jr, MD, Professor of Surgery, Department of Surgery, Louisiana State University, School of Medicine, New Orleans, Louisiana

The role of heredity in pancreatic cancer has not been clearly defined, but there have been case reports of familial clustering. Recent studies have confirmed increased risks in individuals who have a close relative with pancreatic malignancy.

It is unusual to encounter pancreatic cancer in patients younger than 40. The mean age at diagnosis is about 63 years, with a slight male predominance. Mortality rates for pancreatic cancer nearly equal the incidence rate, with only a small percentage of patients surviving 5 years and almost never without surgical intervention. Survival is approximately 4 months for an untreated pancreatic exocrine cancer, 7 months with a bypass procedure, and 16 months following resectional surgery. According to recent statistics, 20% of patients with a diagnosis survive 1 year, with 3% surviving 5 years.

Rodent models of pancreatic cancer have been developed using the rat (azaserine), the Syrian hamster (N-nitrosobis [2-oxypropyl] amine or amine BOP), and the guinea pig (methylnitrosourea). Nitroso compounds are among the most effective carcinogens used in rodent models. Diets high in saturated fats have been observed to promote carcinogenesis in the rat model. Ishizuka and colleagues have shown that neurotensin can stimulate growth in human pancreatic carcinoma.[7] Cholecystokinin (CCK) or its analogue, cerulein, is known to stimulate the growth of exocrine pancreas in laboratory animals. Presumably because of CCK release, diets high in soybean flour and trypsin inhibitors promote carcinogenesis in the rat. CCK and secretin in combination can stimulate carcinogen-induced pancreatic cancer. In studies by Smith and colleagues, CCK stimulated the growth of human pancreatic adenocarcinoma xenografts in the nude mouse.[8] Recently, a potent CCK-receptor antagonist has been shown to inhibit azaserine-induced preneoplastic pancreatic lesions in the rat. However, the role of such antagonists in the clinical management of pancreatic cancer remains to be investigated. Lovastatin, a cholesterol-lowering drug, inhibits pancreatic cancer growth in vitro.

Pathology

More than 90% of pancreatic malignancies arise from ductal epithelium, even though <15% of the pancreas by mass is made up of ductal tissue—a disparity without explanation. Two thirds of tumors are located in the pancreatic head. Most pancreatic tumors are mucin-producing adenocarcinomas, with perineural invasion in 90%, lymph node involvement in 70% to 80%, and venous involvement in 50%. A brisk desmoplastic response is seen in virtually all cases. Peritumoral pancreatitis can make obtaining reliable biopsy material difficult. Other tumors arising from the pancreas include acinar cell carcinoma (5%), cystadenocarcinoma (mucinous), adenosquamous carcinoma, solid microglandular carcinoma, carcinoid, sarcoma, and malignant lymphoma. Cancers arising in the head of the pancreas must be distinguished from peripancreatic lesions arising from the distal common bile duct, the ampulla of Vater, or the duodenum. While ampullary cancer is the most resectable and associated with the most favorable prognosis, survival rates with all three are higher than with pancreatic cancer.

Recent studies have found mutant Kirsten (Ki)-*ras* oncogene in a high percentage of human pancreatic cancers. According to Motojima and colleagues, the prevalence of the mutation in Ki-*ras* codon 12 is 89% for pancreatic lesions, 13% for ampullary lesions, and 20% for those arising from the common bile duct.[9] This finding may be of some help in further classifying difficult tumors. Further biomolecular information relating to mutant genes in pancreatic cancer may provide insight into initiation of carcinogenesis as well as possibly providing markers useful in tumor detection.

Clinical Presentation

The clinical diagnosis of pancreatic cancer is frequently made late in the course of the disease. The presenting symptom triad of weight loss, abdominal pain, and jaundice is almost diagnostic for pancreatic cancer (Table 15-1).[10] Weight loss is a nonspecific symptom—usually gradual and progressive. When it is the sole symptom, several months may ensue before the diagnosis of pancreatic cancer is made. Abdominal pain is present in 65% to 80% of patients and is characterized by a steady, "boring" midepigastric pain that is usually worse at night. The pain may be lessened by assuming the fetal position and aggravated by lying flat or sitting up. Many times the pain is vague and ill defined, contributing to a delay in diagnosis.

Jaundice is the third most frequent presenting symptom, and in many instances may present late. Although jaundice is usually progressive, spontaneous fluctuation has been documented. Usually, jaundice is the only clinical finding associated with a small pancreatic cancer close to the common bile duct. For this reason, unexplained jaundice should be carefully evaluated, since such tumors are more likely to be resectable. Commonly, jaundice is accompanied by pruritus involving the arms, legs, and abdomen, which is generally most troublesome at night. The pruritus is thought to be due to bile salts retained in the skin; levels of the latter correlate with the degree of itching more closely than the absolute serum bilirubin level. According to one theory, bile salts may promote the release of proteases from surrounding cells, which then contribute to the itching. Not all jaundice patients complain of itching, and occasionally pruritus may precede the clinical onset of jaundice. While

Table 15-1. Frequency of Presenting Symptoms in 449 Patients With Pancreatic Carcinoma

Symptom	Number of Patients	Percent of Patients	Patients With Resectable Lesions	
			Number	Percent
Weight loss	327	73%	48	74%
Abdominal pain	293	65	29	45
Jaundice	201	45	45	69
Anorexia	163	36	18	28
Significant gastro-intestinal bleeding	30	7	1	15

From Gray et al.[10]

painless jaundice is still heralded erroneously as the presenting symptom of pancreatic cancer, a patient presenting in this manner is certainly the exception. Less common signs and symptoms include anorexia, ascending cholangitis, and alterations in bowel habit (constipation, diarrhea, malabsorption, bloating, or flatulence). Diabetes mellitus may occur concomitantly. Gastric outlet symptoms may occur secondary to direct invasion of the stomach, pylorus, or duodenum, or possibly as a result of functional gastric motility disturbances. Migratory thrombophlebitis (Trousseau's sign), although more commonly associated with lung cancer, may be an early sign of pancreatic cancer. In the middle ages, melancholia, hypochondria, and hysteria were thought to originate in the pancreas. Psychiatric symptoms, chiefly depression, are occasionally seen in patients with pancreatic cancer. More than half of such patients will have psychiatric symptoms predating the physical signs and symptoms of pancreatic cancer by more than 6 months. With the multitude of nonspecific and vague signs and symptoms, the difficulty of making an early diagnosis of pancreatic cancer is understandable and the physician must maintain a high level of suspicion.

Diagnostic Workup

Moossa has suggested that a high level of suspicion be maintained in patients older than 40 years who present with any of the following clinical symptoms: (1) obstructive jaundice; (2) recent unexplained weight loss >10% of body weight; (3) recent unexplained upper abdominal or lumbar back pain; (4) recent vague, unexplained dyspepsia in a normal upper GI investigation; (5) sudden-onset diabetes mellitus without predisposing factors such as family history or obesity; (6) sudden onset of unexplained steatorrhea; and (7) an attack of idiopathic pancreatitis.[11] If a patient is a heavy smoker, the level of suspicion should be doubled.[11]

The initial diagnostic test of choice is the computed tomography (CT) scan. The newer high-speed scanners are operator independent and not limited by patient size or bowel or stomach gas. Liver metastasis, lymphadenopathy, and perivascular invasion can be demonstrated, but not lesions <2 cm or peritoneal nodules reliably. Information obtained by CT may serve to stage the patient and lead to a nonsurgical approach to management. Findings of distant metastasis, tumor extension to contiguous structures, vascular encasement or invasion, and local lymphadenopathy indicate irresectability. However, CT is less accurate in predicting a resectable tumor. A percutaneous fine needle aspiration (FNA) biopsy may be obtained by CT guidance since tissue confirmation is important, especially in the nonoperative setting.

Ultrasonography (US) is used more commonly in Europe than in the US. It is less expensive than CT, readily available, and can visualize the liver, intrahepatic and extrahepatic biliary tree with a sensitivity and specificity of tumor detection exceeding 90%. Ultrasound studies are hampered by being dependent on the technical skills of the operator, by large patient size, and by bowel and stomach gas. Many times, US is used as a complementary test with CT.

To date, magnetic resonance imaging (MRI) has not been useful in the detection of pancreatic cancer. At this time it offers no advantage over CT, but as expertise in the field develops, a future role may be established.

Endoscopic retrograde cholangiopancreatography (ERCP) is especially useful in determining the presence of bile duct calculi as well as in making the diagnosis of distal common bile duct lesions and obtaining tissue biopsies of duodenal and ampullary cancers.

Small head lesions may be detected by compression or occlusion of the pancreatic duct or common bile duct, or both—the so-called double duct sign (Fig 15-1). The pancreatogram is seldom normal in the presence of pancreatic malignancy. When there is dilatation of the common bile duct secondary to unresectable malignancy, ERCP offers the possibility of papillotomy and placement of an endoprosthesis, thus avoiding surgical decompression of the biliary tree. US has been incorporated into the endoscope, providing a novel approach to the diagnosis of pancreatic neoplasia. Currently at an early stage of development, the technique clearly holds great potential.

FNA cytology guided by CT or US will diagnose pancreatic cancer with a sensitivity of 76% to 90% and a specificity of almost 100% (Fig 15-2).[12] FNA can be particularly useful when surgery is not indicated or desirable, eg, in tail or body lesions, in extensive metastatic disease, and with poor surgical candidates. Warshaw has cautioned against use of FNA in potentially resectable patients after finding positive cytologic evidence in peritoneal washings in six of eight patients following FNA.[13]

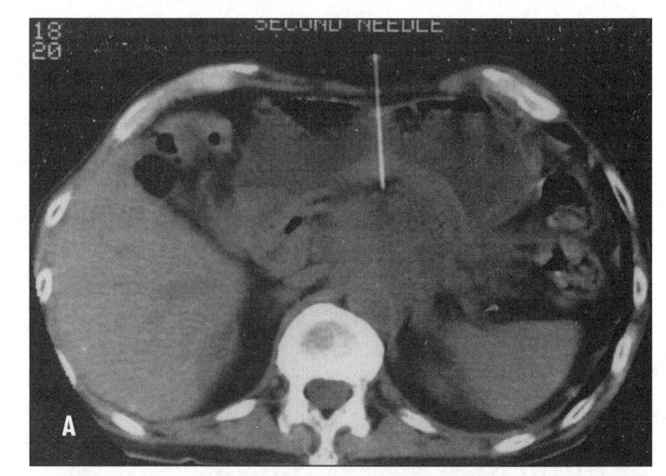

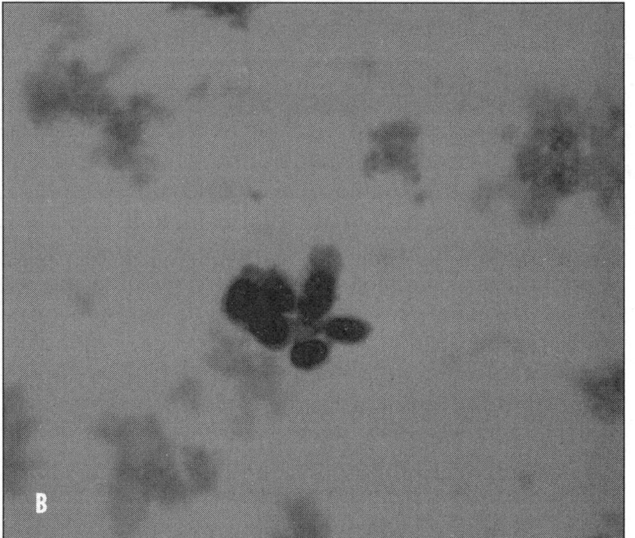

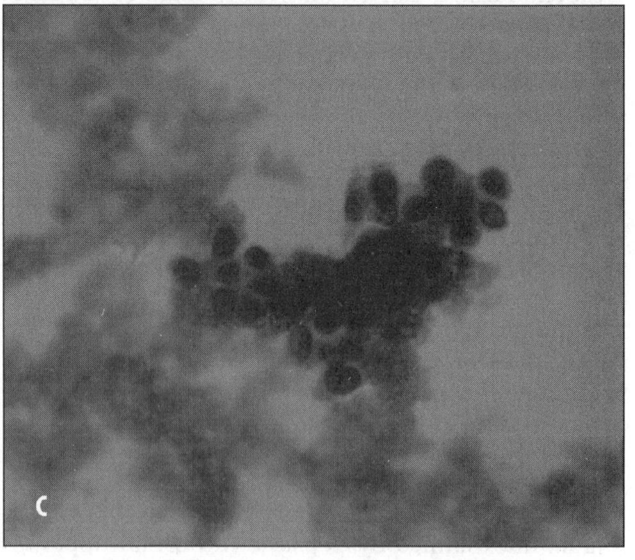

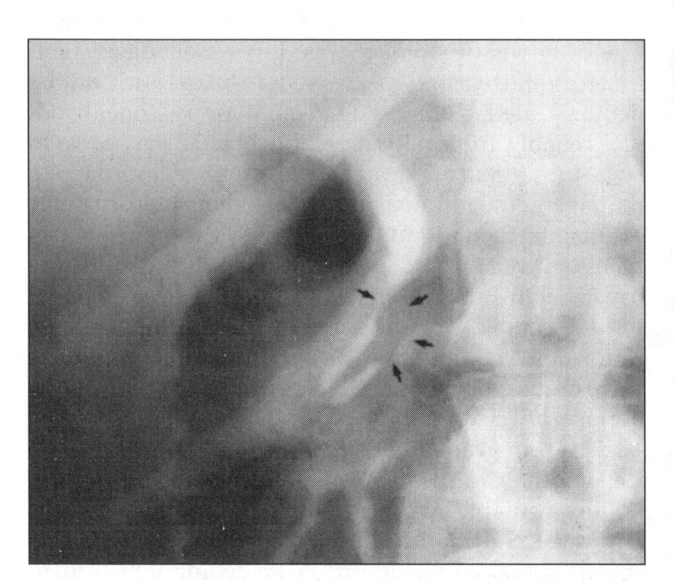

Fig 15-1. Double duct sign on endoscopic cholangiopancreatography is the result of simultaneous obstruction of the common bile duct and pancreatic duct by tumor from the head of the pancreas. This sign is highly suggestive of carcinoma, but has been reported with pancreatitis.

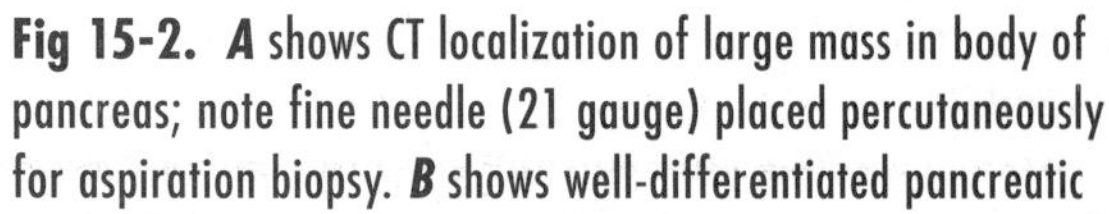

Fig 15-2. ***A*** shows CT localization of large mass in body of pancreas; note fine needle (21 gauge) placed percutaneously for aspiration biopsy. ***B*** shows well-differentiated pancreatic duct adenocarcinoma (Papanicolaou's stain, x200); group of ductal cells with slight nuclear enlargement and disordered architectural features. ***C*** shows a different field from the same specimen as ***A***; well to moderately well-differentiated pancreatic duct carcinoma (Papanicolaou's stain, x400). Variation in tumor cells, sizes, and shapes are present in a larger group with no architectural polarity. From Beazley et al.[12]

Staging

Each diagnostic test may provide staging information that has resulted in fewer diagnostic laparotomies but an increase in the percentage of resectable patients. For those felt to be resectable following CT, ultrasound, or ERCP, other studies might provide additional staging information. Warshaw has proposed using the laparoscope in staging pancreatic cancer, having documented liver metastasis in 23 of 64 patients in whom CT had failed to show hepatic secondary tumors. Simultaneously, unsuspected peritoneal metastases were observed. When laparoscopy, CT, and angiography were all negative, 78% of pancreatic head lesions were resectable as were 100% of ampullary tumors.[14]

Dooley and associates reported similar results combining CT and preoperative angiography in staging patients with periampullary tumors. Major vessel encasement or occlusion, or both, significantly diminished resectability, whereas normal angiography predicted resectability in 77% of patients.[15] Preoperative angiography is important in demonstrating vascular abnormalities in the upper abdomen, most commonly those associated with the anomalous right hepatic artery arising from the superior mesenteric artery, which occurs in 16% to 29% of patients. With this vessel running through the area of the head of the pancreas, dearterialization of the liver and extrahepatic biliary tree is a risk. Staging of pancreatic cancer is shown in Table 15-2.[16]

Table 15-2. TNM Staging of Pancreatic Cancer

Primary Tumor (T)

TX	Primary tumor cannot be assessed
T0	No evidence of primary tumor
T1	Tumor limited to the pancreas
T1a	Tumor 2 cm or less in greatest dimension
T1b	Tumor more than 2 cm in greatest dimension
T2	Tumor extends directly to any of the following: duodenum, bile duct or peripancreatic tissues
T3	Tumor extends directly to any of the following: stomach, spleen, colon or adjacent large vessels

Regional Lymph Nodes (N)

The regional lymph nodes are as follows:

Peripancreatic

Superior:	Lymph nodes superior to the head and body of pancreas
Inferior:	Lymph nodes inferior to the head and body of pancreas
Anterior:	Anterior pancreaticoduodenal, pyloric, and proximal mesenteric lymph nodes
Posterior:	Posterior pancreaticoduodenal, common bile duct or pericholedochal, and proximal mesenteric nodes
Splenic:	Hilum of the spleen and tail of the pancreas

The following nodes are also considered regional:

Hepatic artery

Infrapyloric (for tumors in the head only)
Subpyloric (for tumors in the head only)
Celiac (for tumors in the head only)

Superior mesenteric

Pancreaticolienal (for tumors of the body and tail only)
Splenic (for tumors in the body and tail only)
Retroperitoneal
Lateral aortic

All other lymph nodes are considered distant and should be coded as M1. The peripancreatic lymph nodes are often referred to as the superior pancreatic, inferior pancreatic, anterior pancreatic, posterior pancreatic, and splenic.

NX	Regional lymph nodes cannot be assessed
N0	No regional lymph node metastasis
N1	Regional lymph node metastasis

Distant Metastasis (M)

MX	Presence of distant metastasis cannot be assessed
M0	No distant metastasis
M1	Distant metastasis

Stage Grouping

Stage I	T1	N0	M0
	T2	N0	M0
Stage II	T3	N0	M0
Stage III	Any T	N1	M0
Stage IV	Any T	Any N	M1

From American Joint Committee on Cancer.[16]

Tumor markers have not been helpful in the diagnosis or staging of carcinoma of the pancreas, but may play a role in follow-up management. Carcinoembryonic antigen (CEA) is elevated in a large percentage of cases, but it has a low sensitivity and is elevated in other benign and malignant conditions. CA 19-9 may be slightly more useful in pancreatic cancer than CEA; it is not specific for pancreas and can be elevated in colon and bile duct tumors. Other tumor markers include DU-PAN-2, pancreatic oncofetal antigen, and galactosyltransferase. These tests are neither widely available nor easily obtainable. A National Cancer Institute Conference group concluded that because of the lack of tumor specificity, most tumor markers were unreliable for diagnosis when used by themselves. In addition, it was concluded that the use of multiple markers might increase the sensitivity but usually decreased their specificity.

Treatment

Surgery offers the best chance of a "cure" in pancreatic malignancy. Unfortunately, roughly 80% of individuals on presentation are ineligible for a curative attempt. With recent staging improvements, some authors have reported higher resectability rates in individuals who do proceed to surgery.

In 1899 Halsted performed the first successful resection of a malignant tumor of the ampulla of Vater. In 1914 Herschel performed a one-stage partial pancreaticoduodenectomy, and in 1922 Tet Tetani carried out a pancreaticoduodenectomy in two stages. In 1935 Whipple, Parsons, and Mullins published their report of a two-stage pancreaticoduodenectomy in which the entire duodenum was removed for an ampullary carcinoma.[17] Today, basically the same operation is done in one stage and is known as a Whipple procedure. Priestley and colleagues performed the first total pancreatectomy, with long-term survival, for insulinoma in 1944.[18] Ten years later, Ross reported a total pancreatectomy for carcinoma of the pancreas, demonstrating the multifocal nature of the disease.[19]

Preparation for Surgery

Patients who are potential candidates for the Whipple procedure generally require basic physiologic preparation prior to surgery. Age is not a contraindication to resectional surgery. If the patient's intake has been poor or if he or she has been compromised by nausea and vomiting, adequate preoperative hydration is critical. Volume and electrolyte deficits should all be corrected prior to surgery to minimize the risk of postoperative renal failure. Liver function may have deteriorated secondary to biliary obstruction and occasionally cholangitis. Albumin levels and coagulation studies are easily obtainable measures of liver function. Vitamin K administration and, at times, fresh frozen plasma may be indicated to restore the patient's clotting status. Preoperative external drainage of the obstructed biliary tree has not been found to be helpful since the obstructed biliary tree following drainage rapidly becomes colonized, further compromising hepatic function. At this time, the role of preoperative endoscopic biliary drainage remains to be fully determined.

Recent reports suggest that resection should not be

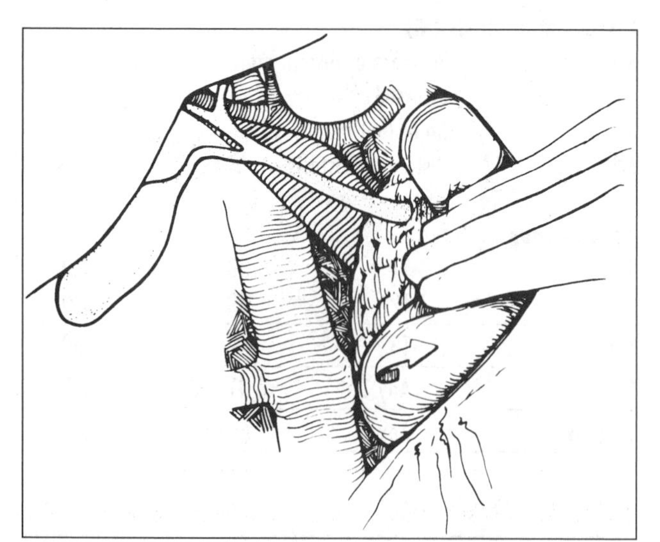

Fig 15-3. A generous and wide Kocher maneuver will permit evaluation of tumor extension especially into the vena cava, duodenum, and portal vein and superior mesenteric artery.

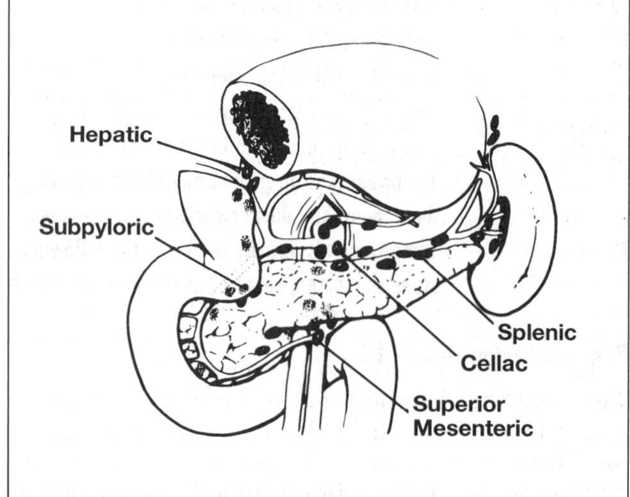

Fig 15-4. Initial exploration of the abdominal cavity for metastatic tumor spread should include all peritoneal surfaces, the liver, base of the transverse mesocolon in addition to regional lymph nodes. From Beazley et al.[12]

contraindicated in patients older than 70, although the operative mortality and morbidity is slightly higher.

Extensive cardiovascular monitoring will ensure adequate preoperative management and be helpful during surgery and postoperatively. Perioperative antibiotics are indicated, as is the placement of an epidural catheter for postoperative pain control and improvement of the patient's ventilatory function.

Resection

Several incisions may be used for the operative approach. Most common is the right subcostal incision for initial exploration, with an extension to the left into a "rooftop" incision. After gaining access to the peritoneal cavity, the surgeon should carefully examine all peritoneal surfaces, the omentum, the liver, and the transverse mesocolon. Metastasis to any of these areas will dictate against pancreatic resection. A Kocher maneuver, mobilizing and reflecting the duodenum and head of the pancreas, may give an indication of tumor extension or fixation to the retroperitoneal structures, vena cava, portal vein, or superior mesenteric artery (Fig 15-3). Next, the lesser sac should be entered through the gastrocolic omentum, to visualize the pancreatic body and tail and gain access to the celiac nodes. Likewise, the hepatoduodenal ligament should be closely examined for metastatic nodes and direct tumor extension (Fig 15-4).[12] Suspicious nodes should be biopsied and evaluated. A rapid cytologic diagnosis can be made by FNA, thus avoiding open biopsy of the primary tumor mass and potential tumor spillage, bleeding, and subsequent pancreatic fistula. Experienced surgeons can differentiate between pancreatic changes and cancer with a high degree of reliability. Howard and Jordan have suggested that a patient with pancreatitis severe enough to be confused with carcinoma would probably benefit from pancreatic resection.[20] Indeed, obtaining a tissue diagnosis is of much more importance in the individual who is not a resectional candidate and requires other therapy.

Figs 15-5 and 15-6 outline the technical steps required to perform resection of the head of the pancreas and duodenum. Particularly important is the maneuver to elevate the neck of the pancreas off the underlying superior mesenteric and portal veins, which is only possible because there are no venous tributaries entering the portal vein on the ventral surface. The "Achilles' heel" of the Whipple procedure is generally felt to be the pancreaticojejunal anastomosis. Of the two major techniques for accomplishing this anastomosis, the Hunt technique, or end-to-end anastomosis, is preferred when the pancreas is soft and friable, while the end-to-side pancreaticojejunostomy is performed when there are fibrotic changes in pancreatic remnant.

A recent technical modification of the "standard"

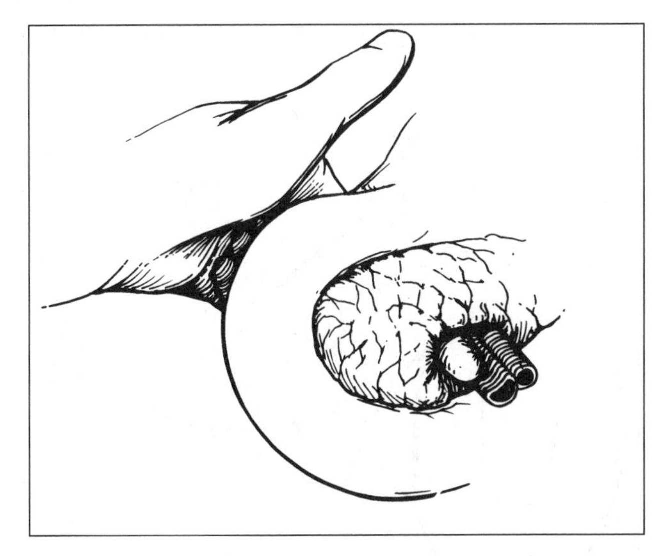

Fig 15-5. If the lesion appears resectable after the Kocher maneuver, the procedure is continued by exposing the portal vein. Access to the portal vein may be gained by following the middle colic vein to the superior mesenteric vein at the inferior pancreatic border. Careful dissection will free the superior mesenteric and portal veins from the overlying pancreatic neck. This maneuver is facilitated by the fact that the pancreatic portal tributaries enter the portal vein medially or laterally and that ventrally the vein surface is usually free of venous branches. Difficulty with this dissection might indicate tumor involvement. Similarly, portal vein exposure may be obtained by dissection behind the first portion of the duodenum and common bile duct.

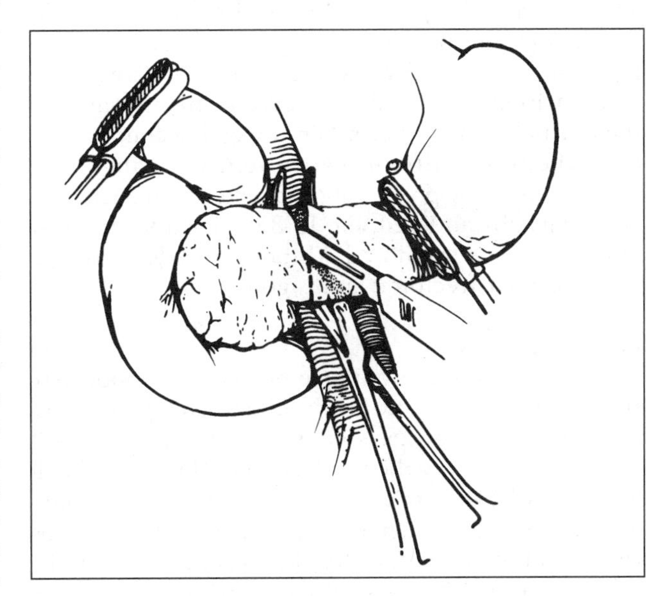

Fig 15-6. After separating the pancreas from the portal vein, while carefully protecting the underlying vein, the pancreas is transected. Ligatures placed in the superior and inferior borders of the cut edge of the pancreas control the pancreaticoduodenal vessels and allow further exposure of the underlying portal vein and its pancreatic venous tributaries as the uncinate lobe is dissected.

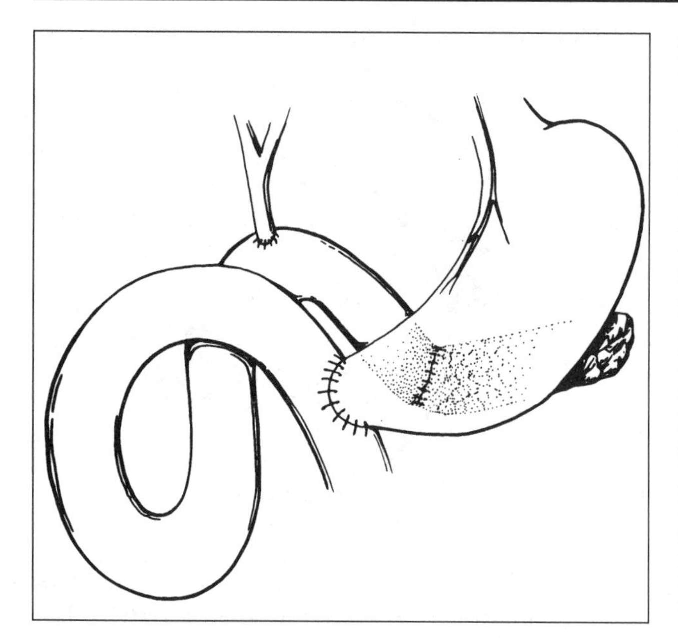

Fig 15-7. A pylorus-sparing pancreatectomy is the technical modification that appears to reduce nutritional morbidity associated with standard classical Whipple resection as well as decreasing duration of surgery.

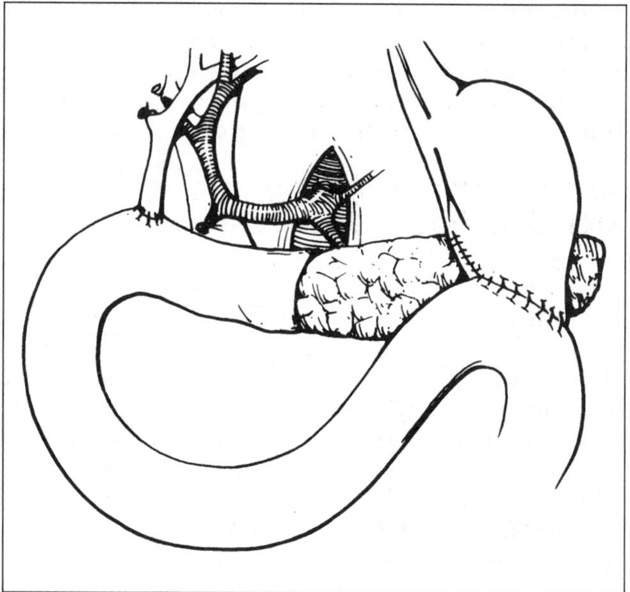

Fig 15-8. After completing the pancreaticojejunostomy, the common bile duct is anastomosed to the jejunal loop followed by a gastrojejunostomy. It is important to include a vagotomy if a limited gastric resection is accomplished. Also, to minimize the risk of stomal ulceration, it is critical to place the gastrostomy distal to the biliary and pancreatic anastomosis. Outlined above is the completed anatomy of a classic Whipple resection.

Whipple is the "pyloric sparing" Whipple, which is accomplished by preserving the first portion of the duodenum and performing an end-to-side duodeno-jejunostomy (Fig 15-7). A vagotomy is not required, and nutrition is generally improved by maintenance of the normal stomach reservoir. A nagging concern has been the possibility of inadvertently leaving some tumor behind by preserving the pylorus; this fear has yet to be substantiated. Fig 15-8 depicts the anatomy of the completed standard Whipple procedure, including partial gastrectomy and vagotomy.[21]

Complications

Complications of the Whipple procedure include sepsis, biliary or pancreatic fistula, and bleeding. The overall morbidity rate varies between 27% and 46%.[22-26] Sepsis is frequently the result of undrained blood collections or leakage from the GI tract. Aggressive management is indicated, which in many instances may be carried out by percutaneous drainage. Pancreatic fistula formation occurs in 10% to 18% of patients, frequently presenting as clinical sepsis, and may be associated with a mortality of 7% to 10%. Many fistulas can be controlled with good drainage, somatostatin administration, and hyperalimentation, with surgical intervention required in <50% of cases. Hemorrhage in the immediate postoperative period is usually related to an uncontrolled blood vessel or disseminated intravascular coagulation. Late bleeding may be a result of sepsis or fistula formation, leading to arterial erosion or ligature slough. Delayed gastric emptying after pancreatectomy, especially following a pyloric-sparing operation is a relatively common nonlife-threatening complication, which may on occasion herald localized peritoneal sepsis. Less frequent complications include intestinal obstruction, mesenteric thrombosis, hepatic failure, cholangitis, pancreatitis, renal failure, and necrotizing fasciitis. In the last decade, operative mortality at major centers has decreased to 2% to 4%, due to better patient selection, improved anesthesia, and fewer surgeons performing more pancreatic surgery. Cameron and colleagues have reported more than 145 consecutive pancreaticoduodenectomies without mortality (Table 15-3).[22-27]

Survival

Until recently, 5-year survival after pancreaticoduodenectomy for cancer was exceedingly rare. Survival rates of 3% to 25% are currently being reported. Occasionally, long-term survivors are reported with a large tumor, but the majority of survivors are those who have small lesions and negative lymph nodes (T1, N0, M0). Mean survival after pancreatic resection is 17 months. A recent study suggested that perioperative transfusion may adversely affect survival after pancreaticoduodenectomy. In addition, tumor DNA ploidy and proliferative index may be as strong or stronger independent survival predictors as tumor size or the number of positive lymph nodes.[28]

Table 15-3. Results of Pancreatic Resections Reported Between 1980 and 1992*

	N	Mortality	Morbidity
Grace et al[24]	45	2.0%	26%
Pellegrini[22]	51	2.0	27
Brooks et al[25]**	28	0	27
Trede et al[26]	133	2.2	–
Miedema et al[23]	279	4.0	46
Cameron et al[27]	145	0	45
Overall	681	2.5%	33%

*Incomplete listing of reports.

**Total pancreatectomy.

Palliative Treatment

Palliation of pancreatic cancer has changed in recent years. Previously, surgery was needed to make the diagnosis of pancreatic cancer and a palliative procedure was usually performed simultaneously. Today, with CT scans, ultrasound, FNA, and the like, the diagnosis can be made without surgical intervention and nonoperative palliative options are available. The results and survival are about the same when surgery is compared with other interventional methods, with total cost being less for the latter. Overall morbidity, as reflected by the need for repeated hospitalizations, is higher for the nonsurgical approach. The most common symptom for which palliation is required is jaundice. Surgical biliary drainage under such conditions will fall into the category of a cholecystoenterostomy, choledochojejunostomy, and very seldom choledochoduodenostomy or choledochogastrostomy. Regardless of the procedure utilized, the effectiveness is equivalent, with survival being approximately 5 to 6 months.

Randomized studies have recently addressed the role of endoscopic biliary stenting in this setting. The success rate is high, and the immediate morbidity and mortality low. There is no survival difference compared with surgical decompression. Twenty to thirty percent of patients require repeat hospitalizations because of ascending cholangitis or technical problems associated with the stent. Stents larger than 10 French bore are preferred because they appear to be associated with fewer problems.

Prophylactic gastric bypass may be employed in patients who do not have outlet obstruction symptoms, as 10% to 15% of patients will alternately develop a gastric outlet problem, generally as a preterminal event. Control of the unrelenting pain associated with unresectable pancreatic cancer is a significant patient care challenge. Some individuals obtain pain relief following biliary decompression, others are controlled by oral analgesics, and still others require parenteral medications. Celiac splanchnic nerve blocks using alcohol may be performed at the time of surgery or later by percutaneous approaches, with relief in up to 75% of patients. Many patients receiving radiation therapy also get pain relief.

Adjuvant Therapy

Adjuvant therapy has been addressed by two trials from the Gastrointestinal Tumor Study Group (GITSG). The first study compared patients who had undergone curative Whipple resections, with one group acting as controls and the second receiving 5-fluorouracil (5-FU) and two courses of radiation therapy (20 Gy each). The median survival for the control group was 11 months, compared with 20 months for the treatment group.[29] A follow-up study, without a control group, confirmed the original observations.[30] As a result of these findings, many patients are currently treated with adjuvant 5-FU and radiation therapy after a "successful" Whipple resection. It is the hope of many that adjuvant therapy will play an increasing role in the management of resected patients.

Chemotherapy

In contrast to adjuvant therapy, treatment of unresectable cancer has been relatively disappointing. While many drugs have been evaluated, no single drug has produced a response rate in excess of 15% or median survival greater than 3 months. As a result of these disappointing findings, multiple drugs have been employed but early results barely exceeded those with 5-FU alone. Clinical trials comparing combinations of mitomycin-C and 5-FU with streptozotocin (SMF) and without streptozotocin (MF) found an objective response rate of 34% in patients receiving SMF and 8% in those receiving MF. While the median survival was identical for both groups, responders had a significantly lengthened median survival. A second trial confirmed these findings comparing SMF with semustine and doxorubicin. Trials of leucovorin and 5-FU have failed to show therapeutic activity in advanced pancreatic cancer. Hexamethylmelamine, mitomycin-C, and 5-FU (HexMF) have been evaluated and found to be an alternative to regimens containing streptozotocin and doxorubicin. "The 17-month survival associated with response to HexMF is better than any described for patients with comparably advanced disease."[31] Presently, clinical trials are beginning to evaluate the use of the new agent taxol in the management of advanced pancreatic cancer.

Radiation Therapy

Although initially considered to be radioresistant, pancreatic exocrine tumors have been responsive to recent improvements in radiation therapy. The results are dose related, with a few radiation cures documented over the years. The proximity of radiosensitive tissues, including the liver, kidney, and duodenum, severely limits the efficacy of external-beam radiation therapy and has led to innovative approaches for delivering high-dose treatment, including precision high-dose external-beam techniques, interstitial or brachytherapy, and intraoperative and adjuvant radiation therapy. There is reported value for all these techniques, but because of the heterogeneity of patients, tumor size, stage of disease, performance status, and volume of the tumor, it is difficult to make a definitive conclusion concerning the superiority of one modality over the others. Titanium clips, which do not interfere with CT studies, can be surgically placed to mark the margins of the tumor, thus enabling the radiation therapist to design fields that will maximize tumor dosage and minimize injury to radiosensitive, normal adjacent structures. Dobelbower and Milligan reported results with this "precision" external-beam approach in 40 patients, 12 of whom also received chemotherapy. They observed a 12-month median survival in patients receiving radiation therapy alone, compared to a 15-month survival in the combination group.[32] Interestingly, two patients survived 5 years and one 9 years, while 22 of the 32 with pain recorded significant pain relief. As mentioned previously, pain relief may be a benefit of radiation therapy.

Endocrine Tumors of the Pancreas

Pancreatic endocrine tumors are rare, occurring in <1 per 100,000. These tumors present variably, generally a reflection of overproduction of a specific hormone. Insulinoma is the most common of the pancreatic endocrine tumors, followed by gastrinoma. Vipoma, glucagonoma, and somatostatinoma are very rare. The malignancy of many of these lesions is not readily apparent on histologic examination and perhaps clinically confirmed only after a delay of years. Functioning endocrine tumors should be diagnosed biochemically, and radiologic procedures used for localization. Because of the vascularity of many tumors, angiography is important, especially in insulinoma, but CT and ultrasound are also useful. Transhepatic portal vein sampling (PVS) can help in localizing tumors that are too diffuse or too small to be visualized by other modalities. Intraoperative ultrasound has become a standard in the surgical management of islet cell tumors, especially insulinoma. Surgery for endocrine pancreatic tumors may be curative as in the easily enucleated solitary insulinoma. On the other hand, major resective procedures may be required to obtain palliation of symptoms. Long-term survival may be achieved by aggressive surgical resection in patients with lymph node or liver metastases. Debulking surgery frequently eliminates or significantly reduces disabling hormonal symptoms. Carty and associates recently reported a 50% longer disease-free interval in 17 patients who underwent aggressive surgical resection of a variety of metastatic pancreatic endocrine tumors.[33]

Insulinoma

The first description of hyperinsulinism, caused by an islet cell tumor, came only 5 years after Banting and Best isolated insulin in 1922. Roscoe Graham was the first surgeon to resect an insulinoma, in 1929. In 1930 Whipple described the triad useful for so many years in making a clinical diagnosis of insulinoma.

Having a malignancy rate of <10%, insulinoma constitutes 75% of all reported islet cell tumors. Although usually solitary, insulinomas can be multiple and are generally associated with multiple endocrine neoplasia type I (MEN-I). The major signs and symptoms of insulinoma are a result of excess insulin secretion and marked hypoglycemia. Neurologic symptoms are common, including loss of consciousness, coma, seizures, confusional states, visual disturbances, and abnormal behavior. It is important that the symptoms be recognized and that hypoglycemia be reversed, because permanent neurologic damage will result from prolonged hypoglycemia.

Whipple's triad is clinically helpful in making a diagnosis of insulinoma. It consists of (1) signs and symptoms of hypoglycemia occurring during periods of fasting or exercise; (2) blood sugar levels <50 mg/dL while symptomatic; and (3) reversal of symptoms on oral or intravenous administration of glucose.[34] Today the diagnosis is made by obtaining simultaneous serum glucose and insulin levels during a suspected hypoglycemic episode or in the fasting patient. The normal ratio of insulin to glucose is <0.4, while insulinoma patients have a ratio >0.4 and frequently close to 1.0. Another diagnostic test is the radioimmunoassay measurement of proinsulin and C-peptide. Proinsulin is the large precursor molecule found in the beta cell, which is cleaved into insulin and a connecting molecule known as C-peptide. Circulating proinsulin and C-peptide, which are secreted in equimolar amounts, are almost always found in the serum of patients with insulinoma. Measurement of serum C-peptide is an indirect determination of endogenous insulin production and can be useful in the investigation of hypoglycemia, especially in patients who are diabetic or suspected of having self-induced hyperinsulinism. Tolbutamide and glucagon may be used as provocative tests for insulinoma if the fasting test does not produce hypoglycemia in the face of strong clinical suspicion. Additionally, intravenous calcium infusion in insulinoma will result in discharge of proinsulin from the neurosecretory granules and subsequent splitting into insulin and C-peptide (effecting a drop in serum glucose levels).

The majority of insulinomas are solitary tumors <1.5 cm in diameter, thus making CT scanning of limited diagnostic usefulness. Similarly, ERCP may not be helpful. It is said that only 20% of insulinomas can be either seen or palpated at the time of surgical exploration, so it is important to attempt preoperative localization. Three tests may be helpful in this regard. Angiography is best for preoperative localization of insulinoma, since these tumors are characteristically hypervascular and show a marked "blush" 60% to 80% of the time. Percutaneous transhepatic selective PVS for hormonal assay is highly sensitive and may assist the surgeon in localizing small lesions to the pancreatic head or tail, and in determining whether there are multiple adenomas or the syndrome of nesidioblastosis or islet cell hyperplasia. If a blind pancreatic resection were to be necessary, supporting positive venous catheterization data are reassuring. The use of intraoperative ultrasound (IOUS) has been helpful in localizing small nonpalpable lesions, as islet cell tumors appear as hyperechogenic masses compared with normal pancreatic tissue. In fact, Norton has stated that "the exploration for occult insulinomas should no longer rely on blind distal or subtotal pancreatectomy, but rather on precise localization of the tumor facilitated by preoperative PVS and IOUS."[35] In benign insulinoma, enucleation is the procedure of choice, especially with head lesion, whereas distal resection appears to be preferred with body and tail tumors. The classical Whipple procedure is used infrequently and usually only in the reoperative setting.

Complications of surgery, including fistula, pancreatitis, sepsis, and bleeding, have been reported in 15% to 30% of patients. In contrast to a high surgical complication rate, operative mortality rate is 0% to 0.2% and most commonly associated with reoperation. Surgical success, normoglycemia, normal glucose tolerance test, and histologic proof of insulinoma are seen in 97% to 99% of patients.

Medical Management

Norton has suggested that definitive cures be reevaluated at 6 months with biochemical tests following a 72-hour fast, although this is generally not done. Multiple insulinomas should suggest MEN-I syndrome. Gastrinoma is the most common accompanying pancreatic lesion in MEN type I syndrome, with insulinoma ranking second. In one large series of insulinomas, MEN-I constituted 7.3% of the total number of cases and 70% of multiple tumors. Patients in whom resection is not curative or who are not candidates for surgery may be treated with diazoxide, which directly inhibits insulin release, and diphenylhydantoin, to reduce the hypoglycemia. Malignant lesions usually respond transiently to the administration of streptozotocin.

Gastrinoma

Gastrinoma, the second most common islet cell tumor, accounts for 15% to 20% of islet cell neoplasms. Although there are six reports beginning in the 1940s and extending into the 1950s describing patients with virulent peptic ulcer diathesis and islet cell tumor, it was Zollinger and Ellison in 1955 who postulated a humoral agent produced by the islet cell and capable of stimulating gastric acid secretion. In his discussion of their famous paper, Lester Dragstedt suggested that the islet cells responsible for this agent might be related to the gastric antral cell known to secrete gastrin.[36] In 1960 Gregory and colleagues isolated a gastric secretagogue from an islet cell tumor surgically removed from a patient with Zollinger-Ellison syndrome.[37] Subsequent work concluded that the tumor's principal secretion was indeed gastrin.

In 1962 a Zollinger-Ellison tumor registry was established and there are now more than 2,000 of these once "rare" tumors in accession. The estimated annual incidence is one in a million people, with the majority in patients aged 40 to 60 years. Males tend to predominate, but in the familial MEN-I gastrinoma, the sexes are nearly equally affected.

Diagnostic Workup

The manifestations of Zollinger-Ellison syndrome (ZE) are the effect of the tumor-secreted gastrin. Because gastrin is the most potent gastric acid stimulus, peptic ulceration is the primary clinical feature associated with gastrinoma. Ulcers may be large and multiple, with 80% to 90% of gastrinoma patients incurring ulcer disease sometime during their clinical course. Gastrin has a trophic effect on GI mucosa, leading to parietal cell hyperplasia, which further enhances acid production. This is radiologically and endoscopically reflected in hypertrophic gastric folds and elevated basal acid secretion.

Approximately one third of gastrinoma patients have diarrhea, and in 50% of them it may be the only symptom. The cause of the diarrhea is unknown, but may be related to massive amounts of gastric acid secreted into the upper GI tract, morphologic alterations in small-bowel mucosa, or intestinal absorptive cell metaplasia leading to fat malabsorption. Many patients with gastrinoma have esophageal symptoms secondary to reflux esophagitis, with dysphagia, ulcer, or stricture.

The preferred modality for diagnosing ZE is elevated blood levels of gastrin. Normal individuals have fasting gastrin levels between 40 and 60 pg/mL, while ZE patients commonly have fasting levels in excess of 200 pg/mL (average, 1,000 to 2,000 pg/mL). Because many ZE patients have nondiagnostic levels of gastrin, provocative testing can be helpful in separating gastrinomas from other causes of hypergastrinemia. An increase in serum gastrin of 200 pg/mL over baseline after intravenous infusion of secretin (two units/kg/kilo over 30 seconds) is considered a positive test. Other substances have been used as provocative agents for gastrin secretion, including bombesin, glucagon, pancreatic polypeptide, and calcium.

Once the biochemical diagnosis of gastrinoma is made, the nature (benign versus malignant), extent, and possible role of surgery must be determined. Ultrasonography of the abdomen is the least expensive and the least invasive diagnostic test, but it is also the least sensitive. CT is much more sensitive, detecting approximately 60% of tumors. MRI will demonstrate gastrinomas by a bright signal intensity on T_2 weighted images, similar to those typical of pheochromocytoma. Currently, though, the sensitivity of MRI does not exceed the sensitivity of CT scanning. Selective angiography and PVS are the most sensitive localizing studies but also the most invasive, with an accuracy approaching approximately 60% to 70%. Duodenal gastrinomas, which account for as many as 50% of lesions, may be localized by endoscopic ultrasound (Fig 15-9).

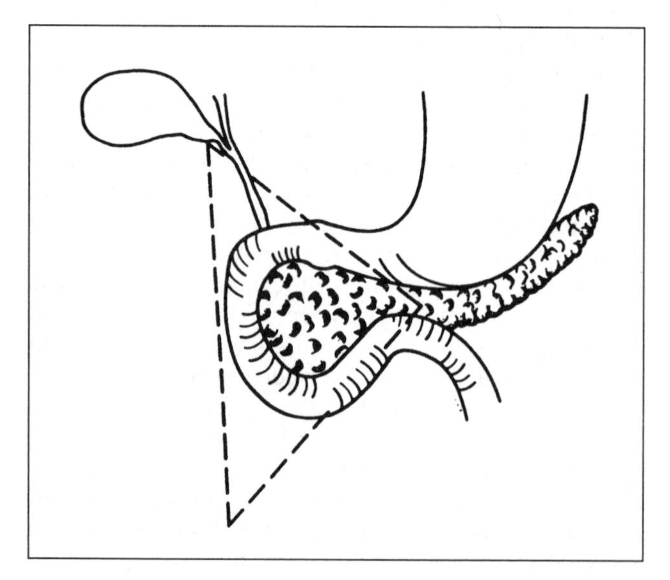

Fig 15-9. The anatomic triangle in which gastrinomas are most frequently found. From Stabile et al.[21]

Treatment

Management of gastrinomas should be individualized, based on the patient's age, general health, compliance, and access to medical surveillance. Additional factors include the biological behavior of the tumor and extent of the localizing data. Gastric acid hypersecretion has been reliably managed with histamine $(H)_2$ receptor antagonists and more recently with hydrogen potassium in adenosine triphosphatase (H^+/K^+=ATPase) inhibitors. More than 50% of gastrinomas are malignant, posing a long-term hazard to the patient. Optimal treatment is complete removal of the tumor; with early diagnosis and good localizing information, 30% to 40% of sporadic gastrinomas can be resected for cure. Gastrinomas associated with MEN-I are usually multiple, multifocal, and unresectable, but correction of the accompanying hyperparathyroidism will reduce gastric acid secretion.

While total gastrectomy is seldom performed any longer for this disorder, patients may benefit from parietal cell vagotomy, which reduces acid secretion as well as the total dosage requirement of H_2 antagonist. Long-term survival after complete resection approaches 100%; after partial resection, 25% to 40%. Even in disseminated disease, long-term survival exceeds 20%.

Many gastrinomas will respond to treatment with streptozotocin with a decrease in serum gastrin and tumor size. Streptozotocin has been used singly and in combination with 5-FU and doxorubicin. There is no hard evidence to document that chemotherapy prolongs the life of a gastrinoma patient. Somatostatin reduces gastrin release by decreasing the responsiveness of the parietal cell to gastrin. Long-term treatment with a somatostatin analogue may play a future role in the clinical management of this disease.

Glucagonoma

Glucagonoma was first described by McGavran and colleagues in 1966, in a patient who had bullous and eczematoid dermatitis of the hands, feet, and legs as well as diabetes mellitus.[39] The patient was originally thought to have inoperable pancreatic cancer, but her long-term survival and subsequent improvement after a second operation were interpreted as the result of a tumor of islet cell origin rather than pancreatic ductal origin. Immunoassay documented the presence of large amounts of glucagon both in the tumor and in the patient's serum. Approximately 75% of glucagonomas are malignant, with liver and peripancreatic nodal spread common. In addition to dermatologic manifestations, most patients exhibit malnutrition with anemia/hypoproteinemia because of the catabolic glycogenolytic and lipolytic actions of glucagon.

Diagnosis and Treatment

A clinical presentation of diabetes, dermatitis, and weight loss suggests glucagonoma. Patients also have thrombotic complications and mental changes, including depression. Most have normochromic normocytic anemia, hypoaminoacidemia, and hyperglucagonemia. A biochemical diagnosis is made from an elevated serum glucagon determination. Localization of lesions may be performed in the same manner in which the other islet cell tumors are localized. Because tumors are generally large, venous catheterization studies are usually unnecessary but may be helpful in selected patients. In the rare instance in which the tumor is localized, dramatic clinical improvement may follow surgical resection. More extensive disease may respond to debulking procedures and subsequent administration of intravenous dimethylriazenoimidazole carboxamide (DTIC), streptozotocin, and 5-FU. The use of somatostatin analogues also may be helpful.

Vipoma

In 1958 a syndrome characterized by severe diarrhea and hypokalemia in association with islet cell adenoma of the pancreas was described by Verner and Morrison.[40] A number of patients have since been described with this syndrome, which has been referred to variously as Verner-Morrison syndrome; watery diarrhea, hypokalemia, and achlorhydria (WDHA) syndrome; and pancreatic cholera. Bloom in 1973 reported a new peptide with vasoactive properties that had been isolated from both the tumor and plasma of patients with Verner-Morrison syndrome.[41] This peptide, known as vasoactive intestinal polypeptide (VIP), is associated with the clinical signs and symptoms of the tumor.

Diagnosis and Treatment

The mean age when vipoma is diagnosed is approximately 47 years; roughly 60% of patients are female. Eighty to ninety percent of tumors are located in the pancreas, although extrapancreatic sites have been described. The most prominent feature of vipoma is the profuse, cholera-like diarrhea that may present for a considerable time prior to diagnosis. Because the stools contain high concentrations of potassium, daily potassium losses may be 20 to 25 times normal. A metabolic acidosis often results from the large fecal loss of bicarbonate. The accompanying weakness, lethargy, and occasional nephropathy are the results of the profound potassium depletion. Usual antidiarrheal agents are ineffective. Sixty percent of patients have an abnormal glucose tolerance test and mild hypercalcemia. When the latter is present, a diagnosis of MEN-I syndrome should be considered. Approximately 50% of vipomas are malignant and have usually metastasized by the time of the clinical diagnosis.

VIP is a highly specific marker for this tumor and should be sought in individuals presenting with massive diarrhea. Markers for other pancreatic tumors should be evaluated. Patients can have the clinical syndrome with low levels of VIP, in which case other serum mediators, such as pancreatic polypeptide and prostaglandin E_2 (PGE_2), may be present. Preoperative localization of VIP-secreting tumors is made essentially in the same manner as that for other islet cell tumors—CT, ultrasound, selective angiography, and percutaneous transhepatic portal venography with selective PVS. Patients considered to have operable tumors may be prepared for surgery by administration of somatostatin analogues. Patients with an inoperable tumor, on the other hand, or significant metastatic disease can be treated with a combination of streptozotocin and 5-FU. Long-term management with somatostatin, with its profound negative effect on diarrhea, is also a possibility. Patients with malignant tumors generally survive about 1 year.

Other Pancreatic Tumors

Pancreatic polypeptide (PP) is found in the F cells of the pancreatic islets, and while its physiologic function is uncertain, it may inhibit exocrine pancreatic secretion and biliary tract motility. In MEN-I families, an exaggerated plasma PP response following meal stimulation has been observed with the trait for MEN-I.[42] Only a few PP tumors have been documented, but without a typical clinical picture, many may have been overlooked.

Carcinoids (Islet Cell Tumors)

Carcinoids arise from the enterochromaffin cells and can occur in most tissues derived from endoderm. Most abdominal carcinoids are found in the midgut, although these tumors may arise in the foregut (pancreas, stomach, and bronchi). Foregut carcinoids generally lack the enzyme aromatic L-amino acid decarboxylase, which converts 5-hydroxytryptophan to 5-hydroxytryptamine (serotonin). The "carcinoid" syndrome may not be seen, or may be atypical, in these patients. In addition to the metabolites of tryptamine, carcinoids of the pancreas may secrete a variety of other peptides. These pancreatic tumors are exceedingly rare and are diagnosed as carcinoids because of their morphologic pattern. However, many may be polypeptide-producing islet cell tumors.

Somatostatin-Secreting Tumor

Somatostatin, which is secreted by the D cells of the pancreatic islet, appears to inhibit the release of all known GI hormones and insulin and also delays gastric emptying. Symptoms generally are related to prolonged exposure to somatostatin and may include diabetes, cholelithiasis, diarrhea, steatorrhea, and gastric hypochlorhydria. A handful of somatostatin-secreting tumors have been described, mostly in women, arising from the head of the pancreas and being malignant. Many patients had liver metastasis at the time of presentation.

Carcinoma of the Gallbladder

Gallbladder carcinoma is the fourth most common GI cancer in the US, representing about 50% of cancers of the extrahepatic biliary tree and approximately 0.5% of all malignancies. There is a slight female predominance, with cases seen most commonly in individuals in their late 60s and early 70s. The incidence of gallbladder cancer is higher in white women than in black women and roughly ten times higher in Mexicans, American Indians, and Alaskan natives. The incidence of gallbladder carcinoma in the presence of gallstones is low, whereas chronic gallstone disease is found in up to 70% to 80% of gallbladder cancer patients. Lund found that the incidence of gallbladder carcinoma in patients with longstanding gallstones is approximately 1%, a rate too low to justify prophylactic cholecystectomy.[43] Polk and others have emphasized the frequency of carcinoma in porcelain (calcified) gallbladders.[44] The risk of carcinoma in this group of patients is extremely high, justifying prophylactic cholecystectomy.

Natural History

Ninety percent of gallbladder neoplasms are adenocarcinomas, usually of the scirrhous type, but mucus-secreting, papillary forms are also seen. Squamous and mixed adenoepidermoid tumors constitute about 5% of gallbladder cancers. A variety of rare lesions, including carcinoid, sarcoma, melanoma, and lymphoma, may also arise from the gallbladder. Tumors initially develop in the mucosa, then infiltrate the gallbladder wall, producing diffuse thickening, and subsequently penetrate into surrounding structures. Gallbladder carcinoma spreads by direct extension and local invasion of the liver and surrounding organs, including the duodenum, colon, and anterior abdominal wall. The common hepatic duct is not infrequently involved by direct extension through Calot's triangle. This presentation can mimic a common hepatic duct tumor or a cancer arising at the confluence of the hepatic ducts. The fact that the gallbladder fossa lies in segment V facilitates early direct liver invasion and involvement of the segmental bile duct. In a patient who is jaundiced, failure to visualize the segment V duct on percutaneous transhepatic cholangiogram is suggestive of a gallbladder carcinoma. Distant hematogenous spread does not occur until the gallbladder carcinoma is locally advanced. At cholecystectomy, approximately 10% of patients are found to have a small invasive lesion confined to the gallbladder. An equal number of patients have early invasive cancers involving the gallbladder and regional lymphatics.

Staging

Patients most likely to be cured are those in whom the tumor is found serendipitously at the time of cholecystectomy for gallstones. Nevin has proposed a staging system for gallbladder carcinoma, with stage I representing an intramucosal lesion unrecognized at the time of surgery and subsequently discovered by the pathologist; stage II involving the mucosa and muscularis; stage III involving all three layers of the gallbladder; stage IV involving all three layers plus the cystic duct lymph node; and stage V involving the liver by direct extension or metastasis.[45]

Clinical Presentation

A change in the pattern of longstanding right upper quadrant symptoms may herald the development of gallbladder carcinoma. Clinical presentation may well depend on the stage of the disease. Symptoms related to stages I and II frequently are attributable to gallstones and range from dyspepsia or biliary colic to acute and chronic cholecystitis. Advanced stages generally produce pain, anorexia, weight loss, and obstructive jaundice. More advanced disease may result in a palpable mass, ascites and duodenal obstruction, and GI bleeding.

Diagnosis

The diagnosis of gallbladder carcinoma may be made in a number of ways, depending on the disease stage. Subclinical disease may be found on histopathologic examination of gallbladder tissue removed for cholecystitis or cholelithiasis, or both. This is the chief reason the gallbladder should be examined "fresh"—while the patient's abdomen is opened—because additional surgery might be indicated if a subclinical mucosal lesion were recognized and the diagnosis made at the time of the initial operation. More extensive disease may present as changes in right upper quadrant pain or acute cholecystitis, and may be diagnosed by conventional techniques such as ultrasound. Patients presenting with an abdominal mass may undergo ultrasound or CT with a potential diagnosis of gallbladder carcinoma in mind. Those presenting with jaundice most likely should have ultrasound, CT, and possibly some attempt to visualize the biliary tree, such as ERCP or percutaneous transhepatic cholangiogram (PTC). ERCP is most helpful when there is an absence of dilated intrahepatic biliary radicals. On examination, irregular filling defects within the gallbladder, nonfilling of the gallbladder, or evidence of infiltration of the common bile duct or extrahepatic bile duct may be observed. Ultrasound may show irregular thickening of the gallbladder wall, a fungating mass within the lumen of the gallbladder, or direct invasion of the adjacent hepatic parenchyma with poor tissue plane definition between the liver and the tumor. PTC in a patient with jaundice may demonstrate distortion, beading, or nonfilling of the bile ducts draining liver segments adjacent to the gallbladder. Collier and colleagues have reported subtle changes in segment V bile ducts in a small series of patients with gallbladder carcinoma.[46] Histologic documentation of malignancy may be obtained by ultrasound- or CT-guided FNA cytology. In advanced cases, this may allow nonoperative palliative means to be used.

Treatment

Removal of all gross disease is possible in only about 25% percent of patients with gallbladder carcinoma. Usually this is achieved by cholecystectomy and tissue removal in Calot's triangle and nodes along the porta hepatis. A more aggressive approach would include a thorough lymphadenectomy of the porta, along with resection of a wedge of the liver abutting the gallbladder bed (Fig 15-10). It is difficult to tell whether a more extensive resection results in increased survival. In a review of 1,486 patients resected for cure, 214 (14.5%) survived at least 5 years, 92% of whom had been treated solely by cholecystectomy.[47] If the unsuspected diagnosis of stage I or II gallbladder carcinoma is made in the postoperative period, further treatment is not necessarily indicated. These patients fare well

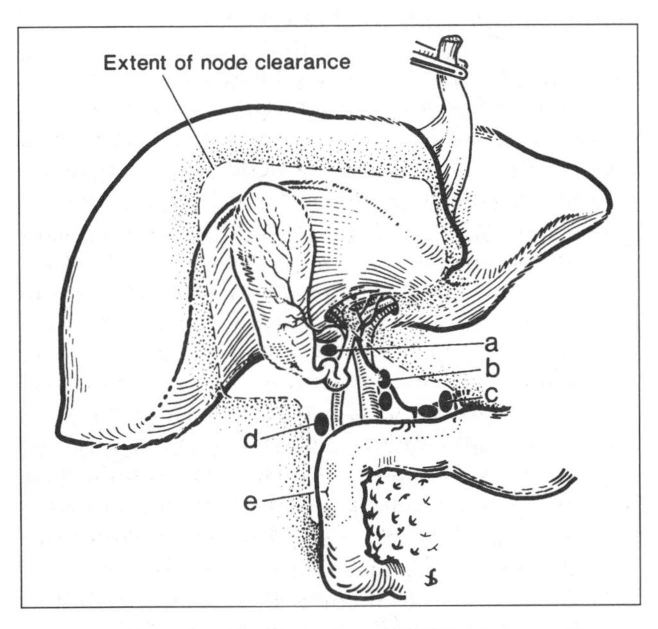

Fig 15-10. Extended cholecystectomy, including portions of liver segments IV and V and dissection of the regional lymph nodes (a-e). From Blumgart.[38]

with cholecystectomy alone. Foster has suggested, however, that if the tumor has invaded beyond the muscularis of the gallbladder, three treatment options are feasible: (1) immediate reoperation and extended resection if obvious spread has not taken place; (2) reoperation after 8 to 12 weeks, an interval that might allow the biologically more aggressive tumors to become manifest; and (3) postoperative radiation therapy in curative doses. There are no comparative data to favor any therapeutic course.

Survival with gallbladder cancer correlates with histologic staging. Early-stage (I and II) lesions have a good prognosis while more advanced disease seldom is associated with long-term survival. Patients usually survive only a few weeks or months, and those with advanced disease may not leave the hospital. Palliative procedures in advanced disease are limited. A large tumor mass generally prevents visualization of the liver hilum, as well as surgical measures to relieve jaundice. In such patients, a segment III hepaticojejunostomy may be an internal bypass option. Otherwise, transhepatic tubes may be required to relieve itching and jaundice. Pain is difficult to control unless related to biliary obstruction. Palliative irradiation may be used, but responses are infrequent and usually short lived. Currently, chemotherapy has little to offer these patients.

Carcinoma of the Bile Ducts

Carcinoma of the bile ducts is relatively uncommon in the US, accounting for one third of tumors arising in the extrahepatic biliary tree and approximately 4,500 new cases annually. In southeast Asia, in contrast, bile duct cancer is the most frequent cause of cholestasis in patients with malignant tumors.

Primary carcinoma of the extrahepatic biliary tract has been classified according to anatomic location: Upper-third lesions occur at the confluence of the hepatic ducts or distally in the common hepatic duct to the junction of the cystic duct. Middle-third lesions occur in the common bile duct between the cystic duct and upper border of the duodenum, and lower-third tumors in the portion between the upper part of the duodenum and the ampulla of Vater. Extrahepatic cholangiocarcinoma assumes three basic morphologic variants: papillary, nodular, and diffuse. The papillary type most commonly appears in the lower third of the common bile duct, while the nodular type (small, well-localized masses) typically occurs in the middle and upper thirds. The diffuse, or sclerosing, type presents as a marked thickening of the duct wall, resulting in luminal narrowing and occasionally mimicking sclerosing cholangitis.[48]

Natural History

As with gallbladder cancer, the vast majority of patients

with bile duct malignancy succumb within 6 to 12 months of the initial diagnosis, most frequently of local tumor extension and secondary obstruction and cholangitis. Lesions arising in the lower third of the common hepatic duct have the best prognosis, presumably because of the technical ease of surgical management. The etiology of cholangiocarcinoma is uncertain; there is a relationship with ulcerative colitis, hepatic fibrosis, polycystic disease and longstanding poorly drained choledochal cysts. In the Far East, *Clonorchis sinensis* and *Opisthorchis viverrini* are the most frequent infectious agents, although more commonly associated with intrahepatic cholangiocarcinoma. The frequency of the triad of bile stasis, infection, and chronic bile duct inflammation as a common denominator in patients at high risk for cholangiocarcinoma is striking. The natural history of untreated bile duct carcinoma is not readily available; however, reports suggest that patients with lesions involving the confluence who are managed nonsurgically generally survive 3 to 5 months from the onset of symptoms.

Diagnosis

Tumors of the extrahepatic biliary tree may be clinically silent and go unrecognized for extended periods. Jaundice, sometimes intermittent, is the most common presenting symptom. Of 94 patients admitted to London's Hammersmith Hospital with cholangiocarcinoma at the confluence of the hepatic ducts, all had liver function tests consistent with obstructive jaundice.[49] Other signs and symptoms include pruritus, anorexia, nausea, and vomiting. Infrequently a patient complaining of fever or malaise may have an elevated alkaline phosphatase value discovered incidentally while in the anicteric state; the diagnosis is subsequently established. Weight loss is a common finding in patients with bile duct tumors; bleeding and melena are unusual symptoms. Liver enlargement with a smooth liver edge is frequently found. Lower bile duct lesions may give rise to a clinically enlarged gallbladder, but a palpable mass in the right upper quadrant should raise the clinical suspicion of gallbladder carcinoma.

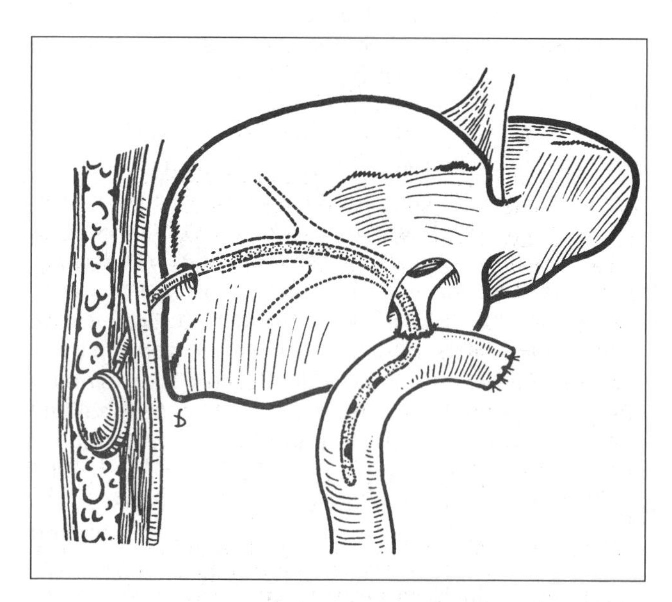

Fig 15-11. Exoendoprosthesis for stenting lesions of the extrahepatic biliary tree; proximal end of tube is buried under the skin in the subcutaneous tissue, and may be attached to a reservoir, allowing access for bile sampling and radiologic studies. From Blumgart.[38]

The most efficient approach to patients suspected of having extrahepatic biliary tract obstruction secondary to bile duct carcinoma consists of ultrasound of the liver, gallbladder, and extrahepatic ducts. Dilated intrahepatic radicals, a normal or absent common bile duct, and a normal gallbladder strongly suggest a diagnosis of hilar or upper-third bile duct obstruction. The next diagnostic procedure should be PTC to visualize the intrahepatic duct and the site of obstruction. Care must be taken to ensure filling of both the left and right branches of the biliary tree so that the operability of tumors at the confluence may be more accurately predicted. Bilateral studies may be required. The segment V duct should be examined carefully, due to frequent involvement in gallbladder carcinoma but infrequent infiltration in bile duct cancer. CT has not been a major clinical aid in hilar tumors but will aid in the diagnosis of lesions in the biliary tree. In many instances, the tumor will have completely obstructed the bile duct on presentation, rendering ERCP of limited diagnostic value, as visualization of only the distal extent of the tumor will be obtained and knowledge of the proximal limit of the tumor is essential for surgical planning.

If confluence of the hepatic ducts is involved and major hepatic resection is being considered, visualization of the portal vein and its branches is mandatory because the tumor may extend posteriorly into the portal vein, which results in a difficult resection or renders resection impossible. Late-phase splenoportography will provide the information required to make a decision concerning resectability.

Treatment

Cancers occurring at or near the confluence have a surgical resectability rate of approximately 20%. In this region, liver resection is generally required for a curative attempt. Contraindications to resection include bilateral ductal involvement beyond second-order hepatic ducts, involvement of the main trunk or portal vein, bilateral involvement of the hepatic arterial or portal venous structures, or a combination of vascular involvement on one side and tumor involvement on the opposite side. Complete tumor excision in the latter instance will result in a poorly vascularized hepatic remnant and possible death. Patients considered ineligible for resection of the confluence because clear surgical margins are unobtainable may have a palliative resection with silastic stenting tubes placed through the subsequent hepaticojejunostomy, allowing postoperative brachytherapy. If resection is not possible, the following therapeutic options should be considered: (1) biliary diversion using percutaneously placed stenting tubes through the liver, tumor, and into the GI tract or surgically placed to exit through the skin in "U-tube" fashion; (2) exoendoprosthesis as described by Voyles[50] (Fig 15-11); (3) hepaticojejunostomy to the segment III duct, as described by Soupault and Couinaud[51]; (4) occasionally, placement of an internal endoscopic stent by way of the ampulla of Vater; and (5) introduction of a permanent expandable metallic biliary stent.

Lower bile duct tumors tend to be papillary and easily visualized by ERCP, which establishes the site of origin and extent of the tumor. These tumors are less frequent than upper bile duct lesions, but are more easily managed by conventional surgical techniques: local resection with establishment of a hepaticojejunostomy by Roux-en-Y loop or by pancreaticoduodenectomy for intrapancreatic bile duct lesions. Frequently it is impossible to clinically differentiate intrapancreatic duct lesions from more common pancreatic cancer. Mortality and morbidity associated with resection of these cancers are considerably lower than for cancer in the hilar region. Resectable cancers in this location have a 5-year survival rate of 15% to 20%, not as high as for duodenal or ampullary carcinoma but superior to survival for pancreatic cancer. Resectable lesions occurring in the hilum of the liver are infrequently cured, but have a median postsurgical survival of 18 to 24 months. The quality of life after resection is higher than in individuals with an unresectable lesion, thus justifying the surgical effort.

Radiation Therapy

The localized nature of bile duct carcinoma permits the use of radiation therapy for both cure and palliation. Radiation therapy is limited by the tolerance of the normal adjacent tissue, but newer, specialized techniques such as wedging and shrinking fields have helped to minimize risk to surrounding vital structures. Doses exceeding 40 Gy appear to be required for tumor control. Generally, radiation therapy is used as palliation or in the postoperative adjuvant setting. Experience with intraoperative radiation therapy for bile duct cancers has been too limited to evaluate. The percutaneous placement of bridging stents through an obstructing biliary tract cancer allows the option of internal radiation or brachytherapy. A number of reports have documented average survival of approximately a year utilizing this innovative approach.

Chemotherapy

Agents used in the treatment of bile duct cancer chiefly have been 5-FU and doxorubicin. Because these cancers are generally slow-growing and many times encased in dense desmoplastic reaction with a relatively limited blood supply, at least on a theoretical basis, dramatic chemotherapeutic responses should not be expected. Partial responses of 20% to 30% have been reported with systemic chemotherapy. No large patient series are available to direct our therapeutic efforts.

References

1. Boring CC, Squires TS, Tong T, Montgomery S. Cancer Statistics, 1994. *CA Cancer J Clin.* 1994;44:7-26.

2. Waterhouse J, Muir C, Correa P, Powell J. Cancer incidence in five continents. *Lyon: International Agency for Research on Cancer*; 1976: Vol 3.

3. Whittemore AS, Paffenbarger RS Jr, Anderson K, Halpern J. Early precursors of pancreatic cancer in college men. *J Chronic Dis.* 1983;36:251-256.

4. Howe G, Jain M, Burch JD, Miller AB. Cigarette smoking and cancer of the pancreas: evidence from a population-based case-control study in Toronto, Canada. *Int J Cancer.* 1991;47:323-328.

5. Burney PGJ, Comstock GW, Morris JS. Serologic precursors of cancer: serum micronutrients and the subsequent risk of pancreatic cancer. *Am J Clin Nutr.* 1989;49:895-900.

6. Mancuso TF, el Attar AA. Cohort study of workers exposed to betanaphthylamine and benzidine. *J Occup Med.* 1967;9:277-285.

7. Ishizuka J, Townsend CM Jr, Thompson JC. Neurotensin regulates growth of human pancreatic cancer. *Southern Surgical Association.* 1992;104:abstr2.

8. Smith JP, Solomon TE, Bagheri S, Kramer S. Cholecystokinin stimulates growth of human pancreatic adenocarcinoma. *Dig Dis Sci.* 1990;35:1377-1384.

9. Motojima K, Tsunoda T, Kakashi K, Nagata Y, Urano T, Shiku H. Distinguishing pancreatic cancer from other periampullary carcinomas by analysis of mutations in Kirsten-*ras* oncogenes. *Ann Surg.* 1991;214:657-662.

10. Gray LW, Crook JN, Cohn I Jr. Carcinoma of the pancreas. *Seventh National Cancer Conference Proceedings.* 1972;530-510.

11. Moosa AR. *Tumors of the Pancreas.* Baltimore, Md: Williams & Wilkins; 1980:433.

12. Beazley RM, McAneny DA, Cohen I Jr. *Progress in Pancreatic Cancer.* Atlanta, Ga: American Cancer Society;1991:4,5.

13. Warshaw AL. Implications of peritoneal cytology for staging of early pancreatic cancer. *Am J Surg.* 1991;161: 26-30.

14. Warshaw AL, Gu Z, Wittenburg J, Waltman AC. Preoperative staging and assessment of resectability of pancreatic cancer. *Arch Surg.* 1990;125:230-233.

15. Dooley WC, Cameron JL, Pitt HA, Lillemore K, Yue NC, Venbrux AC. Is preoperative angiography useful in patients with periampullary tumors. *Ann Surg.* 1990;211:649-655.

16. Beahrs OH, Henson DE, Hutter RVP, Kennedy BJ, eds. *American Joint Committee on Cancer Manual for Staging of Cancer.* 4th ed. Philadelphia, Pa: JB Lippincott Co; 1992.

17. Whipple AO, Parsons WB, Mullins S. Treatment of carcinoma of the ampulla of Vater. *Ann Surg.* 1935;102:763-779.

18. Priestley JT, Comfort MW, Radcliffe J Jr. Total pancreatectomy for hyperinsulinism due to an islet-cell adenoma: survival and cure at 16 months after operation: presentation of metabolic studies. *Ann Surg.* 1944;119:211-221.

19. Ross DE. Cancer of pancreas: a plea for total pancreatectomy. *Am J Surg.* 1954;87:20-33.

20. Howard JM, Jordan GL Jr. Cancer of the pancreas. *Curr Probl Cancer.* 1977;2(3):4-52.

21. Stabile BE, Morrow DJ, Passaro E Jr. The gastrinoma triangle: operative indications. *Am J Surg.* 1984;147:25-31.

22. Pellegrini CA, Heck CF, Raper S, Way LW. An analysis of the reduced morbidity and mortality rates after pancreaticoduodenectomy. *Arch Surg.* 1989;124:778-781.

23. Miedema BW, Sarr MG, van Heerden JA, Nagorney DM, McIlrath DC, Ilstrup D. Complications following pancreaticoduodenectomy: current management. *Arch Surg.* 1992;127:945-950.

24. Grace PA, Pitt HA, Tompkins RK, Den Besten L, Longmire WP Jr. Decreased morbidity and mortality after pancreatoduodenectomy. *Am J Surg.* 1986;151:141-149.

25. Brooks JR, Brooks DC, Levine JD. Total pancreatectomy for ductal cell carcinoma of the pancreas. *Ann Surg.* 1989;209:405-410.

26. Trede M, Schwall G, Saeger HD. Survival after pancreatoduodenectomy: 118 consecutive resections without an operative mortality. *Ann Surg.* 1990;211:447-458.

27. Cameron JL, Pitt HA, Yeo C, Coleman J, Lillemore K. One hundred and forty-five consecutive pancreatoduodenectomies without a mortality. *Ann Surg.* 1993;217:430-438.

28. Allison DC, Bose KK, Hruban RH, et al. Pancreatic cancer cell DNA content correlates with long-term survival after pancreatoduodenectomy. *Ann Surg.* 1991;214:648-656.

29. Kalser MH, Ellenberg SS. Pancreatic cancer: adjuvant combined radiation and chemotherapy following curative resection. *Arch Surg.* 1985;120:899-903.

30. Gastrointestinal Tumor Study Group. Further evidence of effective adjuvant combined radiation and chemotherapy following curative resection of pancreatic cancer. *Cancer.* 1987;59:2006-2010.

31. Bruckner HW, Kalman J, Spigelman M, et al. Primary treatment of regional and disseminated pancreatic cancer with hexamethylmelamine, mitomycin C and 5-fluorouracil infusion. *Oncology.* 1989;46:366-371.

32. Dobelbower RR Jr, Milligan AJ. Treatment of pancreatic cancer by radiation therapy. *World J Surg.* 1984;8:919-928.

33. Carty SE, Jensen RT, Norton JA. Prospective study of aggressive resection of metastatic pancreatic endocrine tumors (MPET). *Surgery.* 1992;112:1024-1032.

34. Whipple AO, Frantz VK. Adenoma of islet cells with hyperinsulinism: a review. *Ann Surg.* 1935;101:1299-1335.

35. Norton JA, Shawker TH, Doppman JL, et al. Localization and surgical treatment of occult insulinomas. *Ann Surg.* 1990;212:615-620.

36. Zollinger RM, Ellison EH. Primary peptic ulcerations of the jejunum associated with islet cell tumors of the pancreas. *Ann Surg.* 1955;142:709-728.

37. Gregory RA, Tracy HJ, French JM, Sircus W. Extraction of a gastrin-like substance from a pancreatic tumour in a case of Zollinger-Ellison syndrome. *Lancet.* 1960;1:1045-1048.

38. Blumgart LH, ed. *Surgery of the Liver and Biliary Tract.* Edinburgh, Scotland: Churchill Livingstone; 1988:824,847.

39. McGavran MH, Unger RH, Recant L, Polk HC, Kilo C, Levin ME. A glucagon-secreting alpha-cell carcinoma of the pancreas. *N Engl J Med.* 1966;274:1408-1413.

40. Verner JV, Morrison AB. Islet cell tumor and a syndrome of refractory watery diarrhea and hypokalemia. *Am J Med.* 1958;25:374-380.

41. Bloom SR, Polak JM, Pearse AGE. Vasoactive intestinal peptide and watery-diarrhoea syndrome. *Lancet.* 1973;2:14-16.

42. Friesen SR, Tomita T, Kimmel JR. Pancreatic polypeptide update: its roles in detection of the trait for multiple endocrine adenopathy syndrome, type I, and pancreatic polypeptide-secreting tumors. *Surgery.* 1983;94:1028-1037.

43. Lund J. Surgical indications in cholelithiasis: prophylactic cholecystectomy elucidated on the basis of long-term follow-up on 526 nonoperated cases. *Ann Surg.* 1960;151:153-162.

44. Polk HC. Carcinoma in the calcified gallbladder. *Gastroenterology.* 1966;50:582-585.

45. Nevin JE, Moran TJ, Kay S, King R. Carcinoma of the gallbladder: staging, treatment, and prognosis. *Cancer.* 1976;37:141-148.

46. Collier NA, Carr D, Hemingway A, Blumgart LH. Preoperative diagnosis and its effect on treatment of carcinoma of gallbladder. *SG&O.* 1984;159:465-470.

47. Foster JH. Carcinoma of the gallbladder. In Way LW, Pellegrini CA, eds. *Surgery of the Gallbladder and Bile Ducts.* Philadelphia, Pa: WB Saunders; 1987:471-485.

48. Weinbren K, Mutum SS. Pathological aspects of cholangiocarcinoma. *J Pathol.* 1983;139:217-238.

49. Blumgart LH, Hadjis NF, Benjamin IS, Beazley RM. Surgical approaches to cholangiocarcinoma at confluence of hepatic ducts. *Lancet.* 1984;1:66-70.

50. Voyles CR. The exoendoprosthesis in proximal bilioenteric anastomoses. *Am J Surg.* 1985;149:80-83.

51. Soupault R, Couinaud CI. Sur un procédé nouveau de dérivation biliaire intra-hépatique: les cholangiojejunostomies gauches sans sacrifice hépatique. *Presse Med.* 1957;65:1157-1159.

16

TUMORS OF THE LIVER

John E. Niederhuber, MD

Primary liver tumors are relatively uncommon in the United States. Worldwide, however, these neoplasms pose a serious health problem. In contrast to an estimated incidence in the US of 3 per 100,000 population, the incidence in areas such as Africa and Asia varies from 30 per 100,000 to >100 per 100,000.[1,2] Although primary liver cancer ranks low on the list of incident cancers in the US, it carries a grave prognosis with a fatality-to-case ratio of 0.8.[1]

Tumors of the liver may be benign or malignant. In recent years, new technologies have contributed significantly to the more precise diagnosis of space-occupying lesions of the liver and have assisted greatly in the staging of these "tumors." In addition, a better understanding of the etiology and natural history of liver tumors has led to a more aggressive, multimodality approach to therapy.

Benign Liver Tumors

It is estimated from autopsy series that 1% to 7% of the population have some type of benign liver tumor.[3,4] As a result, benign lesions become an important factor in the differential diagnosis of any liver mass. By far, the most common benign liver tumor is the hemangioma.[5,6] Other benign tumors include adenoma and focal nodular hyperplasia (Table 16-1).

Hemangioma

Hemangiomas are classified as hemangioendotheliomas, capillary hemangiomas, and cavernous hemangiomas. They are believed to be sequestrations of primordial angioblastic cells. Hemangioendotheliomas are generally found in infants and children, and approximately 50% of cases are associated with cutaneous vascular lesions.[7,8] Most are discovered within the first 6 months of life and may continue to enlarge.

Infantile Hepatic Hemangioendothelioma

Infantile hepatic hemangioendotheliomas are highly vascular, containing multiple arteriovenous fistulas, and may be multicentric.[9] The incidence is twice as common in females as males; most often, this tumor occurs in the right lobe of the liver. Large lesions may cause high-output cardiac failure or obstruction of the biliary system, requiring resection. They have also been reported to regress spontaneously, but mortality rates as high as 70% have been reported in infants presenting with high-output failure.[8] Thrombocytopenia, afibrinogenemia (Kasabach-Merritt syndrome), and anemia are frequently associated with these hemangiomas.[10] Hemangioendotheliomas rarely occur in adults. When they do, lesions are thought to be secondary to chemical exposure such as to vinyl chloride and are almost always malignant.[11]

Infantile hepatic hemangioendotheliomas should be considered whenever cutaneous hemangioma is present, particularly if the cutaneous lesion quickly increases in size and number. Signs of congestive heart failure—tachypnea, cardiomegaly, systolic murmur, jaundice, and hepatomegaly—are common findings.[9] Diagnosis is confirmed by ultrasound and arteriography. Computed tomography (CT) and magnetic resonance imaging (MRI) demonstrate the lesion(s) within the liver. Needle biopsies are unnecessary and never performed because of a high risk of uncontrolled hemorrhage.

Initial treatment focuses on support of the heart with digitalis and diuretics. Prednisolone 2 to 5 mg/kg/day for 1 to 3 weeks has been observed to help reduce the size of cutaneous hemangioma and therefore may be of benefit in treating hepatic lesions. Signs of continued deterioration require aggressive treatment, including hepatic arterial segmental embolization and intraoperative hepatic artery ligation.[9,12,13]

In the past, the approach to these lesions was almost

John E. Niederhuber, MD, Emile Holman Professor and Chair, Department of Surgery, Professor of Microbiology and Immunology, Stanford University School of Medicine, Stanford, California

Table 16-1. Benign Liver Tumors

Type	Affected Population	Distinguishing Characteristics	Therapeutic Options
Hemangioma			
Hemangioendothelioma	Infants	High-output failure thrombocytopenia, afibrinogenemia, anemia, cutaneous hemangioma	Digitalis, diuretics, steroids, arterial embolization, transplantation
Capillary	All ages	Usually asymptomatic	Observation
Cavernous	Adults	Usually asymptomatic (13% symptomatic)	Observation, rarely resection, ? X-ray therapy
Hepatic adenoma	Adult women with history of oral contraceptives	Acute rupture and hemorrhage	Resection
Hepatic adenomatosis (>10 adenomas)	Adult women with history of oral contraceptives	Greater risk of hemorrhage and malignant transformation	Resection, transplantation
Focal nodular hyperplasia	Adult women	Usually asymptomatic	Observation

always surgical, with an effort to identify feeding arteries that could be ligated, including major hepatic arteries.[14] Occasionally, major hepatic resections were attempted. Mortality, as noted, was unacceptably high. With advances in radiologic interventional technology, the current approach is therapeutic embolization of selected feeding arteries. With technical advances, transplantation could prove to be an important consideration in highly selected infants. When this tumor occurs in young adults, it is usually diffuse. Immunohistochemical evaluation using antibodies to factor VIII–related antigen is important in differentiating this tumor from angiosarcoma and cholangiocarcinoma.

Capillary Hemangioma

Capillary hemangiomas are observed in all ages. Rarely are they large enough to produce symptoms and require resection. In the adult, capillary and cavernous hemangiomas are commonly seen on liver imaging and often must be differentiated from potential metastatic lesions.

Cavernous Hemangioma

Cavernous hemangiomas (Fig 16-1) are generally found only in adults, with a mean age at diagnosis of 50 years. Autopsy studies document hemangioma as the most common benign hepatic tumor (incidence of 3% to 7%).[4,6] In adults they are usually small (1 to 2 cm in diameter). It is estimated that multiple lesions are infrequent (approximately 10% of cases), and only 13% of cavernous hemangiomas are symptomatic. Cavernous hemangiomas are lined with a single layer

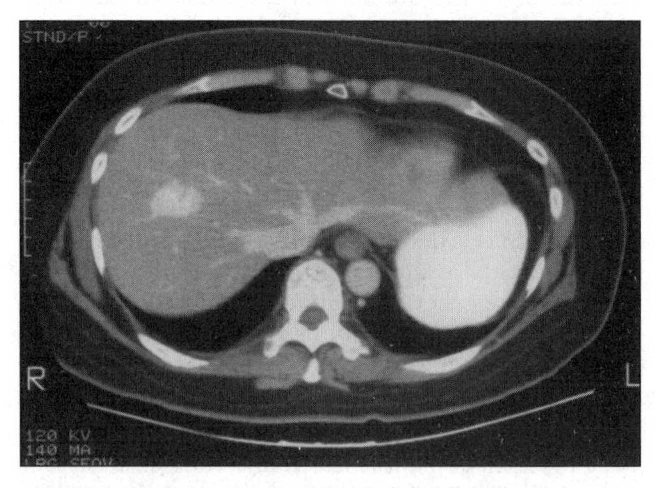

Fig 16-1. Intravenous contrast-enhanced CT demonstrating a cavernous hemangioma of the liver.

of endothelium and generally have some hamartomatous features.

An incidental finding of asymptomatic hepatic hemangioma has increased dramatically with more frequent use of ultrasound and CT during the evaluation of many health problems. As a result, the physician is frequently required to differentiate hemangiomas from possible primary or metastatic cancer involving the liver.

Diagnosis and Management

On ultrasound, there is a homogeneously echogenic mass, usually <5 cm in diameter with posterior enhancements. The mass is well circumscribed with sharp borders.[6] Hemorrhage within the lesion over time may result in fibrosis and calcification, thus altering echogenicity, causing a more solid appearance, and increasing the difficulty of differentiating such lesions from a metastatic tumor. This is especially true with larger hemangiomas. More recently, duplex Doppler ultrasound has been used, and none of the hemangiomas had Doppler shifts >0.7 kHz, whereas solid primary and secondary cancer were usually >15 kHz.[6]

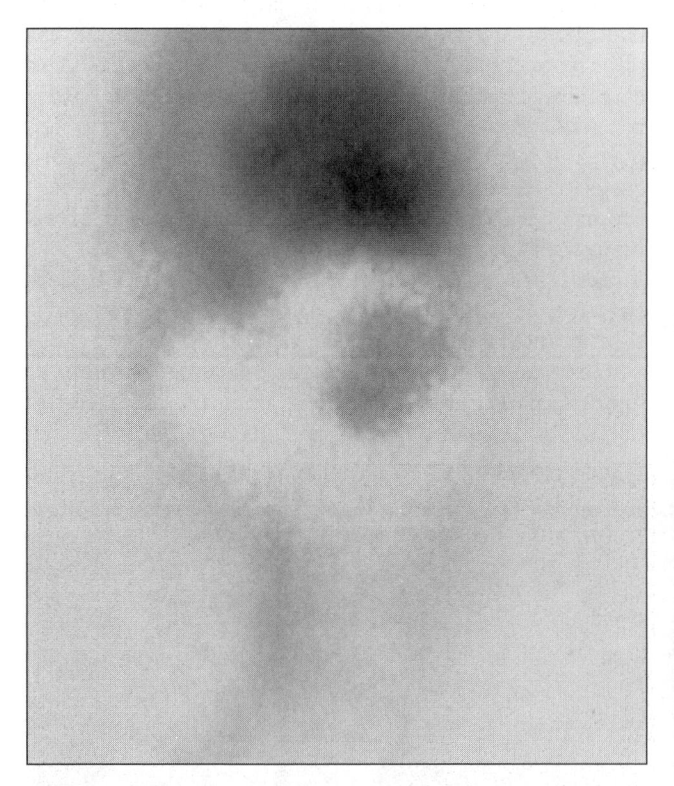

Fig 16-2. ^{99m}Tc-RBC scintigram (lateral projection) demonstrating a cavernous hemangioma. The dark field of uptake is the heart. Below the heart image, the computer has subtracted the counts obtained by injecting ^{99m}Tc-sulfur colloid intravenously. This gives the "white" background of the liver volume containing the uptake of the hemangioma within.

When ultrasound is not diagnostic, ^{99m}Tc-RBC scintigraphy is indicated (Fig 16-2). The accuracy of scintigraphy may be increased when used with single photon emission computed tomography (SPECT). Classically, hemangiomas have decreased radionuclide uptake on the blood flow phase of the study and increased activity on delayed blood pool images at 1 to 2 hours. As with ultrasound, fibrosis within the lesion may be extensive and alter nuclide uptake. A lesion near the hilum may be difficult to evaluate with this technique because of the large portal veins. Hepatomas and metastatic tumors will usually have increased early flow but decreased uptake on delayed images. Selective hepatic artery angiography can also be useful in differentiating hemangiomas from cancers (Fig 16-3). While ^{99m}Tc-RBC scintigraphy and angiography may be diagnostic, it is advisable to include at least one morphologic imaging study in the evaluation process. MRI is one such approach (Fig 16-4), and while all hepatic masses are hyperintense relative to normal tissue on T-2 weighted sequences, it is the degree of this intensity in a fluid-filled lesion that distinguishes it as a hemangioma.[15] Today Gadolinium-enhanced MRI is the test of choice and has virtually replaced all those mentioned above (Figs 16-4 and 16-5A, 5B, 5C).

Observation by scanning, without intervention, is the appropriate management for cavernous hemangioma. At the Mayo Clinic, 36 persons observed for 15 years remained symptom free, with only four hemangiomas

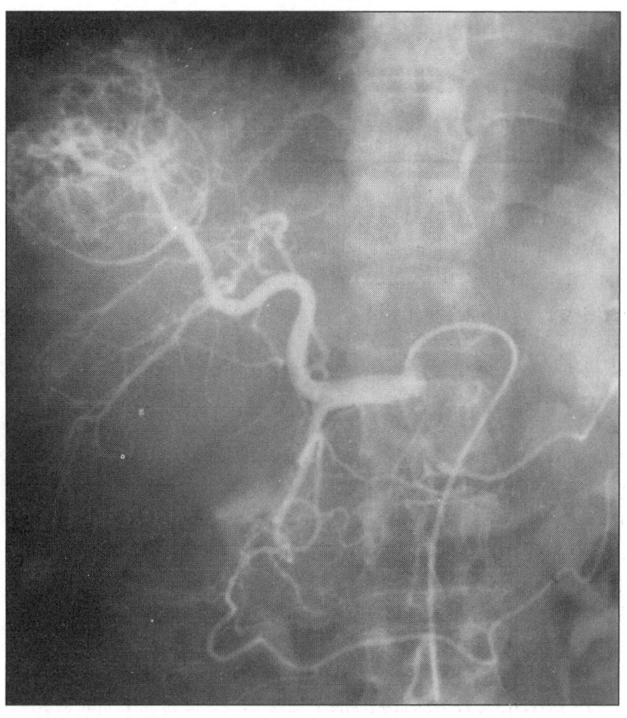

Fig 16-3. Selective hepatic artery angiogram demonstrating a cavernous hemangioma of the liver.

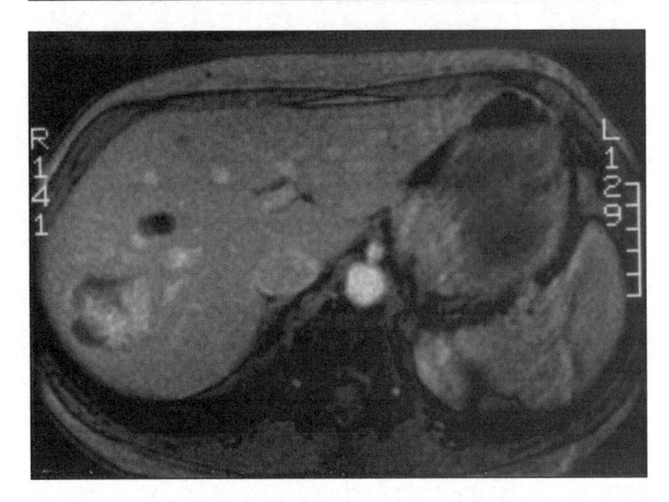

Fig 16-4. MRI demonstrating a cavernous hemangioma. The nonenhanced lesion anterior to the hemangioma is a benign cyst.

showing an increase in size over time.[16] In another report, only one hemangioma increased in size, while 85 remained unchanged during 6 years of observation. There is no evidence of adult hemangiomas becoming malignant. Surgical resection is considered for large symptomatic lesions producing pain, fullness, and other complications such as jaundice, Kasabach-Merritt syndrome, uncontrolled congestive heart failure, or hemorrhage. In two reported series, the incidence of symptomatic hemangiomas was 14% and 20%.[16,17]

Hemorrhage is the most life-threatening complication. Unfortunately, it is difficult to define exact criteria for an unacceptable risk of spontaneous or traumatic rupture. Even so, hemorrhage appears to be exceedingly rare, with only 28 cases reported since 1898.[18] Transcatheter hepatic arterial embolization may be a useful approach during acute hemorrhage or in preparation for resection. In most instances, embolization will not provide definitive therapy because of rapid collateralization. Risks of necrosis and abscess formation following embolization must be considered.

Reports of spontaneous rupture suggest that this rare event occurs in lesions 3 to 25 cm in diameter and probably involves <5% of this subpopulation of larger lesions. In the past, mortality from rupture was reported to be as high as 50%.[18] Changes in management, combining interventional radiology and modern surgical technique, have greatly improved results. In addition to the improved surgical techniques used in actual liver transection, the management of blood replacement (cell-saver and rapid infusers), experience in cardiac surgery, liver transplantation, and modern critical care methods have all contributed to significantly lowering operative risk.

It is of interest that at least 19 persons have been effectively treated with ionizing radiation.[19] There is every indication in these reports that this is a safe and appropriate alternative to surgery for symptomatic lesions. It does, however, carry the risk of radiation hepatitis.

Hepatic Adenoma

Over the past two decades, hepatic adenoma has become more common among women because of the use of oral contraceptives. Prior to the introduction of oral contraceptives in 1960, hepatic adenomas were rare. For example, before 1958, only two cases were reported in a series of 50,000 autopsies conducted over a 36-year period. The Mayo Clinic reported four cases collected between 1907 and 1954.[20,21] In recent reports, 93% of patients with hepatic adenoma gave a history of oral contraceptive use. The incidence was directly associated with duration of oral contraceptive use, as was the most common form of presentation: hemorrhage or rupture, or both.

Hepatic adenomas are found mainly in three groups of patients: oral contraceptive and steroid users, those with diabetes and glycogen storage dis-

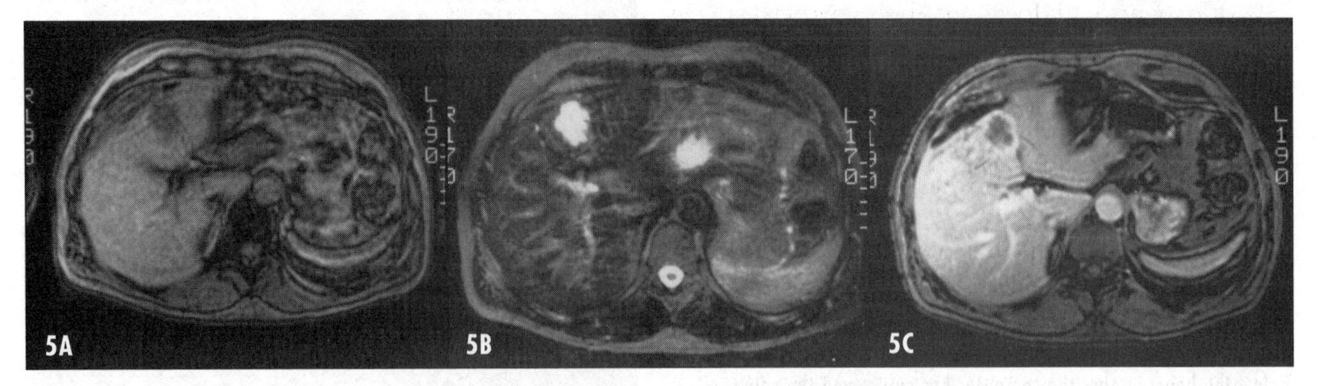

Fig 16-5. ***5A*** T1 weighted MRI image of lesion in left lobe of liver. ***5B*** is T2 weighted image of same lesion. The fluid-like density of the signal raises possibility that lesion is hemangioma. ***5C*** is Gadolinium-enhanced image showing enhanced vascular ring with poorly enhanced central area confirming that lesion is not hemangioma but metastatic tumor from original colon primary.

ease, and those with adenomatosis. The relative risk of developing hepatic adenoma while taking oral contraceptives has been estimated to be 2.5 at 5 years, 7.5 at 9 years, and 25 at ≥10 years.

Hepatic adenomas vary in size, with an average diameter of 8 to 10 cm at the time of diagnosis. They may be contained entirely within the liver parenchyma or project from the capsule as a pedunculated growth. Adenomas are more commonly found in the right lobe (approximately 75% of cases). Adenomas contain areas of hemorrhage and necrosis, but lack bile-duct features. Hemorrhage and necrosis are not found in focal nodular hyperplasia.

Hepatic adenomatosis, defined as >10 adenomas, is a less common problem. While histologically identical, clinical patterns are different. Patients with adenomatosis have a greater risk of hemorrhage and malignant transformation than those with adenoma and are candidates for liver transplantation. Liver resection is the recommended therapy for adenomas. Resection eliminates the estimated 50% risk of rupture and life-threatening hemorrhage and can be accomplished today with minimal morbidity and a <1% risk of operative mortality.

Focal Nodular Hyperplasia

The term *focal nodular hyperplasia* was introduced by Edmondson in 1958 to describe a rare benign liver tumor composed of hepatocytes and Kupffer's cells.[22] These tumors may occur as multiple lesions, and their etiology and natural course remain unknown. It has been suggested that focal nodular hyperplasia is the result of a preexisting arterial malformation, but no direct evidence for this hypothesis exists. The lesions do, however, have a much greater degree of intimal and medial vascular alterations than is seen in adenomas of the liver. Focal nodular hyperplasia has been observed in association with hepatic adenoma and fibrolamellar carcinomas.

Associated hemangiomas have been reported in 23% of patients with focal nodular hyperplasia.[20] No such association with hemangiomas appears to exist with hepatic adenomas. Focal nodular hyperplasia is found primarily in women during their reproductive years. There does not appear to be as direct a relationship with the use of oral contraceptives as exists with hepatic adenomas. Following the introduction of oral contraceptives, however, several incidents of hemorrhage were reported in patients with focal nodular hyperplasia. The main differential diagnosis is with adenomas, and therefore a biopsy of the lesion is important since management will differ.

Pain and colleagues reported on 22 patients with focal nodular hyperplasia (19 female and 3 male) in 1991.[23] Eight were discovered in asymptomatic individuals and 14 were diagnosed because of pain or mass. A report from the Mayo Clinic noted only 4 of 41 patients to be symptomatic, and in three other series about 23% were symptomatic at the time of diagnosis.[24]

Since there is no evidence for malignant transformation and, unlike adenoma, no apparent risk of rupture and hemorrhage, the approach to focal nodular hyperplasia is one of observation once the histologic diagnosis is confirmed. Ultrasound provides a good means of monitoring. If present, oral contraceptive use is discontinued. Resection is reserved for symptomatic patients.

Malignant Liver Tumors

The most common primary malignant liver tumor, accounting for approximately 75% of liver cancers, is hepatocellular carcinoma. Less common are cholangiocarcinomas arising from the bile duct epithelium and rarely tumors with a mixture of bile duct and hepatocellular elements (Table 16-2). As with any organ, rare tumors are found arising from other cellular components of the liver, including angiosarcoma.

Hepatocellular Carcinoma

Hepatocellular cancer is one of the most common and most malignant tumors occurring in the world's male population, and in some areas of Asia and Africa the incidence continues to increase. A number of factors are associated with the etiology of hepatocellular cancer, and the major cause may differ from one part of the world to another. Risk factors include hepatitis B infection, alcohol-induced cirrhosis, aflatoxin-contaminated food, and certain drugs such as anabolic steroids, Thorotrast, and immunosuppressive agents. Pesticides, chlorinated hydrocarbons, aromatic amines, and chlorophenols are some of the chemicals considered to be potential inducers of hepatocellular cancer.

A common feature is the presence of cirrhosis.[25] The risk of developing hepatocellular cancer with nutritional cirrhosis (micronodular) is approximately 10%. With cirrhosis secondary to hepatitis B infection, the incidence increases to 20%; in areas of the world where hepatitis B is endemic, >70% of patients with hepatocellular cancer are hepatitis B positive.[26] With hemochromatosis of the liver the risk of hepatocellular cancer is approximately 13% (all in cirrhotic livers), and with alpha$_1$-antitrypsin deficiency the risk is 40%.[27,28] Parasitic infections involving the liver, such as *Clonorchis sinensis, Opisthorchis felineus,* and schistosomiasis, can cause liver scarring with a risk of subsequent liver tumor formation.

There are several histologic patterns of hepatocellular cancer growth: a diffuse involvement of the liver with multiple tumor nodules, a single tumor mass, and a pattern termed *fibrolamellar* which is not associated with cirrhosis. The latter has a distinct histologic appearance, is thought to be slow-growing,

Table 16-2. Malignant Liver Tumors

Type	Affected Population	Distinguishing Characteristics	Therapeutic Options
Hepatocellular single mass, diffuse, multiple encapsulated	Adult	Most often associated with cirrhosis	Reresection, transplantation, chemotherapy
Fibrolamellar histology		Not associated with cirrhosis	Transplantation
Cholangiocarcinoma	Adult	Frequently CEA producing, indolent and diffuse	Chemotherapy ? transplantation
Cystadenoma	Rare in adults, more common in females	Nodular cyst wall	Resection
Epithelioid hemangioendothelioma	Adult	Multifocal in both lobes	Transplantation

and has a more favorable prognosis when resected or managed by liver transplant.

In 1977, Okuda and colleagues described an encapsulated form of hepatocellular carcinoma.[29] The review of 26 such cases suggested that the encapsulated variety grows slowly as a single focus and metastasizes late. Like fibrolamellar tumors, this variety also has a more favorable prognosis.

Hepatocellular cancer cells resemble normal liver cells with large, round, hyperchromatic nuclei, prominent nucleoli, and abundant granular eosinophilic cytoplasm. These cells are generally arranged in trabeculae that are 2 to 8 cells in width. Like liver cords, the trabeculae are covered with a basement membrane, surrounded outside by endothelial cells. Poorly differentiated tumors lose this organized pattern and demonstrate spindle cells and giant cells.

Diagnosis

Patients usually present with symptoms of upper abdominal pain, often on the right (Fig 16-6). A large tumor of the right lobe may be palpable and produce a detectable friction rub. A few patients are diagnosed during evaluation of abnormal liver function tests, especially an elevated alkaline phosphatase level. The most important tumor marker is alpha-fetoprotein (AFP), with elevated serum levels reported in 75% to 90% of patients with hepatocellular carcinomas.[30] False-positives are occasionally found with embryonal cell carcinoma and pancreatic cancers. AFP-positive tumors have a more aggressive course (median survival of 5 months versus 10.5 months for AFP-negative tumors) and are less responsive to chemotherapy. AFP is an extremely sensitive assay for following patients postresection. A rise in AFP following resection of a primary AFP-positive tumor is pathognomonic of recurrence.

CT arterial portography provides the most critical evaluation today (Fig 16-7). This is usually performed following selective celiac and superior mesenteric angiography, while the catheter is still positioned in the superior mesenteric artery.[31] Sitzmann and colleagues documented that CT arterial portography detected 94% of tumors found at surgery and was sensitive enough to image 82% of lesions <1 cm.[32] MRI may also provide useful information and can generate sagittal as well as planar images.

The imaging information obtained from CT arterial portography, coupled with the angiogram, is critical to determining resectability. However, images displayed as planar slices are not optimal for planning surgery. A three-dimensional display of tumor(s) and their relationship to hepatic veins, portal venous anatomy, and the biliary ducts would be ideal for determining resectability and planning the extent of resection. Toward this goal, a new advance in CT scanning called spiral CT now provides imaging of the liver with high resolution in one breathhold. This method of data acquisition is used with volumetric rendering to produce a three-dimensional model of liver anatomy.[33] The tumor(s) is visualized in three dimen-

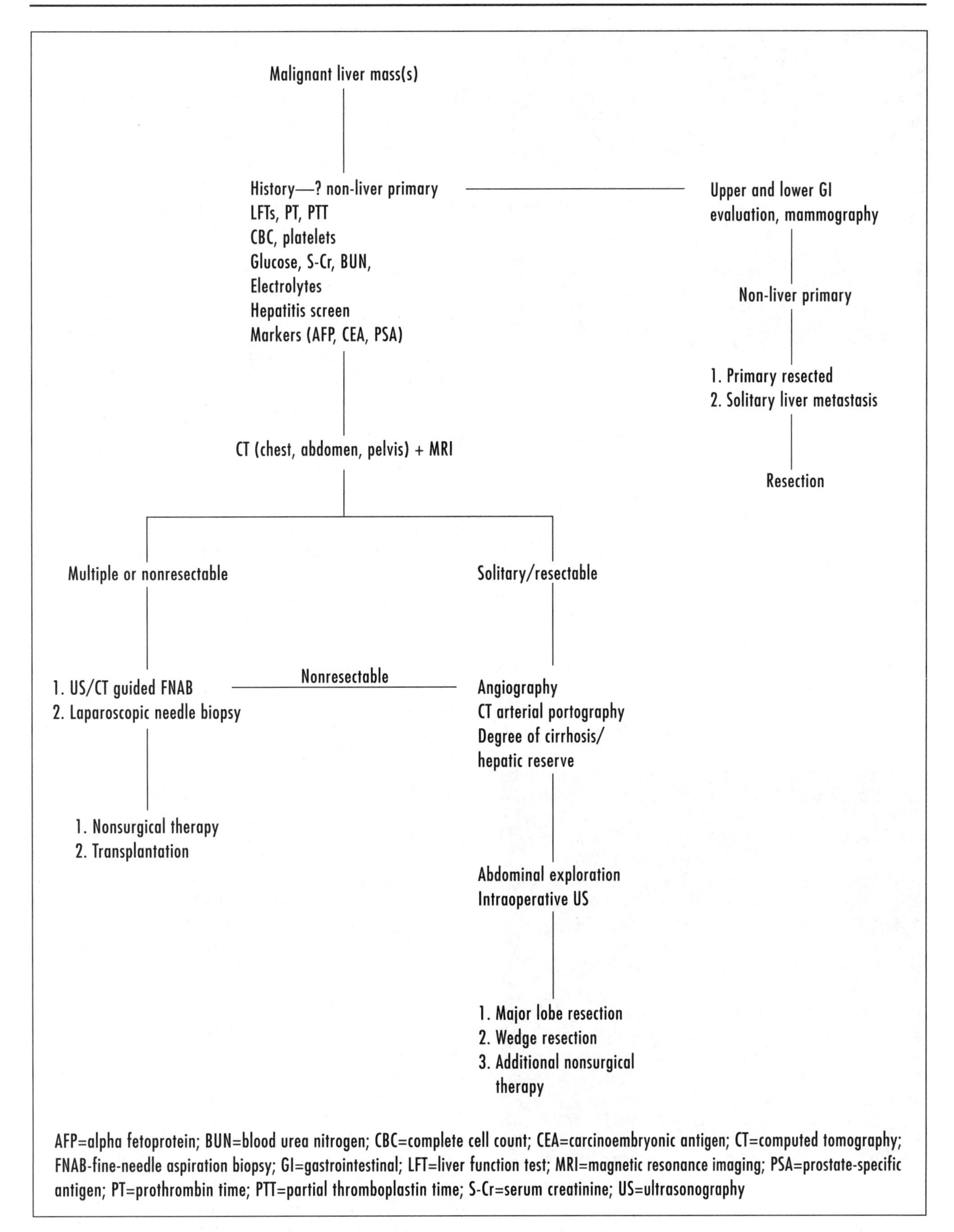

Fig 16-6. Algorithm for evaluating solid liver lesions.

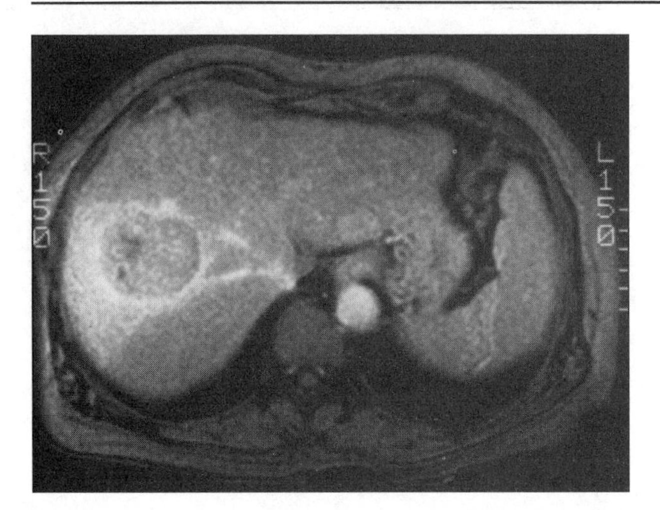

Fig 16-7. Intravenous contrast-enhanced CT demonstrating a hepatocellular carcinoma.

sions as it is situated within the liver parenchyma and as it relates to liver vasculature.

These preoperative images are confirmed at surgery using intraoperative ultrasound. Intraoperative ultrasonography determines the presence or absence of additional tumors and confirms resectability by showing the relationship of the tumor to the major portal and hepatic veins (Fig 16-8).

It is essential in planning resectional therapy to establish whether cirrhosis is present and, if so, the degree of liver impairment. This is important because the patient must have adequate hepatic reserve to survive a major resection. A measure of hepatic reserve is provided by Pugh's modification of the Child's classification.[34] The presence of portal hypertension indicates an unacceptable risk. If jaundice is present, it should be carefully evaluated preoperatively usually by endoscopic retrograde cholangiopancreatography (ERCP) or in selected cirrhotic patients by percutaneous transhepatic cholangiography.

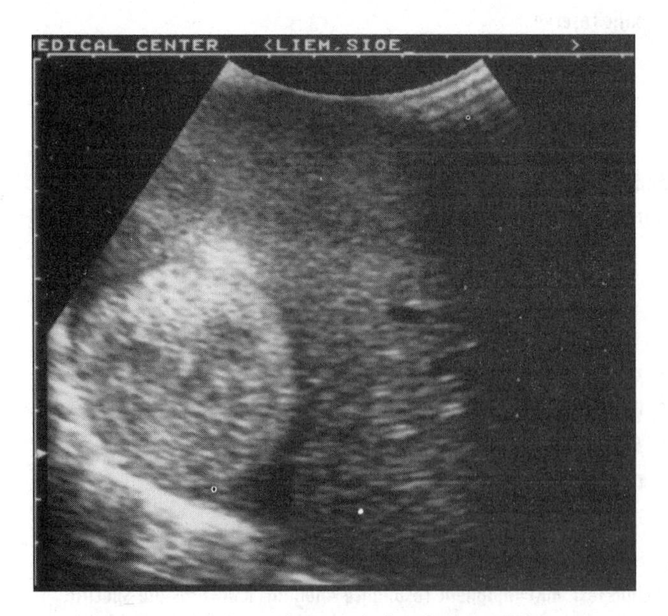

Fig 16-8. Intraoperative ultrasound of an hepatocellular carcinoma. The ultrasound confirms the resectability of the tumor and the absence of additional tumors.

Percutaneous needle biopsy is used only to confirm the diagnosis of unresectable tumors. This avoids any unnecessary complications and the possibility of seeding tumor cells at the time of biopsy.

Staging

There is a strong tendency for hepatocellular cancers to invade liver blood vessels, a fact that increases the importance of various imaging procedures in determining the tumor stage. Table 16-3 summarizes the definitions of the TNM system as agreed to by the American Joint Committee on Cancer and published in the *Manual for the Staging of Cancer* (1992).[35] Regional lymph nodes are those in the hepatoduodenal ligament, periportal (porta hepatic) region, along portal vein and hepatic arteries, and nodes along the hepatic portion of the inferior vena cava. More distant positive nodes are considered M1 disease stage. If tumors are resected, a pathologic TNM stage is obtained and can be augmented by histologic grading of the tumor. G1 is well differentiated, G2 is moderately differentiated, G3 is poorly differentiated, and G4 is undifferentiated.

Surgery

Hepatocellular cancers quite often present as large tumors, and their resection requires removal of significant liver tissue. As a result, it is imperative that the remaining liver be sufficiently functional in the immediate postoperative recovery period. In addition to standard assessment of serum bilirubin and liver transaminases, plasma clotting factors and serum albumin concentration are good indicators of hepatic reserve.

The primary risk factor is the presence or absence of cirrhosis. With cirrhosis, liver function is impaired, there is increased blood loss during surgery, especially in the presence of portal hypertension, and the liver lacks the normal capacity to regenerate. A low white blood cell count and low platelet count may be subtle but early indicators of portal hypertension and hypersplenism.

Without question, liver resection has become a much safer procedure. A better understanding of liver anatomy, experience with liver transplantation, and the availability of cell-savers and rapid transfusers have all contributed to improved survival. Nevertheless, the operative mortality is still 3% to 15%, and significant morbidity occurs in at least one third of resected patients.

Most hepatic surgeons no longer perform this operation using incisions that include a right

Table 16-3. TNM Staging

Primary Tumor (T)

TX	Primary tumor cannot be assessed
T0	No evidence of primary tumor
T1	Solitary tumor ≤2 cm in greatest dimension without vascular invasion
T2	Solitary tumor ≤2 cm in greatest dimension with vascular invasion; or multiple tumors limited to one lobe, none >2 cm in greatest dimension without vascular invasion; or a solitary tumor >2 cm in greatest dimension without vascular invasion
T3	Solitary tumor >2 cm in greatest dimension with vascular invasion; or multiple tumors limited to one lobe, none >2 cm in greatest dimension, with vascular invasion; or multiple tumors limited to one lobe, any >2 cm in greatest dimension, with or without vascular invasion
T4	Multiple tumors in more than one lobe, or tumor(s) involving major branches of the portal or hepatic vein(s)

Regional Lymph Nodes (N)

NX	Regional lymph nodes cannot be assessed
N0	No regional lymph node metastasis
N1	Regional lymph node metastasis

Distant Metastasis (M)

MX	Presence of distant metastasis cannot be assessed
M0	No distant metastasis
M1	Distant metastasis

Stage Grouping

Stage I	T1	N0	M0
Stage II	T2	N0	M0
Stage III	T1	N1	M0
	T2	N1	M0
	T3	N0	M0
	T3	N1	M0
Stage IVA	T4	Any N	M0
Stage IVB	Any T	Any N	M1

From American Joint Committee on Cancer.[35]

thoracotomy. Adequate operative exposure is essential and is best obtained through a generous midline incision or a bilateral subcostal incision. During the initial assessment, evidence of intra-abdominal extrahepatic metastases and for extracapsular extension is sought. Involvement of the diaphragm does not exclude resection but may require excision of a segment of diaphragm. The falciform ligament is divided, and the involved lobe of liver is mobilized. If the operation is to be a right lobectomy or trisegmentectomy, the right lobe is dissected free of the inferior vena cava, carefully ligating and oversewing the numerous small veins between the liver and inferior vena cava.

The hepatic arterial supply and portal venous supply are isolated early in the dissection of the porta hepatis. Generally it is safer to transect the hepatic vein(s) a centimeter or two within the liver parenchyma rather than directly on the cava. A Cavitron ultrasonic dissector and argon beam coagulator facilitate the dissection across the liver parenchyma and significantly minimize blood loss. However, a cirrhotic liver requires careful dissection with frequent placement of suture ligatures. If necessary, the midline incision is easily extended superiorly by a median sternotomy, but sternotomy is rarely needed.

As noted, the anatomic location of the tumor, tumor invasion of the hepatic veins, vena cava, or portal vein, and impaired synthetic function secondary to cirrhosis may preclude resection. In such patients, the question is often raised as to the role of liver transplantation. Several recent reports suggest that regardless of stage, patients receiving transplants do better than those who have undergone resection.[36-38] There is certainly a significant problem with recurrence in the remaining liver of resected patients. This is especially true in cirrhotic livers and probably relates to the multicentricity of hepatocellular cancer in this setting. Tumors with an infiltrative pattern (not circumscribed) on scan, multiple satellite nodules, major-vessel invasion, and elevated AFP levels can be classed as having a poor prognosis with resection. Such tumors, when confined to the liver, may be better managed by transplantation. Even so, relatively few patients would be acceptable transplant candidates. This fact, in conjunction with the scarcity of donor organs, makes it difficult to properly study the role of transplantation in the treatment of hepatocellular cancer.

Prognosis

Earlier reports cited operative mortality in the range of 3% to 15%. In major cancer centers with a high volume of such patients, operative mortality is close to 2% for major lobectomy and <1% for wedge resection.[39] Patient selection is extremely important in achieving safe, low-risk surgery and avoiding discovery of unresectable tumor at laparotomy.

While reports suggest that only 30% of patients explored will be resectable, it is now quite unusual to find an unresectable tumor at laparotomy due to the detailed assessment provided by modern-day imaging. Current information suggests that with resection 30% of patients will survive >5 years. If cirrhosis is present, however, the experience in this country suggests few patients will be alive 5 years postresection.[39]

Other Therapeutic Options

Surgical resection is the treatment of choice for hepatocellular cancer and, along with transplantation, offers the only chance for cure. Unfortunately, resection is not indicated in 85% to 90% of cases, and recurrences may develop requiring nonsurgical therapy. The following three criteria exclude patients from surgery: 1) an unacceptable risk based on the degree of cirrhosis, 2) tumor spread within the liver that precludes adequate surgical margins, and 3) evidence of extrahepatic tumor spread. For these patients, regional chemotherapy, systemic chemotherapy, and external-beam radiation, often in combination, may provide some degree of palliation.

There is an extensive series of reports on systemic chemotherapy for hepatocellular cancer, but the majority involve small numbers of patients often not randomized and are difficult to evaluate. Single agents such as 5-fluorouracil (5-FU) and doxorubicin are the drugs most often used, but responses are infrequent (15% to 20%) and of short duration. Today, combination chemotherapy is the standard and whenever possible should be part of a clinical study. Baker and colleagues reported a 13% response rate using 5-FU and doxorubicin (Adriamycin).[40] Falkson and colleagues reported a phase II trial comparing acivicin versus 4′ deoxydoxorubicin.[41] The results were dismal with no response on acivicin and only two patients responded to 4′ deoxydoxorubicin. Severe toxicity was documented in 23% and 45% respectively. Higher response rates have been achieved with 5-FU plus mitomycin C (38%), with 5-FU plus carmustine (BCNU) (37%), and with VM-26 in combination with Adriamycin and 5-FU (44%).[42] One thing seems clear in reviewing reports of combination therapy for hepatocellular cancer: poor performance status is consistently indicative of a poor response to any systemic therapy.

Even when unresectable, this tumor is often confined to the liver. As a result, there is considerable interest in hepatic arterial infusion (HAI) chemotherapy. In a study by the Gastrointestinal Oncology Service at Memorial Sloan-Kettering Cancer Center, even AFP-positive patients had a 40% response rate and median survival of 14.5 months using fluorodeoxyuridine (FUDR) and mitomycin C.[43] While the presence of cirrhosis is generally associated with shorter survival times, cirrhotic patients often can be treated by HAI therapy. However, they may be more susceptible to toxicity and require careful monitoring.

Other approaches to therapy have evolved along with HAI driven by the poor response to systemic chemotherapy. For example, chemoembolization was developed in Japan.[44] This involves embolizing the tumor with pellets of gelatin sponge permeated with mitomycin C or doxorubicin. Survival was reported to be 44% and 29% at 1 and 2 years, respectively. Clinical trials have indicated that chemoembolization may rival HAI therapy for response and improved survival. Both approaches appear much more efficacious than systemic therapy for disease confined to the liver.

Recently, it has been shown that fatty acid esters such as Lipiodol and Ethiodol are localized in the hypervascular hepatocellular carcinoma for a long time following hepatic artery injection. Studies are investigating the use of chemotherapy-Lipiodol suspensions such as Adriamycin-Lipiodol for efficacy in treating hepatocellular cancer. In one report, a significant amount of Adriamycin remained detectable in tumor resected 1 and 2 months after treatment.[45] Similarly, ^{131}I-Lipiodol or ^{131}I-Ethiodol injected via the hepatic artery can deliver a high dose of radiation to the liver tumor.

While external-beam radiotherapy may provide some palliation by relieving abdominal pain associated with an enlarging tumor mass, there is little long-term benefit. Recently, investigators have used two courses of hyperfractionated external-beam radiation in combination with hepatic arterial administration of FUDR. A 70% response rate was observed in contrast to 15% to 30% responses with external-beam radiation alone.[46]

Radiolabeled antibodies have also been evaluated. For example, ^{131}I- and ^{90}Y-labeled antiferritin antibodies have been used in clinical trials. Investigators have reported tumor targeting of 300μCi ^{131}I-antiferritin with a tumor half-life of 3.5 to 4 days.[47]

Direct attacks on hepatocellular cancer have also involved ultrasonographically guided percutaneous transhepatic ethanol injection. Long-term survivors have been reported.[48] Another method also deserves mention: cryosurgery using subzero temperatures and freeze-thaw cycles. Usually three freeze-thaw cycles are used. Significant survival rates have been reported,[49,50] including a study by Zhou and coworkers, indicating a 5-year survival of 37.5% for hepatocellular cancers <5 cm in diameter.[49]

Other Rare Primary Liver Tumors

Intrahepatic cholangiocarcinomas represent <0.5% of liver tumors. These tumors tend to be slow-growing, can be AFP-positive, and frequently secrete carcinoembryonic antigen (CEA). For these diffuse tumors, the preferred approach has included external-beam radiotherapy and HAI chemotherapy. Some patients have been treated with ^{131}I-labeled anti-CEA antibodies. Overall, the prognosis is poor. Such disease is rarely detected early enough that lobe resection offers a chance for cure. The results of transplantation have been dismal. This differs from the experience with orthotopic liver transplantation for patients with hilar adenocarcinoma of the bile ducts, in which a 64% 2-year survival has been reported.[36-38]

Cystadenomas of the liver are rare. They are best diagnosed by CT and ultrasound, which demonstrate septation and nodularity of the walls. Mucous cystadenomas have malignant potential, and complete excision is indicated. Cystadenocarcinoma is so rare that the presence of a simple cyst is not, in itself, an indication for excision. However, if biopsy of the cystic lesion indicates the presence of carcinoma, then a formal lobectomy of the involved portion of liver is advised.

Ishak and co-workers reported on a series of patients with a malignant liver tumor of endothelial origin termed epithelioid hemangioendothelioma. This tumor was first described by Weiss and Enzinger, and similar cancers have been described in the lung and bone. Epithelioid hemangioendotheliomas are generally multifocal, involving both lobes of the liver.

While the etiology of epithelioid hemangioendothelioma is unknown, reports have suggested an association with oral contraceptive use and with exposure to vinyl chloride. It is generally an indolent tumor and has a better prognosis than primary liver angiosarcoma. As a result, total hepatectomy and orthotopic liver transplantation is the recommended treatment.[51]

Metastatic Tumors

The liver is the most common site of involvement with metastatic tumors, and therefore most solid lesions in the liver are secondary to tumors of other organs. The most common metastatic lesions are from tumors of the gastrointestinal tract, especially colon and rectal cancer. Other cancers frequently metastasizing to the liver include gastric, pancreatic, breast, lung, ovary, kidney, and intestinal carcinoids.

The evaluation of metastatic tumors of the liver is essentially the same as for primary hepatic neoplasms. CT arterial portography and selective celiac and SMA angiography with venous phase films provide the best initial assessment. This defines the extent of metastatic involvement, aids in determining resectability, and combined with other aspects of the CT scan excludes other sites of recurrent tumor.

Significant potential for cure exists when metastases are from colorectal cancer and can be resected. Resection is the ideal approach when there are four or fewer metastatic tumors present. The 5-year survival rate for resected colorectal liver metastases is 33% with a disease-free survival of approximately 25%.[52,53] Patients with Wilm's tumor are excellent candidates for resection of hepatic metastases, but other primary tumors such as gastric, pancreatic, lung, and breast cancer do not appear to benefit from such efforts. The management of various tumors and their metastases to the liver will be addressed more extensively in specific disease-based chapters.

References

1. American Cancer Society. *Cancer Facts and Figures, 1994.* Atlanta, GA: American Cancer Society Inc; 1994.

2. Rustgi VK. Epidemiology of hepatocellular carcinoma. In: Di Bisceglie AM, Rustgi VK, Hoofnagle JH, Dusheiko GM, Lotze MT. Hepatocellular carcinoma. *Ann Intern Med.* 1988;108:390-401.

3. Henson SW Jr, Gray HK, Dockerty MB. Benign tumors of the liver. *Surg Gynecol Obstet.* 1956;103:23-30.

4. Ishak KG, Rabin L. Benign tumors of the liver. *Med Clin North Am.* 1975;59:995-1013.

5. Johnson CM, Sheedy PF II, Stanson AW, Stephens DH, Hattery RR, Adson MA. Computed tomography and angiography of cavernous hemangiomas of the liver. *Radiology.* 1981;138:115-121.

6. Lipman JC, Tumeh SS. The radiology of cavernous hemangioma of the liver. *Crit Rev Diagn Imaging.* 1990; 30:1-18.

7. Joyce AD, Howard ER. Hepatobiliary tumors of childhood: investigation and management. *Prog Pediatr Surg.* 1989;22:69-93.

8. Luks FI, Yazbeck S, Brandt M, Bensoussan AL, Brochu P, Blanchard H. Benign liver tumors in children: a 25-year experience. *J Pediatr Surg.* 1991;26:1326-1330.

9. Becker JM, Heitler MS. Hepatic hemangio-endotheliomas in infancy. *Surg Gynecol and Obstet.* 1989;168: 189-200.

10. Kasabach HH, Merritt KK. Capillary hemangioma with extensive purpura: report of a case. *Am J Dis Child.* 1940;59:1063-1070.

11. Kauppinen T, Riala R, Seitsamo J, Hernberg S. Primary liver cancer and occupational exposures. *Scand J Work Environ Health.* 1992;18:18-25.

12. Johnson DH, Vinson AM, Wirth FH, et al. Management of hepatic hemangioendotheliomas of infancy by transarterial embolization: a report of two cases. *Pediatrics.* 1984;73:546-549.

13. Vomberg PP, Buller HA, Marsman JWP, et al. Hepatic artery embolisation: successful treatment of multinodular hemangiomatosis of the liver. *Eur J Pediatr.* 1986;144: 472-474.

14. Matalo NM, Johnson DG. Surgical treatment of hepatic hemangioma in the newborn. *Arch Surg.* 1973;106:725-727.

15. Stark DD, Felder RC, Wittenberg J, et al. Magnetic resonance imaging of cavernous hemangioma of the liver: tissue-specific characterization. *Am J Roentgenol.* 1985; 145:213-222.

16. Trastek VF, Van Heerden JA, Sheedy PF II, Adson MA. Cavernous hemangiomas of the liver: resect or observe? *Am J Surg.* 1983;145:49-53.

17. Park WC, Phillips R. The role of radiation therapy in the management of hemangiomas of the liver. *JAMA.* 1970;212:1496-1498.

18. Yamamoto T, Kawarada Y, Yano T, Noguchi T, Mizumoto R. Spontaneous rupture of hemangioma of the liver:

treatment with transcatheter hepatic arterial embolization. *Am J Gastroenterol.* 1991;86:1645-1649.

19. McKay MJ, Carr PJ, Langlands AO. Treatment of hepatic cavernous haemangioma with radiation therapy: case report and literature review. *Aust N Z J Surg.* 1989; 59:965-968.

20. Shortell CK, Schwartz SI. Hepatic adenoma and focal nodular hyperplasia. *Surg Gynecol Obstet.* 1991;173:426-431.

21. Foster JH. Benign liver tumours. In: Blumgart LH, ed. *Surgery of the Liver and Biliary Tract.* New York, NY: Churchill Livingstone; 1988:1115-1127.

22. Edmondson HA. Tumors of the liver and intrahepatic bile ducts. In: *Atlas of Tumor Pathology*. Washington DC: Armed Forces Institute of Pathology; 1958: section 7, fasc 25.

23. Pain JA, Gimson AES, Williams R, Howard ER. Focal nodular hyperplasia of the liver: results of treatment and options in management. *Gut.* 1991;32:524-527.

24. Kerlin P, Davis GL, McGill DB, Weiland LH, Adson MA, Sheedy PF II. Hepatic adenoma and focal nodular hyperplasia: clinical pathologic and radiologic features. *Gastroenterology.* 1983;84:994-1002.

25. Adami H-O, Hsing AW, McLaughlin JK, et al. Alcoholism and liver cirrhosis in the etiology of primary liver cancer. *Int J Cancer.* 1992;51:898-902.

26. Blumberg BS, London WT. Hepatitis B virus and the prevention of primary hepatocellular carcinoma. *N Engl J Med.* 1981;304:782-784.

27. Niederau C, Fischer R, Sonnenberg A, Stremmel W, Trampisch HJ, Strohmeyer G. Survival and causes of death in cirrhotic and in noncirrhotic patients with primary hemochromatosis. *N Engl J Med.* 1985;313:1256-1262.

28. Eriksson S, Carlson J, Velez R. Risk of cirrhosis and primary liver cancer in alpha$_1$-anti deficiency. *N Engl J Med.* 1986;314:736-739.

29. Okuda K, Musha H, Nakajima Y, et al. Clinicopathologic features of encapsulated hepatocellular carcinoma: a study of 26 cases. *Cancer.* 1977;40:1240-1245.

30. Waldmann TA, McIntire KR. The use of radioimmunoassay for alpha-fetoprotein in the diagnosis of malignancy. *Cancer.* 1974;34:1510-1515.

31. Miller DL, Simmons JT, Chang R, et al. Hepatic metastases detection: comparison of three CT contrast enhancement methods. *Radiology.* 1987;165:785-790.

32. Sitzmann JV, Coleman J, Pitt HA, et al. Preoperative assessment of malignant hepatic tumors. *Am J Surg.* 1990;159:137-143.

33. Ney DR, Fishman EK, Niederhuber JE. Three-dimensional display of hepatic venous anatomy generated from spiral computed tomography data: preliminary results. *J Digit Imaging.* 1992;5:242-245.

34. Pugh RNH, Murray-Lyon IM, Dawson JL, Pietroni MC, Williams R. Transection of the oesophagus for bleeding oesophageal varices. *Br J Surg.* 1973;60:646-649.

35. Beahrs OH, Henson DE, Hutter RVP, Kennedy BJ, eds. *American Joint Committee on Cancer Manual for Staging of Cancer.* 4th ed. Philadelphia, Pa: JB Lippincott Co; 1992.

36. Olthoff KM, Millis JM, Rosove MH, Goldstein LI, Ramming KP, Busuttil RW. Is liver transplantation justified for the treatment of hepatic malignancies? *Arch Surg.* 1990;125:1261-1268.

37. Haug CE, Jenkins RL, Rohrer RJ, et al. Liver transplantation for primary hepatic cancer. *Transplantation.* 1992;53:376-382.

38. Campbell DA Jr, Merion RM, Ham JM, Turcotte JG. Liver transplantation for hepatic neoplasm. In: Niederhuber JE, ed. *Current Therapy in Oncology.* St Louis, Mo: Mosby Year Book Inc BC Decker; 1993:396-401.

39. Patti MG, Pellegrini CA. Factors affecting morbidity of liver resection. In: Cameron JL, ed. *Current Surgical Therapy.* St Louis, Mo: Mosby Year Book Inc BC Decker; 1992:293-296.

40. Baker LH, Saiki JH, Jones SE, et al. Adriamycin and 5-fluorouracil in the treatment of advanced hepatoma: a Southwest Oncology Group study. *Cancer Treat Rep.* 1977;61:1595-1597.

41. Falkson G, Cnaan A, Simson IW, et al. A randomized phase II study of acivicin and 4' deoxydoxorubicin in patients with hepatocellular carcinoma in an Eastern Cooperative Oncology Group Study. *Am J Clin Oncol.* 1990; 13:510-515.

42. Wanebo HJ, Falkson G, Order SE. Cancer of the hepatobiliary system. In: DeVita VT Jr, Hellman S, Rosenberg SA. *Cancer Principles & Practice of Oncology.* 3rd ed. Philadelphia, Pa: JB Lippincott Co; 1989:836-874.

43. Atiq OT, Kemeny N, Niedzwiecki D, Botet J. Treatment of unresectable primary liver cancer with intrahepatic fluorodeoxyuridine and mitomycin C through an implantable pump. *Cancer.* 1992;69:920-924.

44. Yamada R, Sato M, Kawabata M, Nakatsuka H, Nakamura K, Takashima S. Hepatic artery embolization in 120 patients with unresectable hepatoma. *Radiology.* 1983;148:397-401.

45. Katagiri Y, Mabuchi K, Itakura T, et al. Adriamycin-lipiodol suspension for i.a. chemotherapy of hepatocellular carcinoma. *Cancer Chemother Pharmacol.* 1989;23:238-242.

46. Lawrence TS, Kessler ML, Robertson JM. Conformal high-dose radiation plus intraarterial floxuridine for hepatic cancer. *Oncology.* 1993;7:51-58.

47. Klein JL, Nguyen TH, Laroque P, et al. Yttrium-90 and iodine-131 radioimmunoglobulin therapy of an experimental human hepatoma. *Cancer Res.* 1989;49:6383-6389.

48. Shiina S, Tagawa K, Unuma T, et al. Percutaneous ethanol injection therapy of hepatocellular carcinoma: analysis of 77 patients. *Am J Roentgenol.* 1990;155: 1221-1226.

49. Zhou X-D, Tang Z-Y, Yu Y-Q, Ma Z-C. Clinical evaluation of cryosurgery in the treatment of primary liver cancer: report of 60 cases. *Cancer.* 1988;61:1889-1892.

50. Ravikumar TS, Kane R, Cady B, Jenkins R, Clouse M, Steele G Jr. A 5-year study of cryosurgery in the treatment of liver tumors. *Arch Surg.* 1991;126:1520-1524.

51. Kelleher MB, Iwatsuki S, Sheahan DG. Epithelioid hemangioendothelioma of liver: clinicopathological correlation of 10 cases treated by orthotopic liver transplantation. *Am J Surg Pathol.* 1989;13:999-1008.

52. Adson MA. Diagnosis and surgical treatment of primary and secondary solid hepatic tumors in the adult. *Surg Clin North Am.* 1981;61(1):181-196.

53. Fortner JG, Silva JS, Golbey RB, Cox EB, Maclean BJ. Multivariate analysis of a personal series of 247 consecutive patients with liver metastases from colorectal cancer. *Ann Surg.* 1984;199:306-316.

17

GASTRIC NEOPLASMS

Walter Lawrence, Jr, MD, Alvin Zfass, MD

Clinically significant gastric neoplasms include both benign and malignant lesions. Several varieties of malignant neoplasms begin in the stomach, but the overwhelming majority are primary carcinomas developing in the mucosal glands. Until now these cancers, as well as other lesions considered in the differential diagnosis, were primarily treated surgically. However, the generally poor prognosis of gastric cancer after surgical therapy has naturally led to the current interest in potential benefits from much earlier diagnosis and from other treatment modalities.

This chapter will provide information on the clinical presentation and natural history of gastric cancer, as well as state-of-the-art management approaches. While this disease has a poor prognosis at this time, both epidemiologists and clinical researchers are striving to reduce the incidence of gastric cancer where it is still prevalent as well as to improve the outcome after treatment.

Relevant Anatomy

The Stomach

The stomach is an anatomic structure joined by the esophagus at the diaphragmatic hiatus and the duodenum at the distal pylorus. It serves as a food reservoir and an initiator of the digestive process. The mucosal lining normally differs proximally and distally in the stomach: The proximal stomach mucosa produces acid/peptic juice from the "oxyntic glands," which include the parietal cells (producing acid) and chief cells (pepsin producers). The distal mucosa produces a mucous secretion as well as gastrin, a hormone that plays a controlling role in acid/peptic secretion. External to the mucosa is a submucosal layer that is enveloped by two additional layers of musculature. These layers provide the motility required for the normal functions of the stomach. Prognosis depends on the extent of involvement of these various gastric layers by primary cancer, affecting both the patient evaluation process and treatment decisions.

Adjacent Anatomic Structures

The stomach is anatomically situated in the upper abdomen juxtaposed to the overlying left lobe of the liver anteriorly, the pancreas adjacent to the posterior gastric wall, the spleen (to which it is attached by both mesenteric and venous connections), and the transverse colon and its mesocolon (Fig 17-1). Any of these extragastric structures may be involved by direct extension of large gastric neoplasms, although local extension to the transverse mesocolon or the body of the pancreas occurs more frequently than to other sites because of the anatomic proximity of these structures. Distally, the pyloric boundary of the stomach is anatomically adjacent to the biliary and vascular structures of the porta hepatis. Invasion into this anatomic site, with resulting obstructive jaundice, is a less likely, but possible, manifestation of advanced gastric cancer. Proximally, the stomach joins the esophagus at the diaphragmatic hiatus so that local invasion by gastric cancer into the esophagus is relatively frequent, particularly for cancers that are localized to the proximal portion of the stomach.

Lymphatic Anatomy

As with most malignant neoplasms arising from the epithelium of the gastrointestinal tract, the lymphatic anatomy of the stomach is important because this is a possible site of tumor spread. The gastric lymphatics follow the course of the multiple vascular structures supplying the stomach (Fig 17-2). The most proximal lymph nodes are along the greater and lesser curvatures of the stomach, accompanying the distal

Walter Lawrence, Jr, MD, Professor of Surgery, Division of Surgical Oncology and Director Emeritus, Massey Cancer Center, Medical College of Virginia, Richmond, Virginia

Alvin Zfass, MD, Professor of Medicine, Director of Gastroenterology and Director of Endoscopy, Medical College of Virginia, Richmond, Virginia

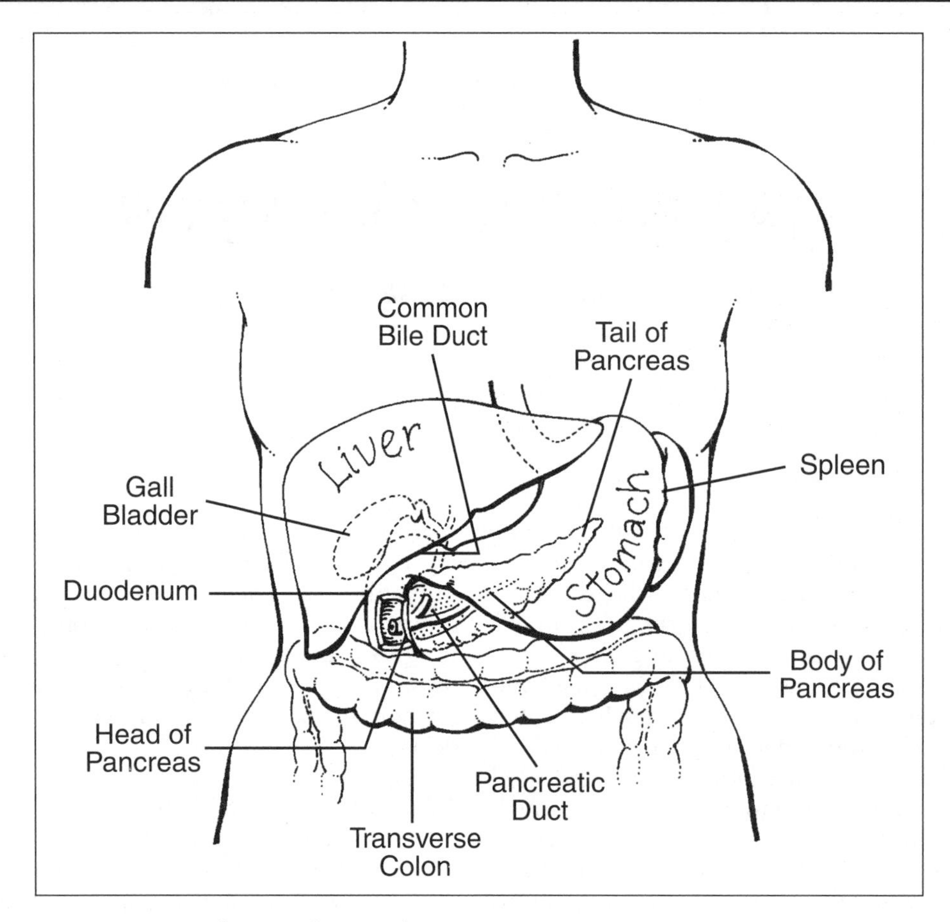

Fig 17-1. Organs adjacent to the stomach.

portions of the left gastric artery and the gastroepiploic vessels. The next somewhat more distant draining lymph nodes are those near the aorta at the origin of the celiac axis (hepatic artery, splenic artery, and left gastric artery origins) and those along the hepatic and splenic arteries themselves. As will be described, lymphatic drainage and extent of lymphatic involvement play a significant role in both the prognosis and the surgical management of gastric cancer.

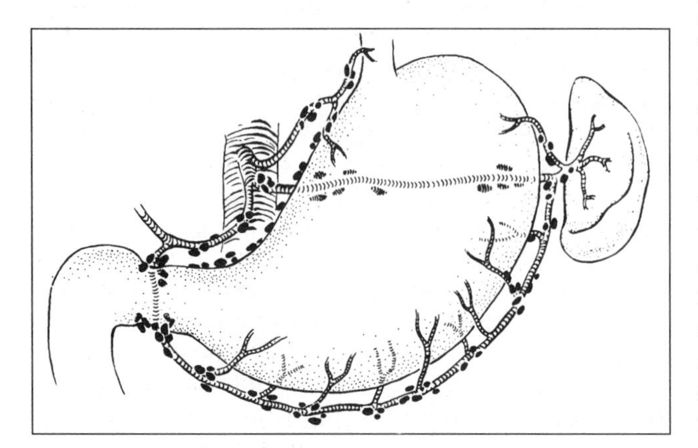

Fig 17-2. Lymphatic drainage of the stomach.

Epidemiology and Etiology

To understand the etiology of any cancer in humans, it is necessary to have demographic information that may provide clues.

Two unusual observations have been made about the epidemiology of gastric cancer. The first is that the mortality of gastric cancer has been decreasing in the United States for more than 50 years (Fig 17-3), even though no major advances in treatment strategy have been made during this period. Second, a wide variation in mortality rates from gastric cancer occurs from country to country. Gastric cancer is a relatively common cause of death in Japan, Chile, and Iceland. The death rate is about five times that in the US.[1] A United Nations estimate of cancer incidence in 24 world areas in 1980 showed that stomach cancer was the most common cancer when combined data (incidences in both men and women) were reviewed.[2] For no apparent reason, the incidence of gastric cancer appears to be greater in countries farther from the equator. Also, in most countries people in lower socioeconomic classes tend to develop the disease more frequently than upper classes. However, there are no rural-urban or occupational differences observed in incidence.

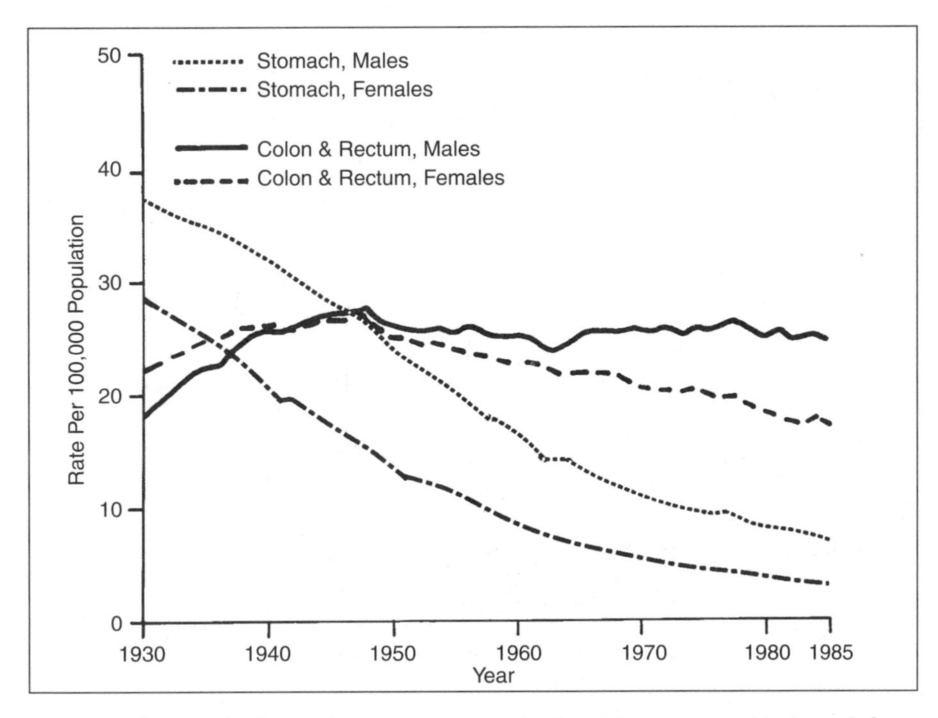

Fig 17-3. Changing death rates for gastric cancer in the United States compared with trends for colon and rectal cancer.

The change in methods of food preservation in the US, with more emphasis on frozen foods over the last several decades, as well as an increased intake of vitamin C may well play a role in the difference in frequency of gastric cancer between the US and many other countries. Much study still needs to be done to delineate those dietary factors that may contribute to these major geographic differences in incidence.[3-5] *Helicobacter pylori* infection also is clearly associated with gastric cancer.[6,7] All of these findings will aid in the development of prevention strategies in those countries where gastric cancer is still a common fatal disease.

Despite the continued decrease in incidence of gastric cancer in the US, it was estimated that there were about 24,000 new cases in 1994 and approximately 14,000 deaths. Gastric cancer is found more commonly in people between 50 and 70 years of age and is predominantly a disease of men rather than women (1.7:1 ratio). In the US, gastric cancer is more common than cancers of the esophagus, small intestine, biliary tract, or liver, but slightly less frequent than pancreatic cancer and much less frequent than colorectal cancer.

The epidemiologic studies described above, and their etiologic implications, are closely tied to various cancer-associated pathologic changes that occur in the stomach. Atrophic gastritis has been increasingly observed in many of the countries where there is a higher incidence of gastric cancer. Also, a progression of the disease from atrophic gastritis to gastric cancer has been demonstrated on repeated biopsies in a selected group of patients.[8] In this same vein, there are data to suggest a higher incidence of gastric cancer in patients with atrophic mucosal changes following a prior distal gastrectomy for benign peptic ulcer disease, particularly after more than a 20-year interval.[9] Serial endoscopic studies with biopsy, following partial gastrectomy, support this concept of evolving neoplastic change in the remaining stomach subsequent to initial gastric resection. Findings of dysplasia on random biopsy indicate a greater likelihood of development of carcinoma in the remaining stomach, and this identifies a subset of patients requiring more aggressive endoscopic surveillance after gastrectomy.[10]

What is the stimulus for this chain of pathologic events from dysplasia or atrophic gastritis to carcinoma? Studies have shown that nitrosamines can produce gastric cancer in experimental animals, and these compounds may be carcinogenic in man as well. It has been shown that nitrosamines can be produced in the stomach from nitrates. The intermediate in the synthesis of nitrosamines from nitrates is nitrites. Nitrites can be produced from nitrates by bacteria in the stomach, but the bacteria with enzymes capable of catalyzing this reaction are killed by the acid environment that is present in a normal stomach. This

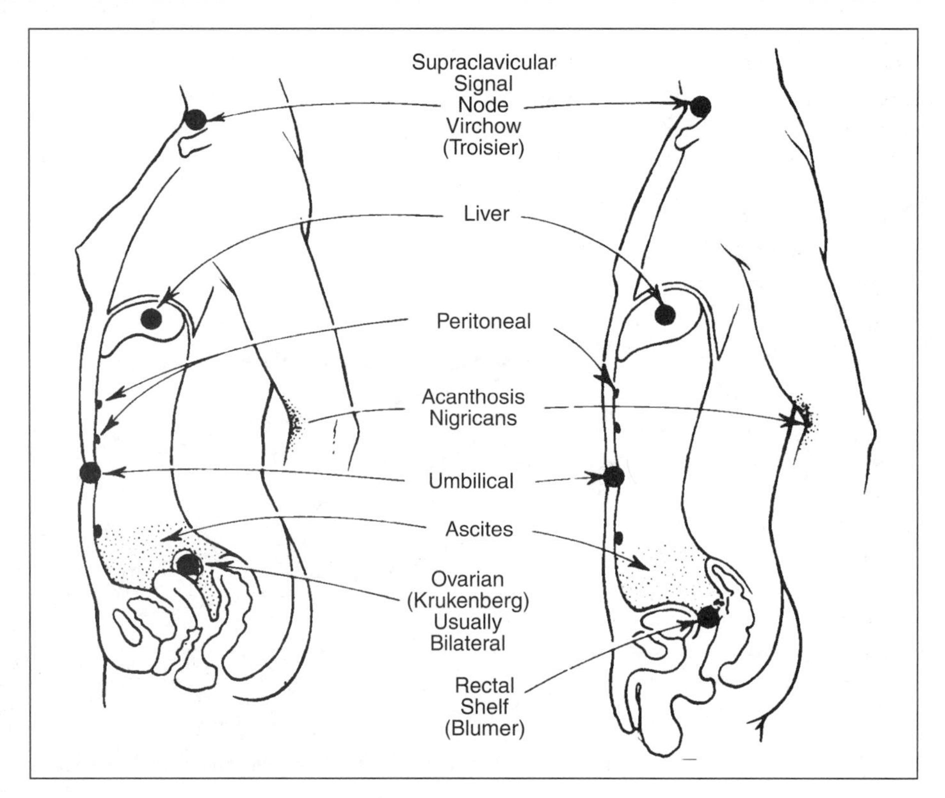

Fig 17-4. Diagram of routes of spread of gastric cancer.

might well explain why gastric cancer develops more frequently in patients with atrophic gastritis and hypochlorhydria. Once nitrites are formed, they quickly combine with amines that are naturally present in gastric juices to form nitrosamines. Changes in methods of food preservation and increased utilization of vitamin C are both factors that would interfere with this proposed mechanism of carcinogenesis for gastric cancer.

Patients who have pernicious anemia, hypochlorhydria, or achlorhydria seem to develop gastric cancer more frequently than others. As noted, atrophic gastritis and intestinal metaplasia have been thought to be major precursor lesions.[1] Adenomatous polyps are not considered major precursor lesions for gastric cancer, but patients with adenomatous polyps do have an increased incidence of gastric cancer.[11] In contrast to their occurrence in the colon, however, adenomatous polyps are uncommon in the stomach and are probably less common than gastric cancer.

There have been reports of a 15% to 20% increased incidence of gastric cancer in persons with blood group A, and this suggests a genetic relationship. A small increased incidence has been noted, also, in the direct relatives of people who had gastric cancer. Napoleon Bonaparte's family is the best-known example of one of the few families that have been reported in which the incidence of gastric cancer is remarkably high. One study of Japanese immigrants, however, has provided evidence to the contrary.[12] Japanese immigrants in the US maintain nearly the same incidence of gastric cancer as seen in the region where they spend their first 20 years of life. In contrast, their offspring have an incidence of gastric cancer that is lower and almost comparable to that of Caucasians living nearby. These findings suggest that there are probably exposures in early life, rather than a genetic influence, that are the major causative factors in gastric cancer.

Epidemiologic research has provided a number of clues that are now being evaluated and subjected to clinical trials. The ultimate objective is the exploitation of this information for the prevention of gastric cancer in those areas where it is still a significant health problem.

Background and Natural History of Gastric Cancer

Gastric cancer includes malignant lymphoma and malignant neoplasms of mesodermal origin (particularly leiomyosarcoma) as well as very rare gastric neoplasms (such as carcinoids, plasmacytoma, metastatic carcinoma). However, this discussion will focus solely on adenocarcinoma arising from the mucosal lining of the stomach. Most adenocarcinomas arise from the distal portion of the stomach and are on the lesser curvature, which is also a common site for benign gastric ulcer. In one large series, 45% of all malignant lesions were primarily in the distal third of the stomach, 33% in the pars media, and 22% in the proximal third. However, there is a recent trend in the US toward an increasing incidence of proximal gastric cancer.[13] This may be related to an increase or reduction in some of the etiologic factors for specific types of gastric cancer. The location of the cancer determines whether surgery is appropriate and the patient's prognosis.

Routes of Spread

Since gastric cancer originates in the mucosal layer of the stomach, lesions described as "early" are grossly and histologically limited to the mucosa or submucosa, a lesion specifically defined as "early gastric cancer." It is presumed that many or all gastric cancers are initially confined to the mucosa, but clinical diagnosis of gastric cancer at this stage has been quite uncommon in the US. In Japan, where screening measures have been more vigorous, cancer of the mucosa has been increasingly identified.[14] Gastric cancer seen in the US usually invades the muscular layers of the gastric wall and is frequently evident on the external serosal surface of the stomach.

Gastric carcinomas can spread in a number of ways (Fig 17-4). They can penetrate the gastric wall and directly invade contiguous anatomic structures. In this way gastric carcinomas can involve the pancreas, spleen, esophagus, colon, duodenum, gallbladder, liver, or the adjacent mesenteries. As noted earlier, local posterior extension to the adjacent body of the pancreas and transverse mesocolon is the most frequent route of local spread. All local extensions occur after growth to and through the serosal surface of the stomach, and all are associated with some diminution in prognosis.

In addition to local extension of the cancer to other anatomic structures, gastric cancers often will spread to the peritoneal surface of the abdominal cavity. This type of spread produces tiny "implants," coalesced peritoneal surface masses, or a reactive ascites, which clearly has the same poor prognostic significance as hematogenous spread of the disease.

Gastric cancer also spreads via lymphatics and does so in almost two thirds of the patients who are surgically explored and have pathologic studies done on lymphatic tissues. The initial regional lymphatics involved are determined somewhat by the anatomic location of the primary lesion. The lymph nodes that are adjacent to the primary lesion are involved first, but regional lymph node spread may be quite extensive and involve the lymphatic chains on both the lesser and greater curvatures of the stomach. The next level of regional lymphatic spread along the hepatic and splenic vessels often follows. More distant lymphatic spread, particularly that detected in the left supraclavicular nodes (Virchow's node), is a classic sign indicating that surgery is not a treatment option.

Gastric carcinomas may spread hematogenously via the portal circulation to the liver and, less often, to other sites during the remainder of the clinical course. Histologic evidence of metastatic spread to the lungs has been identified in 25% of patients at autopsy, for example, whereas on clinical evaluation, hematogenous spread to the lungs and other distant sites is rarely noted.

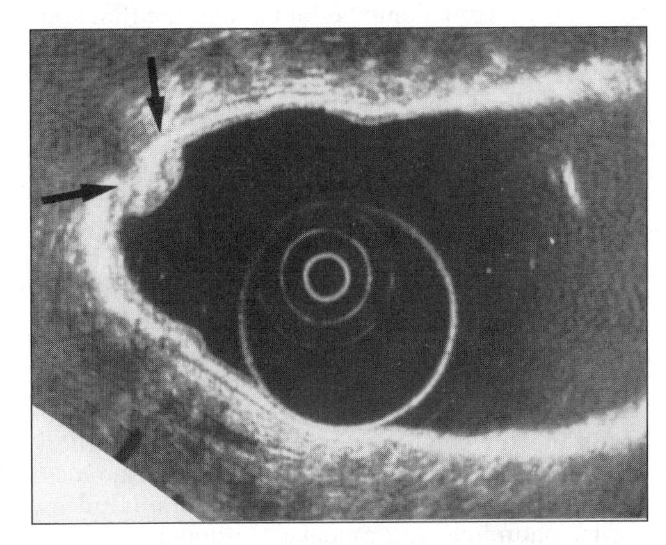

Fig 17-5a. Endoscopic ultrasound image showing a mass of epithelial origin projecting into the lumen. The lesion measures 1.5 cm in diameter and 9 mm in height. There is "heaped up" mucosa and distortion of the echogenic submucosal layer. Adenopathy is not identified. Note the echogenic layers identified (hypoechogenic or hyperechogenic).

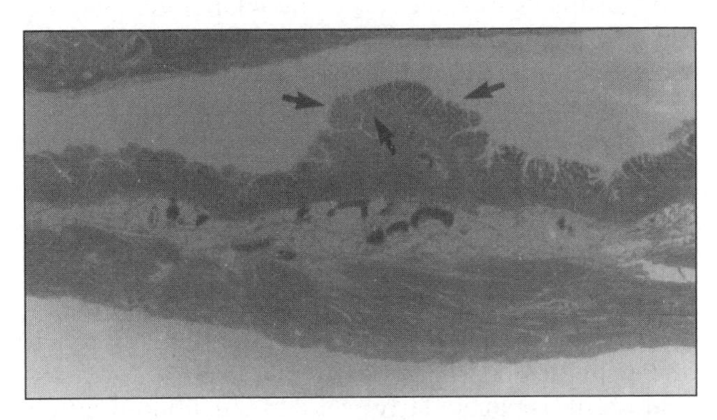

Fig 17-5b. Histologic sample from the same mass. A sharp line of demarcation is obvious between normal mucosa and tumor (arrows). The involved mucosa stains darker. The underlying submucosa and muscularis propria are invaded by tumor.

Clinical Presentation

One of the most difficult aspects of the diagnosis of gastric cancer is the nonspecific nature of the symptoms produced by this disease. The vast majority of gastric cancer patients present with such gastrointestinal complaints as vague epigastric discomfort or indigestion, occasional vomiting, belching, or postprandial fullness and/or early satiety. Five percent to 10% of gastric cancer patients may have complaints similar to those of patients with classic peptic ulcer disease. Another 10% have nonspecific symptoms of chronic disease, such as anemia, weakness, and weight loss. A small number of patients are first seen with an acute intra-abdominal problem, such as massive upper gastrointestinal bleeding, acute obstruction of the esophagus or pylorus, or gastric perforation, often requiring emergency surgery. Diagnosis is difficult, since most of these symptoms can be either manifestations of local or distant extensions of the neoplasm or simply attributed to other noncancerous diseases in the upper abdomen.

As with history taking, physical examination is rarely helpful except in identifying signs of advanced, and often incurable, disease. The only observation on physical examination that may lead to a reasonably early diagnosis of gastric cancer is a positive fecal occult blood test. Other physical signs suggest more advanced disease and include a palpable ovarian mass (from metastasis), hepatomegaly, abdominal mass, ascites, jaundice, and cachexia. Although a patient with a palpable gastric cancer may be suitable for a curative resection, this finding is often associated with a diminished prognosis. Nevertheless, a diagnostic approach to all of these symptoms or signs is clearly necessary.

Diagnostic Workup

With the absence of diagnostic symptoms or signs peculiar to gastric cancer, the physician must evaluate any patient with persistent upper gastrointestinal symptoms—particularly individuals over 40 years of age—for cancer. Diagnosis of a gastric neoplasm can be established by upper gastrointestinal (GI) endoscopy, upper GI radiographic examination, or a combination of the two.

Endoscopy

Upper GI endoscopy in conjunction with targeted or directed biopsy and cytology is the standard approach and provides a precise diagnosis in 95% of cases. Endoscopy is particularly useful in the differentiation of neoplasm from benign gastric ulcer and is very helpful in identifying early, or superficial, cancers. Multiple biopsies are taken from any area of "suspicious mucosa," any ulcerations that are noted, or any polypoid changes.

Upper GI Radiographs

Initial diagnostic evaluation may employ an upper GI series but, more often, double-contrast radiographic studies are useful in selected cases when endoscopic evaluation is considered inadequate. Linitis plastica, the gross description of gastric cancer known also as "leather bottle stomach," has a characteristic radiographic appearance. Occasionally, the submucosal location and extension of this relatively uncommon type of gastric cancer may not be identifiable by endoscopy, biopsy, or cytologic study.

Endoscopic Ultrasound

Endoscopic ultrasound is a relatively new technology that allows the endoscopist to visualize all layers of the gastric wall. The ability to "see" the wall of the stomach and identify the full extent of the neoplasm helps in the diagnosis and also contributes to the TNM staging process (Fig 17-5).

A dedicated instrument for this purpose, with a radial (360°) scanning ultrasound, has been available in Europe for some time, and endoscopic ultrasound technology is now becoming available in a number of centers in the US. Ultrasound probes that can be inserted through the biopsy channels of conventional endoscopes are now available and being evaluated.

Pathologic Classification and Significance in Management and Prognosis

The first classification of gastric cancer, in terms of gross pathology, was constructed by Borrmann in 1926 and is summarized as follows:

- *Type I—Polypoid carcinoma:* clearly demarcated; may be ulcerated; late metastasis; relatively good prognosis.
- *Type II—Ulcerating carcinoma ("ulcero cancer"):* sharply defined margins; difficult to differentiate from benign ulcer on gross examination; requires biopsy; relatively good prognosis.
- *Type III—Ulcerating and infiltrating:* lacks clearcut margins; extensive submucosal infiltration and usually extends to the serosa; most common type of gastric cancer; relatively poor prognosis.
- *Type IV—Diffuse infiltration:* early metastasis, includes linitis plastica ("leather bottle stomach"), has poorest prognosis of all gastric cancers.

Both types I and II appear to be decreasing in incidence in the US, in contrast to types III and IV.

Additional gross classifications include superficial spreading carcinoma (large, ulcerating, and irregular lesions that are confined to the mucosa and submucosa) and "early gastric cancer" (small, usually very early lesions that do not infiltrate beyond the submu-

Table 17-1. TNM Staging for Stomach Cancer

Primary Tumor (T)

TX	Primary tumor cannot be assessed
T0	No evidence of primary tumor
Tis	Carcinoma in situ; intraepithelial tumor without invasion of lamina propria
T1	Tumor invades lamina propria or submucosa
T2	Tumor invades the muscularis propria or the subserosa*
T3	Tumor penetrates the serosa (visceral peritoneum) without invasion of adjacent structures**†
T4	Tumor invades adjacent structures**†

*Note: A tumor may penetrate the muscularis propria with extension into the gastrocolic or gastrohepatic ligaments or into the greater or lesser omentum without perforation of the visceral peritoneum covering these structures. In this case, the tumor is classified T2. If there is perforation of the visceral peritoneum covering the gastric ligaments or omenta, the tumor should be classified T3.

**Note: The adjacent structures of the stomach are the spleen, transverse colon, liver, diaphragm, pancreas, abdominal wall, adrenal gland, kidney, small intestine, and retroperitoneum.

† Note: Intramural extension to the duodenum or esophagus is classified by the depth of greatest invasion in any of these sites, including the stomach.

Regional Lymph Nodes (N)

The regional lympth nodes are the perigastric nodes along the lesser (1, 3, 5) and greater (2, 4a, 4b, 6) curvatures and the nodes located along the left gastric (7) and common hepatic (8), splenic (10, 11), and celiac arteries (9). Involvement of other intra-abdominal lymph nodes, such as hepatoduodenal (12), retropancreatic, mesenteric, and paraaortic, is classified as distant metastasis.

Note: The numerical order corresponds to the proposals of the Japanese Research Society for Gastric Cancer Study in Surgery and Pathology, the Japanese Journal of Surgery, Tokyo 11:127-145, 1982.

NX	Regional lymph node(s) cannot be assessed
N0	No regional lymph node metastasis
N1	Metastasis in perigastric lymph node(s) within 3 cm of the edge of the primary tumor
N2	Metastasis in perigastric lymph node(s) more than 3 cm from the edge of the primary tumor, or in lymph nodes along the left gastric, common hepatic, splenic, or celiac arteries

Distant Metastasis (M)

MX	Presence of distant metastasis cannot be assessed
M0	No distant metastasis
M1	Distant metastasis

Table 17-1 *Continued.* TNM Staging for Stomach Cancer

Histopathologic Type

World Health Organization (WHO)

n	Adenocarcinoma	M81403
n	Papillary adenocarcinoma	M82603
n	Tubular adenocarcinoma	M82113
n	Mucinous adenocarcinoma	M84803
n	Signet ring cell carcinoma	M84903
n	Adenosquamous carcinoma	M85603
n	Squamous cell carcinoma	M80703
n	Carcinoid tumor	M82403
n	Mixed carcinoid-adenocarcinoma	M82443
n	Small cell carcinoma	M80413
n	Undifferentiated carcinoma	M80203
n	Other (specify):________________	

Code Numbers: SNOMED, College of American Pathologists, 1979

Histopathologic Grade (G)

n	GX	Grade cannot be assessed
n	G1	Well differentiated
n	G2	Moderately differentiated
n	G3-4	Poorly differentiated or undifferentiated

Stage Grouping

Stage 0	Tis	N0	M0
Stage IA	T1	N0	M0
Stage IB	T1	N1	M0
	T2	N0	M0
Stage II	T1	N2	M0
	T2	N1	M0
	T3	N0	M0
Stage IIIA	T2	N2	M0
	T3	N1	M0
	T4	N0	M0
Stage IIIB	T3	N2	M0
	T4	N1	M0
Stage IV	T4	N2	M0
	Any T	Any N	M1

From American Joint Committee on Cancer.[18]

cosa). These early cancers with a favorable prognosis constitute up to 35% of some series in Japan but are still quite uncommon in the US.

Histologic Categories

The original histologic classification for gastric cancer was developed by Broder, who described four grades (I-IV) based on the degree of differentiation present. A more recent, commonly used histologic classification was described by Lauren.[15] He discussed two types of lesions: the *intestinal*, a well-differentiated lesion; and the *diffuse* or undifferentiated carcinoma. Epidemiologists prefer this differentiation. It does enable them to demonstrate that the association of atrophic gastritis and gastric cancer in certain countries may be entirely the result of increased numbers of cancers of the intestinal variety. This suggests that the intestinal and the diffuse types of lesions may well have differing causes.

Although adenocarcinoma is by far the most common gastric cancer, several other types of malignant gastric neoplasms are seen and should be mentioned. Malignant lymphoma is the second most common stomach cancer and now accounts for up to 8% of all cancers of this organ. Although this tumor presenting in the stomach may be a manifestation of a systemic process, lymphoma will often have its primary and only site in the stomach. When this is the case, it may present as a discrete polypoid lesion, an ulcerated mass, or as giant rugal folds. Histologic differentiation must be made from pseudolymphoma, an unusual inflammatory process that is sometimes associated with benign gastric ulcer.[16] Extranodal lymphomas arising as primary cancers of the stomach may or may not show regional lymph node metastasis.

The second most common cancer of mesodermal origin in the stomach is leiomyosarcoma, making up 1% to 3% of all gastric cancers.[17] Benign leiomyomas occur much more frequently than leiomyosarcomas. The differentiation of sarcoma from a benign leiomyoma is often made on the basis of the frequency of mitotic figures on histologic sections. Other types of sarcoma are more clearly infiltrative on gross examination. Less frequent sarcomas first appearing in the stomach are liposarcoma, fibrosarcoma, carcinosarcoma, or malignant soft tissue tumors of vascular origin.

Other, rare types of malignant gastric tumors are the carcinoids, plasmacytomas, and metastatic cancers. Carcinoids are generally small, firm, yellow, well-circumscribed submucosal lesions, as they are in other locations. Carcinoid tumors are argentaffin-positive on histologic staining. Some cancers that may rarely metastasize to the stomach arise in the lung, pancreas, prostate, breast, ovary, cervix, liver, and the skin (malignant melanoma).

Staging

Clinical staging of the gastric cancer patient is based on the extent of the disease as shown by both physical examination and by radiologic and endoscopic studies (clinico-diagnostic stage). Endoscopic ultrasound, as noted earlier, may well improve our ability to establish the stage of disease prior to surgical intervention. However, the most accurate staging classification for end-result reporting after surgical treatment is based on the extent of the disease found at the time of surgical exploration of the abdomen and the histologic study of the excised surgical specimen when the cancer can be resected (clinico-pathologic stage). At the time of celiotomy, the operative findings may reveal completely resectable disease, and the tumor-nodes-metastasis (TNM) stage can then be determined from pathologic study of the resected specimen (Table 17-1).

It is apparent that the categorization as stages I through III in the TNM system relates completely to the various features of local and regional extension. Stage IV is reached if one of the following occurs: metastasis to a cervical lymph node, the liver, or the peritoneum, or the appearance of metastatic lesions in less common sites. When the cancer has reached stage IV, palliative treatment is indicated. Such adverse findings are often not apparent until celiotomy is performed, although pretreatment evaluations may allow proper categorization.

The principal factor affecting the TNM classification[18] from the standpoint of the primary tumor is the degree of penetration of the gastric wall by the carcinoma. The size or the location of the primary tumor is of less significance in assigning "T" for the estimation of prognosis. Nodal involvement is a significant prognostic factor in the staging process, ranging from no metastasis to lymph nodes (N0), to lymphatic spread to immediately adjacent nodes (N1), to nodes in the perigastric area on both the lesser and greater curvatures (N2), or to more distant lymph nodes (N3). Patients with distant metastases to the peritoneal surfaces, the liver, or other sites detected at surgery are categorized as M1, a uniformly poor prognostic sign.

Prognostic Factors Influencing Choice of Treament

Prognostic factors relating to the clinical presentation, pathology, and the extent of disease have been evaluated. Patients with a short history of symptoms tend to have a poorer prognosis than those with a longer history, undoubtedly because the cancer growth rate is higher in patients with a short history of symptoms. Patients with the "ulcer" type of symptomatology seem to do better than those presenting

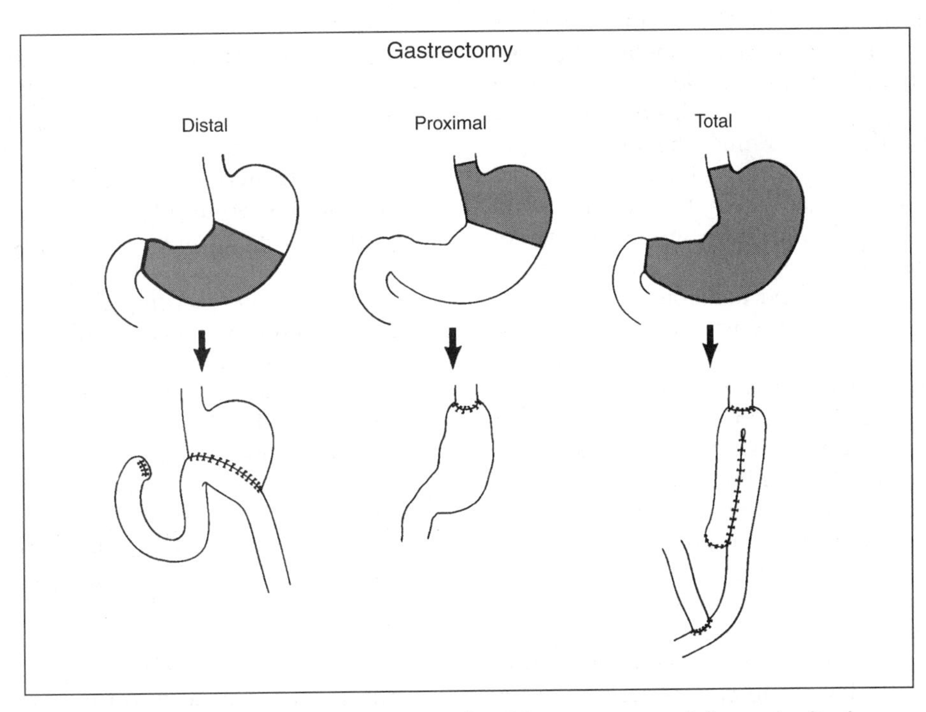

Fig 17-6. Diagrams of operative resections employed for gastric cancer. Left to right: distal gastrectomy, proximal gastrectomy, total gastrectomy (method of reconstruction shown below each procedure).

with the more frequent symptoms of "indigestion." The type of lesion on gross pathology, the location of the cancer in the stomach (distal more favorable than proximal lesions), and the presence or absence of lymphatic metastasis are more important indicators of prognosis than the pattern or duration of symptoms. Actually, the presence or absence of lymphatic metastasis is probably the most significant prognostic variable noted for all patients who have localized lesions suitable for "curative" gastric resection. Only a small proportion of patients demonstrating lymphatic metastasis (approximately 15%) enjoys long-term survival after radical resection that includes the regional lymph nodes. However, patients without lymphatic metastasis who are suitable for curative radical gastrectomy have a reasonably good prognosis; approximately 50% of these patients will have long-term survival. In the subset of this group that have the primary lesion limited to the mucosa or submucosa (early gastric cancer), 5-year survival rates have been reported to be more than 90%.

It is clear that none of the factors discussed above is under the control of the clinician except for the future possibility of effective primary prevention strategies, or secondary prevention by detection of early gastric cancer through screening interventions. The former has occurred fortuitously in the US, to some extent, as evidenced by the marked decrease in incidence over the last several decades despite the fact that this has been a confusing experiment of nature. Early (presymptomatic) diagnosis programs for minimal and superficial lesions are not really feasible now in the US due to the current relatively low frequency of this disease in our population. However, genetic predisposition to gastric cancer at a cellular level of measurement, using the new techniques of molecular biology, may be utilized in the future for selective screening strategies. Such approaches may greatly affect the prognosis of gastric cancer in the US by increasing the proportion of patients who are diagnosed with small, superficial, highly curable lesions.

General Management

Treatment Principles

Currently, surgery is the only effective curative method in the primary treatment of gastric cancer and continues to be the major approach for palliation as well. Despite major improvements over the years in both surgery and postsurgical management, overall survival rates remain quite low for all but those with early gastric cancer.[19-21]

All patients with gastric cancer, except those with evidence of peritoneal metastasis (ascites containing malignant cells or rectal shelf), documented liver metastasis, or other proven distant metastases (usually to cervical lymph nodes) should be subjected to exploratory celiotomy to select both potentially curable patients and those who might benefit from palliative resection. If the cancer is regionally localized at exploration, adequate resection of the primary tumor, as well as actual and potential regional lymphatic extensions, is performed. Unfortunately, fewer than 40% of patients so explored are able to undergo a resection with some hope of cure on the basis of the findings at operation.

In designing a radical gastrectomy for patients with curable gastric cancer, the removal of potential regional lymphatic extensions must be considered. Although the incidence of regional lymphatic spread varies with different gross and histologic types of cancer, the overall incidence of lymphatic spread from carcinoma of the stomach is high—more than 60%. In addition, gross observations often do not reveal whether lymph node metastases are present or not. Potential areas of lymphatic spread must always be considered in the design of radical gastrectomy, since the status of the regional lymphatics can be determined with confidence only after completion of the resection. Unfortunately, removal of histologically involved lymph nodes is often not effective for long-term cancer control, although about 15% of the patients with limited lymphatic spread do have long-term survival in most Western series. Results in Japan are somewhat better than this.[22]

Surgical Options

The major options for surgical resection of gastric cancer are distal subtotal gastric resection, proximal subtotal resection, or total gastrectomy. Restoration of continuity of the alimentary tract is achieved by anastomosis of the small intestine to the gastric remnant (gastroenterostomy), distal stomach to the esophagus (esophagogastrostomy) or small intestine to esophagus (esophagojejunostomy), with or without a jejunal reservoir (Fig 17-6). These procedures may include resection of adjacent organs affected by local extension of the cancer, such as the body and tail of the pancreas, a portion of the liver, transverse colon, or perhaps the duodenum and head of the pancreas. Inclusion of extragastric organs in the resection is an infrequent consideration because involvement of such organs is often accompanied by other gross signs of incurability. The surgeon tends to be discouraged from proceeding with major resection in many instances, particularly when resection would include the head of the pancreas.

Larger lesions of the pars media of the stomach and lesions of the proximal stomach are close to, or involve, the esophagogastric junction. To achieve an adequate margin around the cancer, the proximal line of resection should usually be through the distal esophagus. With either proximal or total gastrectomy for cancer in these sites, an esophageal anastomosis is required. Esophageal anastomosis has been associated with some increase in morbidity and mortality in the past, but less so in recent years.

The presence of microscopic spread beyond the gross margin of a gastric cancer is frequent, so removal of a generous margin of normal stomach around the carcinoma is a standard principle of gastric resection for all malignant lesions. In distal gastric lesions, generous resection of the adjacent first portion of the duodenum is required; in proximal lesions, the removal of a generous margin of distal esophagus is necessary. Frozen section examination of the site of transection usually is obtained at the time of operation in both situations if there is any question regarding the adequacy of resection. Failure to control a potentially curable cancer by not achieving an adequate gross margin around the primary tumor is a serious and often avoidable error.

Although careful abdominal exploration is designed to avoid unnecessary radical surgery when cure is not possible, it is also important for the surgeon to confirm the diagnosis of cancer histologically, if resection proves not to be possible. If a gastric cancer is observed to be resectable on gross evaluation, it does not seem essential to obtain a positive biopsy prior to resection, particularly if the procedure planned is less radical than a total gastrectomy.

Palliative Surgery

A significant number of patients have unfavorable findings at the time of celiotomy, such as serosal implants, liver or ovarian metastasis, or metastasis seen in lymph nodes outside the limits of a radical en bloc resection. This is the case in more than 60% of gastric cancer patients who are operated on with the hope that curative resection is possible. A palliative procedure is then planned, or the abdomen is closed without further surgery except for biopsy confirmation of the findings.

Palliative resection of gastric cancer is always the preferred procedure in these circumstances if this can be accomplished without total gastrectomy, without transection of gross tumor at the site of planned anastomosis, and without major hazards to the patient. If these conditions are met, palliative resection can significantly relieve symptoms in most patients, and it also appears to prolong survival. Palliative nonresectional procedures, such as gastrojejunostomy, gastrostomy, or jejunostomy rarely alleviate symptoms or prolong life expectancy. In carefully selected patients, total gastrectomy may be used for palliation, particularly if the patient is obstructed, or if extensive lymphatic spread is the only finding preventing a curative resection. These patients seem to have a longer survival time after palliative resection than those incurable because of liver or peritoneal metastasis. Considerable judgment is needed in making decisions about the choice of operative procedure when definite signs of incurability are detected at the time of exploration.

Radiation Therapy

Radiation therapy is rarely helpful in patients with gastric cancer that is insuitable for resection, as the usual reason for nonresectability is the lack of anatomic localization of the cancer. Radiation therapy is sometimes used to relieve localized obstruction, particularly in the region of the cardia, and for patients with chronically bleeding cancers that cannot be resected. Radiation is rarely indicated as a palliative tool but may have benefit in highly selected cases. Some surgeons have recently been using intraoperative radiation therapy, along with resection, but this adjuvant technique has not been used long enough to allow for complete evaluation. There has been no evidence to support the simple addition of postoperative radiation by external beam.

Chemotherapy

Many chemotherapeutic drugs have been tried in the past as single agents for the palliation of gastric cancer, but the results were generally disappointing. The antimetabolite 5-fluorouracil (5-FU) was the drug used most frequently as a single agent alone or in combination with palliative radiation therapy. In one large review, approximately 22% of the patients treated with 5-FU had a limited degree of transient improvement and no definite increase in survival time. Many other single agents have been used, with minimal palliative benefit, except for the drug Adriamycin.

There has been more enthusiasm for various combinations of chemotherapeutic agents for patients with advanced gastric cancer. The combination of 5-FU, Adriamycin, and mitomycin-C (FAM) and the combination of 5-FU and methyl CCNU have been associated with objective response rates in the range of 40% in prospective trials. It is still uncertain, however, whether overall survival has been significantly increased as a result of palliative chemotherapy for non-resectable disease.

The overall results of surgical resection for gastric cancer are disappointing enough to encourage aggressive clinical trials of adjuvant chemotherapy for all or selected groups of patients undergoing curative gastrectomy. Earlier results from one or two studies were encouraging, but no clear-cut survival benefit has been demonstrated from any of these adjuvant programs. Further adjuvant trials are clearly indicated.

Prognosis

The prognosis for patients with gastric cancer following either surgical or combined therapy remains poor because almost two thirds of these patients have either physical examination or operative findings that eliminate the possibility of surgical cure. No more than one third of patients who are considered candidates for curative resection live 5 years or more after surgical treatment as the only intervention.[19] This overall success rate of only 10% to 15% for all patients presenting with clinical carcinoma of the stomach is discouraging, particularly since no major improvement in end-results has occurred over the years. The majority of patients who develop regrowth of their cancers following surgical resection usually do so within 3 years of surgery and, in most series, about 90% of patients reaching the 5-year mark remain well indefinitely.

Short- and Long-Term Sequelae

Since the primary treatment of gastric cancer is surgical resection, the short-term sequelae of the surgery described include those complications that follow all major abdominal surgery. In addition, there is always the possibility of leakage from the anastomosis between the esophagus and the stomach or jejunum when the proximal or entire stomach is resected. There is less adequate healing of these structures than usually follows more distal gastroenteric anastomoses. Leak is relatively uncommon (less than 5%), however, and the long-term sequelae of gastrectomy are more significant than the short-term ones.

After recovery from gastrectomy, some patients have various postprandial symptoms associated with the surgical alterations of internal anatomy, the most frequently described symptom complex being the so-called dumping syndrome. This problem may follow either partial gastrectomy or total gastrectomy but is more frequently associated with the latter. The primary cause of such symptomatology is the loss of the pyloric mechanism that normally delays the transit of food stuff into the small intestine, but the usual physiologic explanation is the reaction of the small bowel to hyperosmolar feedings. There is great variability among patients in regard to the development of these symptoms, but it has proven wise to avoid hyperosmolar feedings soon after surgery until the patient has become established on a reasonable diet and has recovered completely from surgery. A diet that tends to reduce such symptoms is a six-feeding, high-protein, low-carbohydrate diet, although all patients do not require this level of attention. In addition, various types of substitute reservoirs constructed after total gastrectomy tend to reduce these symptoms.

Another latent problem following gastrectomy is the development of anemia. The most frequent early cause is partial or total decreased iron absorption secondary to the gastrectomy. Inadequate absorption of vitamin B_{12} due to the loss of intrinsic factor is a later mechanism for anemia following total gastrectomy. However, this does not prove to be a problem until 4 or more years after the procedure. Intrinsic hepatic stores of vitamin B_{12} are available, initially, and this is the reason for the delay in development of B_{12} deficiency and the accompanying neurologic sequelae.

Anti-cancer chemotherapy, when employed, is accompanied by the common side effects of these agents that are described. Radiation therapy causes nausea more frequently in treatment of gastric cancer than cancer of other anatomic sites probably because the liver is included in the radiation field.

Clinical Trials

Most of our information on the choice of surgical procedure for the potential cure or palliation of gastric cancer is based on retrospective review of results of these surgical interventions rather than from well-designed prospective clinical trials. There is an ongoing multinational trial to test the hypothesis advanced by several Japanese surgeons that a more extensive lymphatic dissection than is currently done will improve survival. The results of this trial will not be known for some time. A similar, but smaller, completed trial has shown that a more extensive dissection results in a higher complication rate, longer hospitalization, and no real improvement in survival.[23]

Clinical trial protocols have been employed primarily for the evaluation of the potential benefits of adjuvant chemotherapy following resection for gastric cancer or as therapy for patients who would not benefit from surgical resection. The current use of a number of combinations of agents for palliative care is based on a number of clinical trials showing a modest alteration in clinical course from these combinations, but limited survival benefit. All randomized phase III clinical trials of adjuvant chemotherapy after curative resection of gastric cancer have failed to demonstrate significant survival benefits thus far. This area of study requires further emphasis in the future, but promising leads are limited.

References

1. Correa P. A human model of gastric carcinogenesis (prospectives in cancer research). *Can Res.* 1988;48:3554-3560.

2. Parkin DM, Laara E, Muir CS. Estimates of the worldwide frequency of 16 major cancers in 1980. *Intl J Can.* 1988;41:184-197.

3. Chyou PH, Nomura AM, Hankin JH, Stemmermann GN. A case-cohort study of diet and stomach cancer. *Can Res.* 1990;50:7501-7504.

4. Risch HA, Jain M, Choi NW, et al. Dietary factors and the incidence of cancer of the stomach. *Am J Epidemiol.* 1985;12:947-959.

5. You WC, Blot WJ, Chang Y-S, et al. Allium vegetables and reduced risk of stomach cancer. *J Natl Can Inst.* 1989; 81:162-164.

6. Parsonnet J, Vandersteen D, Goats J, et al. *Helicobacter pylori* infection in intestinal and diffuse type gastric adenocarcinomas. *J Natl Can Inst.* 1991;83:640-643.

7. Talley NJ, Zinsmeister AW, DiMagno EP, et al. Gastric adenocarcinoma and *Helicobacter pylori* infection. *J Natl Can Inst.* 1991;83:1734-1738.

8. Siurula M, Varis K, Wilijasala M. Studies of patients with atrophic gastritis: a 10 to 15-year follow-up. *Scand J Gastroenterol.* 1966;1:40-48.

9. Caygill CPJ, Hill JR, Kirkham JS, et al. Mortality from gastric cancer following gastric surgery for peptic ulcer. *Lancet.* 1986;I:929-931.

10. Greene FL. Neoplastic changes in the stomach after gastrectomy. *Surg Gynecol Obstet.* 1990;171:477-480.

11. Tamasulo J. Gastric polyps. *Cancer.* 1971;27:1346-1355.

12. Haenszel WM, Kurihara M. Studies of Japanese immigrants. I: mortality from cancer and other diseases in the United States. *J Natl Can Inst.* 1968;40-43-68.

13. Meyers WC, Damiano RJ, Postlethwait RW, Rotlo F. Adenocarcinoma of the stomach (changing patterns over the last four decades). *Ann Surg.* 1987;205:1-8.

14. Hisamichi S. Screening for gastric cancer. *World J Surg.* 1989;13:31-37.

15. Lauren P. The two histologic main types of gastric carcinoma: diffuse and so-called intestinal type carcinoma: an attempt at a histochemical classification. *Acta Pathol Microbiol Scand.* 1965;64:31-49.

16. Orr R, Lininger JR, Lawrence W Jr. Gastric pseudolymphoma: a challenging clinical problem. *Ann Surg.* 1984; 100:185-194.

17. Appelman HD, Helwig EB. Sarcomas of the stomach. *Am J Clin Pathol.* 1977;67(1):2-10.

18. Beahrs OH, Henson DE, Hutter RVP, Kennedy BJ, eds. *American Joint Committee on Cancer Manual for Staging of Cancer.* 4th ed. Philadelphia, Pa: JB Lippincott Co; 1992.

19. Adashek K, Sanger J, Longmire WP Jr. Cancer of the stomach: a review of consecutive ten-year intervals. *Ann Surg.* 1979;189:6-10.

20. Bringaze WL, Chappuis CW, Cohn I, Correa P. Early gastric cancer (21-year experience). *Ann Surg.* 1986;204:103-107.

21. Itoh H, Oohata Y, Nakamura K, et al. Complete 10-year post-gastrectomy follow-up of early gastric cancer. *Am J Surg.* 1989;158:14-16.

22. Noguchi Y, Imada T, Matsumo A, et al. Radical surgery for gastric cancer (a review of the Japanese experience). *Cancer.* 1989;64:2053-2062.

23. Dent DM, Madden MV, Price SK. Randomized comparison of R1 and R2 gastrectomy for gastric carcinoma. *Brit J Surg.* 1988;75:110-112.

18

CANCER OF THE ESOPHAGUS

F. Henry Ellis, Jr, MD, PhD, Mark Huberman, MD, Paul Busse, MD, PhD

Carcinoma of the esophagus is a debilitating disease, the treatment of which is difficult and controversial. While not a common disorder in the United States, where there were about 11,000 new cases in 1994,[1] its prevalence has reached almost epidemic proportions in other areas of the world, particularly in China, Japan, the Caspian littoral of Iran, the Transkei district of South Africa, the departments of Brittany and Normandy in northern France, and some Moslem republics in what used to be the Union of Soviet Socialist Republics. While the prognosis for patients with carcinoma of the esophagus is poor—untreated patients surviving an average of only 4 months after diagnosis—it is better than it was in the past, due in part to the various forms of therapy available today. Patients with carcinoma of the esophagus are seeking medical attention earlier than previously, and this development, combined with a more aggressive approach by surgeons, has increased operability and resectability rates and lowered the hospital mortality rate so that there has been an improvement in overall postoperative survival statistics. Resection appears to offer the best palliation of dysphagia and, in addition, results in longer survival. Whether the use of a standard resection alone or the employment of more radical "en bloc" surgical procedures or the use of neoadjuvant therapy will make a significant impact on the long-term results of treatment remains to be seen. Thus far, evidence would suggest that early diagnosis may be the most important factor in achieving satisfactory long-term cure rates, and it would seem appropriate to emphasize close surveillance of patients at high risk for the development of malignant degeneration. Cost-effectiveness considerations make screening for early diagnosis impractical in the US, but screening has been successful in certain endemic areas in other parts of the world, particularly in Linxian County of the Henan Province of China.[2]

F. Henry Ellis, Jr, MD, PhD, Chief Emeritus, Division of Cardiothoracic Surgery, New England Deaconess Hospital, Clinical Professor of Surgery, Harvard Medical School, Boston, Massachusetts

Mark Huberman, MD, Co-Director of Deaconess/Dana Farber Oncology Unit, Assistant Professor of Medicine, Harvard Medical School, Boston, Massachusetts

Paul Busse, MD, PhD, Chief, Division of Radiation Oncology, New England Deaconess Hospital, Boston, Massachusetts

Demographics and Etiology

Carcinoma of the esophagus predominates in elderly men, the male-to-female ratio being approximately 3:1. It is more common in blacks than in whites.[3] While the disease usually develops in the seventh and eighth decades of life, young adults and octogenarians are not exempt.

Death rates among men vary widely in different parts of the world, ranging from 5.9 per 100,000 in the US, where the rate is considerably higher among black males than white males (15.4 versus 5.1), to 161 per 100,000 persons in endemic areas of China.[4]

Surprisingly, these marked geographic differences in prevalence have not helped to define the cause of disease. There are probably a variety of etiologic factors. Genetic factors do not appear to play a role except in individuals with the rare condition of keratosis palmaris et plantaris (tylosis), which is inherited as an autosomal dominant trait. Dietary factors may play a role because concentrations of nitrosamines and their precursors (nitrates and nitrites) are high in food and water samples from areas in China with a high incidence of esophageal carcinoma. In these regions, there is high consumption of moldy and fermented foods that are heavily contaminated by fungi, thus promoting the synthesis of nitrosamines. Nitrosamines and alcoholic beverages have been implicated in the frequency of this disease among the Bantu in South Africa. Alcohol and tobacco, which have been found to contain nitrosamine compounds, have been implicated in the occurrence of carcinoma of the esophagus in the northern coastal region of

France and in the US. Apparently, ethanol and nicotine act synergistically through an unknown mechanism to produce a higher rate of esophageal cancer than is associated with either drug alone. A low socioeconomic status and a deficient diet may be factors common to all high-incidence areas.

Although the precise role of carcinogens in the development of esophageal cancer remains conjectural, the occurrence of certain precancerous lesions has been recognized for some time. The incidence of carcinoma of the esophagus in patients with achalasia is said to be seven times greater than that in healthy individuals,[5] though this has been disputed. Cancer of the esophagus has been shown to occur with increasing frequency in patients with the Paterson-Kelly (Plummer-Vinson) syndrome. Its incidence in patients with caustic esophageal injury who are observed for ≥24 years, has been reported to be 1,000 times greater than in the normal population.[6] Of current interest is the association between adenocarcinoma of the esophagus and Barrett's esophagus, the prevalence varying from 8.6% to nearly 50% depending on the population studied. The risk of carcinoma developing in a patient with benign Barrett's mucosa is difficult to determine, since reported incidence rates have ranged from 1 per 81 to 1 per 441 patient-years of follow-up. The incidence of 1 per 99 patient-years of follow-up, reported by the Lahey Clinic, probably represents a reasonably accurate picture of this risk, as it is based on a substantial number of patients followed closely endoscopically.[7] It represents a risk of developing cancer of the esophagus that is 75 times greater than that in a similar demographic population.

Diagnosis

Clinical Detection

Dysphagia is by far the most frequent complaint of patients with esophageal carcinoma. It is usually apparent initially following ingestion of bulky foods, later with soft foods, and ultimately with liquids. Weight loss, regurgitation, and aspiration pneumonitis may also occur. In patients who do not experience dysphagia, the predominant symptoms are odynophagia (pain on swallowing) and gastroesophageal reflux. The latter symptoms are associated in some patients with minor degrees of blood loss. Massive blood loss is uncommon.

Symptoms and signs suggesting advanced stages of the disease include cervical adenopathy; chronic cough, suggesting tracheal involvement; choking after eating, suggesting a fistula with the tracheobronchial tree; massive hemoptysis or hematemesis or both, suggesting perforation of the lesion into adjacent vascular structures; and hoarseness, suggesting recurrent pharyngeal nerve paralysis. Pain is an unusual symptom and suggests local extension to adjacent structures.

Diagnostic Procedures

Esophageal roentgenography is an essential part of the workup of any patient complaining of difficulty in swallowing. The characteristic finding of an irregular ragged mucosal pattern with luminal narrowing is typical of carcinoma of the esophagus. Unlike benign obstructing lesions, carcinoma is usually not associated with proximal dilatation of the esophagus. Cinefluorography may also be useful in the diagnosis of problem cases. The exact role of computed tomography (CT) and magnetic resonance imaging (MRI) remains controversial, but they may be helpful tools in identifying invasion of tissues outside the confines of the esophagus. CT may be useful in preoperative staging, but has not proved a reliable indicator of nonresectability. Increasing experience with endoscopic esophageal ultrasound suggests that it may be a more valuable preoperative staging technique than other methods as well as a valuable prognostic indicator of survival.

Esophagoscopy is required to confirm the clinical suspicion of carcinoma. The use of fiberoptic instruments has simplified the performance of this study, which must include biopsy to provide histologic material for evaluation. Lesions involving the upper portion of the thoracic esophagus near the tracheal carina necessitate bronchoscopy in addition to esophagoscopy to determine the presence or absence of involvement of the trachea or bronchial tree. The use of supravital staining techniques with such agents as iodine (Lugol's solution), toluidine blue, or indigo carmine may help identify potential biopsy sites during esophagoscopy. The addition of brush biopsy may provide useful material for cytologic study in patients at risk for development of esophageal carcinoma. Another promising technique is the use of radioisotopes in tumor scanning. Materials preferentially absorbed by esophageal cancer cells, such as gallium 67 or cobalt 57, may be useful in early diagnosis.

Classification

Histopathology

Squamous cell carcinoma accounts for approximately two thirds of cases that arise from the surface epithelium of both cervical and intrathoracic esophagus (Table 18-1). Adenocarcinoma, the second most common form of malignancy encountered in the thoracic esophagus, is seen today more frequently than in the past. It usually arises from metaplasia of Barrett's mucosa and now accounts for one third of all cases of malignancy developing in the intrathoracic esophagus among surgically resected patients. Patients in whom "primary" adenocarcinoma of the esophagus is diagnosed may merely represent advanced stages of tumor arising from Barrett's mucosa, with complete replacement of the benign Barrett's mucosa by malignant degeneration. Carcinomas of the cardia, not considered in this chapter, account for almost half of the malignant lesions of the esophagus and the esophagogastric junction (Fig 18-1).[8]

Tumors similar in microscopic appearance to those arising in salivary glands account for most of the remaining glandular tumors of the esophagus. They are considered to arise from the ducts of the esophageal submucous glands. Occasionally, an adenocarcinoma may occur in which squamous differentiation is histologically evident and the term *adenosquamous carcinoma* is applied to them. Carcinosarcoma and pseudosarcoma are less common lesions, usually presenting as bulky intraluminal polypoid growths. Both are slow-growing tumors that warrant aggressive therapy.

Sarcomas represent <1% of all malignant esophageal tumors and include such histologic diagnoses as fibrosarcoma, leiomyosarcoma, and rhabdomyosarcoma. Of the rarer malignant tumors involving the esophagus, primary melanoma is the most common. Verrucous squamous cell carcinoma is also rare, with an indolent biologic behavior that makes it susceptible to cure. Small-cell carcinoma may arise in the esophagus and is considered to be a true apudoma arising from the argyrophil Kulchitsky's cells in the surface epithelium. These tumors are bulky and obstructive and usually occur in the lower esophagus. They are highly malignant lesions. No 5-year survivors have been reported.

Table 18-1. Histopathologic Classifications of Carcinoma of the Esophagus

Squamous cell carcinoma
Adenocarcinoma
Adenoid cystic carcinoma
Mucoepidermoid carcinoma
Adenosquamous carcinoma
Carcinosarcoma and pseudosarcoma
Miscellaneous
Sarcoma
Melanoma
Plasmacytoma
Verrucous carcinoma
Oat cell carcinoma

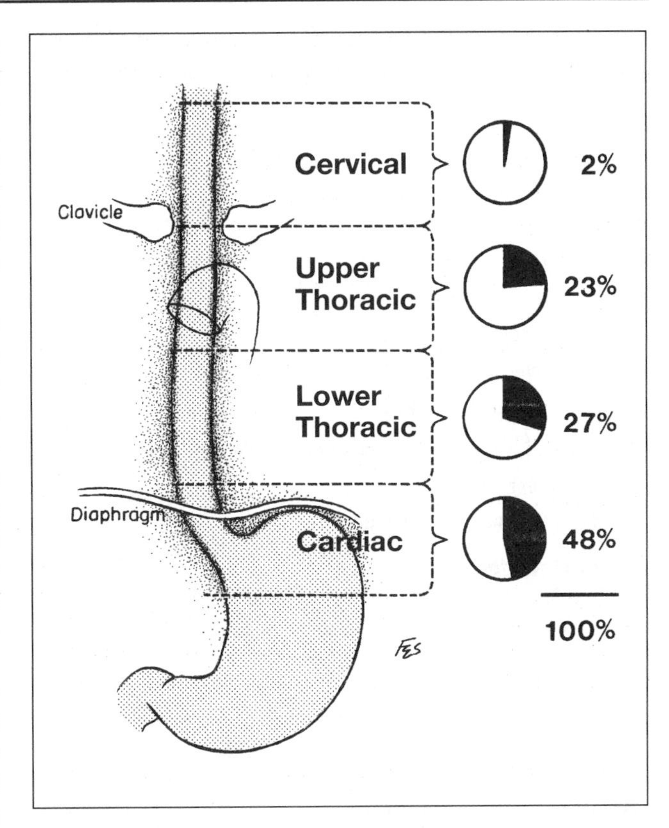

Fig 18-1. Location of surgically treated carcinomas of the esophagus and cardia. Adapted from Ellis.[8]

Staging

The staging of esophageal carcinoma is based on the revised criteria of TNM staging by the American Joint Committee for Cancer (AJCC), published in 1988.[9] This revision represents a joint effort with the Union Internationale Contre le Cancer (UICC) and was designed to provide simplified staging criteria applicable to clinical as well as pathologic staging, and to improve the ability of the staging criteria to provide meaningful prognostic stratification of cases in terms of long-term survival (Tables 18-2 and 18-3).

Treatment

Radiation Therapy

The use of radiation therapy as a single modality in the definitive treatment of esophageal cancer has met with little success despite efforts to increase the total dose to the tumor and reduce the amount of irradiated normal tissue. The median survival for patients treated with radiation is around 12 months, and long-term survivors are few.[10-13] The best results with radiation alone have come from a series reported by Pearson, in which a 5-year survival rate of 17% was achieved after 50 Gy, 2.5 Gy per fraction.[14] It should be noted that these results have not been representa-

Table 18-2. TNM Staging for Cancer of the Esophagus

Primary Tumor (T)

TX	Primary tumor cannot be assessed
T0	No evidence of primary tumor
Tis	Carcinoma in situ
T1	Tumor invades lamina propria or submucosa
T2	Tumor invades muscularis propria
T3	Tumor invades adventitia
T4	Tumor invades adjacent structures

Regional Lymph Nodes (N)

NX	Regional lymph nodes cannot be assessed
N0	No regional lymph node metastasis
N1	Regional lymph node metastasis

Distant Metastasis (M)

MX	Presence of distant metastasis cannot be assessed
M0	No distant metastasis
M1	Distant metastasis

From American Joint Committee on Cancer.[9]

tive of the universal experience. In fact, a review by Earlam and Cunha-Melo of more than 8,400 patients from 49 series concluded that the overall 1-, 2-, and 5-year survival rates were 18%, 8%, and 6%, respectively.[15] Despite these poor results overall, there appears to be a relationship between the T stage and survival. Patients with T1 and T2/T3 tumors had median survival rates of 20 and 8 months, respectively, following radiation alone.[16] In addition to T stage, the authors felt that tumor control may also be related to the total radiation dose up to 60 Gy, after which no further improvement was seen.

Frequently the role of radiation is palliative, particularly for patients who present with severe dysphagia in the setting of extensive regional or metastatic disease. The anticipated lifespan of such patients is short, but complete esophageal obstruction will result if some form of intervention is not undertaken. Radiation therapy will produce some form of improvement in more than 80% of these patients. As with survival, the probability of a favorable response is inversely related to the size of the primary tumor.

Since the radiation dose necessary to either radically treat or achieve palliation exceeds 40 Gy, most patients experience some degree of dysphagia during treatment which is usually self-limiting. Following doses of 60 ≥Gy, esophageal stenosis from benign fibrotic strictures can develop, necessitating dilation. Radiation pneumonitis is an infrequent but troublesome long-term complication that is directly related to the volume of lung irradiated. Recent advances in thoracic imaging and CT image-directed radiation treatment planning have allowed for a reduction in the volume of irradiated normal tissue, which should translate into a decreased incidence of chronic pulmonary and cardiac morbidity.

Table 18-3. Stage Grouping, Cancer of the Esophagus

Stage			
0	Tis	N0	M0
I	T1	N0	M0
IIA	T2	N0	M0
	T3	N0	M0
IIB	T1	N1	M0
	T2	N1	M0
III	T3	N1	M0
	T4	Any N	M0
IV	Any T	Any N	M1

From American Joint Committee on Cancer.[9]

Chemotherapy

The role of chemotherapy in the management of esophageal cancer is continually evolving. There are three situations in which chemotherapy is used: as palliative treatment of advanced esophageal cancer, in which it has, at best, limited benefit; preoperatively, either as sole treatment or in combination with radiation therapy, to reduce the size of the primary tumor and, by so doing, improve resectability rates as well as, it is hoped, to eliminate microscopic metastatic disease; and in conjunction with irradiation as primary therapy for esophageal carcinoma with or without surgery.

In essence, the role of chemotherapy remains investigational as there is no compelling evidence of a significant impact on survival, either in patients with metastatic disease or, when combined with one or two local modalities, in those with localized disease. However, there are data from a randomized trial comparing radiation therapy alone with a combination of chemotherapy plus concomitant radiation therapy that suggest survival benefit for the combined treatment program in localized esophageal cancer.[16]

A number of single agents have demonstrated activity in metastatic esophageal carcinoma, including bleomycin, cisplatin, 5-fluorouracil (5-FU), mitomycin C, doxorubicin (Adriamycin), and methotrexate.[17] In addition, the investigational agents vindesine and mitoquazone (MGBG) have modest activity. Response rates with single agents generally range from 10% to 40%. Combinations of two or more of these drugs have also been evaluated in patients with advanced disease, with response rates in similar ranges of 17% to 50% for studies in which more than

10 patients were treated. However, the impact on survival and symptomatic palliation is unimpressive. The median survival reported in some studies of patients with disseminated disease ranges from 4 to 8 months. Thus, there is currently no standard palliative chemotherapy for metastatic esophageal cancer and new drugs are desperately needed. It should be mentioned that the great majority of the reported chemotherapy experience in advanced esophageal cancer is limited to squamous cell carcinoma. However, in patients with adenocarcinoma, the response rate and drug efficacy are likely to be very similar to that seen in squamous cell carcinoma. This certainly seems to be the case when using preoperative chemotherapy for locoregional disease.

Complications of chemotherapy vary depending on specifics of the drug or drugs used (whether single or in combination), dose, and schedule. In the management of metastatic disease, it is difficult to prove that combination therapy is any better than single-agent therapy. In addition, given the limited efficacy of available agents in this setting, phase I and phase II trials of new drugs will often be the preferred approach in chemotherapy for metastatic disease. The toxicities of chemotherapy are generally well known and include nausea, vomiting, alopecia, stomatitis, diarrhea, and bone marrow suppression. Organ-specific toxicity, such as renal and cardiac dysfunction, depends on the chemotherapeutic agent used.

Surgery

Despite recent improvements, pessimism persists regarding the role of surgery in the management of patients with carcinoma of the esophagus. This negative attitude to the surgical management of the disease is unjustified in light of the marked reduced mortality and morbidity rates in recent years. Furthermore, an aggressive surgical approach provides excellent palliation of dysphagia, increased longevity compared with other forms of therapy, and a reasonable opportunity for cure, particularly in patients with early stages of the disease. Unfortunately, however, three quarters of the patients presenting for resection are already in stage III or stage IV.

While some have espoused a superradical (en bloc) resection for selected patients in the early stages of esophageal carcinoma,[18,19] this approach has not been widely adopted because evidence for its superiority

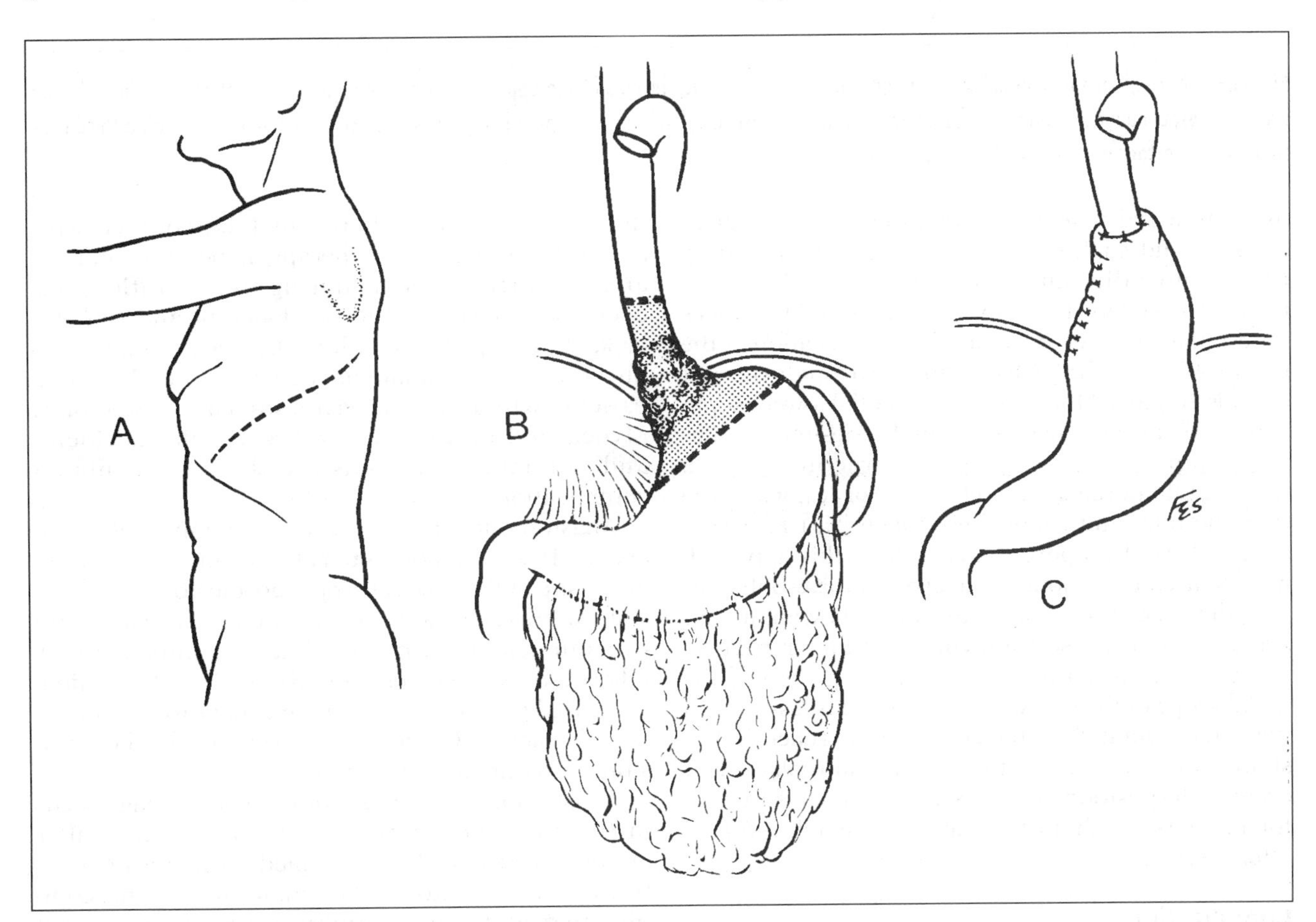

Fig 18-2. Technique of esophagogastrectomy and esophagogastrostomy for carcinoma of the cardia. A, site of incision; B, extent of resection (shaded area); C, completed esophagogastrostomy. Adapted from Ellis and Shahian.[20]

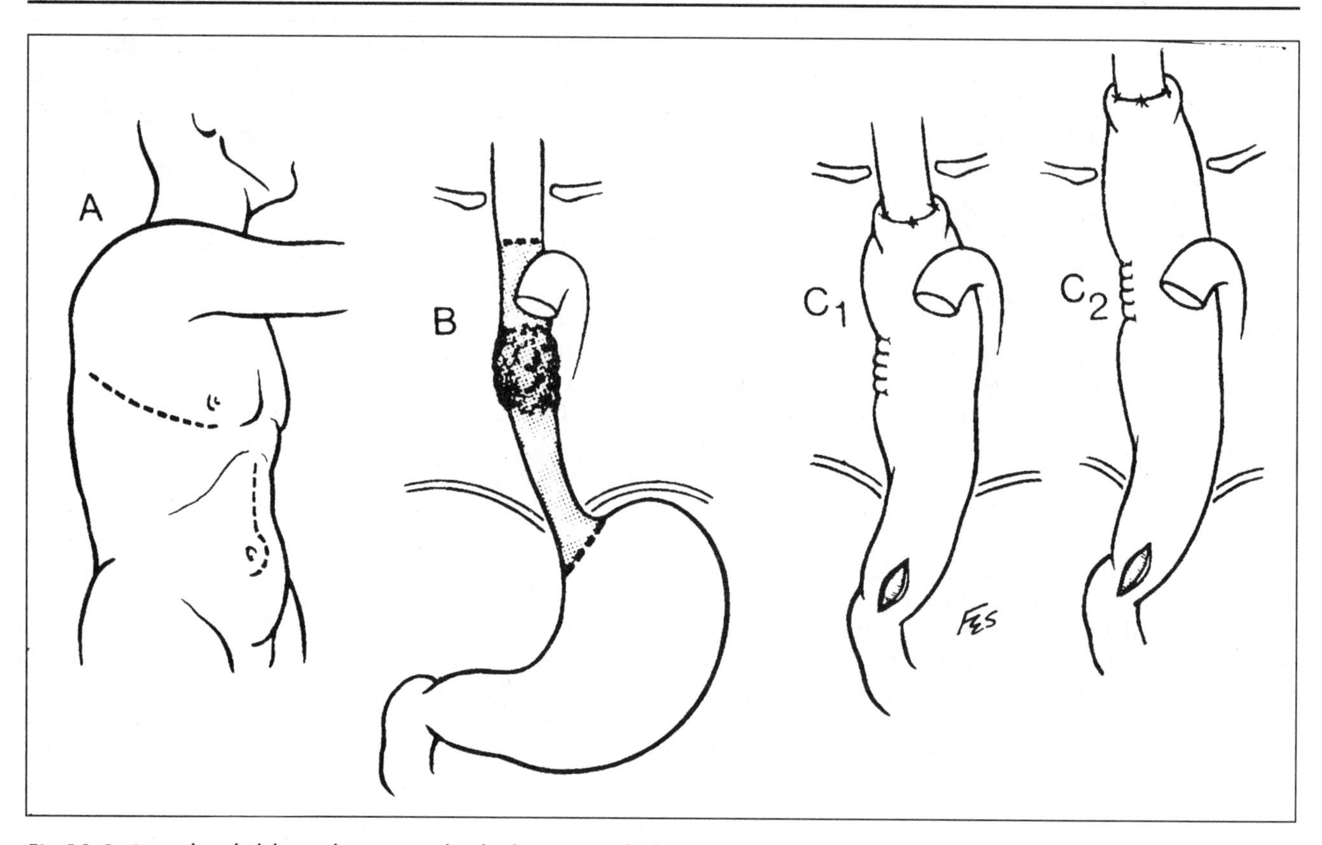

Fig 18-3. A, combined abdominal incision and right thoracotomy for lesions of the upper thoracic esophagus; B, extent of resection (shaded area); C_1, esophagogastrostomy can be performed in the chest; C_2, if submucosal spread is great, a cervical anastomosis through a third incision can be performed. Adapted from Ellis.[21]

over standard resectional techniques is as yet ill defined, and such procedures are accompanied by higher mortality and morbidity rates. Figs 18-2 through 18-4 depict examples of standard techniques for esophagogastrectomy based on the location of the lesion.[20,21] Esophagogastrectomy through the left chest is employed for most lesions in the lower esophagus and cardia, whereas for higher lesions a combined laparotomy and right thoracotomy, or a transhiatal approach, is preferred. For lesions at the thoracic inlet and cervical esophagus, a transhiatal approach is also appropriate. In fact, this approach may be used for lesions at all levels of the esophagus, including the cardia. Survival rates following its use are similar to those following standard resection through a thoracotomy incision, even though the nodal scope of the transhiatal approach is less radical than that obtained by the standard approach.[22] The stomach is preferred as the esophageal replacement organ, interposition being reserved by most surgeons for patients in whom inadequate stomach remains after resection.

Complications

Complications after esophagogastrectomy are much less common now than in the past. Patients are coming for treatment earlier. This fact, coupled with advances in respiratory therapy, hyperalimentation, and anesthetic support during the operation, has decreased markedly the incidence of anastomotic leaks and respiratory failure. Cardiovascular complications predominate as a cause of death among patients who fail to survive esophagogastrectomy. Myocardial infarction, cerebrovascular accident, and pulmonary embolus are the most common complications.

Anastomotic leakage is now uncommon. When it occurs, it is seen more often after colon interposition at the site of the cervical esophagocolostomy. Cervical leaks are usually well managed conservatively with hyperalimentation. Impaired gastric emptying may follow esophagogastrostomy. Mechanical obstruction, decreased gastric tone, pylorospasm, or torsion of the intrathoracic stomach may be responsible and occasionally requires reoperation.

Anastomotic strictures requiring bougienage occur in 10% to 15% of cases and are more common after an anastomotic leak or a stapled anastomosis. Gastroesophageal reflux is a common cause of this complication and can be minimized by conventional antireflux measures. Local recurrence of the cancer at the site of the anastomosis is fortunately uncommon

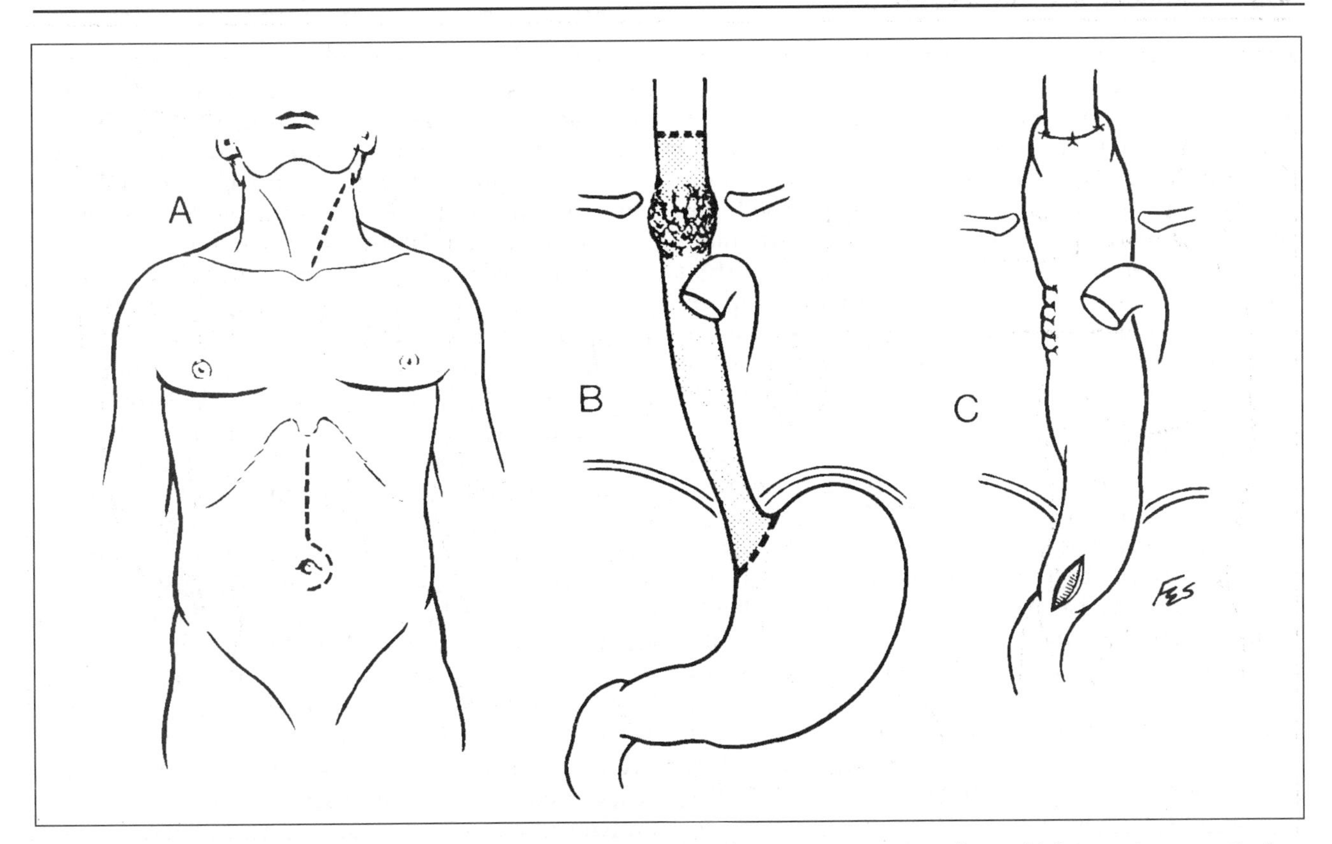

Fig 18-4. For esophagectomy without thoracotomy, the patient is in the supine position. A, upper midline and left cervical incisions (broken lines) are made; B, extent of resection (shaded area) is shown; C, completed anastomosis. Adapted from Ellis.[21]

if an adequate margin (>5 cm) of normal esophagus is included in the resected specimen.

Results

Although the percentage of patients living ≥5 years after surviving resection has changed very little over the past several decades, the overall survival rate of all patients with the disease, including those not operated on and those failing to survive resection, has quadrupled.[23] This is the result of an increase in operability and resectability rates and a marked reduction in hospital mortality rates.

A review of the recent literature on the results of esophagogastrectomy for cancer of the esophagus discloses a wide variation in reported hospital mortality and morbidity rates.[24] There are, however, increasing reports of hospital mortality rates under 5% for these operations. In the experience of one of the authors (FHE Jr), the 30-day mortality rate following 364 esophagogastrectomies for cancer of the esophagus or cardia, performed from January 1970 to July 1992, was 2.5%. Postoperative complications occurred in 25% of patients, with only half of these being considered major (that is, the patient's hospital stay was prolonged).

The 5-year survival rate also varies widely in the literature, averaging 20% to 25%. Akiyama's reported 5-year survival rate of 35% after 354 resections has not been matched by others except in patients with early-stage lesions.[25] The experience at the Lahey Clinic, based on patients operated on between January 1970 and January 1988, revealed an overall 5-year survival rate of 20.8%, with 23.3% of patients surviving 5 years after a curative resection, in which all visible and palpable tumor was removed.[23] Multivariate analysis of factors influencing survival showed that neither duration of symptoms, location of tumor, nor cell type was important. Only the stage of the lesion had prognostic significance, lending further credence to the concept that early diagnosis may be the ultimate key to long-term survival. Most importantly, slightly more than 80% of all patients followed received excellent palliation of dysphagia following resection.

Palliative Procedures

Intubation of the tumor, either perorally or by traction at the time of operation, can provide good palliation of dysphagia in patients with nonresectable tumors, but oral intake thereafter is usually restricted to a liquid or soft diet since patients are unable to tolerate a regular diet. Furthermore, the technique is not without complications, including perforation, hemorrhage, migration of the prosthesis, and even death.[26]

The use of neodymium:yttrium-aluminum-garnet (Nd:Yag) laser coagulation as palliative therapy for obstructing esophageal carcinoma is increasing in patients in whom resection cannot be performed. While both of these procedures give comparable results as far as relief of dysphagia is concerned, the need for retreatment was three times more common with laser therapy, which also is associated with a higher incidence of perforation.[27] Photodynamic therapy, in which patients are presensitized with a hematoporphyrin derivative before treatment with light delivered by an argon-pumped dye laser, has also proved to be an effective alternative to other forms of palliation.[28] Its ultimate role in the management of patients with nonresectable esophageal cancer remains to be determined.

Surgical bypass procedures have, for the most part, been superseded by these new techniques. Feeding jejunostomy or gastrostomy is usually mentioned only to be condemned. These procedures provide no palliation because the swallowing mechanism is not restored and they are not without risk. Occasionally, such procedures may be justified as a temporizing measure between the stages of reconstructive procedures such as colon interposition or as a means of maintaining adequate nutrition for patients undergoing chemotherapy or radiotherapy, either preoperatively or alone, in anticipation of normal alimentation.

Combined Therapy

Preoperative and Postoperative Radiation

The recognition that patients with carcinoma of the esophagus frequently harbor occult regional disease has led to the use of adjuvant therapy in the hope that a reduction in locoregional recurrence might lead to an improvement in overall survival. Data from a number of single institutions are available that retrospectively evaluate either preoperative or postoperative radiation therapy, occasionally with claims of an improvement in survival.[13,29-31] Although some of these studies were quite large, care must be taken in the interpretation of results because of potential sources of bias such as case selection and staging differences.

Two randomized trials have addressed the question of whether preoperative radiation, with doses of 33 and 40 Gy, could improve long-term survival in patients with resectable carcinoma of the esophagus. The first, reported by Launois and associates, randomized 124 patients to either 40 Gy followed by surgery or surgery alone. The resectability rates, incidences of postoperative mortality, and ultimately 5-year survival rates were not significantly different in either arm.[32] A larger trial by the European Organization for Research and Treatment of Cancer (EORTC),[33] with 208 patients, had essentially the same results—ie, no benefit from the use of preoperative radiation therapy. Thus, neither preoperative nor postoperative radiation therapy result in improved cure rates for patients with potentially resectable carcinoma of the esophagus, presumably because of the high incidence of distant regional and metastatic disease, which is unaffected by such therapy.

Preoperative Chemotherapy

The high response rates to chemotherapy noted by various investigators in the initial therapy for locally advanced head and neck cancer stimulated the evaluation of this combined approach in esophageal cancer, its purpose being to reduce the size of the primary tumor and thereby improve resectability as well as to eliminate microscopic metastatic disease. A number of reports in the past 10 years have described results of preoperative chemotherapy with platinum-based combinations of drugs followed by surgical resection in patients with localized esophageal cancer. Response rates to preoperative chemotherapy (generally based on follow-up endoscopy and barium swallow) have ranged from 14% to 76%.[34] Curative resections were accomplished in the majority of patients (35% to 79%). However, pathologic evidence of a complete response to the preoperative chemotherapy was low (0% to 9%), and median survival was in the 9- to 18-month range.

The two randomized trials to date that have compared preoperative platinum-based chemotherapy followed by surgery with a control group treated by surgery alone or preoperative radiation plus surgery have shown no survival benefit for preoperative chemotherapy.[35,36] Currently, there is an ongoing multi-institutional trial in the US of preoperative chemotherapy with cisplatin and 5-FU followed by surgery and then additional chemotherapy, compared with surgery alone. A similar study is under way in Great Britain. Thus far, there is no convincing evidence that preoperative chemotherapy improves the outcome compared with surgical resection alone in the management of esophageal carcinoma.

Preoperative Chemoradiation

The low pathologic complete response rate with preoperative chemotherapeutic regimens necessitates a more active modality if the cure rate of esophageal cancer is to be improved. Preoperative chemotherapy and radiation therapy has been, and continues to be, investigated for treatment of localized esophageal carcinoma. The preoperative chemotherapeutic regimen has generally been infusional 5-FU plus platinum or infusional 5-FU plus mitomycin, although there are variations in the drug combinations.[37-39] These programs have been associated with a higher pathologic complete response rate of about 25% in resected specimens. Median survival rates were in the 12- to 18-month range.

Investigators at the University of Michigan have reviewed their recent experience using concurrent chemotherapy and radiation followed by transhiatal esophagectomy for locoregional disease.[34,40] They reported a median survival of 29 months in 43 patients, including 22 patients with squamous cell carcinoma and 21 with adenocarcinoma. The median survival of patients with adenocarcinoma was better, 32 months as compared with 23 months for squamous cell carcinoma. However, there is no convincing evidence that preoperative chemoradiation is better than surgical resection alone, as randomized studies have not been reported. Thus, the proof of efficacy of this approach awaits results of phase III randomized studies comparing this trimodality approach to surgery alone. Such studies are under way in the US and Europe.

Chemoradiation Therapy Alone

Programs of concomitant chemotherapy and radiation, similar to those described above, have been used without surgery. Results from larger single-institution studies indicate median survival in the 18- to 22-month range.[41,42] However, the incidence of recurrent or persistent locoregional disease was substantial. A randomized phase III trial comparing radiation therapy alone with concomitant radiation plus chemotherapy with 5-FU plus cisplatin was discontinued early because of a significant survival advantage for the combined-modality group at both 12 and 24 months.[16] The 24-month survival rate was 10% for the radiation group and 38% for the combined-modality group. The median survival also favored the combined-modality therapy (8.9 versus 12.5 months). However, the median survival of patients receiving combined-modality therapy was only 12.5 months. In addition, 44% of initial recurrences in patients treated by combined therapy were within the radiation field.

Toxicity of Combined Therapy

The toxicity of simultaneous chemotherapy and radiation therapy is certainly more substantial and frequent than that seen with either modality alone. Thus, significant myelosuppression, including leukopenia and thrombocytopenia, with resulting episodes of febrile neutropenia and infection may occur in a substantial number of patients. Significant gastrointestinal side effects, including nausea and vomiting, oral stomatitis, and substantial esophagitis, are frequent problems. Nutritional support is important in many cases if the patient is not already receiving such care prior to therapy. The frequency and severity of esophagitis is greater than with radiation alone. Other more severe but infrequent esophageal problems include perforation, fistula formation, and fibrosis and stricture. In addition, depending on the specifics of radiation port and chemotherapeutic drugs, pulmonary and skin toxicity might be enhanced.

In summary, the role of chemotherapy whether used by itself as preoperative therapy, combined with radiation to be followed by surgery, or combined with radiation without surgery, is far from clear. The percentage of patients who are free of recurrence at 5 years remains small. Much of the information based on single-institution experiences holds the potential for strong patient selection bias. Further information from randomized studies comparing combined-modality therapy with local therapy alone is necessary. It is clear that chemotherapeutic programs used to date have not made a major impact on the treatment of carcinoma of the esophagus. Substantial improvement will come only when more effective systemic therapy is available to interdigitate with local therapy to control both locoregional and systemic disease.

Summary

Carcinoma of the esophagus, while not one of the more common malignancies in the US, remains a devastating disorder with a suboptimal cure rate regardless of the therapeutic modality employed. Surgery remains the mainstay of therapy and a standard esophagogastrectomy with use of the stomach as an esophageal substitute is preferred. Radical "en bloc" procedures have yet to be proved more effective in extending survival.

Standard esophagogastrectomy is now applicable to the majority of patients at low mortality and morbidity rates and provides excellent palliation of dysphagia. Five-year survival rates are acceptable, particularly for patients with stage I or stage II disease. Despite the fact that there has been little improvement in the 5-year survival of patients surviving resection, the overall survival rate of all patients with the disease, including those not operated on and those failing to survive resection, has quadrupled over the past several decades.

Patients with nonresectable disease can obtain palliation by a variety of invasive procedures, such as prosthetic intubation, brachytherapy, and laser and photodynamic therapy. Neoadjuvant therapy employing preoperative chemotherapy, radiation therapy, or both has not yet been shown to improve long-term survival, as compared with surgery alone, although a 25% to 33% pathologic complete response rate is usually observed in patients so treated with a prolongation of postoperative survival. This therapeutic approach warrants continued evaluation that should be confined to larger institutions capable of conducting appropriately designed neoadjuvant protocols.

Lack of evidence in support of the superiority of either ultra-radical operations or combined therapy, coupled with the excellent survival data following resection for early lesions (stages 0 and I), suggests that early diagnosis is the key to improved cure rates. This justifies close endoscopic surveillance of patients at risk for the development of esophageal carcinoma, particularly patients with benign Barrett's esophagus.

References

1. Boring CE, Squires TS, Tong T, Montgomery S. Cancer statistics 1994. *CA Cancer J Clin.* 1994;44:7-26.

2. Coordinating Group for Research on Esophageal Cancer, Linhsien County, Honan. Early diagnosis and surgical treatment of esophageal cancer under rural conditions. *Chin Med J (Engl).* 1976; 2:113-116.

3. Garfinkel L, Poindexter CE, Silverberg E. Cancer in black Americans. *CA Cancer J Clin.* 1980;30:39-44.

4. Qui S, Yang G. Precursor lesions of esophageal cancer in high-risk populations in Henan Province, China. *Cancer.* 1988;62:551-557.

5. Wychulis AR, Woolam GL, Andersen HA, Ellis FH Jr. Achalasia and carcinoma of the esophagus. *JAMA.* 1971; 215:1638-1641.

6. Kiviranta UK. Corrosion carcinoma of the esophagus: 381 cases of corrosion and 9 cases of corrosion carcinoma. *Acta Otolaryngol (Stockh).* 1952;42:89-95.

7. Williamson WA, Ellis FH Jr, Gibb SP, et al. Barrett's esophagus: prevalence and incidence of adenocarcinoma. *Arch Intern Med.* 1991;151:2212-2216.

8. Ellis FH Jr. Esophageal carcinoma. In: Glenn GJ, Cady B, eds. *General Surgical Oncology.* Philadelphia, Pa: WB Saunders Co; 1992:89.

9. Beahrs OH, Henson DE, Hutter RVP, Kennedy BJ, eds. *American Joint Committee on Cancer Manual for Staging of Cancer.* 4th ed. Philadelphia, Pa: JB Lippincott Co; 1992.

10. Beatty JD, DeBoer G, Rider WD. Carcinoma of the esophagus: pretreatment assessment, correlation of radiation treatment parameters with survival, and identification and management of radiation treatment failure. *Cancer.* 1979;43:2254-2267.

11. Newaishy GA, Read GA, Duncan W, Kerr GR. Results of radical radiotherapy of squamous cell carcinoma of the oesophagus. *Clin Radiol.* 1982;33:347-352.

12. Schuchmann GF, Heydorn WH, Hall RV, et al. Treatment of esophageal carcinoma: a retrospective review. *J Thorac Cardiovasc Surg.* 1980;79:67-73.

13. van Andel JG, Dees J, Dijkhuis CM, et al. Carcinoma of the esophagus: results of treatment. *Ann Surg.* 1979;190:684-689.

14. Pearson JG. The present status and future potential of radiotherapy in the management of esophageal cancer. *Cancer.* 1977;39:882-890.

15. Earlam R, Cunha-Melo JR. Oesophageal squamous cell carcinoma: II. A critical review of radiotherapy. *Br J Surg.* 1980;67:457-461.

16. Herskovic A, Martz K, Al-Sarraf M, et al. Combined chemotherapy and radiotherapy compared with radiotherapy alone in patients with cancer of the esophagus. *N Engl J Med.* 1992;326:1593-1598.

17. DeVita VT Jr, Hellman S, Rosenberg SA, eds. *Cancer: Principles and Practice of Oncology.* 3rd ed. Philadelphia, Pa: JB Lippincott Co; 1989.

18. Skinner DB. En bloc resection for neoplasms of the esophagus and cardia. *J Thorac Cardiovasc Surg.* 1983;85: 59-71.

19. DeMeester TR, Zaninotto G, Johansson K-E. Selective therapeutic approach to cancer of the lower esophagus and cardia. *J Thorac Cardiovasc Surg.* 1988;95:42-54.

20. Ellis FH Jr, Shahian DM. Tumors of the esophagus. In: Glenn WWL, Baue AE, Geha AS, Hammond GL, Laks H, eds. *Thoracic and Cardiovascular Surgery.* 4th ed. Norwalk, Conn: Appleton & Lange; 1983:560-576.

21. Ellis FH Jr. Esophagogastrectomy for carcinoma: technical considerations based on anatomic location of lesion. *Surg Clin North Am.* 1980;60:265-279.

22. Shahian DM, Neptune WB, Ellis FH Jr, Watkins E Jr. Transthoracic versus extrathoracic esophagectomy: mortality, morbidity, and long term survival. *Ann Thorac Surg.* 1986;41:237-246.

23. Ellis FH Jr. Treatment of carcinoma of the esophagus or cardia. *Mayo Clin Proc.* 1989;64:945-955.

24. Ellis FH Jr. Esophageal carcinoma. In: Glenn GJ, Cady B, eds. *General Surgical Oncology.* Philadelphia, Pa: WB Saunders Co; 1992:96.

25. Akiyama H, Tsurumaru M, Kawamura T, Ono Y. Principles of surgical treatment for carcinoma of the esophagus: analysis of lymph node involvement. *Ann Surg.* 1981; 194:438-446.

26. Cusumano A, Ruol A, Segalin A, et al. Push-through intubation: effective palliation in 409 patients with cancer of the esophagus and cardia. *Ann Thorac Surg.* 1992;53:1010-1014.

27. Low DE, Pagliero KM. Prospective randomized clinical trial comparing brachytherapy and laser photoablation for palliation of esophageal cancer. *J Thorac Cardiovasc Surg.* 1992;104:173-179.

28. Marcus SL, Dugan MH. Global status of clinical photodynamic therapy: the registration process for a new therapy. *Lasers Surg Med.* 1992;12:318-324.

29. Langer M, Choi NC, Orlow E, Grillo H, Wilkins EW Jr. Radiation therapy alone or in combination with surgery in the treatment of carcinoma of the esophagus. *Cancer.* 1986;58:1208-1213.

30. Drucker MH, Mansour KA, Hatcher CR Jr, Symbas PN. Esophageal carcinoma: an aggressive approach. *Ann Thorac Surg.* 1979;28:133-138.

31. Kasai M, Mori S, Watanabe T. Follow-up results after resection of thoracic esophageal carcinoma. *World J Surg.* 1978;2:543-551.

32. Launois B, Delarue D, Campion JP, Kerbaol M. Preoperative radiotherapy for carcinoma of the esophagus. *Surg Gynecol Obstet.* 1981;153:690-692.

33. Gignoux M, Roussel A, Paillot B, et al. The value of preoperative radiotherapy in esophageal cancer: results of a study of the EORTC. *World J Surg.* 1987;11:426-432.

34. Forastiere AA. Combined modality treatment of esophageal cancer. *J Infusional Chemotherap.* 1992;2:21-26.

35. Kelsen DP, Minsky B, Smith M, et al. Preoperative therapy for esophageal cancer: a randomized comparison of chemotherapy versus radiation therapy. *J Clin Oncol.* 1990;8:1352-1361.

36. Roth JA, Pass HI, Flanagan MM, Graeber GM, Rosenberg JC, Steinberg S. Randomized clinical trial of preoperative and postoperative adjuvant chemotherapy with cisplatin, vindesine, and bleomycin for carcinoma of the esophagus. *J Thorac Cardiovasc Surg.* 1988;96:242-248.

37. Steiger Z, Franklin R, Wilson RF, et al. Eradication and palliation of squamous cell carcinoma of the esophagus with chemotherapy, radiotherapy, and surgical therapy. *J Thorac Cardiovasc Surg.* 1981;82:713-719.

38. Leichman L, Steiger Z, Seydel HG, et al. Preoperative chemotherapy and radiation therapy for patients with cancer of the esophagus: a potentially curative approach. *J Clin Oncol.* 1984;2:75-79.

39. Poplin E, Fleming T, Leichman L, et al. Combined therapies for squamous-cell carcinoma of the esophagus, a Southwest Oncology Group Study (SWOG 8037). *J Clin Oncol.* 1987;5:622-628.

40. Forastiere AA, Orringer MB, Perez-Tamayo C, et al. Concurrent chemotherapy and radiation therapy followed by transhiatal esophagectomy for local-regional cancer of the esophagus. *J Clin Oncol.* 1990;8:119-127.

41. Coia LR, Engstrom PF, Paul AR, Stafford PM, Hanks GE. Long-term results of infusional 5-FU, mitomycin-C, and radiation as primary management of esophageal carcinoma. *Int J Radiat Oncol Biol Phys.* 1991;20:29-36.

42. Leichman L, Herskovic A, Leichman CG, et al. Nonoperative therapy for squamous-cell cancer of the esophagus. *J Clin Oncol.* 1987;5:365-370.

19

MALIGNANT MELANOMA

Marshall M. Urist, MD, Donald M. Miller, MD, PhD, William A. Maddox, MD

Melanomas develop by malignant transformation of the melanocyte, a cell of neural crest origin that produces melanin pigment. Historically, the first published instance of a patient with melanoma was by John Hunter (1728-1793) in 1787. The patient was a 35-year-old man with a secondary deposit in the neck. René Laennec, in an unpublished memoir presented to the Faculty of Medicine in 1806, first described melanoma as a disease entity.

This cancer arises most commonly in the skin but is found as a primary melanoma in the uveal tract (choroid, iris, ciliary body), upper aerodigestive tract, anal canal, rectum, and vagina. Melanoma accounts for 3% of all cancers in the United States and is increasing in incidence. The worldwide incidence is also on the rise, a development that cannot be explained by any major change in diagnostic criteria.

Among Americans it is estimated that 32,000 new cases of melanomas occurred in 1994, with about an additional 8,000 new cases of in situ melanoma.[1] Recent research has advanced our understanding of cutaneous melanoma and its biology, natural history, and treatment.[2] In the past, melanoma was notorious for a poor prognosis. The current 5-year survival rate of 84% represents a marked improvement over the 60% rate for the period 1960 to 1963.[3]

Epidemiology and Risk Factors

Although the etiology of melanoma is unknown, major risk factors have been identified.[4] Melanoma is extremely uncommon before puberty and increases in incidence with age. It occurs slightly more frequently in males and is uncommon in the black race. Immunosuppression is considered a risk factor. The risk of developing a second primary melanoma is 3% to 5%.

Epidemiologic studies suggest that sunlight (ultraviolet radiation) is the most common environmental factor in the pathogenesis of melanoma. The body of evidence in support of this hypothesis depends on intermittent exposure to sun, especially before the age of 20. The classic patient at risk is fair-skinned, redheaded, and freckled. He or she is easily prone to first- and second-degree sunburns and experiences little tanning of the skin.[5]

Dysplastic nevi are larger (usually >6 mm in greatest diameter) than common melanocytic nevi and have clinical features such as haphazard pigmentation with irregular borders (Fig 19-1—Color plate following page 372). The presence of these lesions portends increased incidence of melanoma, either in the dysplastic nevus or more commonly in skin without a dysplastic nevus.[6]

Congenital moles are pigmented nevi present at birth or soon after, also referred to as "Spitz" nevi. A detailed description of the clinical presentation, microscopic characteristics, and clinical course of 13 patients was published by Spitz.[7] Congenital nevi vary in size from <1 cm to large areas of the trunk referred to as "giant congenital nevi." The microscopic findings are of melanoma except for giant cells in the epidermis and dermis. Prior to puberty, congenital nevi are generally associated with a benign course; in adults, the same microscopic characteristics have a poorer prognosis.

Recognition—Biopsy

The increasing occurrence of melanoma has caused public concern for cutaneous nevi. Physicians, nurses, patients, family members, and others should be inquisitive of the nature of skin lesions. Classic melanoma

Marshall M. Urist, MD, Professor of Surgery, Director, Division of General Surgery and Chief, Section of Surgical Oncology, University of Alabama School of Medicine, Birmingham, Alabama

Donald M. Miller, MD, PhD, Professor and Director, Division of Hematology/Oncology, University of Alabama School of Medicine, Birmingham, Alabama

William A. Maddox, MD, Clinical Professor of Surgery, Division of General Surgery, Section of Surgical Oncology, University of Alabama School of Medicine, Birmingham, Alabama

arises in a pigmented lesion that is asymptomatic, with irregular borders, color variation or dark-black, and variable diameter. A change in color, size (especially rapid growth), and shape, with an extension of pigmentation outside the prior smooth margin of a mole, should prompt a suspicion of melanoma. A raised area within a previously flat mole with ulceration, bleeding, crusting, or pruritus should be considered a melanoma until proven otherwise.

Once a suspicious lesion for melanoma is identified, histologic proof is necessary. The biopsy may be excisional or core-punch but must adequately represent the full thickness and levels of invasion of the lesion. These histopathologic features are essential for staging and determining clinical management. Shave biopsies or electrodesiccation of a suspected melanoma is inappropriate.

Growth Patterns

There are four major growth patterns of melanoma: superficial spreading melanoma, nodular melanoma, lentigo maligna melanoma, and acral lentiginous melanoma (Fig 19-2—Color plate section following page 372). Each pattern has unique growth, histologic, and clinical features.

Superficial Spreading Melanoma

This tumor, which constitutes 70% of all melanomas, is characterized by a horizontal or radial extension along the dermo-epidermal junction. It is associated with a relatively better prognosis. The lesions arise in a flat nevus with slowly expanding radial growth or more rapid vertical growth. They are increasingly more common among young adults. They may have irregular leading edges due to lateral extension. The surface may be irregular with various colors ranging from black-to-brown or reddish-pink to white patches of regression.

Nodular Melanoma

Nodular melanomas make up 15% to 30% of melanoma cases, occurring more commonly among older men. They have vertical growth patterns, frequently without a recognizable antecedent mole. The color is often blue and black but may be amelanotic. They may be polypoid, and this thickness portends a poor prognosis.

Lentigo Maligna Melanomas

This melanoma (1% to 5% of cases) begins as a lentigo maligna (in situ melanoma), which appears as a slowly expanding black-to-tan lesion with >3-cm irregular borders. They are typically located on the face and neck of elderly, severely suntanned whites. About 5% of these melanomas are invasive, with vertical growth in a portion of the lesion that frequently becomes much darker and tends to ulcerate.[8]

Acral Lentiginous Melanoma

Acral lentiginous melanomas occur on the palms and soles or under nail beds. Although this growth pattern constitutes only 2% to 8% of melanomas in whites, it constitutes 35% to 60% of melanomas in dark-skinned patients, particularly blacks. Histologically, atypical melanocytes extend along the dermo-epidermal junction as a manifestation of the lentiginous radial growth phase. Initially the melanin can be seen through the epidermis as flat stains, and later a vertical growth phase may appear.

Subungual melanoma, considered to be a variant of acral lentiginous melanoma, occurs about equally among whites and blacks. This variant appears as brown or black discoloration under the nail bed, commonly in the great toe and thumb. The course is indolent, and with ulceration the lesion can be mistaken for a chronic paronychia. Subungual hematoma is the most important benign lesion to distinguish from subungual melanoma.[9]

Staging

Clinical staging of the primary tumor is extremely inaccurate. Biopsy and pathologic interpretation are necessary for proper staging.

Pathologic staging of the primary melanoma is based on a microscopic assessment of thickness[10] and level of invasion (Clark's levels I to V).[11] Therefore, evaluation of the entire tumor is advised rather than a wedge or a punch biopsy. Regional nodes should be evaluated by physical examination. Enlarged regional nodes should be noted for staging. If the primary melanoma is not available, it is coded TX. If no primary tumor is found, it is coded T0.

The staging system adapted by the American Joint Committee on Cancer is based on tumor microstaging of the primary melanoma and the known pattern of metastasis. This staging applies only to malignant melanoma of the skin (excluding eyelids).[12] The staging system is summarized in Table 19-1 and illustrated in Fig 19-3.

Evaluation for Metastasis

Although melanoma can metastasize to virtually any organ or tissue of the body, knowledge of the patterns of metastasis will help focus on the sites most likely to harbor spread. Regional nodal basins are the most common metastatic sites, followed by regional skin, subcutaneous tissue, and lung. Other common sites are the liver, brain, and bone. Although metastasis of cancer to small bowel is relatively uncommon, it occurs most frequently with melanoma, often resulting in obstruction, bleeding, or both. The surgeon usually restricts the metastatic workup in the absence of symptoms or signs suggestive of spread.

A practical metastatic survey should include the following:

1. A careful history and physical examination addressing all symptoms and signs, with biopsy of any suspicious subcutaneous or skin metastases or second primary melanomas;

2. Chest radiograph for metastases to the lung and computed tomographic (CT) scan of the chest, if needed, for evaluation;

3. Serum alkaline phosphatase and lactic dehydrogenase levels to evaluate possible hepatic spread (if levels are elevated and accompanied by symptoms of weight loss, anorexia, or abdominal pain, a liver ultrasound and/or CT scan may be helpful);

4. Brain CT or magnetic resonance imaging (MRI) scan to evaluate symptoms or signs of altered central nervous system (CNS) function; and

5. Nuclear bone scan to evaluate recent persistent localized bone pain, with or without elevated serum alkaline phosphatase levels.

Clinical follow-up after treatment of the primary melanoma is based on the same principles of response to clinical symptoms and physical findings at examination. Patients with early, Stage I, <0.75-mm thick melanoma are at low risk, warranting merely biannual examination. For melanomas of >0.75-mm thickness, the patient should be examined more frequently, every 3 to 4 months during the first 2 years, every 6 months in the third year, and once yearly throughout the patient's lifetime.

Prognostic Factors

The surgical management of melanoma is based on the knowledge of factors predicting the risk of local recurrence and metastatic disease and on the potential morbidity of a surgical procedure. Implicit in the staging system is consideration of multiple prognostic factors related to the cancer and stage of disease. Balch and colleagues performed univariant and multivariant analyses of clinical and pathologic factors in 8,500 patients grouped according to the stage of melanoma.[13]

Stages I and II Melanomas: 6,515 Patients

Prognostic factors included primary lesion site, median age, sex, tumor thickness (0 to 3.99 mm), level of invasion, ulceration (present or absent), and growth pattern. Total vertical height (tumor thickness) is the most important prognostic factor. Other prognostic variables generally derive their predictive ability from secondary correlation with tumor thickness. This study allowed derivation of a simple nonlinear mathematical model that describes the relationship between tumor thickness and 10-year mortality rate (Fig 19-4).

Stage III Melanoma: 1,698 Patients

Twelve prognostic features of melanoma were analyzed by multifactorial analysis in 1,698 patients with simultaneous or delayed nodal metastases. The number of positive nodes, primary melanoma site, and ulceration of the primary tumor were dominant variables.

Table 19-1. TNM Staging of Cutaneous Melanoma (Excluding Eyelid)

Stage		Criteria
I	pT1	Localized melanoma ≤0.75 mm in thickness and invading papillary dermis (Clark's level II)
	pT2	Localized melanoma >0.75 to 1.5 mm in thickness and/or invades to the papillary-reticular dermal interface (Clark's level III)
II	pT3a	Melanoma >1.5 mm but not more than 3 mm thickness (Clark's level IV)
	pT3b	Melanoma > 3 mm thickness but not more than 4 mm thickness (Clark's level IV)
	pT4a	Tumor >4.0 mm thickness and/or invades subcutaneous tissue (Clark's level V)
	pT4b	Satellite(s) within 2 cm of primary tumor
III	Any pT	(N1) Metastasis ≤3 cm in any regional lymph node(s) (N2a) Metastasis >3 cm in any regional lymph node(s) (N2b) In-transit metastases (>2 cm from primary) (N2c) Both (N2a and N2b)
IV	Any pT	(Any N) M1a Metastasis in skin, subcutaneous tissue, or lymph node beyond regional lymph node M1b Visceral metastasis

Adapted from Beahrs et al.[12]

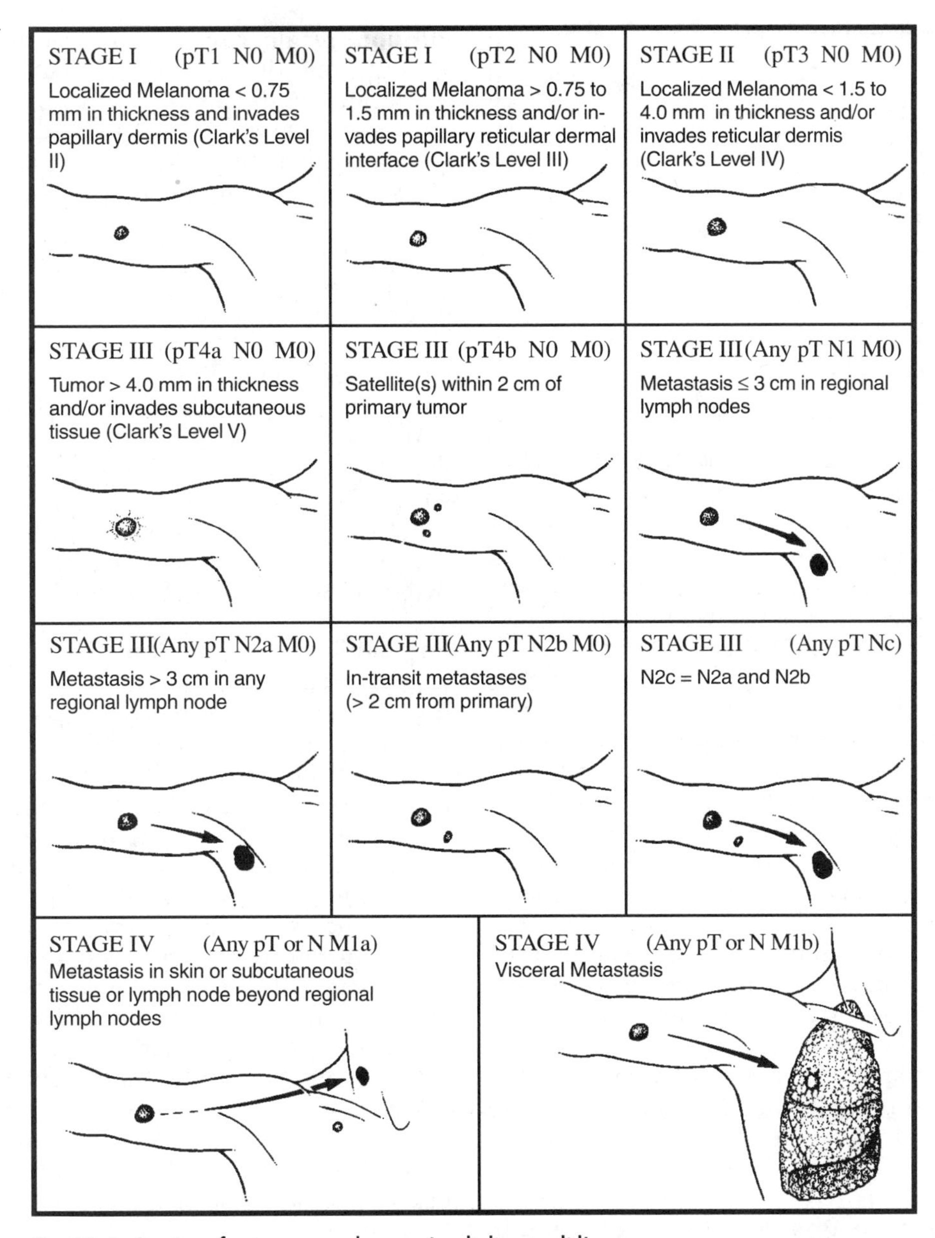

Fig 19-3. Staging of cutaneous melanoma (excluding eyelid).

Stage IV Melanoma: 200 Patients

The appearance of a metastasis at any distant site carries a very poor prognosis, especially in the case of visceral metastases. Clinical and pathologic factors in 200 patients with distant metastasis were analyzed. The median survival time for these patients was 6 months.

Principles of Treatment

For pathologic stages I and II melanoma, tumor thickness and/or level of invasion is the primary criterion for determining the surgical approach to the primary site and regional lymph nodes. For stage III patients with or without clinical evidence of metastasis to regional lymph nodes or subcutaneous tissues, a therapeutic nodal dissection along with resection of the primary site is recommended. Surgical resection of solitary visceral metastases to distant sites is usually indicated for local disease control and expectant palliation.

Resection of Primary (Stages I and II) Melanoma

The extent of surgical removal of the primary melanoma was excessive for many years and local recurrences were rare. The World Health Organization (WHO) Melanoma Group performed a prospective randomized study for stage I melanomas.[14] Invasive melanomas of 0- to 1-mm and 1- to 2-mm thickness were randomized to 1-cm margin removal (n = 305)

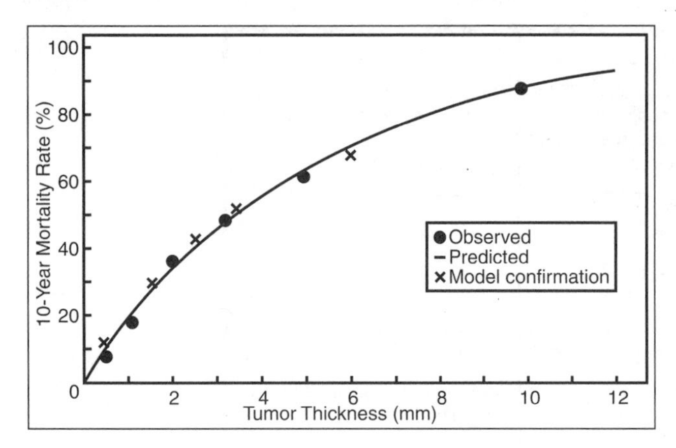

Fig 19-4. Observed and predicted 10-year mortality rates based on a mathematical model derived from tumor thickness.

or 3-cm margin removal (n = 307). Major prognostic criteria were well balanced. Subsequent development of metastatic disease in regional lymph nodes or distant sites was not different. Disease-free survival at 55 months was similar in the two groups. There were no local recurrences for patients with melanomas <1 mm thick. Three local recurrences appeared in patients with 1- to 2-mm thick lesions who received 1-cm margin resection and no local recurrences for 1- to 2-mm thick melanomas who received 3-cm margin excision. These results strongly suggest that 1-cm wide resection of stage I melanomas <1.0 mm thick is sufficient.

A North American study in progress randomized 1- to 4-mm thick melanoma for 2- or 4-cm margin resection. Preliminary results indicate no significant difference in local recurrence at 6 years. If thickness, as well as other factors predicting local recurrence, is considered, it appears that 1-cm margin excision for stage I melanoma (<1.5 mm thick) and 2-cm margin excision for melanoma 1.5 to 4 mm thick are adequate.[15]

Elective Lymph Node Dissection for Stages I and II Melanoma

The surgical management of the clinically negative regional nodal basin for primary melanoma is still controversial. Until the past decade, clinical decisions relative to management of the at-risk nodal basin were made in response to published retrospective reviews showing conflicting results. The development of histologic staging and identification of other predictive factors (see section on staging) related to the primary melanoma allowed retrospective reviews of archival pathologic material and comparison of retrospective surgical results based on previously unidentified risk factors.[2] These studies have progressively altered staging of melanoma. It is now evident that patients with melanomas <1 mm thick should not have elective lymph node dissection (ELND) because of the paucity of occult node metastases. In addition, primary melanomas >4 mm thick, even without clinically involved regional node metastasis, are at such high risk of distant metastasis that a regional node dissection is indicated only for possible expectant palliation. An intergroup clinical trial to test ELND for 1- to 4-mm thick melanomas versus delay of regional lymph node dissection until metastatic lymph nodes are evident has closed, but the length of follow-up is insufficient for analysis. Randomized trials by WHO[16] and the Mayo Clinic[17] did not show improved survival for patients with melanoma of extremities having ELND, compared with similar patients treated by wide excisions alone.

Morton and colleagues have developed a methodology (dye-directed selective lymphadenectomy) by which regional nodal status of patients at risk for occult lymph node metastasis can be further evaluated for ELND.[18] This may prove to be a useful method to select patients for ELND.

Surgical Resection for Stage III Melanoma

Stage III melanomas (>4-mm thickness, with or without clinically detectable regional spread) have a guarded prognosis due to the high probability of occult distant disease. Resection of the primary melanoma with in-continuity removal of subcutaneous tissue and fascia over muscle and the contiguous nodal basin is recommended when considered feasible, to decrease the risk of leaving (in-transit) satellite metastasis. Women with a small number of dermal in-transit metastasis and absence of regional nodal metastasis have a relatively better prognosis. Patients with enlarged regional lymph nodes have about an 85% chance of harboring distant metastases, and the survival rate at 10 years is <10%. Isolated limb perfusion with chemotherapy and hyperthermia is the most effective treatment for lesions on an extremity. Surgical resection of a limited number of indolent metastases may be helpful.

Surgical Resection for Stage IV Melanoma

Treatment goals for distant metastases are palliation, prolongation of life, or clinical staging to determine any subsequent treatment. The more common distant sites of metastasis for which resection should be considered are solitary pulmonary metastases, cerebral metastases, and gastrointestinal (stomach, colon, small bowel) metastases causing obstruction or bleeding. Approximately 60% of patients who die from melanoma have gastrointestinal metastases at autopsy.

Radiotherapy

While radiotherapy is seldom efficacious for eradication of melanoma, it often causes tumor shrinkage and may be useful as palliative therapy. Dosage schedules can be varied for patient convenience.

Chemotherapy

While the majority of patients with stage I melanoma can be cured with surgery, the results of chemotherapy for metastatic melanoma have been disappointing. The chemotherapeutic agent most widely used for the treatment of melanoma for the past 20 years is dacarbazine (DTIC). Although it is considered the best single agent, response rates are between 15% and 20% in most series.[19] These responses occur most commonly in soft tissue disease and have an average duration of 3 to 6 months. Complete remissions occur in <5% of patients. More recently, a number of combination drug regimens have been developed that appear to be somewhat more effective. The combination of DTIC, carmustine, cisplatin, and tamoxifen has been associated with an overall response rate of 50% in previously untreated patients, with a complete response rate of 15%.[20] The median survival of responders was 10.8 months. The most common site of failure was the CNS. Other workers have investigated the use of a three-drug regimen containing cisplatin, vinblastine, and DTIC for metastatic melanoma. This regimen has an overall response rate of 40%, with a complete response rate of 4%. The median duration of response is 9 months, with a median survival time of 12 months for responders.

A number of phase I studies are ongoing, including a trial documenting several partial responses to treatment of melanoma with taxol.[21] The use of adjuvant chemotherapy for malignant melanoma remains controversial. There are no proven treatment regimens that significantly reduce the likelihood of recurrent disease. A number of ongoing trials are investigating combinations of DTIC and biomodulators, such as interferon and interleukin-2 (IL-2).

Immunotherapy

The lack of effective chemotherapy for metastatic melanoma and the development of recombinant DNA technology have led to studies of a variety of immunologic and biologic agents. Recombinant α-interferon has produced response rates of 15% to 20% with an occasional long-term complete response.[22] Combinations of interferons with cytotoxic agents have caused only modest improvements in response rate. Clinical trials with IL-2 and adoptive immunotherapy have documented antitumor activity, although the overall response rate has been somewhat disappointing. While toxic effects of high-dose IL-2 are severe, significant response rates have been reported in many patients treated by bolus injection.

Adoptive immunotherapy is currently being tested through the use of lymphocytes isolated from tumor sites (tumor-infiltrating lymphocytes or TILS), which are further expanded by treatment with IL-2 or other biomodulators.[23,24] Substantial antitumor activity has been noted in animal trials, and phase I trials using this approach are ongoing.

Another area of investigation is the use of monoclonal antibodies targeted at antigens expressed on the surface of melanoma.[25] These antibodies can be either used to activate the host immune system or conjugated to a cytotoxic agent, with direct delivery of the agent to the tumor site. A number of partial responses have been reported with this approach, and the toxicity has been relatively mild. Studies are currently under way testing the utility of chimeric monoclonal antibodies genetically constructed with the mouse antigen-binding regions linked to the human immunoglobulin sequences, in order to eliminate the human antimouse immunogenic response.

Gene therapy for malignant melanoma is also being tested at the National Cancer Institute.[26,27] Tumor-infiltrating lymphocytes are transfected with tumor necrosis factor, with the goal of causing local cell lysis after "homing" of the TILS. This approach, while still at an early stage, has considerable theoretical promise as a means of targeted therapy.

Summary

Cutaneous melanoma accounts for 3% of all cancers and is increasing in incidence. Diagnosis is established by full-thickness biopsy of any suspicious mole that is changing in size or color or becomes ulcerated.

Dominant prognostic factors are tumor thickness, regional lymph node metastases, dermal or subcutaneous metastases, and distant metastases. Metastatic survey should include a careful history and physical examination, chest radiograph, and liver function tests. Additional tests are warranted only to clarify any findings suggestive of metastasis. Treatment is primarily surgical. For stage I melanomas (<0.75 mm thick), resection 1 cm wide of tumor margin is sufficient. For thicknesses of >0.75 to 1.5 mm, resection 1 to 2 cm skin wide of tumor is adequate. Elective lymph node dissection is not indicated. Stage II melanomas should have resection 2 cm skin wide of tumor; elective regional lymph node dissection is optional. For Stage III melanomas, resection of 2 to 3 cm of normal skin wide of the tumor site is performed. When regional lymph nodes are enlarged, in-continuity removal of subcutaneous tissue, fascia, and regional nodes is recommended. Stage IV melanomas require surgical excision of isolated accessible metastasis for palliation.

Response rates to combination chemotherapy have been encouraging; however, the median survival is still short. Immunotherapy is being studied with varied approaches and some encouraging results. Gene therapy may hold promise for future improvements in therapy.

References

1. Boring CC, Squires TS, Tong T, Montgomery S. Cancer statistics. *CA Cancer J Clin.* 1994;44:7-26.

2. Balch CM, Soong S-J, Milton GW, et al. A comparison of prognostic factors and surgical results in 1,786 patients with localized (stage I) melanoma treated in Alabama, USA, and New South Wales, Australia. *Ann Surg.* 1982;196:677-684.

3. Miller BA, Ries LAG, Hankey BF, et al. *SEER Cancer Statistics Review 1973-90.* Bethesda, Md: National Cancer Institute; 1993. Dept. of Health and Human Services publication NIH 93-2789.

4. Koh HK. Cutaneous melanoma. *N Engl J Med.* 1991; 325:171-182.

5. Elwood JM. Melanoma and sun exposure: contrasts between intermittent and chronic exposure. *World J Surg.* 1992;16:157-165.

6. Rigel DS, Rivers JK, Kopf AW, et al. Dysplastic nevi: markers for increased risk of melanoma. *Cancer.* 1989; 63:386-389.

7. Spitz S. Melanomas of childhood. *Am J Pathol.* 1948; 24:591-609.

8. McGovern VJ, Shaw HM, Milton GW, et al. Is malignant melanoma arising in a Hutchinson's melanotic freckle a separate entity? *Histopathology.* 1980;4:235-242.

9. Krementz ET, Reed RJ, Coleman WP III, Sutherland CM, Carter RD, Campbell M. Acral lentiginous melanoma: a clinicopathologic entity. *Ann Surg.* 1982;195:632-645.

10. Breslow A. Thickness, cross-sectional areas, and depth of invasion in the prognosis of cutaneous melanoma. *Ann Surg.* 1970;172:902-908.

11. Clark WH Jr, From L, Bernardino EA, Mihm MC. The histogenesis and biologic behavior of primary human malignant melanomas of the skin. *Cancer Res.* 1969;29:705-726.

12. Beahrs OH, Henson DE, Hutter RVP, Kennedy BJ, eds. *American Joint Committee on Cancer Manual for Staging of Cancer.* 4th ed. Philadelphia, Pa: JB Lippincott Co; 1992.

13. Balch CM, Soong S-J, Shaw HM, Urist MM, McCarthy WH. An analysis of prognostic factors in 8500 patients with cutaneous melanoma. In: Balch CM, Houghton AN, Milton GW, Sober AJ, Soong S-J, eds. *Cutaneous Melanoma.* 2nd ed. Philadelphia, Pa: JB Lippincott Company; 1992:165-187.

14. Veronesi U, Cascinelli N, Adamus J, et al. Thin stage I primary cutaneous malignant melanoma: comparison of excision with margins of 1 or 3 cm. *N Engl J Med.* 1988; 318:1159-1162.

15. Balch CM, et al. Efficacy of 2 cm surgical margins for intermediate thickness melanoma (1-4): results of a multi-institutional randomized surgical trial. *Ann Surg.* In press.

16. Veronesi U, Adamus J, Bandiera DC, et al. Delayed regional lymph node dissection in stage I melanoma of the skin of the lower extremities. *Cancer.* 1982;49:2420-2430.

17. Sim FH, Taylor WF, Pritchard DJ, Soule EH. Lymphadenectomy in the management of stage I malignant melanoma: a prospective randomized study. *Mayo Clin Proc.* 1986;61:697-705.

18. Morton DL, Wen D-R, Wong JH, et al. Technical details of intraoperative lymphatic mapping for early stage melanoma. *Arch Surg.* 1992;127:392-399.

19. McClay EF, Mastrangelo MJ. Systemic chemotherapy for metastatic melanoma. *Semin Oncol.* 1988;15:569-577.

20. McClay EF, Mastrangelo MJ, Berd D, Bellet RE. Effective combination chemo/hormonal therapy for malignant melanoma: experience with three consecutive trials. *Int J Cancer.* 1992;50:553-556.

21. Legha SS, Ring S, Papadopoulos N, Raber M, Benjamin RS. A phase II trial of taxol in metastatic melanoma. *Cancer.* 1990;65:2478-2481.

22. Kirkwood JM. Studies of interferons in the therapy of melanoma. *Semin Oncol.* 1991;18(suppl 7):83-90.

23. Whiteside TL. Cancer therapy with tumor-infiltrating lymphocytes: evaluation of potential and limitations. *In Vivo.* 1991;5:553-559.

24. Hayakawa K, Salmeron MA, Parkinson DR, et al. Study of tumor-infiltrating lymphocytes for adoptive therapy of renal cell carcinoma (RCC) and metastatic melanoma: sequential proliferation of cytotoxic natural killer and non-cytotoxic T cells in RCC. *J Immunother.* 1991;10:313-325.

25. Mittelman A, Chen ZJ, Kageshita T, et al. Active specific immunotherapy in patients with melanoma: a clinical trial with mouse antiidiotypic monoclonal antibodies elicited with syngeneic anti-high-molecular-weight/melanoma-associated antigen monoclonal antibodies. *J Clin Invest.* 1990;86:2136-2144.

26. Rosenberg SA, Aebersold P, Cornetta K, et al. Gene transfer into humans: immunotherapy of patients with advanced melanoma, using tumor-infiltrating lymphocytes modified by retroviral gene transduction. *N Engl J Med.* 1990;323:570-578.

27. Cournoyer D, Caskey CT. Gene transfer into humans: a first step. *N Engl J Med.* 1990;323:601-603.

20

UROLOGIC AND MALE GENITAL CANCERS

Vahan S. Kassabian, MD, FRCS, Sam D. Graham, Jr, MD

Perspective

Cancers that occur in the urinary system, including the male genital tract, are among the most common malignancies in men. They account for approximately one third of all new cancers, if the common nonmelanoma skin cancer is excluded. Surgery is the mainstay of treatment, but radiation therapy, chemotherapy, hormone therapy, and immunotherapy play important roles in the management of many of these tumors.

During the past decade, therapy for testicular cancer is easily the "success story" in urology. Because of intense chemotherapeutic agents and improved surgical techniques, most testicular cancers can now be cured with little morbidity. Nevertheless, some refinements are merited, for example, to decrease the toxicity associated with chemotherapy.

Advances in the management of Wilms' tumor are more impressive and remain an excellent example of how surgery, radiation therapy, and chemotherapy can be combined to maximum benefit.

The treatment of metastatic renal cell carcinoma is still not very successful. Most patients will still succumb to their disease, although immunotherapy seems to prolong survival.

With the advent of prostate-specific antigen and transrectal ultrasound of the prostate, prostatic cancer is being diagnosed more frequently and at an earlier stage. It is hoped this will translate to a better cure rate, but results will not be available for some time. Although prostatic cancer has surpassed all other tumors as the most frequent in men, and as the second most common killer among neoplasms, some patients may be overtreated who otherwise will die of other causes. With the increasing life expectancy of Americans, prostatic cancer will be an even more frequent finding, but the controversy regarding early detection and the best treatment for localized prostatic cancer must be resolved.

Bladder cancer management has become more refined, especially for superficial tumors, but metastasis is still associated with a poor prognosis. New surgical techniques have enabled patients with localized cancer who undergo cystectomy to improve their quality of life with the formation of either continent urinary reservoirs or orthotopic bladder substitutes.

The future is promising in terms of greater knowledge of genetic and molecular biology so that we can better understand carcinogenesis and the potential prospects for manipulation to alter the natural history of different cancers.

Adult Kidney Tumors

Epidemiology

Approximately 11,300 died in 1994 from kidney cancer. An estimated 27,600 new cases were diagnosed, representing 2% of all new cancers. The average age at the time of diagnosis ranges from 55 to 60 years. Renal cell carcinoma occurs in >95% of solid renal tumors, affecting men about twice as often as women.

Etiology

The etiology of renal cell carcinoma is obscure. Renal cell carcinoma is known to arise from the proximal convoluted tubule, and abnormalities on the short arm of chromosome 3 have been implicated in the sporadic and familial types of renal cell carcinoma as well as abnormalities of the common p53 gene which are also found in other cancers.[2,3]

No specific agent has been definitively identified as a cause of renal carcinoma, but epidemiologic studies have incriminated tobacco.[1] Familial renal cell carcinoma has been reported. Patients with von Hippel-Lindau disease have a higher incidence of renal cell

Vahan S. Kassabian, MD, FRCS, Assistant Professor, Department of Urology, The Emory Clinic, Atlanta, Georgia

Sam D. Graham, Jr, MD, Chief of Urology, The Emory Clinic, Atlanta, Georgia

carcinoma[4] as do patients with acquired cystic disease who undergo dialysis as a result of renal failure.

Detection and Diagnosis

Clinical Diagnosis

Early-stage renal cell carcinoma is usually "silent," with symptoms denoting more advanced disease. The typical triad of hematuria, palpable flank mass, and flank pain is associated with an advanced tumor. Polycythemia and fever occasionally occur. Renal cell carcinoma is also known to secrete certain hormones, including parathyroid hormone and erythropoietin, causing hypercalcemia and erythrocytosis, respectively. Stauffer's syndrome is a reversible hepatorenal condition with abnormal results on liver function studies in the absence of hepatic metastasis. Stauffer's syndrome is not necessarily associated with a poor prognosis, unless it persists after resection of all known tumor.

Approximately 30% of patients present with metastases at the time of diagnosis. The most common are lung and bone metastases and lymphadenopathy.

The increased use and improvements in the quality of ultrasound, abdominal CT, and other imaging modalities have significantly increased the early detection of clinically asymptomatic and unsuspected cases.

Diagnostic Procedures

Ultrasound can help differentiate cystic from solid lesions. CT scans are useful in both the diagnosis and staging of renal cell carcinoma. The density, size of tumor, extent of local invasion, vena cava or renal vein involvement, and metastasis to lymph nodes, liver, or lung all can be seen on abdominal CT. Magnetic resonance imaging (MRI) is significantly superior only for the visualization of thrombus in the renal vein or vena cava. In most cases, it can replace vena cava angiography. With gadolinium injection, MRI can also be as useful as CT with contrast to delineate tumors.

Needle aspiration of vascular cystic masses in which the diagnosis is uncertain, including cytologic examination of the fluid, may be a useful adjunct but is rarely needed. Selective renal arteriography is unnecessary, unless renal-sparing procedures are anticipated. Excretory urography and nephrotomography are not needed in the workup; if ordered for other reasons such as hematuria, they might reveal evidence of a space-occupying mass with pelvocalyceal displacement and alteration of the renal contour.

Classification

Anatomic Staging

The primary tumor, nodal involvement, and distal metastasis (TNM) system favored by the American Joint Committee on Cancer (AJCC)[5] and the International Union Against Cancer (UICC)[6] is gradually being adopted, but it may be simplified if the T stages and alphabetic designations are matched.

Tumor stage grouping (Table 20-1) is as follows: T1, tumor confined to the kidney and capsule; T2, tumor >2.5 cm, limited to the kidney; T3, tumor extending into major veins or exhibiting perinephric invasion; and T4, tumor invading beyond Gerota's fascia.

Histopathology

More than 95% of parenchymal tumors are adenocarcinomas and are referred to as hypernephroma, renal cell carcinoma, clear cell cancer, or Grawitz's tumor. These tumors locally infiltrate the capsule; are highly angioinvasive, spreading to the renal vein and vena cava; and result in widespread hematogenous and lymphatic metastases, especially to the lung, liver, nodes, and bone. The tumor biology differs from most tumors in terms of metastasis to unusual sites, such as the testes and skin. Spontaneous regression and delayed metastases have been reported, but are rare.

Clinical Staging

Recommended Procedures

The following is the recommended sequence for clinical staging:

1. Ultrasound.
2. Abdominal CT scan, with and without intravenous contrast.
3. Radiologic metastatic survey, including chest x-ray (bone scan is usually unnecessary unless alkaline phosphatase values are elevated).
4. Laboratory tests, including complete blood count (CBC) and sequential multiple analysis (SMA-12), particularly liver chemistry tests.

Optional Procedures

Excretory urography is unnecessary unless ordered for other reasons such as hematuria or to delineate contralateral kidney function. Nuclear renal scans are important if renal insufficiency and the threat of dialysis exists following nephrectomy. MRI is useful in the presence of thrombus in the vena cava. Lymphangiography is unreliable for high para-aortic and paracaval nodes.

Principles of Treatment

Surgery

Radical nephrectomy, in which the kidney, perinephric fat, Gerota's capsule, and regional nodes are removed, is preferred for all resectable lesions in stages A to C.[7] In advanced cases of renal cell carcinoma, palliative nephrectomy is indicated for intractable bleeding and pain control. Occasional cures are reported with nephrectomy and resection of a solitary metastasis, especially in soft tissue such as

Table 20-1. TNM Staging for Kidney Cancer

Primary Tumor (T)

TX	Primary tumor cannot be assessed
T0	No evidence of primary tumor
T1	Tumor 2.5 cm or less in greatest dimension limited to the kidney
T2	Tumor more than 2.5 cm in greatest dimension limited to the kidney
T3	Tumor extends into major veins or invades adrenal gland or perinephric tissues but not beyond Gerota's fascia
T3a	Tumor invades adrenal gland or perinephric tissues but not beyond Gerota's fascia
T3b	Tumor grossly extends into the renal vein(s) or vena cava below the diaphragm
T3c	Tumor grossly extends into the vena cava above the diaphragm
T4	Tumor invades beyond Gerota's fascia

Regional Lymph Nodes (N)

The regional lymph nodes are the abdominal para-aortic, paracaval, and renal hilar. Laterality does not affect the N classification. The significance of the regional lymph node metastasis in staging kidney cancer lies in the number and size and not in whether unilateral or contralateral.

NX	Regional lymph nodes cannot be assessed
N0	No regional lymph node metastasis
N1	Metastasis in a single lymph node, 2 cm or less in greatest dimension
N2	Metastasis in a single lymph node, more than 2 cm but not more than 5 cm in greatest dimension or multiple lymph nodes, none more than 5 cm in greatest dimension
N3	Metastasis in a lymph node more than 5 cm in greatest dimension

Note: Laterality does not affect the N classification.

Distant Metastasis (M)

MX	Presence of distant metastasis cannot be assessed
M0	No distant metastasis
M1	Distant metastasis

Table 20-1 *Continued.* TNM Staging for Kidney Cancer

Stage Grouping

Stage I	T1	N0	M0
Stage II	T2	N0	M0
Stage III	T1	N1	M0
	T2	N1	M0
	T3a	N0	M0
	T3a	N1	M0
	T3b	N0	M0
	T3b	N1	M0
	T3c	N0	M0
	T3c	N1	M0
Stage IV	T4	Any N	M0
	Any T	N2	M0
	Any T	N3	M0
	Any T	Any N	M1

From American Joint Committee on Cancer.[5]

lung. The presence of tumor in the renal vein or vena cava, or both, does not preclude surgical resection for cure. For bilateral tumors, which occur in approximately 1% of cases, treatment consists of nephrectomy (larger lesion) and partial nephrectomy (smaller lesion), or bilateral partial nephrectomy, if feasible. Bench surgery may be required for these procedures, involving surgical excision of the involved kidney and removing the tumor followed by autotransplantation of the residual kidney. Occasionally, bilateral nephrectomies are indicated. The patient is then placed on chronic hemodialysis or peritoneal dialysis. While some centers have reported good results with renal transplantation in these patients, other centers have stopped performing renal transplantation in patients with a history of renal cell carcinoma.

Radiotherapy

Radiotherapy is of little use in treating the kidney, and although renal cell carcinoma is somewhat radiosensitive, the limiting dose to the remaining normal kidney is 20 Gy before nephritis ensues; bowel complications are also possible with higher dosages. Postoperative radiation therapy has not been very effective in the past for residual or recurrent carcinoma.[8]

Chemotherapy

Single-agent and combination chemotherapy has been evaluated to a limited degree, and response rates have been low. Vinblastine is the most extensively studied, but it appears that no single agent or combination regimen is associated with a response >10%.[9]

Hormonal Therapy

The basis for hormone treatment of advanced renal cell carcinoma was a demonstration of efficacy against an estrogen-induced clear cell tumor in the adult Syrian hamster.[10] Hence, progesterone has been used in metastatic renal cell carcinoma, and although it continues to be used in the absence of more effective agents, no proper study has proved the efficacy of these agents in the management of advanced renal carcinoma.

Immunotherapy

Immunotherapy is a novel approach to the treatment of metastatic renal cell carcinoma; the most effective combination therapy and dosage adjustments to increase efficacy and decrease toxicity are still being researched. Immunotherapy can be classified into active and passive categories. Active immunotherapy refers to immunization of the tumor-bearing host with substances that attempt to induce in the host a state of immune response to the tumor. Passive, or adoptive, immunotherapy involves the transfer to the tumor-bearing host of active immunologic reagents, such as cells with antitumor activity. Initially, nonspecific immune stimulators, such as BCG (bacillus Calmette-Guérin), *Corynebacterium parvum,* and levamisole, were used. Xenogeneic immune ribonucleic acid (RNA) was also used initially without much long-term promise. Coumarin and cimetidine were initially promising but proved not to be very efficacious.

In the past decade, recombinant DNA techniques have enabled the production of large quantities of purified lymphokines (cytokines), which are biologic substances involved in the regulation of the immune system. The first of these lymphokines was interferon. Although interferons have unquestionable activity against renal cell carcinoma, most responders are patients with limited metastases to the lung.[11] Interleukin-2 (IL-2) is an important discovery in the field of immunotherapy. Initial reports from the National Cancer Institute were very promising,[12] showing a 33% total response rate with IL-2, while others reported only a 16% objective response.[13] Side effects of IL-2 therapy have been well documented, and include chills, fever, malaise, nausea, vomiting, and diarrhea, with the most serious being renal and cardiopulmonary failure. IL-2 has been used in combination with interferon to improve the response rate and possibly lower the toxicity; a study at UCLA reported an objective response rate of 30% using the combination.[14] IL-2 has also been used in combination with tumor-infiltrating lymphocytes (TIL). TIL are grown selectively from single-cell tumor suspensions cultured in IL-2 to achieve greater specificity

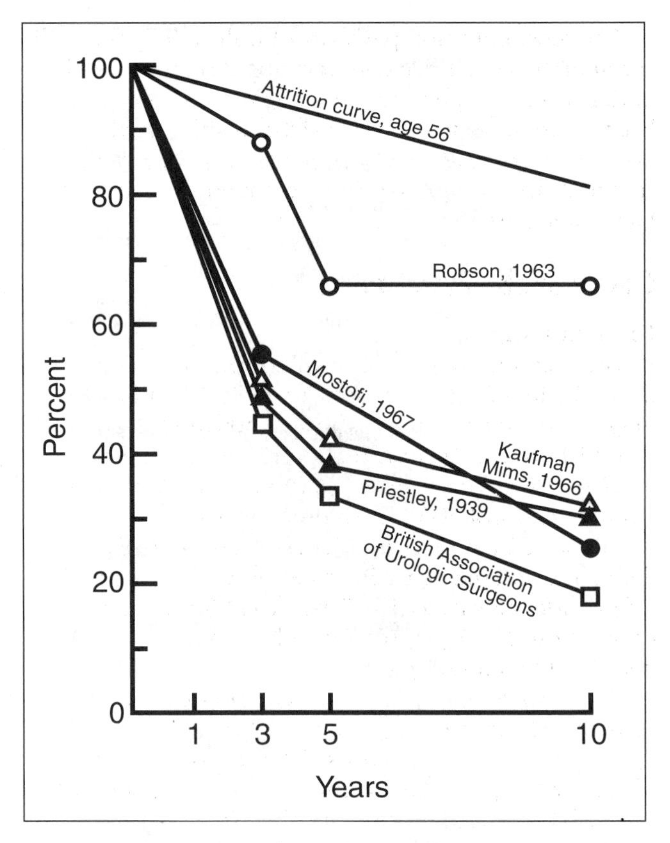

Fig 20-1. Crude survival curves of several large series of renal carcinomas, treated surgically and followed up for 10 years. From Kaufman JJ, Mims M. In: Ravitch MM, Elleson EH, Julian OC, et al, eds. *Current Problems in Surgery.* Chicago, Ill: Year Book Medical Publishers; 1966.

and potent antitumor effects. This approach, at least initially, has not proven more effective than other IL-2-based therapy.

In general, response rates with most immunotherapy protocols average approximately 20% and survival can be improved by several months, especially in patients with good performance status.

Results and Prognosis

Five-year survival rates for stage I renal cell carcinoma treated with nephrectomy are 60% to 80%. For stage II, survival is approximately 50% to 80%; for stage III, 5-year rates are approximately 50% to 60% for renal vein involvement only, 3% to 50% for vena caval involvement only, and 15% to 35% for regional lymph node involvement. For stage IV, survival at 5 years is close to 0%. The best results were reported by Robson (Fig 20-1)[15] and are attributed to radical nephrectomy, including the removal of the ipsilateral adrenal gland, lymph node dissection, and primary ligation of the renal pedicle before tumor manipulation and, of course, removal of Gerota's fascia. Survival improves with earlier diagnosis of incidental carcinomas.

The most common pathway of failure for renal cell carcinoma is widespread metastatic disease, via either nodal spread or hematogenous spread to bone, lung, liver, brain, and virtually any visceral site. Local recurrence is uncommon, unless the tumor is incompletely resected, tumor spillage has occurred, or the tumor has penetrated the renal capsule.

Cancer of the Prostate

Epidemiology

Prostate carcinoma is the most common male cancer in the United States, accounting for 32% of all newly diagnosed cancers, and is the second leading cause of death by cancer, accounting for 13% of cancer deaths in men. With the aging population in the US, the frequency will probably continue to grow.

The median age at incidence is 70, with the incidence rate increasing with each decade after age 50. The incidence rate is 107.7 per 100,000 for the male population, 107.3 per 100,000 white males, and 145.8 per 100,000 nonwhite males.[16]

There were approximately 200,000 new cases of prostate carcinoma in the United States in 1994 and approximately 38,000 deaths.[17] The autopsy incidence of histologic prostate cancer increases substantially with each decade of life from the 50s (5.3%-14%) to the 90s (40%-80%).[18] The prevalence of microscopic lesions at autopsy is identical throughout the world, but the incidence of clinical cancer is quite different. Furthermore, the rate of clinical cancer in Japanese men is quite low; however, after two generations, the clinical rate of Japanese immigrants to the US approaches that of white American males.[19,20]

Etiology

The precise etiology of prostate cancer is unknown, although there is some hormonal relationship and possibly a multistep process involved in the transformation of a benign epithelial cell to adenocarcinoma.

Environmental and familial factors may contribute to an increased incidence. Workers in certain industries have an excess in mortality from prostatic carcinoma, including those who are exposed to cadmium, workers in tire and rubber manufacturing, farmers, mechanics, and sheet metal workers.[21] High fat diets have also been implicated in the increased risk of prostate cancer.[22]

Presentation and Diagnosis

Clinical Presentation

Approximately 58% of patients have clinically localized cancer when first diagnosed.[16] Most of these patients will be asymptomatic or have symptoms of lower urinary tract obstruction. Marked irritative symptoms and the absence of infection should prompt a search for this malignancy.

Advanced presentation includes symptoms of bladder outlet obstruction, with urinary retention, urethral obstruction with possible anuria, azotemia, uremia, anemia, and anorexia. Bone pain is the most frequent complaint of patients presenting with metastatic disease. Spinal cord compression from vertebral metastasis is fortunately a rare occurrence.

Diagnosis

Digital rectal examination (DRE) remains the gold standard for detection of prostatic carcinoma, with 50% of palpable nodules found to be malignant.[23]

Prostate-specific antigen (PSA) is a prostatic marker useful for the early detection of prostate cancer. If the PSA is elevated to >10 ng/mL (Hybritech assay), there is an approximately 66% chance that a biopsy will be positive for carcinoma. If the PSA is between 4 and 10 ng/mL, there is an approximately 22% positive biopsy rate.[24] The role of PSA in screening is still unsettled and its use in the diagnosis of prostate cancer is evolving.

The role of transrectal ultrasonography (TRUS) in the early detection of prostate cancer remains controversial. TRUS is most useful in evaluating prostate size and for the precise biopsy of lesions that may or may not be palpable; it is helpful as a second-line investigation if either the PSA or DRE is abnormal.

Diagnosis is made by histologic or cytologic examination. Core biopsy is used in the US, usually with a spring-driven 18-gauge needle that delivers uniform cores with little displacement of the prostate gland and without the need of an anesthetic agent.

The patient undergoing transurethral resection of the prostate for presumed benign disease will occasionally be found to have unsuspected carcinoma. Historically the frequency was approximately 10%, but with the advent of PSA and transrectal ultrasound, the proportion of stage A patients has decreased.

Prostatic acid phosphatase (PAP) is not as useful as PSA in the diagnosis of patients with prostate cancer. It should still be performed at the time of diagnosis because elevated values usually signify metastatic disease, at least to the lymph nodes, especially if the enzymatic assay is used.

Early Detection

Men older than age 50 and men at high risk older than age 40 should receive a careful rectal examination during an annual or routine physical examination and should have a PSA test performed. Several years are still needed to determine the impact of early detection on the natural history and survival of prostate cancer.

Classification

Anatomic Staging

The American Urologic System consists of ABCD stages that have been translated into TNM categories

Table 20-2. TNM Staging for Prostate Cancer

Primary Tumor (T)

TX	Primary tumor cannot be assessed
T0	No evidence of primary tumor
T1	Clinically inapparent tumor not palpable or visible by imaging
T1a	Tumor incidental histologic finding in 5% or less of tissue resected
T1b	Tumor incidental histologic finding in more than 5% of tissue resected
T1c	Tumor identified by needle biopsy (eg, because of elevated PSA)
T2	Tumor confined within the prostate*
T2a	Tumor involves half of a lobe or less
T2b	Tumor involves more than half of a lobe, but not both lobes
T2c	Tumor involves both lobes
T3	Tumor extends through the prostatic capsule**
T3a	Unilateral extracapsular extension
T3b	Bilateral extracapsular extension
T3c	Tumor invades the seminal vesicle(s)
T4	Tumor is fixed or invades adjacent structures other than the seminal vesicles
T4a	Tumor invades any of: bladder neck, external sphincter, or rectum
T4b	Tumor invades levator muscles and/or is fixed to the pelvic wall

*Note: Tumor found in one or both lobes by needle biopsy, but not palpable or visible by imaging, is classified T1c.

**Note: Invasion into the prostatic apex or into (but not beyond) the prostatic capsule is not classified as T3, but as T2.

Regional Lymph Nodes (N)

The regional lymph nodes are the nodes of the true pelvis, which essentially are the pelvic nodes below the bifurcation of the common iliac arteries. They include the following groups (laterality does not affect the N classification): pelvic, NOS, hypogastric, obturator, iliac (internal, external, NOS), periprostatic, and sacral (lateral, presacral, promontory [Gerota's], or NOS)

Some Distant Lymph Nodes

Distant lymph nodes are outside the confines of the true pelvis. They can be imaged using ultrasound, computed tomography, magnetic resonance imaging, or lymphangiography. Aortic (para-aortic, peri-aortic, lumbar), common iliac, inguinal, superficial inguinal (femoral), supraclavicular, cervical, scalene

Table 20-2 *Continued.* TNM Staging for Prostate Cancer

NX	Regional lymph nodes cannot be assessed
N0	No regional lymph node metastasis
N1	Metastasis in a single lymph node, 2 cm or less in greatest dimension
N2	Metastasis in a single lymph node, more than 2 cm but not more than 5 cm in greatest dimension; or multiple lymph node metastases, none more than 5 cm in greatest dimension
N3	Metastasis in a lymph node more than 5 cm in greatest dimension

Distant Metastasis* (M)

MX	Presence of distant metastasis cannot be assessed
M0	No distant metastasis
M1	Distant metastasis
M1a	Nonregional lymph node(s)
M1b	Bone(s)
M1c	Other site(s)

Stage Grouping

Stage 0	T1a	N0	M0	G1
Stage I	T1a	N0	M0	G2, 3-4
	T1b	N0	M0	Any G
	T1c	N0	M0	Any G
	T1	N0	M0	Any G
Stage II	T2	N0	M0	Any G
Stage III	T3	N0	M0	Any G
Stage IV	T4	N0	M0	Any G
	Any T	N1	M0	Any G
	Any T	N2	M0	Any G
	Any T	N3	M0	Any G
	Any T	Any N	M1	Any G

From American Joint Committee on Cancer.[5]

by the AJCC[5] and the UICC.[6] The TNM classification for prostatic cancer is outlined in Table 20-2.

Stage Grouping

Incidental finding by transurethrally resected prostate specimens in clinically unsuspected carcinoma is either stage A1 (three or fewer foci, well differentiated) or stage A2 (diffuse or more than three foci, poorly differentiated, and more extensive than A1).

Clinically palpable lesions in the prostate are stage B1 (<1.5 cm, involving one lobe) and stage B2 (>1.5 cm, diffuse involvement).

Extension beyond the prostatic capsule, without evidence of metastasis, is stage C.

Metastatic carcinoma is stage D1 (involvement of the pelvic lymph nodes below the aortic bifurcation) and stage D2 (lymph node involvement above the aortic bifurcation and/or distant metastases to other sites).

Histopathology

Most prostatic carcinomas are adenocarcinomas. Multiple grading systems are available. The most frequently used, the Gleason grading system, is based on the tumor's glandular differentiation and growth pattern. Scores range from 2 to 10, and have been shown to be predictive of associated lymph node metastases.[25]

Clinical Staging

Clinical staging is generally accomplished using the following procedures: A CBC and SMA-12 are obtained in all patients. An elevated serum PAP is very suggestive of metastatic disease. The PSA is roughly proportional to prostatic volume. A PSA greater than 40 to 50 ng/mL (Yang assay) is usually associated with locally advanced or metastatic disease.[26]

Recommended Procedures

A radioisotopic bone scan is more sensitive than a skeletal survey and is obtained to rule out metastatic disease.

Optional and Investigative Procedures

CT scan of the pelvis is usually recommended only in patients who have elevated PAP and a normal bone scan or very high PSA to detect large pelvic lymphadenopathy. If large lymph nodes are found, percutaneous fine-needle biopsy of the nodes can be obtained with CT scan guidance. MRI of the pelvis should not be performed routinely; it is not more useful in identifying lymphadenopathy, but may be slightly more sensitive than CT scan in detecting extracapsular extension or seminal vesicle invasion. Lymphangiography is rarely used today, but can determine the extent of periaortic and advanced lymphadenopathy. Biopsy of other nodes and bone marrow aspiration in search of metastatic disease are rarely performed.

Principles of Treatment

Surgery

Radical prostatectomy is usually performed by the retropubic route. The prostate gland, seminal vesicles, and a narrow cuff of bladder neck are removed. Pelvic lymph nodes should be resected and sampled for staging. This treatment is effective for a localized lesion in a healthy man with an otherwise 10-year life expectancy. Patients with stage A2, B1, and B2 disease and younger patients with A1 disease are considered candidates for surgical cure. While patients with A1 disease were traditionally considered to have a benign course, up to 16% of these patients were found recently to have progressed.[27] The nerve-sparing operation of Walsh, in which capsular and periprostatic nerves are spared, has preserved potency in most patients, resulted in good cancer control, and represents a major advance.[28]

The radical perineal prostatectomy has seen some resurgence in the past few years with the advent of laparoscopic pelvic lymph node dissection. The perineal approach usually entails less blood loss and a faster recuperative period. Lymph node sampling is not possible, and exposure is more limited. It is an excellent approach for small tumors with low PSA when the chance of lymph node involvement is low.

Pelvic lymphadenectomy has not been determined to be of therapeutic value,[29] but allows for more precise staging because pelvic lymph nodes are generally the first site of metastatic spread. Laparoscopic pelvic lymph node dissection is as precise as open lymphadenectomy, but usually entails a longer operative time and requires certain acquired technical skills. The laparoscopic approach can be used in patients with suspected pelvic lymph node involvement and in those in whom radical prostatectomy is not an option.

Radiotherapy

Locally invasive cancers, or stages B and C, are treatable with supervoltage irradiation as are A2 and some A1 cancers; this applies to cancers within the capsule and those with extracapsular spread.[29] Highly focused modern techniques enable delivery of 60 to 70 Gy to the prostate cancer with minimal morbidity.[30]

The major issue of radiotherapy is whether pelvic and para-aortic lymph nodes should be irradiated. Most centers will treat pelvic lymph nodes. A common approach that has lost popularity is the operative implantation of gold seeds directly into the prostate followed by external beam radiation therapy.[31] An alternate approach to prostate cancer management is to utilize iodine 125 seed implants at the time of pelvic lymphadenectomy, extending the dissection to the high common iliac nodes and lower para-aortic area.[32] Few centers use this method today.

Radiation therapy is effective in treating pain due to metastatic bone disease, with moderate doses often providing prompt relief. For extensive bone metastases, hemibody radiation in a single dose of 7 to 8 Gy can provide dramatic pain relief in 70% to 80% of patients within 24 hours.[33]

Prior to estrogen therapy, pretreatment of the normal breasts with a modest dose (15 Gy) of radiation prevents nipple tenderness, but not necessarily gynecomastia.

Hormonal Therapy

For almost 50 years, the workup for metastatic prostate cancer has centered around orchiectomy or the administration of estrogens. Both will remove 90% to 95% of circulating testosterone. Median survival is 1 to 3 years in ambulatory patients.[34] Estrogen administration may result in thromboembolic and cardiovascular complications.

Luteinizing hormone-releasing hormone (LHRH) agonists have been shown to be equivalent to orchiectomy or diethylstilbestrol (DES).[35] However, they are expensive and associated with a flare phenomenon characterized by an increase in bone pain and outlet obstruction. Flutamide, a nonsteroidal antiandrogen approved in the US for use with an LHRH agonist, blocks the uptake and/or nuclear binding of androgens in target tissues. Combined androgen ablation using a LHRH agonist and flutamide has been shown to produce significantly better results, particularly in patients with minimal disease.[36] Other drugs that can be used for ablation of both testicular and adrenal androgens include cyproterone acetate, megestrol acetate, aminoglutethimide, and ketoconazole.

Chemotherapy

No standard effective chemotherapy regimen exists for cases refractory to hormone therapy. Clinical investigation is underway in this area.[37,38]

Results and Prognosis

In terms of early survival, both surgery and radiation therapy appear to be equivalent especially for early stage disease. Unfortunately, there is no randomized study that compares radiation therapy to radical prostatectomy for early stage adenocarcinoma of the prostate. Both surgery and radiation therapy have improved techniques and hopefully prostate specific antigen may, in the future, help answer some of the questions regarding these two modes of therapy.

Fifteen-year survival rates in patients with carcinoma clinically confined to the prostate gland and treated with radical prostatectomy is equivalent to rates in age-matched control populations.[39] Moreover, with the improvement in surgical technique brought about by Walsh, postoperative potency is 50% to 70%,[40] while the incontinence rate has dropped to <5%.[41]

Of 900 patients with locally invasive cancer (stages B2 and C) who have been followed for 15 years, disease-specific survival rates after supervoltage therapy are 66% for T1, 46% for T2, and 30% for T3 tumors.[42] Additional advantages of supervoltage therapy are maintenance of potency, in approximately 75% of cases, and low incontinence rate.[32] With the use of PSA, there is usually no biologic recurrence in the first year after radiation therapy, but by the third year, biologic recurrences may occur in approximately 90% of patients.[43]

The most common form of radioisotopic interstitial injection was implantation of gold seeds, followed by external beam radiation therapy. A large study reported 15-year actuarial survival rates that were similar to those of external beam radiation therapy for clinical stage A, B, and B/C patients.[31]

Iodine 125 seeds were used at Memorial Sloan-Kettering Cancer Center in the 1970s; 40% of TB1 and 70% of TB tumors had progressed at 10-year follow-up.[44]

Other seeds have been used, including palladium and iridium 192, but no long-term results are available. Newer techniques, such as ultrasound-guided perineal implantations, seem to achieve a better distribution of seeds with less morbidity, but it is unlikely that these developments will prove to be improvements of current forms of radiation therapy.

Patients who die of metastatic prostate cancer often demonstrate excellent local control of the disease. Metastasis to bone with bone marrow replacement is the predominant event leading to death, although other organs may be affected.

Bladder Cancer

Epidemiology

Bladder carcinoma is the most frequent malignant tumor of the urinary tract, with approximately 51,200 new cases in 1994. Most bladder tumors are found on the lateral and posterior walls of the bladder as well as the trigone. The tumor occurs most commonly in the sixth and seventh decade, accounting for 6% of all cancer cases in men and 2% in women. It accounts for 2% of all cancer deaths in the US, with 7,000 men and 3,600 women (2:1 ratio) dying from bladder cancer in 1994.[17]

Etiology

Aniline dye used in the textile, rubber, and cable industries is an etiologic factor. There is a long latency period (6 to 20 years) from exposure until tumor transformation in humans. Beta-naphthylamine, 4-amino-diphenyl, and tobacco tar can cause tumors in animals. In humans, cigarette smoking is associated with a sixfold higher incidence of bladder tumor.

Chronic bladder infections, calculous disease, and *Schistosoma haematobium* may cause squamous cell carcinoma. Adenocarcinoma may occur in exstrophy of the bladder or in a urachal remnant.[45]

Table 20-3. TNM Staging for Bladder Cancer

Primary Tumor (T)

TX	Primary tumor cannot be assessed
T0	No evidence of primary tumor
Ta	Noninvasive papillary carcinoma
Tis	Carcinoma in situ: "flat tumor"
T1	Tumor invades subepithelial connective tissue
T2	Tumor invades superficial muscle (inner half)
T3	Tumor invades deep muscle or perivesical fat
T3a	Tumor invades deep muscle (outer half)
T3b	Tumor invades perivesical fat
i.	microscopically
ii.	macroscopically (extravesical mass)
T4	Tumor invades any of the following: prostate, uterus, vagina, pelvic wall, or abdominal wall
T4a	Tumor invades the prostate, uterus, or vagina
T4b	Tumor invades pelvic wall or abdominal wall

Regional Lymph Nodes (N)

Regional lymph nodes are those within the true pelvis; all others are distant nodes.

NX	Regional lymph nodes cannot be assessed
N0	No regional lymph node metastasis
N1	Metastasis in a single lymph node, 2 cm or less in greatest dimension
N2	Metastasis in a single lymph node, more than 2 cm but not more than 5 cm in greatest dimension; or multiple lymph nodes, none more than 5 cm in greatest dimension
N3	Metastasis in a lymph node more than 5 cm in greatest dimension

Distant Metastasis (M)

MX	Presence of distant metastasis cannot be assessed
M0	No distant metastasis
M1	Distant metastasis

Table 20-3 *Continued.* TNM Staging for Bladder Cancer

Stage Grouping

Stage 0a	Ta	N0	M0
Stage 0is	Tis	N0	M0
Stage I	T1	N0	M0
Stage II	T2	N0	M0
	T3a	N0	M0
Stage III	T3b	N0	M0
	T4a	N0	M0
Stage IV	T4b	N0	M0
	Any T	N1	M0
	Any T	N2	M0
	Any T	N3	M0
	Any T	Any N	M1

From American Joint Committee on Cancer.[5]

Detection and Diagnosis

Clinical Detection

Gross hematuria is the most common clinical finding and the first sign in approximately 75% of patients. Microscopic hematuria is present in most cases. Frequency, bladder irritability, and dysuria occur in about one third of patients and increase in the later stages of the disease. Intermittent bleeding is characteristic and delays diagnosis because the patient and the physician may defer workup if the urine clears.

The presence of unexplained gross or microscopic hematuria requires evaluation. Cytologic analysis of urine is recommended in high-risk populations, such as workers exposed to carcinogens.

Diagnostic Procedures

Urinalysis often shows microhematuria when urine is grossly clear. Excretory urogram (IVP) is used to evaluate the upper urinary tracts and bladder filling. Cystoscopy is usually diagnostic. Deoxyribonucleic acid (DNA) ploidy by cytology and flow cytometry is helpful in diagnosing and screening high-risk patients and in follow-up. The yield from this study can be increased by brisk lavage of the bladder with normal saline. Cytology may be of screening value in industry and can detect lesions at an early stage in follow-up.

Pelvic CT aids in staging. Other imaging techniques, especially endorectal MRI, seem to be better than CT scan alone, at least in early studies. Flow cytometry of urine may be of value for diagnosis and prognosis.

Classification

The basis of staging of bladder cancer is depth of tumor penetration into the bladder wall, the single most important factor in predicting the prognosis of a lesion. The presence of multiple tumors without invasion and the location of the lesion might be important in determining the mode of therapy. Tumors might seed downward from a renal pelvic or ureteral primary neoplasm.[45,46] Metastasis occurs by lymphatic and hematogenous routes; common sites are regional lymph nodes, liver, lung, and bones.[47]

Bimanual assessment under anesthesia is reflected in the clinical classification. Modification of staging by endoscopic biopsy depends on depth of biopsy in muscle.

Table 20-3 outlines the American Joint Committee on Cancer (AJCC) TNM staging system for bladder cancer. There is concurrence between the AJCC and the UICC (International Union Against Cancer) classifications. Translations of the TNM system[5] into the ABCD American Urologic Association (Jewett-Strong-Marshall) staging system are possible (see Table 20-4).

Histopathology

Transitional cell carcinoma is the most common carcinoma of the bladder in the US (85% of cases), although squamous cell carcinoma (5%) and adenocarcinoma (<1%) may also occur. The histologic appearance, or grade, of the tumor may provide some indication of its potential to infiltrate and spread. Most noninvasive tumors are low grade (I-II), while invasive lesions are usually high grade (III-IV). Carcinoma in situ is a flat (nonpapillary) grade III tumor with an especially ominous prognosis if associated with an otherwise noninvasive tumor. Tumor grade also correlates with exfoliation of the tumor cells that are picked up on cytology or flow cytometry.

Table 20-4. Classification and Staging of Bladder Cancer

	American Urologic Association	American Joint Committee on Cancer
No evidence of tumor	0	To
Noninvasive papillary carcinoma	0	Ta
Carcinoma in situ	0	Tis
Submucosal invasion	A	T1
Invasion of superficial muscle	B1	T2
Invasion of deep muscle	B2	T3A
Invasion of perivesical fat	C	T3B
Invasion of contiguous organ	D1	T4
prostate, uterine, vagina	D1	T4A
pelvic or abdominal wall	D1	T4B
Regional lymph node metastases (below aortic bifurcation)	D1	N1-3
Juxtaregional lymph node metastases (above aortic bifurcation)	D2	N1-3
Distant metastasis	D2	M1

Clinical Staging

Clinical staging of transitional cell carcinoma is necessary to plan treatment. Despite the elegant staging systems available, treatment decisions are based on (1) superficial disease (confined to mucosa); (2) muscle-invasive disease (confined to the bladder); and (3) systemic disease.

Recommended Procedures

The following is the sequence of recommended procedures for staging workup (see Fig 20-2):

1. Cystoscopy, with biopsy or resection into muscle. In addition, biopsies of the bladder or prostatic urethra are usually indicated, especially with concern over multifocal disease. A barbotage specimen may be sent for cytology and flow cytometry.

2. Bimanual examination to stage the tumor.

3. Excretory urography or retrograde pyelogram to determine ureteral obstruction and extension.

If the tumor is invasive, additional studies are required, including:

4. Radiographic survey (chest film and abdominal and pelvic CT scan). Bone scan is useful only if bony metastases are clinically suspected.

5. Laboratory tests, including CBC and SMA-12.

Optional and Investigative Procedures

MRI, especially endorectal MRI, seems to better delineate muscle-invasive disease and may occasionally differentiate between a stage B and C lesion. Studies are under way to determine its usefulness. Laparotomy or pelvic exploration will evaluate the extent of the lymph node involvement.

Principles of Treatment

General Principles

The following factors must be considered before determining the mode and extent of therapy: anatomic and histologic classification (stage and grade); location of tumor; general health; associated genitourinary problems (prostatism, urinary tract infection, ureteral obstruction, compromised renal

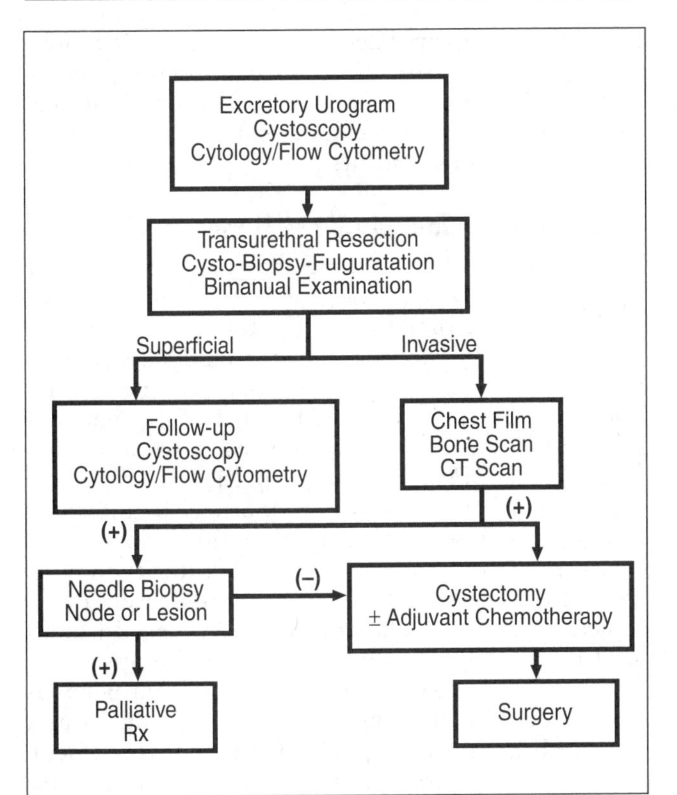

Fig 20-2. Carcinoma of the bladder: clinical evaluation and treatment. This plan may be altered because of factors such as patient's age and general health.

function); patient's ability to tolerate and to care for any urinary diversion; history of tumor recurrence (an increased rate may influence the therapy plan); previous surgery or radiation therapy; and training, experience, and skill of the surgeon, medical oncologist, or radiation therapist.

Surgery

Endoscopic resection and fulguration are used to diagnose, stage, and treat tumors of the bladder. It can also be used to control bleeding in patients who are poor operative risks or who have advanced disease. Treatment with a neodymium-yttrium-aluminum-garnet (Nd:YAG) laser is also a possibility; it is associated with less bleeding, but pathology specimens are not available for analysis. Segmental bladder resection is reserved for large single lesions occurring for the first time, usually at the bladder dome or, in some patients, the lateral wall. Patients who are at too high a risk for total cystectomy may undergo segmental bladder resection, which may also be used in some cases of adenocarcinoma of the urachus. Recurrence rates as high as 70% are seen in superficial tumors and may be treated with repeated endoscopic procedures, intravesical chemotherapy, or both.

Radical cystectomy requires resection of local pelvic lymph nodes, prostate, seminal vesicles, uterus, ovaries, and fallopian tubes in women. Penile urethrotomy is indicated in the presence of disease at the bladder neck or prostatic urethra. Cystectomy is indicated when the tumor is invasive into at least the muscle, or superficial but uncontrollable with conservative modalities, and when the patient has a good life expectancy with no metastasis outside the pelvic area. The second step of the surgery requires a form of urinary diversion. The standard is the ileal conduit, but continent urinary diversion to an abdominal stoma or orthotopic bladder substitutes can be used in highly motivated patients.

Preferred Surgical Procedures by Classification

For superficial-stage (Ta, T1) tumors, consider endoscopic resection and fulguration; segmental bladder resection in selected cases; and total cystectomy in patients who do not respond to conservative methods (intravesical chemotherapy or immunotherapy).

For deep-stage (T2, T3) tumors, total cystectomy with urinary diversion, including urethrectomy for lesions near or distal to the bladder neck, is warranted. Segmental bladder resection may be considered in a few selected cases.

For metastatic disease, urinary diversion is occasionally recommended for palliation.[48]

Radiotherapy

Radiation therapy as definitive therapy is seldom recommended due to the low response and survival rates. Radiation has been examined in the adjuvant setting prior to radical cystectomy,[49] but no additional benefit has been seen on longer follow-up.

In locally invasive disease and in nonoperative patients, radiation therapy can be used palliatively to control pain and bleeding.

Intravesical Chemotherapy or Immunotherapy

Intravesical chemotherapy or immunotherapy is indicated in patients with superficial disease who are at high risk of recurrence by virtue of recurrent tumors, multiple tumors, high-grade tumors, or carcinoma in situ.

Bacillus Calmette-Guerin (BCG) therapy is believed to exert antitumor effects through nonspecific immune responses. It appears to be the most effective agent for intravesical use, but the optimum strain, dose, and frequency have yet to be determined. It is usually administered once a week for 6 weeks, and long-term studies have reported favorable responses in 50% to 89% of patients.[50]

There are many forms of intravesical chemotherapy, including thiotepa, epodyl, doxorubicin (Adriamycin), and mitomycin C. The most effective of these is mitomycin C, which some studies suggest may be as effective as BCG[51]; it certainly is less toxic. Intravesical interferon has also been used with favorable responses, but the limiting factor is cost.

Hematoporphyrin Derivative (Photodynamic) Phototherapy

Hematoporphyrin derivative is a mixture of porphyrins that are highly concentrated in neoplastic and dysplastic tissues. Light with a wave length of 630 nm is used to irradiate the tissues, preferentially destroying tumor cells rather than normal cells via the release of singlet oxygen, causing mitochondrial poisoning. Responses are good with superficial, but not large or invasive, tumors.[52] The disadvantages of phototherapy include generalized cutaneous photosensitivity, requiring the patient to avoid sunlight for 6 to 8 weeks. In addition, local symptoms can be severe and scarring of the bladder can occur. This form of therapy is still experimental.

Chemotherapy

The most useful current regimen for metastatic transitional cell carcinoma of the bladder consists of methotrexate, vinblastine, Adriamycin, and cisplatin (M-VAC). Encouraging initial reports were followed by news of only 20% survival, with a median survival of 13 months.[53] Patients with only nodal metastases respond better and longer; M-VAC therapy appears to be ineffective against carcinoma in situ. It is extremely toxic, requiring frequent hospitalizations for cytopenic sepsis. Another available, but also toxic, regimen is CISCA (cisplatin, cyclophosphamide, and Adriamycin). There is very little difference between the two therapies, and both have a low durable response rate with very high toxicity.

Results and Prognosis

Currently, patients with superficial disease have an excellent prognosis (5-year survival of up to 85% to 90%) and a 10% chance of progression overall. Factors such as tumor size, number of tumors, time of recurrence, grade, histologic stage, presence of carcinoma in situ, and detection of normal cell antigens all have some bearing on prognosis. Muscle-invading disease is currently treated by cystectomy with a 5-year survival rate of 55% to 60%. Systemic disease is associated with a poor prognosis (see Table 20-3).

Patterns of Failure

In the past, when radiation therapy was more widely used, local failure was high. Local recurrence is still possible and is seen with conservative procedures designed to preserve bladder function and invasive disease. The most common site of relapse postcystectomy is at distant metastases.

Clinical investigations are under way to determine better and safer dosages and regimens for intravesical agents in superficial disease. For advanced disease, better chemotherapeutic agents are being studied, none show much promise. New surgical techniques are being attempted, especially in the field of continent stomas and orthotopic bladder substitutes as well as artificial bladder substitutes.

Urothelial Carcinoma of the Upper Tract

Transitional cell carcinoma may also occur in the upper urinary tract, including the renal calices, pelvis, and ureter. The biology of these tumors is similar to transitional cell carcinoma in the bladder. Operable tumors warrant consideration of nephroureterectomy. The entire ureter is removed because of the tendency for transitional cell tumors to seed down along the ureter into the bladder or to be multifocal.[54,55] Partial ureterectomy with reimplantation may be indicated in low-stage, low-grade distal ureteral tumors. Bilateral tumors or tumors in solitary kidneys may be treated endoscopically, or with partial resection or topical or systemic chemotherapy. Advanced lesions are treated with cisplatin-based chemotherapy.

Transitional cell carcinoma of the renal pelvis is associated with the following 5-year survival rates: 52% with noninvasive papillary lesions, 16.7% with papillary lesions with parenchymal infiltration, 7.1% with nonpapillary lesions with infiltration, and 4.3% with venous or lymphatic involvement.[55] Squamous cell carcinoma of the upper urinary tract has a poor prognosis. Carcinoma of the upper urinary tract has a higher local recurrence rate than bladder carcinoma.

Embryonal Kidney Tumors (Wilms' Tumor)

Epidemiology

The origin of this large malignant tumor of childhood is mesodermal. Sixty-five percent occur before the third year, and 75% occur before the fifth year. There is an equal incidence for both sexes, and bilateral involvement is present in <7% of patients.

Detection and Diagnosis

Clinical Detection

A palpable abdominal mass is seen in approximately 50% of patients. Other presenting signs are hematuria (approximately 20%), pain (approximately 30%), and hypertension (approximately 75%).

Wilms' tumor must be differentiated from hydronephrosis, neuroblastoma, multicystic kidney disease, polycystic kidney, and other rare tumors, both benign and malignant.

Diagnostic Procedures

Excretory urogram with tomography is still commonly used for the diagnosis of Wilms' tumor. Ultrasound can rule out hydronephrosis or cystic disease, but CT scan and MRI are important in the staging of Wilms' tumor.

Arteriography is rarely recommended, as is inferior venacavography. Retrograde pyelogram is rarely needed, but is indicated in the presence of hematuria, especially when the kidney is not visualized on IVP. Because of the high incidence of central nervous system metastasis, imaging of the brain on radionuclear scan or CT is indicated if a rhabdoid tumor is found. A bone scan should be done where clear cell sarcoma is used due to the high incidence of bony metastasis.

Classification

Anatomic Staging

The National Wilms' Tumor Study (NWTS) classification, based on surgical and pathologic findings, is the most widely used system.[56] In stage I, the tumor is confined within the intact capsule of the kidney, and completely excised without evidence of tumor at its margin. In stage II, the tumor extends beyond the kidney, but is completely excised grossly; the tumor invades into perinephric fat; and lymph nodes and veins must be resected with a clear margin. Stage II also applies if the tumor has been biopsied or if there is local spillage. Stage III is residual, nonhematogenous tumor confined to the abdomen, indicating tumor rupture at surgery; peritoneal implants; juxtaregional nodes in pelvis; or incomplete resection. Stage IV indicates hematogenous metastases beyond stage III. Stage V indicates bilateral renal involvement at diagnosis.

Histologic Types

Two general types are identifiable: favorable and unfavorable. The latter has focal and diffuse anaplasia and sarcomatous features associated with brain and skeletal metastases.

Recommended Procedures

The following is the sequence of recommended staging workup procedures:

1. Ultrasound of abdomen.
2. Excretory urography, including tomography.
3. CT or MRI for staging and evaluation.
4. Chest films. The lungs are an important metastatic pathway, and suspicious lesions may require CT for confirmation.
5. Laboratory survey, including CBC and SMA-12.
6. Laparotomy to determine primary tumor and nodal extent and for definitive surgical treatment.

Optional and Investigative Procedures

Aortography and renal arteriography may be difficult to perform in children. Retrograde pyelography can be helpful, but is seldom needed. As mentioned previously, bone scan or imaging of the brain may be needed depending on the specific pathologic findings.

Principles of Treatment

Surgery

Transperitoneal nephrectomy should be performed as soon as possible. Local lymphadenectomy is rarely required. The flank approach is contraindicated, because neither the contralateral kidney nor the entire abdomen can be explored.

Radiotherapy

Low-dose radiation therapy is used in stage III or IV patients with favorable histology or in patients with any stage of clear cell sarcoma. It is usually administered after surgery and before chemotherapy. Complications of radiation include minimal scoliosis, radiation nephritis, and occasionally temporary bone marrow suppression.

Chemotherapy

Combination cyclic chemotherapy, consisting of vincristine, Adriamycin, and actinomycin D, is useful.

Treatment According to Stages

Treatment is based on the NWTS Study-4 protocol (Table 20-5).[57] For stage I, chemotherapy is used following nephrectomy. For stage II favorable histology, surgery is followed by more intense chemotherapy. For stage III favorable histology or stage IV favorable histology, surgery is followed by radiation therapy and subsequently by intense chemotherapy. For high-risk patients or patients with clear cell sarcoma of any stage, surgery is followed by radiation therapy and then intense chemotherapy. For stage V disease, aggressive chemotherapy and conservative surgery seem to be the mainstay in the care of synchronous bilateral Wilms' tumor.

Results and Prognosis

The 4-year postnephrectomy survival rate is >85% in patients with favorable histology at any stage. Those with stages I to III unfavorable histology have an almost 70% survival, and those with unfavorable histology in stage IV have approximately 55% survival.

Future Considerations

Conservative surgery seems to be promising if coupled with aggressive chemotherapy. Future goals will include an effort to minimize the morbidity of chemotherapy and radiation therapy, especially for patients with a favorable prognosis. In patients with an unfavorable histology, who still account for most failures, more intense or refined treatments are needed.

Table 20-5. National Wilms' Tumor Study-4 Protocol

Disease	Initial Therapy	Radiotherapy	Chemotherapy Regimen
Stage I/FH	Surgery	None	AMD + VCR (24 wk)
Stage I/anaplastic			Pulsed, intensive AMD + VCR (15 wk)*
Stage II/FH	Surgery	None	AMD + VCR (22 and 65 wk) Pulsed, intensive AMD + VCR (24 and 60 wk)*
Stage III/FH	Surgery	10.8 Gy	AMD + VCR + ADR (26 and 65 wk) Pulsed, intensive AMD + VCR + ADR (24 and 52 wk)*
High risk (clear cell sarcoma, all stages) and stage IV/FH	Surgery	Yes +	AMD + VCR + ADR (26 and 65 wk) Pulsed, intensive AMD + VCR + ADR (24 and 52 wk)*

* Latest National Wilms' Tumor Study protocol for dosage and length of treatment.

\+ Patients with clear cell sarcoma receive 10.8 Gy, and those with stage IV cancer of favorable histologic type are given 10.8 Gy if the primary tumor would qualify as stage III were there no metastasis.

ADR=doxorubicin; AMD=actinomycin D; FH=favorable histologic type; VCR=vincristine.

Adapted from Mesrobian.[57]

Testis Cancer

Epidemiology and Etiology

Testis cancer represents only about 1% of all cancers in males, but is the most common solid malignancy in men between the ages of 20 and 34. The average rate among American black men is 0.7 per 100,000, or approximately one eighth the rate in white American males. There were approximately 6,800 new cases in the US in 1994 and approximately 325 deaths.

A significantly increased incidence of carcinoma is found in cryptorchid testes. The relative risk of testicular cancer in patients with cryptorchidism is thought to be between three and 14 times the normal expected incidence.[58]

Roughly 25% of patients with bilateral cryptorchidism and a history of testis tumor on one side develop a tumor on the contralateral testis, in contrast to only 1% of patients with naturally descended testes in the scrotum.[59]

Experimental and clinical evidence supports the importance of congenital factors in the etiology of testicular cancer, in an alteration in the primordial germ cell line, caused by either cryptorchidism, gonadal dysgenesis, or hereditary and environmental factors.

Detection and Diagnosis

Clinical Detection

Typically, there are no early symptoms. Usually, a testicular mass is found and approximately 96% of solid tumors of the testes are malignant. Most are usually painless or associated with nonspecific complaints, such as a heavy feeling in the testicle, whereas pain usually means hemorrhage in the tumor.

The differential diagnosis includes epididymitis; spermatocele; hydrocele; benign tumor of the testis; a tumor of the epididymis or tunica albuginea, which is very rare; or simple orchitis, infarction, or trauma.

Early detection is accomplished best by self-examination of the testis and is recommended for patients with a prior history of testicular malignancy.

Generalized symptoms are usually indicative of metastasis, such as pulmonary metastasis, causing dyspnea or hemoptysis; abdominal mass; or ureteral obstruction by lymph node involvement.

Diagnostic Procedures

The physician should palpate the testes and surrounding structures for a testicular mass, examine the breasts for signs of gynecomastia, transilluminate intrascrotal lesions, and perform abdominal examination for pal-

Table 20-6. TNM Staging for Testis Cancer

Primary Tumor (T)

The extent of primary tumor is classified after radical orchiectomy.

pTX	Primary tumor cannot be assessed (If no radical orchiectomy has been performed, TX is used.)
pT0	No evidence of primary tumor (e.g., histologic scar in testis)
pTis	Intratubular tumor: preinvasive cancer
pT1	Tumor limited to the testis, including the rete testis
pT2	Tumor invades beyond the tunica albuginea or into the epididymis
pT3	Tumor invades the spermatic cord
pT4	Tumor invades the scrotum

Regional Lymph Nodes (N)

NX	Regional lymph nodes cannot be assessed
N0	No regional lymph node metastasis
N1	Metastasis in a single lymph node, 2 cm or less in greatest dimension
N2	Metastasis in a single lymph node, more than 2 cm but not more than 5 cm in greatest dimension; or multiple lymph nodes, none more than 5 cm in greatest dimension
N3	Metastasis in a lymph node more than 5 cm in greatest dimension

Distant Metastasis (M)

MX	Presence of distant metastasis cannot be assessed
M0	No distant metastasis
M1	Distant metasatis

Stage Grouping

Stage 0	pTis	N0	M0
Stage I	Any pT	N0	M0
Stage II	Any pT	N1	M0
	Any pT	N2	M0
	Any pT	N3	M0
Stage III	Any pT	Any N	M1

From American Joint Committee on Cancer.[5]

pable mass, as well as look for adenopathy in the supraclavicular region, axillae, and inguinal regions.

Ultrasound of the scrotum is usually unnecessary if a solid tumor is felt to originate from the testicle on physical examination, but is helpful in equivocal cases. CT of the abdomen and pelvis and a plain chest x-ray are standard, with or without CT of the chest. Radioimmunoassay (RIA) for serum alpha-fetoprotein (AFP) and beta-subunit human chorionic gonadotropin (beta-hCG) should be performed.[60]

Excretory urogram can be performed, if there is hydronephrosis secondary to para-aortic or paracaval lymph node involvement. Pedal lymphangiography may be performed,[61] but the advent of refined CT scans has replaced lymphangiography.

Classification

Anatomic Staging

Anatomic classification and expansion of histologic typing have occurred because both are important factors in the prognosis and treatment of testis cancer. The AJCC and UICC have published a TNM classification which is outlined in Table 20-6.[5,6]

Stage Grouping

Stage grouping is an older approach. In stage A, tumor is confined to the testis. Involvement of retroperitoneal lymph nodes is found in the following stages: stage B1, minimal (<6 positive nodes and no node >2 cm in diameter); stage B2, moderate (>6 positive nodes or any node >2 cm but <5 cm in diameter); stage B3, massive (nodal mass >5 cm); and stage C, metastasis to nodes above the diaphragm or to distant sites.[62]

Histopathology

There are two theories on the histogenesis of testicular tumors: the holistic, or single germ cell origin, theory (Fig 20-3) is favored over the dual origin theory,

Table 20-7. Representative Distributions

Germinal Origin (97%)
- Seminoma (pure)—47.7%[62]
- Typical (classical)
- Anaplastic
- Spermatocystic (atypical)
  - Embryonal carcinoma—20% to 25%
  - Teratoma—5% to 9%
  - Teratoma with malignant areas—25% to 30%
- (Teratocarcinoma)
  - Choriocarcinoma—1% to 3%

Nongerminal Origin (3%)
- Interstitial cell tumors
- Gonadal-stromal tumors

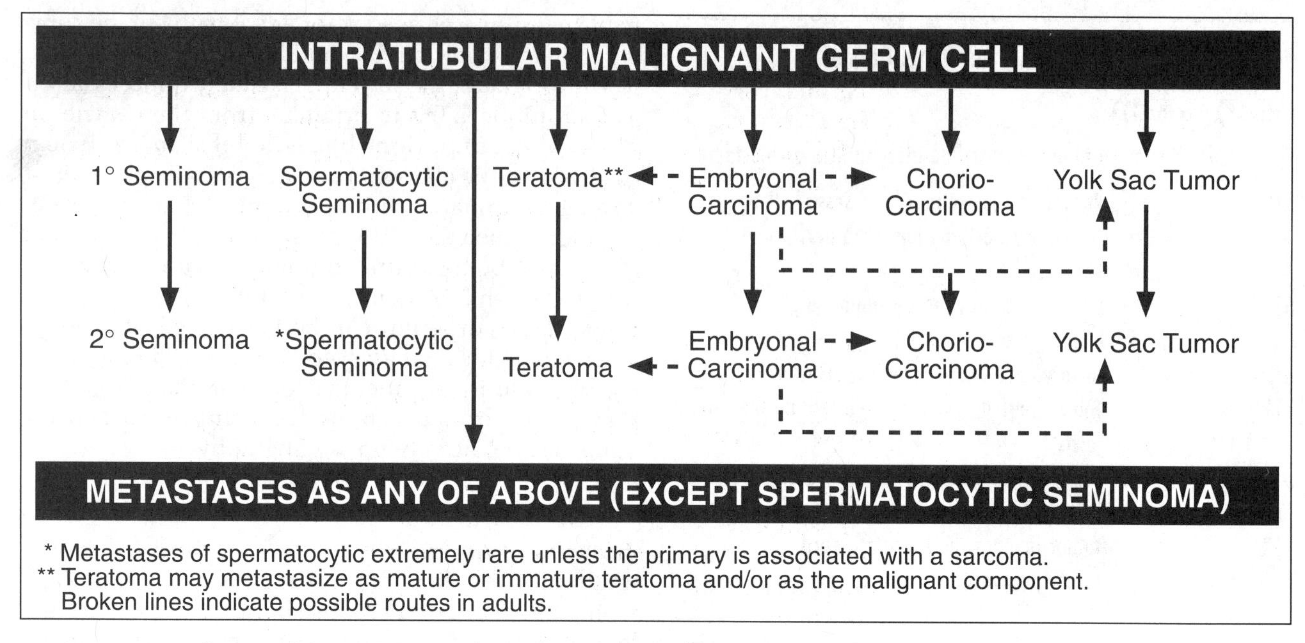

Fig 20-3. Germ cell tumor of the testis. Histogenic routes. Source: Mostofi.[63]

which hypothesizes a separate origin for seminomas and teratomatous cancers.[63] A representation of the dual origin for the derivation of testicular tumors is depicted in Table 20-7.[63]

Diagnosis and Clinical Staging

The following procedures are recommended for clinical staging:

1. Clinical evaluation and scrotal ultrasound in equivocal cases.

2. Radiographic surveys, usually limited to CT of the abdomen and pelvis, and chest x-ray with or without tomograms, versus a CT of the chest.

3. Laboratory survey, including CBC and SMA-12.

4. Beta-hCG and AFP are necessary before surgery and reflect the type of tumor found; both values are also helpful in follow-up.

5. The most important is the actual pathology and the presence or absence of invasion of the cord, epididymis, tunica albuginea, rete testis, scrotum, lymphatics, or blood vessels. This will dictate the prognosis and treatment.

In patients in whom testicular tumor is a possibility, inguinal exploration with high ligation of the cord, followed by orchiectomy, is carried out. Vascular control should be achieved prior to manipulation of the tumor, and an open biopsy, as well as scrotal exploration, is contraindicated.

Principles of Treatment

Surgery

If the pathology sample reveals nonseminomatous elements, including embryonal carcinoma, teratocarcinoma, adult teratoma, or seminoma with an elevated AFP level, or a seminoma with persistent beta-hCG levels after orchiectomy, a bilateral retroperitoneal lymph node dissection is usually carried out for a T, N1 or N2, M0 patient. Observation certainly is an option for clinical N0 patients.

In the presence of bulky nodal involvement for N3 or M-positive patients, chemotherapy-induced debulking should precede surgery. A surgical lymphadenectomy provides debulking and staging information needed for planning further therapy. For metastatic disease limited to the lungs or abdomen, surgery may be deferred after a complete response to chemotherapy, and careful follow-up employed but only as part of a clinical trial.

Radiotherapy

Seminomas

Irradiation of the retroperitoneal and homolateral iliac nodes to the level of the diaphragm is the usual form of treatment for small to moderate lymph node involvement of the retroperitoneum. Surveillance of stage I seminomas is usually not recommended, since the success of radiation therapy is high and morbidity low.

Prophylactic mediastinal irradiation does not significantly improve survival, and may prevent the optimal use of subsequent chemotherapy.[64] Careful follow-up is necessary.

Nonseminomas

Cytoreductive surgery and chemotherapy have largely replaced radiation therapy as the treatment of low-stage nonseminomatous tumor of the testes. Occasionally, radiation therapy may be helpful in localized metastatic disease that cannot be excised and does not respond to chemotherapy.

Chemotherapy

Seminomas

Chemotherapy is useful for cases unresponsive to radiation therapy and for bulky metastatic disease.[65] Patients with advanced seminoma seem to have chemosensitive tumors; potential cure with chemotherapy is comparable to the observed rate for patients with nonseminomatous germ cell tumors. More than 85% of patients have achieved continuous disease-free status with cisplatin combination chemotherapy. If the patient responds initially to chemotherapy for advanced seminoma, no further treatment should be instituted if a complete response is confirmed radiographically. With a small residual mass, close and careful observation is favored over consolidation with radiation therapy or surgical excision.[66]

Nonseminomas

Dramatic progress in combining chemotherapeutic agents has markedly affected the survival of patients with metastatic disease. Two schools of thought have emerged historically, one from Memorial Sloan-Kettering Cancer Center, using VAB (vinblastine, actinomycin D, and bleomycin) protocols, with the addition of cisplatin on the VAB VI protocols initiated in 1979. The other school of thought, from Indiana University, included the PVB (platinum, vinblastine, and bleomycin) protocols. Recently, etoposide (VP-16), as a single agent, has shown activity in patients with testicular cancer.

It has been shown that three cycles may be as good as four, and VP-16 has replaced vinblastine because of the neurotoxicity associated with the latter. Currently, BEP (bleomycin, etoposide, and platinum) is the standard for patients with disseminated germ cell tumor.

Should there be residual carcinoma following chemotherapy, salvage chemotherapy or surgical resection should be considered. Salvage chemotherapy usually includes ifosfamide or VP-16, if not used in the initial chemotherapeutic regimen. Conversely, if VP-16 was used, vinblastine should be used as a second-line chemotherapeutic agent.

Third-line chemotherapy for patients unresponsive to first- and second-line regimens includes autologous bone marrow transplantation with high-dose chemotherapy regimens, usually with carboplatin rather than cisplatin.

Results and Prognosis

The dramatic response to single-agent and combination drug regimens has made even advanced cases of testis cancer curable. Radiation therapy still has a curative role in seminomas, but has been almost replaced by chemotherapy in nonseminomatous tumors. Tumor markers aid in early diagnosis and are equally important in follow-up, because they may be the earliest indication of recurrent tumors.

Seminomas

Radiation therapy results in a >95% survival in patients with clinical stage I seminoma. In patients with small to moderate retroperitoneal lymph nodes treated by radiation therapy, the expected survival is between 80% and 90%. In advanced seminoma, >85% of patients have achieved continuous disease-free status with cisplatin combination chemotherapy (American Cancer Society, 1987).

Nonseminomas

In patients treated with orchiectomy and retroperitoneal lymph node dissection in pathologic stage I nonseminoma, the 5-year survival rate is >90%. Patients with small to moderate retroperitoneal lymph nodes have a >80% survival at 5 years. Those with metastatic or bulky disease achieve complete remission in 50% to 75% of cases, and another 10% to 15% of patients can be made disease-free by surgical removal of residual tumor; however, relapses occur in 10% to 20% of patients who have achieved a complete remission. It appears that almost all relapses occur within 18 months of the initial chemotherapy protocol.

Clinical Investigations

The major thrust of current investigations is to preserve high cure rates while decreasing the toxicity of the chemotherapeutic regimen, by either replacing drugs with less toxic alternatives or decreasing the number of cycles.

For Localized Disease

While the search for new tumor markers is being carried out, surgical techniques are being improved to decrease morbidity, especially anejaculation.

For Advanced and Metastatic Stages

Alterations of drug dosages and intervals of therapy, as well as drug combinations, are being evaluated to decrease the significant toxicity associated with combined chemotherapy without adversely affecting the level of efficacy achieved with current combination regimens.

References

1. Kantor AF. Current concepts in the epidemiology and etiology of primary renal cell carcinoma. *J Urol.* 1977; 117:415-417.

2. Reiter RE, Anglard P, Liu S, Gnarra JR, Linehan WM. Chromosome 17p deletions and p53 mutations in renal cell carcinoma. *Cancer.* 1993; 53(13):3092-7.

3. Gnarra JR, Glenn GM, Latif F, Anglard P, Lerman MI, Zbar B, Linehan WM. Molecular genetic studies as sporadic and familial renal cell carcinoma. *Urol Clin North Ame.* 1993; 2:207-16.

4. Lauritsen JG. Lindau's disease: a study of one family through six generations. *Acta Chir Scand.* 1973; 139:482-486.

5. Beahrs OH, Henson DE, Hutter RVP, Kennedy BJ, eds. *American Joint Committee on Cancer Manual for Staging of Cancer.* 4th ed. Philadelphia, Pa: JB Lippincott Co; 1992.

6. Hermanek P, Sobin LH, eds. *TNM Classification of Malignant Tumours.* 4th ed. 2nd rev. Berlin: Springer-Verlag; 1992.

7. Robson CJ, Churchill BM, Anderson W. The results of radical nephrectomy for renal cell carcinoma. *Trans Am Assoc Genitourin Surg.* 1968;60:122-129.

8. Flocks RH, Kadesky MC. Malignant neoplasms of the kidney: an analysis of 353 patients followed 5 years or more. *J Urol.* 1958; 79:196-201.

9. Yagoda A. Chemotherapy of renal cell carcinoma, 1985-1989. *Semin Urol.* 1989; 7:199.

10. Kirkman H, Bacon RL. Renal adenomas and carcinomas in diethylstilbestrol treated male golden hamsters. *Anat Rec.* 1949;103:475. Abstract.

11. Sarna G, Figlin R, deKernion J. Interferon in renal cell carcinoma: the UCLA experience. *Cancer.* 1987; 59:610-612.

12. Rosenberg SA, Lotze MT, Muul LM, et al. Observations on the systemic administration of autologous lymphokine-activated killer cells and recombinant interleukin-2 to patients with metastatic cancer. *N Engl J Med.* 1985; 313:1485-1492.

13. Fisher RI, Coltman CA, Jr, Doroshow JH, et al. Metastatic renal cancer treated with interleukin-2 and lymphokine-activated killer cells: a phase II clinical trial. *Ann Intern Med.* 1988; 108:518-523.

14. deKernion JB, Belldegrun A. Renal tumors. In: Walsh PC, Retik AB, Stamey TA, Vaughan ED Jr, eds. *Campbell's Urology.* 6th ed. Philadelphia, Pa: WB Saunders Co; 1992; 2: 1053-1093.

15. Robson CJ. Radical nephrectomy for renal cell carcinoma. *J Urol.* 1963; 89:37-42.

16. Miller BA, Ries LAG, Hankey BF, Kosary CL, Harras A, Devesa SS, Edwards BK, eds. SEER Cancer Statistics Review: 1973-1990, National Cancer Institute. NIH Pub. No. 93-2789, 1993.

17. Boring CC, Squires TS, Tong T, Montgomery S. Cancer Statistics 1994. *CA Cancer J Clin.* 1994;44:7-26.

18. Sheldon CA, Williams RD, Fraley EE. Incidental carcinoma of the prostate: review of the literature and critical reappraisal of classification. *J Urol.* 1980; 124:626-631.

19. Chiarodo A. National Cancer Institute roundtable on prostate cancer: future research directions. *Cancer Res.* 1991; 51:2498-2505.

20. Muir CS, Nectoux J, Staszewski J. The epidemiology of prostate cancer: geographic distribution and time trends. *Acta Oncol.* 1991; 30:133-140.

21. Carter BS, et al. Epidemiologic evidence regarding predisposing factors to prostate cancer. *Prostate.* 1989; 16:187-197.

22. LaVecchia C. Cancers associated with high fat diets. *Monogr Natl Cancer Inst.* 1992; 12:79-85

23. Jewett HJ, Bridge RW, Gray GF, Shelley WM. The palpable nodule of prostatic cancer: results 15 years after radical excision. *JAMA.* 1968; 203:403-406.

24. Catalona WJ, Smith DS, Ratliff TL, et al. Measurement of prostate-specific antigen in serum as a screening test for prostate cancer. *N Engl J Med.* 1991; 324:1156-1161.

25. Paulson DF. Uro-oncology research group. The impact of current staging procedures in assessing disease extent of prostatic adenocarcinoma. *J Urol.* 1979; 121:300-302.

26. Palken M, Cobb OE, Warren BH, Hoak DC. Prostate cancer: correlation of digital rectal examination, transrectal ultrasound and prostate specific antigen levels with tumor volumes in radical prostatectomy specimens. *J Urol.* 1990; 143:1155-1162.

27. Epstein JI, Paull G, Eggleston JC, Walsh PC. Prognosis of untreated stage A1 prostatic carcinoma: a study of 94 cases with extended followup. *J Urol.* 1986; 136:837-839.

28. Walsh PC, Lepor H. The role of radical prostatectomy in the management of prostatic cancer. *Cancer.* 1987; 60(suppl):526-537.

29. Catalona WJ, Scott WW. Carcinoma of the prostate. In: Walsh PC, Gittes RF, Perlmutter AD, Stamey TA, eds. *Campbell's Urology.* 5th ed. Philadelphia, Pa: WB Saunders Co; 1986;2:1463-1534.

30. Kiesling VJ, McAninch JW, Goebel JL, Agee RE. External beam radiotherapy for adenocarcinoma of the prostate: a clinical followup. *J Urol.* 1980; 124:851-854.

31. Scardino PT, Wheeler TM. Local control of prostate cancer with radiotherapy: frequency and prognostic significance of positive results of postirradiation prostate biopsy. Bethesda, Md: US Dept Health and Human Services, Public Health Service; 1988; National Cancer Institute monograph. 7:95.

32. Batata MA, Hilaris BS, Chu FCH, et al. Radiation therapy in adenocarcinoma of the prostate with pelvic lymph node involvement at lymphadenectomy. *Int J Radiat Oncol Biol Phys.* 1980; 6:149-153.

33. Salazar OM, Rubin P, Hendrickson FR, et al. Single half-body irradiation for the palliation of multiple bone metastases from solid tumors: a preliminary report. *Int J Radiat Oncol Biol Phys.* 1981; 7:773-781.

34. DeVoogt HJ, Suciu S, Sylvester R, et al. Multivariant analysis of prognostic factors in patients with advanced prostate cancer: results from 2 year European Organization for Research on Treatment of Cancer trials. *J Urol.* 1989; 141:883-888.

35. Leuprolide study group: leuprolide versus diethylstilbestrol for metastatic prostate cancer. *N Engl J Med.* 1984; 311:1281-1286.

36. Crawford ED, Eisenberger MA, McLeod DG, et al. A controlled trial of leuprolide with and without flutamide in prostatic carcinoma. *N Engl J Med.* 1989; 321:419-424.

37. Paulson DF. *Urology.* Multimodal therapy of prostate cancer. 1981; 17(4, suppl):53-56.

38. Schmitt JD, Scott WW, Gibbons R, et al. Chemotherapy programs of the National Prostatic Cancer Project (NPCP). *Cancer.* 1980; 45:1937-1946.

39. Consensus conference. The management of clinically localized prostate cancer. *JAMA.* 1987; 258: 2727-2730.

40. Walsh PC, Donker PJ. Impotence following radical prostatectomy: insight into etiology and prevention. *J Urol.* 1982; 128:492-497.

41. Drago JR, Badalament RA, Nesbitt JA, York JP. Radical nerve-sparing prostatectomy with epidural anaesthesia in 100 patients. *Br J Urol.* 1990; 65:517-519

42. Bagshaw MA. The challenge of radiation treatment of carcinoma of the prostate. In: Lepor H, Lawson RK, eds. *Prostate Diseases*. Philadelphia, Pa: WB Saunders Co; 1993: 326-346.

43. Stamey TA, Kabalin JN, Ferrari M. Prostate specific antigen in the diagnosis and treatment of adenocarcinoma of the prostate: III. Radiation treated patients. *J Urol.* 1989; 141:1084-1087.

44. Whitmore WF Jr, Hilaris B. Treatment of localized prostate cancer by interstitial $_{125}$I. In: Karr JP, Yamanaka H, eds. *Prostate Cancer: The Second Tokyo Symposium.* New York, NY: Elsevier Science Publishing Co; 1989: 344-360.

45. deKernion JB, Skinner DG. Epidemiology, diagnosis and staging of bladder cancer. In: Skinner DG, deKernion JB, eds. *Genitourinary Cancer.* Philadelphia, Pa: WB Saunders Co; 1978: 213-231.

46. Prout GR Jr. Classification and staging of bladder carcinoma. *Cancer.* 1980; 45(suppl):1832-1841.

47. Smith JA, Whitmore WF Jr. Regional lymph node metastasis from bladder cancer. *J Urol.* 1981; 126:591-593.

48. Whitmore WF Jr, Marshall VF. Radical total cystectomy for cancer of the bladder: 230 consecutive cases 5 years later. *J Urol.* 1962; 87:853-868.

49. Wallace DM, Bloom HJG. The management of deeply infiltrating (T_3) bladder carcinoma: controlled trial of radical radiotherapy versus preoperative radiotherapy and radical cystectomy (first report). *Br J Urol.* 1976; 48:587-594.

50. Coplen DE, Marcus MD, Myers JA, Ratliff TL, Catalona WJ. Long-term followup of patients treated with one or two 6-week courses of intravesical bacillus Calmette-Guerin: analysis of possible predictors of response free of tumor. *J Urol.* 1990; 144:652-657.

51. Soloway MS. Intravesical and systemic chemotherapy in the management of superficial bladder cancer. *Urol Clin North Am.* 1984; 11:623-635.

52. Benson RC Jr. Endoscopic management of bladder cancer with hematoporphyrin derivative phototherapy. *Urol Clin North Am.* 1984; 11:637-642.

53. Sternberg CN, Yagoda A, Scher HI, et al. Methotrexate, vinblastine, doxorubicin and Cisplatin for advanced transitional cell carcinoma of the urothelium: efficacy and patterns of response and relapse. *Cancer.* 1989; 64:2448-2458.

54. Catalona WJ. Urothelial tumors of the urinary tract. In: Walsh PC, Retik AB, Stamey TA, Vaughan ED Jr, eds. *Campbell's Urology.* 6th ed. Philadelphia, Pa: WB Saunders Co; 1992; 2:1094-1158.

55. McDonald JR, Priestly JT. Carcinoma of the renal pelvis: histologic study of 75 cases with special reference to prognosis. *J Urol.* 1944; 51:245-258.

56. D'Angio GJ, Breslow N, Beckwith JB, et al. Treatment of Wilms' tumor: results of the Third National Wilms' Tumor Study. *Cancer.* 1989; 64:349-360.

57. Mesrobian HGJ. Wilms tumor: past, present, future. *J Urol.* 1988; 140:231-238.

58. Farrer JH, Walker AH, Rajfer J. Management of the postpubertal cryptorchid testes: a statistical review. *J Urol.* 1985; 134:1071-1076.

59. Campbell HE. The incidence of malignant growth of the undescended testicle: a reply and reevaluation. *J Urol.* 1959; 81:663-668.

60. Javadpour N. The role of biologic tumor markers in testicular cancer. *Cancer.* 1980; 45(suppl):1755-1761.

61. Wallace N. Lymphography in the management of testicular tumours. *Clin Radiol.* 1969; 20:453-458.

62. Smith RB. Diagnosis and staging of testicular tumors. In: Skinner DG, deKernion JB, eds. *Genitourinary Cancer.* Philadelphia, Pa: WB Saunders Co; 1978: 448-459.

63. Mostofi FK. Pathology of germ cell tumors of testes: a progress report. *Cancer.* 1980; 45(suppl):1735-1754.

64. Thomas GM, Rider WD, Dembo AJ. Seminoma of the testis: results of treatment and patterns of failure after radiation therapy. *Int J Radiat Oncol Biol Phys.* 1982; 8:165-174.

65. Yagoda A, Vugrin D. Theoretical considerations in the treatment of seminoma. *Semin Oncol.* 1979; 6:74-81.

66. Fossa S, Borge L, Aass N, et al. The treatment of advanced metastatic seminoma: experience in 55 cases. *J Clin Oncol.* 1987; 5:1071-1077.

21

BASAL CELL AND SQUAMOUS CELL CARCINOMA OF THE SKIN

Robert J. Friedman, MD, MSc, Darrell S. Rigel, MD, Robert Nossa, BA, Robert Dorf, BA

Basal Cell Carcinoma

Definition

Basal cell carcinoma (BCC), or basal cell epithelioma, is a malignant neoplasm of the skin that arises from the basal cells of the epidermis and its appendages. It is characterized by slow local growth capable of causing extensive tissue destruction. Although metastases are rare, these neoplasms can be fatal if left untreated.

Epidemiology

Basal cell carcinoma is the most common cancer in man, accounting for 75% of all nonmelanoma skin cancers and almost one quarter of all cancers diagnosed in the United States.[1] Basal cell carcinoma occurs primarily on skin exposed to ultraviolet radiation, a fact that has been recognized for many years. It rarely develops in dark skinned persons; when it does, the areas of the head and neck exposed to the sun are affected primarily.[2,3] Although historically there has been a male preponderance, BCC currently affects men only slightly more than women.[1] Once infrequent before the age of 40, BCCs are becoming more common in people still in their 20s. This steady increase is presumably due to changes in fashion and lifestyle, leading to increased sun exposure, possibly coupled with depletion of the ozone layer, which prevents much of the ultraviolet light from reaching earth.[4]

Robert J. Friedman, MD, MSc (Med), Clinical Assistant Professor, Department of Dermatology, NYU School of Medicine, New York University, New York, New York

Darrell S. Rigel, MD, Clinical Associate Professor, Department of Dermatology, NYU School of Medicine, New York University, New York, New York

Robert Nossa, BA, State University of New York at Stony Brook, College of Medicine, Stony Brook, New York

Robert Dorf, BA, Research Fellow, Dermpath Labs, Scarsdale, New York

Pathogenesis

The most frequently implicated factor in the pathogenesis of BCC is exposure of the skin to ultraviolet light (UVL). The most damaging radiation lies in the 290- to 320-nm (UVB) range.[5] Demographically, the people at greatest risk of developing skin cancer are those living near the equator or in ozone-depleted areas such as Norway.[4,6]

Cumulative exposure to UVL over many years is necessary for the development of skin cancer. Therefore, individuals with outdoor professions or extensive outdoor recreation are at risk of BCC.[7] Light- skinned people who tend to burn easily have a definite propensity for acquiring BCC. One study correlates heavy freckling or moles with a diameter of >5 cm in children with a tendency to develop BCC in adulthood.[8] The risk of BCC is substantially decreased in dark-skinned people and those who tan easily.[2,8,9] In mice, the use of UV-absorbing sunscreens suppresses the development of UV-associated cancers of the skin.[10]

Ionizing radiation is an etiologic factor in BCCs with a long latency period.[11] Davis and colleagues stated that the latency period of skin cancer varies inversely with the dose of radiation received.[11] The neoplasm is usually located on the irradiated area. However, facial skin seems to be more susceptible to damage caused by ionizing radiation.[11] As with carcinomas caused by UVL, damage to deoxyribonucleic acid (DNA) probably plays a critical role.[12,13] Chemical factors associated with the development of BCC include arsenic and topically applied nitrogen mustard.

The immune system plays a role in the pathogenesis of skin cancer that is not well understood. Immunosuppressed patients with lymphoma or leukemia,[14] patients who have undergone renal transplants,[1] and nontransplant patients on immunosuppressive medication[15,16] all have marked increases in the incidence of squamous cell carcinoma (SCC), but only a slight variation in BCC development. Whether immune suppression per se affects the biology of BCC is currently not known. Basal cell carcinomas can develop in patients infected with human immunodeficiency virus (HIV)[17,18]; in one patient the metastasis of BCC has been reported.[18]

Biologic Behavior

The stroma is critical for both initiating and maintaining the development of BCC. Transplantations of neoplasms devoid of stroma are usually unsuccessful.[1,19] This stromal dependence is best exemplified by the low incidence rate of metastatic BCC.

Tumor development also depends on a sufficient blood supply. Basal cell carcinomas can elicit angiogenic factors, which account for the telangiectatic vessels characteristically seen on the tumor's surface. Large BCCs often have necrotic centers due to an exceeding radial distance from its blood supply.[1,20] The growth rate of BCCs is generally slow, the result of opposing forces of growth and tumor regression. The dominant phase dictates the rate at which the tumor enlarges.[21] Many studies indicate that collagenase may contribute to the spread of BCC.[22]

Metastatic BCC is rare, with incidence rates varying from 0.0028% to 0.1%.[1,23] It occurs most commonly via lymphatic spread to regional nodes and hematogenous spread to long bones and lungs. When metastasis is present, the primary lesion usually is located on the head and neck area and has been long-standing. Basal cell carcinoma may invade both the vasculature and periosteum. Although the adenoid and basosquamous (metatypical) variants of BCC metastasize most often, all the histologic subtypes have the potential to do so.

In contrast to low rates of metastasis, BCCs are locally invasive and destructive. Basal cell carcinoma follows the path of least resistance, which explains why invasion of bone, cartilage, and muscle is a late event. When an invasive BCC reaches these areas it tends to migrate along the perichondrium, periosteum, fascia, or tarsal plate.[24-26] This type of spread accounts for high recurrence rates on the eyelid, nose, and scalp.[24,27-29]

Embryonic fusion planes offer little resistance and can lead to deep invasion and tumor spread with extraordinarily high rates of recurrence following therapy. The most susceptible areas include the inner canthus, philtrum, mid-lower chin, nasolabial groove, preauricular area, and the retroauricular sulcus.[24-26,30]

Basal cell carcinomas usually do not penetrate the subcutis because of an insufficient vascular supply. Perineural spread is uncommon and usually seen with recurrent aggressive lesions.[31,32] The patient may feel numbness, tingling, or pain, and experience motor weakness or paralysis.

Clinical Manifestations

Nodular (or noduloulcerative) BCC is the most common type of primary lesion. It usually presents as a flesh-colored or pink translucent nodule with superimposed telangiectasis. Ulceration may accompany growth of the tumor (Fig 21-1—Color plate following page 372). The occasional presence of melanin accounts for the variable amount of visible pigment and may make the lesion appear black, resembling a melanocytic neoplasm (Fig 21-2—Color plate following page 372). Over many years, these tumors can grow and invade deeply, destroying an eyelid, nose, or ear (Fig 21-3—Color plate following page 372). The destruction may be so extensive that the ulcer's primary cause is not easily discernible. Close inspection of the ulcer's periphery, however, often reveals a pearly telangiectatic rolled border.

The superficial multicentric variant of BCC is most often found on the trunk and extremities, although it may also occur in the head and neck region. The lesion is usually an erythematous, slightly scaly patch that typically has a rolled translucent border. Atrophy and pigmentary alterations appear in areas in which regression has occurred. Lesions vary in size and may be single or multiple. Their appearance may resemble benign inflammatory processes such as nummular dermatitis and psoriasis. Early radial growth is responsible for the large size of these tumors; however, they also can penetrate vertically, forming nodules and ulceration. A high recurrence rate following surgical removal is caused by persistent subclinical centrifugal extension of the lesions.

The morpheaform type of BCC presents as an indurated sclerotic plaque of varying size with occasional telangiectases, resembling a lesion of morphea (Fig 21-4—Color plate following page 372). Clinically and histologically it can also mimic metastatic carcinoma. Morpheaform BCCs infiltrate aggressively and subclinically, tending to recur after seemingly adequate treatment. Cystic BCCs are characterized by clear bluish cystic lesions containing a clear fluid that can be expressed with manipulation. When present on the face they resemble hidrocystomas. Occasionally the cystic changes that can be seen histologically are quite subtle clinically, thus giving the tumor the appearance of a common nodular BCC.

Basal cell carcinoma with squamous metaplasia (basosquamous or metatypical carcinoma) is a histologic classification, although it is clinically more aggressive than other BCCs. Some believe that its characteristics are more like those of squamous cell carcinoma, with an increased incidence of metastasis and postoperative recurrences.[33,34] The primary tumor in such cases is probably composed of relatively more squamoid cells. The estimated incidence of metastasis for this type of BCC is 9.7%.[33]

There are conflicting opinions about the role of irradiation in the induction of basosquamous carcinoma.[35,36] Some believe that the metatypical histologic features gradually evolve with each successive recurrence of BCC.[33-35]

The fibroepithelioma of Pinkus is a rare variant of BCC usually found on the lower back. The lesion, a firm smooth nodule classically pedunculated, resembles a fibroma.

Staging

The American Joint Committee on Cancer includes a TNM (tumor, node, metastasis) staging system that applies to both basal cell and squamous cell carcinoma, with instructions for clinical and pathologic staging of the disease.[37] *Clinical* staging is based on physical examination and palpation of the lesion and lymph nodes. In the case of fixed lesions, underlying bony structures should be imaged, especially if these lesions occur on the scalp. *Pathologic* staging requires resection of the entire site and confirmation of any lymph node involvement. For both clinical and pathologic staging, complete excision of the site and microscopic verification is necessary to determine the histologic type (Table 21-1).

Treatment Overview

The most important goal in the management of a patient with BCC is complete elimination of the lesion. Also important are the need for conservation of normal structure and function as well as an optimal cosmetic result. Although often stressed, the latter should not take precedence over the total removal of the lesion, since in the long run the cosmetic defect would be even larger if more procedures were required. One study revealed a high incidence of recurrent BCCs in young women for whom cosmetic outcome was given priority over adequate treatment.[38]

Although BCCs enlarge slowly and seldom metastasize, their potential for aggressive local growth should not be underestimated when determining the treatment approach. The decision to perform repeated desiccation and curettage, rather than surgically remove a recurrent BCC, could eventually result in extensive tissue destruction if the tumor depth is not sufficiently appreciated.

The anatomic location and type of tumor also should be considered when selecting the appropriate treatment. A clinician inexperienced in performing the optimal procedure for a particular patient should make a referral to an appropriately skilled expert. When multiple treatment options are suitable, the clinician should select the one with which he or she has the most experience.

Adequate treatment of BCCs requires a good working knowledge of the pathologic pattern of the neoplasm, along with its varying modes of extension. While some BCCs are small and superficial and behave in essentially a "biologically benign" manner as long as they are conservatively removed, others behave more aggressively and require more radical treatment. Examples of the latter include BCCs that

Table 21-1. TNM Staging of Basal Cell and Squamous Cell Carcinoma of the Skin (Excluding Eyelid, Vulva, and Penis)

Primary Tumor (T)

TX	Primary tumor cannot be assessed
T0	No evidence of primary tumor
Tis	Carcinoma in situ
T1	Tumor ≤2 cm in greatest dimension
T2	Tumor >2 cm in greatest dimension but not >5 cm in greatest dimension
T3	Tumor >5 cm in greatest dimension
T4	Tumor invades deep extradermal structures (eg, cartilage, skeletal muscle, or bone)

Note: In the case of multiple simultaneous tumors, the tumor with the highest T category will be classified and the number of separate tumors will be indicated in parentheses; eg, T2(5).

Regional Lymph Nodes (N)

NX	Regional lymph nodes cannot be assessed
N0	No regional lymph node metastasis
N1	Regional lymph node metastasis

Distant Metastasis (M)

MX	Presence of distant metastasis cannot be assessed
M0	No distant metastasis
M1	Distant metastasis

Stage Grouping

Stage 0	Tis	N0	M0
Stage I	T1	N0	M0
Stage II	T2	N0	M0
	T3	N0	M0
Stage III	T4	N0	M0
	Any T	N1	M0
Stage IV	Any T	Any N	M1

Histopathologic Grade (G)

GX	Grade cannot be assessed
G1	Well differentiated
G2	Moderately differentiated
G3	Poorly differentiated
G4	Undifferentiated

From American Joint Committee on Cancer.[37]

ulcerate early in their evolution, particularly those located on the nasolabial fold or ear. Further, basal cell carcinomas having infiltrative (morpheic) features and those that invade deeper structures such as cartilage or bone require wider, deeper, and generally more extensive surgical extirpation.

Excisional surgery, cryosurgery, and curettage with and without electrodesiccation often can be used for circumscribed, noninfiltrating BCCs. Mohs micrographic surgery (microscopically controlled excisional surgery) is the method of choice for most recurrent BCCs and for those with a morpheaform pattern, particularly if the tumor is located on the face. Radiotherapy is best suited for older patients, in particular those with extensive lesions and those with lesions on the ear, lower limbs, or eyelids. Radiotherapy is not indicated for recurrent lesions or morpheaform lesions.

Prevention is significant in the management of skin cancer patients, who should be informed about the potential hazards of excessive sun exposure and the importance of regular sunscreen use.

Curettage and Electrodesiccation

Curettage and electrodesiccation is the method dermatologists most commonly use in the treatment of BCCs. Some authors contend that the procedure should be repeated a fixed number of times.[39,40] However, treating deeper than is required to eradicate the tumor will only contribute to poor cosmesis. Some investigators have omitted electrodesiccation to optimize the cosmetic result and achieved cure rates only slightly lower than with the combination of curettage and electrodesiccation.[41] Although the omission decreases the incidence of hypertrophic scarring, it does not prevent postinflammatory pigmentary alterations.

Cure rates using curettage and electrodesiccation have been reported as high,[40-42] but only certain lesions are amenable to this form of therapy. Curettage and electrodesiccation should not be considered for BCCs arising in areas characterized by a high rate of recurrence (eg, eyelids, nose, lips, ears, scalp, temple, and embryonic fusion planes) because there is no definitive proof that the tumor is destroyed. Silverman and co-workers stated that BCCs <6 mm in diameter regardless of anatomic site are effectively treated by curettage and electrodesiccation.[43] Alternative forms of treatment should be considered for lesions >1 cm in diameter.[42]

Excision

Surgical excision provides a specimen that can be histologically evaluated. If performed skillfully, it can produce a cosmetically good result and speedy healing. Theoretically, excision is appropriate for most BCCs but it takes more time and requires more experience than electrodesiccation and curettage. It may also sacrifice normal tissue in the process. The cure rates are inferior to those for Mohs surgery in the treatment of recurrent BCCs,[44] morpheaform BCCs,[45] some large superficial multicentric BCCs (SMBCCs),[46] and BCCs in high-risk areas.[47] Wolf and Zitelli have shown that for nonmorpheaform BCCs with a distinct border and a diameter ≤2 cm, 4-mm clear margins were necessary to eliminate 98% of the lesions.[48] They reported that the subclinical extension of the neoplasms was not uniform in all directions; in BCCs >2 cm in diameter, subclinical spread was so irregular that the investigators could not offer advice regarding an appropriate margin.

The question as to the proper depth of the excision remains unanswered. For small primary BCCs, excision into fat is generally appropriate since spread into the subcutis is rare. However, large, recurrent, or high-risk BCCs may infiltrate deeper into the subcutaneous tissue.

Mohs Micrographic Surgery

Mohs micrographic surgery permits the best histologic verification of complete removal and allows maximum conservation of tissue.[49,50] It is the preferred treatment for large penetrating tumors; for morpheaform, recurrent, poorly delineated, high-risk, and incompletely removed BCCs; and for those sites in which tissue conservation is imperative.[32,44,45,49,50]

Mohs surgery is more time-consuming than routine surgery and is not always as easily accessible. Although this technique was developed to treat the most aggressive BCCs, other surgical specialists may need to be consulted for help either in removing deeply invasive tumors or in repairing the surgical defect.[51,52]

Radiation Therapy

Radiation therapy is helpful in the treatment of some BCCs. Its major advantage is that normal tissue is spared, obviating the need for complicated surgical procedures. It is often preferred for BCCs of the nose, ear, and periocular area since reconstructive surgery is not required and functional integrity (eg, of the lacrimal duct) is preserved.[53,54] Its use offers elderly patients an alternative to a surgical procedure they may not be willing to undergo.[54] Radiation therapy also has been used for palliation in inoperable BCCs and can improve the patient's quality of life.[55] However, it should not be used in young patients because of potential late radiation sequelae.

The 5-year cure rate for primary BCCs treated with radiation is 90% to 95%.[47,53,54] Although one dose of x-ray can adequately treat a small BCC (≤1 cm), appropriate treatment usually consists of fractionated doses given over several sessions to maximize cure and cosmesis.[53,54] The skin of the head and neck endures the effects of radiation therapy better than that of the trunk and extremities. Cure rates for recurrent BCCs are poorer than for primary lesions, probably due to the subclinical spread of the neoplasm.[54]

Complications of radiation therapy include scarring, cutaneous necrosis, and chronic radiation dermatitis.[54,55] Whereas surgical scars improve with time, cosmesis deteriorates after radiation therapy. At 9 to 12 years, only 50% of patients achieve satisfactory cosmetic results.

Cryosurgery

Cryosurgery has become an accepted treatment for certain BCCs. A liquid nitrogen spray unit is required; cotton-tipped swabs in liquid nitrogen are not acceptable. A double freeze-thaw cycle to a tissue temperature of -50°C is required to sufficiently destroy the tumor. A margin of normal-appearing skin also should be frozen to ensure eradication of subclinical disease.[56,57]

Cryosurgery is not advised for BCCs of the scalp. Lesions on the lower legs treated with cryosurgery heal slowly and often yield poor cosmetic results. Cryosurgery is recommended for BCCs of the eyelid because the procedure preserves normal tissue and obviates the need for reconstructive surgery.[57] Potential complications include loss of eyelashes, scarring, hypopigmentation, and increased eyelid thickness. In this anatomic area, cure rates as high as 97% have been reported for BCCs <1 cm in diameter; the cure rate decreases with larger and recurrent lesions. Cure rates for cryosurgery of BCCs in other areas are excellent (97% to 98%) for tumors <2 cm in diameter. Larger tumors and morpheaform, recurrent, and high-risk BCCs are more likely to recur after therapy.[57]

Cryosurgery is not advised for BCCs attached to the periosteum. Patients with blood dyscrasias, dysglobulinemia, cold intolerance, or autoimmune disease, and those who are receiving immunosuppressive therapy or renal dialysis should not receive cryosurgery. Complications include tissue depression, hypertrophic scarring, and postinflammatory pigmentary changes. The occurrence of pain early during the thaw can be avoided by preoperative infiltration of the treatment area with epinephrine-free lidocaine. Blistering, crusting, and swelling also can develop, but these effects usually resolve within a few weeks.

Lasers

The carbon dioxide (CO_2) laser has several advantages over conventional surgery. The sealing of small blood vessels and nerves provides a relatively bloodless surgical field and reduced postoperative pain.[58,59] It can be used in the focused cutting mode or in the defocused vaporizing mode in combination with curettage to treat large or multiple SMBCCs.[59]

Interferon

Interferon has been used as an alternative therapy for noduloulcerative and superficial BCCs. A study of 172 patients receiving intralesional injections of interferon alfa-2b resulted in an 81% cure rate after a follow-up period of 1 year.[60] Single doses of 1.5 million IU were administered 3 times a week for 3 weeks, resulting in a total dose of 13.5 million IU. Attempts using lower doses were unsuccessful. Side effects from this therapy include fever, malaise, myalgias, chills, transient leukopenia, and itching at the site of injection.

Retinoids

Experience with the use of retinoids is limited, most often in patients with the basal cell nevus syndrome.[61,62] Partial regression of BCC has resulted from the use of 4.5 mg/kg/day of isotretinoin and 1 mg/kg/day of etretinate. High-dose isotretinoin (1.5 mg/kg/day) has a preventive effect.[1,61,63] However, side effects limit the use of these agents for long periods, and discontinuation of therapy can lead to relapse.

Chemotherapy

Chemotherapy is appropriate for locally aggressive or metastatic tumors. Disseminated disease is otherwise associated with a poor prognosis, with an average survival of 10 to 20 months.[34,64] A complete systemic workup is required when evaluating a patient for metastasis. This includes a thorough medical history, physical examination, complete blood counts, liver profile, chest x-ray, bone and liver scans, and computed tomographic (CT) scans, when appropriate.

For metastatic disease limited to the regional nodes, surgery with or without radiation is indicated.[65] Systemic chemotherapy, occasionally in combination with radiation, should be used in cases with more extensive metastases, including those involving bone. Cisplatin, bleomycin, cyclophosphamide, 5-fluorouracil, and vinblastine have been studied; cisplatin has been the most effective and is associated with the longest remission.[65] Cisplatin, doxorubicin, and radiation therapy can achieve palliation in widely disseminated or inoperable BCC.

Follow-up

It is imperative to regularly examine patients with BCC. Although most recurrences appear within 5 years, many can develop later. Subsequent new primary BCCs can also appear; 20% to 30% develop within 1 year of treatment of the original lesion.[66,67]

Finally, it is important to advise patients to avoid excessive sun exposure and to apply a sunscreen with a sun protective factor (SPF) of 15 at regular intervals whenever they are exposed to direct or reflected sunlight.

Squamous Cell Carcinoma

Definition

Squamous cell carcinoma is a malignant tumor of the keratinizing cells of the epidermis. SCC has a greater propensity than BCC to metastasize to regional lymph nodes and distant sites.

Epidemiology

Squamous cell carcinoma is the second most common skin cancer in humans, with nearly 100,000 cases diagnosed in the US each year. It is a disease of older people, with the risk of occurrence increasing dramatically with age.[68,69] Men outnumber women in ratios varying by study between 1.4 to 1 and 3.1 to 1.[70,71] In a large retrospective study, the mean ages at diagnosis of SCC were 68.1 and 72.7 years for men and women, respectively.[72] Most studies reported very few, if any, occurrences of SCC under the age of 40.[73]

Many studies have effectively proven that SCC depends on the total accumulated dose of solar radiation (Fig 21-5—Color plate following page 372).[71,74,75] The relative risk of SCC increases between 3 and 5.5 times for individuals who are exposed to excessive solar radiation.[74] It is also clear that skin pigmentation protects against the induction of skin cancer. People of Celtic descent, with fair complexions, poor tanning ability, and a predisposition to sunburn, are at increased risk for developing SCC. Marks and coworkers stated that chronic sun exposure in childhood and adolescence is directly related to solar keratoses and subsequent SCC in adulthood.[75]

It has been suggested that the use of oral psoralen and ultraviolet A (UVA) radiation for the treatment of psoriasis may be associated with the development of SCC in these patients.[76,77] In the past few years, commercial tanning booths designed for the year-round maintenance of a "beautiful tan" have proliferated. The lamps in most tanning booths emit primarily in the UVA spectrum.[78] In a study by Van Weelden and associates, UVA was proven to be carcinogenic in mice.[79] However, no study has conclusively found a correlation between UVA and cancer in a human model. The UVA spectrum has also been found to induce alterations in the immune system.[78] It remains to be seen whether the incidence of SCC in tanning booth patrons will increase. Other predisposing factors for SCC are exposure to chemical carcinogens (arsenic and organic hydrocarbons) and ionizing radiation.[72]

Pathogenesis

The factors that initiate or promote the development of SCC are similar to those for BCC. In a recent review of 106 patients, the causes of the SCC included previous exposure to radiation (notably on the hands of radiologists and dentists), burn scars, chronic inflammatory dermatoses, ulcers, osteomyelitis, and arsenic ingestion.[73] The evidence for an association with sunlight (UVL) is even stronger for SCC than for BCC.[74] The rate at which solar keratoses undergo malignant transformation has been estimated to be as high as 20%.[80] However, Marks and colleagues demonstrated that the risk of malignant transformation of solar keratosis to SCC within 1 year was <1 in 1,000.[81] Heritable conditions associated with SCC include xeroderma pigmentosum, and oculocutaneous albinism. In addition, SCC may develop in areas of chronic inflammation, such as lesions of discoid lupus erythematosus, chronic osteomyelitis, acne conglobata, lupus vulgaris, hidradenitis suppurativa, pilonidal sinus, thermal burns, and leg ulcers.[82-84]

Immune suppression also may play a role in pathogenesis. Patients receiving immunosuppressive therapy and renal transplant patients are prone to SCC.[15,16] Skin cancers in these patients appear primarily on sun-exposed skin. This correlation suggests that immune suppression and UVL act as cofactors in the development of SCC. People infected with HIV tend to have significantly higher occurrences of SCC.[85] However, the exact correlation between HIV and incidence of SCC has not yet been determined.

An animal model has been developed in which UVB can induce a selective state of immunosuppression that allows tumors to persist.[86] The UVL exposure appears to interfere with antigen processing by Langerhans cells, which in turn gives rise to T suppressor cells that lead to a state of immune tolerance.

Recent research has focused on the role of human papillomavirus (HPV), specifically HPV-5, HPV-16, and HPV-18, in the development of SCC.[87] Eliezri and associates found a direct correlation between the venereal spread of HPV-16 and the initiation of SCC.[88]

Biologic Behavior

The biologic behavior of SCC is determined by a number of variables. The overall invasiveness and depth of the neoplasm is significant when determining the risk of recurrence. Only SCCs that penetrate to the reticular dermis and subcutis recur. Immerman and co-workers observed a 20% incidence of recurrence in 86 patients with invasive SCC.[89] Patients with moderately or poorly differentiated neoplasms had a greater degree of recurrence.

Dzubow and colleagues found that in both sexes, lower extremities were the most likely site of recurrence after Mohs surgery.[90]

Squamous cell carcinoma in situ includes Bowen's disease, erythroplasia of Queyrat, and, some believe, bowenoid papulosis. Squamous cell carcinoma in situ also may arise in association with preexisting actinic/arsenical keratosis. These lesions are considered "biologically benign," without competence for metastasis, as long as they are completely removed or otherwise destroyed.

Invasive SCC can metastasize. The most common type arises on sun-damaged skin, often associated with actinic keratosis and solar elastosis. The incidence of metastasis of such lesions is low (3% to 5%). A higher incidence (10% to 30%) is associated with SCCs arising on mucosal surface (eg, lip, external genitalia) and on sites of prior injury (eg, burn sites, other scars, vaccination sites, and sites of chronic ulceration).

The tendency for regional lymph node metastasis is also variable. Tumors arising in areas of chronic inflammation—Bowen's disease, discoid lupus erythematosus, lichen sclerosus et atrophicus, chronic osteomyelitis, radiation dermatitis, chronic draining sinuses, and ulcers—have a 10% to 30% rate of metastasis.[91] The incidence of metastasis from SCC not due to preexisting inflammatory or degenerative conditions varies from 0.5% to 16%.[92] Although actinically induced tumors behave in a more biologically benign fashion than de novo SCCs, all lesions have the potential to become invasive locally and to metastasize to draining lymph nodes. Friedman and co-workers demonstrated that all trunk and extremity primary SCCs that later developed local or nodal recurrence were at least 4 mm deep and penetrated into the reticular dermis or subcutis.[93] Every fatal lesion was at least 10 mm deep and invaded the subcutis.

The extent of cellular differentiation also determines the metastatic potential. Tumors that invade regional lymph nodes tend to be more anaplastic than those that have not metastasized.

Squamous cell carcinomas arising in nonglabrous mucocutaneous sites (lip, vulva, penis, perianal area) are more likely to metastasize than those involving glabrous areas of the skin.[91] The incidence of metastasis for SCC varies from 0.5% for patients with primary cutaneous SCC to 11% for patients with mucocutaneous labial lesions. Some 10% to 40% of cases of SCC develop at sites of preexisting inflammatory conditions. Squamous cell carcinomas developing at burn scar sites reportedly have a metastatic rate of 18%, those with chronic osteomyelitis a rate of 31%, those induced by radiation a 20% rate, and those arising in discoid lupus erythematosus a 30% rate.[91,94-96] Tumors are more likely to disseminate to regional lymph nodes than to organs, although intravascular metastases to viscera have appeared in as many as 5% to 10% of all metastatic cases.[97]

Distant metastases may also occur via perineural involvement. In one study,[98] 14% of SCCs showed perineural spread, while other investigators have found rates as high as 36%.[99] Regional lymph node and distant metastases were increased in patients with perineural involvement. Squamous cell carcinomas of the head and neck may metastasize to cervical lymph nodes and distantly to the central nervous system, the latter either hematogenously or via the perineural space, which directly connects to the subarachnoid space. Areas of the body that tend to develop SCCs with neural involvement include the midface, lip, and areas involving the mandibular branch of the trigeminal nerve.[98] Although these patients are generally asymptomatic, they show a lower 10-year survival (23% vs 88%) and a higher local recurrence rate (47% vs 7.3%) than those without neural involvement.[98] Despite poor prognosis, Mohs micrographic surgery can occasionally achieve successful treatment in such patients.[100]

Clinical Manifestations

Squamous cell carcinoma occurs within, and may be confined to, the epidermis. Intraepidermal, or in situ, SCC may occur in preexisting thermal keratosis, hydrocarbon keratosis, and arsenical keratosis. There are morphologic variants of in situ SCC, including Bowen's disease, bowenoid papulosis, and erythroplasia of Queyrat.[84] Intraepidermal SCC remains within the epidermis for a variable time, but may breach the dermoepidermal junction and become an invasive SCC with the propensity to metastasize.

An intraepidermal carcinoma or a premalignant lesion usually precedes invasive SCC clinically. Squamous cell carcinoma other than that arising from an in situ tumor is rarely seen on skin that appears normal.[84] Although there are no specific characteristics on which to base a definitive diagnosis of SCC, most lesions consist of plaques that may be covered with scale (Fig 21-6—Color plate following page 372), crust, or ulceration. They usually lack the pearly rolled border and superficial telangiectases found in BCCs. Although most are reddish, SCCs that are hyperkeratotic or that occur on mucocutaneous surfaces may be white. The clinical differential diagnosis includes other tumors (BCC, keratoacanthoma, adnexal neoplasm); precancerous lesions (actinic keratosis, Bowen's disease); and some inflammatory diseases (psoriasis, infections, pseudo-epitheliomatous hyperplasia).

Squamous cell carcinoma of the nose was studied by Binder and colleagues, who found that 21 of 114 patients had involvement of underlying cartilage and bone.[101] In 77% of these 21 individuals, lesions were >3 cm in diameter and symptoms had been present for >1 year. The incidence of nodal metastasis in this study was 8%.[101] Other studies have shown metastatic rates as high as 21%.[35] Every patient in Binder's study who developed metastases had involvement of the cervical lymph nodes (ipsilateral in 6 cases, bilateral in 2, and contralateral in 1), had symptoms for at least 1 year, and had cartilage or bone involvement; most had a primary lesion >3 cm in diameter. Only one patient developed distant metastases.

The majority of SCCs on the lip arise from the lower lip in an area of chronic actinic cheilitis. The reported risk of metastasis from SCC of the lip has ranged from 5% to 37%.[84]

Squamous cell carcinoma can also occur on the nail bed, nail folds, and matrix (Fig 21-7—Color plate following page 372); >100 cases had been reported by 1984.[102] The patient usually has symptoms of swelling, redness, and discomfort. If the nail matrix is affected, atrophy or loss of the nail plate can result. The differential diagnosis of these lesions includes paronychia, pyogenic granuloma, verrucae, nail dystrophies, and tumors such as glomus, keratoacanthoma, and melanoma. There have been two reports of metastasis to regional lymph nodes from subungual SCC, while the incidence is 30% for hand tumors that have extended to bone or tendon.[102]

Small SCCs appearing on the trunk and extremities are easily treated, although advanced lesions are aggressive. Factors associated with a poor prognosis included a low degree of histologic differentiation, location on the sacrum or perineum, and degree of lymphatic metastasis. SCCs of the trunk and extremities usually spread to the axillary and inguinal lymph nodes, whereas hand and foot tumors metastasize to epitrochlear and popliteal nodes, respectively. Cutaneous and subcutaneous metastatic nodules were found in transit between the primary lesion and the draining lymph nodes in 11 patients. Fourteen patients showed evidence of visceral metastasis. These were curable surgically in the absence of bone and lymph node involvement. There was no therapeutic advantage to prophylactic node dissection.

Squamous cell carcinoma of the penis is rare; its incidence is <1% of all cancers in males.[103] Incidence rates are higher in Uganda, Mexico, China, India, and Puerto Rico. The patient is invariably uncircumcised and often has phimosis and poor hygiene. SCC of the penis may develop within lesions of leukoplakia, erythroplasia of Queyrat, and balanitis xerotica obliterans. Verrucous carcinoma of the penis (Buschke-Lowenstein tumor) is histologically well differentiated, with features of a wart, but it behaves clinically like an aggressive SCC; it may induce malignant transformation of the tumor and development of metastasis.

Penile SCC usually occurs between the ages of 40 and 60. It may present with a penile nodule, ulceration, discharge, edema, or inguinal adenopathy. The most common site of involvement is the glans (Fig 21-8—Color plate following page 372). However, it can develop anywhere along the shaft. Metastasis to inguinal lymph nodes has been reported in 33% to 50% of patients at the time of first examination.[84]

Verrucous carcinoma is a subtype of low-grade SCC that can affect the cutaneous and mucosal surfaces.[104,105] This lesion occurs most often in middle-aged and elderly men. It is characterized by a warty exophytic neoplasm containing sinuses with a greasy, malodorous discharge. In a study of 46 patients with cutaneous verrucous carcinoma, only one developed inguinal lymph node metastasis, and no patient had disseminated or fatal disease after a 19-year follow-up period.[105]

Staging

See staging section under "Basal Cell Carcinoma."

Treatment Overview

Many of the treatments for BCC are appropriate for SCC. The type of therapy should be selected on the basis of size of the lesion, anatomic location, depth of invasion, degree of cellular differentiation, and history of previous treatment.

There are essentially three approaches to treatment of SCC: (1) curettage and electrodesiccation/cryosurgery; (2) excisional surgery/Mohs micrographically controlled surgery; and (3) radiotherapy. Curettage and electrodesiccation can be used for small lesions arising in solar-altered (keratotic) skin. There is a 5-year cure rate of >95%. Excisional surgery is indicated for larger, ill-defined lesions, as well as for more extensive lesions that have invaded deeper structures. Rarely, regional lymph node dissection may be required in SCCs that have metastasized there. Radiotherapy is indicated for head and neck SCCs in which there is no spread to bone or cartilage and there is no evidence of metastasis.

Curettage and Electrodesiccation

Squamous cell carcinomas <2 cm in diameter are amenable to this form of therapy. Honeycutt and Jansen reported a 99% cure rate for 281 SCCs after a 4-year follow-up.[106] Two recurrences were noted in lesions >2 cm in diameter. However, in a separate study involving 29 cases of SCC on the lower lip, there were three recurrences, all in lesions <2 cm in diameter. Others have reported 5-year cures ranging from 97% to 98.8% in selected cases.[107,108]

Excision

Surgical excision is another well-accepted treatment modality. Freeman and co-workers reported a 91% 5-year cure rate in a high-risk group of 91 patients with SCC not amenable to curettage and electrodesiccation.[107] Lesions of the scalp, forehead, and distal extremities >3 cm in diameter are best treated by excision because of the poor healing qualities of the thin layers of subcutaneous tissue overlying bone.[84] Carcinomas of the eyelid and lip commissures are usually excised because function and cosmesis can be better preserved. Carcinomas of the penis, vulva, and anus are usually treated by excision because of the frequent need for lymph node dissection and because of poor tolerance of these areas to irradiation.[84] Surgical excision is the treatment of choice for verrucous carcinoma.[109,110]

Mohs Micrographic Surgery

Mohs surgery is useful for SCCs that fall into one of the following groups: (1) residual SCC following recurrence of a previously treated lesion; (2) recurrent SCC; (3) clinically ill-defined SCCs; (4) SCCs invading bone or cartilage; (5) carcinoma arising in late radiation dermatitis; and (6) other SCCs arising in areas at high risk for recurrence.

Mohs micrographic surgery accomplished a 94.8% 5-year cure rate for primary cutaneous SCC.[111] The cure rate varied with the degree of histologic differentiation (98.9% for grade I to 45.2% for grade IV) and lesion size (99.5% for lesions <1 cm to 58.9% for lesions >3 cm in diameter). Successful treatment also depended on anatomic location: forehead, 84.3%; leg, 85.6%; and foot and toes, 71.4%. Dzubow and colleagues reported on 414 cases of primary cutaneous SCC and found a 5-year mortality-table-adjusted cure rate of 93.3%.[90] The number of surgical stages correlated significantly with recurrence rate. This modality is especially useful when the preservation of the maximum amount of tissue for function and cosmesis is necessary.[112,113]

Radiation Therapy

As with BCC, radiation therapy is excellent for elderly patients with SCC who are unwilling to undergo surgery. It is especially suitable for lesions of the nose, lip, eyelid, and region of the canthus. Radiation therapy in a fractionated dose schedule is associated with a better cosmetic result and probably an enhanced therapeutic effect.

The use of radiation therapy for verrucous carcinoma has been controversial because of the potential for anaplastic transformation and/or a high rate of metastasis.[114]

Cryotherapy

Cryotherapy for SCC is useful in selected patients. Lesions having a diameter between 0.5 and 2.0 cm with well-defined borders are amenable to this modality. This technique boasts exceptional cosmetic results and has achieved 5-year cure rates as high as 96.1%.[115]

Other Modalities

New or experimental treatments include the neodymium-yttrium-aluminum-garnet (Nd:YAG) laser, CO_2 laser, photodynamic therapy, retinoids, 5-fluorouracil given either topically or systematically, and a combination of cisplatin and 5-fluorouracil.[116-118]

Follow-up

Invasive SCC can be a potentially lethal neoplasm and warrants close follow-up. The association between solar radiation and the development of SCC is firmly established and it is important to advise patients to avoid excessive exposure to the sun and to always use a sun block with an SPF ≥15.

References

1. Miller SJ. Biology of basal cell carcinoma. *J Am Acad Dermatol.* 1991;24:1-13, 161-175.
2. Brody I. Contributions to the histogenesis of basal cell carcinoma. *J Ultrastruct Res.* 1970;33:60-79.
3. Graham HD, Mentz HA, Butcher RB. Basal cell carcinoma of the head and neck. *J La State Med Soc.* 1989;141:11-15.
4. Moan J, Dahlback A, Henrikson T, Magnus K. Biological amplification factor for sunlight-induced nonmelanoma skin cancer at high latitudes. *Cancer Res.* 1989;49:5207-5212.
5. Black HS, Chan JT. Experimental ultraviolet light carcinogenesis. *Photochem Photobiol.* 1977;29:183-199.
6. Fears TR, Scotto J, Schneiderman MA. Mathematical models of age and ultraviolet effects on the incidence of skin cancer among whites in the United States. *Am J Epidemiol.* 1977;105:420-427.
7. Marks R, Jolley D, Dorevitch AP, Selwood TS. The incidence of non-melanocytic skin cancers in an Australian population: results of a five-year prospective study. *Med Aust.* 1989;150:475-478.
8. Kricker A, Armstrong BK, English DR, Heenan PJ. Pigmentary and cutaneous risk factors for non-melanocytic skin cancer: a case-control study. *Int J Cancer.* 1991;48:650-662.
9. Vitaliano PP, Urbach F. Relative importance of risk factors in nonmelanoma carcinoma. *Arch Dermatol.* 1980;116:454-456.
10. Kligman LH, Akin FJ, Klingman AM. Sunscreens prevent ultraviolet photocarcinogenesis. *J Am Acad Dermatol.* 1980;3:30-35.
11. Davis MM, Hanke W, Zollinger TW, Montebello JF, Hornback NB, Norins AL. Skin cancer in patients with chronic radiation dermatitis. *J Am Acad Dermatol.* 1989;20:608-616.
12. Lehmann AR, Kirk-Bell S, Arlett CF, et al. Repair of ultraviolet light damage in a variety of human fibroblast cell strains. *Cancer Res.* 1977;37:904-910.
13. Kraemer KH. Cancer prone genodermatoses and DNA repair. *Prog Dermatol.* 1981;15:2-6.
14. Cohen C. Multiple cutaneous carcinomas and lymphomas of the skin. *Arch Dermatol.* 1980;116:687-689.
15. Halgrimson CG, Penn I, Booth A, et al. Eight to ten-year follow-up in early cases of renal homotransplantation. *Transplant Proc.* 1973;5:787-791.
16. Marshall V. Premalignant and malignant skin tumors in immunosuppressed patients. *Transplantation.* 1974; 17:272-275.
17. Fisher BK, Warner LC. Cutaneous manifestations of the acquired immunodeficiency syndrome: update 1987. *Int J Dermatol.* 1987;26:615-630.
18. Sitz KV, Koppen M, Johnson DF. Metastatic basal cell carcinoma in acquired immunodeficiency syndrome-related complex. *JAMA.* 1987;257:340-343.
19. Van Scott EJ, Reinertson RP. The modulating influence of stromal environment on epithelial cells studied in human autotransplants. *J Invest Dermatol.* 1961;36:109-131.
20. Wolf JE Jr, Hubler WR Jr. Tumor angiogenic factor and human skin tumors. *Arch Dermatol.* 1975;111:321-327.
21. Franchimont C, Pierard GE, van Cauwenberge D, Damseaux M, Lapiere CM. Episodic progression and regres-

sion of basal cell carcinomas. *Br J Dermatol.* 1982;106:305-310.

22. Barsky SH, Grossman DA, Bhuta S. Desmoplastic basal cell carcinomas possess unique basement membrane-degrading properties. *J Invest Dermatol.* 1987;88:324-329.

23. Von Domarus H, Stevens PJ. Metastatic basal cell carcinoma: report of five cases and review of 170 cases in the literature. *J Am Acad Dermatol.* 1984;10:1043-1060.

24. Mora RG, Robins P. Basal-cell carcinoma in the center of the face: special diagnostic, prognostic, and therapeutic considerations. *J Dermatol Surg Oncol.* 1978;4:315-321.

25. Bailin PL, Levine HL, Wood BG, Tucker HM. Cutaneous carcinoma of the auricular and periauricular region. *Arch Otolaryngol Head Neck Surg.* 1980;106:692-696.

26. Levine HL, Bailin PL. Basal cell carcinoma of the head and neck: identification of the high risk patient. *Laryngoscope.* 1980;90:955-961.

27. Binstock JH, Stegman SJ, Tromovitch TA. Large, aggressive basal-cell carcinomas of the scalp. *J Dermatol Surg Oncol.* 1981;7:565-569.

28. Roenigk RK, Ratz JL, Bailin PL, et al. Trends in the presentation and treatment of basal cell carcinomas. *J Dermatol Surg Oncol.* 1986;12:860-986.

29. Rosen HM. Periorbital basal cell carcinoma requiring ablative craniofacial surgery. *Arch Dermatol.* 1987;123:376-378.

30. Gullane PJ. Extensive facial malignancies: concepts and management. *J Otolaryngol.* 1986;15:44-48.

31. Mark G. Basal cell carcinoma with intraneural invasion. *Cancer.* 1977;40:2181-2187.

32. Hanke CW, Wolf RL, Hochman SA, O'Brien JJ. Perineural spread of basal-cell carcinoma. *J Dermatol Surg Oncol.* 1983;9:742-747.

33. Borel DM. Cutaneous basosquamous carcinoma: review of the literature and report of 35 cases. *Arch Pathol.* 1973;95:293-297.

34. Farmer ER, Helwig EB. Metastatic basal cell carcinoma: a clinicopathologic study of 17 cases. *Cancer.* 1980;46:748-757.

35. Conley J. Cancer of the skin of the nose. *Arch Otolaryngol.* 1966;84:55-60.

36. Schuller DE, Berg JW, Sherman G. Krause CJ. Cutaneous basosquamous carcinoma of the head and neck: a comparative analysis. *Otolaryngol Head Neck Surg.* 1979;87:420-427.

37. Beahrs OH, Henson DE, Hutter RVP, Kennedy BJ, eds. *American Joint Committee on Cancer Manual for Staging of Cancer.* 4th ed. Philadelphia, Pa: JB Lippincott Co; 1992.

38. Robins P, Albom MJ. Recurrent basal cell carcinoma in young women. *J Dermatol Surg Oncol.* 1975;1:49-51.

39. Knox JM, Freeman RG, Heaton CL. Curettage and electrodesiccation in the treatment of skin cancer. *South Med J.* 1962;55:1212-1215.

40. Kopf AW, Bart RS, Schrager D, Lazar M, Popkin GL. Curettage-electrodesiccation treatment of basal cell carcinomas. *Arch Dermatol.* 1977;113:439-443.

41. McDaniel WE. Therapy for basal cell epitheliomas by curettage only: further study. *Arch Dermatol.* 1983;119:901-903.

42. Salasche SJ. Status of curettage and desiccation in the treatment of primary basal cell carcinoma. *J Am Acad Dermatol.* 1984;10:285.

43. Silverman MK, Kopf AW, Grin CM, Bart RS, Levenstein MJ. Recurrence rates of treated basal cell carcinomas II curettage and electrodesiccation. *J Dermatol Surg Oncol.* 1991;17:720-726.

44. Menn H, Robins P, Kopf AW, Bart RS. The recurrent basal cell epithelioma: a study of 100 cases of recurrent, retreated basal epitheliomas. *Arch Dermatol.* 1971;103:628-631.

45. Salasche SJ, Amonette RA. Morpheaform basal-cell epitheliomas: a study of subclinical extensions in a series of 51 cases. *J Dermatol Surg Oncol.* 1981;7:387-394.

46. Sloane JP. The value of typing basal cell carcinomas in predicting recurrence after surgical excision. *Br J Dermatol.* 1977;96:127-132.

47. Dublin N, Kopf AW. Multivariate risk score for recurrence of cutaneous basal cell carcinomas. *Arch Dermatol.* 1983;119:373-377.

48. Wolf JE, Zitelli JA. Surgical margins for basal cell carcinoma. *Arch Dermatol.* 1987;123:340-344.

49. Robins P. Chemosurgery: my 15 years of experience. *J Dermatol Surg Oncol.* 1981; 7:779-789.

50. Rowe DE, Carroll RJ, Day CL Jr. Mohs surgery is the treatment of choice for recurrent (previously treated) basal cell carcinoma. *J Dermatol Surg Oncol.* 1989;15:424-431.

51. Riefkohl R, Pollack S, Georgiade GS. A rationale for the treatment of difficult basal cell and squamous cell carcinomas of the skin. *Ann Plast Surg.* 1985;15:99-104.

52. Baker SR, Swanson NA, Grekin RC. An interdisciplinary approach to the management of basal cell carcinoma of the head and neck. *J Dermatol Surg Oncol.* 1987;13:1095-1106.

53. Chahbaziam CM, Brown GS. Radiation therapy for carcinoma of the skin of the face and neck: special considerations. *JAMA.* 1980;244:1135.

54. Gladstein AH, Kopf AW, Bart RS. Radiotherapy of cutaneous malignancies. In: Goldschmidt H, ed. *Physical Modalities in Dermatologic Therapy: Radiotherapy, Electrosurgery, Phototherapy, Cryosurgery.* New York, NY: Springer-Verlag; 1978:95-121.

55. Hunter RD, Easson EC, Pointon RCS, eds. *Skin in the Radiotherapy of Malignant Disease.* New York, NY: Springer-Verlag; 1987:135.

56. McLean DI, Haynes HA, McCarthy PL, Baden HP. Cryotherapy of basal-cell carcinoma by a simple method of standardized freeze-thaw cycles. *J Dermatol Surg Oncol.* 1978;4:175-177.

57. Zacarian SA. Cryosurgery for Cancer of the Skin. In: *Cryosurgery for Skin Cancer and Cutaneous Disorders.* St Louis, Mo: CV Mosby Co; 1985.

58. Sacchini V, Lovo GF, Arioli N, Nava M, Bandieramonte G. Carbon dioxide laser in scalp tumor surgery. *Lasers Surg Med.* 1984;4:261-269.

59. Wheeland RG, Bailin PL, Ratz JL, Roenigk RK. Carbon dioxide laser vaporization and curettage in the treatment of large multiple superficial basal cell carcinomas. *J Dermatol Surg Oncol.* 1987;13:119-125.

60. Cornell RC, Greenway HT, Tucker SB, et al. Intralesional interferon therapy for basal cell carcinoma. *J Am Acad Dermatol.* 1990; 23:694-700.

61. Cristofolini M, Zumiani G, Scappini P, Piscioli F. Aromatic retinoid in the chemoprevention of the progression of nevoid basal-cell carcinoma syndrome. *J Dermatol Surg Oncol.* 1984;10:778-781.

62. Hodak E, Ginzburg A, David M, Sandbank M. Etretinate treatment of nevoid basal cell carcinoma syndrome: therapeutic and chemopreventive effect. *Int J Dermatol.* 1987;26:606-609.

63. Peck GL. Topical tretinoin in actinic keratosis and basal cell carcinoma. *J Am Acad Dermatol.* 1986;15:829-835.

64. Safao B, Good RA. Basal cell carcinoma with metastasis: review of literature. *Arch Pathol Lab Med.* 1977;101:327-331.

65. Coker DD, Elias EG, Viravathana T, McCrea E, Hafiz M. Chemotherapy for metastatic basal cell carcinoma. *Arch Dermatol.* 1983;119:44-50.

66. Epstein E. Value of follow-up after treatment of basal cell carcinoma. *Arch Dermatol.* 1973;108:798-800.

67. Robinson JK. Risk of developing another basal cell carcinoma: a 5-year prospective study. *Cancer.* 1987;60:118-120.

68. Osterlind A, Hou-Jensen K, Jensen OM. Incidence of cutaneous melanoma in Denmark, 1978-1982. Anatomic site distribution, histologic types, and comparison with non-melanoma skin cancer. *Br J Cancer.* 1988;9-88:385-391.

69. Glass AG, Hoover RN. The emerging epidemic of melanoma and squamous cell skin cancer. *JAMA.* 1989; 262:2097-2100.

70. Levi F, LaVecchia CL, Te VC, Mezzanotte G. Descriptive epidemiology of skin cancer in the Swiss canton of Vaud. *Int J Cancer.* 1988;42:811-816.

71. Gallagher RP, Ma B, McLean DI, et al. Trends in basal cell carcinoma, squamous cell carcinoma and melanoma of the skin from 1973 through 1987. *J Am Acad Dermatol.* 1990;23:413-421.

72. Aubry F, MacGibbon B. Risk factors of squamous cell carcinoma of the skin. *Cancer.* 1985;55:907-911.

73. Shiu MH, Chu F, Fortner JG. Treatment of regionally advanced epidermoid carcinoma of the extremity and trunk. *Surg Gynecol Obstet.* 1980;150:558-562.

74. Green A, Battistutta D, Incidence and determinants of skin cancer in a high-risk Australian population. *Int J Cancer.* 1990; 46:356-361.

75. Marks R, Jolley D, Lectsas S, Foley P. The role of childhood exposure to sunlight in the development of solar keratoses and non-melanocytic skin cancer. *Med J Aust.* 1990;152:62-66.

76. Stern RS, Laird N, Melski J, Parrish JA. Fitzpatrick TB, Bleich HL. Cutaneous squamous-cell carcinoma in patients treated with PUnA. *N Engl J Med.* 1984;310:1156-1161.

77. Gupta AK, Anderson TF. Psoralen photochemotherapy. *J Am Acad Dermatol.* 1987;17:703-734.

78. Rivers JK, Norris PG, Murphy GM, et al. UVA sunbeds: tanning, photoprotection, immunological changes and acute adverse effects. *Br J Dermatol.* 1989;120:767-777.

79. Van Weelden H, Van der Putte SC, Toonstra J, Van der Leun JC. UVA-induced tumors in pigmented hairless mice and the carcinogenic risks of tanning with UVA. *Arch Dermatol.* 1990;282:289-294.

80. Bendl BJ, Graham JH. New concepts on the origin of squamous cell carcinomas of the skin: solar (senile) keratosis with squamous cell carcinoma: a clinicopathologic and histochemical study. *Proc Natl Cancer Conf.* 1971;6:471-488.

81. Marks R, Rennie G, Selwood TS. Malignant transformation of solar keratoses to squamous cell carcinoma. *Lancet.* 1988;1:795-796.

82. Horton CE, Crawford HH, Love HG, Loeffler RA. The malignant potential of burn scar. *Plast Reconstr Surg.* 1958;22:348-353.

83. Sehgal VN, Reddy BSN, Koranne RV, et al. Squamous cell carcinoma complicating chronic discoid lupus erythematosus. *J Dermatol.* 1983;10:81-84.

84. Stoll HL Jr, Schwartz RA. Squamous cell carcinoma. In: Fitzpatrick TB, Eisen AZ, Wolff K, Freedberg LM, Austen KF, eds. *Dermatology in General Medicine.* 3rd ed. New York, NY: McGraw-Hill Book Co; 1987:746-758.

85. Dover JS, Johnson RA. Cutaneous manifestations of human immunodeficiency virus infections, I. *Arch Dermatol.* 1991;127:1383-1391.

86. Kripke ML. Role of UVL-induced immunosuppression in experimental photocarcinogenesis. *Prog Dermatol.* 1982;16:1-6.

87. Pfister H. Human papillomaviruses and impaired immunity vs. epidermodysplasia verruciformis. *Arch Dermatol.* 1987;123:1469-1470.

88. Eliezri YD, Silverstein SJ, Nuovo GJ. Occurence of human papillomavirus type 16 DNA in cutaneous squamous and basal cell neoplasms. *J Am Acad Dermatol.* 1990;23:836-842.

89. Immerman SC, Scanlon EF, Christ M, Knox KL. Recurrent squamous cell carcinoma of the skin. *Cancer.* 1983; 51:1537-1540.

90. Dzubow LM, Rigel DS, Robins P. Risk factors for local recurrence of primary cutaneous squamous cell carcinomas. *Arch Dermatol.* 1982;118:900-902.

91. Moller R, Reymann F, Hou-Jensen K. Metastases in dermatological patients with squamous cell carcinoma. *Arch Dermatol.* 1979;115:703-705.

92. Dinehart SM, Pollack SV. Metastases from squamous cell carcinoma of the skin and lip. *J Am Acad Dermatol.* 1989;21:241-248.

93. Friedman HI, Cooper PH, Wanebo HJ. Prognostic and therapeutic use of microstaging of cutaneous squamous cell carcinoma of the trunk and extremities. *Cancer.* 1985; 56:1099-1105.

94. Sedlin ED, Fleming JL. Epidermal carinoma arising in chronic osteomyelitis foci. *J Bone Joint Surg.* 1963;45:827-837.

95. Arons MS, Lynch JB, Lewis SR, Blocker TG Jr. Scar tissue carcinoma, I: a clinical study with special reference to burn scar carcinoma. *Ann Surg.* 1965;161:170-188.

96. Martin H, Strong E, Spiro RH. Radiation-induced skin cancer of the head and neck. *Cancer.* 1970;25:61-71.

97. Epstein E, Epstein N, Bragg K, Linden G. Metastases from squamous cell carcinomas of the skin. *Arch Dermatol.* 1968;97:245-251.

98. Goepfert H, Dichtel WJ, Medina JE, Lindberg RD, Luna MD. Perineural invasion in squamous cell skin carcinoma of the head and neck. *Am J Surg.* 1984;148:542-547.

99. Carter RL, Foster CS, Dinsdale EA, Pittam MR. Perineural spread by squamous cell carcinomas of the head and neck: a morphological study using antiaxonal and antimyelin monoclonal antibodies. *J Clin Pathol.* 1983; 36:269-275.

100. Cottel IW. Perineural invasion by squamous-cell carcinoma. *J Dermatol Surg Oncol.* 1982;8:589-600.

101. Binder SC, Cady B, Catlin D. Epidermoid carcinoma of the skin of the nose. *Am J Surg.* 1968;116:506-512.

102. Mikhail GR. Subungual epidermoid carcinoma. *J Am Acad Dermatol.* 1984;11:291-298.

103. Hoppmann HJ, Fraley EE. Squamous cell carcinoma of

the penis. *J Urol.* 1978;120:393-398.

104. Jones MJ, Levin HS, Ballard LA Jr. Verrucous squamous cell carcinoma of the vagina: report of a case and review of the literature. *Cleve Clin.* 1981;48:305-313.

105. Kao GF, Graham JH, Helwig EB. Carcinoma cuniculatum (verrucous carcinoma of the skin): a clinicopathologic study of 46 cases with ultrastructural observations. *Cancer.* 1982;49:2395-2403.

106. Honeycutt WM, Jansen GT. Treatment of squamous cell carcinoma of the skin. *Arch Dermatol.* 1973;108:670-672.

107. Freeman RG, Knox JM, Heaton CL. The treatment of skin cancer: a statistical study of 1,341 skin tumors comparing results obtained with irradiation, surgery, and curettage followed by electrodesiccation. *Cancer.* 1964;17: 535-538.

108. Chernosky ME. Squamous cell and basal cell carcinomas: preliminary study of 3,817 primary skin cancers. *South Med J.* 1978;71:802-803.

109. Johnson DE, Lo RK, Srigley J, Ayala AG. Verrucous carcinoma of the penis. *J Urol.* 1985;133:216-218.

110. Tornes K, Bang G, Koppang HS, et al. Oral verrucous carcinoma. *Int J Oral Surg.* 1985;14:485-492.

111. Mohs FE. Carcoma of the skin: a summary of results in chemosurgery. In: *Chemosurgery: Microscopically Controlled Surgery for Skin Cancer.* Springfield, Ill: Charles C Thomas; 1978:153.

112. Mohs FE, Sahl WJ. Chemosurgery for verrucous carcinoma. *J Dermatol Surg Oncol.* 1979;5:302-306.

113. Swanson NA, Taylor WB. Plantar verrucous carcinoma. *Arch Dermatol.* 1980;116:794-797.

114. Smith RRL, Kuhajda FP, Harris AE. Anaplastherapy. *Am J Otolaryngol.* 1985;6:448-452.

115. Kuflik EG, Gage AA. The five year cure rate achieved by cryosurgery for skin cancer. *J Am Acad Dermatol.* 1991; 24:1002-1004.

116. Meyskens FL Jr, Gilmartin E, Alberts DS, et al. Activity of isotretinoin against squamous cell cancers and preneoplastic lesions. *Cancer Treat Rep.* 1982;66:1315-1319.

117. Brunner R, Landthaler M, Haina D, Waidelich W, Braun-Falco O. Treatment of benign, semimalignant, and malignant skin tumors with the Nd:YAG laser. *Lasers Surg Med.* 1985;5:105-110.

118. Odom RB. Fluorouracil. In: Epstein E, Epstein NE Jr, eds. *Skin Surgery.* 6th ed. Philadephia, Pa: WB Saunders; 1987:396-400.

22

CANCER OF THE THYROID AND PARATHYROID GLANDS

J. Shelton Horsley, III, MD, Melvin J. Fratkin, MD

Thyroid cancer is a heterogenous group of malignant diseases that affects all ages but is more serious in the elderly. Its behavior varies across a broad spectrum from the nearly uniformly lethal anaplastic carcinoma to the rather benignly behaving papillary carcinoma of the young. Parathyroid cancer, although rare, is usually symptomatic, presenting with clinical manifestations of hyperparathyroidism.

Thyroid

Anatomy

The thyroid gland is located in the anterior midline of the neck. It has two lateral lobes and a connecting strip—the isthmus—which overlies the trachea. It is covered by the skin and platysma muscle and lies posterior to the sternohyoid and sternothyroid muscles. The lateral boundaries are the sternocleidomastoid muscles on either side. The main arterial blood supply is the superior thyroid artery arising from the external carotid artery and the inferior thyroid artery, from the thyrocervical trunk, which enters near the middle of the gland. The deep thyroid veins—superior, middle, and inferior—typically drain into the internal jugular vein. The inferior thyroid veins may join to form the thyroidea ima vein and empty into the innominate vein.

The lymphatic drainage of the thyroid gland is extensive. It may extend vertically as far as the upper neck and down into the mediastinum, horizontally to the lateral neck, into the retropharyngial area, or to the opposite side of the neck (Fig 22-1).[1]

J. Shelton Horsley, III, MD, Professor of Surgery, Ella Gordon Valentine American Cancer Society Professor of Clinical Oncology, Division of Surgical Oncology, Department of Surgery, Medical College of Virginia, Virginia Commonwealth University, Richmond, Virginia

Melvin J. Fratkin, MD, Professor of Radiology and Medicine, Department of Radiology, Nuclear Medicine Division, Medical College of Virginia, Virginia Commonwealth University, Richmond, Virginia

The recurrent laryngeal nerves arise from the vagus nerves. The right recurrent laryngeal nerve originates where the vagus nerve crosses the first portion of the subclavian artery and curves around the artery and ascends laterally to the trachea, entering the larynx posterior to the thyroid at the cricothyroid articulation. The left recurrent laryngeal nerve leaves the vagus nerve as it crosses over the arch of the aorta, hooks around the aorta, and ascends laterally to the trachea to enter the larynx. The recurrent laryngeal nerves in the area of the lower pole of the thyroid gland are 1 to 2 cm lateral to the trachea and are closely associated with the inferior thyroid artery, where it enters the mid-portion of the gland. They supply motor branches to the laryngeal muscles.

The superior laryngeal nerves arise from the vagus nerve near the base of the skull, descend medially to the carotid vessels and divide into two branches at the level of the hyoid cornu. The internal branch is sensory to the hypopharynx, and the external is the motor branch innervating the cricothyroid muscle. Both branches are closely adjacent to the superior thyroid artery and may be injured when that artery is ligated, particularly when the ligature is placed high above its entrance into the thyroid gland.

Epidemiology and Risk Factors

Cancer of the thyroid occurred in about 13,000 citizens of the United States in 1994.[2] It is more common in females (9,600) than males (3,400). There are about 1,025 projected deaths, 625 females and 400 males. Thyroid cancer accounts for 90% of all endocrine gland malignancies. The majority of cases occur between ages 25 and 65 years. However, thyroid cancer does occur in the very young and in the elderly. The highest risk ages for differentiated thyroid cancer are in the fourth or fifth decades. Autopsy studies of patients dying of other diseases show a thyroid cancer prevalence of between 5% and 10%. These small, occult, usually papillary, cancers are of little or no clinical significance and do not correlate with an increased

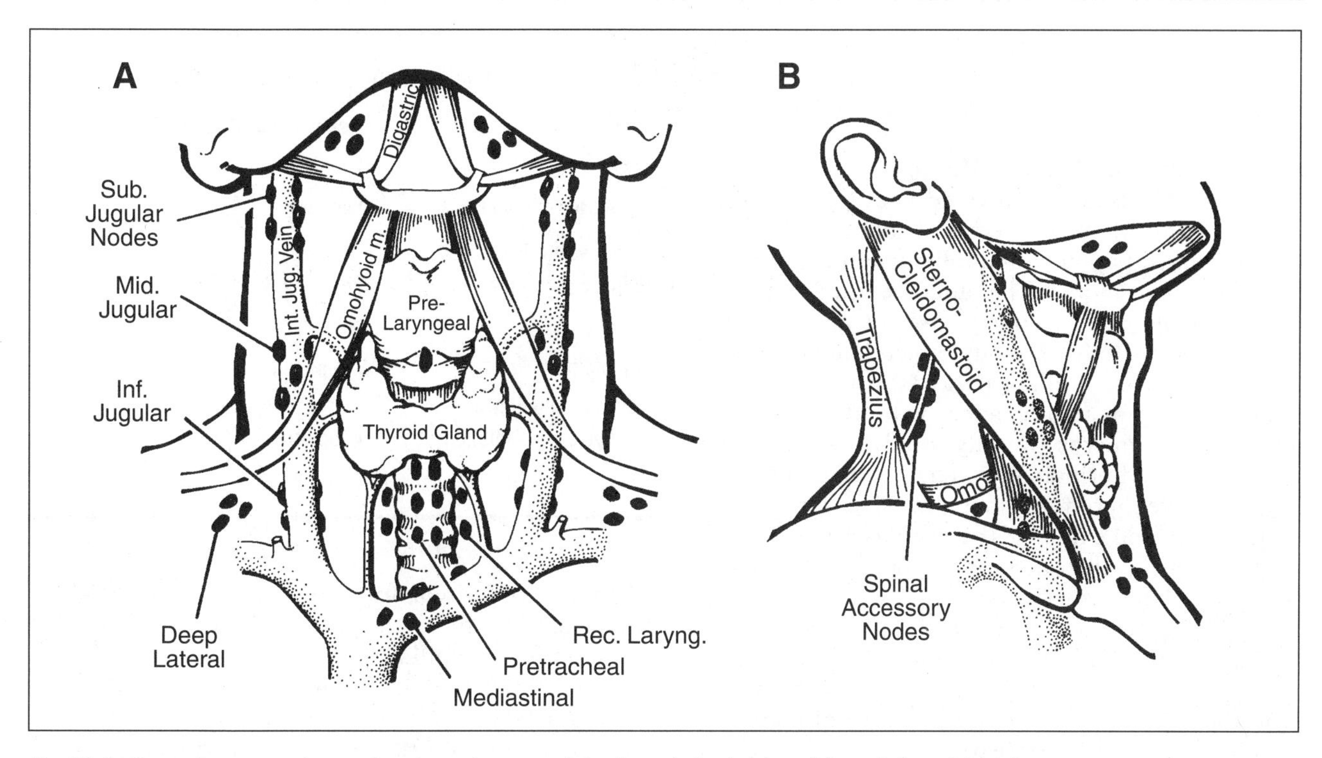

Fig 22-1. Surgical anatomy showing lymphatic drainage of the thyroid gland. Adapted from Cady and Rossi.[1]

clinical incidence or mortality from thyroid cancer.

There is an epidemiologic association of thyroid cancer with childhood radiation.[3] In 1950 carcinoma of the thyroid was reported in 9 of 28 children who had previously undergone radiation for thymic enlargement. Subsequent larger studies in the 1970s confirmed the association between childhood therapeutic radiation of the head/neck region and thyroid malignancy. A reasonable estimate of risk suggests approximately 2 to 5 cases per million children exposed per rad per year. However, only 10% to 15% of patients with differentiated thyroid cancer have a history of significant past radiation exposure. If a large group of children who have received radiation exposure in the range of 10 to 1,200 rads is followed, about 10% will develop differentiated thyroid cancer. Typically, these will be papillary, small, sometimes only a microscopic focus, and have a favorable prognosis. There is also a significant incidence (30%) of benign abnormalities found in these patients by palpation and/or thyroid scans. Where the radiation dose is higher—over 2,000 rads—the risk of thyroid cancer declines because the gland is sterilized. With less than this dose, the DNA of thyroid epithelial cells is damaged and leads to mutations. Impaired thyroid hormone secretion results in an increase of thyroid-stimulating hormone (TSH), which may play a role in promoting cancer development after radiation-induced cellular damage.

Iodine deficiency has been implicated in development of endemic goiter and a higher incidence of follicular carcinoma of the thyroid. With the iodination of salt over the past 50 years in the US, the incidence of follicular carcinomas has decreased, and now papillary cancers are the predominant cell type. In geographic regions where iodine deficiency and goiter are prevalent, such as in Switzerland, follicular carcinoma is more common. It is postulated that this is secondary to chronic stimulation of the follicular cells by prolonged elevated TSH levels.

A history of nodular goiter is present in a large majority (80%) of patients with anaplastic carcinomas. However, in the US, palpable thyroid nodules are present in 4% to 7% of the general adult population and in 20% to 30% of the population exposed to radiation. Thyroid cancer is found in a small percentage of patients with thyroid nodules and no significant radiation exposure. However, it occurs in 30% to 50% of thyroid glands in patients previously exposed to radiation who have a palpable nodule.[4]

One type of thyroid cancer, medullary carcinoma, is influenced by genetic factors, although the exact mechanism is still controversial. In 20% of the patients this tumor is inherited as an autosomal dominant trait. It occurs in three familiar situations: familial medullary thyroid carcinoma and multiple endocrine neoplasia (MEN) types 2a and 2b.[5]

Thyroiditis does not seem to predispose to carcinoma. However, with severe Hashimoto's thyroiditis, there is an increased incidence of lymphoma. The risk factors for thyroid cancer are listed in Table 22-1.[6]

Table 22-1. Factors Predisposing to Thyroid Cancer

Factor	Associated Malignancy
TSH	Papillary
Low-dose radiation	Papillary
Iodine deficiency	Follicular
Iodine abundance	Papillary
Genetic	Medullary
Thyroiditis	Lymphoma
Preexisting goiter or neoplasia ± radiation	Anaplastic

Adapted from Jackson and Cobb.[6]

Background and Natural History

The natural history of thyroid cancer depends, in part, on the histologic type of malignancy: well-differentiated papillary and follicular, medullary, and anaplastic carcinoma. The outcome of differentiated thyroid malignancy is largely based on age at the time of diagnosis with further outcome related to size and extent of disease in older patients. It is confusing to many physicians that a cancer with identical pathologic features microscopically could differ so much in outcome based principally on age at diagnosis. Even more perplexing is the fact that size, lymph node metastases, and extent of the primary lesion have little relevance to the outcome in younger patients but strongly relate to survival in older patients.[7]

Regional lymphatic involvement is common in papillary and medullary carcinoma of the thyroid. Follicular carcinoma metastasizes by the hematogenous route. The predominant feature of anaplastic carcinoma is locally invasive disease. Knowledge of the natural history of these four major types of thyroid cancer and an appreciation of the importance of influencing the outcome of prognostic factors provide the physician with the clinical acumen to appropriately evaluate and manage patients with thyroid malignancy.

Clinical Presentation

The majority of patients with thyroid malignancy present with an asymptomatic thyroid nodule discovered when the neck is examined during the course of a routine physical examination or evaluation for an unrelated medical problem. In most cases the malignant nodule is a well-differentiated (papillary or follicular) carcinoma, is less than 3 cm, is firm and mobile rather than hard and fixed, and is contained within an otherwise normal or nonpalpable thyroid gland. Thyroid malignancy, however, may present as a dominant nodule in a multinodular goiter. The presence of bilateral discrete thyroid nodules suggests familial medullary carcinoma, especially when associated with findings of MEN—pheochromocytoma, hyperparathyroidism, or ganglioneuromas—or with a family history of thyroid cancer. An invasive thyroid cancer, frequently anaplastic carcinoma but rarely well-differentiated carcinoma, presents as a fixed or rapidly enlarging neck mass and may be associated with symptoms of hoarseness, dysphagia, stridor, or neck pain. On occasion, the predominant finding (but rarely the only finding) is cervical lymphadenopathy. In patients with well-differentiated thyroid cancer initial evaluation reveals a small, but variable prevalence of distant metastatic disease with approximately 85% of metastases involving lung and/or bone. Distant metastases occur in an average of 4% (1% to 8%) of patients with papillary carcinoma and 16% (3% to 33%) of patients with follicular carcinoma.[8] Patients with thyroid cancer are euthyroid when initially seen. Rarely, extensive intra-glandular involvement produces sufficient replacement of normal thyroid tissue to produce hypothyroidism; a few cases of large follicular carcinomas have been associated with hyperthyroidism.

Thyroid nodular disease challenges the clinician: (1) to determine which thyroid nodule is malignant in a population of predominantly benign nodules; (2) to establish the diagnosis with a cost-effective work-up and with as little patient morbidity as possible; (3) to decide what is the appropriate surgical procedure and whether adjuvant therapy is indicated; and (4) to plan and provide long-term management.

Diagnostic Work-Up

The clinical presentation of a patient with a thyroid nodule offers little definitive data to distinguish benignity from malignancy. A history of radiation exposure during infancy or childhood is an important risk factor, but most patients with thyroid malignancy have not been exposed to radiation doses associated with later development of cancer. Thyroid malignancy, with the exception of anaplastic carcinoma, usually is not locally invasive and cannot be distinguished by palpation from a benign nodule. At times it is even difficult to be certain that the palpated neck mass is thyroid tissue. The usual findings of an aggressive malignant lesion—a rapidly enlarging, fixed, or painful mass—also occur with benign thyroid disease: hemorrhagic/cystic degeneration of benign nodule, chronic fibrous thyroiditis, or subacute thyroiditis. Cervical lymphadenopathy is an important finding and may be clinically palpable in 25% of patients with papillary carcinoma,[9] but less frequently in other types of thyroid malignancy. Distant metastatic disease is infrequently present at initial diagnosis, and, if present, usually is asymptomatic. Thus, after a careful and thorough history and physical examination, thyroid malignancy may be suspected but not excluded.

Blood tests offer little or no value in diagnosing thyroid malignancy except for medullary carcinoma of the thyroid gland. Thyroid hormone assays and TSH measurement provide no differential diagnostic information. Benign and malignant thyroid nodules rarely alter overall thyroid hormone production and secretion. Papillary and follicular carcinoma secrete thyroglobulin, the glycoprotein that provides tyrosyl groups for thyroid hormonogenesis. Serum thyroglobulin levels increase in benign thyroid disease associated with glandular enlargement, hyperthyroidism, and thyroiditis, and hence do not distinguish benign from malignant thyroid disease.[10] Calcitonin, secreted by thyroid C-cells or parafollicular cells, is significantly elevated in patients with thyroid medullary carcinoma. A low prevalence of this histologic type of thyroid carcinoma precludes the cost-effective use of screening calcitonin measurements in patients with thyroid nodules.

Thyroid gland imaging and biopsy, singly or in combination, provide the necessary data to discriminate thyroid nodule benignity from malignancy in nearly all cases. Radioiodine imaging of the thyroid gland using gamma camera scintigraphy with pinhole collimation in multiple views accurately depicts nodular function. Malignant thyroid nodules, such as well-differentiated carcinoma, accumulate very little radioiodine; medullary and anaplastic carcinoma accumulate no radioiodine. They both appear as nonfunctioning or "cold" nodules. Unfortunately, most benign nodules are cold. A hyperfunctioning or "hot" nodule essentially excludes malignancy. Thyroid sonography characterizes a thyroid nodule as a cystic, complex (solid with cystic component), or solid lesion. The uncommon, pure thyroid cyst is benign; otherwise, sonography is not diagnostic, as both benign and malignant nodules have a complex or solid pattern. Magnetic resonance imaging (MRI) and transmission computed tomography (CT), while providing high resolution images of the neck with exquisite anatomic detail, cannot directly distinguish between cancer and benign nodules.[11]

Fine (23- or 25-gauge) needle aspiration biopsy (FNAB) of the thyroid gland has gained widespread use, is easy to perform, and is associated with only mild patient discomfort limited to the few moments required to complete the aspiration. Diagnostic accuracy depends on the experience of the cytopathologist but approaches 90%.[12] The procedure is less accurate in patients with cystic or hemorrhagic lesions if the solid component of the nodule is not sampled. On occasion the aspirate provides insufficient cellular

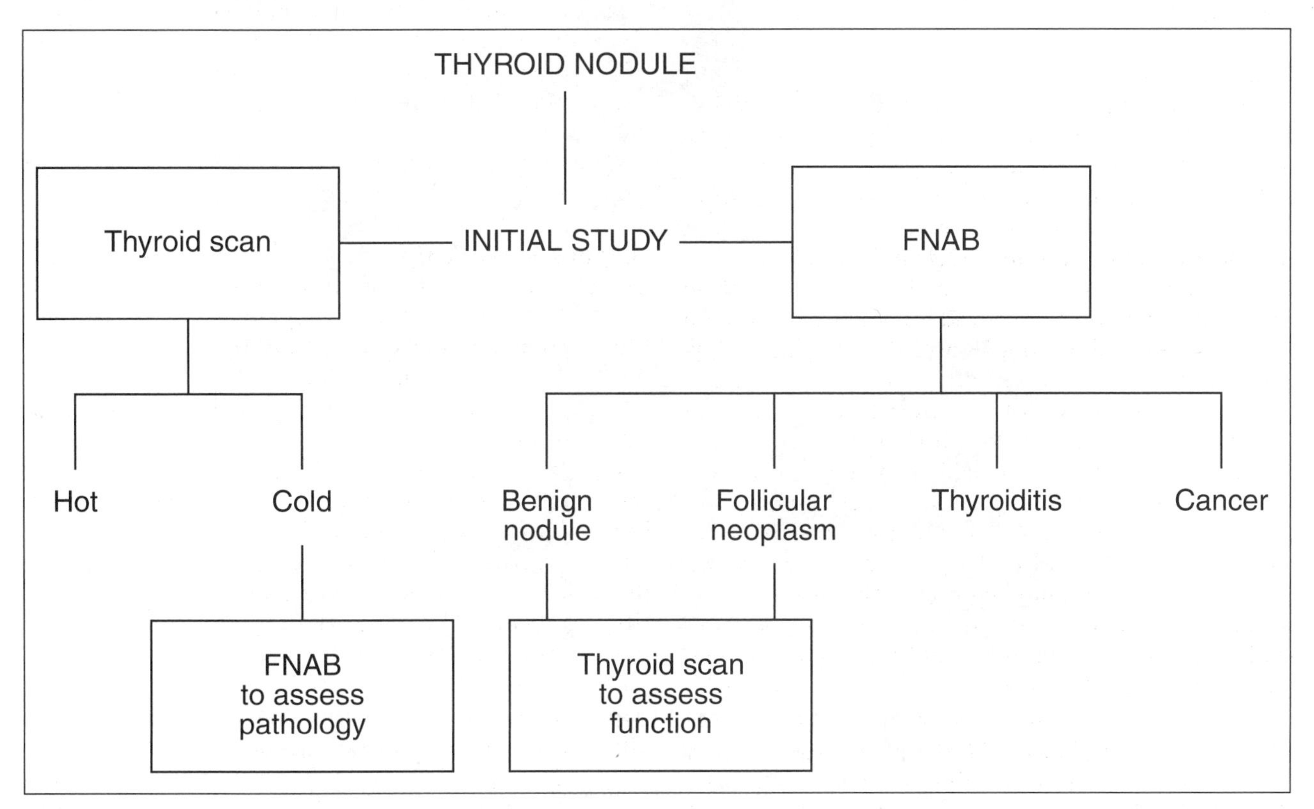

Fig 22-2. Algorithm for using combination of functional and cytologic studies in the diagnosis of thyroid nodules.

material for a cytologic diagnosis. Cytologic evaluation is unable to distinguish a benign follicular adenoma from a follicular carcinoma because the aspirate does not provide material to assess vascular or capsular invasion, the discriminating feature of follicular cell type malignancy. Flow cytometric DNA measurement and analysis of DNA ploidy patterns of biopsied specimens, while a predictor of survival in proven carcinoma, cannot separate benign from malignant follicular neoplasms.[13]

No single clinical test will provide a definitive pathologic tissue diagnosis in all patients presenting with a thyroid nodule. In most patients, a combination of radioiodine thyroid imaging and FNAB are necessary to diagnose thyroid cancer (Figs 22-2 and 22-3). Approximately 85% of solitary nodules and dominant nodules in multi-nodular goiters are cold and require an FNAB. Similarly, about 80% of FNAB aspirates are benign adenomatous nodules or follicular neoplasms that require radioiodine imaging to assess the functional state of the nodule. Whereas a cytologic diagnosis of adenomatous nodule has excluded malignancy, a hot nodule must be ruled out prior to treatment with thyroid hormone suppressive therapy; demonstration that a follicular neoplasm is hyperfunctioning essentially excludes malignancy. In a small percent of cases thyroid lobectomy is required to definitively establish the pathology of a thyroid nodule.

Staging System

The histologic diagnosis, age of the patient, and extent of disease are of critical importance in predicting the behavior and prognosis of thyroid cancer. The clinical staging of a malignant tumor of the thyroid depends on inspection and palpation of the thyroid gland and regional lymph nodes in the neck. Other evaluative tests are usually not required. If there is advanced local disease, CT examination of the thyroid area may be helpful. At initial presentation, distant metastases are uncommon and rarely occur in sites other than the lung. Chest x-ray is usually adequate for initial staging, although chest CT imaging is more sensitive in detecting pulmonary metastases. Routine imaging of the liver and bone are not necessary. Selective CT scanning or MRI is only indicated when there is strong suspicion of distant metastases based on clinical findings. Radioiodine imaging for metastatic disease is not efficacious prior to thyroidectomy.

The traditional staging system based on anatomic

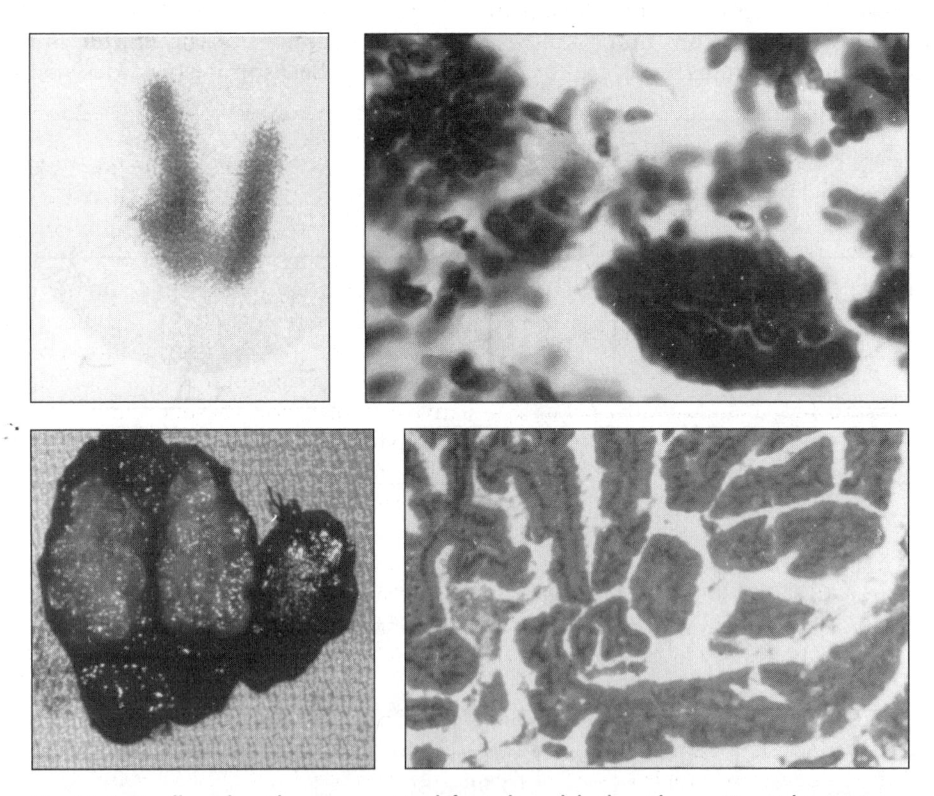

Fig 22-3. Papillary thyroid carcinoma. (Top left) Radionuclide thyroid scan. (Top right) FNAB specimen. (Bottom left) Gross specimen. (Bottom right) Histologic section. Microscopic sections courtesy of WJ Frable, MD, Director Surgical Pathology, Medical College of Virginia/VCU, Richmond, Va.

extent of disease—tumor/node/metastases (TNM)—is inadequate in many respects for staging the unique types of thyroid malignancy. The important prognostic factors of age and histologic types of thyroid cancer must be considered. Additional prognostic variables have been studied by univariate and multifactorial statistical analyses, and many prognostic scoring systems with variable weighting of parameters have been proposed. Table 22-2 describes the Mayo Clinic prognostic scoring system and outcome experience for papillary thyroid cancer.[14] The modified TNM staging system for the four major histologic types of thyroid malignancy recommended by the American Joint Committee on Cancer is outlined in Table 22-3.[15] None of the proposed staging systems enjoys universal acceptance or approval.

Table 22-2. Mayo Clinic Prognostic Index for Papillary Thyroid Cancer

Variables	Score
Age ≤ 39 years	3.1
≥ 40 years	0.08 x age
Tumor size	0.3 x cm
Extrathyroid invasion	1.0
Incomplete resection	1.0
Distant metastases	3.0

Total Score	10-year Recurrence (%)	20-year Cause-Specific Mortality (%)
< 6.0	3	1
6.0-6.9	18	13
7.0-7.9	40	45
≥ 8.0	60	76

Table 22-3. TNM Staging for Thyroid Cancer*

Papillary or Follicular

	Under 45 Years	45 Years and Older
Stage I	Any T, Any N, M0	T1, N0, M0
Stage II	Any T, Any N, M1	T2, N0, M0
		T3, N0, M0
Stage III		T4, N0, M0
		Any T, N1, M0
Stage IV		Any T, Any N, M1

Medullary

Stage I	T1	N0	M0
Stage II	T2	N0	M0
	T3	N0	M0
	T4	N0	M0
Stage III	Any T	N1	M0
Stage IV	Any T	Any N	M1

Undifferentiated

(All cases are stage IV.)

Stage IV	Any T	Any N	Any M

*Separate stage groupings are recommended for papillary and follicular, medullary, and undifferentiated.

From American Joint Committee on Cancer.[15]

Pathologic Classification

The vast majority of thyroid cancers are of glandular-epithelial origin and are well-differentiated (Table 22-4). The differentiated cancers—papillary and follicular carcinoma—represent 90% of all thyroid malignancies. The most common type of thyroid cancer is the papillary variety (60%), which may have varying proportions of follicular features. It may, however, have predominantly follicular features and has been called a mixed papillary-follicular adenocarcinoma. As there appears to be no difference in prognosis based on the mixture of cell types—principally papillary, principally follicular, or equally mixed—the tumors are classified as papillary. Mitoses are infrequent. However, multifocality (30% to 80%), squamous metaplasia, psammoma bodies, and lymphatic invasion are commonly found. Metastasis to regional nodes in the neck can even occur with the small occult papillary thyroid cancers.

The follicular cancers make up approximately 30% of thyroid cancers. They are purely follicular. Often there is difficulty in differentiation of a follicular adenoma from a follicular carcinoma. The carcinoma has invasion of blood vessels and/or the tumor capsule. Occasionally, metastases are found with follicular adenomas, but more extensive study of the primary tumor usually reveals invasion of the pseudocapsule. Lymph node metastases are infrequent. This type of thyroid cancer typically spreads by the bloodstream.

Hürthle cell, or oxyphil cell tumors, are derived from the follicular cell. Invasion of the pseudocapsule and/or vascular invasions are the criteria for malignancy as in other follicular neoplasms.

Medullary carcinomas make up approximately 5% of all thyroid cancers. This is a tumor of the C cells of the thyroid gland that secrete calcitonin. Approximately 20% of these patients show an autosomal dominant inheritance pattern. In patients with MEN, the cancer is present in both thyroid lobes. On the other hand, sporadic (nonfamilial) medullary carci-

Table 22-4. Pathologic Classification of Thyroid Cancer

Well-Differentiated Carcinoma (95%)
Papillary
Follicular
Hürthle cell
Medullary
Undifferentiated (Anaplastic) Carcinoma (5%)
Spindle cell
Giant cell
Other Thyroid Malignancies (<1%)
Lymphoma
Sarcoma
Metastases

noma is unilateral. Patients with MEN type 2a have medullary thyroid carcinoma, pheochromocytoma, and hyperparathyroidism; MEN 2b is characterized by pheochromocytoma, multiple mucosal neuromas, ganglioneuromatosis, and a typical phenotype. Medullary thyroid cancer metastasizes both by lymphatics and blood stream.

Fortunately, anaplastic carcinoma of the thyroid is decreasing in incidence. These are undifferentiated and display spindle or giant cells. The decrease may be due to better diagnostic techniques to differentiate between this cancer and medullary carcinomas and lymphomas. Occasionally these highly malignant neoplasms arise from long-standing untreated thyroid tumors, particularly in the elderly.

Other malignant tumors of the thyroid are sarcomas, lymphomas, and metastatic cancers. The most common primary sites for metastases to the thyroid gland are lung, breast, kidney, and melanoma. Direct extension from adjacent squamous cell carcinomas of the head and neck may also occur.

Prognostic Factors Influencing Outcome

Prognosis of the differentiated thyroid cancers is strongly related to the age of the patient. All patients under 40 years of age and women under 50 years will infrequently die of thyroid cancer. With each decade over 50 years, the outlook worsens. Elderly patients have a poorer prognosis as do patients whose primary thyroid cancers are large (>5 cm).

The usual criteria of tumor size, metastases to regional lymph nodes, and local extent of disease do not relate to outcome in younger patients (<40 years) but do affect the outcome with increasing importance in the older patient. The radiation-induced thyroid cancer is a well-differentiated papillary or papillary-follicular cancer, is usually small, and has an overall good prognosis. The occult papillary cancers of the thyroid by definition are less than 1.0 to 1.5 cm, sometimes multiple, and have no clinical significance. Metastatic cervical lymphadenopathy in papillary thyroid cancer has little or no deleterious effect on the outcome. However, the prognosis is worse in follicular carcinoma with regional metastatic cervical lymphadenopathy.

Several groups have published prognostic criteria for differentiated thyroid carcinomas that are helpful in predicting outcome. Those patients in the low-risk group are younger (men <40 and women <50 years), patients with well-differentiated (tumor grade 0 to +1), smaller (<5 cm) tumors confined to the gland with no distant metastases. The more common low-risk group, constituting 89% of the patients, has a death rate of only 2%. The less prevalent high-risk group has a 46% mortality.[16] Scoring of selected weighted risk factors demonstrates a progression from excellent to poor outcome (Table 22-2).

Medullary cancers of the thyroid can metastasize by both lymphatics and bloodstream. The growth rate is considerably slower than anaplastic carcinoma, but the outlook is not good, with only a 50% 10-year survival rate. The prognosis is worse for the older patient and patients with MEN 2b, large tumors, regional lymph node metastases, and distant metastases. In familial cases, the cure rate is high (95%) in patients with elevated calcitonin levels when the tumor is not palpable, but low (17%) if the tumor is palpable.[5]

The prognosis for undifferentiated or anaplastic thyroid cancer is dismal. All of these cancers are classified as Stage IV regardless of the extent of the disease. Most studies show a 2-year survival rate near zero. Fortunately, the incidence has been decreasing over the past several decades.

General Management

Initial Management

All suspicious nodules of the thyroid gland should be explored surgically. Complete removal of the lobe containing the lesion should be the minimum operation performed. Simple excision of the nodule should not be done. The entire specimen is sent to the pathologist for evaluation and frozen section.

If the nodule is benign on frozen section, or the pathologist cannot be certain of malignancy (follicular adenoma versus carcinoma) or the diagnosis is well-differentiated malignancy <2 cm in diameter, the involved lobe is removed. The contralateral lobe is exposed, carefully inspected, and palpated. If a nodule or tumor is found, this lobe should also be removed. If the contralateral lobe grossly appears benign, some still favor total thyroidectomy, others subtotal removal of the contralateral gland, and still others leave the opposite lobe intact. Certainly, subtotal removal of the remaining lobe seems to be all that can be justified for differentiated cancer confined to the gland, since local recurrence is not reduced by performing a total thyroidectomy.[17,18] Total thyroidectomy increases the chance of permanent hypoparathyroidism, a troublesome complication for the patient. However, if the diagnosis is follicular cancer or findings indicate a greater risk for recurrence or metastases such as large size (>5 cm), extraglandular extension, or age >50 years, a total thyroidectomy is indicated. This also facilitates the postoperative use of radioactive iodine for diagnosis and treatment of possible ^{131}I avid or functioning residual and/or metastatic disease.

In medullary cancers the disease is frequently bilateral, particularly in the familial situations. The anaplastic carcinomas are often unresectable at presentation. If they can be removed by total thyroidectomy, this should be performed.

The extent of neck dissection depends on the histologic type of thyroid malignancy. For the well-differentiated thyroid cancers—papillary and follicular—the central and cervical nodes are carefully palpated preoperatively and at the time of surgical exploration. They are removed if palpable. This is done locally or by a modified neck dissection, leaving intact the sternocleidomastoid muscle, the internal jugular vein, and the spinal accessory nerves typically removed with the standard neck dissection. However, with medullary and undifferentiated carcinomas, a unilateral neck dissection of the standard variety is routinely advocated because of the frequent extensive nodal involvement with regional metastases.

Thyroid hormone therapy is mandatory for all patients following thyroidectomy in full hormonal replacement doses to provide patients with normal thyroid function and suppression of TSH to eliminate the potential growth of any residual tissue from chronic TSH stimulation. If postoperative radioiodine studies are planned, thyroid hormone therapy is withheld for 6 weeks.

Post-thyroidectomy Management

Well-differentiated thyroid cancer, while "nonfunctioning" on radioiodine imaging in comparison with normal thyroid tissue, usually is able to concentrate iodide. The uptake and retention of iodide provides for diagnostic and therapeutic application of radioiodine in the postoperative evaluation and management of patients with papillary and follicular thyroid cancer. Therapy with radioiodine is efficacious in completing a less-than-total surgical resection of the thyroid gland and in treating residual and metastatic thyroid malignancy. Radionuclide scintigraphy with millicurie doses of ^{131}I will reveal thyroid bed uptake of radioiodine after thyroid surgery including patients who have had a total thyroidectomy by macroscopic assessment of the surgeon.[19] Post-thyroidectomy diagnostic radioiodine imaging should be performed in

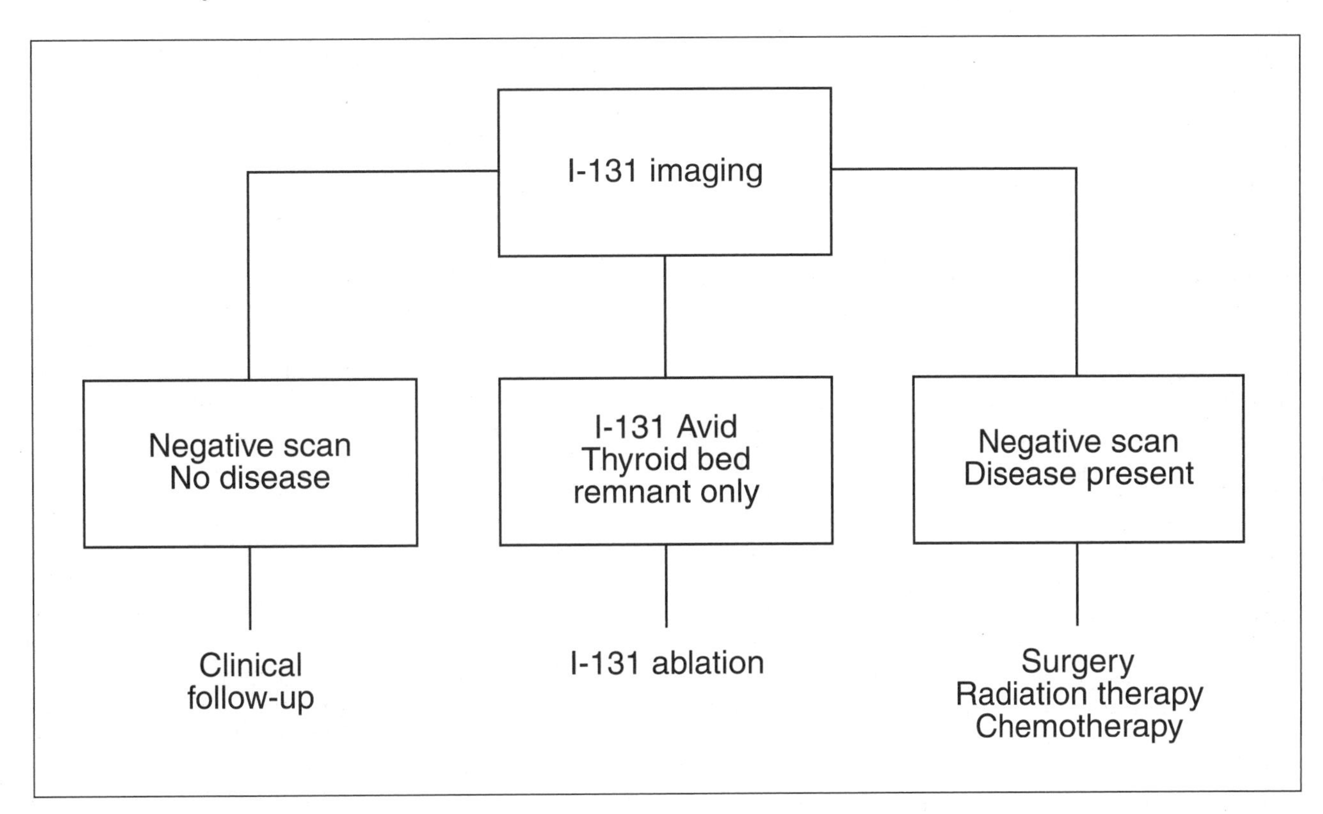

Fig 22-4. Therapeutic guide based on post thyroidectomy thyroid imaging results.

all patients with well-differentiated thyroid malignancy. Thyroid hormone must be withheld for an appropriate period of time prior to the radioiodine studies: 6 weeks for levothyroxine and 2 weeks for liothyronine. As thyroid hormone levels diminish, TSH reaches peak levels, which ensures maximal stimulation of any residual thyroid tissue. The results of radioiodine uptake and imaging serve as a guide for patient management (Fig 22-4). If a significant thyroid bed remnant is present, most thyroidologists recommend ^{131}I ablation of residual normal thyroid tissue for the following reasons: 1) to increase the sensitivity in detecting functioning residual or metastatic disease on subsequent post-thyroid ablation ^{131}I imaging; 2) to improve the specificity of serum thyroglobulin measurement as a biochemical marker of thyroid malignancy; and 3) to therapeutically irradiate any undetected microscopic foci of thyroid malignancy in the thyroid bed remnant, cervical lymph nodes, and possible distant micrometastases.

Three to 6 months after ^{131}I treatment to ablate the thyroid gland remnant, radioiodine imaging is repeated after withdrawal of thyroid hormone. Whole-body radioiodine scan findings provide the basis for subsequent patient management (Fig 22-5). If ^{131}I avid residual or metastatic disease is demonstrated, the patient is hospitalized for radiation isolation and treatment with several hundred millicuries of radioiodine. Annual radioiodine imaging and therapy continue until no abnormal ^{131}I uptake is detectable or there is evidence of bone marrow suppression, precluding further systemic radiation therapy. When radioiodine imaging is negative and there is no other evidence of thyroid malignancy (physical examination, radiographs, thyroglobulin), the patient is evaluated annually for life. When the whole body radioiodine scan shows no functioning malignancy, but residual, recurrent, or metastatic disease is present, surgery, external radiation therapy, and chemotherapy are therapeutic options.

There is no accepted role for radioiodine imaging or treatment in the management of nonpapillary and follicular thyroid carcinomas because they are incapable of concentrating ^{131}I.

Long-term evaluation of patients with well-differentiated thyroid malignancy must be individualized, and the potential risk of recurrence should be considered. The optimal versus the most cost-effective use of diagnostic tests has not been established.[10] Whereas most recurrences occur within 5 years after initial treatment, metastatic or local recurrent disease may present 10 to 25 years later. Radioiodine imaging every few years is expensive and inconvenient for the patient. Thyroglobulin measurement is an accepted alternative, since it is a sensitive and specific biochemical marker of recurrent malignant disease, especially after complete elimination of all normal thyroid gland tissue. However, about 10% of patients have cir-

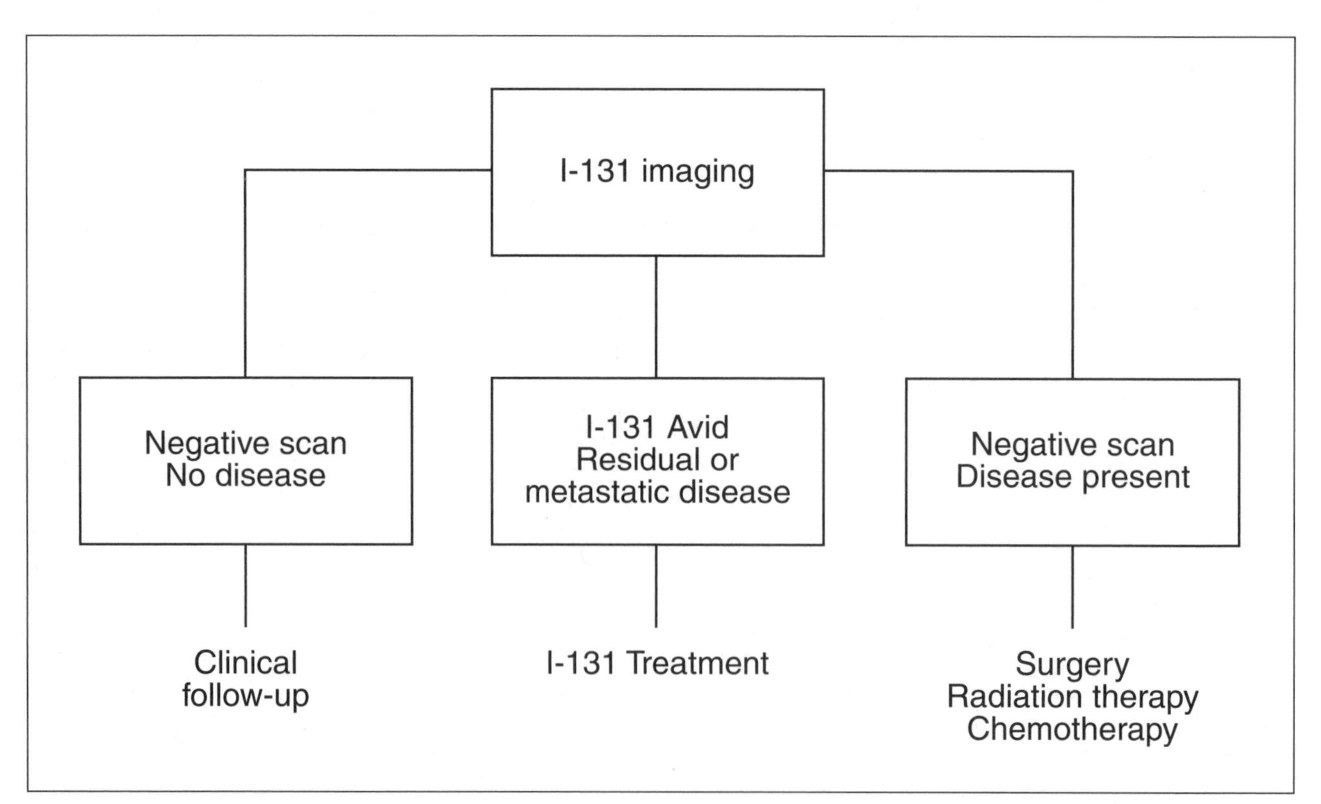

Fig 22-5. Management guide for thyroid cancer after I-131 therapy to ablate post surgical thyroid gland remnant.

culating endogenous thyroglobulin antibodies that interfere with the measurement of thyroglobulin.[20] Periodic chest radiographs are a prudent and probably cost-effective procedure to screen for pulmonary metastases, especially in higher risk patients. Computed tomography or magnetic resonance imaging of the neck is valuable when recurrent cervical disease is suspected and is especially helpful if surgical resection is planned. Routine CT or MR examinations of the neck and chest are not indicated nor are routine bone imaging or skeletal surveys cost effective in screening for skeletal metastases. Whenever clinical examination, thyroglobulin levels, or a radiographic imaging procedure suggests recurrent disease, radioiodine imaging is indicated to assess the feasibility of ^{131}I therapy.

Thyroidologists, endocrinologists, nuclear medicine physicians, and surgeons differ in their recommendations for long-term surveillance and management of patients with well-differentiated thyroid carcinoma. The disease course is highly variable and dependent on the risk for recurrence. The authors recommend recent comprehensive reviews for the reader who is interested in the details and controversies regarding long-term care of papillary and follicular carcinoma patients.[8,10,21-24]

Measurement of serum calcitonin concentration offers a sensitive and specific test for recurrent medullary carcinoma of the thyroid gland. A persistently elevated level indicates residual or metastatic disease that then requires an attempt to localize the disease with CT, sonography, and/or special radionuclide imaging procedures.[25] If these studies demonstrate no residual or metastatic disease, C-cell (hyperplasia or residual tumor) within an incompletely resected thyroid gland may be the source of calcitonin secretion. Radioiodine ablation of the thyroid gland remnant has reduced postoperative persistently elevated calcitonin levels, presumably by irradiation of microscopic disease from adjacent ^{131}I-containing thyroid follicular cells.[26]

Anaplastic thyroid carcinoma unfortunately offers no opportunity for long-term management, as it is usually fatal secondary to uncontrolled local disease within a year of diagnosis.

Results

Results of Surgery

The results of therapy for thyroid cancer depend on histologic type, age, and extent of disease at the time of diagnosis. Patients with well-differentiated thyroid carcinoma, in general, do well. Low-risk papillary thyroid carcinoma patients, which represent the majority of patients, have a death rate of only 1% to 2%, whereas those at high risk have a mortality of 46% to 76%.[14,16] The extent of surgery necessary to achieve these results is debatable, with strong proponents for lobectomy, subtotal thyroidectomy, and total thyroidectomy. When patients are grouped according to risk, the effect of surgery on outcome is clearer. For low-risk patients, surgery greater than ipsilateral lobectomy shows no improvement in cause-specific survival, but the risk of developing local recurrence is reduced from 14% to 4%. In high-risk patients, subtotal thyroidectomy compared to lobectomy improves survival and reduces local recurrence threefold. Total thyroidectomy neither improves survival nor reduces local recurrences when compared with subtotal thyroidectomy in low-risk and high-risk patient groups.[23] The prognosis for patients with well-differentiated, noninvasive follicular carcinoma is excellent. When distant metastases are present, mortality is about 75% within 10 years.[24]

Total thyroidectomy is recommended for medullary thyroid carcinoma. In general, 10-year adjusted survival rates are about 65% with variable biologic behavior related to the type of medullary cancer. Death due to MEN 2b medullary carcinoma occurs in 50% to 60% of patients; sporadic cases, 30% to 45%; MEN 2a patients, 5% to 10%.[27]

Anaplastic carcinoma is usually fatal within 2 years. The extent of surgery with or without radiotherapy and chemotherapy, singly or in combination, appears to have no significant effect on outcome.

Results of Post-Thyroidectomy Therapy

Radioiodine treatment, in contrast to external beam radiotherapy, provides systemic rather than local irradiation and thereby offers the potential for cure of disseminated metastatic thyroid cancer. After nearly 50 years of experience using ^{131}I in the treatment of well-differentiated thyroid cancer, appropriate therapeutic regimens and efficacy of treatment are still being debated in the scientific literature. The controversies persist in part because treatment has been based on empirically administered doses of ^{131}I rather than on radiodosimetry. The radiation dose delivered to normal and malignant thyroid tissue is directly dependent on the concentration and retention of ^{131}I and inversely related to the amount of functioning thyroid tissue. Quantitative measurement of these radiodosimetric parameters is difficult but possible with today's gamma camera/computer imaging systems. With calculation of ^{131}I dosimetry and standardization of treatment to 30,000 rads rather than to an empiric administered dose of radioiodine (30 to 150 mCi), ablation of the post-thyroidectomy thyroid remnant occurs in 80% of patients and in 94% of cases when the mass of thyroid residua is <2 g.[28]

The therapeutic value, however, of ablating the thyroid bed remnant after apparent curative surgery is a controversial issue.[23] In patients with cervical ^{131}I uptake after thyroidectomy, the incidence of local cervical recurrence is reduced with radioiodine therapy.[9] However, when radioiodine therapy is used in patients without evidence of microscopic residual disease, radioiodine-ablated patients, compared with thyroidectomy alone, have no significant differences in local recurrence or long-term survival. While the therapeutic indication for thyroid remnant ablation is debatable, there is general agreement in the use of radioiodine imaging and thyroglobulin measurement in the postoperative evaluation and follow-up of well-differentiated thyroid cancer patients. The highest sensitivity and specificity for these studies occur when there is essentially no residual normal thyroid tissue, which usually requires ^{131}I ablation following thyroid surgery. Resolution of this controversial issue of radioiodine ablation after thyroidectomy for papillary and follicular carcinoma, especially in low-risk patients, will require a randomized clinical trial. Such a trial probably will never be conducted because of the need for a very large number of patients and prolonged follow-up due to the indolent course of this type of malignancy.

No controversy exists regarding the use of radioiodine therapy for residual and metastatic thyroid disease. However, differences in patient selection, ^{131}I treatment protocols, and follow-up evaluation fuel the debate regarding the effectiveness of radioiodine therapy. When performed, calculation of lesion radiation dose from administered ^{131}I shows an anticipated dose/response relationship: 8,500 or more rads to nodal metastases is associated with 80% to 90% successful treatment; with less than 8,000 rads, only 20% of metastases respond to ^{131}I, and no metastases respond to a dose of less than 3,500 rads.[28] Dosimetric studies are in general agreement, but are limited in the number of patients studied and duration of follow-up. Therefore, the effectiveness of ^{131}I therapy of thyroid cancer is based on treatment regimens without knowledge of lesion radiation dose. Despite this major shortcoming, the extensive experience over many years with the use of empirically administered fixed doses of ^{131}I based on location of disease (neck, lung, bone) clearly shows the beneficial effects of radioiodine therapy. In patients with residual microscopic disease, therapy reduces the incidence of recurrent disease. Radioiodine treatment, in patients with gross residual local tumor and metastatic disease, provides palliation and prolongs survival. The relative risk of death is about three times greater when the metastases fail to take up radioiodine.[29] In cases of ^{131}I avid metastases, about 70% of lymph nodal, nearly 50% of pulmonary, but less than 10% of skeletal lesions resolve following radioiodine treatment.[8] When metastatic disease is initially eradicated, survival is three times as long as in patients not freed of their disease with ^{131}I therapy.[30] In a small percentage of patients with distant metastatic disease, radioiodine therapy cures the disease, primarily in those with microscopic or micronodular pulmonary metastases.

Randomized, prospective studies are not available to compare the effectiveness of radioiodine therapy versus external beam radiation treatment. Radiotherapy (at least 5,000 rads) is efficacious in controlling local disease and is beneficial in treating symptomatic distant metastases. Primary indications for external beam radiation therapy include rapidly growing or large, inoperable tumors, and expanding lesions that threaten adjacent vital structures. Radioiodine is not recommended in these situations because of treatment preparation delay (thyroid hormone withdrawal), uncertainty of lesion ^{131}I uptake capacity, and relatively slow therapeutic response in comparison with external radiotherapy.

Recurrent or metastatic thyroid malignancy that is unresectable and not amenable to radiation therapy, radioiodine, or external beam should be considered for chemotherapy. Experience with chemotherapy is limited, but doxorubicin is the most effective single agent. Defining response as a reduction in tumor size, chemotherapy is efficacious in about one-third of patients. The median survival of responders is 15 to 20 months as compared to 3 to 5 months for nonresponders.[31] Combination therapy with doxorubicin and cisplatin has a similar response rate as single drug therapy, but a few long-term complete responses have been noted.[32] In general, response rates are best with well-differentiated and poorest with anaplastic carcinoma.

Parathyroid

Anatomy

The parathyroid glands (Fig 22-6) are typically (80%) four in number and are closely associated with the thyroid gland.[1] Occasionally there may be three glands or five or more. The superior thyroid glands are most often located in the region of the intersection between the laryngeal nerve and the inferior thyroid artery. The most common location of the inferior glands is more central, close to the lower thyroid pole, or in the upper thymus. Aberrations are found on occasion, such as location of the lower parathyroid glands high in the neck because of failure to descend during embryologic development. They may be found in the thymus or in the anterior mediastinum.

Epidemiology and Risk Factors

The occurrence of parathyroid carcinoma is rare. A recent review of functioning parathyroid carcinomas reported in the English literature from 1981 to 1989 had only 163 cases.[33] The incidence of parathyroid carcinoma in patients with primary hyperparathyroidism is low, less than 1%. Its etiology is obscure. It

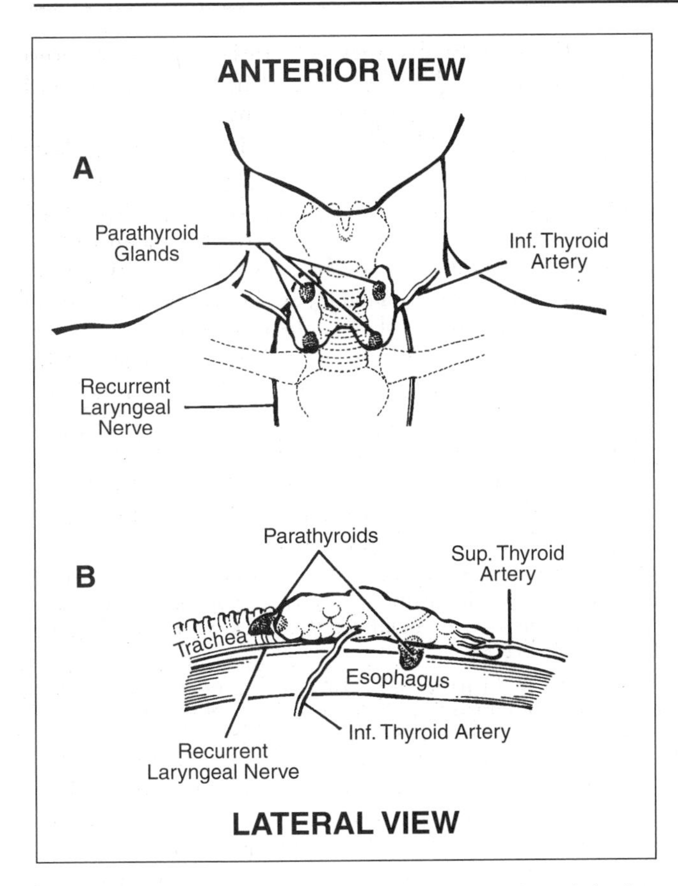

Fig 22-6. Surgical anatomy of the thyroid and parathyroid gland. A, anterior view; B, lateral view. There are two major arteries to each thyroid lobe: the superior thyroid artery and the inferior thyroid artery. The superior parathyroid glands are superior and lateral to both the recurrent laryngeal nerve and the inferior thyroid artery. The inferior parathyroid glands are inferior and medial to both the recurrent laryngeal nerve and the inferior thyroid artery. The inferior thyroid artery is usually superficial to the recurrent laryngeal nerve, but this anatomic relationship may vary. From Norton et al.[5]

may be associated with familial hyperparathyroidism or MEN type 1 syndrome. There is an increased incidence reported in patients receiving irradiation to the head and neck.

Clinical Presentation

The usual presentation for parathyroid carcinoma is that of hyperparathyroidism, characterized by markedly elevated serum calcium and parathormone (PTH), a palpable mass, and rather severe clinical manifestations.[5] Parathyroid carcinoma occurs at a female-to-male ratio of 1.2:1. Rarely are the patients asymptomatic. These carcinomas are only detected by elevated serum calcium on biochemical screening.

Diagnostic Work-Up

The diagnosis of parathyroid carcinoma is suggested by its clinical presentation. Ultrasound demonstrating invasion may be helpful. At the time of surgical exploration the finding of a firm gland encased in dense pale white fibrous tissue adherent to surrounding structures and/or invasion of the thyroid gland with cervical adenopathy may be encountered. When the preoperative diagnosis is strongly suspected, a chest x-ray and a CT scan of the neck and mediastinum may detect metastases.

General Management

The treatment is surgical resection. Preoperative therapy is primarily hydration with normal saline and furosemide (Lasix) for the elevated serum calcium. The operative approach should be an en bloc resection, which usually necessitates thyroid lobectomy, excision of tracheoesophageal tissue and lymph nodes and the adjoining thymus. If the recurrent laryngeal nerve is involved, it should be resected. Most surgeons advocate neck dissection only for those patients with grossly enlarged nodes. With this approach one can expect a 5-year survival rate of 25% to 50%.[1]

Results

Parathyroid carcinoma is slow growing but tenacious. Most patients die of the metabolic complications of hyperparathyroidism rather than from the recurrence of the carcinoma per se. Therefore, an aggressive approach to eliminate all PTH-secreting malignant tissue by resection of contiguous structures such as tracheal wall and esophagus is justified. Recurrent and metastatic deposits (lung) that can be removed should be resected for similar reasons.

Medical therapy to control recurrent disease with its accompanying hypercalcemia consists of hydration and therapy with Lasix, Mithramycin, and/or the new intravenous phosphonate derivatives.

References

1. Cady B, Rossi RL. *Surgery of Thyroid and Parathyroid Glands.* 3rd ed. Philadelphia, Pa: WB Saunders Co; 1991:23-30, 309-312.

2. Boring CC, Squires TS, Tong MS, Mongomery S. Cancer Statistics 1994. *CA Cancer J Clin.* 1994;44:7-26.

3. Robbins J, moderator. NIH conference. Thyroid cancer: a lethal endocrine neoplasm. *Ann Intern Med.* 1991;115:133-147.

4. Rojeski MT, Gharib H. Nodular thyroid disease: evaluation and management. *N Engl J Med.* 1985;313:428-436.

5. Norton JA, Doppman JL, Jensen RT. Cancer of the endocrine system. In: DeVita VT, Hellman S, Rosenberg SA, eds. *Cancer Principles and Practices of Oncology.* 3rd ed. Philadelphia, Pa: JB Lippincott Co;1989:1269-1287.

6. Jackson IMD, Cobb WE. Disorders of the thyroid. In: Kohler PO, ed. *Clinical Endocrinology.* New York, NY: John Wiley Co;1986.

7. Cady B. Head, neck and thyroid cancer. In: Holleb AI, Fink DJ, Murphy GP, *American Cancer Society Textbook of Clinical Oncology.* 1st ed. Atlanta, Ga: American Cancer Society;1991:323-328.

8. Maxon HR, Smith HS. Radioiodine-131 in the diagnosis and treatment of metastatic well-differentiated thyroid cancer. *Endocrinol Metab Clin N Amer.* 1990;19:685-718.

9. Mazzaferri EL, Young RL, Oertel JE, et al. Papillary thyroid carcinoma: the impact of therapy in 576 patients. *Medicine.* 1977;56:171-196.

10. Ross DS. Long-term management of differentiated thyroid cancer. *Endocrinol Metab Clin N Amer.* 1990;19:719-739.

11. Shulkin BL, Shapiro B. The role of imaging tests in the diagnosis of thyroid carcinoma. *Endocrinol Metab Clin N Amer.* 1990;19:523-543.

12. Altavilla G, Pascale M, Nenci I. Fine needle aspiration cytology of thyroid gland diseases. *Acta Cytologica.* 1990;34:251-256.

13. Grant CS, Hay ID, Ryan JJ, et al. Diagnostic and prognostic utility of flow cytometric DNA measurements in follicular thyroid tumors. *World J Surg.* 1990;14:283-290.

14. Hay ID, Taylor WF, Bergstralh EJ. The "MACIS" score: a reliable prognostic index for papillary thyroid cancer. *Thyroid.* 1992;1(suppl 1):S-3.

15. Beahrs OH, Henson DE, Hutter RVP, Kennedy BJ, eds. *American Joint Committee on Cancer Manual for Staging of Cancer.* 4th ed. Philadelphia, Pa: JB Lippincott Co;1992.

16. Cady B, Rossi R. An expanded view of risk-group definition in differentiated thyroid carcinoma. *Surgery.* 1988;104:947-953.

17. Cohn KH, Backdahl M, Forsslund G, et al. Biologic considerations and operative strategy in papillary thyroid carcinoma: arguments against the routine performance of total thyroidectomy. *Surgery.* 1984;86:957-970.

18. Grant CS, Hay ID, Gough IR, et al. Local recurrence in papillary thyroid carcinoma: is extent of surgical resection important? *Surgery.* 1988;104:954-962.

19. Fratkin MJ, Newsome HH, Sharpe AR, et al. Cervical distribution of iodine 131 following total thyroidectomy for thyroid cancer. *Arch Surg.* 1983;118:864-867.

20. Moser E, Braun S, Kirsch CM, et al. Time course of thyroglobulin auto-antibodies in patients with differentiated thyroid carcinoma after radioiodine therapy. *Nucl Med Comm.* 1984;5:317-321.

21. Hurley JR, Becker DV. The use of radioiodine in the management of thyroid cancer. In: Freeman LM, Weissman HS, eds. *Nuclear Medicine Annual.* New York, NY: Raven Press;1983:329-384.

22. DeGroot LJ, Kaplan EL, McCormick M, et al. Natural history, treatment, and course of papillary thyroid carcinoma. *J Clin Endocrinol Metab.* 1990;71:414-424.

23. Hay ID. Papillary thyroid carcinoma. *Endocrinol Metab Clin N Amer.* 1990;19:545-576.

24. Cooper DS, Schneyer CR. Follicular and Hürthle cell carcinoma of the thyroid. *Endocrinol Metab Clin N Amer.* 1990;19:577-591.

25. Gauer A, Raue F, Gagel RF. Changing concepts in the management of hereditary and sporadic medullary thyroid carcinoma. *Endocrinol Metab Clin N Amer.* 1990;19:613-635.

26. Deftos LJ, Stein MF. Radioiodine as an adjunct to surgical treatment of medullary thyroid carcinoma. *J Clin Endocrinol Metab.* 1980;50:967-968.

27. Sizemore GW. Medullary carcinoma of the thyroid gland. *Semin Oncol.* 1987;14:306-314.

28. Maxon HR, Englaro EE, Thomas SR, et al. Radioiodine-131 therapy for well-differentiated thyroid cancer—a quantitative radiation dosimetric approach: outcome and validation in 85 patients. *J Nucl Med.* 1992;33:1132-1136.

29. Schlumberger M, Tubiana M, deVathaire F, et al. Long-term results of treatment of 283 patients with lung and bone metastases from differentiated thyroid carcinoma. *J Clin Endocrinol Metab.* 1986;63:960-967.

30. Beierwaltes WH, Nishiyama RH, Thompson NW, et al. Survival time and "cure" in papillary and follicular thyroid carcinoma with distant metastases: statistics following University of Michigan therapy. *J Nucl Med.* 1982;23:561-568.

31. Ahuja S, Ernst A. Chemotherapy of thyroid carcinoma. *J Endocrinol Invest.* 1987;10:303-310.

32. Shimaoka K, Schoenfeld DA, Dewys WD, et al. A randomized trial of doxorubicin versus doxorubicin plus cisplatin in patients with advanced thyroid carcinoma. *Cancer.* 1985;56:2155-2160.

33. Obara T, Fujimoto Y. Diagnosis and treatment of patients with parathyroid carcinoma: an update and review. *World J Surg.* 1991;15:738-744.

23

CANCER OF THE HEAD AND NECK

Ashok R. Shaha, MD, FACS, Elliot W. Strong, MD, FACS

Cancer of the head and neck, which constitutes approximately 4% of all cancers in the United States, generally affects the elderly and is notoriously associated with long-term habits of cigarette smoking and alcohol consumption.

The management of head and neck tumors presents considerable functional and esthetic problems, especially relating to the loss of function of the mandible and larynx. The eventual outcome of treatment has been improved by major advances in plastic surgery, including the use of myocutaneous flaps and free microvascular tissue transfer. In addition, the roles of chemotherapy and radiation therapy have been better defined over the past 10 years. Despite these advances, a significant challenge remains the treatment of loco-regional recurrence. Most of the time, the success of salvage therapy for tumor recurrence is poor. Most patients with loco-regional recurrence develop progressive recurrent disease that is associated with significant suffering.

Finally, effective management consists of a true multidisciplinary approach involving the head and neck surgeon, neurosurgeon, plastic surgeon, chemotherapist, radiation therapist, oral surgeon, maxillofacial prosthodontist, speech therapist, nutritionist, social worker, clinical nurse, pain service, and neurology service.

Topographic Anatomy of Head and Neck

The main areas of the upper aerodigestive tract involved in head and neck tumors are the oral cavity, pharynx, paranasal sinuses, and larynx (Fig 23-1).[1,2] Tumors of salivary glands form an integral part of head and neck cancer, as do lesions of the skin of the face and neck and cervical lymph nodes.

The oral cavity extends from the skin-vermilion junction of the lips to the junction of the hard and soft palate above and the line of circumvallate papillae below, and is divided into specific areas including the lip, buccal mucosa, lower and upper alveolar ridges, retromolar gingiva (retromolar trigone), floor of the mouth, hard palate, and anterior two thirds of the tongue (oral tongue). The main routes of drainage from the oral cavity are into the first station cervical lymph nodes which are the jugulo digastric-jugulo omohyoid, upper deep cervical, lower deep cervical, and submaxillary and submental lymph nodes. Some of the primary sites drain bilaterally.

The pharynx is divided into the oropharynx, nasopharynx, and hypopharynx (Table 23-1). The oropharynx includes the base of the tongue, vallecula, soft palate, tonsil and tonsillar fossa, and posterior pharyngeal wall. The region of the nasopharynx extends from the level of the junction of the hard and soft palate to the base of the skull. The hypopharynx includes three areas: the piriform sinus, the posterior pharyngeal wall extending from the level of the floor of the vallecula to the level of the cricoarytenoid joints, and the postcricoid area which extends from the level of the arytenoid cartilages to the inferior border of the cricoid cartilage. The main routes of lymphatic drainage from both the pharynx and the oral cavity are into the first station cervical lymph nodes, which are the jugulo-digastric, jugulo-omohyoid, upper deep cervical, lower deep cervical, and submaxillary and submental lymph nodes. Some primary sites drain bilaterally. Tumor (T) staging of lesions of the oropharynx, nasopharynx, and hypopharynx is different from that of tumors of the oral cavity, mainly because of the inability to measure the exact extent of the lesion.

Anatomically, lesions of the larynx are divided into the supraglottis, glottis, and subglottis. Tumors of the subglottic region are very rare (approximately 1% of laryngeal tumors); such tumors generally begin on the

Ashok R. Shaha, MD, FACS, Head & Neck Service, Department of Surgery, Memorial Sloan-Kettering Cancer Center, New York, New York

Elliot W. Strong, MD, FACS, Head & Neck Service, Department of Surgery, Memorial Sloan-Kettering Cancer Center, New York, New York

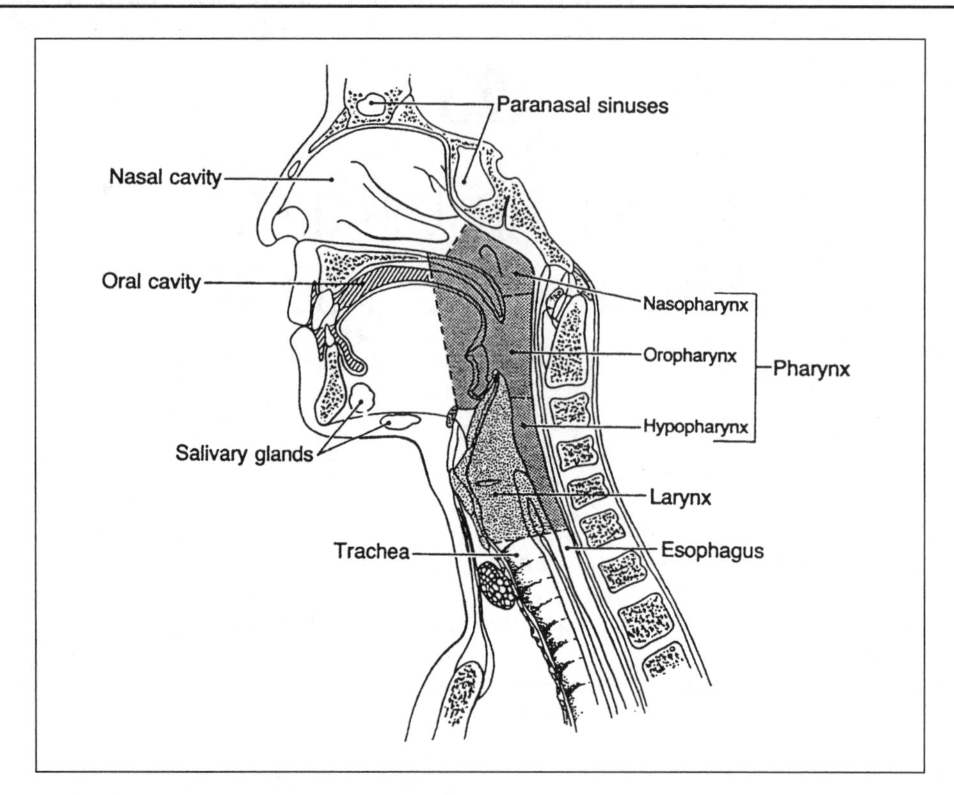

Fig 23-1. Sagittal section of the upper aerodigestive tract.[2]

vocal cord and extend to the subglottic region. The true vocal cord (glottis) has minimal lymphatic supply. However, when tumors of the glottic larynx extend to the supraglottic or subglottic area, they have a high propensity to metastasize to the tracheoesophageal groove lymph node and jugular chain of lymph nodes. The region of the supraglottic larynx has a rich lymphatic drainage, and there is a propensity for supraglottic tumors to metastasize bilaterally.

Cancer of the maxillary sinus is the most common paranasal sinus tumor. Other sites of tumor in this region include the ethmoid sinuses, nasal cavity, and sphenoid sinus. Neoplasms of the sphenoid and frontal sinuses are very rare. Ohngren's line, a theoretic plane joining the medial canthus of the eye with the angle of the mandible, may be used to divide the maxillary antrum into an antero-inferior (infrastructure) and supero-posterior portion (suprastructure). Approximately 15% of patients with tumors of the maxillary sinus will present with metastatis to regional lymph nodes, mainly the submental and high jugulo-digastric lymph nodes.

The major salivary glands are the parotid, submaxillary, and sublingual. Tumors arising in minor salivary glands (mucus-secreting glands in the lining membrane of the aerodigestive tract) are not included in the staging system.

The cervical lymph nodes can be divided into various groups (Figs 23-2 and 23-3): preauricular and parotid group, submental and submandibular group, deep jugular lymph nodes, supraclavicular lymph nodes, lymph nodes along the accessory nerve in the posterior triangle, occipital group, and lymph nodes in the tracheoesophageal groove and superior mediastinum.[3] More than 50 years ago, at Memorial Sloan-Kettering Cancer Center, cervical lymph nodes were grouped into five levels,[3,4] a classification that remains anatomically sound and clinically reproducible and has particular reference to metastasis of tumors of the upper aerodigestive tract. Fig 23-4 identifies levels I through V: I, lymph nodes in the submandibular triangle; II, upper jugular; III, mid-jugular; IV, low jugular; and V, posterior nodes. The tracheoesophageal groove lymph nodes are labeled as level VI and lymph nodes in the superior mediastinum are labeled as level VII.

Over the past few decades, the management of cervical lymph node metastasis has undergone many changes. For more than three quarters of a century, the classic radical neck dissection, popularized in 1906 by George Crile, stood the test of time. However, with a better understanding of the patterns of cervical lymph node metastasis, we are in a position to appreciate the biology of tumor spread, and a more tailored surgical procedure can be performed in most instances.

Epidemiology and Risk Factors

Tumors of the head and neck account for about 4% of the overall incidence of cancer in the US with approximately 42,000 new cases of head and neck cancer and

Table 23-1. Subsites in Head and Neck Areas

Oral Cavity
Lips: upper
lower
Buccal mucosa
Floor of mouth
Oral tongue
Hard palate
Gingivae: upper
lower
retromolar trigone

Oropharynx
Faucial arch
Tonsillar fossa, tonsil
Base of tongue
Pharyngeal wall

Nasopharynx
Posterosuperior wall
Lateral wall

Hypopharynx
Piriform fossa
Postcricoid area
Posterior wall

Larynx
Supraglottis: Ventricular bands (false cords)
Arytenoids
Suprahyoid epiglottis (both lingual and laryngeal aspects)
Infrahyoid epiglottis
Glottis: True vocal cords, including anterior and posterior commissures
Subglottis

From American Joint Committee on Cancer[1]

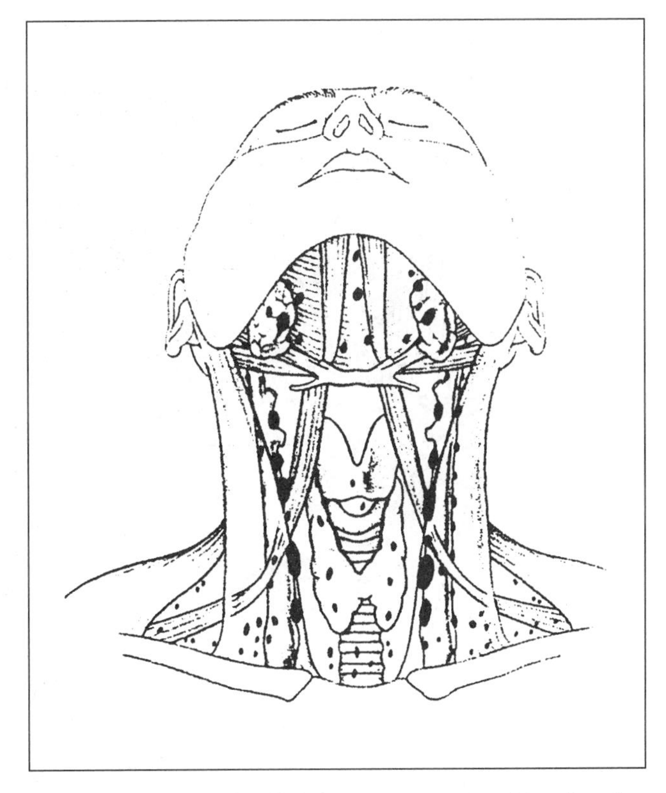

Fig 23-2. Anterior view of the neck showing regional lymph node groups.[3]

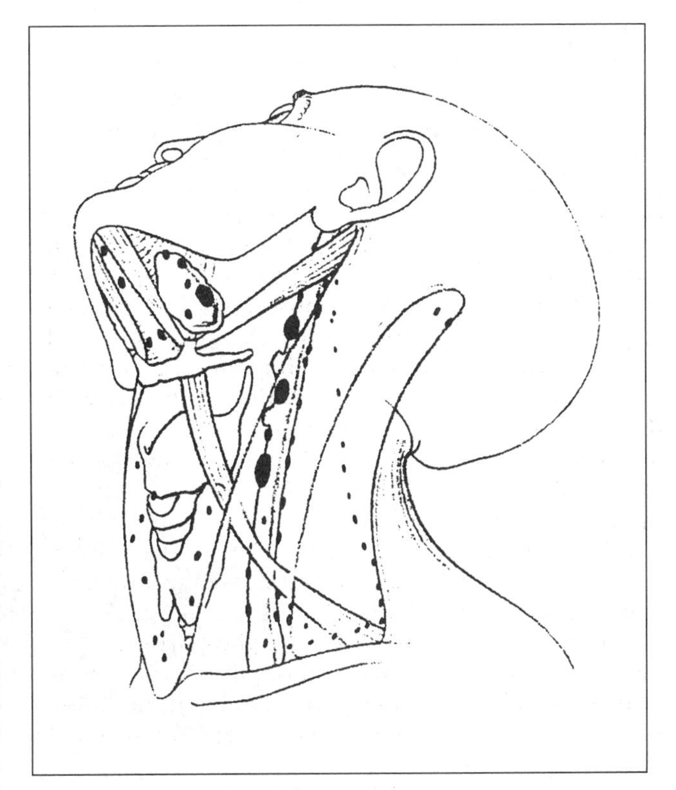

Fig 23-3. Lateral view of the neck showing regional lymph node groups.[3]

an additional 25,500 larynx and thyroid cancers were estimated for 1994 (Fig 23-5), and approximately 13,000 deaths (Fig 23-6).[5] Worldwide, approximately 500,000 new cases of head and neck cancer are projected annually. Tumors of the upper aerodigestive tract occur mostly in the fifth and sixth decades of life and predominantly affect men, although recently there seems to be a gradual increase in incidence in women. Over the past decade, we have seen patients at a much younger age, in the third and fourth decades, suffering from head and neck cancer, especially cancers of the

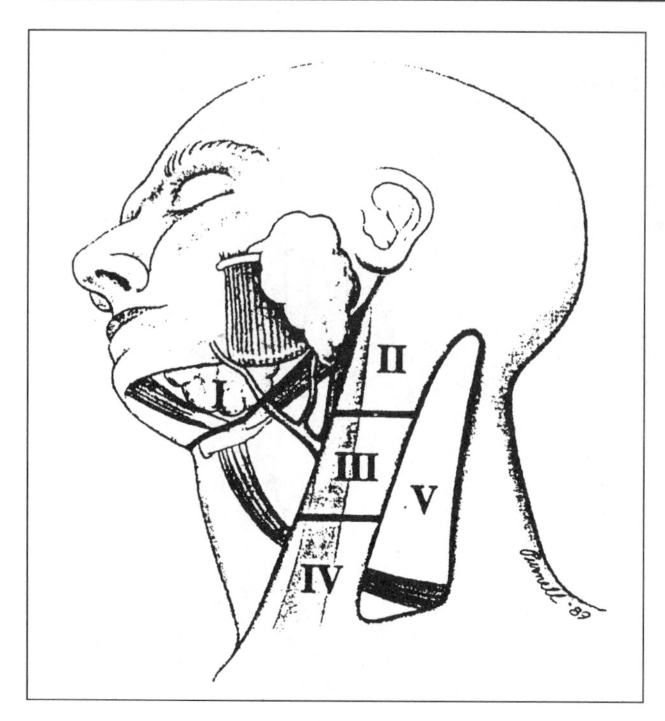

Fig 23-4. Diagram of the neck showing levels of lymph nodes.[3] Level I, submandibular; Level II, high jugular; Level III, mid jugular; Level IV, low jugular; Level V, posterior jugular. Levels VI (tracheoesophageal) and VII, (superior mediastinal) are not shown in the diagram.

oral cavity and tongue. Approximately half of all squamous cell carcinomas of the upper aerodigestive tract occur in the oral cavity. Head and neck cancer is more prevalent in certain regions of the world. Cancers of the nasopharynx and hypopharynx are extremely common in Hong Kong and south China, while tumors of the oral cavity and base of the tongue are fairly common in Bombay, India.

The most important risk factors are tobacco and alcohol. Alcohol definitely potentiates the carcinogenic risk associated with tobacco. A strong association has been shown between smokeless tobacco and oral carcinogenesis. Approximately 80% to 85% of patients presenting with head and neck cancer or tumor of the upper aerodigestive tract report a significant history of tobacco and alcohol consumption. Combined tobacco and alcohol consumption appears to have a synergistic effect, with a very high relative risk of development of head and neck cancer. Recent experimental evidence suggests that ethanol suppresses the efficiency of deoxyribonucleic acid (DNA) repair after exposure to nitrosamine compounds. In India, chewing betel nut with lime and catechu (in the form of pan) is a common habit that is correlated with a high incidence of oral cancer, especially cancer of the cheek. Chronic snuff use and marijuana smoking have also received attention recently as etiologic factors in the development of head and neck cancer.

Dietary factors include nutritional deficiency, especially in alcoholics. Plummer-Vinson syndrome, which includes esophageal web, iron deficiency anemia, and dysphagia, is associated with a high incidence of postcricoid carcinoma, especially in Europe. Nasopharyngeal cancer, which is very common in Southeast Asia and China, appears to have significant genetic and viral association. However, the nitrosamine-rich diet in endemic areas may contribute to the development of this tumor. The application of vitamin A as a major preventive substance probably favors its role as a nutritional influence on carcinogenesis. Epidemiologic data suggests a protective role for dietary carotenoids and an inverse association between consumption of fruits and vegetables and the incidence of head and neck cancer.

Occupational risks include nickel refining, woodworking, and exposure to textile fibers. To date, the

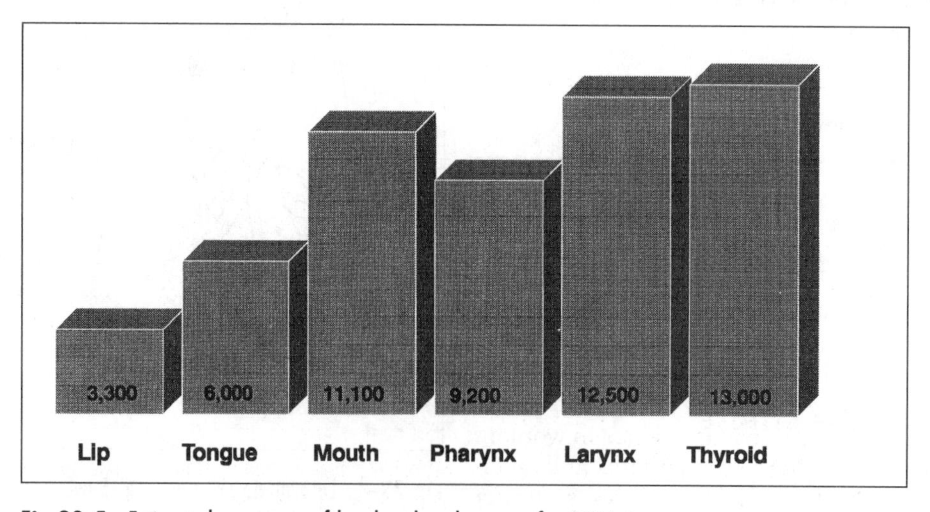

Fig 23-5. Estimated new cases of head and neck cancer for 1994.[5]

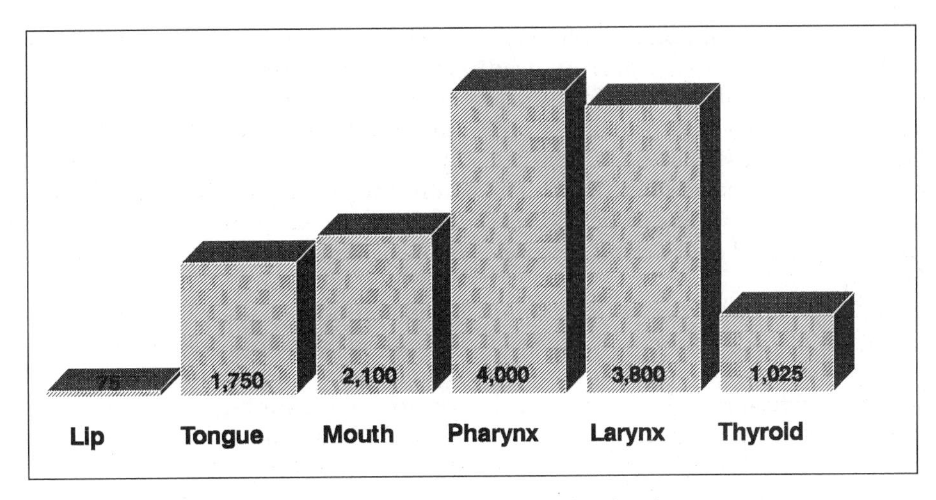

Fig 23-6. Estimated number of deaths in 1994 due to head and neck cancer.[5]

relation between asbestos exposure and cancer of the larynx has not been confirmed.

Genetic Factors

A genetic predisposition to head and neck cancer has been suggested by its sporadic occurrence in young adults and in nonusers of tobacco and alcohol. Mutagen-induced chromosomal fragility is an independent risk factor and correlates with the prospective development of second primary tumors. A subset of patients may have genetic factors that increase their cancer susceptibility to the influence of tobacco and alcohol.[6] Bloom syndrome and Li-Fraumeni syndrome have been associated with head and neck cancer in some patients with minimal tobacco exposure, which may indicate increased susceptibility to environmental carcinogens in these patients. Patients with head and neck cancer appear more sensitive to the mutagenic effect of bleomycin. This may represent mutagen sensitivity in these individuals.

Viruses

Increasing evidence suggests a role for viruses in the development of head and neck cancer. Epstein-Barr (EB) virus is associated with nasopharyngeal cancer. DNA from EB virus is found in nasopharyngeal tissues, and elevated titers of IgG and IgA antibodies are seen in all patients with nasopharyngeal cancer.[7] Elevated titers have been used as a marker to screen populations in high-risk areas and as an indicator of the likelihood of relapse. DNA from human papillomavirus has been detected in head and neck tissue.

Natural History of the Disease

Even though the diagnosis of head and neck cancer is relatively easy, only one third of patients present at an early stage (I or II). Approximately half the patients present with locally advanced disease, either at the primary site or with cervical lymph node metastasis (Fig 23-7). The presence of distant metastasis at the time of presentation is not very common. With improved loco-regional control and long-term follow-up, approximately 20% of patients are reported to develop distant metastasis. The pattern of lymph node metastasis from primary tumors of the head and neck is better understood in recent years as a result of the research of Shah and colleagues.[8] We are now able to define lymph node involvement in specific tumors of the upper aerodigestive tract (Tables 23-2 and 23-3).

The sites of distant metastasis are well recognized in the head and neck primary tumors. The most common metastatic site is the lung; however, it is important to recognize that a solitary pulmonary nodule in a patient with head and neck cancer is generally a second primary tumor in the lung rather than metastatic

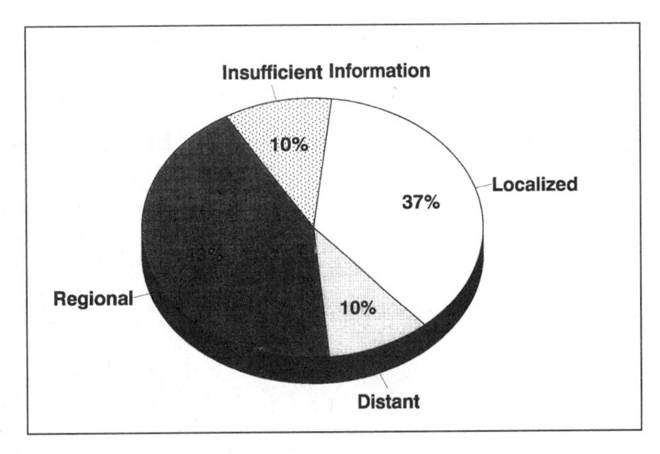

Fig 23-7. Distribution by stage of tumors of the oral cavity and pharynx (1983-1987).[5]

cancer. The presence of diffuse pulmonary nodules is most likely suggestive of metastatic cancer from head and neck tumors. Other sites of metastatic disease include mediastinal lymph nodes, the liver, and brain. The incidence of distant metastasis varies with the primary site, and is highest with cancers of the nasopharynx and hypopharynx. There appears to be a direct correlation between bulky nodal disease and development of distant metastasis.

Aberrant metastatic spread may occur in patients who were treated previously for tumors in the head and neck region. Patients who have had a neck dissection or who have received radiation therapy are at increased risk of developing aberrant metastasis both to the head and neck and to subcutaneous and cutaneous sites. Recently, perineural spread was reported, most often with large skin cancers, salivary tumors, and some tumors of the oral cavity, spreading along the inferior alveolar nerve. In many cases, the concept of perineural spread has clarified the presence of metastasis to the base of the skull. Direct invasion of surrounding nerves is also common in head and neck tumors. Tumors of the oral cavity and metastatic disease in the neck may involve the surrounding cranial nerves, such as the hypoglossal, lingual, vagus and sympathetic trunk. Large parotid tumors with high-grade malignancy are known to involve the facial nerve, causing facial palsy.

Table 23-2. Distribution and Histologic Confirmation of Metastatic Disease by Site

Primary Site	Number of Patients	Number of RNDs	Positive Nodes in Elective RNDs	Positive Nodes in Therapeutic RNDs
Oral cavity	501	516	34%	76%
Oropharynx	207	213	31	84
Hypopharynx	126	128	17	97
Larynx	247	262	37	84
Total	1,081	1,119	33	82

Results in 1,081 patients undergoing 1,119 elective and therapeutic RNDs.
RND = radical neck dissection. From Shah.[8]

Table 23-3. Percentage of Metastatic Lymph Nodes Involved in Elective and Therapeutic RNDs

	Primary Site							
Level of metastatic lymph nodes	Oral Cavity		Oropharynx		Hypopharynx		Larynx	
	Elective	Therapeutic	Elective	Therapeutic	Elective	Therapeutic	Elective	Therapeutic
I	58%	61%	7%	17%	0%	10%	14%	8%
II	51	57	80	85	75	78	52	68
III	26	44	60	50	75	75	55	70
IV	9	20	27	33	0	47	24	35
V	2	4	7	11	0	11	7	5

RND = radical neck dissection
From Shah.[8]

Clinical Presentation

Of several warning signs promulgated by the American Cancer Society, at least three pertain to the head and neck: dysphagia, chronic ulcer, and lump in the neck. Despite these obvious and common findings, two of every three patients with head and neck cancer still present at an advanced stage, primarily because of neglect on their parts and, on several occasions, misdiagnosis by the primary physician. In an elderly person who presents with head and neck complaints, it is extremely important to rule out the presence of malignancy and maintain close observation.

Symptoms vary from site to site. Some tumors may become symptomatic at an early stage, such as hoarseness with tumors of the vocal cord, while others, such as tumors of the nasopharynx or hypopharynx, may not be suspected at all. Common symptoms in patients with cancer of the oral cavity include a painful ulceration, slurred speech, bleeding in the oral cavity, and an exophytic mass. The diagnosis of oral cancer is occasionally made on routine examination by a dentist or oral surgeon.

A patient with early nasopharyngeal cancer may present with unilateral otitis media. Tumors of the oropharynx and laryngopharynx are associated with odynophagia, dysphagia, change of voice, and occasionally, airway obstruction. Unexplained weight loss is an important finding in patients with head and neck cancer. Occasionally, the patient may neglect to treat change of voice or minor airway distress until they present to the emergency room with acute airway obstruction requiring emergency airway intervention.

Tumors of the nasal cavity and paranasal sinuses may remain undetected for a long time and be mistaken for sinusitis or allergic rhinitis. Recurrent epistaxis, malar swelling, and diplopia are common symptoms in advanced maxillary sinus tumor. These symptoms may remain undiagnosed for a long time. Pain, a late symptom in head and neck tumors, generally is mediated by the trigeminal or glossopharyngeal nerve. The glossopharyngeal and vagus nerves transmit pain from pharyngeal and laryngeal tumors as referred pain to the ear. Hypopharyngeal neoplasms or tumors of the base of the tongue may cause otalgia through Arnold's nerve, the auricular branch of the vagus nerve. In advanced stages, the patient may present with acute airway distress as described above or with intense pain, severe dysphagia and weight loss, obvious involvement of the skin of the face and neck, and occasionally mandibular involvement with loose teeth. Advanced tumors of the oral cavity may extend to the skin and subcutaneous tissue complicated by orocutaneous fistula.

Synchronous and Metachronous Second Primary Tumors

There is a substantial risk of a second primary tumor in patients with head and neck cancer. Factors such as smoking and alcohol intake have a carcinogenic effect on the entire surface of the upper aerodigestive tract. While a patient may present at any time with one primary cancer, there is about a 15% incidence of a synchronous second primary tumor, including cancer of the lung or esophagus. The incidence of metachronous cancer is approximately 4% annually on follow-up. This is the main reason a patient with head and neck cancer should always remain under close observation and cancer surveillance.[2] The increased risk of a second primary cancer requires very close follow-up in patients with head and neck cancer and thorough evaluation of the entire upper aerodigestive tract, including a chest x-ray and barium swallow or esophagoscopy for unexplained weight loss.

Standard surveillance of patients with head and neck cancer includes a monthly follow-up in the first year, bimonthly follow-up in the second year, every 3 months in the third year, and subsequently every 6 to 12 months. A chest x-ray is routinely performed initially every 4 to 6 months and, after 2 to 3 years, annually. It is important to evaluate the chest x-ray critically and compare the films with previous radiographs for any abnormality in the lung fields.

Diagnostic Workup

The diagnostic workup in a patient with head and neck cancer can be divided into history and physical findings, biopsy including fine-needle aspiration (FNA), imaging studies including a panoramic x-ray of the mandible, computed tomographic (CT) scan, ultrasonogram, and magnetic resonance imaging (MRI). Specific symptoms that may not be appreciated by the patient such as otalgia, odynophagia, hoarseness of voice, and sore throat should be carefully evaluated. A thorough head and neck examination with the use of mirror and fiberoptic rigid telescope or fiberoptic nasopharyngolaryngoscope is important.

Radiologic Studies

The use of routine x-rays of the head and neck is not crucial; however, airway films or the chest x-ray will reveal any asymmetry of the vocal cords and any pathologic abnormality in the lungs. A plain film of the paranasal sinus will reveal gross abnormality in one of the maxillary sinus. However, with the routine use of CT and MRI, tumors of the base of the skull and base of the tongue can be better delineated. The CT scan is also of great help in evaluating clinically nonpalpable cervical lymph nodes. Tumors of the deep lobe of the parotid and parapharyngeal areas can be better defined by either CT scan or MRI.

Biopsy Techniques

It is very important to make a correct diagnosis before initiating treatment for head and neck tumors. Even though the role of the pathologist is extremely important in the appropriate interpretation of biopsy material, the technique of performing biopsy is also very important. Various techniques commonly utilized in the head and neck include punch biopsy, incisional biopsy, excisional biopsy, curettage, and needle aspiration biopsy. Fine needle aspiration yields a specimen for cytologic diagnosis, while other techniques provide tissue for histologic diagnosis.

The most common technique for obtaining a mucosal biopsy in the head and neck is punch biopsy. Various punch biopsy forceps are used; the most common is the cup forceps.[9] Even though it is generally recommended that a biopsy be performed on the periphery of the lesion, we feel a small portion of the exophytic lesion is satisfactory to make a diagnosis, especially for squamous cell carcinoma. We rarely use stitches after the biopsy. Local pressure for a few minutes will generally stop bleeding from the biopsy site. If there is infection or necrotic material, the biopsy should be performed on a fleshy, nonulcerated region.

Biopsies of lesions of the larynx or pharynx are generally performed endoscopically under anesthesia. If the patient is to be brought to the operating room for proper evaluation of the extent of the tumor and biopsy, then it is appropriate to perform direct laryngoscopy, pharyngoscopy, and esophagoscopy. If the chest x-ray is normal, we generally do not perform routine bronchoscopy and selective bronchial washings.

If a lesion in the oral cavity is small, it may be more appropriate to perform an excisional biopsy with satisfactory margins. In patients with diffuse areas of leukoplakia or erythroplakia in the oral cavity, surface staining with vital dyes such as toluidine blue may be helpful. The dye is an acidophilic, metachromatic nuclear stain that colors the areas of squamous cell carcinoma.

The incisional biopsy is best used for lesions of the skin and soft tissue masses. Frozen sections are routinely utilized under general anesthesia to obtain adequate sampling and enhance diagnosis. Biopsy of irradiated lesions is always difficult because of mucosal edema and radiation changes.

Needle biopsy has been popular in this country since the landmark article in 1930 by Hayes Martin.[10] Unfortunately, for the fear of needle tract implantation it was not routinely used until the 1970s. With the advent of Papanicolaou (Pap) stain, the cytologic diagnosis can be made based on FNA. The FNA has become extremely popular and is used for almost all head and neck masses. The technique of FNA has been described extensively in the literature, and every individual dealing with head and neck tumors should be conversant with the technique (Fig 23-8).[9] FNA is extremely useful in cervical lymphadenopathy, thyroid tumors, and salivary tumors.

In the evaluation of cervical lymphadenopathy, an algorithmic approach can be used in patients presenting with suspicious malignant pathology (Fig 23-9). An FNA finding of cervical lymph node metastasis can be interpreted as metastatic squamous cell carcinoma, metastatic adenocarcinoma, metastatic thyroid carcinoma, or suspicion of lymphoma.[11] The final diagnosis of lymphoma is based on open biopsy. Open biopsy is also important for T&B marker studies and electron microscopic studies. FNA has become the first diagnostic test in the evaluation of the thyroid mass. It appears to be the most cost-effective, and its accuracy in detecting thyroid tumors exceeds 80%. Results of FNA of the thyroid can be considered malignant, suspicious, benign, or indeterminate. The diagnosis of follicular neoplasm based on a cellular smear generally requires operative exploration. The diagnoses of benign follicular adenoma and follicular carcinoma cannot be made based on FNA alone, since the entire capsule needs to be evaluated after excision of the thyroid mass.

The role of FNA in salivary gland lesions is controversial, as most of these lesions can be easily evaluated clinically and approached surgically by superficial parotidectomy. However, in certain tumors involving the tail of the parotid in which a clinical diagnosis may be uncertain, FNA is of great help in distinguishing salivary from nonsalivary pathology. On average, the accuracy of FNA in detecting salivary lesions exceeds 80% (Table 23-4).[12]

Even though there are many pitfalls in the evaluation of FNA in the head and neck, clearly this appears

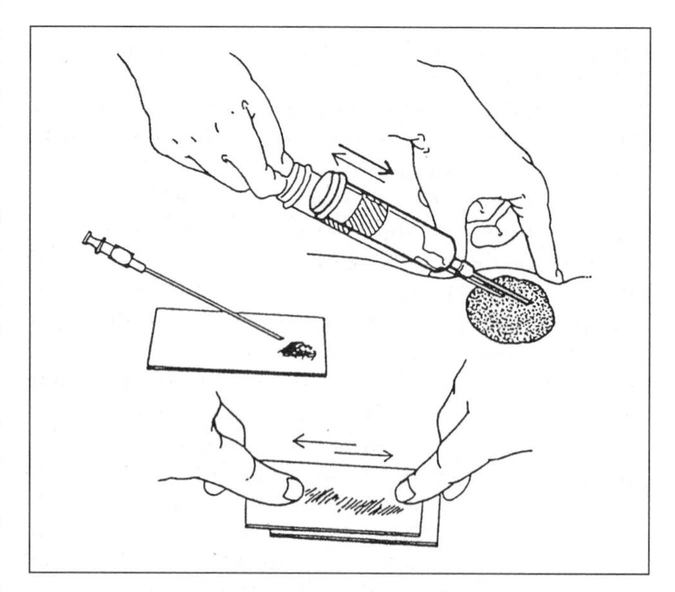

Fig 23-8. Technique of fine needle aspiration.[9]

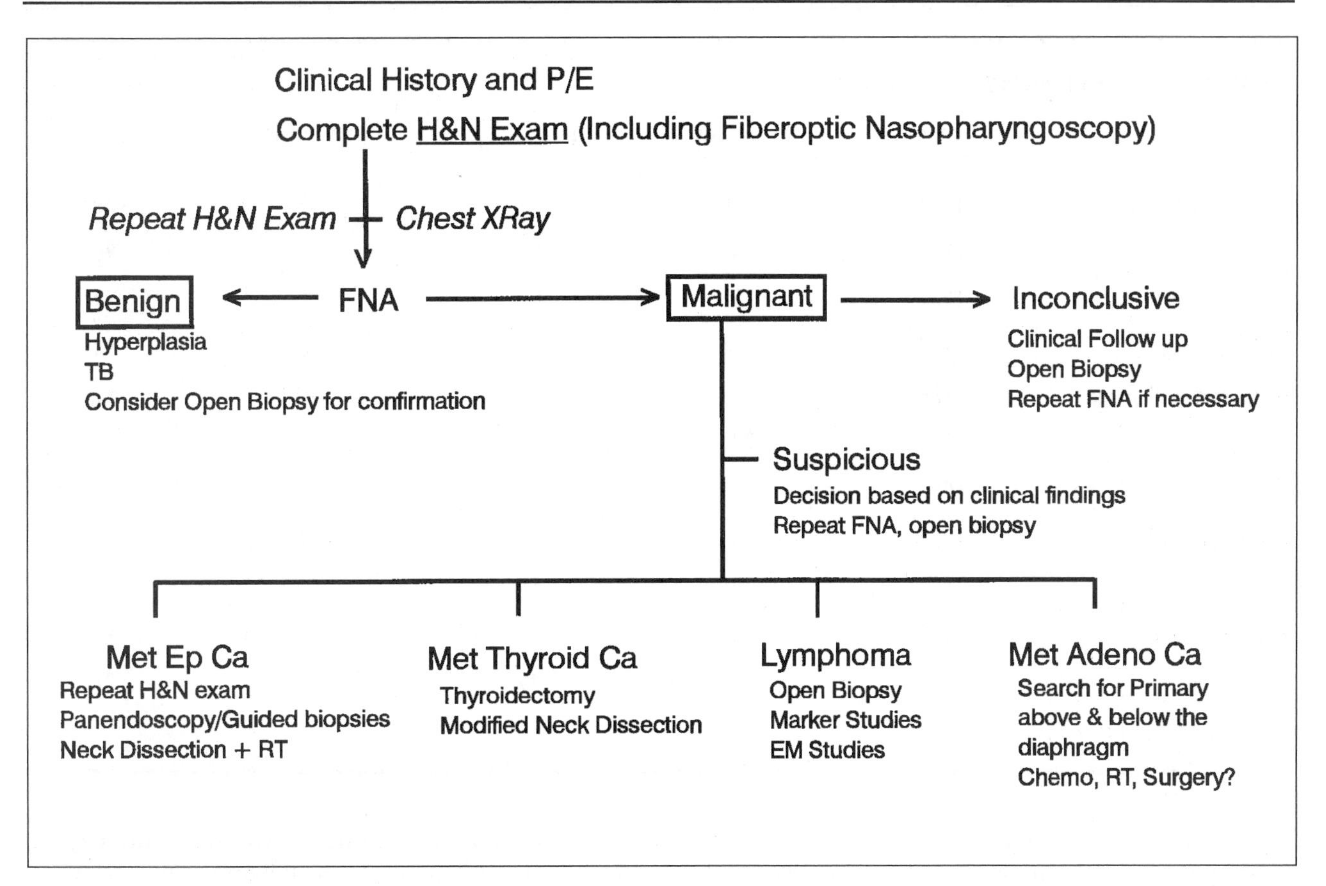

Fig 23-9. Algorithmic approach to the management of cervical lymphadenopathy.[11]

to be one of the most important diagnostic tests available today. The clinical correlation must be made with the results of the FNA and whenever the FNA does not corroborate the clinical findings, further investigation should be performed including open biopsy based on clinical judgment.

Staging System

In 1992, the American Joint Committee on Cancer in collaboration with the International Union Against Cancer (UICC) updated the TNM staging system for the head and neck.[1] Essentially, this is a TNM staging in which tumors are classified T1 to T4 (Table 23-5); nodal disease is described as N1, N2, or N3 (Table 23-6); and distant metastases are noted as M1. The stage grouping (I to IV) is also very important (Table 23-7). The TNM staging system for cervical lymph nodes is depicted in Fig 23-10. Stages I and II tumors are generally considered to be early cancers with a more favorable prognosis than advanced (stage III and IV) cancers. Most protocol studies and randomized prospective trials of the head and neck include patients with advanced cancer. Recently, the radiologic evaluation was included as a part of the initial work-up and integral part of the staging system.

Pathologic Classification

Since the upper aerodigestive tract is lined mainly by squamous epithelium, the most common tumors in the head and neck are squamous cell carcinomas. However, other tumors, such as adenocarcinomas originating in minor salivary glands are also seen occasionally. Other rare tumors, such as soft tissue sarcomas, including leiomyosarcoma, rhabdomyosarcoma, and fibrosarcoma are also encountered. It is important for a person evaluating head and neck cancer to understand and appreciate the importance of leukoplakia and erythroplakia. Leukoplakia is a clinical term that describes a white patch in the oral cavity. Approximately 2% to 5% of patients with leukoplakia will develop squamous carcinoma long-term. In contrast, the incidence of squamous carcinoma in erythroplakia is approximately 30%. Both leukoplakia and erythroplakia are considered highly premalignant, and patients with these conditions should be kept under close observation.[8] Any suspicious area in this region should be biopsied. Vital dyes, such as toluidine blue, have been used to evaluate suspicious areas in leukoplakia. The transformation of leukoplakia to infiltrating carcinoma undergoes a number of stages, including carcinoma in situ.

Table 23-4. Needle Biopsy in Salivary Lesions

Author	Year	No. of Cases	Sensitivity	Specificity	Accuracy
Enroth and Zajicek	1970	690	64%	95%	89%
Kline et al	1981	47	100	95	96
Sismanis et al	1981	51	85	96	92
Qizilbash et al	1985	101	88	100	98
Lindberg and Akerman	1986	461	67	85	81
O'Dwyer et al	1986	341	73	94	93
Layfield et al	1987	171	91	98	92
Nettle and Orell	1989	106	80	99	94
Jayram et al	1989	195	81	94	88
Rodriguez et al	1989	64	85	97	93
Shaha et al	1990	160	95	98	97

From Shah et al.[12]

Verrucous carcinoma is a clinical diagnosis characterized by an exophytic tumor of wart-like appearance that is very well differentiated microscopically and is sometimes difficult to diagnose based on histology alone. These tumors are commonly seen in the mucosa of the cheek and larynx. Surgical excision has been the preferred form of treatment, although radiotherapy occasionally produces good results. Exophytic tumors and ulcerating or infiltrating carcinomas are other varieties noted in the head and neck region. Lymphoepithelial masses are poorly differentiated squamous cell carcinomas with lymphoid stroma, most commonly noted in the nasopharynx and tonsil. These tumors are more radiosensitive.

The prognostic factors related to pathology include the differentiation of the tumor and the depth of invasion. In recent studies involving mucosal sites in the head and neck area, such as the tongue and floor of the mouth, a direct relation was demonstrated between the depth of invasion and the incidence of metastasis to the lymph node and survival.[13]

Table 23-5. TNM Staging of Head and Neck Tumors (Primary Tumor [T])

Lip and Oral Cavity	
T1	Tumor ≤2 cm in greatest dimension
T2	Tumor >2 cm but ≤4 cm in greatest dimension
T3	Tumor >4 cm in greatest dimension
T4	(Lip) tumor invades adjacent structures, eg, through cortical bone, tongue, skin of neck
T4	(Oral cavity) tumor invades adjacent structures, eg, through cortical bone, into deep (extrinsic) muscle of tongue, maxillary sinus, skin
Oropharynx	
T1	Tumor ≤2 cm in greatest dimension
T2	Tumor >2 cm but ≤4 cm in greatest dimension
T3	Tumor >4 cm in greatest dimension
T4	Tumor invades adjacent structures, eg, through cortical bone, soft tissues of neck, deep (extrinsic) muscle of tongue

Continued

Table 23-5 *Continued.* TNM Staging of Head and Neck Tumors

Nasopharynx	
T1	Tumor limited to one subsite of nasopharynx
T2	Tumor invades more than one subsite of nasopharynx
T3	Tumor invades nasal cavity and/or nasopharynx
T4	Tumor invades skull and/or cranial nerve(s)
Hypopharynx	
T1	Tumor limited to one subsite of hypopharynx
T2	Tumor invades more than one subsite of hypopharynx or an adjacent site, without fixation of hemilarynx
T3	Tumor invades more than one subsite of hypopharynx or an adjacent site, with fixation of hemilarynx
T4	Tumor invades adjacent structures, eg, cartilage or soft tissues of neck
Supraglottis	
T1	Tumor limited to one subsite of supraglottis with normal vocal cord mobility
T2	Tumor invades more than one subsite of supraglottis or glottis, with normal vocal cord mobility
T3	Tumor limited to larynx with vocal cord fixation and/or invades postcricoid area, medial wall of piriform sinus, or pre-epiglottic tissues
T4	Tumor invades through thyroid cartilage, and/or extends to other tissues beyond the larynx, eg, to the oropharynx, soft tissues of neck
Glottis	
T1	Tumor limited to vocal cord(s) (may involve anterior or posterior commissures) with normal mobility
T1a	Tumor limited to one vocal cord
T1b	Tumor involves both vocal cords
T2	Tumor extends to supraglottis and/or subglottis, and/or with impaired vocal cord mobility
T3	Tumor limited to the larynx with vocal cord fixation
T4	Tumor invades through thyroid cartilage and/or extends to other tissues beyond the larynx, eg, oropharynx, soft tissues of neck
Subglottis	
T1	Tumor limited to the subglottis
T2	Tumor extends to vocal cord(s) with normal or impaired mobility
T3	Tumor limited to larynx with vocal cord fixation
T4	Tumor invades through cricoid or thyroid cartilage and/or extends to other tissues beyond the larynx, eg, oropharynx, soft tissues of neck
Maxillary Sinus	
T1	Tumor limited to the antral mucosa with no erosion or destruction of bone
T2	Tumor with erosion or destruction of the infrastructure including the hard palate and/or the middle nasal meatus
T3	Tumor invades any of the following: skin of cheek, posterior wall of the maxillary sinus, floor or medial wall of orbit, anterior ethmoid sinus
T4	Tumor invades orbital contents and/or any of the following: cribriform plate, posterior ethmoid or sphenoid sinuses, nasopharynx, soft palate, pterygomaxillary or temporal fossae or base of skull
Salivary Glands	
T1	Tumor ≤2 cm in greatest dimension
T2	Tumor >2 cm but ≤4 cm in greatest dimension
T3	Tumor >4 cm but ≤6 cm in greatest dimension
T4	Tumor >6 cm in greatest dimension

From American Joint Committee on Cancer.[1]

Treatment

The management of head and neck cancer requires a detailed evaluation of the extent of disease and a multidisciplinary approach. Therapeutic modalities include surgery, radiation therapy, chemotherapy, and immunotherapy. At present, the role of immunotherapy is investigational. There have been randomized as well as nonrandomized trials utilizing chemotherapy in the head and neck, and various chemotherapeutic agents have been found to be very useful. However, no difference in survival has been demonstrated with preoperative chemotherapy or with neo-adjuvant chemotherapy. Therefore, the main treatment modalities for head and neck cancer remain surgery and radiation therapy.

Decisions regarding the appropriate treatment are based on such tumor factors as site, histology, size, depth of invasion, disease stage, previous treatment, and the need for reconstructive surgery. Patient factors include impact on quality of life, medical condition, patient preference, treatment cost, convenience, and compliance. Physician factors include the availability of necessary personnel, a comprehensive multidisciplinary team, physician preference, and the institutional practice. Clearly, considering these various parameters, individual patients require tailored treatment approach.

Table 23-6. TNM Staging of Head and Neck Tumors (Lymph Node [N])

NX	Regional lymph nodes cannot be assessed
N0	No regional lymph node metastasis
N1	Metastasis in a single ipsilateral lymph node, ≤3 cm in greatest dimension
N2	Metastasis in a single ipsilateral lymph node, >3 cm but ≤6 cm in greatest dimension, or multiple ipsilateral lymph nodes, none >6 cm in greatest dimension, or bilateral or contralateral lymph nodes, none >6 cm in greatest dimension
N2a	Metastasis in a single ipsilateral lymph node >3 cm but ≤6 cm in greatest dimension
N2b	Metastasis in multiple ipsilateral lymph nodes, none >6 cm in greatest dimension
N2c	Metastasis in bilateral or contralateral lymph nodes, none >6 cm in greatest dimension
N3	Metastasis in a lymph node >6 cm in greatest dimension

From American Joint Committee on Cancer.[1]

Table 23-7. Stage Grouping of Head and Neck Tumors

Stage 0	Tis	N0	M0
Stage I	T1	N0	M0
Stage II	T2	N0	M0
Stage III	T3	N0	M0
	T1	N1	M0
	T2	N1	M0
	T3	N1	M0
Stage IV	T4	N0	M0
	T4	N1	M0
	Any T	N2	M0
	Any T	N3	M0
	Any T	Any N	M1

From American Joint Committee on Cancer.[1]

Early-stage (stages I and II) tumors of the head and neck can best be treated with either surgery or radiation therapy, with almost equally good control rates. For small lesions of the oral cavity, we generally prefer wide local excision rather than radiation therapy. Since radiation therapy can be given only once, we prefer to utilize it in more advanced conditions or for recurrent tumors. However, certain lesions, such as early laryngeal cancers, are best treated with radiation therapy to better preserve voice function, and surgery is reserved for salvage from recurrent disease.[14]

Radiation therapy clearly has complications: xerostomia, dental problems, and occasionally osteoradionecrosis. The current practice in the management of advanced cancers of the head and neck is a multimodality approach involving surgery followed by radiation therapy. Preoperative radiation therapy, which was practiced in the mid-1970s, did not show any therapeutic advantage and was associated with increased problems of wound healing and an increased risk of surgical complications.

In stages III and IV cancers, postoperative radiation therapy improves local control and survival, with 5-year survival rates increasing from 31% to 59%. Postoperative radiation therapy also improves survival in patients with extracapsular nodal disease and in those with positive surgical margins. Chemotherapy has been evaluated for organ preservation, with trials focusing on the larynx.[15] A large randomized trial recently confirmed that laryngeal preservation was feasible in 64% of patients who received induction chemotherapy followed by radiation therapy, although the survival rates were not significantly different from

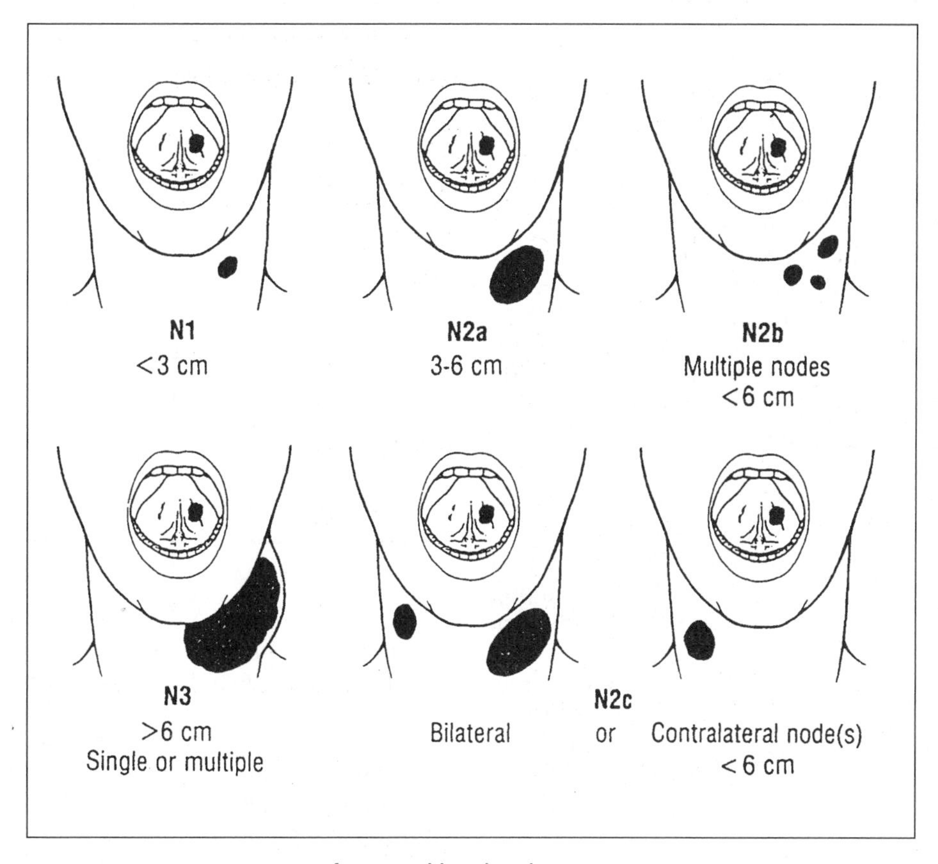

Fig 23-10. TNM staging system for cervical lymph nodes.[3]

those of patients treated with laryngectomy and radiation. Organ preservation at other sites of head and neck cancer is currently under investigation.

Unknown Primary Tumors

An unknown primary tumor is defined as the presence of metastatic cancer in the neck while the primary tumor remains undetected. A thorough evaluation of the head and neck region is quite essential. With the advent of fiberoptic telescopes and nasopharyngoscopes, the nasopharynx and certain critical areas of the upper aerodigestive tract can be evaluated readily. Examination under anesthesia and guided or random biopsies are routinely performed in patients with an unknown primary tumor. The panendoscopy or triscopy includes evaluation of the larynx, pharynx, esophagus, and lungs under general anesthesia. "Blind" biopsies or random biopsies should be routinely performed of the nasopharynx, base of the tongue, tonsil, piriform sinus, and epiglottis. Recently directed biopsies of the likely site of the primary tumor have been suggested, depending on the location of the metastasis to the neck. An open biopsy of the neck should be considered, depending on FNA findings and evaluation of the primary tumor. Open biopsy may be performed prior to the therapeutic decision and neck dissection. One should be prepared to proceed with the neck dissection if open biopsy is performed. However, in most cases of a neck mass, open biopsy is not done for fear of infection, tumor spread into the subcutaneous tissue, and occasionally the patient's being lost to follow-up.

The standard treatment of metastatic carcinoma with an unknown primary tumor still remains neck dissection followed by radiation therapy. There appears to be considerable controversy over the portals to be included in postoperative radiotherapy. Whether the nasopharynx should be included or not remains controversial. However, if the metastatic tumor involves the upper part of the neck, the nasopharynx should be routinely included in the radiation portals. After appropriate management of the unknown primary tumor, recurrence ranges from 11% to 14%. The prognosis depends on the extracapsular spread of disease, the histologic features of the metastatic cancer, squamous carcinoma vs adenocarcinoma vs anaplastic carcinoma, and tumor grade. Metastatic adenocarcinoma of the neck generally originates in structures below the clavicle, such as the lung, breast, stomach, pancreas, and ovary. Occasionally, the primary tumor may be located in the salivary gland.[16] Metastatic adenocarcinoma to the supraclavicular region presenting as Virchow's lymph node is generally considered to be a systemic disease and best treated by chemotherapy. The role of neck dissection in metastatic adenocarcinoma is extremely limited, being reserved for pressure symptoms or fungating pathology.

Neck

The management of the neck comprises elective treatment for N0 disease and management of N+ disease. For the past half-century, radical neck dissection, as described by George Crile in 1906 and popularized by Hayes Martin, has been considered standard treatment for N+ neck. The standard neck dissection procedure included removal of all lymph nodes in the neck from levels I to V, with removal of the internal jugular vein, spinal accessory nerve, and sternocleidomastoid muscle. The main argument against radical neck dissection was the loss of shoulder function due to sacrifice of the spinal accessory nerve. The modified neck dissection was popularized in the mid-1960s by O'Suarez and Bocca. In the US, it was popularized by Richard Jesse, Allando Ballantine, and Robert Byers.

Various modifications of neck dissection were practiced and there was considerable confusion regarding the nomenclature. The American Academy of Otolaryngology–Head and Neck Surgery has made recent efforts to standardize the nomenclature of neck dissection (Table 23-8).[17] The bilateral simultaneous radical neck dissection is associated with a mortality rate of approximately 17%. Today it would be a rare event, necessitating bilateral standard radical neck dissection. We would consider performing a staged radical neck dissection or radical neck dissection on one side with a modified neck dissection on the other side.

Almost all patients with N+ disease will require postoperative radiation therapy. Local recurrence with neck dissection alone was 30%, 50%, and 70% in N1, N2, and N3 disease, respectively. Clearly, there is an increasing need for postoperative radiation therapy in the management of cervical lymph node metastasis. The radical neck dissection remains the surgical mainstay in patients with N2 or N3 disease. In selected N1 disease, especially if the tumor is in the submandibular region or away from the accessory nerve, efforts should be made to preserve the accessory nerve and consequently the shoulder function.

The management of N0 neck has become both controversial and of interest to most surgeons. If the risk of micrometastasis is >20%, elective treatment of N0 neck should be considered, which may be either surgery or irradiation. We generally avoid routine use of radiation therapy for N0 neck because of complications related to radiation therapy as well as long-term consequences. Since the incidence of microscopic disease is only 15% to 20%, we feel that in the remaining 80% of patients this is overtreatment, and we would rather reserve radiation therapy for local recurrence or further metastatic disease in the neck.

Table 23-8. Neck Dissection Classification

1. Radical neck dissection
2. Modified radical neck dissection
3. Selective neck dissection
   a. Supraomohyoid neck dissection
   b. Posterolateral neck dissection
   c. Anterior compartment neck dissection
   d. Lateral neck dissection
4. Extended radical neck dissection

The supraomohyoid neck dissection, which includes removal of lymph nodes at levels I, II, and III, has become a routine staging procedure for most tumors of the oral cavity.[8] Radiation therapy is reserved for those with multiple nodal metastases or extracapsular spread. Our indications for postoperative radiation therapy in cervical metastasis include multiple lymph node metastasis, extracapsular extension of the disease, a lymph node >3 cm, and critical areas such as level IV or V.[3] Local control in the neck can be achieved in >70% of patients with N2 or N3 disease if surgery is followed by radiation therapy.

Nasopharynx

Approximately 75% of patients with nasopharyngeal cancer present with nodal metastasis. Radiation therapy is the choice of treatment for most nasopharyngeal cancers.[7] Interestingly, even massive nodal disease responds well to radiation therapy alone. Lymphoepithelioma is highly radiosensitive. Neck dissection may be performed for persistent nodal disease after radiation therapy. The 5-year survival rate exceeds 70%, and a dose >7,000 cGy is generally recommended. Recently, interstitial implantation has been used in the management of persistent or recurrent nasopharyngeal cancer. The role of surgery in nasopharyngeal cancer is limited to localized recurrent disease. Exposure and access to the nasopharynx is difficult; in most cases, the tumor is removed either piecemeal or with close margins. Survival is clearly different between World Health Organization (WHO) type 1 and type 3 nasopharyngeal carcinoma, with type 3 or (lymphoepithelioma) responding best to the treatment. The relation of EB virus to nasopharyngeal cancer is the subject of ongoing studies. EB virus titer is also used as a prognostic indicator in the follow-up of these patients.

Oral Cavity

The most common sites of tumors in the oral cavity are the floor of the mouth and the tongue. The treatment decision for tumors of the oral cavity depends on T stage, size, site (anterior or posterior in the oral cavity), proximity to the mandible, direct involvement of the mandible, and incidence of micrometastasis or gross metastasis to the neck. Early cancers of the oral cavity can be treated equally well with surgery or radiation therapy. However, small lesions can be easily excised through the open mouth with minimal compromise in speech or swallowing function. Small cancers of the lip can easily be excised in the fashion of a V excision, with primary reconstruction or with local flaps. However, patients with advanced lip cancer will require complex reconstruction of the lip such as Abbe-Estlander or Karapandzic flaps. Early lesions of the tongue can be easily excised with primary closure. Small lesions on the floor of the mouth can be easily excised through open mouth, and the defect may be left open to heal by secondary intention or skin grafted. Whenever a lesion near the opening of the submandibular salivary duct is excised, consideration should be given to excision of the submandibular salivary gland due to future problems related to obstructive sialadenitis. In certain select cases, the duct may be transposed. Tumors close to the mandible warrant consideration of excision of a portion of the mandible via a marginal or segmental mandibulectomy, depending on the extent of mandibular invasion.[18]

Advanced lesions of the oral cavity will be difficult to control with external radiation therapy alone and may require brachytherapy. However, the high incidence of mandibular complications must be kept in mind prior to consideration of radiation therapy alone. In the treatment of tongue cancer, consideration should be given to the high incidence of metastasis to cervical lymph nodes. The incidence of micrometastasis for T1, T2, and T3 tongue cancer varies from 30% to 65%. Tumors of the posterior oral cavity and posterior portion of the lateral aspect of the tongue can be easily resected by either cheek flap or mandibulotomy. Recently, the mandibular swing approach has become popular as an adjunct to better exposure of tumors in the posterior oral cavity with preservation of function and cosmesis.

Trismus and osteoradionecrosis are major complications of radiation therapy for tumors of the oral cavity. Both are difficult to manage and lead to poor functional outcome. Trismus is best prevented by regular exercises and close observation; during radiation therapy, patients should undertake intensive oral exercises and remain under the close observation of the treating physician. Dental evaluation and management of infected or loose teeth should be undertaken prior to radiation therapy. Fluoride therapy during and after irradiation should be utilized under care of a dentist.

Oropharynx

In the oropharynx, tumors are commonly found on the tonsils and base of the tongue. Most tumors of the tonsil present with lymph node metastasis. Early tonsillar lesions can be treated with radiation therapy. However, with advanced lesions, especially metastatic disease to the neck, surgical resection followed by postoperative radiation therapy produces the optimal survival results. The surgical approach to both the tonsil and the base of the tongue can be achieved by paramedian mandibulotomy. We feel paramedian mandibulotomy is preferred to midline mandibulotomy because of the space between the incisor and canine teeth, adequate soft tissue coverage of the alveolar margin, easy fixation of the body of the mandible with miniplate, and noninvolvement of the fracture site in the postoperative radiation therapy portals.

Recently, tumors of the base of the tongue have been managed with a combination of external radiation and brachytherapy with interstitial implantation. However, complications including necrosis of the base of the tongue and edema warrant further evaluation. Local control and cure rates have been reported to exceed 80%. Overall cure rates in patients with oropharyngeal cancer are about 40%. Stages I and II cancers of the oropharynx have 5-year survival rates of 50% to 60% after radiotherapy with surgical salvage. Lesions requiring combined treatment include stages III and IV disease, which have a 5-year survival rate of 46%.

Mandible

Considerations in the management of the mandible include the spread of oral cancers to the mandible, marginal mandibulectomy, mandibulotomy, and the role of segmental mandibulectomy and mandibular reconstruction. Preoperative evaluation of the mandible is very important in the management of cancers of the oral cavity, especially those that are either adherent to the medial aspect of the mandible or very close to the mandible. There is no definitive investigation that can evaluate the mandible with absolute accuracy. At present, the best "test" remains the clinical evaluation, especially with tumors adherent or close to the mandible, mainly because minimal bony invasion is extremely difficult to evaluate by any test. Common tests, including dental x-rays, panoramic x-ray of the mandible, CT scan, bone scan, and MRI, all have a high incidence of false-positive results. Dental fillings lead to considerable artifacts on CT scan. When there is destruction of the mandible, panoramic x-ray is helpful to evaluate the extent of mandibular resection required during surgery. However, the best judgment and surgical decision is still based on the clinical examination, especially as to whether marginal versus segmental mandibulectomy should be performed.[19]

Our understanding of tumor spread from the oral cavity has evolved. In the past, tumors of the oral cavity were believed to spread through the mandibular periosteum and the bone to the cervical lymph nodes. It is apparent now that there are no direct lymphatics from the oral cavity to the cervical lymph nodes going through the mandible. The way the tumor spreads from the oral cavity to the mandible is by direct extension through the alveolar ridge, through the pores on the alveolar border of the mandible or through the dental socket. Clearly, the edentulous mandible is at high risk for direct invasion by tumors of the floor of the mouth. Tumors involving the retromolar region are also at high risk for direct invasion of the mandible.

Over the past two decades, there has been a considerable switch from routine segmental mandibulectomy, which was used for access, to conservation of the mandible either by marginal mandibulectomy or the mandibular swing approach. Marginal mandibulectomy can be performed via a horizontal, vertical, or oblique cut (Fig 23-11). We routinely use the oblique method to maintain a strong remaining mandible. The oblique cut also gives adequate clearance of the tumor, especially if the tumor invades the diaphragm of the floor of the mouth. The defect after marginal mandibulectomy can be easily covered either by advancement of the mucosa or by split-thickness skin graft. In smaller defects, the area can be left open to heal by secondary intention.

The mandibular swing, or mandibulotomy, approach has become popular in recent years. The main indications for this approach are tumors involving the base of the tongue and the oropharynx. If the tumor is away from the mandible, segmental mandibulectomy should not be used merely to achieve access. Under such circumstances, the mandibulotomy approach is excellent. Median mandibulotomy in a stepladder fashion or a paramedian incision between the canine and incisor teeth can be used. The swing is performed by incising the mucosa on the medial aspect of the mandible on the floor of the mouth, and the tumor can be easily resected. This approach is also excellent for resection of tumors in the parapharyngeal area, including deep lobe parotid tumors. The cosmetic and functional outcomes of this approach are excellent, as demonstrated by Spiro and colleagues. Unfortunately, a substantial number of patients present with tumors of the oral cavity at advanced stages so that segmental mandibulectomy is necessary.

Increased attention has been paid recently to mandibular reconstruction, especially after resection of the arch of the mandible. The cosmetic and functional results of resection of the arch of the mandible need to be considered prior to resection of the tumor. In the past decade, primary mandibular reconstruction has become popular with the advent of free microvascular flaps.[20] Even though use of trays, iliac crest, or metallic plates was common in the past, the state-of-the-art reconstructive technique is to use microvascular flap. The common flaps utilized are the fibula, iliac crest, or scapula. The choice of donor site depends on the practice of the institution and the individual microvascular surgeon. Under difficult circumstances, reconstruction may be performed with the A-O plates; however, success with the A-O plates is limited, and the extrusion rate is very high. There appears to be very little deleterious effect of radiation on the free microvascular flap. Osseo-integrated implants on these reconstructed mandibles can provide better cosmetic and functional results.

Osteoradionecrosis is a long-standing problem in the management of tumors of the oral cavity. Clearly, the pre-radiation therapy dental evaluation is important and every patient should be referred to the dental service and followed regularly. The fluoride treatment is extremely important, as is extraction of poor dentition. Nevertheless, a substantial number of patients will develop osteoradionecrosis. Management remains controversial. Recently, it was shown that

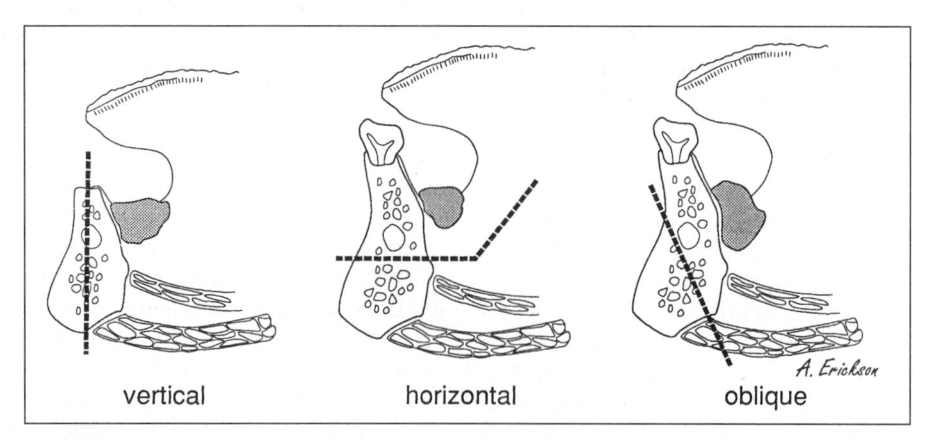

Fig 23-11. Various types of marginal mandibulectomies: vertical, horizontal, and oblique cuts.[18]

hyperbaric oxygen is helpful. However, if the bone is necrotic and the sequestrum is present, it definitely needs to be removed. Occasionally, a microvascular flap may be utilized for resection and reconstruction of the osteoradionecrotic mandible.

Larynx

The management of early vocal cord cancers has become controversial. Even though standard treatment used to be radiation therapy or limited surgery, recently endoscopic excision with carbon dioxide (CO_2) laser of small lesions of the mobile vocal cord have shown equally good results. However, careful case observation, expertise with the technique, and close patient observation are essential in the management of patients with this approach. Partial laryngectomy is used for patients with T2 or early T3 glottic lesions. The cure rates of early glottic cancers exceed 90% to 95% with either treatment, and surgical salvage may be utilized in patients who fail on radiation therapy. Even though partial laryngectomy can be performed in radiation therapy failures, it is important to document the initial extent of disease prior to radiation therapy, should any consideration be given to partial laryngectomy subsequently.

Lesions of the supraglottic larynx generally present in advanced stages because of minimal symptoms. In addition, the incidence of microscopic or bilateral metastasis is high. Treatment generally involves the primary tumor and the lymph node metastasis. A careful selection process should be involved in the management of supraglottic cancers, especially for supraglottic laryngectomy. The pulmonary status needs to be evaluated properly to avoid long term aspiration problems and resultant pulmonary complications. Radiation therapy may be used as a definitive treatment modality in selected supraglottic cancers, especially suprahyoid epiglottic cancers.

Advanced lesions of the larynx are generally treated by total laryngectomy with postoperative radiation therapy. In a few select centers, with proper case selection, a subtotal laryngectomy (Pearson procedure) has been utilized. However, with the availability of total laryngectomy and voice rehabilitation, the role of the Pearson procedure is questioned by many surgeons. In most instances of advanced laryngeal cancer, consideration is given to modified neck dissection including levels II, III, and IV (anterolateral selective neck dissection).[17] Combined treatment using surgery and radiotherapy is associated with a 60% survival rate in patients with stage III and IV laryngeal cancer. In some centers, radical radiation and salvage surgery (RRSS) is practiced in patients with advanced laryngeal cancer in an effort to preserve voice function.

Recently, a multi-institutional randomized Veterans Administration study has evaluated the role of induction chemotherapy followed by radiation therapy in replacing total laryngectomy and preserving laryngeal function.[15] The chemotherapy included cis-platinum and 5-fluorouracil. A complete or partial response to chemotherapy was reported in 85% of patients, who went on to receive radiation therapy. No survival advantage was noted in either group. However, laryngectomy was avoided in 64% of patients receiving chemotherapy and radiation therapy. Recently, some concern has been raised in utilizing this approach in patients with T4 cancers or cartilage destruction.

A problem clinicians commonly face is follow-up in patients with previous radiation therapy. The evaluation of the larynx after radiation therapy for edema is difficult, and the early detection of recurrent cancer may be almost impossible.

Hypopharynx

Most patients with hypopharyngeal cancer present in advanced stages, both at the primary site and with metastatic disease in the neck. Generally these patients will require combined-modality treatment. Occasionally, an early T1 cancer of the piriform sinus may be managed with partial pharyngectomy or radiation therapy. However, most patients will require total laryngopharyngectomy. Reconstruction of the pharyngeal defect includes a myocutaneous flap for patch pharyngoplasty, gastric pull-up if the entire circumferential pharynx is removed, or microvascular reconstruction with a jejunal flap. Neck dissection is routinely performed in conjunction with resection of hypopharyngeal tumors. The incidence of nodal metastasis exceeds 80%. Postoperative radiation therapy is routinely used. Chemotherapeutic protocols, in an attempt to save the larynx, have been used with less than enthusiastic response. The cure rate for advanced lesions of the hypopharynx is approximately 25% at 5 years. Distant metastasis, which may occur in >20% of patients, is more commonly noted in those presenting with advanced metastatic disease in the neck. Generally, patients with advanced hypopharyngeal and cervicoesophageal lesions have a dismal prognosis.

Recurrent Head and Neck Cancer

The treatment of recurrent head and neck cancer depends on previous treatment and the initial extent of disease. Tumors of the anterior floor of the mouth with well-localized recurrent disease can be satisfactorily resected by radical surgical extirpation with appropriate reconstruction. It is extremely important in patients undergoing an initial nonsurgical approach to evaluate the resectability of the tumor at the beginning of treatment. Resection of a recurrent tumor should encompass the entire area of the initial extent of the tumor rather than solely the recurrent disease or tumor nidus. A problem in patients receiving curative radiation therapy is evaluating the exact extent of the disease and resection margins. Invariably tumors recur at the margins of the resection area. Relative contraindications to surgery include invasion of the skull base, involvement of the common or internal carotid artery or prevertebral fascia, and tumor adherent to the vertebral bodies.

Advanced, Inoperable Cancers

In the evaluation of advanced cancer, it is extremely important for the surgeon to distinguish operable from inoperable cancers. The surgeon should document the inoperability of the tumor and obtain a second opinion if necessary. The best approach under these circumstances is either use one of the investigational protocols or consider new modalities such as hyperfractionation radiation therapy or chemosensitizers such as cis-platinum or mitomycin C. Since the patient has advanced, inoperable cancer, strong consideration should be given to best palliative efforts, which will include avoidance of airway problems, managing nutrition, and consideration of combined modality including radiation and chemotherapy.[21] It is quite tempting to consider surgical intervention at the conclusion of chemoradiotherapy; however, due consideration must be given to the possibility of local control and problems related to the radicality of surgery. Patients falling in this category are usually assessed by the hospital tumor board or multimodality conference. Randomized trials of induction or adjuvant chemotherapy are summarized in Table 23-9.

Newer Approaches

In recent years, many new radiotherapeutic approaches have been investigated, including concomitant chemotherapy plus radiation therapy and altered fractionation radiation therapy.[21] It is postulated that cells with intrinsic or acquired resistance to radiation will become radiosensitive in the presence of chemotherapy. Unfortunately, most randomized trials have reported increased toxicity with concomitant therapy. Altered schedules of radiation therapy as a single treatment are also being evaluated. These newer pilot studies seem to be quite promising and need further investigation.

Prevention

The main etiologic factors in head and neck cancer remain tobacco and alcohol. Sincere efforts to control tobacco exposure have been undertaken by governmental agencies. Probably the best place to implement this policy is with teenagers in high schools. The recent introduction of smoking cessation programs and nicotine patches has been of great help for some patients. Early intervention may reduce the risk of progression to malignancy or development of second primary tumors. Trials of vitamin A analogs have shown promise in controlling preneoplastic mucosal lesions and prevention of subsequent second primary tumors. The use of cis-retinoic acid has been associated with a lower incidence of second primary cancers; at present, however, these investigational treatment modalities should be used only on a protocol basis.

The most common premalignant lesion in the head and neck is leukoplakia. The ability of retinoids to reverse leukoplakia has been studied intensively, with response rates ranging from 55% to 100%. Unfortunately, the effect of 13-cis-retinoic acid in the reduction of leukoplakia has not been long-lasting. Within 3 months of cessation of therapy, most responding lesions showed progression. There also were substantial side effects. It appears that low-dose 13-cis-retinoic acid has much better effect than beta carotene. However, both low-dose isotretinoin and beta carotene were very well tolerated in investigational series.[22,23]

Salivary Tumors

The salivary glands can be divided into major and minor types. Major salivary glands include the parotid, submandibular, and sublingual salivary glands. Malignant tumors of the salivary glands are rare and constitute about 7% of tumors of the head and neck area. However, benign neoplasms of the parotid gland are common. There are 500 to 700 minor salivary glands, distributed throughout the mucosa of the upper aerodigestive tract.[24] Approximately 50% are located on the hard palate which accounts for the common dictum that a lesion on the hard palate should be considered a minor salivary tumor unless proved otherwise. Even though the etiologic factors leading to salivary tumors are not known, there may be some genetic predisposition and an increased risk in patients exposed to ionizing radiation.

The parotid gland is the largest salivary gland and forms the main bulk of salivary neoplasms. It is divided into the superficial and deep lobes by the presence of the facial nerve. The superficial lobe constitutes approximately 80% of the gland, while the deeper lobe is only 15% to 20%. Tumors of the deep lobe of the parotid are rare. The surgery of the parotid involves critical and crucial dissection and preservation of the facial nerve. The parotid duct (Stensen's duct) arises in the anterior part of the gland and runs obliquely and inferiorly toward the second upper molar tooth on the surface of the masseter muscle.

The anatomy of the facial nerve is extremely important for the head and neck surgeon. The main trunk of the facial nerve can be located at the confluence of three important anatomic structures: the posterior belly of the digastric muscle, the tip of the mastoid process, and the bony auditory canal. At the junction

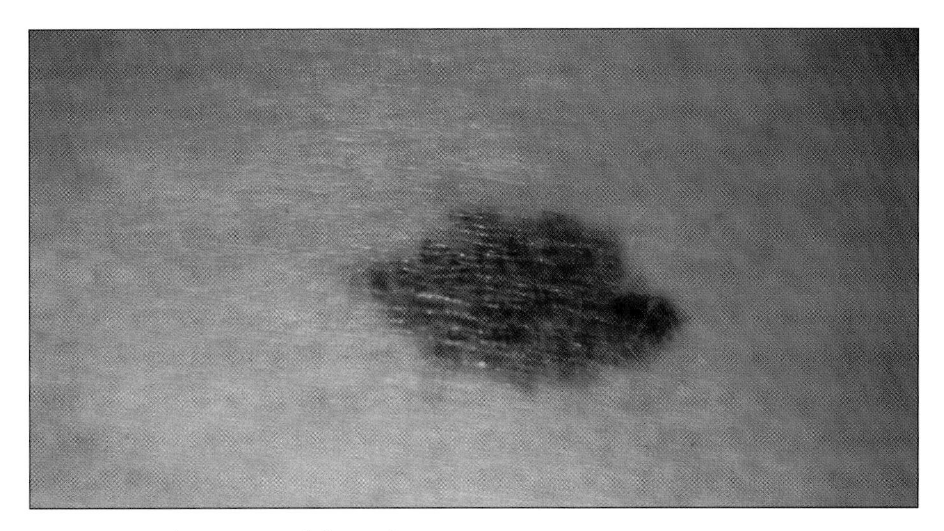

Fig 19-1. Dysplastic nevus (of the trunk).

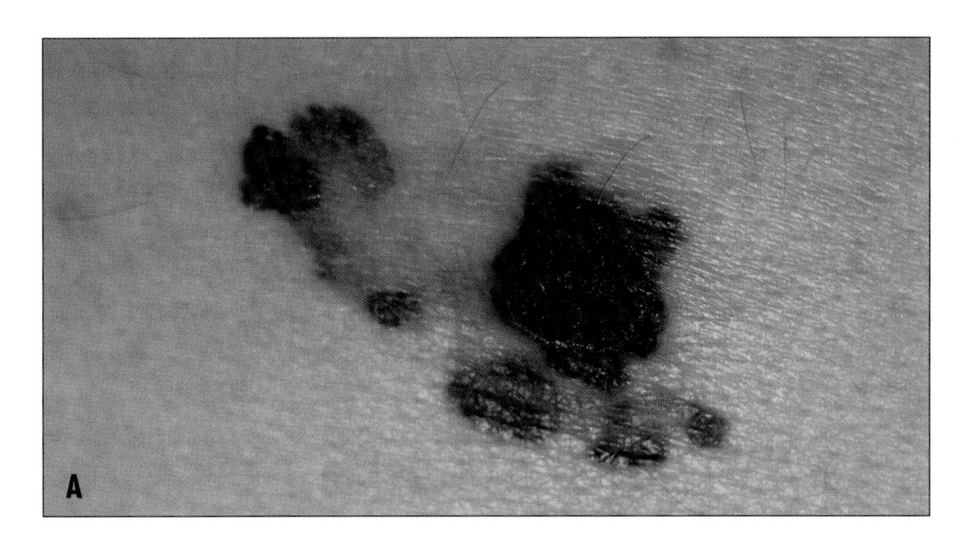

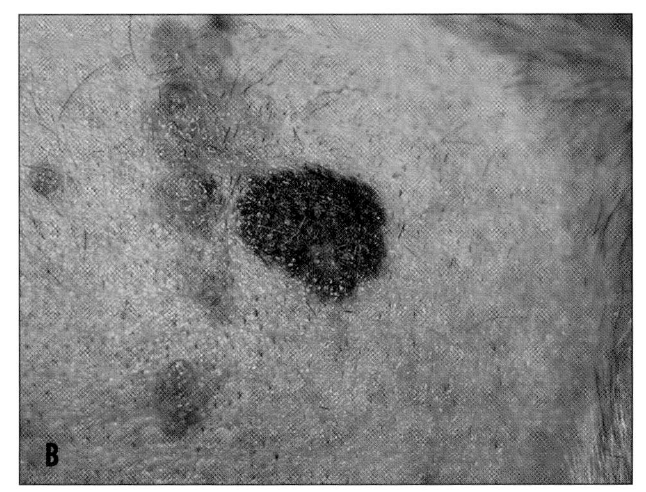

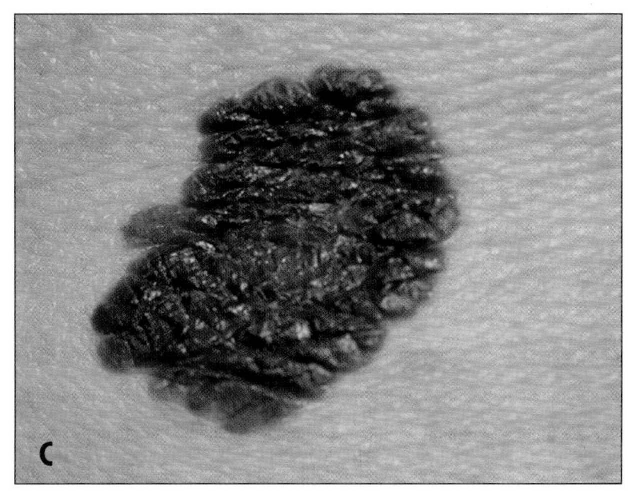

Fig 19-2. Growth patterns of melanomas: ***A*** shows superficial spreading melanoma; ***B***, the same growth pattern in the scalp; ***C***, superficial spreading melanoma of the trunk (Clark's level III).

(Continued on next page)

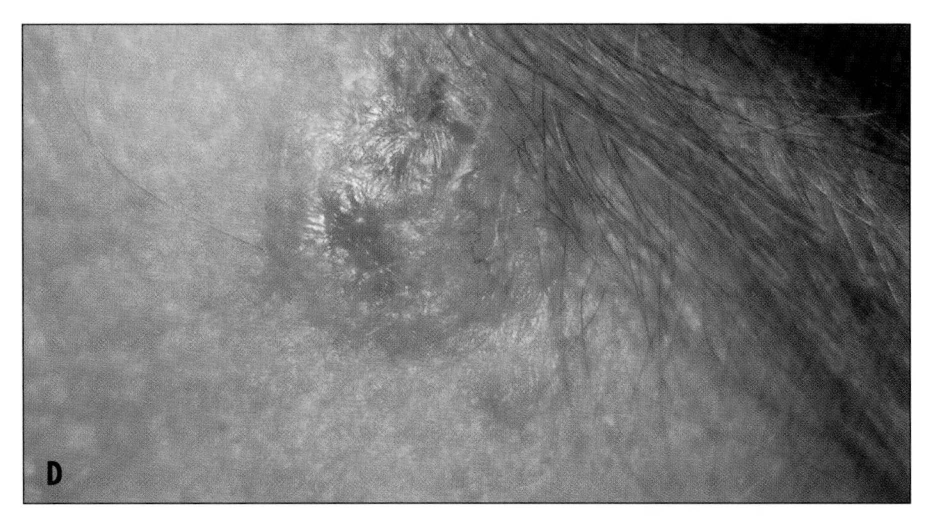

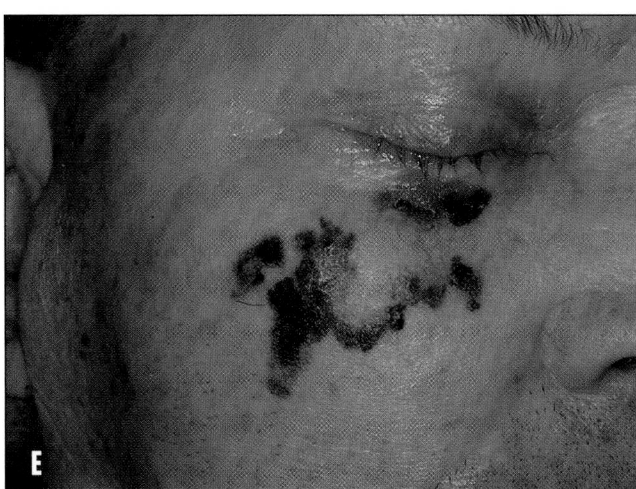

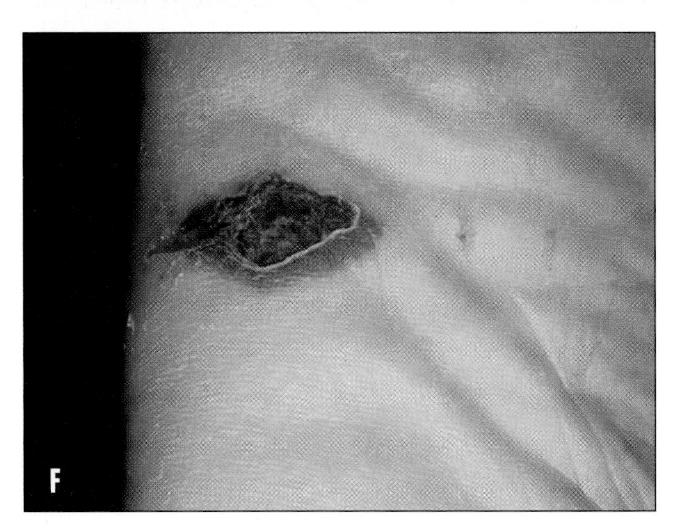

Fig 19-2 ***Continued.*** Growth patterns of melanomas: ***D*** shows amelanotic nodular melanoma of the forehead. ***E*** shows lentigo maligna melanoma of the cheek. ***F*** shows acral lentiginous melanoma of the foot.

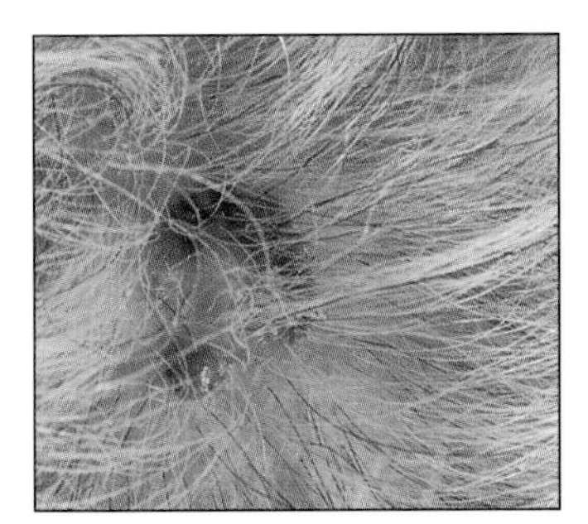

Fig 21-1. Ulcerated BCC measuring >2 cm in diameter is characterized by a centrally ulcerated nodule and a rolled, pearly border. This lesion grew slowly over many years.

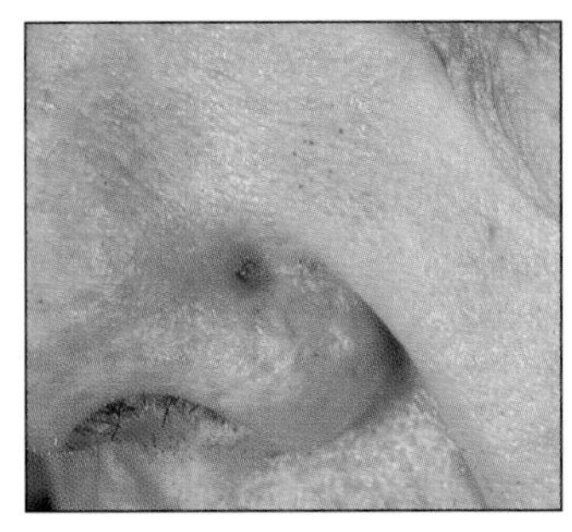

Fig 21-2. Pigmented BCC on scalp of 70-year-old white man. This 1.4-cm pigmented lesion is difficult to distinguish from malignant melanoma. A rolled, pearly border is a clue to the diagnosis of pigmented BCC.

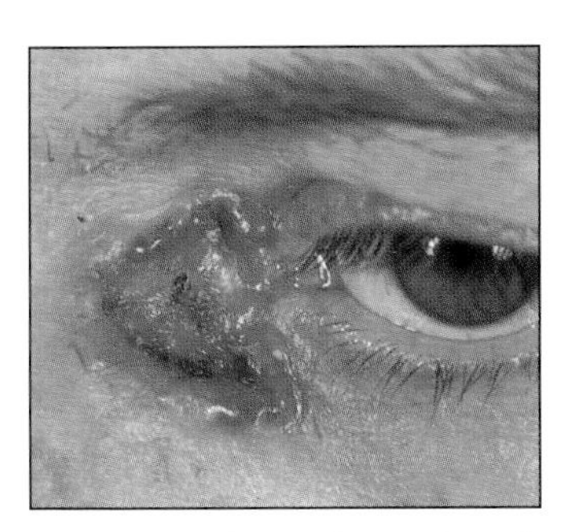

Fig 21-3. Large fungating, ulcerated BCC. This advanced neoplasm has been present for many years and has nearly replaced a large portion of the nose in this elderly white man.

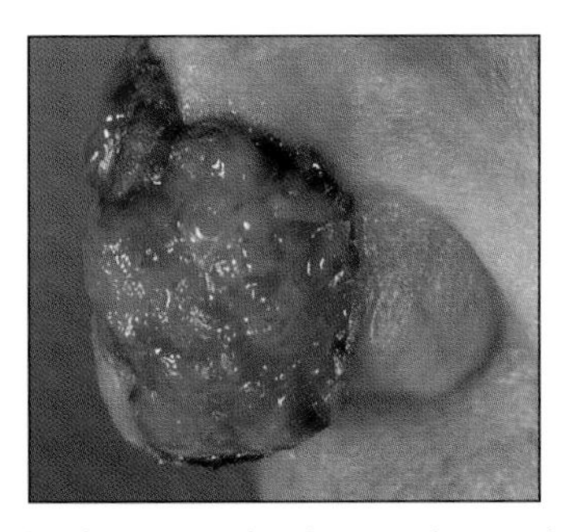

Fig 21-4. Morpheaform BCC. This depressed 7-mm lesion was present for many years on the left ala of a 50-year-old white woman.

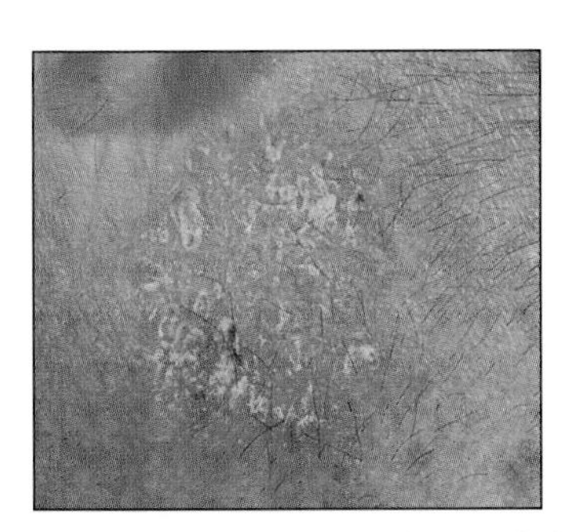

Fig 21-5. Multiple SCC on markedly sun-damaged skin in an elderly man. Many of the lesions present are actinic keratoses. The patient has at least 1 SCC of the helix of the ear. A second lesion is present in the left malar region.

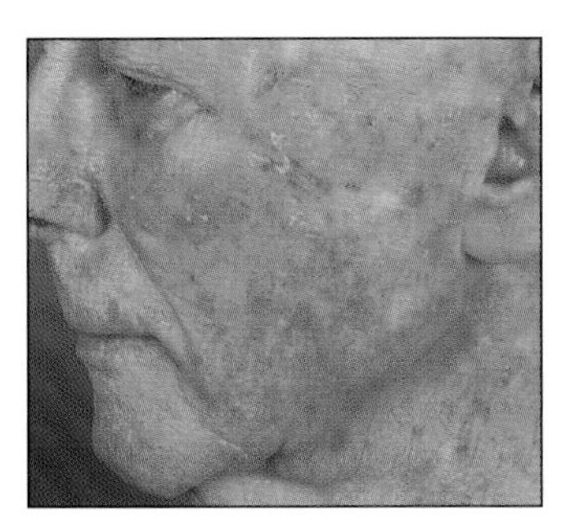

Fig 21-6. In situ SCC in an elderly white man. This scaly, slightly elevated plaque is located on the side of the neck and has been present for many years.

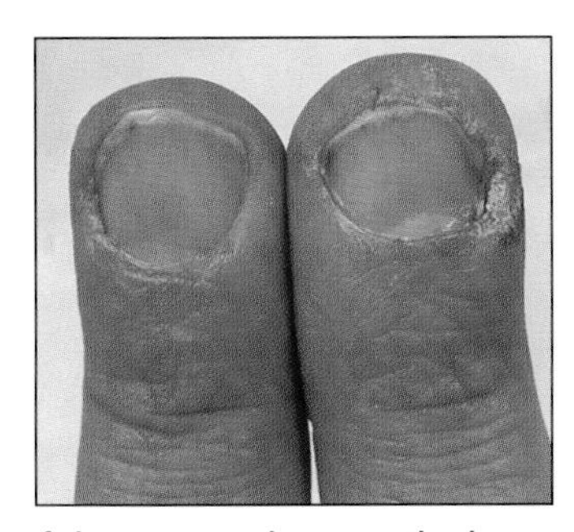

Fig 21-7. SCC of the periungual region. This biopsy-proven carcinoma arose on the site of a previous wart infection.

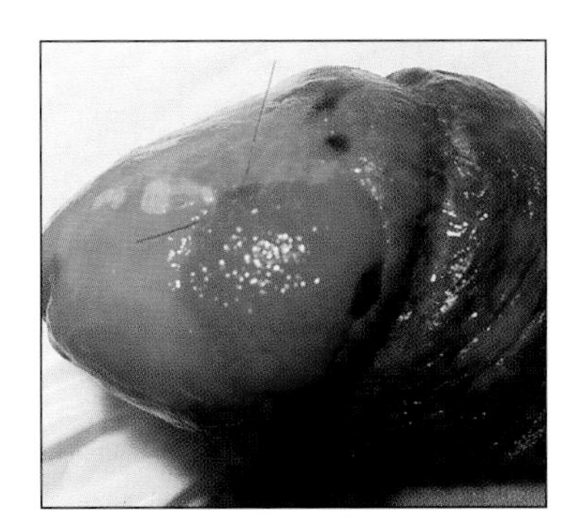

Fig 21-8. Invasive SCC of the glans penis.

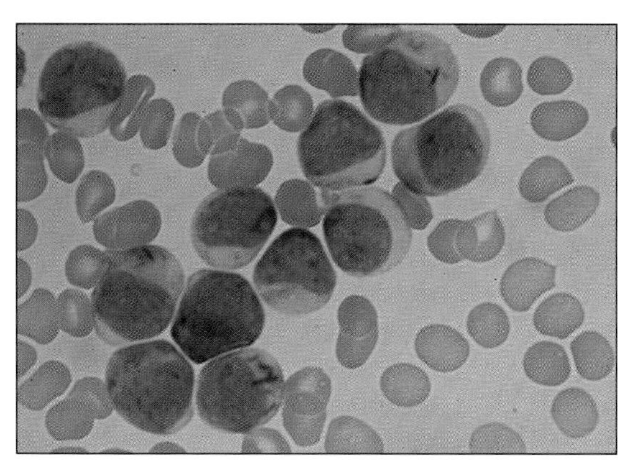

A. M2—peripheral blood (PB): myeloblasts stained with myeloperoxidase highlighting granules and Auer rods. Note prominent nucleoli.

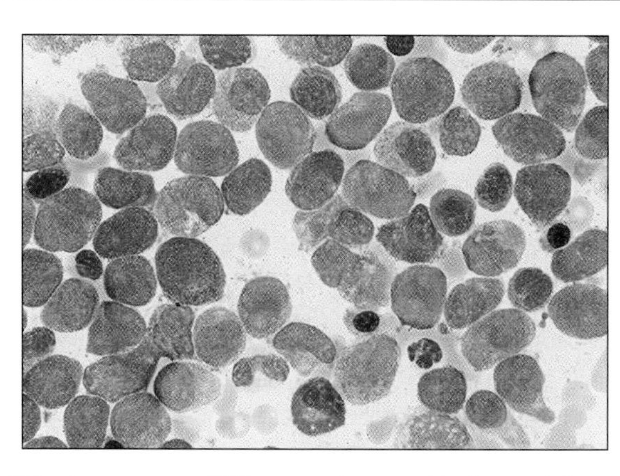

B. M3—bone marrow (BM): promyelocytes with abnormal, heavy reddish granules. Some tumor cells contain more than one Auer rod.

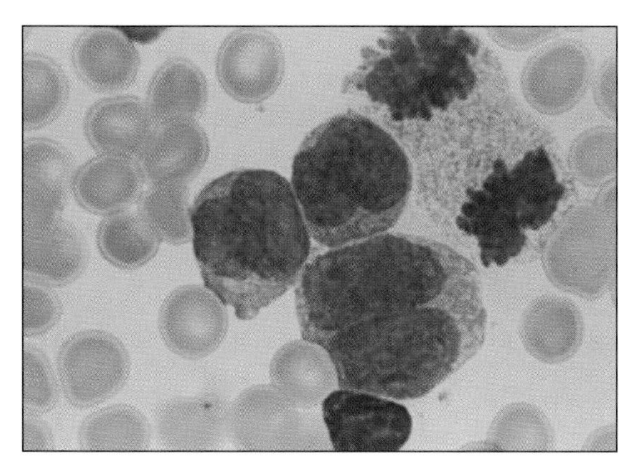

C. M3—microgranular variant (PB): In this morphologic variant of M3 the cells have bi-lobed or folded nuclei and subtle granulation that may remain undetected unless myeloperoxidase staining or electron microscopy is performed.

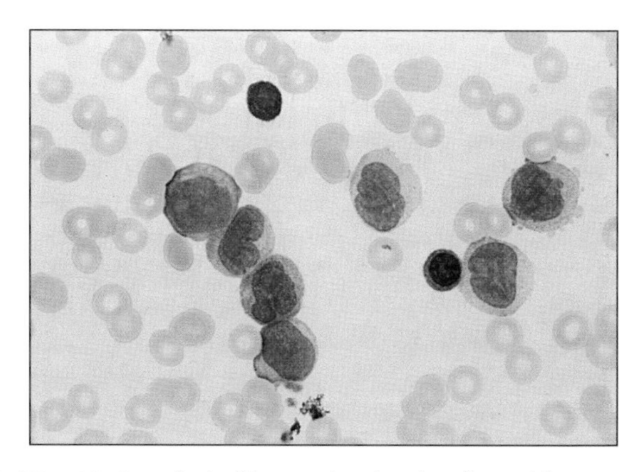

D. M5—PB: Note the highly convoluted nuclei of monoblasts.

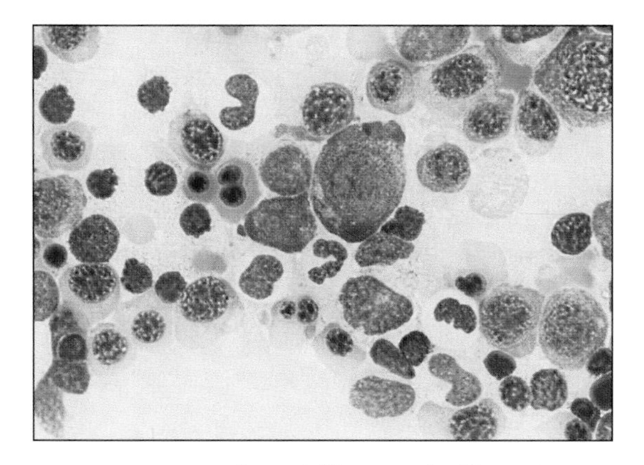

E. M6—BM: Gigantic and megaloblastic erythroblasts of Diguglielmo's disease. Note marked erythroid dysplasia. Other diagnostic features (not shown) include pulverized nuclei and cytoplasmic vacuoles.

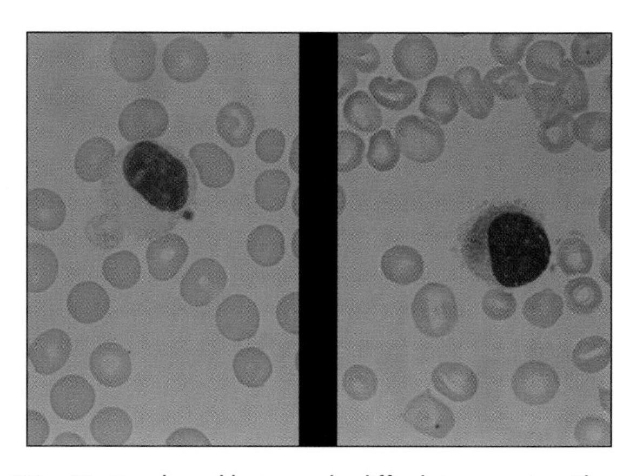

F. M7—PB: Megakaryoblasts may be difficult to recognize. The cytoplasm is grey-blue with occasional blebbing.

Fig 30-1. Morphology of some FAB subtypes in AML.

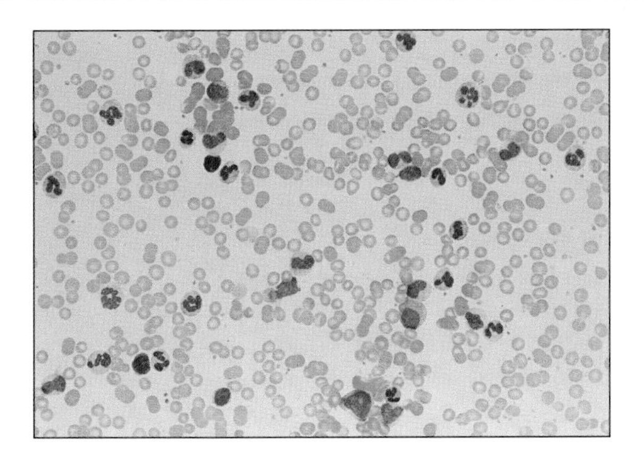

Fig 30-3a. CML—stable phase (PB). Note leukocytosis with orderly maturation from immature to more mature WBC. Occasionally a basophil is detected.

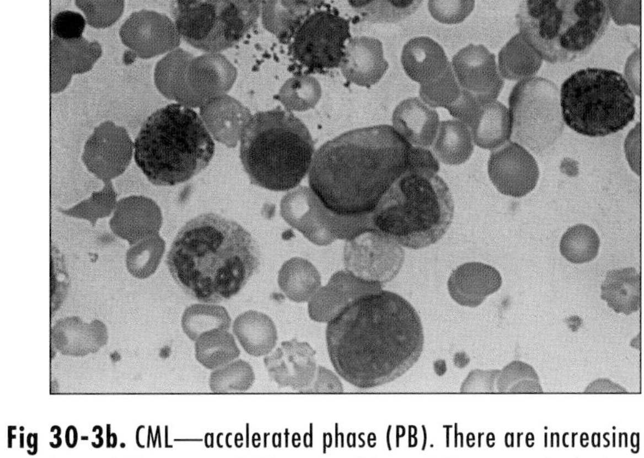

Fig 30-3b. CML—accelerated phase (PB). There are increasing numbers of blasts (myeloblasts) and basophils, some of which are hypogranulated.

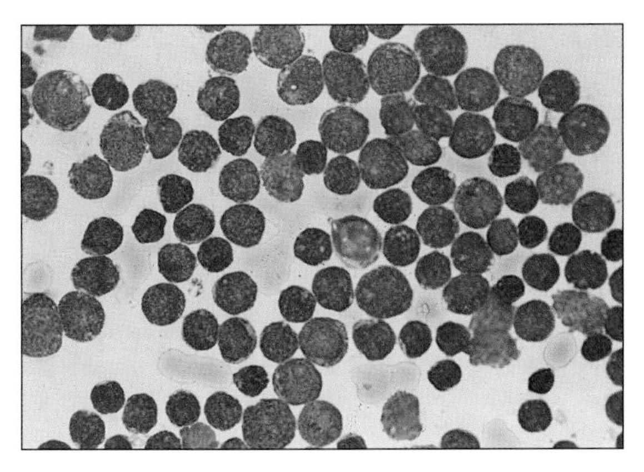

Fig 30-5a. ALL-L1 (BM). Uniform population of small lymphoblasts with scant cytoplasm and subtle vacuolization.

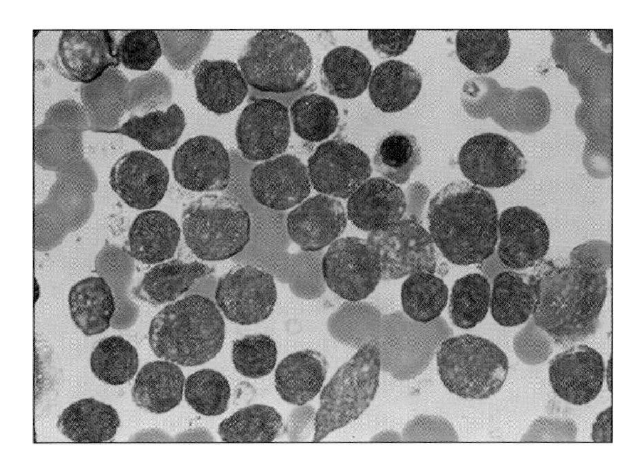

Fig 30-5b. ALL-L2 (BM). Lymphoblasts of varying sizes.

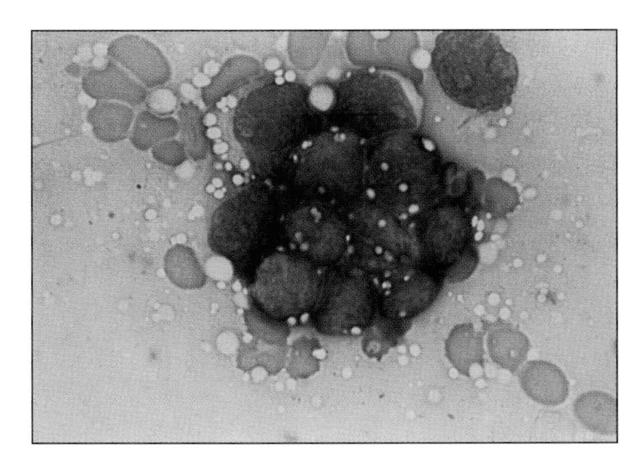

Fig 30-5c. L3 ALL (BM). Lymphoblasts are large with dark blue cytoplasm and prominent vacuolization. They are indistinct from tumor cells in Burkitt's lymphoma.

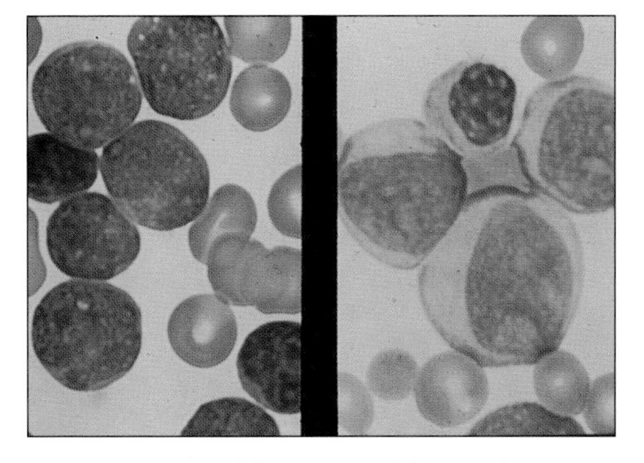

Fig 30-6. Lymphoblast (left) versus myeloblast (right). Myeloblasts in general have more cytoplasm than lymphoblasts (lighter blue). Nucleoli are prominent in the former cells and more subtle in the latter.

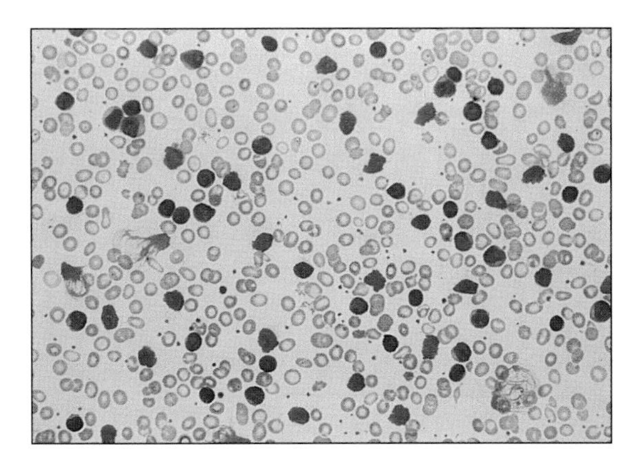

Fig 30-7. Chronic lymphocytic leukemia (PB). Lymphocytosis consisting of mature lymphocytes. Occasional "smudge" cell is noted.

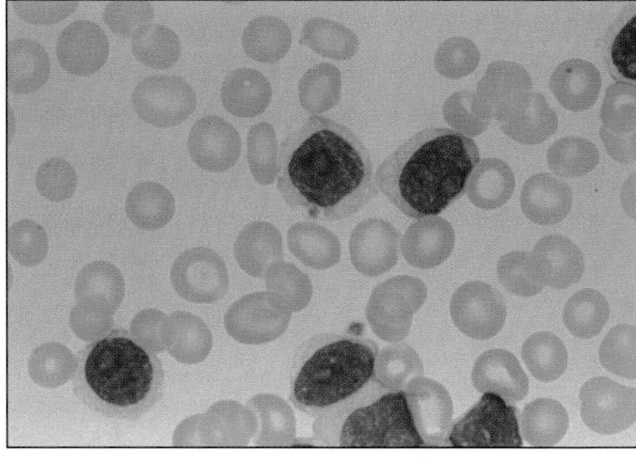

Fig 30-8. Prolymphocytic leukemia (PB). Prolymphocytes are larger than normal lymphocytes and have more generous cytoplasm. Nucleoli are prominent.

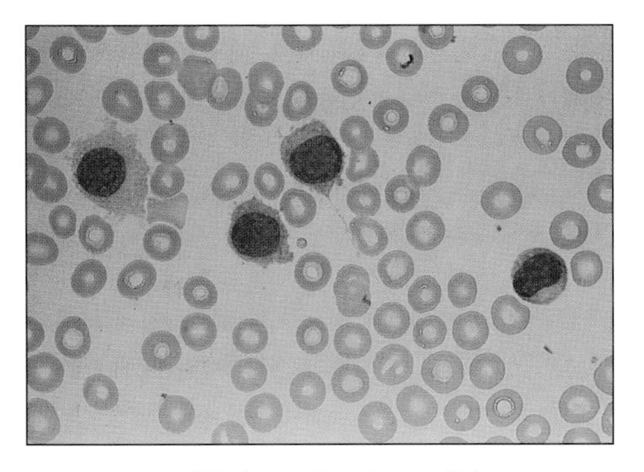

Fig 30-9a. Hairy cell leukemia (PB). Hairy cells have prominent cytoplasmic projections. Nuclei are round or folded.

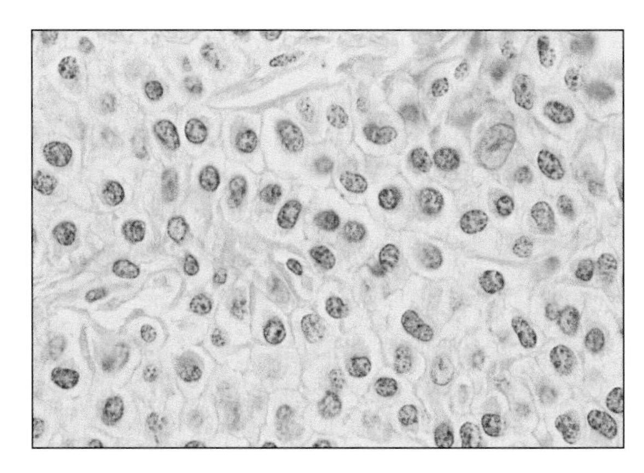

Fig 30-9b. Histologic section of hairy cells demonstrates characteristic "fried egg" appearance. Nuclei are separated by generous amounts of cytoplasm.

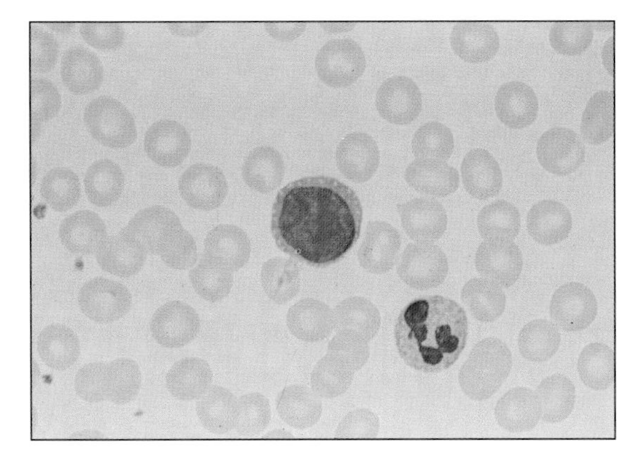

Fig 30-10. Sezary cells (PB) may have convoluted or rounded nuclei and a "ring of pearl" pattern of vacuolization in the cytoplasm.

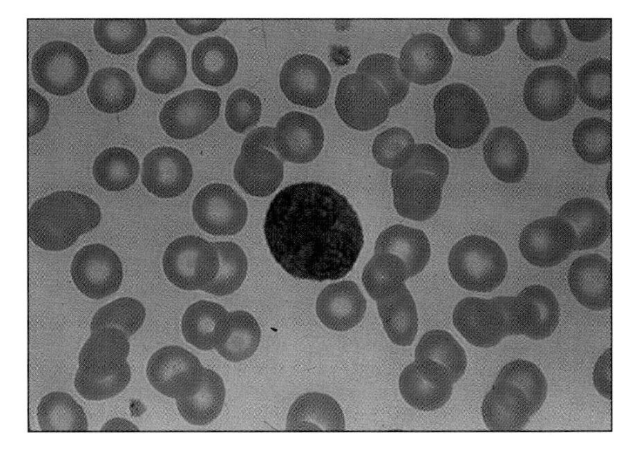

Fig 30-11. Circulating tumor cells in adult T-cell leukemia-lymphoma have deep blue cytoplasm and very folded nuclei.

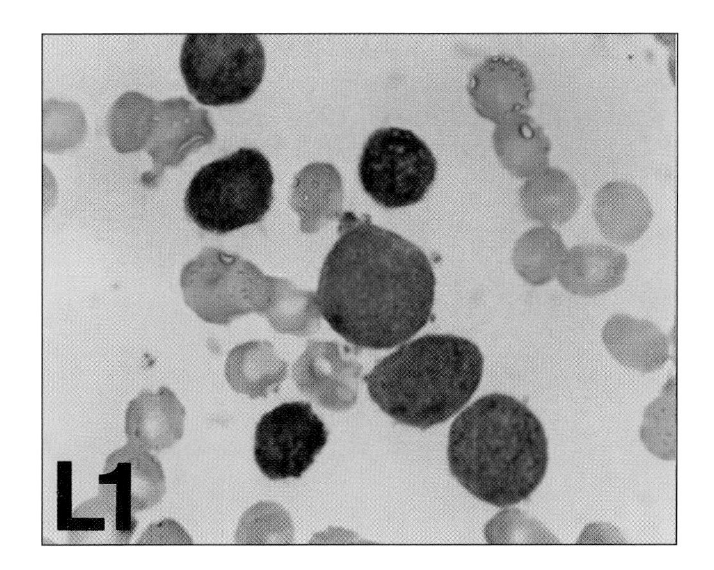

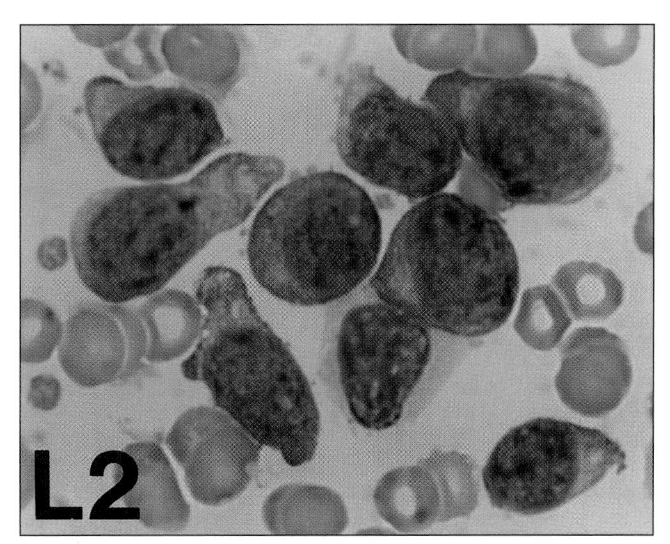

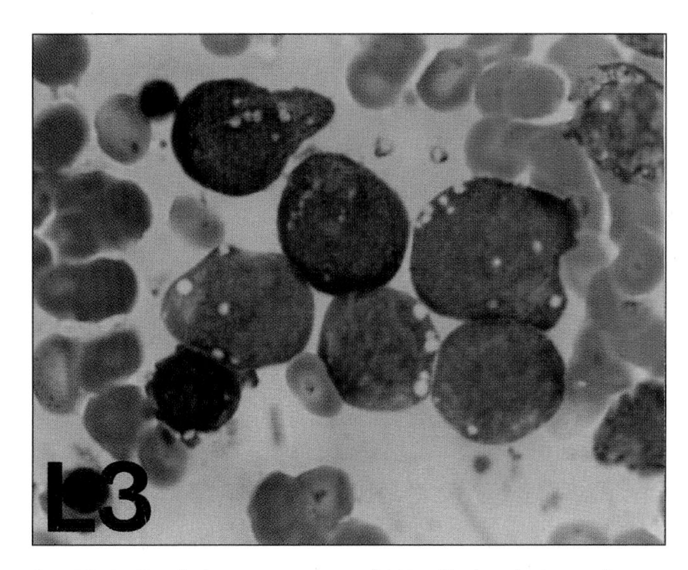

Fig 31-1. Morphologic appearance of ALL cells classified according to the FAB system: L1 to L3.

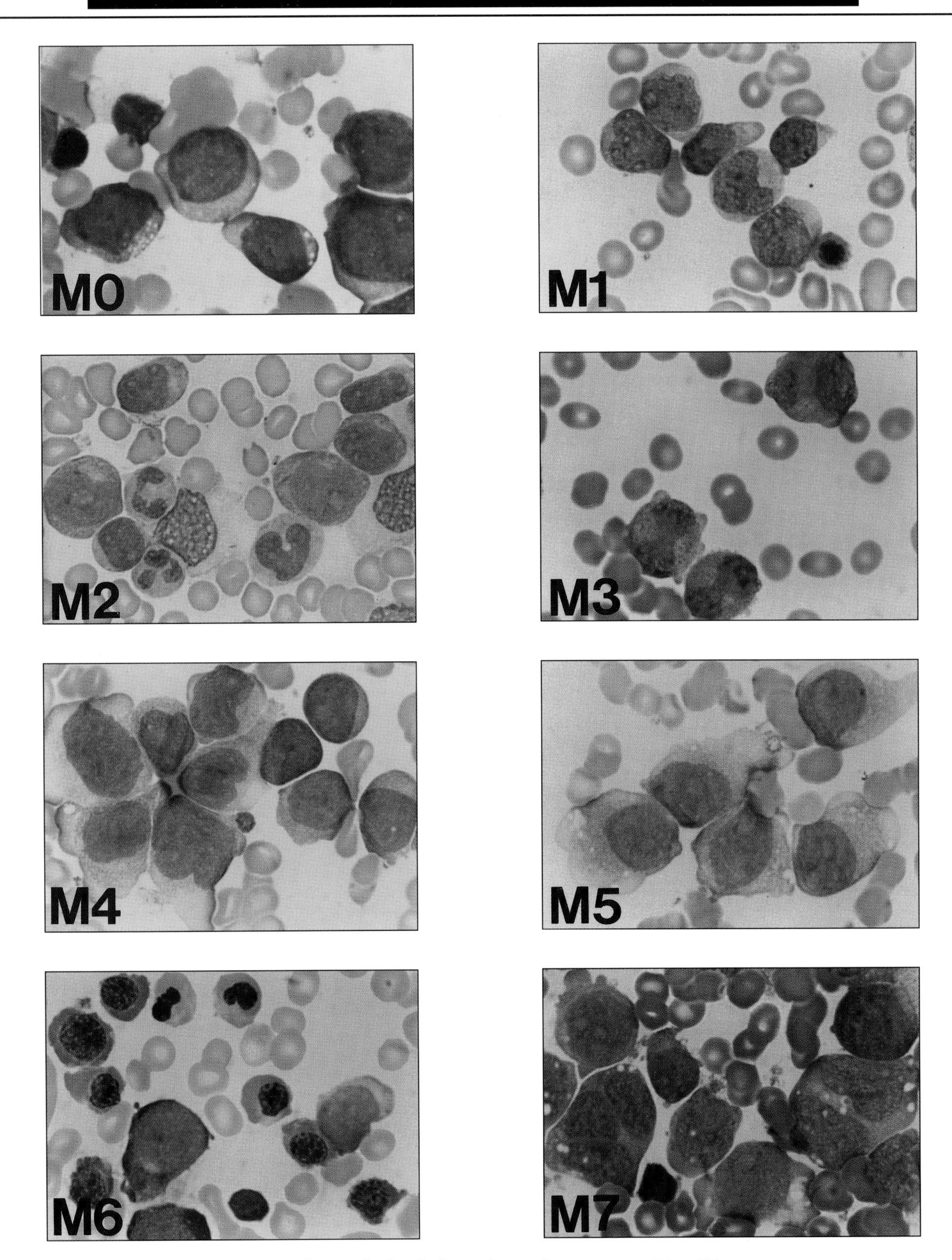

Fig 31-2. Morphologic appearance of AML cells classified according to the FAB system: M0 to M7.

Table 23-9. Randomized Trials of Induction and/or Adjuvant Chemotherapy

Study	Patients Analyzed	Drugs	Response Rate to CT (Complete Response)	Local Therapy	Outcome	Comments
Jacobs	443	Cisplatin, bleomycin	37% (3%)	S/XRT	No significant difference in survival	Induction and adjuvant CT, survival benefit for N2 disease by subset analysis, decreased distant metastases with adjuvant CT
Shuller	158	Cisplatin, methotrexate, bleomycin, vincristin	70% (19%)	S/XRT	No significant difference in survival	Induction CT, decreased distant metastases
VA larynx study	332	Cisplatin, 5-FU	86% (31%)	XRT vs S/XRT	No significant difference in survival	Induction CT, decreased distant metastases, larynx preservation
Laramore	448	Cisplatin, 5-FU	NA	S/XRT	No significant difference in survival	CT adjuvant to surgery, decreased incidence of distant metastases

CT = chemotherapy; 5-FU = 5 fluorouracil; NA = not applicable; S/XRT = local therapy with surgery and/or radiotherapy; VA = Veteran's Administration

From Vokes and Weichselbaum.[21]

of these three points, the facial nerve emerges from the stylomastoid foramen and enters the substance of the parotid gland and bifurcates into two main branches: the zygomaticotemporal (upper) branch and the cervicomandibular (lower) branch. The buccal branch may arise from either division. Eventually, the nerve divides into five main branches: the temporal, zygomatico-orbital, buccal, mandibular (ramus mandibularis), and cervical. The two most important branches of the facial nerve are the orbital branch, supplying the eyelids, and the mandibular branch, innervating the lip. Injury to these branches during surgery leads to considerable cosmetic and functional disability.

The submandibular gland lies in the submandibular triangle on the surface of the hyoglossal muscle above the digastric. The three nerves in close proximity to the submandibular gland are the lingual, hypoglossal, and mandibular division of the facial nerve. Proper evaluation of these nerves is extremely important in the management of malignant tumors of the submandibular salivary gland. The submandibular duct (Wharton's duct) runs forward from the deeper portion of the submandibular salivary gland under the mylohyoid muscle to the floor of the mouth, where it opens lateral to the frenulum. Tumors of the sublingual gland may be easily mistaken for tumors of the floor of the mouth.

Approximately 75% of tumors of the parotid gland are benign, while 50% of tumors of the submandibular salivary gland are malignant. In contrast, approximately 80% of tumors of minor salivary glands are malignant.

Diagnostic Workup

The diagnostic workup includes sialogram, CT sialogram, FNA, CT scan, and MRI scan. The sialogram and CT sialogram were once popular, but are fairly nonspecific. The same information can be easily obtained today from a CT scan. Imaging with a CT or MRI scan is helpful, especially to evaluate the extent of disease, lymph node involvement, and location of the tumor.

Fine needle aspiration of the salivary glands has become controversial. There appears to be considerable reluctance to use FNA for the evaluation of salivary lesions. In most cases, the diagnosis of the salivary gland neoplasm and the therapeutic decisions can be easily made clinically. There are many pitfalls of FNA, especially in distinguishing between malignant pathologies, and occasionally, a benign mixed tumor may be interpreted cytologically as an adenoid cystic carcinoma or an inflammation. However, FNA has been helpful in lesions of the tail of the parotid, where a distinction can be made between salivary and nonsalivary pathology.

A preoperative suspicion of salivary neoplasm will prepare the operating surgeon mentally for discussion with the patient regarding facial nerve injury or sacrifice. If the diagnosis of malignancy can be established on FNA, the surgeon can better prepare the patient with the understanding of facial nerve involvement in the tumor. Even though there are many cytologic pitfalls in the use of FNA, the technique is simple and easy to perform. FNA also renders important information prior to surgical undertaking, especially in patients in whom the clinical diagnosis is unclear.

Benign Parotid Tumors

Common benign tumors seen in the parotid gland include benign mixed tumor, Warthin's tumor, oncocytoma, and benign lymphoepithelial lesions.

Approximately 80% of benign lesions of the parotid are benign mixed tumors. They are also called pleomorphic adenoma and include various histologic components: myxoid, chondroid, fibroid, and mucoid elements. The tumor generally grows slowly, but occasionally may represent with rapid growth and malignant transformation. The incidence of a benign mixed tumor's becoming malignant is about 1% to 7% (carcinoma ex-pleomorphic adenoma). The facial nerve is commonly involved in malignant mixed tumor; however, even in large benign mixed tumors, facial nerve function is generally intact. The clinical presentation of a benign mixed tumor is a solitary, well-defined, well-encircled mass in the superficial lobe of the parotid. Occasionally, the tumor may extend into the deep lobe. The most appropriate and optimal surgery for benign mixed tumor is superficial or subtotal parotidectomy, dissection of the facial nerve, and preservation of the branches of the facial nerve.

Tumors of the deep lobe of the parotid may be difficult to excise and essentially will result in enucleation; however, facial nerve function can still be preserved by careful dissection and separation of the facial nerve and its branches. Local recurrence is high in patients who have undergone inadequate surgery in the form of enucleation or local excision.

It is important to remember that any tumor in the parotid area is considered a parotid tumor unless proved otherwise, and all patients should be brought to the operating room for appropriate surgical intervention, which includes standard parotid incision, identification and dissection of the facial nerve and its branches, and removal of the parotid tumor. Occasionally, for a very large deep-lobe parotid tumor presenting as a parapharyngeal mass, a mandibulotomy may be necessary.

Warthin's tumor, also called papillary cystadenoma lymphomatosum, originates in the periparotid or intraparotid lymph nodes surrounding the parotid gland, and accounts for approximately 10% to 15% of benign parotid tumors. Ten percent of these tumors are multifocal, and 10% may be bilateral. The risk of malignant transformation is extremely rare, and the diagnosis of Warthin's tumor can be easily made with FNA.

Oncocytomas are rare, fleshy, slow-growing, benign tumors of the parotid that constitute approximately 1% of salivary gland tumors.

With the increasing incidence of acquired immunodeficiency syndrome (AIDS) and human immunodeficiency virus (HIV) positivity, benign lymphoepithelial lesions are seen more frequently. They are also commonly seen in patients with AIDS-related complex (ARC). These lesions represent involvement of the periparotid and intraparotid lymph nodes. Generally the patient presents with a large mass in the tail of the parotid, which may be cystic. The long duration of the mass (4 to 6 months), the history of HIV positivity, and the characteristic clinical appearance and cystic consistency almost certainly establish the diagnosis of benign lymphoepithelial lesion of the parotid. CT has been used to document multiple cystic areas and bilaterality. Since the natural history of this disease is not known, there is a tendency toward conservative treatment, including multiple needle aspirations and close observation. However, if the patient is symptomatic and has no obvious stigmata of AIDS, one may consider surgical excision, which appears to produce excellent results.

Malignant Parotid Tumors

Adenoid cystic carcinomas constitute approximately 10% of parotid malignancies. This tumor exhibits an unpredictable behavior due to local extension beyond the gross lesion, perineural involvement, and a high incidence of local recurrence. Distant metastases are also fairly common, mostly to the lung, where they may remain dormant for a long time. A "Swiss-cheese"-like histopathologic appearance is characteristic.

Mucoepidermoid carcinomas constitute approximately 44% of parotid malignancies. These tumors originate in the salivary duct epithelium and are classified as low or high grade. Low-grade lesions clinically mimic benign mixed tumors. A standard superficial parotidectomy is adequate for low-grade mucoepidermoid carcinomas. The incidence of local recurrence and distant metastasis is small. High-grade tumors can invade the facial nerve, and there is an approximately 50% incidence of lymph node metastasis at the time of presentation.

Malignant mixed tumors, which represent approximately 17% of parotid malignancies, may originate in slow-growing benign mixed tumors.[24,25] Approximately 25% of patients present with regional lymph node involvement. There is commonly a long-term history of benign mixed tumor showing rapid growth of recent origin with fixation to the deeper structures and to the skin, occasionally with ulceration. The facial nerve may be involved in the malignant pathology.

Table 23-10. Involvement of Cervical Lymph Nodes by Metastasis of Primary Carcinoma in Parotid, Submandibular, and Minor Salivary Glands

Time of Appearance	Parotid (n = 623)	Submandibular (n = 129)	Minor Glands (n = 526)
Initially	20%	33%	13%
Subsequently	5	4	9
Total	25	37	22

From Shah and Ihde.[24]

Treatment

Enucleation of the parotid tumor is uniformly condemned and contraindicated. The minimal operation for a lesion involving the parotid gland is superficial parotidectomy. Most tumors are located in the superficial lobe of the parotid and can be easily approached by this procedure. Surgical considerations include identification and careful preservation of the facial nerve. Tumors of the deep lobe constitute a challenge regarding both the surgical approach and preservation of the facial nerve. Generally the facial nerve is wrapped around the lesion, and careful dissection and identification of branches of the facial nerve is extremely crucial. In most cases, a deep-lobe parotid tumor can be removed without injury to the branches of the facial nerve. Occasionally, though, if the bulk of the deep-lobe tumor is against the pharyngeal wall, a mandibulotomy approach may be necessary for better exposure of the parapharyngeal area.

The management of the facial nerve in malignant parotid tumors has become a clinical concern. In general, if the facial nerve is not paralyzed preoperatively and there is no direct extension of the disease into the facial nerve at the time of surgery, every effort should be made to preserve it. There are very few instances of malignant parotid tumors in which a normally functioning facial nerve would be sacrificed.

The management of malignant submandibular tumors is more complex due to the proximity of the lingual and hypoglossal nerves. Block dissection of the submandibular salivary gland tumor will entail removal of the entire contents of the submandibular triangle. If the tumor is adherent to the mandible, mandibular resection may be necessary or excision of the outer periosteum. A supraomohyoid neck dissection may be considered, along with excision of the malignant submandibular salivary gland tumor.

The principle of management of malignant tumors of minor salivary glands remains wide local excision. Involvement of the hard palate would generally require a through-and-through excision of the hard palate or infrastructure partial maxillectomy with a dental obturator.

The approach to cervical lymph nodes in malignant salivary tumors remains controversial. The incidence of cervical lymph node involvement is approximately 25%, and most metastases are noted at the time of initial presentation (Table 23-10).[24] Elective supraomohyoid neck dissection may be considered in high-grade, high-stage malignant tumors. However, in the absence of grossly enlarged lymph nodes, elective neck dissection should not be considered. If suspicious lymph nodes are encountered at the time of primary surgery, a modified neck dissection may be performed. When there are grossly enlarged nodes at the initial presentation, radical neck dissection should be considered.[24,25] The determinate cure rates in patients with malignant tumors of various salivary glands is shown in Table 23-11.[25]

Radiation Therapy

Indications for radiation therapy in salivary gland tumors include advanced inoperable cancer; high-grade, high-stage primary tumor; tumors with positive margins; advanced tumor stage; high-grade histology; deep-lobe parotid tumors; presence of cervical lymph node metastasis; and tumor spillage at the

Table 23-11. Determinate "Cure" Rates in Patients With Malignant Tumors

Interval (years)	Parotid (n = 623)	Submandibular (n = 129)	Minor Glands (n = 52)
5	55%	31%	48%
10	47	22	37
15	40	15	23
20	33	14	15

From Spiro.[25]

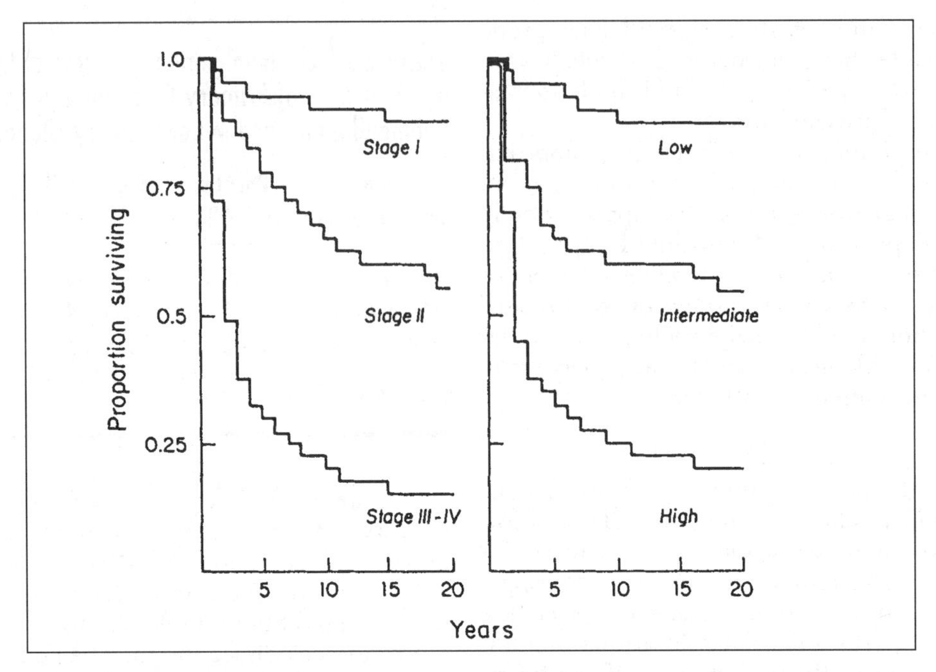

Fig 23-12. Significant differences in survival were observed when previously untreated patients with salivary tumors were grouped according to the clinical stage (*p* <0001) (left). Survival differences were similar when patients with adenocarcinoma, mucoepidermoid carcinoma, or squamous carcinoma were analyzed by histologic grade (p <0001)(right).[25]

time of surgery. The use of fast neutrons for advanced salivary gland neoplasms is under investigation and has shown promising initial results. Since the incidence of local recurrence in adenoid cystic carcinoma remains high, postoperative radiation therapy should be considered in high-stage lesions.

Prognosis

Tumor stage remains the most important prognostic factor in salivary gland neoplasms. The overall 10-year survival rates for stages I, II, and III are approximately 90%, 65%, and 22%, respectively (Fig 23-12).[25] Grade is also an important prognostic factor: the 10-year survival rate for low-grade tumors is 90%, compared with 25% for high-grade tumors (Fig 23-12). Overall, the management of salivary gland neoplasms still is based on adequate and appropriate surgical extirpation.

References

1. Beahrs OH, Henson DE, Hutter RVP, Kennedy BJ, eds. American Joint Committee on Cancer. *Manual for Staging of Cancer.* 4th ed. Philadelphia, Pa: JB Lippincott Co; 1992:27-62.

2. Vokes EE, Weichselbaum RR, Lippman SM, Hong WK. Head and neck cancer. *N Engl J Med.* 1993;328:184-194.

3. Shah JP, Medina J, Shaha AR, Schantz SP, Marti JR. Cervical lymph node metastasis. *Curr Probl Surg.* 1993; 30:273-344.

4. Shah JP. Cervical lymph node metastases: diagnostic, therapeutic and prognostic implications. *Oncology.* 1990; 4:61-76.

5. Boring CC, Squire TS, Tong T. Cancer statistics, 1994. *CA Cancer J Clin.* 1994;44:7-26.

6. Davidson BJ, Hsu TC, Schantz SP. The genetics of tobacco-induced cancer susceptibility. *Cancer Epidemiol Biomarkers Prev.* 1991;1:83-89.

7. Niedobitek G, Hausmann M, Herbst H, et al. Epstein-Barr virus and carcinomas: undifferentiated carcinomas but not squamous cell carcinomas of the nasopharynx are regularly associated with the virus. *J Path.* 1991;165:17-24.

8. Shah JP. Patterns of cervical lymph node metastasis from squamous carcinoma of the upper aerodigestive tract. *Am J Surg.* 1990;160:405-409.

9. Shah JP. *Color Atlas of Head & Neck Surgery.* Orlando, Fl: Grune & Stratton Inc; 1987.

10. Martin HE, Ellis EB. Biopsy by needle puncture and aspiration. *Ann Surg.* 1930;92:169-181.

11. Shaha AR, Webber C, Marti J. Fine-needle aspiration in the diagnosis of cervical adenopathy. *Am J Surg.* 1986; 152:420-423.

12. Shaha AR, Webber C, DiMaio T, Jaffe BM. Needle aspiration biopsy in salivary gland lesions. *Am J Surg.* 1990; 160:373-376.

13. Spiro RH, Huvos AG, Wong GY, Spiro JD, Gnecco CA, Strong EW. Predictive value of tumor thickness in squamous carcinoma confined to the tongue and floor of the mouth. *Am J Surg.* 1986;152:345-350.

14. Mendenhall WM, Parsons JT, Stringer SP, Cassisi NJ, Million RR. The role of radiation therapy in laryngeal cancer. *CA Cancer J Clin.* 1990;40:150-165.

15. Department of Veterans Affairs Laryngeal Cancer Study Group. Induction chemotherapy plus radiation compared with surgery plus radiation in patients with advanced laryngeal cancer. *N Engl J Med.* 1991;324:1685-1690.

16. Lee NK, Byers RM, Abbruzzese JL, Wolf P. Metastatic adenocarcinoma to the neck from an unknown primary source. *Am J Surg.* 1991;162:306-309.

17. Robbins KT, Medina JE, Wolfe GT, Levine PA, Sessions RB, Pruet CW. Standardizing neck dissection terminology. *Arch Otolaryngol Head Neck Surg.* 1991;117:601-605.

18. Shaha AR. Marginal mandibulectomy for carcinoma of the floor of the mouth. *J Surg Oncol.* 1992;49:116-119.

19. Shaha AR. Preoperative evaluation of the mandible in patients with carcinoma of the floor of mouth. *Head Neck.* 1991;13:398-402.

20. Hidalgo D. Aesthetic mandibular reconstruction. *Plast Reconstr Surg.* 1991;88:574-585.

21. Vokes EE, Weichselbaum RR. Chemoradiotherapy for head and neck cancer. *PPO Updates*, vol 7, no 6. Philadelphia, Pa: JB Lippincott Co; 1993.

22. Lippman SM, Batsakis JG, Toth BB, et al. Comparison of low-dose isotretinoin with beta carotene to prevent oral carcinogenesis. *N Engl J Med.* 1993;328:15-20.

23. Hong WK, Lippman SM, Itri LM, et al. Prevention of second primary tumors with isotretinoin in squamous-cell carcinoma of the head and neck. *N Engl J Med.* 1990; 323:795-801.

24. Shah JP, Ihde JK. Salivary gland tumors. *Curr Probl Surg.* 1990;27:775-883.

25. Spiro RH. Salivary neoplasms: overview of a 35-year experience with 2,807 patients. *Head Neck Surg.* 1986;8: 177-184.

24

TUMORS OF THE CENTRAL NERVOUS SYSTEM

Kamal Thapar, MD, Edward R. Laws, Jr, MD

Patients afflicted with tumors of the central nervous system (CNS) have generally been regarded with pessimism, viewed as helpless captives of an intellectually humiliating, physically crippling, and inextricably fatal process. Furthermore, brain tumors have invoked special philosophical and emotional sentiments, for they attack the very organ of our humanity, and have therefore been perceived as especially devastating by patients, their families, and their physicians. While these statements reflect some of the inescapable realities of contemporary neuro-oncology, the grounds for pessimism are gradually dissipating, as these statements are applicable to a shrinking proportion of patients with CNS tumors. In fact, approximately 50% of patients with CNS tumors can now be successfully treated, and the excellent long-term prognosis they enjoy serves as the ultimate accolade for the dramatic recent advances witnessed in radiologic imaging, neurosurgical technique, and adjuvant therapy.

This chapter reviews principles of diagnosis and therapy for primary and metastatic tumors of the CNS. Because the clinical presentation, culpable pathologies, therapeutic considerations, and prognostic issues depend so heavily on the level of neuroaxis involvement and whether the tumor is primary or metastatic, this discussion of CNS tumors is divided into three parts: primary brain tumors, primary intraspinal tumors, and metastatic tumors to the CNS. Tumors of the pituitary gland constitute another important form of intracranial neoplasia, and they are discussed in Chapter 25.

It is essential to recognize that the CNS is an environment of special vulnerability. Thus, tumors arising therein are governed by unique therapeutic considerations, which, in concept and in practice, deviate considerably from the oncologic issues imposed by tumors arising elsewhere. Designations such as "benign" or "malignant," however absolute for tumors arising in other organ systems, are only relative distinctions for CNS neoplasms. When situated within eloquent sites of the CNS, the local recurrence of a histologically benign, although physically ineradicable, tumor will eventually prove just as lethal as a similarly placed, histologically malignant tumor. Because the CNS lacks a lymphatic system, histologically malignant CNS tumors, although locally invasive, almost never metastasize systemically. For these reasons and others, classic oncologic concepts predicated on histologic grade, nodal status, and staging strategies, although highly valuable and predictive for cancers arising elsewhere, are not entirely applicable to tumors of the CNS. Instead, the approach to, and prognosis for, CNS tumors depend on at least four important variables: tumor histopathology, anatomic location, patient age, and neurologic status. As will be seen, these variables are critical in governing the nature, extent, and outcome of therapy for tumors of the CNS.

Part I: Primary Brain Tumors

Epidemiology

Primary brain tumors contribute significantly to morbidity and mortality in every age group. Their age-related incidence is bimodal, with an early peak in infancy and childhood, a gradual rise in young adulthood, and a broader, sustained peak from the fifth to the eighth decades. In infants and young children, brain tumors are the second most common form of cancer, after leukemia. In adults, primary brain tumors rank thirteenth in frequency of all adult cancers. Depending on the age of the population studied, primary brain tumors have an annual incidence rate of between 4.8 and 19.6 per 100,000 population, which translates to an average of 17,500 new cases

Kamal Thapar, MD, Division of Neurosurgery, University of Toronto, Toronto, Ontario, Canada

Edward R. Laws, Jr, MD, Professor of Neurological Surgery and Medicine, University of Virginia, Charlottesville, Virginia

annually in the United States.[1] These figures underscore the fact that brain tumors are sufficiently prevalent that virtually every physician, regardless of specialty, will encounter brain tumor patients in some aspect of clinical practice.

Etiology and Pathogenesis

Although primary brain tumors have been subject to considerable study, etiologic and pathophysiologic details concerning their genesis remain obscure. In small discrete subgroups of patients, definite genetic predispositions to brain tumor development have been identified. Neurofibromatosis (NF), the most common member of these, is an autosomal dominant condition and occurs in two distinct forms (NF1 and NF2). Although these two conditions are phenotypically and cytogenetically distinct, both share an increased risk for CNS tumor development. Optic nerve gliomas and intraspinal neurofibromas occur with increased frequency in NF1. Patients with NF2 have, by definition, bilateral eighth cranial nerve neurinomas (schwannomas), but are also at increased risk for the development of meningiomas and schwannomas anywhere in the neuroaxis. Other predisposing neurologic conditions and their respective CNS tumors include von Hippel-Lindau disease (hemangioblastomas), tuberous sclerosis (astrocytomas), Turcot syndrome (gliomas and medulloblastomas), Li-Fraumeni syndrome (gliomas), and multiple endocrine neoplasia type 1 syndrome (pituitary adenomas).[2] As these genetic syndromes are either uncommon or absolute rarities, the vast majority of CNS tumors appear spontaneous, without any characterizable genetic link. It is to be acknowledged, however, that epidemiologic studies have repeatedly identified clustering of certain brain tumors (gliomas and, very rarely, meningiomas, medulloblastomas, and paragangliomas) within families. In one recent survey, almost 7% of newly diagnosed patients with glial tumors, and without any of the above-mentioned neurogenic conditions, had a blood relative with a positive and pathologically verifiable history of a glial tumor.[3]

The possibility that certain environmental carcinogens may be associated with CNS tumor development has remained a smoldering concern for some time. Sustained exposure to vinyl chlorides, polycyclic hydrocarbons, nitrosoureas, and certain pesticides has been implicated in the development of astrocytic tumors. In this regard, variable statistical associations between brain tumor occurrence and workers in the rubber, petrochemical, and farming industries have been raised. However, the credibility of these associations is uncertain, as results of epidemiologic surveys have been conflicting.

Although viruses have shown direct transforming capability in rat and primate brain tumor models, there is currently little evidence to support an oncogenic role for viruses in human brain tumors. There are, however, some interesting associations. The most provocative of these concerns the finding that tumoral DNA from patients with primary CNS lymphoma frequently contains integrated genomic sequences of the Epstein-Barr virus.[4] This finding alone is insufficient to constitute a direct cause-and-effect relationship, but it is sufficiently strong that a viral etiology for human brain tumors cannot be entirely ignored. The accumulated data concerning the molecular biology of human brain tumors are now legion. Although this aspect of brain tumor biology is of considerable conceptual importance, space does not permit its discussion here, and the interested reader is referred to a recent review.[2]

Classification of Brain Tumors

Brain tumors are routinely classified on the basis of both cellular origin and histologic grade (Table 24-1). With regard to cellular origin, it is of interest that neurons, despite their extreme tissue density in the CNS (numbering about 100 billion in the adult brain) and their overall importance to brain function, have no significant reproductive capabilities and are therefore rarely the cellular substrate of neoplastic transformation. Alternatively, the enigmatic glial cells, which numerically exceed the number of neurons and contribute to the structural and metabolic integrity of the latter, have a marked propensity for neoplastic transformation, and are the cellular substrate for almost half of all primary brain tumors (astrocytomas, oligodendrogliomas, ependymomas, and glioblastoma multiforme). The remaining brain tumors take origin from a variety of other supporting elements of the CNS: meninges (meningiomas), choroid plexus (choroid plexus papillomas), nerve sheath tumors (neurinomas), and blood vessels (hemangioblastoma). Finally, there is a class of primary brain tumors that are derivatives of primitive embryonal cells. Such cells normally maintain a temporary presence in the developing brain; however, their abnormal persistence in the mature brain, either in their undifferentiated form or as dysplastic inclusions ("primitive cell rests"), results in the formation of various primitive neoplasms. Examples of primitive tumors in undifferentiated form are the primitive neuroectodermal tumors (PNET) and embryonal tumors of the pineal gland. Tumors resulting from germinal malmigration include craniopharyngioma, teratoma, and the dermoid/epidermoid cyst. The intracranial location and relative frequency of major forms of CNS neoplasia are depicted in Fig 24-1[5] and Table 24-2,[6] respectively.

Attempts to categorize brain tumors exclusively on the basis of cellular origin and histologic grade must be regarded with some caution, as tumor location,

Table 24-1. Abbreviated WHO Histologic Classification of CNS Tumors

1. Tumors of neuroepithelial tissue
- A. Astrocytic tumors
  - Low-grade astrocytoma
    - Pilocytic
    - Protoplasmic
    - Gemistocytic
  - Anaplastic astrocytoma
- B. Oligodendroglial tumors
  - Low-grade oligodendroglioma
  - Mixed oligodendroglioma
  - Anaplastic oligodendroglioma
- C. Ependymal tumors
  - Low-grade ependymoma
  - Anaplastic ependymoma
- D. Tumors of choroid plexus
  - Choroid plexus papilloma
  - Choroid plexus carcinoma
- E. Pineal cell tumors
  - Pineocytoma
  - Pineoblastoma
- F. Poorly differentiated embryonal tumors
  - Glioblastoma
  - Medulloblastoma

2. Tumors of nerve sheath cells
- Schwannoma
- Neurofibroma

3. Tumors of meningeal and related tissue
- A. Benign meningiomas
  - Meningothelial
  - Fibrous
  - Transitional
- B. Malignant meningioma
  - Hemangiopericytoma
- C. Meningeal sarcomas

4. Primary CNS lymphoma

5. Germ cell tumors
- Germinoma
- Embryonal carcinoma
- Endodermal sinus tumor
- Choriocarcinoma
- Teratoma
  - Mature
  - Immature

6. Other tumors of disordered embryogenesis
- Craniopharyngioma
- Epidermoid tumor
- Dermoid tumor
- Colloid cyst of the third ventricle

7. Pituitary tumors
- Anterior lobe
  - Adenoma
  - Carcinoma
- Posterior lobe
  - Choristoma

8. Local extension from regional tumors
- Chordoma
- Glomus jugulare tumor

Modified from Zulch et al.[54]

independent of pathology, is often a critical factor governing therapy and prognosis. Both these parameters can to some degree be integrated by considering brain tumors within three broad classes: intra-axial lesions, extra-axial lesions, and tumors arising from primitive tissues. The nature, diagnosis, and management of the more common tumors within these categories are reviewed below.

Diagnosis and Therapy of Brain Tumors: General Aspects

Before considering specific brain tumors in detail, some of the basic pathophysiologic, diagnostic, and therapeutic considerations applicable to all brain tumors are presented.

Clinical Features

Despite their pathologic diversity, the clinical effects

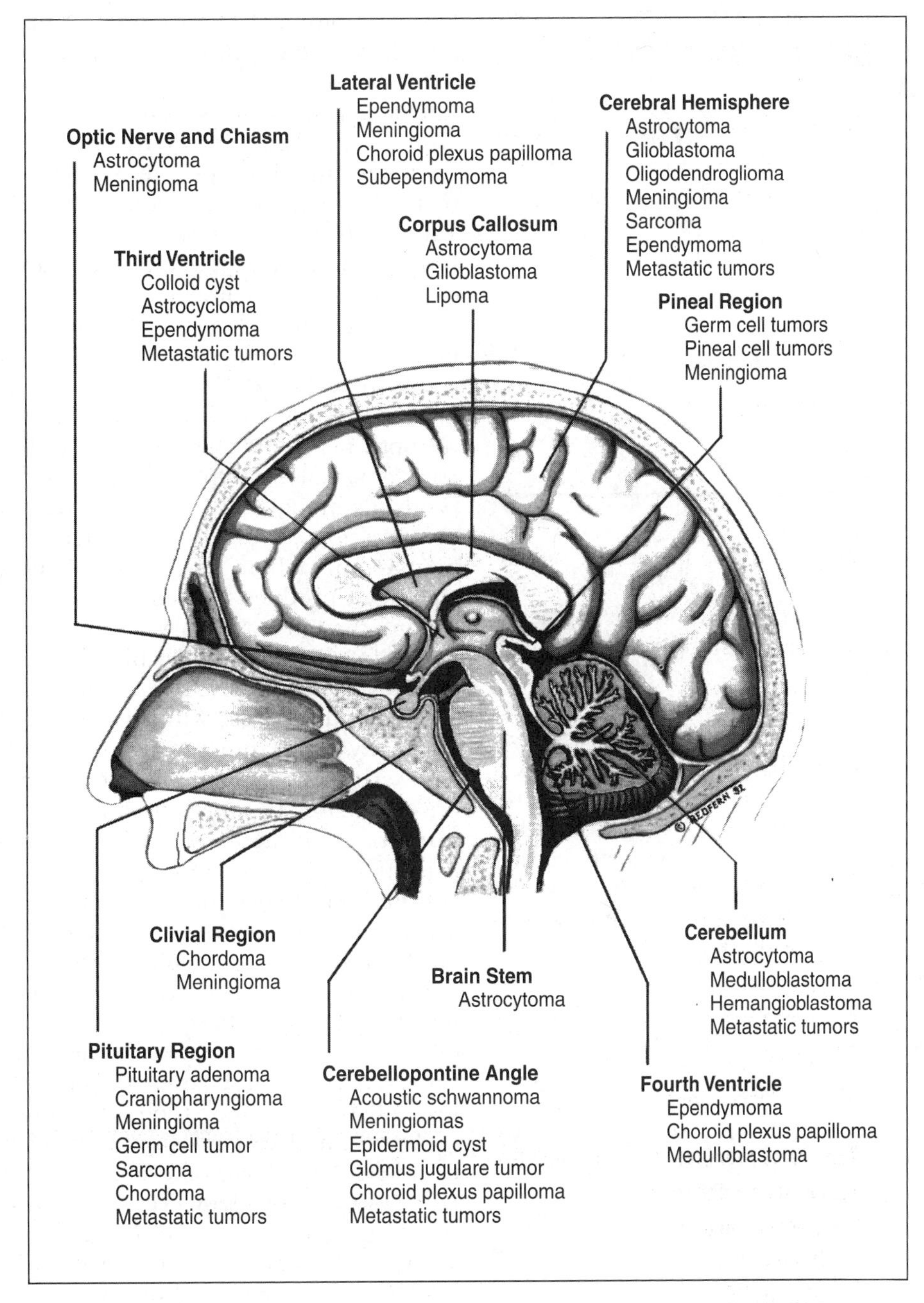

Fig 24-1. Topologic distribution and preferred sites of primary CNS tumors. Modified from Burger et al.[5]

of brain tumors are mediated through relatively few pathophysiologic mechanisms. One of the most essential concepts pertaining to brain tumor pathophysiology is that brain tumors occur within the rigid and unyielding confines of the skull. As the volume of the cranial cavity is constant, any expanding intracranial mass will necessarily generate a proportionate rise in intracranial pressure (ICP). When compensatory mechanisms have been exceeded, continued growth will be at the expense of the brain's volumetric requirements—a critical circumstance resulting in brain distortions, herniations, and ultimately death. Initially, though, the brain has a surprising tolerance to the compressive and infiltrative effects of brain tumors, and there may be few early symptoms. In time, all brain tumors may be expected to produce symptoms by one or more of the following mechanisms: (1) increased ICP due to tumor mass, brain edema, or obstruction of cerebrospinal fluid (CSF) pathways; (2) local destruction, compression, or dis-

Table 24-2. Frequency Distribution of Primary Intracranial Tumors

Tumor Type	Relative Frequency
Glioma (all types)	50%
Meningioma	20
Pituitary adenoma	10
Neurinoma	6
Craniopharyngioma	3
Medulloblastoma	3
All other primary CNS tumors	8

From Berens et al.[53]

tortion of brain substance resulting in specific neurologic deficits; (3) compression or distortion of cranial nerves, resulting in characteristic cranial nerve palsies; and (4) local electrochemical instability, resulting in seizures.

Brain tumor symptoms are of two basic types: nonfocal symptoms related to the generalized effect of increased ICP, and site-specific focal symptoms referable to dysfunction of the particular area of brain substance affected. Elevations in ICP are responsible for many of the nonspecific symptoms produced by brain tumors. Headache is one such symptom that commonly accompanies brain tumors. When produced by an intracranial tumor, the headache tends to have a number of characteristic features. It is often a "pressure"-type headache of moderate severity, typically generalized or retro-orbital, and often worse in the early morning. Such headaches tend to be aggravated by coughing, straining, stooping forward, or any other Valsalva-type maneuver. It is caused by irritation of pain-sensitive structures (dura and blood vessels). Nausea and vomiting are also commonly seen, with the latter often described as "projectile," especially in children. The effects of elevated ICP on the optic nerve result in blurred vision, an enlarged blind spot, and papilledema. The sixth cranial nerve, because of its long intracranial course, is highly susceptible to ICP elevations, and its functional impairment results in lateral rectus weakness and diplopia. Finally, in young children, elevated ICP may result in diastases of cranial sutures and enlarging head size.

Site-specific focal symptoms are variable, depending on the neuroanatomic structure(s) involved, and are characterized by a gradual and progressive loss of neurologic function. Lesions affecting the motor cortex will produce a contralateral hemiparesis. Involvement of the sensory cortex will impair one or more sensory modalities. Impairment of memory, judgment, and personality is typical of frontal and temporal lobe lesions. Dominant hemispheric frontal and temporal lobe lesions can produce a variety of language and speech deficits. Occipital lobe lesions cause contralateral homonymous hemianopic visual deficits. Tumors of the posterior fossa often present with cerebellar dysfunction: ipsilateral incoordination (cerebellar hemisphere) and ataxia (cerebellar vermis). Tumors in the region of the hypothalamus and pituitary gland can produce a wide range of systemic endocrine abnormalities.

When brain tumors impinge on cranial nerves, they produce a range of symptoms that are of exquisite localizing value: Basal anterior fossa lesions produce anosmia (cranial nerve I). Parasellar lesions affecting the optic nerve and chiasm produce characteristic patterns of visual loss. Optic nerve compression generally produces monocular visual loss whereas chiasmatic compression is typically associated with a bitemporal hemianopic deficit. Lesions involving the cavernous sinus can produce palsies of the cranial nerves traversing therein (CN III, IV, V, VI). Tumors in the posterior fossa can produce facial numbness (CN V), facial weakness (CN VII), hearing disturbances (CN VIII), and difficulties with swallowing (CN IX, X).

Finally, brain tumors can cause partial or generalized seizure activity. In fact, the occurrence of recent-onset seizures in an adult should be considered the result of an intracranial mass until proven otherwise. Although seizures can occur in the context of any supratentorial structural abnormality (neoplastic or otherwise), their occurrence with brain tumors is usually the result of longstanding compression or irritation of brain tissue that is immediately adjacent to the neoplastic focus. Since the epileptogenicity of compressed or infiltrated brain is a phenomenon that develops over time, longstanding seizures often tend to signify a biologically benign tumor, though not invariably.

A presumptive diagnosis of brain tumor usually can be made on the basis of a thorough history and physical examination. However, an anatomic diagnosis rests on neuroradiologic imaging studies. In this regard, magnetic resonance imaging (MRI) has evolved as the most recent and most informative means of providing a precise anatomic diagnosis. Given its superior imaging capabilities, especially when enhanced by the paramagnetic contrast agent gadolinium, MRI should detect virtually all tumors greater than a few millimeters in size. For larger tumors, MRI has the particular appeal of defining, in vivid multiplanar detail, critical anatomic relationships between the tumor and surrounding neurovascular structures (Fig 24-2).

Computed tomographic (CT) scanning of the head remains a widely accessible, convenient, and effective means of detecting brain tumors. Although its imaging capabilities are inferior to MRI, CT scanning of the brain can still identify approximately 95% of brain

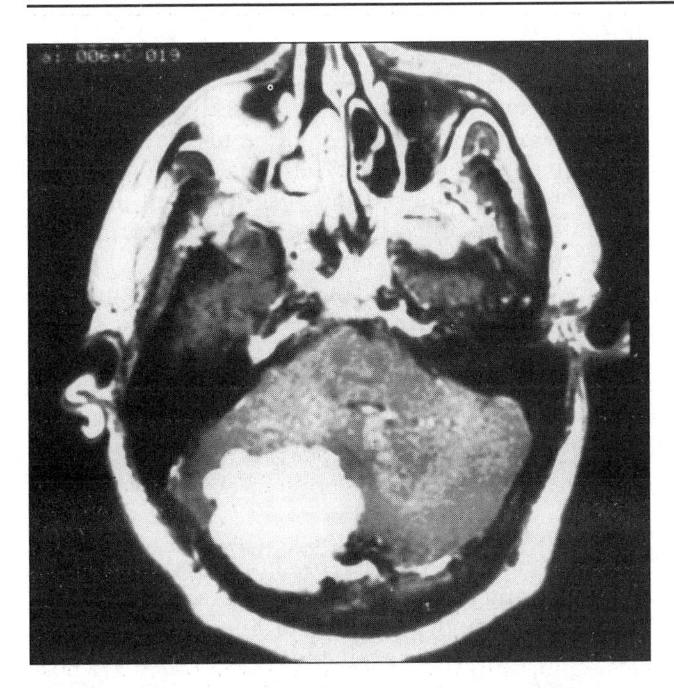

Fig 24-2. Gadolinium-enhanced MRI scan of a posterior fossa meningioma. The white mass in the cerebellum is the tumor.

tumors, and is therefore an accepted alternative when MRI is unavailable or technically not possible.

For the majority of intracranial tumors, MRI or CT scanning provides sufficient information on which to base therapeutic strategies. Occasionally, additional procedures may be required to further delineate the nature of the tumor and identify possible operative hazards. Angiography is useful in certain tumors (meningiomas, hemangioblastomas, glomus tumors) when extreme vascularity is anticipated, and precise knowledge of feeding arteries and draining veins permits a safer and more complete surgical resection. It also identifies those tumors amenable to preoperative embolization, a procedure increasingly used to reduce tumoral vascularity and facilitate surgical resection.

Aside from pituitary tumors, in which hormonal assays are diagnostically and prognostically important, measurement of tumor markers in the blood or CSF has a very limited role in CNS neoplasia. Only certain tumors of the pineal region liberate tumor markers, including alpha-fetoprotein (AFP), beta subunit of human chorionic gonadotropin (β-hCG), and placental alkaline phosphatase (PLAP). Their diagnostic use and limitations are discussed below (see section on pineal region tumors).

Treatment

Surgery

Surgical resection is the most important form of initial therapy for virtually all primary brain tumors. It fulfills three essential and immediate goals: (1) it establishes a tissue diagnosis; (2) it quickly relieves intracranial pressure and mass effect, thus improving neurologic function; and (3) it achieves oncologic cytoreduction, which may prolong life in and of itself, and/or enhance the efficacy and safety of adjuvant therapies such as irradiation.

Technological and conceptual advances in neurosurgery continue to be made, and have enabled safer and more effective forms of therapy. Tumors previously considered inaccessible, such as those situated in deep or eloquent brain regions, can now be confidently approached with the aid of the operating microscope, micro-instrumentation, and microtechnique. Few intracranial tumors can escape the direct surgical access afforded by the contemporary neurosurgical armaments of lasers, ultrasonic aspirators, intraoperative ultrasound, and computer-interactive image-based stereotaxic resection procedures. Collectively, these innovations have added considerable dimension to the repertoire of surgical strategies available to the brain tumor patient.

For most benign extra-axial lesions (meningiomas and acoustic neurinomas), the goal of surgery is total excision and potential cure. The challenge in such cases is to remove the tumor as completely as possible, while minimizing operative trauma to adjacent neural structures. This usually can be achieved, particularly with the use of intraoperative electrophysiologic monitoring techniques that can alert the surgeon to vulnerable neural structures at risk during the course of tumor resection.

For the infiltrative intra-axial malignant brain tumors, the majority of which are glial in origin, surgery provides both a tissue diagnosis and a measure of temporary control by reducing mass effect and ICP. Because of their locally aggressive nature, malignant brain tumors are currently beyond cure, and their control requires multimodal strategies. Although there is some controversy over the role of aggressive surgery in the management of these lesions, most neuro-oncologists agree that "cytoreduction" and elimination of tumor burden are reasonable surgical goals, provided they are achieved without imposing a neurologic deficit.

The mortality and morbidity for cranial operations have diminished considerably over recent decades. Thirty-day mortality rates for brain tumor resections are generally <3% in most recently reported series. The postoperative complication rate depends on the nature of the tumor and its location. Serious complications (hemorrhage at the operative site, infection, and permanent neurologic injury) are uncommon, collectively occurring in <10% of cases overall.

Corticosteroids and Brain Edema

By mechanisms as yet unclear, both benign and malignant brain tumors frequently invoke vasogenic edema of surrounding peritumoral brain tissue. At times, brain swelling can be massive, contributing significantly to overall mass effect and clinically accelerating any neurologic deficits imposed by the tumor alone. For these reasons, corticosteroids have assumed an important therapeutic role as anti-inflammatory agents capable of prompt and effective reduction in peritumoral edema. That steroids alone can often produce immediate and dramatic improvements in clinical status and neurologic function, underscores the pathophysiologic contribution of brain edema to the overall deleterious effects of brain tumors. Steroids are generally used perioperatively, and are gradually tapered following tumor resection. They also serve a palliative function in patients with recurrent and progressive malignant tumors, in whom they can, at least temporarily, maximize residual neurologic function.

Radiation Therapy

Radiotherapy is of proven effectiveness for most malignant brain tumors. Once the pathological diagnosis of brain malignancy has been established and maximal surgical resection undertaken, radiotherapy is usually indicated. Although the various histologic entities show individual differences in radiosensitivity, the short-term (1-5 years) survival advantage accrued from radiation therapy for most CNS tumors is unquestionable.[6] The major factor limiting its long-term effectiveness is the level of tumoricidal radiation doses, which often exceeds thresholds of CNS tolerance. Even when prescribed radiation doses are within established tolerance levels (40-60 Gy), the brain is vulnerable to a variety of toxic effects. Acute reactions, occurring during or immediately after radiation therapy, are the result of acute brain swelling and manifest as an increase in neurologic deficit. Fortunately, these reactions respond well to steroids and are generally reversible. A similar but delayed postirradiation syndrome is seen 1 to 3 months after radiation, and it too is reversible with steroids. The least common, but most severe and irreversible, brain reaction is known as radiation necrosis and can follow cranial irradiation by months to years. This is a dose-dependent progressive brain reaction and presumably is the result of direct toxicity of the brain and its microvasculature. Affected patients present with insidiously progressive deterioration, focal neurologic signs, and dementia. It can be difficult to distinguish radiation necrosis from recurrent tumor, since the two can have similar clinical and imaging characteristics. In this circumstance, therapy may include steroids or a salvage decompressive procedure. However, many affected patients are frequently in terminal stages of their disease, and conservative palliation is therefore most often appropriate.

As patients with CNS tumors survive longer, a number of additional long-term complications of irradiation are of increasing concern. These include hypopituitarism, radiation-induced occlusive disease of cerebral vessels, and radiation-induced oncogenesis. Radiation-induced tumors (meningiomas, sarcomas, and gliomas) are a rare and late complication, generally occurring decades after cranial irradiation. Finally, irradiation of the spinal axis for primary and secondary tumors can cause transient and permanent myelopathies, as well as a motor neuron-type syndrome. Of greatest concern are the risks of radiation in young children. These include learning disabilities, hypopituitarism, myelopathy, and spinal deformities, in addition to the adverse effects discussed above. As myelinization of the CNS is generally complete by 2 to 3 years of age, radiation therapy prior to this age can be especially devastating, and is generally avoided.

Chemotherapy

Despite periodic episodes of short-lived optimism, chemotherapy has yet to make a dramatic impact in the management of malignant brain tumors. Virtually every antitumor agent available for use in hematologic and systemic malignancies has been studied against brain tumors. Aside from some recent successes in certain pediatric neoplasms such as medulloblastoma,[7] chemotherapy has not proven of consistent benefit for the majority of brain tumor patients.[8] On purely oncologic grounds, brain tumors, with their highly localized position, relatively small tumor burden, and nonmetastasizing nature, might be expected to show a favorable response to chemotherapy. These factors are overshadowed by the unique complexity of the CNS, where the blood-brain barrier severely restricts access to most antitumor agents. Although the integrity of this pharmacologic-physiologic barrier is variably impaired with different brain tumors, penetration by most chemotherapeutic agents is still limited. There are, however, a small number of nonpolar, lipid-soluble agents of low molecular weight capable of free transit through an intact blood-brain barrier. These include nitrosoureas, hydroxyureas, and diazoquinone (AZQ). Access to other, less permeable agents (methotrexate, vincristine, cisplatin) can sometimes be facilitated with osmotic blood-brain barrier disruption, intrathecal delivery, and intra-arterial delivery.[9] Of these six agents, nitrosoureas and hydroxyureas have been studied most vigorously. A recent meta-analysis of prospective randomized trials conducted over the past decade has shown that chemotherapy following surgery and irradiation for malignant gliomas does provide modest survival increments. The mean 24-month survival rate was 23.4% in the chemotherapy group, compared with 15.9% in those with radiation and surgery alone.[10] However, these small, albeit statistically significant gains can often be obscured by other variables such as age and performance status at presentation.

Other Adjuvant Therapies

Almost without exception, local tumor recurrence eventually develops in virtually all malignant brain tumor patients despite aggressive multimodality therapy (surgery, radiotherapy, and chemotherapy). Adjuvant strategies to control local tumor growth have evolved considerably over the past decade, and include alternative methods of radiation delivery and immunotherapy. Of these, interstitial brachytherapy and stereotaxic radiosurgery are gaining increasing prominence, although immunotherapy has had minor success in selected patients. All these modalities are existing options for selected patients, and their roles will likely expand in the foreseeable future.

Alternate Methods of Radiation Delivery

The positive correlation between tumor control and increasing radiation dose has led to the development of alternative techniques of radiation delivery which maximize exposure to tumor volume, yet minimize toxicity to adjacent brain tissue. Although interstitial brachytherapy and stereotaxic radiosurgery exploit different principles of radiation physics, both techniques deliver a controlled, concentrated, and highly discrete radiation dose to the tumor, which is designed to rapidly dissipate at the tumor margins. Interstitial brachytherapy involves the stereotaxic deposition of removable radioactive implants (iodine^{125} or iridium^{192}) directly within the tumor, at predetermined sites of optimum dosimetry. For a period of 3 to 6 days, continuous interstitial radiation delivers cumulative doses of 30 to 120 Gy to the tumor, but because of rapid "falloff," surrounding brain tissue is spared. As well, the radiobiology of low dose-rate radiation (ie, radiation delivered over days instead of over minutes as in conventional fractionated radiation) is such that sublethal radiation damage can be better repaired by normal tissue than tumor tissue. Thus, the therapeutic window between normal and tumor tissue is further improved. Brachytherapy is most applicable to localized, non-midline tumors <5 cm in diameter. In patients with recurrent GBM or anaplastic astrocytoma, brachytherapy has provided median survival of 54 weeks and 81 weeks, respectively, from the time of recurrence.[11] Encouraging preliminary results have also been observed in other glial tumors, meningiomas, acoustic neurinomas, and chordomas.

Stereotaxic radiosurgery is a technique in which tumor necrosis is induced by the delivery of a large external radiation dose in a single, highly focused fraction, via very small and well-collimated radiation beams. This is currently performed with one of three technologies, each differing in radiation source, method of radiation delivery, and availability. The gamma knife uses high-energy photon beams emanating from 201 stationary and independent cobalt^{60} sources, each directed at a specific "isocenter," and finely focused by a collimating helmet. Less expensive and more widely available are linear accelerator-based radiosurgery systems. These deliver high-energy photon beams to the target volume from a mobile source, in a series of non-coplanar converging arcs which discretely intersect at the target site. The most expensive and least available instrumentation is proton beam therapy, in which heavy charged particle beams (protons or helium ions) are emitted from a synchrocyclotron, enter the skull through a small number of portals, and deposit their energy at the target site by way of the Bragg peak effect. For more than a decade, a wide variety of metastatic and primary brain tumors (gliomas, craniopharyngiomas, acoustic neurinomas, pituitary tumors, pineal tumors, vascular tumors, and others) have been treated by radiosurgery. As reviewed by Larson and coworkers,[12] most reports indicated a favorable response. However, small patient numbers and limited follow-up raise questions about response consistency and durability. Because the popularity and availability of radiosurgery units are rapidly increasing, data concerning radiosurgical indications and outcomes are on the immediate horizon.

Immunotherapy

Of the existing therapies available to brain tumor patients, immunotherapy is the most infrequently used, most poorly characterized, and of least proven benefit. Nevertheless, it continues to generate considerable theoretical appeal, especially with the emerging evidence implicating aberrant immune regulation as potentially permissive to the maintenance and/or progression of cancer. The observation that malignant glioma patients have a marked depression of immune competence affecting both cellular and humoral mechanisms, lends credibility to the potential roles of biological response modifiers in the treatment of these tumors. Immunotherapeutic strategies used for CNS tumors, primarily malignant gliomas, have assumed the form of active, restorative, adoptive, and passive immunotherapy. These include immunization with cell wall fractions of bacillus Calmette-Guerin (BCG); intratumoral and intrathecal administration of beta interferon; deposition of autologous lymphocyte activated killer (LAK) cells into the tumor bed; and the use of monoclonal antibodies.[8,9,12,13] Preliminary studies with each modality have shown some promise, although any survival advantage provided by them has been modest, at best.

Primary Intra-Axial Brain Tumors

Gliomas

As a group, glial neoplasms are the most common primary brain tumors, accounting for 40% to 50% of all primary intracranial neoplasms. Glial cells are of three basic types: astrocytes, oligodendroglial cells, and ependymal cells. Each is a product of different developmental lineage, each maintains different functional and morphologic characteristics, and each is susceptible to neoplastic transformation. Their respective tumors—astrocytomas, oligodendrogliomas, and ependymomas—are, by virtue of their divergent developmental lineages, sufficiently different from clinical, pathological, and prognostic standpoints that they are considered separately.

Astrocytic Tumors

From the standpoint of biological behavior, astrocytic tumors can range from indolent foci of atypical astrocytes having minimal proliferative capacity, to wildly aggressive, necrotic masses with chaotically brisk kinetic profiles. Insofar as these are extremes of the broad biologic spectrum encompassing astrocytic tumors, a number of classification schemes have managed to translate these differences in biological behavior into the practical context of histologic grade. Regardless of the exact classification system used, there are four essential elements to be evaluated when classifying astrocytic tumors: nuclear atypia, mitotic activity, endothelial proliferation, and necrosis. Daumas-Duport and colleagues have devised a simple and prognostically valid classification scheme that incorporates these pathologic criteria.[14] Tumors are given a numerical grade (I to IV) based on the cumulative number of features present: grade I: absence of all features; grade II: any one feature present; grade III: any two features present; and grade IV: any three features present. Grades I and II are referred to as low-grade astrocytomas; grade III tumors are known as malignant astrocytomas; and grade IV lesions are designated as glioblastoma multiforme. A higher histologic grade is associated with an increasingly aggressive tumor. This is illustrated in a recent retrospective review, with the median survivals being inversely proportional to tumor grade: 4 years for grade II lesions, 1.6 years for grade III tumors, and 0.7 years for grade IV disease.[15]

Low-Grade Astrocytomas

Low-grade astrocytomas represent approximately one third of all gliomas. They are proportionally more common in children, in whom they represent 55% of glial tumors, in comparison with 30% of glial tumors in adults. In all age groups, the majority of these lesions occur within the cerebral hemispheres, although the brain stem and cerebellum are additional favored sites in children. Most supratentorial low-grade astrocytomas (90%) present with seizures as their initial manifestation. Headache and focal neurologic deficits are also seen, though less commonly. On CT, they appear as a nonenhancing low-density area, which may be associated with mass effect of varying degree, although MRI better approximates their full extent. Because low-grade astrocytomas are metabolically less active than surrounding brain tissue, positron emission tomographic (PET) scanning for glucose metabolism detects these lesions as "cold spots," compared with the "hot spots" of higher-grade tumors. As aggressiveness can be inferred from such metabolic imaging studies, PET scanning is most helpful when conventional imaging studies are inconclusive as to whether the lesion is high or low grade.

A major conceptual barrier that continues to overshadow therapeutic considerations for low-grade astrocytomas concerns our limited knowledge of their natural history. Despite the benignity implied in the term "low grade," these are nearly always infiltrative lesions, which extend, often imperceptibly, into adjacent brain substance that is considered to be clinically, radiographically, and functionally unaffected. They are generally progressive, with "estimated" untreated (biopsy proven) 5- and 10- year median survival rates of 32% and 11% respectively.[14-16] Up to half of these low-grade tumors can be expected to dedifferentiate into higher-grade lesions (grade III or IV), usually 3 to 4 years after diagnosis.[15] The cellular composition of low-grade astrocytomas also impacts on prognosis, with tumors composed of pilocytic astrocytes having a better prognosis than those composed of gemistocytic astrocytes. The latter are more aggressive and more prone to dedifferentiation. Surgical resection appears to be beneficial, with a trend toward higher survival rates in patients receiving gross "total" resection, versus those only partially resected.[15] The role of adjuvant radiotherapy is unclear, although it appears to be of greatest benefit in those patients with partially resected tumors.

With these considerations in mind, therapy must be individualized, taking into account patient age, tumor size and mass effect, tumor location, and the neurologic status of the patient. For small and eloquently placed lesions in neurologically intact patients, a conservative approach appears justified. In these cases, a stereotaxic biopsy will provide a confirmatory tissue diagnosis, and definitive resection may be delayed until tumor growth or dedifferentiation, as determined by serial MRI and PET scanning, warrants a more surgically aggressive approach. For large cerebral tumors with associated mass effect, regardless of location, and tumors of any size in noneloquent sites, surgical resection should be the initial consideration. In these cases, gross total resection should be attempted, provided that this can be achieved without producing a neurologic deficit. Radiation therapy is generally reserved for cases of incomplete tumor removal. When tumor excision is complete, extremely high 5- and 10- year survival rates have been reported, sometimes approaching 100% for pilocytic astrocytomas. The combination of partial resection and radiotherapy yields 5- and 10-year survival rates of 60% and 35%, respectively.[15]

Other Low-Grade Astrocytomas

Pilocytic astrocytomas are a special subgroup of low-grade astrocytomas characterized by a slow and relatively benign clinical course. The term *pilocytic* refers to a distinct histologic pattern, and can be seen in astrocytomas arising anywhere within the CNS. Although all pilocytic astrocytomas have a better prognosis than their nonpilocytic counterparts, two specific entities deserve special mention: pilocytic astrocytomas of the cerebellum and of the optic nerve.

Cerebellar Astrocytomas These neoplasms are predominantly tumors in children, in whom they represent 25% of all posterior fossa tumors. About 25% of cerebellar pilocytic astrocytomas are seen in late adolescence or early adulthood (median age, 18 years). The majority of these tumors are situated laterally in the cerebellar hemisphere, although midline and paramedian tumors involving the vermis are also common. Most tumors are cystic, consisting of an eccentrically placed tumor mass (mural nodule), surrounded by a protein-rich fluid-filled cyst. Occasionally, tumor cells may infiltrate the cyst wall, and less often the cerebellar parenchyma. Patients present with typical cerebellar findings, and many with symptoms of increased ICP due to obstructive hydrocephalus. CT or MRI will reveal a cystic cerebellar mass with a contrast-enhancing mural nodule and varying degrees of hydrocephalus. Complete surgical excision is almost always possible and is curative in the majority of cases. Radiation therapy is not indicated. Recurrence is a problem in fewer than 10% of patients and is best managed with repeat resection.

Astrocytomas of the Optic Nerve[17,18] Most optic nerve gliomas occur in the first decade of life, and only occasionally do they occur after age 20. Most are histologically benign, slow-growing, low-grade lesions. When arising in adults, optic nerve gliomas tend to be more aggressive and often frankly malignant. Twenty to thirty percent of affected individuals have NF1. Although the natural history of most optic nerve astrocytomas is generally one of quiescence or very slow growth, the clinical course can be unpredictable—some tumors proliferate rapidly and can quickly cause patient demise. At the time of diagnosis, only 30% of tumors are confined to one optic nerve. The remainder involve the chiasm alone, the optic nerve and chiasm, or the chiasm and extrachiasmic structures (hypothalamus, thalamus, optic tract, internal capsule, and ventricular system).

Tumors involving the intraorbital portion of the optic nerve cause progressive, painless unilateral proptosis, accompanied by varying degrees of visual loss. Tumors involving the chiasm usually produce bilateral visual disturbances of varying degrees (hemianopsia or homonymous defects). Chiasmatic tumors can extend into the hypothalamus, causing endocrine disturbances (precocious puberty, diabetes insipidus), or into the ventricular system, causing hydrocephalus and symptoms related to elevated ICP.

Therapeutic options for these tumors include observation alone, surgical resection, radiation therapy, or surgery followed by radiation. There is some debate concerning the ideal time for surgical intervention and some uncertainty as to the role of radiation as either a primary or adjuvant therapy. The clearest indication for surgical resection is disfiguring proptosis, where the viability of the globe is jeopardized, or severe visual loss occurring with a tumor confined to the optic nerve. In this situation, excision of the involved optic nerve and associated tumor is generally curative. For chiasmatic gliomas, especially those extending into extrachiasmatic structures, there is less consensus as to optimal treatment. Most are approached surgically, a histologic diagnosis is obtained, and some degree of surgical resection may be carried out. If there is significant residual tumor (which is often the case), radiation is considered. Such a strategy has been shown to effect stabilization and improvement in both vision and other neurologic symptoms.[18] Assuming the tumor does not dedifferentiate into a more malignant form, the long-term outcome is favorable. However, various series indicate that 10% and 25% of patients will eventually succumb to recurrent local disease.[18]

Malignant Astrocytoma and Glioblastoma Multiforme (GBM)

Most of the pessimism, yet much of the challenge confronting contemporary neuro-oncology, is directed at these two entities, which assume positions of extreme aggressiveness in the contexts of brain tumors, in particular, and human malignancy, in general. Returning to the concept that astrocytic tumors encompass a graded biologic spectrum beginning with pilocytic low-grade astrocytomas at the well-differentiated extreme, anaplastic astrocytomas assume intermediate positions of aggressiveness, and glioblastoma multiforme represents the most florid product of malignant transformation. The histologic features of these two entities disclose their malignant intent, with degrees of nuclear atypia, mitotic activity, endothelial proliferation, and necrosis closely paralleling biological behavior. Necrosis is generally considered the histologic hallmark of GBM, and is frequently the factor distinguishing it from anaplastic astrocytoma.

Together, anaplastic astrocytoma and GBM account for more than half of all astrocytic tumors, with the latter being the single most common primary intracranial tumor. The mean age of presentation for anaplastic astrocytomas is 45 years, whereas GBM typically presents in older patients, between 45 and 65 years of age. Although either tumor can arise anywhere within the neuroaxis, the cerebral hemispheres are the most common sites of origin. The unrelenting local aggressiveness of these lesions is illustrated by their kinetic profiles, in which cell cycle durations of 2.5 days and estimated doubling times as brief as one week have been noted.[19] Despite their local aggressiveness, neither has significant extraneural metastatic potential. Fewer than 1% of patients with surgically resected malignant astrocytoma will develop extraneural metastases (lungs, lymph nodes, and bone marrow being the most common sites). There is, however, some potential for metastatic spread within the neuroaxis, as free tumor cells can be found within the CSF in up to 20% of GBM patients, and a similar percentage of patients will show leptomeningeal invasion at autopsy. Because the survival of these patients is so short-term, dissemination within the CSF space is rarely of clinical significance.

These tumors share similar clinical profiles, presenting with progressive symptoms of focal neurologic dysfunction and/or global ICP elevations. Headaches, cognitive dysfunction, dysphasia, extremity weakness, and seizures are the most common features, although other site-specific symptoms can occur, depending on the precise location of the tumor. MRI or CT will clearly define the extent of the tumor, and the associated peritumoral edema and mass effect that typically accompany these lesions. A feature common to many anaplastic astrocytomas and almost all GBMs is their inhomogeneous radiographic appearance. When studied with CT contrast agents, these lesions demonstrate ring-like or nodular enhancement patterns, imparting the multi-compartmentalized radiographic appearance characteristic of malignant tumors.

Therapeutic strategies for malignant astrocytic tumors have been, and continue to be, undermined by two major obstacles: their infiltrative nature, which precludes complete excision, and their seemingly obstinate resilience to virtually all forms of adjuvant therapy. Acknowledging these therapeutic constraints, the primary goals of therapy for malignant astrocytic tumors are establishing a histologic diagnosis and increasing the duration of high-quality survival. As an initial step, corticosteroids will provide prompt and often dramatic symptomatic improvement in the majority of patients. Cytoreductive surgery, though not curative, still has a crucial role. It provides a definitive histologic diagnosis, offers immediate palliation to the effects of elevated ICP and focal neural compression, confers a two-log reduction in tumor burden, and serves as a necessary prerequisite to the efficacy of a variety of adjuvant therapies.[20] Some degree of cytoreductive surgery should therefore be considered in most patients, provided that it can be achieved without compromising existing neurologic function. For those lesions in eloquent or inaccessible locations (deep cerebral or brain stem lesions), a stereotaxic biopsy will safely provide a tissue diagnosis on which further therapy can be based.

Although survival is positively correlated with the degree of tumor resection, all malignant astrocytomas will eventually recur. In the case of glioblastoma, the median survival with decompressive surgery alone is only 4 months. Therefore, some form of adjuvant therapy is necessary to forestall recurrence. Radiotherapy has become standard in the postoperative care of malignant astrocytic tumors, resulting in increased quality and duration of survival, at all intervals during the first 18 months following diagnosis.[9,20] Seventy percent of patients with anaplastic astrocytoma survive 1 year, 40% survive 2 years, and only 10% to 20% of patients are alive at 5 years. Expectedly, GBM patients have an even grimmer prognosis, with about 50% of aggressively treated patients surviving 1 year, <15% alive at 2 years, and rare long-term survival.[21,22] Factors associated with a more favorable outcome include younger age at diagnosis, a high neurologic performance level at diagnosis, extensive resection at the time of surgery, and lower histologic grade. Postoperatively, most patients will, for some period of time, enjoy "useful" survival, although only a minority return to gainful employment.

Recurrent tumors require individual evaluation. When tumor recurrence is accompanied by significant intellectual and functional decay, patients benefit most from compassionate care, in which patient comfort, not survival, becomes the primary consideration. In younger patients, and in those with a high level of functioning, repeat resection can extend survival for 40 weeks or longer.[20] After reoperation, many of these patients may also be candidates for adjuvant therapies such as interstitial brachytherapy, photodynamic therapy, or chemotherapy (with nitrosoureas, hydroxyureas, procarbazine, and vincristine). As noted earlier, interstitial brachytherapy has been of benefit in selected patients, increasing median survival from time of recurrence to 54 and 81 weeks for glioblastoma and malignant astrocytoma, respectively.[11] The benefits of the other two modalities, though impressive in isolated cases, is generally modest.

Brain Stem Gliomas

Gliomas of the brain stem are predominantly tumors of childhood and adolescence; >75% of cases occur in patients younger than 20 years. In this age group, brain stem gliomas are relatively common, being the third or fourth most common tumor type, and constitute 15% to 25% of all primary pediatric brain tumors.[23] Of the tumor types represented in the brain stem, astrocytomas of varying grades constitute the overwhelming majority, followed by glioblastomas and rarely ependymomas. Despite this relatively narrow pathological spectrum, there is considerable heterogeneity with respect to growth patterns, surgical options, and prognosis. In an attempt to integrate these factors, Epstein and Wisoff have proposed a five-category classification scheme for brain stem tumors, designating them as either diffuse, focal, cystic, exophytic, or cervicomedullary. Their preliminary results suggest that cervicomedullary, exophytic, and cystic tumors have the most favorable outcome, whereas many focal and all diffuse tumors fare poorly.[24] The overall prognosis for brain stem gliomas is relatively poor. However, depending on the histologic grade, preoperative neurologic status, and the tumor class as proposed by Epstein and Wisoff, some patients do better than others, and occasionally gratifying results can be obtained.

Brain stem gliomas present with features of progressive brain stem dysfunction. Unilateral cranial nerve palsies, especially of the sixth and seventh nerves, are often the initial findings. Then, depending on the brain stem and cranial nerve structures involved, drowsiness, ataxia, long tract signs, nausea and vomiting, dysarthria, and difficulty swallowing can all eventually occur. Hydrocephalus and related symptoms are seen in up to half of patients and are referable to compression of the fourth ventricle or cerebral aqueduct. Gadolinium-enhanced MRI is the imaging modality of choice, and is critical for therapeutic planning. The important considerations pertain to the gross morphology of the tumor and whether it is diffusely intrinsic to the brain stem, or whether there is an exophytic or cystic component. Furthermore, MRI will usually exclude other conditions occasionally confused with brain stem gliomas such as meningiomas, clival chordomas, brain stem abscesses, or vascular malformations.

Radiation therapy is the principal form of treatment for brain stem gliomas, and is often administered without a confirmatory tissue diagnosis. In one retrospective pediatric series, radiation therapy improved neurologic symptoms in 75% of patients and was accompanied by an overall 5-year survival rate of 23% for gliomas of the midbrain, pons, and medulla.[25] Aside from shunting for hydrocephalus, the relative role of surgery in the management of brain stem gliomas is unclear and controversial; surgery is currently of unproven benefit. Malignant tumors, regardless of intervention, are uniformly fatal, typically within 12 to 18 months of diagnosis.[23,24] All diffuse and many focal tumors have an anaplastic component and generally fall in this category. Lower-grade tumors, especially those at the cervicomedullary junction and, to a lesser and variable extent, cystic and exophytic tumors at more rostral brain stem sites, are more amenable to partial resection. However, the extent to which "reduction in tumor burden" actually enhances survival is uncertain, and further study is required before precise surgical indications can be defined.

Oligodendrogliomas

Oligodendrogliomas are usually low-grade neoplasms and account for <5% of all intracranial tumors. They arise as neoplastic derivatives of the oligodendroglial cell, which is responsible for axonal myelination within the CNS. These are primarily tumors of the adult brain, although they may occasionally be seen in children. The mean age at presentation ranges from 38 to 45 years, and most series identify a slight male preponderance. Eighty percent of oligodendrogliomas are located within the cerebral hemispheres, with the frontal lobes being a favored location. They can extend into the third or lateral ventricles, sometimes presenting primarily as a ventricular mass. Less frequently, oligodendrogliomas can originate within the posterior fossa or spinal cord. Ventricular extension accounts for the 10% incidence of intraneural metastatic dissemination seen with these tumors. Extraneural metastases very rarely occur, although deposits in bone, lymph nodes, and the lungs have been reported.

Histologically, oligodendrogliomas are composed of a monotonously uniform cell population, with individual cells resembling "fried eggs." More than a third of oligodendrogliomas have intermixed astrocytic or ependymal elements and are therefore designated as "mixed gliomas." Like astrocytomas, oligodendrogliomas can vary in aggressiveness, and several grading schemes have attempted to identify histological correlates that would be of prognostic significance. Possibly the most important of these are necrosis and pleomorphism, although increased cellularity, endothelial proliferation, and increased nuclear to cytoplasmic ratio should all alert the pathologist to the possibility of a more aggressive tumor.[15]

A history of seizures, usually of long duration, is the classic presentation pattern of oligodendrogliomas. Occasionally, oligodendrogliomas can present acutely, usually the result of hemorrhage within the tumor, or obstructive hydrocephalus from intraventricular extensions. The radiologic hallmark of this tumor is calcification, which is identified on CT in >90% of cases.

Oligodendrogliomas are treated surgically, the objective being gross total removal. This can be achieved in approximately one third of patients. In the remainder, the infiltrative nature of the tumor or its eloquent locale limits complete excision. The role of adjuvant radiotherapy is controversial, although a number of reports have shown benefit, particularly in incompletely resected lesions. The combination of surgery and irradiation provide 5- and 10-year survival rates of 83%-100% and 45%-55%, respectively.[15] As these data indicate, despite long intervals of quiescence, the majority of oligodendrogliomas eventually recur, often dedifferentiating into a more aggressive tumor.

Ependymomas

Ependymomas are tumors derived from the ependymal cells normally lining the ventricular chambers and central canal of the spinal cord. Their incidence is bimodal, with an early major peak at the median age of 5 years, and a second smaller peak at the median age of 34 years. They account for approximately 10% and 5% of all intracranial tumors in the pediatric and adult populations, respectively. In both childhood and adult series, a 3:2 male preponderance is generally seen. Insofar as the normal ependymal lining spans the entire longitudinal extent of the neuroaxis, ependymomas can originate at virtually any level of the CNS: the supratentorial, infratentorial, or spinal compartments. Supratentorial ependymomas are more common in adults, while the infratentorial site dominates in the pediatric population. In all age groups, spinal ependymomas are one of the two most common intramedullary spinal tumors (see Part II).

One third of all intracranial ependymomas are located supratentorially. Given their cell of origin, most supratentorial ependymomas arise in close proximity to the ventricular system, although only half have an obvious intraventricular component. The supratentorial intraventricular tumors most commonly take origin from the trigone of the lateral ventricle, the frontal horn of the lateral ventricle, and the posterior portion of the third ventricle. With progressive growth, they tend to fill the ventricular cavity, and often extend beyond ventricular walls into brain parenchyma.

Most intracranial ependymomas are infratentorial. In children, ependymomas are the third most common infratentorial tumor, preceded in frequency only by cerebellar astrocytomas and medulloblastomas. These posterior fossa ependymomas arise from the midline floor of the fourth ventricle. They have an exophytic growth pattern, forming a discrete cauliflower-type mass that occupies and distends the fourth ventricle. With continued growth, the tumor gains access to the subarachnoid space via the foramina of Luschka and Magendie, encasing the brain stem and upper cervical cord and ultimately disseminating into remote areas of the subarachnoid space.

Most ependymomas are histologically benign, but like other neoplasms of glial lineage, they encompass a spectrum of histologic grades and clinical aggressiveness. From a practical standpoint, ependymomas are either low- or high-grade. The former is more common, well differentiated, has minimal pleomorphism, few mitotic figures, and a more favorable prognosis. The latter has all the cellular hallmarks of malignancy, including necrosis, and the compatible clinical profile of aggressive and rapid growth. The overall incidence of subarachnoid seeding is approximately 10%.[6] Those at highest risk have infratentorial high-grade ependymomas, in whom the incidence of subarachnoid seeding approaches 26%. For high-grade supratentorial lesions and low-grade infratentorial lesions, the incidence of subarachnoid seeding is low (4%).

The clinical presentation depends primarily on the tumor site. Both supratentorial and infratentorial tumors having a ventricular component, when sufficiently large, will obstruct the circulation of CSF, causing hydrocephalus. Infratentorial tumors may also be accompanied by ataxia, vertigo, and neck stiffness, whereas supratentorial extraventricular tumors can present with focal neurologic deficits and seizures. MRI or CT will provide the anatomic diagnosis and also identify any associated hydrocephalus. Calcification occurs in >50% of ependymomas and, if present, facilitates its radiologic diagnosis.

Surgical excision followed by irradiation is the recommended therapy for ependymomas. The surgical strategy for all tumors is gross total removal. In supratentorial lesions, complete excision may be limited because of infiltration into eloquent brain, whereas in infratentorial lesions, invasive attachment to the floor of the fourth ventricle is usually the limiting factor. All patients receive postoperative radiotherapy. Evidence of dissemination, as determined by positive CSF cytologic or myelographic findings, warrants additional radiation of the spinal axis. The dose and extent of irradiation is also modified by histologic grade, with anaplastic astrocytomas generally receiving more intensive radiotherapy regimens.

The prognosis for ependymomas is improving, with 5-year survival rates exceeding 80%.[9,26] Ten-year survival rates vary from 40% to 60%. At the time of recurrence, >50% of ependymomas have dedifferentiated into higher-grade lesions. At present, chemotherapy is not of proven benefit for newly diagnosed ependymomas, although platinum-based regimens have shown some initial promise for recurrent tumors.

Hemangioblastomas

Hemangioblastomas are benign neoplasms of uncertain origin, which engender interest because of their curability, their association with a multisystem genetic disorder (Von Hippel-Lindau syndrome), and their peculiar ability to cause polycythemia by liberating erythropoietin. Although they account for only 2% of all intracranial tumors, they are the most common adult intra-axial tumor of the posterior fossa. They are slightly more common in males and generally occur between the third and fifth decades. Most hemangioblastomas occur within the posterior fossa, primarily in the cerebellar hemisphere or vermis, but occasionally in the medulla or pons. Less frequently, they arise outside the posterior fossa, in the supratentorial or spinal compartment. Most hemangioblastomas arise as solitary, sporadic lesions without a hereditary basis. The remainder can be solitary or multiple and arise as a manifestation of von Hippel-Lindau syndrome. This is an autosomal dominant disorder of variable penetrance, linked to a locus on chromosome 3, which encompasses an array of pathologic processes, including retinal angiomas, adrenal pheochromocytomas, pancreatic and renal cysts, and renal cell carcinoma.[2]

More than 80% of hemangioblastomas occur in the cerebellum, where grossly they consist of a solid, highly vascular tumor component (mural nodule) attached to the wall of a surrounding cyst. Both the tumor nodule and the associated cyst are well demarcated from surrounding brain tissue. Histologically, the tumor is a vascular conglomerate of endothelial cells, pericytes, and stromal cells.

The clinical presentation is typical of any gradually progressive cerebellar mass: headache, ataxia, vomiting, vertigo, and varying degrees of obstructive hydrocephalus. Up to 20% of patients have polycythemia, due to the autonomous secretion of erythropoietin by the tumor. CT and MRI will disclose the cystic nature of the lesion and the extent of the vascular tumor nodule. Hemangioblastomas have a characteristic angiographic pattern; hence, vertebral angiography is also used to further secure the correct preoperative diagnosis. The diagnostic evaluation should also include an assessment of family history of von Hippel-Lindau syndrome, which may be subtle, owing to the variable penetrance of this disorder.

Complete surgical excision is both possible and curative for the majority of hemangioblastomas when they are located entirely within the cerebellum. For tumors involving the brain stem, complete removal is more hazardous, but can be still achieved in a substantial proportion of patients. The most important surgical principle for these lesions is that unless the mural nodule (which represents the tumor core) is removed, recurrence is virtually guaranteed. Radiation therapy has been of some benefit for incompletely excised or recurrent tumors. Because hemangioblastomas occurring in the context of von Hippel-Lindau syndrome are known to be multicentric, new tumors can occasionally develop at the operative site or elsewhere in the neuroaxis, often years after the initial resection.

Choroid Plexus Papillomas and Carcinomas

The choroid plexus of the ventricular chambers is rarely a substrate for neoplastic transformation. Hence, choroid plexus papillomas and choroid plexus carcinomas account for <1% of all intracranial tumors. Although generally perceived as pediatric tumors, more than half arise in the adult. These tumors arise in four specific brain locations: the lateral ventricle (43%), the fourth ventricle (39%), third ventricle (9%), and the cerebellopontine angle (9 percent). There are three notable pathophysiologic features shared by these tumors: spontaneous hemorrhage; excess CSF production and/or deficient CSF absorption, resulting in hydrocephalus; and dissemination within the CSF in up to 20% of cases. Aside from the occasional acute presentation relating to tumoral hemorrhage, most patients present with progressive symptoms of elevated ICP related to hydrocephalus. Focal cerebellar findings usually accompany lesions situated in the posterior fossa. CT typically show a calcified, contrast-enhancing intraventricular tumor. Hydrocephalus is invariably present. It is usually not possible to distinguish papillomas from carcinomas on the basis of imaging studies, although the latter are reputed to have a more heterogeneous appearance. CSF cytology and myelography are used for postoperative staging.

Therapy for these tumors is complete surgical excision followed by whole-brain irradiation and irradiation of the spinal axis if CSF cytology or myelography is positive. The radiosensitivity of these tumors has been questioned, as the efficacy of radiation therapy has not been formally evaluated. The prognosis for benign papillomas is excellent, provided complete removal is achieved. The prognosis for choroid plexus carcinomas is very poor, with the expected survival generally less than a year.

Primary Central Nervous System Lymphoma

Primary central nervous system lymphomas (PCNSL), that is, those lymphomas arising in the CNS in the absence of systemic lymphoma, were generally considered rare, accounting for 1% to 2% of all intracranial tumors and typically affecting the elderly. During the past decade, there has been a dramatic rise in the incidence of this entity, partly because of its frequent occurrence in immunodeficient states (acquired immunodeficiency syndrome [AIDS], transplant recipients), but also because of an increased, though unexplained, occurrence in immunocompetent individuals. At the Memorial Sloan-Kettering Cancer Center, PCNSL accounted for 0.9% of all primary brain tumors during the period 1965-1984. From 1985 onward, this rate has increased to 15%, and is even higher if immunocompromised patients are considered.[27]

Although PCNSL can affect normal immunocompetent individuals of any age, sporadic cases still most commonly occur in the fifth to seventh decades, with a male to female ratio of 2:1. In addition, there are four populations at specific risk: AIDS patients, transplant recipients, congenitally immunodeficient patients, and patients with collagen-vascular disorders. In comparison to immunocompetent patients, the risk in transplant recipients and AIDS patients increases 100- and 1,000-fold, respectively. The pathophysiologic basis for development of PCNSL is unknown. In immunodeficient patients, infection with Epstein-Barr or other lymphotropic viruses have been speculated as a possible transforming event. Most PCNSL are B-cell lymphomas, indistinguishable pathologically from B-cell lymphomas originating systemically.

Forty percent of PCNSL begin as solitary cerebral lesions, but eventually most patients develop multiple lesions. Although PCNSL can occur anywhere within the neuroaxis, these tumors typically assume a periventricular position, involving the deep white matter, basal ganglia, corpus callosum, and thalamus. In about 20% of patients, infiltration of the posterior vitreous or retina may coexist. Isolated spinal lesions are rare.

The clinical features of PCNSL are variable, but generally evolve over a period of a few months. Some patients present with generalized symptoms of elevated ICP (headaches, nausea and vomiting, and generalized seizures). Depending on the location of the tumor(s), an equal number will present with focal motor, sensory, or visual symptoms, or a change in mental status. Uveitis occurs in approximately 15% of affected individuals, sometimes preceding cerebral symptoms by months to years. Although PCNSL have no pathognomonic radiologic features, their appearance on CT or MRI imaging can be highly suggestive, especially in the context of an immunodeficient state. Their deep cerebral and periventricular location, multiplicity, and enhancement patterns (either diffuse or ringlike) often prompt the correct diagnosis in most cases.

Management of these lesions begins with confirmatory tissue diagnosis, followed by clinical staging and a combination of radiation and chemotherapy. Surgical resection adds little to life expectancy in this disease; therefore, stereotaxic biopsy is the safest and easiest means of obtaining a tissue diagnosis. Clinical staging includes determination of human immunodeficiency (HIV) status, slit-lamp examination of the eye, and, when safe to do so, a lumbar puncture for CSF cytology. As the secondary cerebral lesions of systemic lymphoma are generally meningeal and rarely intraparenchymal, differentiation of systemic lymphoma with cerebral metastases from primary cerebral lymphoma rarely poses a problem. Steroid therapy is initially very effective in reducing tumor size, and its cytotoxic effect can cause the disappearance of PCNSL after just a few doses. This has occasionally been a problem when steroids are instituted prior to biopsy, as tumor regression can be so dramatic that targeting the lesion for biopsy becomes impossible. However, the effectiveness of steroids generally diminishes as the disease progresses. Earlier protocols have advocated immediate radiation therapy after diagnosis; however, there is increasing use of preradiation chemotherapy. The combination of systemic methotrexate and high-dose cytosine arabinoside, followed by cranial irradiation, has improved median survival to 42 months, in comparison to a median survival of 10 to 14 months with radiation alone.[27] The radiation ports should include the orbits if retinal or vitreous disease is present, and also the spinal axis if CSF cytologic findings suggest meningeal disease. Relapse is not unusual, with the majority manifesting as a local recurrence in most instances.

Extra-axial Primary Brain Tumors

Meningiomas

Meningiomas are the most common of benign intracranial neoplasms, and the second most common primary CNS tumor overall. They account for 20% of all primary brain tumors, and in fortuitous contrast to glial tumors, their complete surgical removal is both possible and curative. Meningiomas are primarily adult tumors, as evidenced by their peak occurrence at 45 years of age. Females are more commonly affected than males by a ratio of 3:2. In particular, women with breast cancer have an even stronger, though unexplained, association with meningiomas. Meningiomas also occur in the context of NF2, in which they can occur anywhere in the neuroaxis and are often multiple. Patients with a prior history of cranial irradiation have a fourfold higher risk of developing meningiomas, although the latency period is usually quite long (15 to 20 years).

Meningiomas are of leptomeningeal origin, arising from arachnoid cap cells (cells lining the outer layer of the arachnoid membrane). Meningiomas can arise at virtually any extra-axial site within the CNS. However, 90% are intracranial, and 90% of these are in the supratentorial compartment. The three most common intracranial sites are adjacent to the superior sagittal sinus (parasagittal-falcine meningiomas); over the cerebral convexities (convexity meningiomas), and along the sphenoid ridge (sphenoidal meningiomas). These sites account for approximately 60% of intracranial meningiomas. Most remaining meningiomas arise along the skull base (olfactory groove, tuberculum sellae, tentorial, and petroclival meningiomas). Less common sites include the optic nerve sheath, the lateral ventricle, and the region of the pineal gland. Infratentorial meningiomas, accounting for 10% of meningiomas, arise over the cerebellar convexity, within the cerebellopontine angle, along the clivus, or in the region of the foramen magnum.

Most meningiomas are slow-growing, well-demarcated, globular masses that are firmly attached to a dural base. With progressive enlargement, normal adjacent brain becomes compressed. Gross brain invasion is not a feature of a benign tumor, and its presence constitutes prima facie evidence of a malignant meningioma. Benign meningiomas do, however, regularly invade the dura, dural sinuses, and adjacent bony structures, but this is not considered a feature of malignancy. In addition to compressive effects, meningiomas generate symptoms by two additional mechanisms: brain edema and a local bony reaction known as hyperostosis. Vasogenic edema of peritumoral brain tissue commonly accompanies symptomatic meningiomas. The amount of brain swelling can be considerable, and it is often a significant component of overall mass effect. The presence of peritumoral edema on imaging studies is also considered a sign of recent tumor growth, and is frequently used as a guide in distinguishing enlarging meningiomas requiring treatment, from incidental tumors best managed by observation.

By virtue of bony invasion or simply noninvasive proximity to calvarial surfaces, meningiomas are known to invoke a local osteoblastic response termed hyperostosis. Affected bone undergoes an exuberant osteoblastic proliferation, resulting in profuse local thickening of the skull. Hyperostosis can contribute to local pressure effects, particularly with meningiomas involving the skull base, where pressure on the globe can cause exophthalmos and encroachment on the bony neural foramina can cause cranial nerve palsies. In cases in which the meningioma grows as a carpet in wide apposition to the dura and skull base (en plaque meningioma), hyperostosis is especially prominent.

Meningiomas are classified pathologically on the basis of four histological patterns: meningothelial, transitional, fibrous, and angioblastic. The first three, unified by their benign behavior, account for the majority of meningiomas. The angioblastic pattern, which includes the hemangiopericytoma variant, is the least common, but most aggressive form.[28] Between 1% and 10% of meningiomas are malignant, as determined by the following indices: brain invasion, increased and atypical mitotic figures, increased cellularity, a papillary histologic pattern, and distant metastases. Overall, metastatic dissemination is rare, occurring in <0.1% of cases. When metastases do occur, they most commonly arise from malignant meningiomas, especially the hemangiopericytic variant, although they have been reported with all forms of meningioma. The most common recipient sites include the lung, liver, lymph nodes, and bone.

The clinical presentation of meningiomas varies according to location and rate of growth. Progressively enlarging and eloquently located lesions will produce the full range of site-specific neurological signs. In convexity and parasagittal lesions, leg or extremity weakness may occur, whereas in skull base meningiomas, cranial nerve palsies often predominate. Seizures are particularly common, occurring in >50% of patients. When located in silent brain areas, some meningiomas can become enormous before causing clinical symptoms. Alternatively, meningiomas can be discovered incidentally in the form of quiescent masses that show no appreciable growth over time. Meningiomas usually have a characteristic radiologic appearance as well-circumscribed, extra-axial, homogeneously enhancing, dural-based masses (Fig 24-2). Peritumoral edema and mass effect are common, particularly in symptomatic lesions. Intratumoral calcification is seen in about 20% of cases.

The most appealing aspect of meningiomas is the prospect of long-term cure, which often accompanies complete surgical resection. In contrast to gliomas, which have inherent therapeutic resistance, meningiomas muster very little oncologic resistance, but can impose therapeutic limitations on the basis of their location. Some meningiomas are so insinuated among delicate neural and vascular structures that their safe removal can be a formidable, if not impossible, surgical challenge. Surgical cure of meningiomas requires complete removal of tumor tissue, including infiltrated dura and bone. As meningiomas will eventually reconstitute themselves from seemingly insignificant amounts of residual tissue, complete surgical resection is the single most important determinant of both curability and disease-free survival. Because the likelihood of complete surgical removal depends so heavily on surgical accessibility, meningiomas at different intracranial sites will have correspondingly different surgical cure rates. Favorably situated lesions (convexity, anterior falcine, and lateral sphenoid wing meningiomas) are usually amenable to complete removal. Alternatively, certain basal meningiomas, particularly those involving the cavernous sinus and petroclival regions, are much more difficult to fully and safely excise. Because many meningiomas are associated with considerable peritumoral edema, steroids are an important perioperative adjunct to surgical therapy.

The prognosis for completely excised benign meningiomas is excellent, with 10-year disease-free survival rates of 80% to 90% for all meningiomas, independent of location. Partially resected benign meningiomas are more prone to recurrence, with 10-year progression-free survival rates of 50% to 70%.[9] Although the clinical course of patients with malignant meningioma can vary, recurrence rates for malignant meningiomas are higher, and the disease-free interval shorter; 65% will recur within 5 years, and almost 80% will recur in 10 years.[9,28] Furthermore, malignant meningiomas, especially hemangiopericytomas, are more prone to metastatic dissemination over time, with 13% and 33% giving rise to remote metastases at 5 and 10 years, respectively.[28]

Radiation therapy has a restricted role in the management of meningiomas. For completely excised benign meningiomas, the prognosis with surgery alone is so favorable that radiation therapy is not indicated. In the case of recurrent tumors, repeat resection is usually advisable. Although radiation therapy has proven of some benefit in forestalling recurrence in partially resected meningiomas, the results are not so uniformly impressive as to advocate its routine use.

The decision to use radiation for residual benign meningiomas is one of experienced judgment, and is based on the anticipated resectability of a future recurrence. If one anticipates a delayed recurrence at an easily accessible site, then radiation can be deferred. Alternatively, if a rapid and uncontrollable recurrence at an inaccessible site is anticipated, then radiation therapy should be used. It is important to remember that while radiation therapy may delay recurrence, it does not eliminate the need for future surgery, and among other risks, it can render future surgical efforts more difficult. When used for partially resected benign meningiomas, one retrospective study has shown radiation to reduce recurrence from 60% to 32%, and almost double the time to recurrence.[29] Because of their higher recurrence rates, all malignant meningiomas should receive postoperative radiation.

Acoustic Neurinomas ("Schwannomas")

Acoustic neurinomas are histologically benign tumors derived from Schwann cells that normally invest the vestibular component of the eighth cranial nerve. Acoustic neurinomas are the most common tumor of the cerebellopontine angle, and account for approximately 8% of intracranial tumors. They occur in males and females with equal frequency, and usually present during the fourth to sixth decades. Although the overwhelming majority occur on a sporadic nonhereditary basis, approximately 5% of acoustic neurinomas occur in the context of neurofibromatosis. In the "central" form of neurofibromatosis (NF2), >90% of affected individuals will have bilateral acoustic neurinomas. In contrast, only 2% of individuals with peripheral neurofibromatosis (NF1) develop acoustic neurinomas, virtually all of which are unilateral.

Acoustic neurinomas arise from either the superior or inferior vestibular nerves, at the interface of CNS oligodendroglial cells and peripheral nervous system Schwann cells. This transition zone is located within the internal auditory canal and is the usual starting point for most acoustic neuromas. With progressive growth, the tumor follows a path of least resistance, eventually mushrooming into the cerebellopontine angle. The facial nerve becomes compressed and is usually stretched over and adherent to the tumor capsule. Eventually, the tumor will encroach on the brain stem and compress the trigeminal nerve superiorly and the ninth, tenth, and eleventh cranial nerves interiorly. When the tumor mass exceeds 3 or 4 cm, distortion of the cerebellar hemisphere leads to compression of the fourth ventricle and hydrocephalus. Although the majority of acoustic neurinomas are slow-growing progressive lesions, others can remain quiescent and unchanged for long periods of time.

Patients typically present with progressive unilateral sensorineural hearing loss. Additional symptoms commonly include tinnitus, vertigo, and unsteadiness. If the tumor is sufficiently large, compression of the trigeminal and lower cranial nerves will cause facial numbness and difficulty swallowing, respectively. Despite the regularity with which acoustic neurinomas compress and stretch the facial nerve, facial weakness is generally a late feature. An audiologic diagnosis of acoustic neurinoma can be obtained with brain stem auditory evoked potentials, which are abnormal in 95% of affected individuals. A radiologic diagnosis is provided with gadolinium-enhanced MRI, which will readily identify even the smallest tumors.

Surgical removal is the principal therapeutic option for patients with acoustic neurinomas. Patient age, tumor size, and degree of hearing loss are important considerations that govern both the type and goal of surgical intervention. Complete removal can be achieved in most cases. However, preservation of existing hearing becomes increasingly difficult with increasing tumor size. Despite surgical strategies to conserve hearing, preservation of serviceable hearing can be achieved in approximately 50% to 75% of small tumors (<1 cm), 25% of medium-sized lesions (1 to 2.5 cm), and rarely in tumors >2.5 cm. In most centers, acoustic neurinoma surgery is conducted by the combined expertise of a neurosurgical and neuro-otological team, as this permits the most versatile use of available operative approaches. Because the facial nerve is almost always adherent to the tumor capsule, inadvertent injury to the facial nerve is of paramount operative concern. Greatly facilitated by intraoperative electrophysiologic monitoring, most experienced centers report preservation of facial nerve function in >90% of cases. As the majority of surgical resections are both complete and curative, no further therapy is required. For incompletely resected lesions, radiotherapy is beneficial in increasing relapse-free survival. In one recent retrospective study, symptomatic recurrence was reduced from 46% to 3% when incomplete resection was followed by radiotherapy.[30]

Because acoustic neurinomas can be so slow-growing, not all patients require immediate surgical therapy. This is especially true in the elderly or medically debilitated patient, in whom a more conservative approach is often justified. When presenting with tumors <2.5 cm and hearing loss alone, these patients can be managed expectantly, with surgery being delayed until documented tumor growth. For larger tumors, in those with additional neurologic symptoms or mass effect, and those with documented growth, surgical resection is usually required. There is a role in these patients for partial resection, which shortens the procedure considerably and reduces the risk of anesthetic and operative complications, while ameliorating the tumor's compressive effects. Depending on the extent of resection, radiation therapy is often used in these cases. Of course, each case is approached individually, as some elderly patients are of sufficient good health that complete resection can be safely achieved. Stereotaxic radiosurgery is a relatively new treatment option for acoustic neurinomas. Early experience has shown that neural preservation (hearing and facial nerve function) is comparable to that achieved with surgery. However, the likelihood of long-term tumor control is uncertain.[31]

Patients with bilateral acoustic neurinoma require special consideration. Because they have progressive bilateral hearing loss, and surgery often accelerates the process, there is some merit in delaying surgery. Paradoxically, the likelihood of hearing preservation is best when tumors are small; therefore, early surgery is also desirable. With these competing considerations in mind, therapeutic strategies must be individually tailored to each patient, with an emphasis on hearing conservation, at least unilaterally, for the longest time possible. Regardless of the surgical strategy used, auditory rehabilitation in the context of lip reading and sign language should begin as soon as the diagnosis is made. These skills are more easily acquired in individuals with some residual hearing.

Congenital and Primitive Tumors

Craniopharyngiomas

Craniopharyngiomas[32] are histologically benign tumors thought to arise from remnants of Rathke's pouch. These embryonic squamous cell "rests" extend from the tuber cinereum to the pituitary gland, along the track of an incompletely involuted hypophyseal-pharyngeal duct. Correspondingly, craniopharyngiomas arise anywhere along this same path. As histologically benign tumors, craniopharyngiomas illustrate the unique vulnerability of the intracranial environment to lesions of seemingly minor oncologic potential. By virtue of their location, craniopharyngiomas can simultaneously compromise a number of important intracranial structures, produce a variety of deleterious clinical effects (visual loss, endocrine disturbance, increased ICP), and afford considerable resistance to successful treatment.

Craniopharyngiomas represent approximately 3% of all intracranial tumors. Their incidence is bimodal, with a major early peak between 5 and 10 years of age, and a smaller peak between 50 and 60 years of age. A slight male preponderance has generally been noted.

Most craniopharyngiomas assume a primary suprasellar location. This is a strategic anatomic position from which a growing mass can compress the optic apparatus, involve the pituitary gland and stalk, extend into the ventricular system, and permeate CSF spaces to gain access to the middle and posterior cranial fossae. About 25% of craniopharyngiomas originate within the sella, producing sellar enlargement in a fashion similar to that produced by pituitary adenomas. Most craniopharyngiomas are cystic, containing a viscid admixture of shimmering cholesterol crystals and calcific desquamated debris, which has classically been described as "machinery oil" in appearance and consistency. These tumors often invoke an intense glial reaction, so they are surrounded by a layer of gliotic tissue, and are often quite adherent to major blood vessels.

Based on their location and gross pathology, craniopharyngiomas produce a characteristic constellation of symptoms and signs. In all age groups, clinical symptoms can be categorized as endocrine dysfunction, visual complaints, cognitive changes, or symptoms related to elevation of ICP. Endocrine symptoms are common in children, often causing growth failure and, less often, diabetes insipidus and primary amenorrhea. Adults usually present with some degree of hypopituitarism. Visual complaints referable to chiasmatic or optic nerve compression occur in patients of all ages, although children are more tolerant of, and more difficult to test for, visual field deficits. Cognitive symptoms in the form of memory loss, dementia, and psychiatric symptoms are seen primarily in adults. Symptoms referable to elevations in ICP are not uncommon, and usually are the result of obstructive hydrocephalus. With CT or MRI, craniopharyngiomas appear as partially calcified suprasellar or intrasellar masses with both solid and cystic components. Additional tests should be performed to document visual performance and endocrine status.

The optimal management of craniopharyngiomas is the subject of considerable debate. Much of the controversy emanates from two opposing philosophies concerning the resectability of the tumor. On the conservative side, craniopharyngiomas are considered too intimately related to vital neurovascular structures that radical excision can be achieved only at the unacceptable expense of irreparable neural and endocrine injury. A safer subtotal resection is therefore advocated, with the adjuvant use of some form of radiotherapy.[33] On the other extreme are those who view craniopharyngiomas as completely excisable lesions, believing that radical and complete excision can be safely undertaken, particularly with the benefit of contemporary surgical technology.[34] They also emphasize that most partially resected tumors will recur within 3 years, and that radical removal is the only means to achieve long-term cure. Perhaps the most pragmatic approach to these difficult tumors is one in which each case is individually appraised as to operative risk and potential for surgical cure. Radical resection is always desirable, provided it can be achieved with a minimum of operative risk. Alternatively, if the tumor is tenaciously attached to the hypothalamus and other perichiasmatic structures and the potential for operative injury is high, a less aggressive, though incomplete, resection is always preferable. Regardless of the extent of resection, all patients should have postoperative endocrine evaluations, and hormonal replacement therapy as needed.

For completely resected lesions, no adjuvant therapy is required. The outlook for these patients is favorable, although late recurrence occurs in up to 25% of patients, despite "total" resection.[33] For incompletely resected tumors, symptomatic recurrence is virtually guaranteed, so radiation therapy is required to forestall recurrence. The combination of partial resection and conventional radiation therapy has been of proven benefit in many series. In one recent series, "radical subtotal resection" followed by radiation therapy resulted in remission (clinical improvement, stable neurologic status, and reduction in tumor size) in 91% of patients after a mean follow-up of 4 years.[35] Another retrospective study suggested that partial resection followed by radiation supports a 10-year survival of 78%.[36] When recurrence does manifest, repeat surgery is frequently required.

Although the complications of radiation therapy have been outlined above, it is important to emphasize that the developing brain is particularly vulnerable to the effects of radiation. To circumvent these deleterious effects, there is increasing interest in intracavitary radiation and stereotaxic radiosurgical techniques for craniopharyngiomas, especially those with recurring cystic components. Instillation of intracavitary phosphorus 32 or yttrium 90 in colloidal suspension has proven effective in selected cases of craniopharyngioma. Radiosurgery has also caused involution of small recurrent cystic craniopharyngiomas, and will likely become an increasingly popular option for recurrent tumors refractory to surgical therapy.[33]

Medulloblastomas

When originally described more than 65 years ago, medulloblastomas were uniformly fatal tumors, notorious for prompt, aggressive, and lethal recurrence despite the best of surgical efforts.[6,7,9] Evolution of therapeutic strategies during the past three decades has dramatically improved the outlook for patients with medulloblastoma, securing these tumors the most impressive survival change of any pediatric brain tumor.

Medulloblastoma is the most common malignant primary CNS tumor of childhood, accounting for 20% of primary brain tumors in the pediatric population. It is not exclusively a childhood tumor, as 20% of cases occur during late adolescence or early adulthood. This is reflected in its bimodal incidence, showing a major early peak between 5 and 8 years of age, and a smaller peak between 20 and 30 years. Most series suggest that males are afflicted almost twice as frequently as females.

Medulloblastomas are thought to arise from primitive neuroepithelial cells of the external granular layer of the cerebellum. Normally, these embryonal cells involute and disappear by 18 months of age. Their abnormal persistence in the form of embryonal cell "rests" is the presumed basis for the development of these primitive tumors. Medulloblastomas are highly cellular tumors, composed of sheets of small round anaplastic cells with pleomorphic nuclei and numerous mitotic figures. This histologic picture is not unique to medulloblastomas, however, because a number of embryonal tumors (neuroblastoma, retinoblastoma, pineoblastoma) situated elsewhere are indistinguishable histologically. Consequently, this group of primitive tumors, unified by histologic features but diverse in location, is collectively referred to as primitive neuroectodermal tumors (PNET). Medulloblastoma is the most common form of PNET.

Anatomically, most medulloblastomas arise from the inferior medullary velum, a midline structure that contributes to the roof of the fourth ventricle. Initially, these tumors fill and expand the fourth ventricle, frequently infiltrating the walls and floor. Permeating along CSF pathways, they ascend superiorly into the cerebral aqueduct, descend interiorly to the cisterna magna, and extend laterally via the foramina of Luschka into the cerebellopontine angle. By this point, CSF circulation has generally been blocked, with obstructive hydrocephalus as the result.

An important biological feature of medulloblastomas is their propensity for metastatic dissemination through CSF pathways. More than half of cases studied at autopsy will disclose intraneural metastatic deposits, and 10% to 30% of patients will have occult or symptomatic CSF dissemination at the time of diagnosis. Most of these deposits will be spinal "drop mets"; however, rostral dissemination into the supratentorial compartment can also occur. Extraneural deposits occur in 5% of patients, mostly to bone and less often to lymph nodes and liver. Ventriculoperitoneal shunting has been implicated in facilitating systemic dissemination.

Medulloblastomas present with progressive features of an expanding posterior fossa mass. Symptoms relating to hydrocephalus and elevated ICP frequently predominate initially, followed eventually by more specific posterior fossa symptoms (ataxia, nystagmus, and rarely cranial nerve palsies). Herniation and impaction of the cerebellar tonsils can cause neck stiffness and head tilt. With CT scanning, most medulloblastomas appear as large contrast-enhancing posterior fossa masses associated with moderate peritumoral edema. Hydrocephalus of some degree is usually present.

The treatment protocol for medulloblastomas begins with surgical resection, followed by postoperative staging and irradiation of the the entire neuroaxis.[7] Gross total resection should be attempted, and can be achieved in about 50% of cases. In the remainder, tumor invasion into the brain stem precludes complete removal. Insofar as tumor removal alone frequently restores CSF circulation, shunting can generally be avoided. Postoperative staging is required to determine the extent of occult spinal disease. Usually 2 weeks following surgery, a myelogram and CSF cytologic studies are performed. Radiation therapy is essential for every patient: 54 Gy to the posterior fossa and tumor bed, 35 Gy to the remaining brain, 24 Gy to the spinal axis, and a local boost to any spinal deposit. Radiation is avoided in children younger than 2 years, in whom chemotherapy is substituted as a temporizing measure.

The prognosis for medulloblastoma is influenced by a number of factors, which distinguish patients as being either a "good" or "poor" risk.[7] Favorable prognostic factors include age >2 years, undisseminated local disease, and >75% tumor resection. In comparison, the poor-risk group has the following prognostic features: age <2 years, leptomeningeal disease, metastatic disease, and <75% tumor resection. In good-risk patients, the 5-year disease-free survival rate exceeds 60% and 70% in most recent series. For poor-risk patients, the 5-year disease-free survival rate is approximately 45%. Chemotherapy for medulloblastoma, until recently, has generally been considered a measure of last resort, being used primarily for recurrent tumors or salvage cases. It now appears that the "up front" addition of multiagent chemotherapy (CCNU, cisplatin, vincristine) can very substantially increase disease-free intervals, particularly in "poor risk" patients. This chemotherapeutic protocol, when given to "poor risk" patients, increased the 5-year disease-free survival to 71% with the result that poor-risk patients treated with chemotherapy (after surgery and irradiation) had a better outcome than good-risk patients treated with surgery and irradiation alone.[7] Medulloblastomas are clearly responsive to some chemotherapeutic agents, and it is likely that chemotherapy will assume an increasingly important role in some, and possibly all, medulloblastomas.

Epidermoid and Dermoid Tumors "Cysts"

Imperfect embryogenesis of the CNS, particularly at the critical time of neural tube closure (third to fifth week of gestation), can result in the formation of a number of rare but interesting tumors. Known as inclusion tumors, these entities arise from misplaced tissue. Depending on the germinal composition of the latter, tumors may be composed of one germ layer (epidermoids, dermoids, lipomas), two germ layers (teratoids), or all three germ layers (teratomas).

Dermoid and epidermoid tumors, which arise from ectopic epithelial tissue, together account for approximately 2% of intracranial tumors. Epidermoid tumors are composed of desquamated epidermal cellular debris, keratin, and cholesterol, and are generally confined within a soft, irregular, stratified squamous epithelial capsule. Despite their origin during early gestation, epidermoid tumors generally do not become symptomatic until the third or fourth decade of life. They grow by combination of progressive desquamation and accumulation of normally growing epidermal cells. They have a predilection for basal regions of the brain, and tend to enlarge along CSF pathways, insinuating themselves among cranial nerve and vascular structures. Common locations include the cerebellopontine angle, suprasellar region, fourth ventricular region, and inside the diploe of the skull. Epidermoid tumors can cause symptoms by local mass effect or recurrent bouts of aseptic meningitis. The latter are due to leakage of irritative cyst contents (cholesterol, fatty acids, and other debris) into the CSF.

Despite similarities in embryologic origin, dermoid tumors differ from epidermoids on the basis of histology, location, and an earlier age of clinical presentation. Occurring with one tenth the frequency of epidermoids, dermoids share the same stratified squamous epithelial composition; however, it is admixed with an additional underlying array of mature dermal elements: hair, hair follicles, sweat glands, and sebaceous glands. Dermoids usually have a midline position with most occurring in the posterior fossa (midline cerebellar) or suprasellar region. Some dermoids, particularly those of the cerebellum, may be associated with a dermal sinus tract extending to the skin surface. If this tract is patent, communication with the skin surface can give rise to repeated episodes of bacterial meningitis.

Because both dermoid and epidermoid tumors are benign, complete surgical excision of the tumor capsule and contents is curative. Unfortunately, these tumors often adhere so tenaciously to surrounding neural and vascular structures that complete removal is not always possible. Despite residual tumor remnants, most patients are cured and symptomatic recurrence is infrequent.

Pineal Region Tumors

Tumors of the pineal region are rare (1% of all intracranial tumors).[37-39] In the pediatric population, they constitute 5% to 8% of intracranial tumors. Males are much more commonly affected than females.

Pathologically, pineal region tumors can be divided into those arising from germ cells; from pineal parenchymal cells; and from supporting structures (meningiomas, gliomas, cavernous angiomas, arachnoid cysts). Only germ cell and pineal parenchymal tumors are discussed here, for their occurrence is specific to the pineal region.

Germ Cell Tumors

Germ cell tumors account for >50% of all pineal region tumors. As implied in their name, these tumors have an embryologic basis, either the result of germinal malmigration and/or the persistence of embryonic cell "rests" located in the pineal region. There are five distinct, but embryologically interrelated germ cell entities, each a neoplastic counterpart of a sequential stage in normal embryogenesis. In order of increasing aggressiveness, these entities include germinoma, teratoma, embryonal carcinoma, endodermal sinus tumor, and choriocarcinoma.

More than 60% of germ cell tumors are germinomas. These are identical to seminomas and dysgerminomas arising in the testicle and ovary, respectively. Intracranial germinomas can be regarded as low- or intermediate-grade tumors and often are only superficially invasive of brain parenchyma. Metastatic dissemination is uncommon, occurring within the spinal axis and systemically in up to 10% and 3% of cases, respectively. Their most notable biologic feature, however, is their exquisite radiosensitivity. In addition to their pineal location, germinomas can involve the hypothalamus and anterior third ventricle, where they have been referred to as "ectopic pinealomas" or suprasellar germinomas.

Except for the mature form of teratoma, the remaining germ cell tumors are aggressive, highly malignant, and generally incurable. Teratomas can be either mature or immature. The former is a derivative of fully differentiated tissues, and is generally slow-growing and oncologically benign. The immature teratoma is derived from primitive, undifferentiated embryonal tissues, and is aggressive, rapid-growing, and carries a poor prognosis.

Because of their rarity, uniformly grave prognosis, and similarities in management, the remaining nongermatomatous germ cell tumors are considered together. Embryonal carcinoma is one of the most primitive neoplasms known, arising from pluripotential epithelial cells of the embryo proper. Endodermal sinus tumors arise from germ cells normally destined for extraembryonic differentiation into yolk sac tissues. Pineal choriocarcinomas are similar to the better known uterine choriocarcinomas, which occur in the context of gestational trophoblastic disease. These are all highly malignant tumors that, in approximately 25% of cases, disseminate throughout the craniospinal axis. Systemic spread occurs in <5% of cases. The combination of surgery and radiation therapy rarely increases median survival beyond 1 year.

Pineal Parenchymal Tumors

These tumors exist in two forms: the better differentiated, less aggressive pineocytoma and the poorly differentiated, highly malignant pineoblastoma. The former takes its origin from pinealocytes (the primary parenchymal cell of the pineal gland) and generally occurs in late adolescence or adulthood. The latter is of primitive neuroectodermal origin, highly infiltrative, generally found in younger patients, and has both morphologic and biologic similarity to cerebellar medulloblastomas. Both tumors, particularly the pineoblastoma, have a tendency for craniospinal dissemination.

Tumors arising in the pineal region produce a characteristic clinical picture. The proximity of the pineal gland to the ventricular system (sylvian aqueduct and third ventricle) makes obstructive hydrocephalus a predictable consequence of growing tumors in this location. Gait ataxia, either on the basis of hydrocephalus or cerebellar compression, may also be present. Compression of the posterior midbrain results in a number of distinctive ocular abnormalities: Parinaud's syndrome (paralysis of upward gaze, light-near pupillary dissociation, and convergence nystagmus) and the sylvian aqueduct syndrome (paralysis of downward and horizontal gaze superimposed on Parinaud's syndrome). Endocrine symptoms are present in up to 10% of children, especially in germinomas, in which hypothalamic invasion can cause diabetes insipidus, hypopituitarism, and rarely precocious puberty.

MRI can provide a detailed anatomic diagnosis, revealing the nature of the mass and the degree of associated hydrocephalus. Although some pineal region tumors have distinguishing radiologic features, it is often impossible to make a definitive diagnosis of a particular tumor type.

Acknowledging the limitations of radiologic imaging studies to reliably predict tumor histology, there has been increasing interest in biochemical tumor markers as more accurate predictors of tumor type. AFP, β-hCG, and PLAP, as measured in both the serum and CSF, are most commonly used in this regard. Elevations of AFP suggest an endodermal sinus tumor, or a mixed germ cell tumor containing endodermal sinus elements. Elevations of β-hCG suggest a choriocarcinoma or a mixed germ cell tumor containing choriocarcinomatous elements. When neither AFP nor β-hCG is elevated, a diagnosis of pure germinoma, pineal parenchymal tumor, or pure teratoma is suggested. However, some germinomas and teratomas may show variable elevations of β-hCG and AFP, respectively. Very high levels of PLAP suggest a diagnosis of germinoma; however, moderate elevations are compatible with any of the germ cell entities. Immunoreactive S-antigen is a relatively new marker liberated by cells with retinal photoreceptor differentiation and is under investigation as a potential marker for pineal parenchymal tumors. Despite their theoretical appeal, these tumor markers lack sufficient sensitivity and specificity to reliably predict tumor histology, or routinely differentiate malignant lesions from less aggressive ones. When elevated, these markers are useful for gauging responses to therapy and early detection of recurrences.

Opinion remains divided as to the ideal management of pineal region tumors. The principal points of controversy concern the necessity of obtaining a tissue diagnosis prior to instituting therapy, the extent to which surgical resection provides a survival advantage, and the benefit of prophylactic spinal irradiation in forestalling symptomatic metastatic dissemination within the spinal axis.[39] After the exclusion of truly benign and surgically excisable lesions (dermoids, meningiomas, vascular lesions) on the basis of imaging studies, some physicians favor an initial empiric approach and initiate therapy without a tissue diagnosis.[37] Hydrocephalus, if present, is treated by shunting, and the tumor is treated with a trial of radiation therapy. Subsequent reduction in tumor size, on the basis of imaging studies, is taken as evidence of a radiosensitive tumor (germinoma, occasionally pineocytoma) and validates radiation therapy alone as adequate initial treatment. If, however, the tumor fails to regress with radiation, surgical excision is undertaken. Most radioresistant lesions are malignant nongermatomatous germ cell tumors or pineoblastomas, with an expected survival of only 1 to 2 years. The results of this conservative approach are impressive, as responsive tumors (presumably germinomas only) have a 5-year survival rate of 70% and a mean survival period exceeding 17 years.[37]

At the other end of the spectrum, there is an increasing number of physicians who advocate a more aggressive initial approach, feeling that optimal therapy is predicated on a precise tissue diagnosis, surgical reduction of tumor burden, and the adjuvant, not primary, use of radiation therapy.[38,39] They emphasize that contemporary neurosurgical techniques permit safe access and gross total removal of many (if not the majority of) pineal region tumors. Furthermore, a definitive tissue diagnosis and reduction in tumor bulk are of paramount importance to the rational use of chemotherapy, a modality that has yet to be consistently applied to pineal region tumors. In the surgical series of Bruce and Stein,[38] the results of operative treatment and radiotherapy appear comparable, but not superior to those achieved with shunting and radiotherapy. The 2-year survival of germinomas and pineal cell tumors was 83% and 75%, respectively. Of the nongerminomatous germ cell tumors, the mean survival at 1 year was only 33%. Although controversial, irradiation of the spinal axis is usually reserved for tumors with demonstrated seeding, as evidenced by positive CSF cytology or myelography.

The effectiveness of chemotherapy for malignant germ cell tumors of the testes has rejuvenated interest in its application in nongerminomatous germ cell tumors of the pineal region, which, despite surgical resection and radiotherapy, have a uniformly bad prognosis. Because the blood-brain barrier does not extend to the pineal gland, chemotherapeutic access should theoretically be less of an obstacle than with other intracranial tumors. Platinum-based regimens, either alone or with vinblastine and bleomycin, have shown some early benefit.

Chordomas

Chordomas[40-42] are uncommon tumors of bone, presumed to arise as neoplastic derivatives of embryonal notochord remnants. Accordingly, they can arise at any site along the axial skeleton, although the preferred locations are the clivus (35%), sacrum (50%), and nonsacral spine (15%). At all sites, men are affected twice as frequently as women, and curiously, despite their presumed embryologic origins, chordomas only rarely affect individuals younger than 20 years. Although chordomas are considered histologically benign, this aspect of their biology has been overemphasized, for their locally destructive nature, inexorably progressive course, and variable metastatic potential legitimize them as truly malignant neoplasms. Spinal chordomas are considered in Part II, as the following discussion pertains to those arising intracranially.

Cranial chordomas account for <1% of intracranial neoplasms. They typically involve an extensive area of the skull base, and virtually always are related in some way to the clivus. Tumors arising at the most rostral extreme of the clivus (basisphenoidal chordomas) can present as sellar or parasellar masses with associated endocrine disturbances and chiasmal compression. Those arising in the middle or inferior regions of the clivus typically involve multiple cranial nerves and compress brain stem structures. In up to a third of cases, clival chordomas grow in a ventral or extracranial direction to involve the nasopharynx and paranasal sinuses. Regardless of location, all chordomas are locally invasive, beginning first with expansile bony destruction at the site of origin, followed by infiltration and transgression of the dura, with eventual widespread intracranial extension and encasement of vital cranial nerve and brain stem structures. Metastatic dissemination is usually a very late occurrence and is seen in 10% to 20% of cases. Blood-borne deposits have been identified in the liver, lungs, heart, peritoneum, lymph nodes, and bone.

The radiographic appearance of chordoma, as determined by CT and MRI scans, is fairly characteristic, consisting of a destructive process of the skull base in association with a coarsely calcified soft-tissue mass.

The combination of surgery and irradiation is standard therapy for chordomas. However, both have significant limitations, as evidenced by the recurrence of local disease in most treated patients. The intimate relationship between the tumor and critical neural structures, compounded by problems of surgical accessibility, has rendered complete and curative resections difficult if not impossible. The problem of accessibility has, to some extent, been circumvented with the development of elaborate skull base surgical techniques. However, the results of such radical procedures are still under evaluation.[38] Radiation therapy appears to offer some measure of temporary tumor control, but because tumoricidal doses generally exceed levels of CNS tolerance, tumor recurrence has proven to be inevitable. Attempts at increasing local irradiation with brachytherapy and radiosurgery are currently being evaluated.

The mean survival of patients with chordomas ranged from 4.2 to 5.2 years. The average time to first recurrence is approximately 3 years.[42] A variant of chordoma that contains conspicuous foci of cartilaginous material intertwined between tumor cells is known as the chondroid chordoma. This variant is seen in approximately one third of clival chordomas and although its clinical presentation is indistinguishable from the standard chordoma, the prognosis is much more favorable. The mean survival of patients with chondroid chordomas is almost 16 years.[42]

Part II: Primary Intraspinal Tumors

Primary tumors involving the spinal cord occur with one sixth the frequency of primary brain neoplasms. Although virtually every histologic type of primary intraspinal tumor also has an intracranial counterpart, the balance between malignant and benign tumors is much more favorable in the spinal compartment, where complete surgical excision is both possible and curative for the majority of primary neoplasms. In contrast to the benignity of many primary intraspinal neoplasms, the spinal canal is host to a variety of metastatic tumors. Metastatic dissemination to the spine can be expected in up to 10% of cancer patients, thus accounting for the fact that metastatic lesions represent more than half of all intraspinal tumors. Because the diagnosis, management, and goals of therapy differ for metastatic lesions, they will be discussed separately in Part III.

Primary intraspinal tumors approach an annual incidence of 2 per 100,000 population, and occur more frequently in adults than in children. Aside from the genetic predisposition imposed by NF1 (spinal neurofibromas); NF2 (spinal neurinomas; rarely, spinal cord astrocytomas and meningiomas); and von Hippel-Lindau syndrome (hemangioblastomas), the cause of most primary intraspinal tumors is unknown. Except for the striking and unexplained female predisposition for spinal meningiomas, the remaining primary intraspinal tumors affect males and females with roughly equal frequency.

It is both classical and convenient to categorize intraspinal tumors into three broad groups, based on their anatomic location with respect to the spinal cord proper and the overlying dural coverings. Tumors are either intramedullary (arising within the spinal cord substance); extramedullary-intradural (outside the spinal cord, but within the dura); and extradural (outside both spinal cord and dura). These three locations, and the tumor types commonly found in each, are depicted in Fig 24-3.[43]

Intramedullary Tumors

Intramedullary tumors[44-46] are the least common form of intraspinal tumor in adults, but the favored type in children. Overall, these tumors account for 5% to 10% of intraspinal tumors. Astrocytomas and ependymomas are the dominant tumor types, occurring with roughly equal frequency overall and affecting a population from infancy to middle age. Proportionately, astrocytomas are more common than ependymomas in children; the reverse is true in adults. Less common intramedullary tumors include hemangioblastomas, epidermoid and dermoid tumors, and teratomas.

Astrocytomas can occur anywhere along the longitudinal extent of the spinal cord, with the thoracic and cervical regions being most commonly affected. Most spinal cord astrocytomas have a longitudinal span of several cord segments, but on occasion, notably in children, they can span the full length of the cord. All spinal astrocytomas are infiltrative lesions, but unlike their cerebral counterparts, the vast majority are low grade, slow growing, and comparable to grades I and II tumors of the brain. They are frequently associated with a fluid-filled cyst or syrinx at their rostral or caudal end. Spinal cord astrocytomas are always infiltrative lesions with indistinct margins and a progressive nature. Accordingly, complete and curative resection is generally not possible in the majority of adult astrocytomas.[44] In the pediatric population, the constitution of spinal cord astrocytomas may be different, as a number of series have suggested that complete excision is technically possible, and associated with an impressive survival advantage.[45,46] Approximately 15% of spinal cord astrocytomas are malignant, have poorly differentiated histologic features, and are associated with metastatic seeding throughout the neuroaxis. In this circumstance, increasing histologic grade is accompanied by a precipitous decline in survival.

Ependymomas of the spinal cord are generally well-differentiated, slow-growing lesions with a notable predilection for the conus medullaris and filum terminale, although they occur at all levels of the spinal cord. These tumors tend to be more discrete, better encapsulated, more often cystic, and

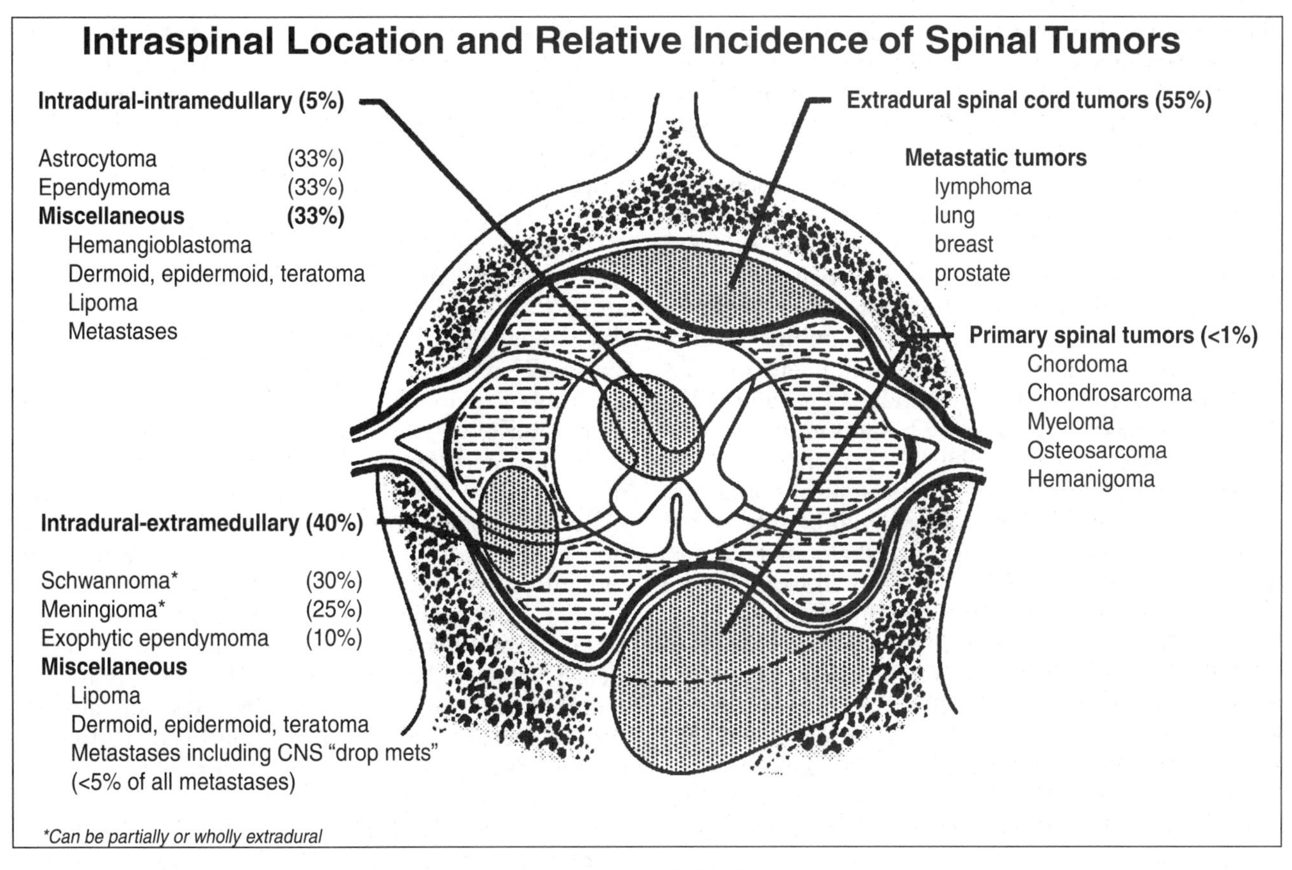

Fig 24-3. Primary and metastatic tumors of the spine and spinal cord. Modified from Poirier et al.[43]

considerably less infiltrative than astrocytomas. These gross morphologic features, coupled with their almost uniform low-grade behavior, facilitate their complete and curative excision in many cases.

Intraspinal hemangiomas, whether sporadic or associated with von Hippel-Lindau syndrome, account for only 1% to 3% of all primary spinal cord tumors. Approximately 25% of spinal hemangioblastoma patients will have evidence of von Hippel-Lindau syndrome. These tumors are most often intramedullary, although occasionally they may take origin from a dorsal nerve root and assume a primarily extramedullary location. The thoracic cord is most commonly involved, followed in frequency by the cervical and lumbar segments. Like their posterior fossa counterparts, spinal hemangioblastomas are highly vascular, consisting of the same serpiginous collection of blood vessels. More than half of these tumors have an associated syrinx, analogous to the cyst of cerebellar hemangioblastomas. As hemangioblastomas are discrete and noninfiltrative, complete excision is often possible.

The remaining intramedullary tumors consist of epidermoid and dermoid tumors, teratomas, lipomas, and neuroenteric cysts. These are all very rare, and can occur in both the intramedullary or extramedullary compartment. As these are all developmental in origin, they have minimal oncologic potential. Both epidermoid and dermoid tumors contain irritative debris which, when leaked into the CSF, can invoke a chemical meningitis. With repeated episodes, a dense chronic arachnoiditis can develop, which can be the source of very significant chronic pain. Finally, dermoid tumors may be associated with a dermal sinus tract, which, if patent, can give rise to repeated episodes of bacterial meningitis. Because these tumors are well encapsulated as a rule, surgical resection is generally followed by long-term cure.

Extramedullary-Intradural Tumors

The most common class of primary intraspinal tumors in the adult, extramedullary-intradural tumors account for approximately 45% of all spinal tumors. These are extra-axial in position and, in contrast to intramedullary tumors, impose their clinical effects by compression rather than invasion of the spinal cord. Schwannomas and meningiomas are the dominant lesions in this class. Other tumors in the extramedullary-intradural compartment are uncommon and include occasional extramedullary hemangioblastomas; "drop metastases" from malignant brain tumors (medulloblastomas, ependymomas); and, rarely, the same developmental entities encountered in the intramedullary compartment (discussed above).

Schwannomas, synonymous with neurilemomas and neurinomas, and similar to neurofibromas, are soft globular masses typically arising from the sensory or dorsal nerve root at any segmental level. They are fairly equally distributed along the entire length of the spinal canal, from the foramen magnum to the cauda equina. Usually they remain entirely confined to the spinal canal, although occasionally they may straddle the intervertebral foramen, extending into paraspinal structures in a so-called dumbbell configuration. In neurofibromatosis, simultaneous involvement of multiple segmental levels is characteristic. Schwannomas are uniformly benign and complete curative resection is the rule.

Only slightly less common than schwannomas are meningiomas. Like their intracranial counterparts, spinal meningiomas are dural-based globular lesions. They occur 10 times more frequently in women than men, and are typically diagnosed during middle age. The majority are located in the thoracic segments of the spine; the cervical region and the foramen magnum are other common sites. Spinal meningiomas are invariably benign, usually very slow-growing, and have generally been present for several years before symptoms arise. Although complete removal is often technically more difficult than with schwannomas, it can be achieved in the vast majority of spinal meningiomas.

Extradural Tumors and Spinal Chordomas

The extradural spinal compartment is rarely the site for primary tumors.[47] Aside from the occasional meningioma or schwannoma that may be wholly extradural, or the rare intrinsic vertebral body tumor (chordoma, chondrosarcoma, or osteosarcoma), tumors of the extradural space are usually due to metastasis. Of these primary tumors, spinal chordomas will be discussed here, with the other entities being discussed elsewhere in this chapter.

Like their cranial counterparts, spinal chordomas are rare, slow-growing, and locally invasive neoplasms presumably derived from notochordal remnants. Although they have been described in all age groups, most are detected between the fifth and seventh decades (median age, 51 years). As mentioned, chordomas arise predominantly at the extremes of the axial skeleton. Not only are spinal chordomas more common than cranial chordomas, they also are much more prone to metastatic dissemination. Up to 40% of spinal chordomas will disseminate hematogenously, with the lung, bone, liver, and soft tissue sites being most common recipient locations.[47]

Although many of the diagnostic and therapeutic principles in the management of chordomas are common to other intraspinal tumors, there are some special considerations. Given that chordomas arise from the vertebral bodies and tend to involve the spinal cord and nerve roots secondarily, they often reach considerable size before causing neurologic symptoms. Accordingly, they often present initially with site-specific visceral symptoms referable to compression of extraneural structures. Chordomas of the sacrum typically present with local symptoms of rectal dysfunction (change in bowel habit, tenesmus, rectal bleeding). Digital examination of the rectum almost always reveals a palpable presacral mass. Occasionally, a sacral chordoma will present with an externally palpable sacral deformity. Chordomas of the lumbar region may have symptoms of a retroperitoneal mass, whereas those involving cervical vertebrae may present with dysphagia and other symptoms of a retropharyngeal mass. All chordomas can produce neurologic symptoms. Depending on the location of the chordoma, such symptoms include pain, radiculopathy, and, for cervical, thoracic, and upper lumbar lesions, spinal cord compression (see below).

The locally invasive nature of these lesions is clearly visualized on imaging studies. On plain films, sacral lesions are characterized by expansile destruction of sacral segments in association with the soft tissue shadow of a large presacral mass. Subtle, peripheral calcification is often seen. Lesions involving true vertebrae arise as multifocal lytic changes involving a single vertebral body, often with a rim of peripheral sclerosis, and varying degrees of vertebral collapse. CT and MRI will reveal the full extent of the paraspinal mass, as well as the degree of spinal cord and nerve root involvement. Often a CT-guided needle biopsy provides a confirmatory histologic diagnosis.

Surgical resection followed by irradiation is standard therapy. Unlike many primary intradural tumors, which can be adequately excised via a laminectomy, spinal chordomas often require extensive surgical approaches. Authorities increasingly advocate radical and en bloc resections as the only means of achieving long-term tumor control. For sacral chordomas, combined anterior and posterior approaches are usually required. Depending on the tumor size and the particular perineal structures involved, resection may include all or part of the sacrum, associated sacral nerve roots, and, if necessary, the rectum. The implications of such radical resections are highly significant and must be kept in mind; the most extensive resection would be associated with loss of bladder control, loss of anorectal function and colostomy, loss of sexual function, and, depending on the number of sacral nerve roots resected, varying degrees of leg and gluteal weakness. For chordomas involving the true vertebrae, transthoracic or transabdominal approaches are often used. Under the best circumstances, radical resection of spinal chordomas followed by radiation therapy provides 5-year survival rates of 50%.[47]

Clinical Features of Intraspinal Tumors

Because the prognosis for recovery from spinal tumors depends heavily on the neurologic status at the time of diagnosis, prompt recognition of early symptoms is of paramount importance. Intraspinal tumors present with the combination of pain and disturbances of sensory, motor, and autonomic function, which are of such exquisite localizing value that the presence, segmental location, and intraspinal site of many tumors can be readily identified on the basis of a careful history and neurologic exam. Nevertheless, most patients have endured years of symptoms and misdiagnosis prior to definitive identification of the tumor.

Specific clinical features of a spinal cord tumor depend primarily on its longitudinal location (cervical, thoracic, lumbar, or cauda equina), but also on its intraspinal compartment (intramedullary or extramedullary). A brief overview of the cardinal symptoms follow.

Pain

Spontaneous pain is a common early feature for most tumors and typically is worse at night. Intramedullary tumors are typically associated with "central pain," characterized as a deep, poorly localized, burning pain in the spine region. Extramedullary tumors produce knifelike radicular pain, which radiates into an extremity, is intensified with coughing or straining, and is referable to nerve root compression. The radicular pain of thoracic neoplasms can sometimes mimic pain arising from gallbladder disease or other intrabdominal or intrathoracic processes.

Sensory Changes

Because intramedullary tumors usually originate in the vicinity of the central canal and grow centrifugally, crossing fibers of the spinothalamic tract conveying pain and temperature are compromised initially. This leads to the characteristic "suspended" or dissociated sensory disturbance, resulting in pain and temperature sensory loss, but preservation of proprioception and light touch. Because sensation to the sacral region is represented peripherally in the spinothalamic tract, sacral sensation is typically intact (sacral sparing). In contrast, extramedullary tumors usually produce sensory loss in the distribution of the involved nerve root(s), or a more diffuse sensory loss in the context of a partial or complete Brown-Séquard syndrome. Tumors involving the conus medullaris or cauda equina are classically associated with "saddle anesthesia," referring to diminished sensation in the perianal, perineal, and genital areas.

Motor Changes

Untreated, all intraspinal tumors will eventually impair motor function. Intramedullary tumors can involve the anterior horn cells, producing lower motor neuron changes (weakness, atrophy, hyporeflexia) at the level of the lesion. They can also involve the descending corticospinal tract and produce upper motor neuron changes (weakness, spasticity, hyperreflexia) at levels below the lesion. The motor changes of extramedullary lesions classically begin with segmental weakness at the lesion site, progressing to a hemicord syndrome (Brown-Séquard) and later a transverse cord syndrome. The weakness is of upper motor neuron type, and is generally preceded by spasticity, leg stiffness, and gait disturbance.

Autonomic Changes

All spinal tumors can produce autonomic dysfunction. Disturbances of bladder, bowel, and sexual function usually occur late, and are least likely to be reversed with treatment. Tumors involving the conus medullaris and cauda equina tend to cause autonomic symptoms sooner than those compressing the spinal cord proper. Rarely, a Horner's syndrome can be seen with intramedullary lesions involving the C8-T2 regions.

Other Symptoms

An unexplained feature of intramedullary cord tumors is hydrocephalus and elevations of ICP. Occurring in up to 10% of pediatric patients, these unusual findings have been attributed to the liberation of oncotically active proteins into the CSF by the tumor.[45] Additional common pediatric symptoms include torticollis with cervical tumors and scoliosis with thoracic lesions. Finally, spinal tumors can very rarely present with a sudden ictus related to acute intratumoral or subarachnoid hemorrhage.

Diagnosis

The history and neurologic examination generally provides a good indication of the level of spinal axis involvement. Enhanced MRI scanning will identify the tumor, its spinal level, and the occupied intraspinal compartment. Plain films of the spine, although useful in the evaluation of metastatic spinal tumors, have limited utility in the evaluation of primary neoplasms. The most common plain film abnormalities include enlarged foramina, bony erosion, spinal canal widening, scoliosis, and the occasionally occult dysraphic state, usually in association with developmental tumors. Lumbar puncture and CSF examination have been largely eliminated in the diagnosis and management of primary spinal tumors.

Treatment and Prognosis

Surgery is the initial and principal form of therapy for all primary intraspinal tumors. As the overwhelming majority are benign lesions, complete and curative resection is the surgical objective in most cases. Corticosteroids are used perioperatively, especially when considerable intramedullary dissection is anticipated. Except for the occasional extramedullary tumor, wholly situated anterior to the spinal cord, most primary tumors are approached through a posterior (laminectomy) route. In most centers, intraoperative electrophysiologic monitoring of the spinal cord is routinely used for all intraspinal tumors. Such monitoring provides a continuous functional assessment of spinal cord sensory tracts during tumor resection. By alerting the surgeon to spinal cord structures at risk of inadvertent operative injury, electrophysiologic monitoring increases, by some measure, the safety of the operative procedure. Intraoperative ultrasonography often can be valuable in locating intramedullary tumors and associated cysts, minimizing unnecessary exploration of the cord. Postoperatively, there may be a slight, transient increase in neurologic deficit for intramedullary tumors; however, gradual and occasionally dramatic improvement is the rule. Physiotherapy and rehabilitation are important components of postoperative care, and are useful in maximizing neurologic function and recovery.

Astrocytomas are the only primary intraspinal tumors for which the curability and value of radical surgical resection are disputed. Until recently, there was an emerging opinion that spinal cord astrocytomas, despite their infiltrative nature and often ill-defined margins, were amenable to complete and curative removal. The results of long-term follow-up of "completely removed" adult astrocytomas have not been compatible with this view, however, and the high frequency of treatment failure has reestablished these tumors as progressive and generally incurable. The current consensus is that extensive debulking of astrocytomas may prolong the disease-free interval, but attempts at curative removal are generally futile. In a recent series, almost 37% of low-grade adult astrocytomas treated with aggressive resection and radiation therapy were associated with fatal recurrence during a mean follow-up of 38 months. All patients with high-grade astrocytomas, despite the extent of resection, irradiation, or chemotherapy, died within 1 year. The effectiveness of radiation therapy for spinal cord astrocytomas of any grade is uncertain.[44]

Astrocytomas in childhood appear to behave more favorably, having a better correlation between the extent of tumor resection and disease-free survival, and accordingly there is a more compelling argument in favor of radical resection. Radical resection alone has a 5-year survival rate of 90%.[46] The Mayo Clinic experience suggests that radical resection and radiation therapy is associated with longer survival than lesser resections and irradiation: mean survivals of 173.5 months versus 66.6 months, respectively.[45] Again, the value of radiation therapy in the pediatric population is uncertain. Some use it routinely, while others are less convinced of its efficacy, resorting to it only after surgical resection of a recurrence.

Ependymomas, hemangioblastomas, and the developmental tumors are more often discrete masses and can usually be completely excised. Clinical deficits are usually improved or stabilized with tumor removal. When completely removed, the long-term outlook is excellent, with recurrence being unusual. Radiation therapy is not required in completely excised tumors, although its role in partially removed benign tumors is unclear. Many surgeons prefer to avoid irradiation and treat recurrences by repeat surgery.

Extramedullary tumors can be completely removed and cured in most cases. Preoperative deficits, depending on their severity and duration, improve rapidly during the first few postoperative months. Recurrence is unusual, although a realistic concern in partially resected lesions. Meningiomas, because of the greater technical demands to effect complete excision, are more likely to recur than schwannomas; however, the recurrence rate on long-term follow-up is <10%. The value of adjuvant radiation therapy for incompletely removed or recurrent extramedullary tumors is uncertain.

Part III: Tumors Metastatic to the CNS

Survival and quality of life with many forms of cancer have been favorably altered with contemporary therapy. This extended longevity has not been without consequence; for example, metastatic complications represent an escalating clinical problem. Metastases to the brain and spinal cord are among the more common and most serious complications of metastatic cancer. The former is a metastatic site in 20% of cancer patients, and the latter in 10%.[48,49] While most CNS metastases occur in the setting of advanced disease, they may also be the first sign of malignancy, or a prelude to relapse. Because all metastases to the CNS either threaten life or jeopardize quality of survival, prompt diagnosis and therapy is often critical.

Brain Metastases

Of the 20% of cancer patients expected to develop brain metastases, the majority will be symptomatic.[48,50] The most culpable primary tumors giving rise to intracranial deposits are bronchogenic carcinoma (especially small-cell carcinomas), breast cancer, renal cell carcinoma, melanoma, and gastrointestinal (GI) malignancies. In up to 10% of cases, brain metastases occur in the absence of a prior cancer history and are therefore the initial manifestation of an otherwise silent primary tumor.

Metastatic tumors gain access to the brain by hematogenous dissemination. Correspondingly, their distribution in the brain is roughly proportional to the blood supply of the specific brain area. The vascular territory of the middle cerebral artery is therefore favored, with most lesions located in the frontal or parietal lobes. Most cerebral metastases are relatively superficial and situated at the well-vascularized interface of the gray and white matter. About 20% of metastatic lesions occur in the posterior fossa, primarily in the cerebellum. In approximately half of all cases, multiple metastatic lesions are present.

Although the most common and clinically significant site for metastases is the brain parenchyma, the skull and pituitary gland are also relatively commonly affected. The skull is a predominant location for metastases emanating from prostate cancer, breast cancer, lymphoma, melanoma, and osteogenic sarcoma. Metastases to the pituitary gland are discussed in Chapter 25.

Clinical Features

Metastatic brain tumors present with the same clinical features common to any intracranial mass, but are distinguished by a much more rapid evolution of symptoms, often measurable in days to weeks. This accelerated clinical course is due to the tremendous accumulation of peritumoral brain swelling, which typically accompanies even the smallest of metastatic deposits. Progressive symptoms of elevated ICP, focal neurologic deficits, and seizures are the usual presenting features. Obstructive hydrocephalus may be an early consequence of cerebellar metastases and often is followed by abrupt clinical deterioration. Approximately 10% of all metastatic brain tumors have a sudden apoplectic presentation as the result of intratumoral hemorrhage. Spontaneous hemorrhage can occur with any metastatic neoplasm; however, melanoma, renal cell carcinoma, and choriocarcinoma have the greatest inherent hemorrhagic propensity.

Contrast-enhanced CT will identify the majority of brain metastases as either ring-enhancing or diffusely enhancing lesions, typically surrounded by a zone of edema that is out of proportion to the size of the lesion. Mass effect of varying degrees can be seen. Acute hemorrhage within the tumor may occasionally obscure the diagnosis of an underlying neoplasm. In general, MRI is more sensitive in identifying multiple lesions.

Multiple brain lesions occurring in the setting of a positive cancer history is virtually certain evidence of a metastatic process. However, solitary brain metastases can occasionally be a diagnostic problem, especially in the absence of a known cancer history. As a number of entities share similar radiologic profiles (primary brain tumors, brain abcesses, cerebral infarcts and hemorrhages), they must all be carefully considered in the differential diagnosis. A presumptive diagnosis of brain metastasis can often be corroborated by reviewing the chest x-ray, with 60% of patients having metastatic brain tumors also showing primary or metastatic disease in the chest. For most patients with a known cancer history, there is >90% certainty that a solitary contrast-enhancing brain lesion is a metastatic deposit. The one caveat to this association occurs in women with breast cancer. Because breast cancer patients have an unusually high incidence of benign (and potentially curable) meningiomas, solitary brain masses in these patients should never be presumed to be metastatic without histologic confirmation.[48]

Management

The median survival of untreated brain metastases is approximately 1 month, with the majority of patients dying as a direct result of the brain lesion. Therefore, some form of treatment is indicated in all patients, except possibly those in the terminal stages of advanced metastatic disease. Therapy for brain metastases includes corticosteroids, surgical excision in selected cases, and cranial irradiation in almost all cases.

Corticosteroids

Because peritumoral brain swelling contributes so heavily to both the clinical presentation and overall mass effect of these lesions, steroids often have a very dramatic clinical effect. It is not unusual for steroids to reverse hemiparesis or increase alertness in a somnolent patient, even after a few doses. Despite this initial responsiveness, steroids alone rarely extend median survival beyond 2 months.

Radiotherapy

Cranial irradiation in combination with steroid therapy provides a median survival of only 3 to 6 months. Because death in >50% of patients so treated is the result of systemic disease and not directly the result of brain lesions, this form of therapy is adequate palliation for many patients. Alternatively, a significant proportion of patients managed in this way will sustain a neurologic death as a direct result of the cerebral lesions. It is for this subgroup of patients that the combination of radiation therapy and steroids is inadequate. Furthermore, there are differences in radiosensitivity among the various metastatic tumors. Lymphomas and small-cell carcinomas of the lung are the most radiosensitive; other lung, breast, and GI malignancies are of intermediate sensitivity, while melanoma and renal cell carcinoma are relatively radioresistant. Finally, patients occasionally present in an acute neurologic crisis, with acutely unstable ICP elevations and impending brain herniation. Primary radiotherapy has no immediate role, as intensive therapy with steroids, mannitol, hyperventilation, and emergency surgery is frequently necessary to revive these patients. So while primary radiotherapy is adequate palliation for patients likely to succumb to systemic disease, its primary therapeutic value diminishes in patients not at immediate risk from their primary tumor, in circumstances of severe and symptomatic ICP elevations, and in those cases of radioresistant metastases. It is in these patient groups that surgical resection becomes a serious consideration.

Surgical Therapy

Surgical excision of brain metastases has historically been an area of controversy. However, recent reports increasingly suggest that surgical removal of solitary brain metastases has a favorable impact on survival. These impressions were recently confirmed by a small prospective randomized trial comparing surgical resection and radiotherapy versus radiotherapy alone.[50] A significant survival advantage accrued in the surgical group, in whom median survival was 40 weeks, compared with 15 weeks in those treated with radiation alone. Furthermore, the quality of life was better, and local recurrence was seen less often and after longer symptom-free intervals. Tumor removal often effected prompt amelioration of edema, obviating the need for long-term steroid therapy. Therefore, surgery should be considered in all patients with solitary brain metastases in whom systemic disease is controlled or limited to the primary site. Although 50% of brain metastases are solitary, half of these cases will not be surgical candidates because of tumor inaccessibility, extensive systemic metastases, or other medical problems. Therefore, a realistic surgical benefit can be expected in approximately 25% of patients with metastatic brain deposits.[48] Regardless of the completeness of resection, all patients receive postoperative radiotherapy. The independent prognostic factors favoring a better prognosis for brain metastases include younger age, higher Karnofsky performance, a solitary brain lesion, and minimal systemic disease.

Patients with multiple brain metastases are ordinarily not considered surgical candidates. Rarely, it may be reasonable to remove one of several brain metastases if it is highly symptomatic or likely to cause premature death.

Other Therapeutic Options

Despite the survival increments achieved with steroids, radiotherapy, and surgery, the overall prognosis for patients with brain metastases remains poor. As a result, alternative therapeutic options continue to be explored. Chemotherapy has shown modest benefit for brain metastases in patients with small-cell carcinoma, breast carcinoma, and melanoma. Minor successes have been noted with alternative forms of radiation delivery, such as stereotaxic radiosurgery and interstitial brachytherapy. Although chemotherapy, radiosurgery, and brachytherapy may eventually prove useful in selected patient groups, their current status is still investigational in patients with brain metastases.

Metastatic Tumors of the Spine and Spinal Cord in Adults

Metastatic involvement of the spine and spinal cord is a common and frequently devastating complication of disseminated cancer.[49] With a symptomatic occurrence in 10% of the cancer population, spinal metastases have steadily eclipsed all primary intraspinal tumors in frequency, and currently represent 55% of all spinal neoplasms. The principal consequence of spinal metastases is epidural spinal cord compression, which, if unrecognized, promptly leads to permanent paralysis and loss of bladder and bowel control. Therefore, metastatic spinal cord compression constitutes a genuine oncologic emergency in which immediate action can often restore, minimize, or prevent permanent neurologic injury.

The most common primary tumors that metastasize to the spine are carcinomas of the lung, breast, prostate, and kidney and lymphoma. In about 10% of cases, the primary tumor is never identified. There are three commonly accepted mechanisms by which metastatic tumors reach the spinal axis. The most common means of access is direct arterial dissemination from the primary site to the vertebral body. Spinal cord compression occurs secondarily by direct tumoral extension into the epidural space, and/or destruction of the vertebral body leading to cord compromise on the basis of spinal instability. The second means of spinal access is retrograde spread via the vertebral venous plexus (Batson's plexus). This is a low-pressure, valveless collection of veins that perforate abundantly into the epidural space and vertebral bodies. This is a particularly favored route for prostatic tumors. The least common metastatic route in adults is direct invasion from a paravertebral primary tumor to the epidural space via the intervertebral foramen. Lymphomas and several pediatric tumors follow this course.

The overwhelming majority of spinal metastases are in the epidural compartment (Fig 24-3),[43] although rarely the location is intramedullary (<5% of cases). Although the spinal cord exhibits surprising tolerance to primary intraspinal tumors because of their slow growth and intradural location, the spinal cord is much less tolerant to rapidly growing lesions in the extradural compartment. Once an established extradural metastasis begins to compress the spinal cord, functional disturbances rapidly ensue, which, without treatment, abruptly accelerate to an irreparable state of functional cord transection. Vascular congestion, edema, focal hemorrhage, and axonal disruption are typical pathologic findings with this degree of spinal cord compression.

The thoracic spine is the most frequent site of involvement (70% of cases), followed by the lumbosacral spine (20%) and the cervical spine (10%). A large proportion of metastases involve the vertebral body and compress the cord from an anterior direction. This topologic arrangement between cord and tumor has important implications with regard to surgical accessibility. Multiple noncontiguous sites of cord compression occur in up to 30% of cases, thus emphasizing the need for thorough clinical and radiologic (MRI) appraisal of the entire spinal axis.

Clinical Features

Back pain is the commonest, earliest, and most prominent symptom in patients with spinal cord metastases. Present in 95% of cases, back pain should be of particularly ominous concern in any patient with a known cancer history. *It is axiomatic that any cancer patient presenting with new-onset back pain be considered to have spinal metastases until proven otherwise.* Pain usually precedes neurologic signs by days, weeks, or months and can be local, radicular, or both. Local pain is related to stretching of the periosteum and is generally a constant, progressive dull ache which is characteristically worse at night or with recumbency. If the diagnosis is not suspected at this stage, pain will be followed by weakness, sensory loss, and sphincter disturbance, which in short order will progress relentlessly to dense paraplegia and permanent loss of sphincter control. The premium on early diagnosis cannot be overemphasized. Patients treated while still ambulatory are likely to remain so. In those in whom paraplegia and sphincteric loss is established, no form of therapy is likely to retrieve neurologic function.

Diagnosis

Patients suspected of spinal cord compression should have a careful neurologic examination. Not only is the latter critical to appropriate selection of radiologic studies, but the timing, nature, and outcome of therapy are all predicated on the patient's neurologic status.

In patients presenting only with pain, plain films of the spine are an inexpensive, readily available, and important first step. Positive findings will be present in up to 80% of patients with spinal metastases. The most common findings are pedicular erosion, vertebral collapse, pathologic fracture dislocation, and a soft tissue shadow suggestive of a paraspinal mass. If plain films are negative, a radioisotope bone scan is the next appropriate test, and metastases will be demonstrated in approximately 20% of patients with negative plain films. If either the plain films or radioisotope scan is positive, or if the patient has neurologic findings, MRI or CT/myelography must be undertaken. There is increasing preference for the former because of its noninvasive nature and the small risk of neurologic deterioration associated with the latter. Whichever study is used, it should encompass the entire spinal axis and clearly demonstrate the site of the compression, including its upper and lower extent, and presence or absence of multiple lesions. In patients with neurologic findings, and especially those with progressive neurologic deficits, these investigations must be performed emergently.

Treatment and Prognosis

Treatment of spinal metastases involves relief from pain, restoration of neurologic function, and preservation of spinal stability. Because cure is beyond expectation, therapy for spinal metastases is palliative. Nevertheless, relief from pain and restoration of mobility contribute immeasurably to the remaining life of the cancer patient and greatly lessen the burden of care. Treatment strategies are individualized and frequently call on the multidisciplinary expertise of the oncologist, radiation therapist, neurosurgeon, and orthopedic surgeon. Treatment options include radiation therapy, either with or without surgical decompression. High-dose steroids are used adjunctively, although their effectiveness in this setting has not been conclusively shown.

Radiation therapy is the initial treatment of choice for most spinal metastases. It is best suited for patients suffering from pain, but without rapidly progressive neurologic deficits or spinal instability. Depending on the radiosensitivity of the tumor, moderate degrees of pain relief can be anticipated. Even in patients with mild neurologic deficits, many radiotherapists advocate beginning with radiotherapy. In cases such as these, the surgeon should be already familiar with the patient in the event of ongoing deterioration.

Although absolute consensus is lacking, surgery is generally reserved for the following scenarios: (1) spinal cord compression in patients having already received maximal radiotherapy; (2) patients with a worsening neurologic deficit during radiotherapy; (3) patients with spinal cord compression on the basis of spinal instability; (4) patients with rapidly progressing neurologic deficits in whom irreparable neurologic injury will likely supervene before the benefits of radiation are realized; (5) patients in whom spinal cord compression occurs in the absence of a cancer history and a tissue diagnosis is required; and (6) patients with spinal cord compression due to tumors known to be radioresistant.

Until recently, most surgical efforts consisted of posterior decompression via laminectomy. Results have been poor, with neurologic improvement occurring in only 30% of patients. The failure of posterior approaches is understandable, as most metastases originate in the vertebral body and compress the cord from a ventral direction. Therefore, access to the tumor mass is limited and frequently impossible by a posterior route alone. Contemporary surgical strategies are much more flexible, as anterior lesions are now approached through anterior (transthoracic, transabdominal, retroperitoneal) approaches, and posteriorly situated lesions are approached through various posterior approaches. Furthermore, better understanding of spinal biomechanics and availability of reconstructive instrumentation for restoring spinal stability have permitted more radical and more effective decompressive procedures.

The most important determinant of outcome is the neurologic status of the patient. According to a recent review of patients treated with radiotherapy alone, 80% of ambulatory patients remained so after therapy and 30% of nonambulatory patients regained gait.[49] In various reports, pain and neurologic function improve in 57% to 97% of operated patients. In one report, 28% of patients were ambulatory preoperatively, and 80% after decompressive surgery. The median postoperative survival was 16 months.[49] Operative mortality approaches 10% in patients treated with radical resections and spinal reconstruction, and is therefore a major consideration given the frequently fragile condition of many cancer patients. Regardless of the therapeutic strategy used, early diagnosis and treatment are the basis for optimal results.

Metastatic Tumors of the Spine and Spinal Cord in Children

From the standpoints of culpable primary tumors, mechanisms of metastatic dissemination, degree of spinal column involvement, surgical strategies, and results of therapy, metastatic spinal tumors in the pediatric population differ considerably from those seen in the adults.[51] Spinal secondaries in the child most commonly arise from sarcomas (40%) and less often from neuroblastomas (27%), lymphomas (6%) and leukemias (6%).[51] Whereas spinal metastases in the adult most often occur in the setting of advanced malignancy, in one third of pediatric patients, spinal cord metastases are presenting features of malignancy. In adults, most metastatic tumors access the spinal compartment by a vascular route, whereas direct extension from an adjacent primary is the principal mode of spinal access in the pediatric population. Furthermore, most pediatric metastases grow through the intervertebral foramen, compress the spinal cord from a posterolateral direction, are not associated with extensive vertebral column destruction or instability. Thus, they generally can be removed through a simple laminectomy. The outcome of therapy (surgery, radiation, and occasionally chemotherapy) is more favorable in children: 96% of patients can expect improvement or stabilization of existing neurologic deficits.[51] In the same report, 60% of nonambulatory patients regained the ability to walk after treatment. For these reasons, an aggressive approach to metastatic spinal disease in the pediatric population is justified. However, the merits of early diagnosis and treatment are just as applicable to children as they are for adults.

Leptomeningeal Carcinomatosis (Carcinomatous Meningitis)

Leptomeningeal carcinomatosis is a term used to describe widespread, multifocal, and metastatic seeding of the meninges and CSF pathways of the CNS.[52] Although considerably less common than solid metastases to either the brain or spinal cord, neoplastic meningitis is still a major contributor to morbidity and mortality in cancer patients. Autopsy studies indicate that at least 8% of cancer patients have metastatic seeding of CSF pathways; however, the exact incidence of clinically apparent seeding is uncertain, but is known to differ among various tumor types. The most common primary tumors responsible for leptomeningeal carcinomatosis include carcinomas of the breast and lung (small cell), non-Hodgkin's lymphoma, melanomas, and adult acute leukemias. Much less commonly, primary intracranial tumors (medulloblastoma, pineal region tumors, ependymomas, glioblastomas) exhibit secondary meningeal involvement.

Systemic cancers gain meningeal access by a variety of routes. Hematogenous spread and direct extension from preexisting parenchymal lesions are thought to be the most common initiating events. Infiltration along spinal and cranial nerve sheaths also has been proposed. Once within the CSF, exfoliated tumor cells are propelled widely in the subarachnoid space by pulsatile CSF flow. Clumps of cells can aggregate and adhere at virtually any meningeal site and give rise to new metastatic deposits. The heaviest sites of infiltration include the basal cisterns and the cauda equina, presumably due to low CSF flow rate in the former and the effect of gravity on the latter. Tumors grow in a sheetlike fashion along the base of the brain and spinal cord, encasing cranial and spinal nerves and often invoking a local inflammatory response of the involved meninges.

The clinical features of leptomeningeal carcinomatosis reflect the diffuse involvement of the CNS: (1) hydrocephalus and elevated ICP due to obstruction of CSF pathways; (2) cranial and spinal nerve dysfunction due to tumor encasement; (3) focal signs of brain or spinal cord dysfunction, including seizures; and (4) signs of meningeal irritation. The most important and most common diagnostic clue is the multiplicity of signs and symptoms referable to a multifocal process. Accordingly, the majority of patients present with a combination of headache, neck stiffness, cranial nerve palsies, and spinal root or cord dysfunction. Mental status changes, ranging from confusion to encephalopathy, also are seen.

In virtually all patients with leptomeningeal carcinomatosis, CSF studies are abnormal. Malignant cells in the CSF can be detected in >90% of cases, although several lumbar punctures may be required to establish their presence. CSF pressure and protein content are usually elevated, and CSF glucose is often decreased (25% of cases). A variety of CSF biochemical markers have been identified in patients with neoplastic meningitis, but their utility is limited by poor specificity and sensitivity. These markers include carcinoembryonic antigen (CEA), beta-glucuronidase, lactate dehydrogenase (LDH), and beta-2-microglobulin. Although the diagnosis of this condition is confirmed by CSF examination, many patients, particularly those with focal findings suggestive of an intracranial mass, are investigated first with CT or MRI of the head. Cranial imaging is abnormal in 25% to 60% of cases, with the most common abnormalities being hydrocephalus and nodular enhancement of basal cisterns and ependymal surfaces of the ventricles. If spinal symptoms are present, myelography or spinal MRI is required to demonstrate lesions in spinal compartment.

Without treatment, most patients with leptomeningeal carcinomatosis experience progressive neurologic decline, leading to death within 4 to 6 weeks. Therefore, except for patients at imminent risk of demise from widespread systemic disease, some form of therapy is often beneficial for many patients. As a principle of therapy, neoplastic meningitis is a diffuse disorder; therefore, therapy must be equally diffuse and directed at the entire neuroaxis. Current treatment protocols consist of radiotherapy to symptomatic sites with concurrent intrathecal chemotherapy. Methotrexate, thiotepa, and cytosine arabinoside are equally effective and are the usual agents of choice. The most convenient method of delivery is intraventricular, through a surgically placed intraventricular fluid access device known as an Ommaya reservoir. In general, fixed neurologic deficits, such as dense cranial nerve palsies and paraplegia, do not resolve with therapy. Lesser deficits either stabilize or show some improvement. Median survival with such therapy is approximately 6 months, with most patients succumbing to systemic disease. Patients with breast cancer and lymphomas generally show the most gratifying benefit. Monoclonal antibodies conjugated with radionucleotides, delivered intrathecally and directed against various tumor cell antigens, have shown some preliminary promise as a potential future option for patients with leptomeningeal carcinomatosis.[13,52]

References

1. Boring CC, Squires TS, Tong T, Montgomery S. Cancer Statistics, 1994. *CA Cancer J Clin* 1994; 44:7-26.

2. Thapar K, Fukuyama K, Rutka J. Neurogenetics and the molecular biology of human brain tumors. In: Laws ER, Kaye A, eds. *Encyclopedia of Human Brain Tumors*. New York, NY: Churchill Livingstone (in press).

3. Ikizler Y, van Meyel DJ, Ramsay GL, et al. Gliomas in families. *Can J Neurol Sci.* 1992;19:492-497.

4. O'Neill BP, Illig JJ. Primary central nervous system lymphoma. *Mayo Clin Proc.* 1989;64:1005-1020.

5. Burger PC, Scheithauer BW, Vogel FS. *Surgical Pathology of the Nervous System and Its Coverings*. 3rd ed. New York, NY: Churchill Livingstone;1991.

6. Leibel SA, Sheline GE. Radiation therapy for neoplasms of the brain. *J Neurosurg.* 1987;66:1-22.

7. Packer RJ, Sutton LN, Goldwein JW, et al. Improved survival with the use of adjuvant chemotherapy in the treatment of medulloblastoma. *J Neurosurg.* 1991;74:433-440.

8. Chatel M, Lebrun C, Frenay M. Chemotherapy and immunotherapy in adult malignant gliomas. *Curr Opin Oncol.* 1993;5:464-473.

9. Black PM. Brain tumors. *N Engl J Med.* 1991;324:1555-1564.

10. Fine H, Dear K, Loeffler J, Canellos GP. Meta-analysis of radiotherapy with and without adjuvant chemotherapy for malignant gliomas in adults. *Proc Am Soc Clin Oncol.* 1991;10:125. Abstract.

11. Larson DA, Gutin PH, Leibel SA, Philips TL, Sneed PK, Wara WM. Stereotaxic irradiation of brain tumors. *Cancer.* 1990;65(3 suppl):792-799.

12. Packer RJ, Kramer ED, Ryan JA. Biologic and immune modulating agents in the treatment of childhood brain tumors. *Neurol Clin.* 1991;9:405-422.

13. Schuster JM, Bigner DM. Immunotherapy and monoclonal antibody therapies. *Curr Opin Oncol.* 1992;4(3):547-552.

14. Daumas-Duport C, Scheithauer B, O'Fallon J, Kelly P. Grading of astrocytomas: a simple and reproducible method. *Cancer.* 1988;62:2152-2165.

15. Guthrie BL, Laws ER. Supratentorial low-grade gliomas. *Neurosurg Clin N Am.* 1990;1(1):37-48.

16. Shaw EG, Daumas-Duport C, Scheithauer BW, et al. Radiation therapy in the management of low-grade supratentorial astrocytomas. *J Neurosurg.* 1989;70:853-861.

17. Wisoff JH. Management of optic pathway tumors of childhood. *Neurosurg Clin N Am.* 1992;3(4):791-802.

18. Kovalic JJ, Grigsby PW, Shepard MJ, Fineberg BB, Thomas PR. Radiation therapy for gliomas of the optic nerve and chiasm. *Int J Radiat Oncol Biol Phys.* 1990;18(4):927-932.

19. Hoshino T. A commentary on the biology and growth kinetics of low-grade and high-grade gliomas. *J Neurosurg* 1984;61:895-900.

20. Salcman M. Malignant gliomas: management. *Neurosurg Clin N Am.* 1990;1(1):49-63.

21. Salcman M. Survival in glioblastoma: historical perspective. *Neurosurgery.* 1980;7:435-439.

22. Salcman M. Epidemiology and factors affecting survival. In: Apuzzo MLJ, ed. *Malignant Cerebral Glioma.* Park Ridge, Ill: American Association of Neurological Surgeons; 1990:95-110.

23. Hoffman HJ, Goumnerova L. Pediatric brainstem gliomas. In: Wilkins RH, Rengachary SS, eds. *Neurosurgery Update II: Vascular, Spinal, Pediatric, and Functional Neurosurgery.* New York, NY: McGraw-Hill Health Professions Division; 1991:327-435.

24. Epstein F, Wisoff JH. Surgical management of brainstem tumors of childhood and adolescence. *Neurosurg Clin N Am.* 1990;1(1):111-121.

25. Grigsby PW, Thomas PRM, Schwartz HG, Fineberg B. Irradiation of primary thalamic and brainstem tumors in a

pediatric population: a 33-year experience. *Cancer.* 1987; 60:2901-2906.

26. Wallner KE, Wara WM, Sheline GE, Davis RL. Intracranial ependymomas: results of treatment with partial or whole brain irradiation without spinal irradiation. *Int J Radiat Oncol Biol Phys.* 1986;12:1937-1941.

27. DeAngelis LM. Primary central nervous system lymphoma: a new clinical challenge. *Neurology.* 1991;41: 619-621.

28. Guthrie BL, Ebersold MJ, Scheithauer BW, Shaw EG. Meningeal hemangiopericytoma: histopathological features, treatment, and long-term follow-up of 44 cases. *Neurosurgery.* 1989;25:514-522.

29. Barbaro NM, Gutin PH, Wilson CB, Sheline GE, Boldrey EB, Wara WM. Radiation therapy in the treatment of partially resected meningiomas. *Neurosurgery.* 1987;20:525-528.

30. Wallner KE, Sheline GE, Pitts LH, Wara WM, Davis RL, Boldrey EB. Efficacy of irradiation for incompletely excised acoustic neurilemomas. *J Neurosurg.* 1987;67:858-863.

31. Linskey ME, Lundsford LD, Flickinger JC. Radiosurgery for acoustic neuromas: early experience. *Neurosurgery.* 1990;26(5):736-745.

32. Laws ER Jr. Craniopharyngioma: diagnosis and treatment. *The Endocrinologist.* 1992;2(3):184-188.

33. Coffey RJ, Lunsford LD. The role of stereotactic techniques in the management of craniopharyngiomas. *Neurosurg Clin N Am.* 1990;1(1):161-172.

34. Hoffman HJ. Craniopharyngiomas: the role for resection. *Neurosurg Clin N Am.* 1990;1(1):173-180.

35. Baskin DS, Wilson CB. Surgical management of craniopharyngiomas: a review of 74 cases. *J Neurosurg.* 1986;65: 22-27.

36. Sung DI, Chang CH, Harisiadis L, Carmel PW. Treatment results of craniopharyngiomas. *Cancer.* 1981;47:847-852.

37. Abay EO II, Laws ER Jr, Grado GL, et al. Pineal tumors in children and adolescence: treatment by CSF shunting and radiotherapy. *J Neurosurg.* 1981;55:889-895.

38. Bruce JN, Stein BM. Pineal tumors. *Neurosurg Clin N Am.* 1990;1:123-138.

39. Baumgartner JE, Edwards MSB. Pineal tumors. *Neurosurg Clin N Am.* 1992;3(4):853-862.

40. Sen CN, Sekhar LN, Schramm VL, Janecka IP. Chordoma and chondrosarcoma of the cranial base: an 8-year experience. *Neurosurgery.* 1989;25:931-940.

41. Laws ER. Clivus chordomas. In: Sekhar LN, Janecka IP, eds. *Surgery of Cranial Base Tumors.* New York, NY: Raven; 1993:679-685.

42. Black KL. Chordomas of the clival region. *Contemp Neurosurg.* 1990;12;(13):1-7.

43. Poirier J, Gray F, Escourelle R. *Manual of Basic Neuropathology.* 2nd ed. Philadelphia, Pa: WB Saunders Co; 1990.

44. Cooper PR. Outcome after operative treatment of intramedullary spinal cord tumors in adults: intermediate and long-term results in 51 patients. *Neurosurgery.* 1989;25:855-859.

45. Reimer R, Onofrio BM. Astrocytomas of the spinal cord in children and adolescents. *J Neurosurg.* 1985;63:669-675.

46. Epstein FJ, Farmer JP. Pediatric spinal cord tumor surgery. *Neurosurg Clin N Am.* 1990;1(3):569-591.

47. Sundaresan N, Krol G, Hughes JEO. Primary malignant tumors of the spine. In: Youmans JR, ed. *Neurological Surgery.* 3rd ed. Philadelphia, PA:WB Saunders;1990: 3548-3573.

48. Patchell RA. Brain metastases. *Neurol Clin.* 1991;9: 817-824.

49. Grant R, Papadopoulos SM, Greenberg HS. Metastatic epidural spinal cord compression. *Neurol Clin.* 1991;9: 825-841.

50. Patchell RA, Tibbs PA, Walsh JW, et al. A randomized trial of surgery in the treatment of single metastases to the brain. *N Engl J Med.* 1990;322:494-500.

51. Raffel C, Neave VCD, Lavine S, McComb JG. Treatment of spinal cord compression by epidural malignancy in childhood. *Neurosurgery.* 1991;28:349-352.

52. Chamberlain MC. Current concepts in leptomeningeal metastases. *Curr Opin Oncol.* 1992;4:533-539.

53. Berens ME, Rutka JT, Rosenblum ML. Brain tumor epidemiology, growth, and invasion. *Neurosurg Clin N Am.* 1990;1:1-18.

54. Zulch KJ, et al. Histological Typing of Tumors of the CNS. *International Classification of Tumors.* Geneva: World Health Organization (WHO). 1979;(21):19-24.

25

TUMORS OF THE PITUITARY GLAND

Kamal Thapar, MD, Edward R. Laws, Jr, MD

Tumors of the pituitary gland constitute a class of neoplasms with a biology that deviates considerably, from both clinical and conceptual standpoints, from that of tumors arising in other organ systems. This uniqueness is derived, in part, from the capacity of many pituitary tumors to secrete pituitary hormones in excess, permitting them to generate some of the most dramatic and colorful clinical syndromes known to medicine. Furthermore, from an oncologic standpoint, pituitary tumors are conceptually different from other neoplasms arising elsewhere. As suggested by several unselected autopsy series, neoplastic transformation occurs with surprising regularity in the pituitary; however, *malignant* transformation in the pituitary is exceedingly rare.[1-3] Thus, pituitary tumors are almost always benign lesions with limited proliferative potential and negligible metastatic potential. Even so, the "benign" histology of pituitary adenomas is often an all too beguiling feature of their biology, for the regularity with which they encroach on critical neural structures, coupled with the distressing endocrinopathies they frequently induce, legitimizes pituitary adenomas as both a frequent and a significant source of patient morbidity and occasionally patient mortality.

Finally, unlike tumors arising in other intracranial structures, or in other organ systems, pituitary tumors impose a different set of diagnostic imperatives, requiring both an anatomic and an endocrine diagnosis. Thus, optimal management of pituitary tumors relies on a thorough appreciation of several interacting factors: the proximity of the tumor to critical neural structures, and the neurologic and endocrine status of the patient. While this frequently relies on a comprehensive interdisciplinary approach, the outcomes are encouraging: tumors of the pituitary have become eminently treatable conditions, with the majority of patients enjoying long-term survival or cure.

The Pituitary Gland: Regional Anatomy and Physiology

One of the most clinically satisfying aspects of pituitary oncology relates to the precision with which symptoms localize the lesion and the predictable correlations that exist between endocrinologic function, clinical phenotype, and tumor morphology. Recognition of these neurologic, endocrinologic, and pathologic correlates is predicated on some appreciation of the normal anatomic and physiologic relationships of the pituitary. This chapter will therefore begin with some of these introductory concepts.

The pituitary gland is a composite neuroendocrine structure consisting of two lobes, each differing in embryologic origin, structure, function, and pathologic processes. The larger anterior lobe, or adenohypophysis, is the site of meticulously regulated hormone secretion and synthesis, and is also the primary site of clinically significant pathology. It consists of a regimented topologic arrangement of five distinct cell types, each engaged in the production of a different hormonal product. These five cell types are categorized as somatotrophs, lactotrophs, corticotrophs, thyrotrophs, and gonadotrophs, and are distinguished functionally by the ability to secrete growth hormone (GH), prolactin (PRL), corticotropin (ACTH), thyroid-stimulating hormone (TSH), and gonadotropins (luteinizing hormone [LH] and follicle-stimulating hormone [FSH]), respectively. The secretory and proliferative capabilities of these cells are governed by a

Kamal Thapar, MD, Division of Neurosurgery, University of Toronto, Toronto, Ontario, Canada

Edward R. Laws, Jr, MD, Professor of Neurological Surgery and Medicine, University of Virginia, Charlottesville, Virginia

precise balance between hypothalamic trophic influences and negative feedback effects imposed by target organ hormones. Although susceptibilities vary, neoplastic transformation can, in a multistep multicausal fashion, occur in any one of these cell types. The resulting adenoma retains the secretory capability, morphologic characteristics, and nomenclature of the cell of origin. That virtually no human tissue escapes, either directly or indirectly, the sustaining or adaptive effects of anterior pituitary hormonal products explains the protean clinical manifestations accompanying hormonally active pituitary adenomas.

In addition to the five distinct hormonally active cell populations described above, a sixth cell type is speculated to be randomly dispersed within the normal pituitary. Known as null cells, these are hormonally inactive cells whose functional contribution to the pituitary remain obscure. They too may be susceptible to neoplastic transformation, giving rise to a common class of pituitary tumors known as null cell adenomas. As null cells do not produce measurable amounts of any known hormonal product, these cells and their respective tumors are designated as nonfunctioning.

The posterior lobe of the pituitary, or neurohypophysis, is an extension of the central nervous system (CNS), and is composed of interlacing nerve fibers and specialized glial elements known as pituicytes. Vasopressin and oxytocin are the principal hormones released by the posterior pituitary. The former is the essential regulator of water and osmolar homeostasis, and the latter is important during labor and lactation. Although the posterior pituitary is occasionally the site of metastatic tumors, it is rarely the site of clinically significant primary tumors.

Many of the neurologic manifestations of pituitary tumors have a predictable neuro-anatomic basis and are easily explained by appreciating parasellar anatomic relationships (Fig 25-1). The pituitary gland is intimately nestled at the base of the brain, situated within the bony confines of the dura-lined sella turcica. Attached to the hypothalamus by the pituitary stalk, the pituitary gland is surrounded by a number of critical and delicate neural structures. Its superior relations include the optic nerves and chiasm, hypothalamus, frontal lobe cortex, and anterior wall of the third ventricle. It is related laterally to the cavernous

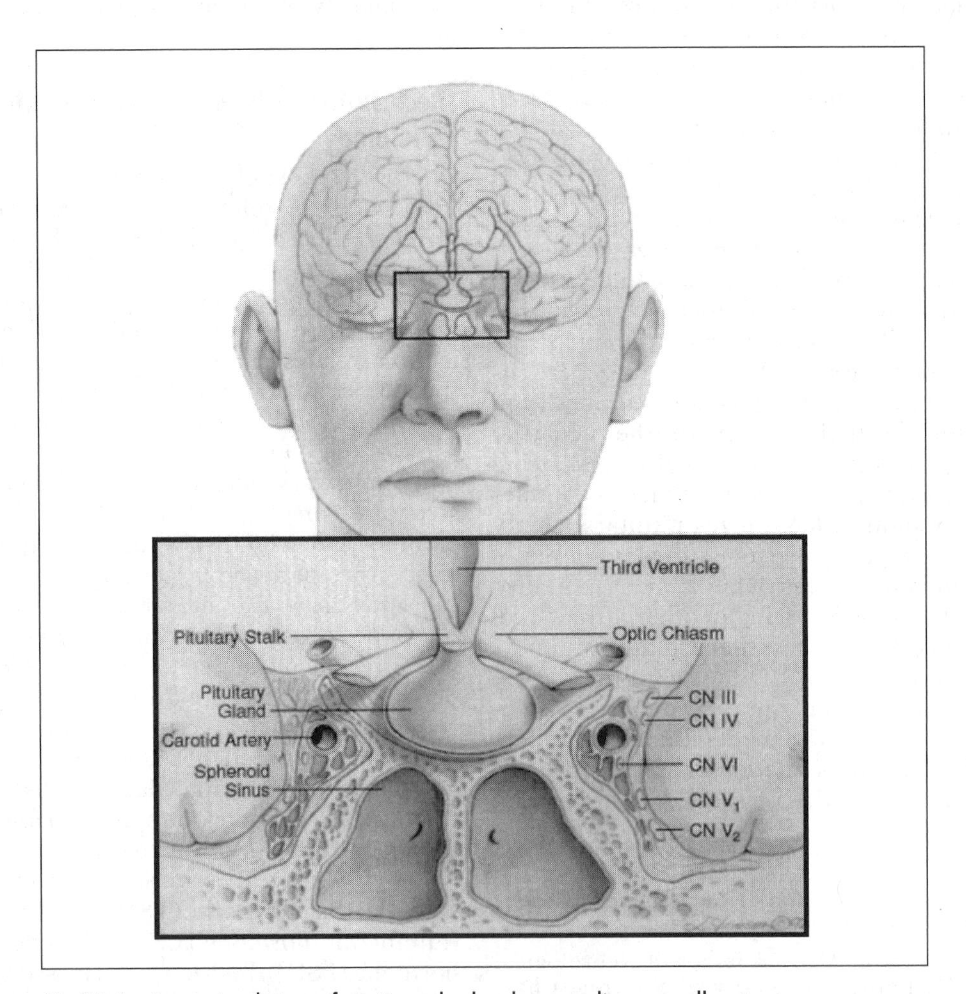

Fig 25-1. Anatomic relations of pituitary gland and surrounding parasellar structures.

sinus, containing cranial nerves and the cavernous segment of the internal carotid artery. Thus, depending on the direction of growth, an expanding pituitary mass is strategically placed to compromise the function of any of these structures (see discussion of clinical features below).

Pituitary Adenomas: General Features

Epidemiology

Pituitary adenomas are common lesions, accounting for up to 15% of all primary intracranial neoplasms treated surgically.[1] Depending on the population studied, the reported incidence rates range from 1 to 14.7 per 100,000 population annually. By this measure, pituitary adenomas represent the third most common primary intracranial neoplasm encountered in neurosurgical practice, following gliomas and meningiomas. It is quite likely that these figures considerably underrepresent the true incidence of pituitary adenomas, as the prevalence in several unselected autopsy series approaches 25%.[1,3] From this perspective, adenomatous transformation in the pituitary appears to be a very common event, although one that does not always become clinically apparent. There is a tendency for pituitary tumors to become more common with age, with the highest incidence occurring between the third and sixth decades. A female preponderance appears to exist, with women of childbearing years being at greatest risk for tumor development. The basis for this increased susceptibility in women is uncertain. Attempts to implicate oral contraceptive use as a potential predisposing or causative factor in pituitary tumorigenesis have been largely dismissed with case-controlled studies. Others contend that the increased frequency of pituitary tumors in premenopausal women is more apparent than real, as manifestations of pituitary dysfunction, specifically menstrual dysfunction, are more conspicuous and generally prompt earlier and more frequent diagnosis. This view is also supported by autopsy studies, in which the prevalence of pituitary tumors appears to be equally distributed between the sexes.[1]

Etiology, Pathogenesis, and Molecular Biology of Pituitary Adenomas

Despite exhaustive laboratory and epidemiologic studies, no environmental, pharmacologic, or physiologic agent has been identified definitively as being causative for pituitary tumorigenesis. A single known genetic predisposition for pituitary tumors exists in the form of hereditary multiple endocrine neoplasia type 1 (MEN1) syndrome. This is an autosomal dominant condition characterized by the spontaneous and simultaneous development of tumors of the pituitary, pancreatic islet cells, and parathyroid glands. Pituitary tumors develop in approximately 25% of these MEN1 patients, and most commonly occur as macroadenomas associated with GH or PRL hypersecretion, or both.[1,4] The nature of this genetic defect has been defined recently on a molecular basis, and involves allelic loss of a putative tumor suppressor gene at the 11q13 locus.[5] The behavior of this MEN1 gene is typical of a recessive oncogene, with susceptible individuals exhibiting a hereditary germ line mutation of one of the two 11q13 locus alleles. Subsequent mutation, deactivation, or loss of the remaining normal allele in susceptible tissue, such as the pituitary gland, initiates a series of poorly understood tumor-promoting events, ultimately leading to the development of the various tumors constituting the MEN1 syndrome. Tumor suppressor gene loss at 11q13 appears to be a tumorigenic mechanism applicable only to pituitary adenomas occurring in the context of MEN1; sporadic pituitary adenomas rarely exhibit similar genomic aberrations at this locus.[6]

Excluding the 3% of surgically resected pituitary adenomas with a hereditary origin (ie, in the context of MEN1), the overwhelming majority of pituitary tumors are acquired lesions, and seemingly without well-defined etiologic correlates. Current concepts of pituitary tumorigenesis suggest transformation in the pituitary to be a multistep process, which, in its most abbreviated form, begins with an irreversible "initiation" phase, followed by a "promotion" or tumor maintenance phase. A fundamental question regarding the pathogenesis of pituitary adenomas relates to the issue of whether transformation in the pituitary is the result of an inductive effect of aberrant hypothalamic trophic influences or simply an intrinsic abnormality of an isolated adenohypophyseal cell. Although hypothalamic dysfunction was historically considered an important initiator/mediator of the tumorigenic process, and continues to have conceptual and experimental support, compelling evidence of a clinical, pathologic, and molecular nature has provided increasing appeal for tumorigenic mechanisms occurring at the level of a single, susceptible adenohypophyseal cell, and in relative autonomy of hypothalamic trophic influence. Pituitary adenomas appear to arise as the result of an intrinsic pituitary cell defect, rather than of aberrant hypothalamic overstimulation, based on the following considerations: many pituitary adenomas can be cured by surgical resection, and these tumors are rarely accompanied by a zone of peritumoral hyperplasia. Further support of a de novo adenohypophyseal origin for pituitary adenomas was provided by a number of recent molecular studies concerning the clonal origins of pituitary adenomas. Using the technique of allelic X-chromosome inactivation analysis, which assesses restriction fragment length polymorphisms and differential methylation patterns of X-linked genes, a monoclonal constitution for both functioning and nonfunctioning pituitary adenomas has been confirmed.[7] This validation of a monoclonal origin for pituitary adenomas has been a conceptually important advance, indicating that these tumors are monoclonal expansions of a single, somatically mutated adenohypophyseal cell.

Various types of structural genomic alterations have been thought to contribute to somatic mutation and subsequent transformation in the pituitary. In addition to tumor suppressor gene inactivation at 11q13, as mentioned above, genomic and oncogene-activating mutations have been identified in a minority of pituitary adenomas. Amplification of v-*fos*[8] and point mutations of H-*ras*[9] oncogenes have been shown in isolated cases of prolactinoma. Mutations of the *gsp* oncogene have been identified in up to 40% of growth hormone-producing pituitary adenomas.[10] The biological implications of oncogene activation, in terms of prognosis and biological behavior, have yet to be fully characterized for pituitary tumors. A number of growth factors have also been identified in the pituitary, and it is thought that growth factor-mediated autocrine and paracrine stimulation may be an important component of pituitary tumorigenesis. The role of growth factors and oncogenes in pituitary tumor development has been summarized in a recent review.[2]

Clinical Presentation

Pituitary tumors are recognized clinically by one or more of three highly predictable patterns of presentation: symptoms of pituitary hypersecretion, symptoms of pituitary hyposecretion, or neurologic symptoms of a sellar mass. In about 70% of cases, the clinical picture is dominated by features of anterior pituitary hypersecretion, resulting in a characteristic hypersecretory syndrome. Acromegaly, Cushing's disease, amenorrhea-galactorrhea syndrome, and, rarely, secondary hyperthyroidism represent the classical paradigms of GH, ACTH, PRL, and TSH hypersecretion, respectively. Alternatively, pituitary tumors can present with symptoms of partial or total hypopituitarism (fatigue, weakness, hypogonadism, regression of secondary sexual characteristics, hypothyroidism). This usually occurs insidiously in association with pituitary macroadenomas that have achieved sufficient size to compress and impair the secretory capability of the adjacent nontumorous pituitary. In the face of chronic and progressive compression, the various secretory elements of the pituitary differ in their functional reserve: the gonadotrophs are most vulnerable, and usually are affected first, followed sequentially by thyrotrophs and somatotrophs, with corticotrophs demonstrating the greatest functional resilience. Pituitary insufficiency can also occur acutely in the context of *pituitary apoplexy*, in which sudden intratumoral hemorrhage or infarction can occasionally produce the life-threatening combination of acute hypopituitarism and an expanding intracranial mass.

The third pattern of presentation is one dominated by neurologic symptoms, either in isolation or coexisting with one or more of the endocrinologic perturbations described above. As alluded to earlier, a progressively enlarging pituitary mass will generate a constellation of neurologic signs and symptoms, depending on its growth trajectory and the critical neural structures in the vicinity that have been compromised. Headache may be an early finding and is attributed to stretching of the enveloping dura or diaphragma sellae. The single most common objective neurologic feature, however, is visual loss, and relates to suprasellar extension of the tumor, with compression of the optic nerves and chiasm. The classic pattern of visual loss is a bitemporal hemianopic field defect, often in association with diminished visual acuity. Large pituitary adenomas can encroach on the hypothalamus, causing alterations of sleep, alertness, behavior, eating, and emotion. Transgression of the lamina terminalis can bring these tumors into the region of the third ventricle, where obstruction to effluent cerebrospinal fluid (CSF) flow can result in obstructive hydrocephalus. Lateral extension of the tumor into the region of the cavernous sinus occurs commonly. With progressive cavernous sinus invasion, the cranial nerves transiting the sinus can occasionally become affected. In this regard, ptosis (cranial nerve III), facial pain or sensory changes (cranial nerve V), and diplopia (cranial nerves III, IV, and VI) are the most characteristic features of cavernous sinus involvement. Finally, some pituitary adenomas can assume gigantic proportions, extending well into the anterior, middle, and occasionally posterior cranial fossae, where they can produce the full spectrum of focal neurologic signs and symptoms. In such circumstances, the epicenter of these lesions can be so far displaced from the sella that their pituitary origin may not be immediately apparent.

An important mass-related, but nonspecific, feature of pituitary adenomas and other mass lesions of the sellar region is hyperprolactinemia. Prolactin secretion is under the inhibitory control of various hypothalamic "prolactin inhibitory factors" (dopamine being the most important). Dopamine released from the hypothalamus descends via the portal vessels to the anterior lobe, where it inhibits the release of PRL by normal lactotrophs. Processes which impair the hypothalamic release of dopamine (eg, compressive or destructive hypothalamic lesions) or impair its adenohypophyseal transfer (eg, compressive or destructive lesions of the pituitary stalk) place pituitary lactotrophs in a disinhibited state. Loss of such hypothalamic suppression induces nontumorous lactotrophs of the pituitary to increase their output of PRL, resulting in moderate elevations in blood PRL levels. Termed the "stalk section" effect, this phenomenon may elevate PRL levels to 150 ng/mL (normal, <25 ng/mL). Only when PRL levels exceed this threshold can they be attributed to autonomous PRL production by a PRL-secreting pituitary tumor. Lesser elevations may be due to a PRL-producing tumor, or any of a variety of other neoplastic and nonneoplastic processes occurring in the sellar region.

It is important to recognize that although pituitary adenomas are the dominant form of neoplastic pathology arising in the sella, other neoplastic and inflammatory processes may also occur in this region. Although many of these conditions are rare, and some have stereotypic clinical and radiologic features, others may masquerade clinically and radiologically as pituitary adenomas. The differential diagnosis of a sellar region mass suspected of being a pituitary adenoma is listed in Table 25-1.

Table 25-1. Differential Diagnosis of Neoplasms and "Tumor-like" Masses of the Sellar Region

Tumors of adenohypophyseal origin
- Pituitary adenoma
- Pituitary carcinoma

Tumors of neurohypophyseal origin
- Granular cell tumor
- Hamartomas
- Astrocytomas

Tumors of nonpituitary origin
- Craniopharyngioma
- Germ cell tumors
- Glioma (hypothalamic, optic nerve/chiasm, infundibulum)
- Meningioma
- Hemangiopericytoma
- Chordoma
- Hemangioblastoma
- Giant-cell tumor of bone
- Chondroma
- Fibrous dysplasia
- Sarcoma (chondrosarcoma, osteosarcoma, fibrosarcoma)
- Postirradiation sarcoma
- Paraganglioma
- Schwannoma
- Glomangioma
- Primary lymphoma

Cysts
- Rathke's cleft cyst
- Arachnoid cyst
- Epidermoid cyst
- Dermoid cyst
- Empty-sella syndrome

Metastatic tumors
- Carcinoma
- Plasmacytoma
- Lymphoma
- Leukemia

Inflammatory conditions
- Infection/abscess
- Mucocele
- Lymphocytic hypophysitis
- Sarcoidosis
- Langerhans cell histiocytosis
- Giant cell granuloma

Vascular Lesions
- Internal carotid artery aneurysms
- Cavernous angioma

Classification

While pituitary tumors have been subject to a variety of classification schemes, only two have proven consistently informative. The first is a radiologic classification, based on tumor size and geometry. The second is a pathologic classification, based on the immunohistochemical character, ultrastructural morphology, and cytogenesis of the tumor. The two classification schemes, therefore, address different but complementary aspects of the clinical problem. Since both classifications furnish practical, pathologic, and conceptual data relevant to the understanding and management of pituitary tumors, both will be reviewed.

Known as the Hardy classification, the radiologic classification distinguishes tumors on the basis of size and gross patho-anatomic features (Fig 25-2). First, tumors are classified according to size, with tumors <10 mm recognized as *microadenomas* and those >10 mm designated as *macroadenomas*. On the basis of sellar radiology, five classes of tumors have been identified. Microadenomas are designated as either grade 0 or grade I tumors, depending on whether the sella appears normal and whether minor focal sellar changes are present. Macroadenomas causing diffuse sellar enlargement, focal sellar erosion, and extensive sellar and skull base destruction are referred to as grades II, III, and IV, respectively. Macroadenomas are further subclassified by the degree of suprasellar extension. The Hardy classification has proven useful in surgical planning, identifying operative risk and determining the potential for surgical cure.

Regardless of the presence or nature of secretory capabilities, all pituitary tumors are morphologically similar at the light microscopic level. Although not truly encapsulated, microadenomas are delineated from the surrounding normal adenohypophysis by a

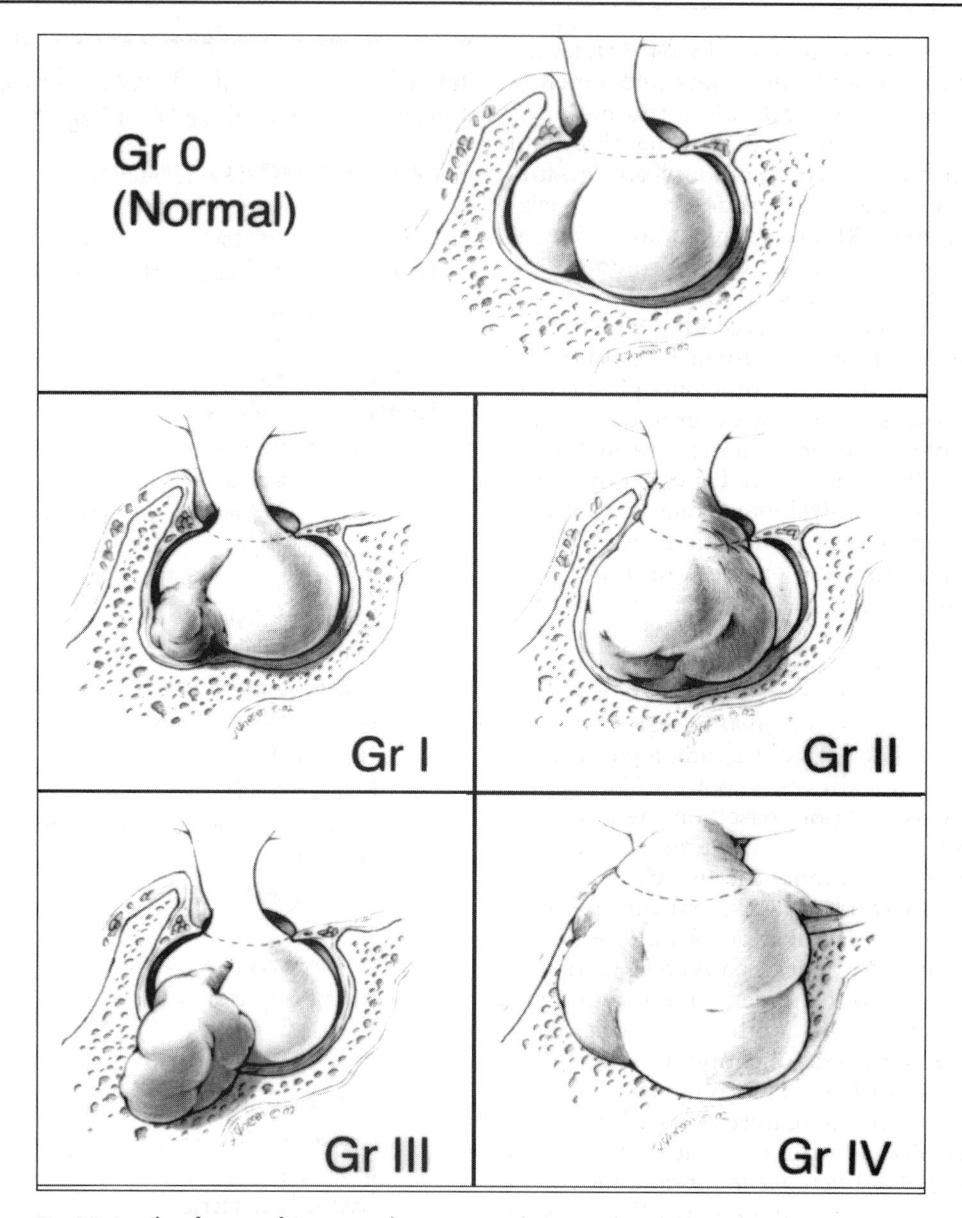

Fig 25-2. Classification of Pituitary Adenomas According to Radiographic Appearance (Hardy Classification)

Grade 0 Intrapituitary adenoma (microadenoma): diameter <1 cm, normal sella

Grade I Intrapituitary adenoma: diameter <1 cm, focal bulging or other minor change in sellar appearance

Grade II Intrasellar adenoma (macroadenoma): diameter >1 cm, enlarged sella, no erosion

Grade III Diffuse adenoma (macroadenoma): diameter >1 cm, enlarged sella, localized erosion, destruction

Grade IV Invasive adenoma: diameter >1 cm, extensive destruction of bony structures, "ghost" sella

Tumors subclassified by the degree of suprasellar extension:

A: Extension to suprasellar cistern only
B: Extension to recesses of third ventricle
C: Extension to involve whole anterior third ventricle

reticulin pseudocapsule. Histologically, they lack the septate acinar structure of the normal pituitary, and appear as a uniform population of polygonal cells arranged in sheets, cords, or nests. Nuclear pleomorphism, increased mitotic activity, and even focal necrosis can be seen to a variable degree; however, none is a reliable index of biologic aggressiveness or potential for recurrence.

By convention, pituitary tumors have been classified pathologically according to cytoplasmic staining affinities, as determined by the application of a few simple histologic stains. Under such a scheme, three traditional morphologic entities emerged: *acidophilic*, *basophilic*, and *chromophobic*. The acidophilic adenomas were assumed to be the exclusive pathologic substrate for acromegaly. The basophilic adenomas were thought to specifically cause Cushing's disease. The chromophobic category was reserved for tumors that failed to stain with acidic or basic dyes, and were therefore assumed to be hormonally inactive. Although the simplicity of this method engendered its appeal for many years, the evolution of immunohistochemical and ultrastructural methods has demonstrated that cytoplasmic staining affinities correlate poorly with reliable cell-type recognition and secretory activity. The current standard for classifying pituitary tumors relies on immunohistochemistry and electron microscopy to categorize tumors on the basis of hormonal content, ultrastructural morphology, and cytogenesis. This functional classification, assembled by Kovacs and Horvath, identifies 17 distinct anterior pituitary tumor types, each with its own structural, functional, and biological character. This classification, in abbreviated form, is presented in Table 25-2. While details of the classification are beyond the scope of this chapter, important clinicopathologic correlates derived from this classification are integrated into the discussion of the various clinical entities below.

Table 25-2. Pathologic Classification of Pituitary Adenomas

Tumor Type	Incidence
Hormonally active adenomas	**75%**
GH-producing adenomas	17%
PRL-producing adenomas	30%
Mixed GH and PRL-producing adenomas	10%
ACTH-producing adenomas	14%
TSH-producing adenomas	1%
Plurihormonal adenomas	3%
Hormonally silent adenomas	**25%**
Null cell adenomas	17%
Oncocytomas	6%
Gonadotroph adenomas	2%

ACTH=corticotropin

From Kovacs and Horvath.[1]

General Principles of Diagnosis and Therapy for Pituitary Tumors

Because pituitary tumors are clinically and endocrinologically heterogeneous, diagnostic parameters, therapeutic options, and long-term outcome vary among the major tumor types. These practical differences notwithstanding, there are common diagnostic and therapeutic principles applicable to all pituitary tumors, which are presented here. Specific details concerning the management of individual tumor types are discussed subsequently.

Diagnosis

Pituitary tumors represent a clinical problem that stands at the interface of a number of medical and surgical disciplines. The evaluation of patients suspected of having pituitary adenomas, therefore, rests on a comprehensive interdisciplinary effort. In the patient with endocrinologic or neurologic findings, or both, suggestive of a pituitary adenoma, the diagnostic process begins with a determination of an endocrinologic diagnosis and an anatomic diagnosis. Guided by findings in the history and physical examination, the clinician may make an endocrine diagnosis by measuring pituitary and/or target-organ hormones in basal and provoked states. These are very sensitive indicators of disturbed pathophysiologic activity, and allow for differentiation of the various pituitary adenoma subtypes. A useful initial screening should include measurements of PRL, GH, plasma cortisol, ACTH, LH/FSH, thyroxine, and TSH. This initial survey estimates the integrity of the various hypothalamic-pituitary-target organ axes, identifying states of relative excess or deficiency. However, further provocative, dynamic, and special hormonal assays may be required to precisely define a specific endocrinopathy.[11]

Anatomic diagnosis, once based on plain skull radiographs, is now routinely achieved with magnetic resonance imaging (MRI). High-resolution MRI with gadolinium enhancement has virtually supplanted computed tomography (CT) in the diagnosis of pituitary tumors. The superior resolution capabilities of MRI are particularly evident in cases of microadenoma, in which lesions as small as 3 mm can be routinely detected. While diagnostic sensitivity is generally less of an issue for macroadenomas, the merit of MRI for these larger tumors lies in its capacity to iden-

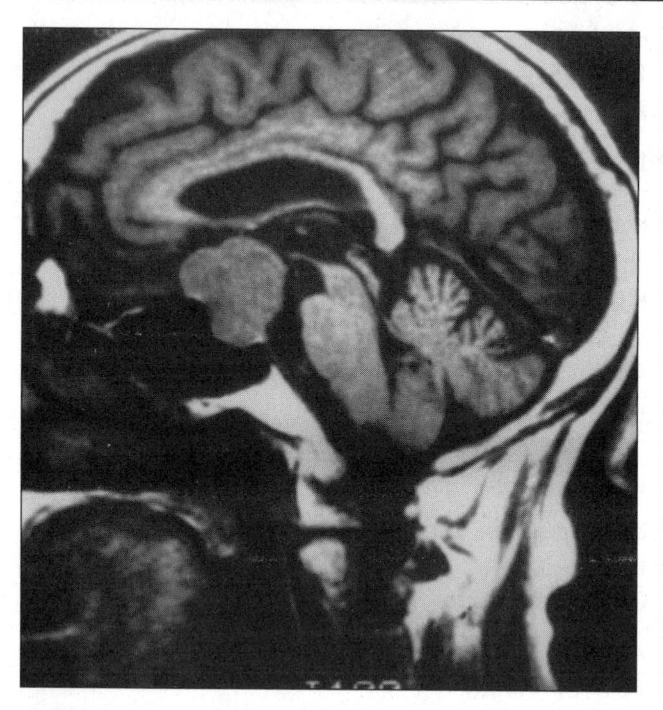

Fig 25-3. Lateral MRI scan of a clinically nonfunctioning pituitary macroadenoma arising from the sella (Hardy grade IVB).

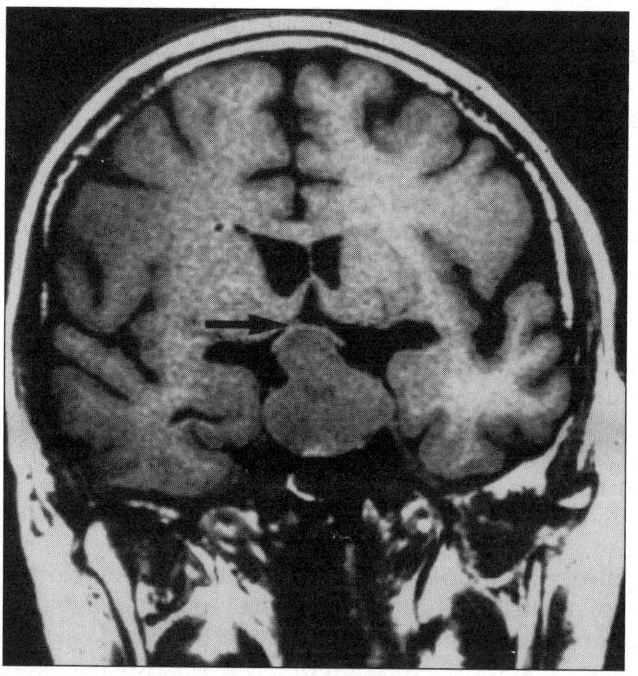

Fig 25-4. Coronal view of a large pituitary macroadenoma (Hardy grade IVB). The patient presented with bitemporal visual loss. The optic chiasm can be seen draped over the superior aspect of the tumor (arrow).

tify critical spatial relationships between the tumor and surrounding neurovascular structures (Fig 25-3, 25-4) In this regard, the position of the carotid arteries, the status of the optic chiasm, and the extent of suprasellar and parasellar tumor extension are of particular operative concern and are clearly delineated by MRI.

Because visual compromise is a complicating feature of many pituitary tumors, a complete neuro-ophthalmologic evaluation is mandatory in all patients with visual complaints and all patients with tumors extending beyond the confines of the sella. Visual field deficits are formally recorded with either manual or automated perimetry. These determinations are frequently performed serially to document disease progression and responses to therapeutic intervention.

Treatment

Once the diagnosis of a pituitary adenoma has been established on clinical, biochemical, and radiologic grounds, an assessment of therapeutic options is made. Therapy for pituitary tumors should be directed at achieving the following goals: (1) reversal of endocrinopathy and restoration of normal pituitary function, and (2) removal of tumor mass and restoration of normal neurologic function.

Fortunately, absolute realization of these goals has become increasingly feasible, due to the evolution of microsurgical techniques, development of receptor-mediated pharmacotherapy, and refinements in the delivery of radiation therapy. Each of these treatment modalities has specific merits and limitations that must be collectively considered and thoughtfully individualized to each patient with a pituitary tumor.

Transsphenoidal Microsurgery

While there is some emerging latitude for the initial use of nonsurgical therapies in selected cases of pituitary adenoma, surgery remains the initial treatment of choice for the overwhelming majority of pituitary tumors. The increased efficacy and safety of pituitary surgery can be ascribed to the development of the transseptal transsphenoidal microsurgical approach, which is the most direct and least traumatic corridor of surgical access to the pituitary. Currently, >95% of pituitary tumors are approached transsphenoidally, with conventional transcranial approaches reserved for the few cases in which anatomic features or the sella or unusual intracranial tumor extensions limit transsphenoidal accessibility. For the majority of pituitary microadenomas, and for many macroadenomas, transsphenoidal surgery alone is curative, obviating the need for adjuvant pharmacologic or radiation therapy. As precise definitions of "cure" differ among the various hypersecretory syndromes, details of surgical efficacy are best discussed below in the context of the individual tumor types.

Operative mortality and morbidity rates, as determined from several cumulative series, are 0.5% and 2.2%, respectively. Potential complications reflect the critical nature of the operative field. The most devastating of these includes traumatic or hemorrhagic hypothalamic injury, resulting in coma and death. Equally severe are injuries or lacerations of the carotid arteries, resulting in cerebral hemorrhage or ischemia. Traction injuries, ischemia, or direct trauma to the optic nerve and chiasm can result in blindness. Transgression of the arachnoid membrane can result in CSF rhinorrhea and predispose to meningitis. Fortunately, such complications are rare and their occurrence can be anticipated and minimized with attention to meticulous surgical technique. A relatively common and usually transient postoperative complication of pituitary surgery is diabetes insipidus. This is the result of damage to the infundibulum or posterior pituitary gland, structures highly susceptible to transient functional injury in response to even the most modest surgical manipulation. The result is a state of relative vasopressin deficiency, characterized by excretion of large amounts of dilute urine. If unrecognized, dehydration and hypernatremia may become extreme, even life threatening. Appropriate therapy includes early recognition, careful fluid management, and the judicious use of synthetic vasopressin. The condition is very rarely permanent, and usually resolves by the tenth postoperative day.

Permanent, postoperative hypopituitarism is uncommon following transsphenoidal surgery. It occurs least frequently after the removal of a microadenoma (<5% of cases). The incidence increases with the size and invasiveness of the tumor, and is highest in patients in whom preoperative anterior pituitary failure already exists. Fortunately, the morbidity of postoperative hypopituitarism can be minimized and adequately managed with endocrine replacement therapy.

Pharmacologic Therapy

The secretory activity of neoplastic pituitary cells does not entirely escape physiologic regulatory controls. This observation establishes the susceptibility to, and therapeutic rationale for, pharmacologic manipulation of these regulatory mechanisms as a form of medical therapy for pituitary adenomas. Two classes of pharmacologic agents have emerged as primary or adjuvant therapies for pituitary tumors: dopamine agonists and somatostatin analogues. The prototypical and most widely used dopamine agonist is bromocriptine, which mediates its clinical effect by amplifying existing inhibitory dopaminergic hypothalamic-pituitary pathways. Dopamine is the native physiologic inhibitor of prolactin secretion. By saturating dopamine receptors on the tumor cell surface, bromocriptine effectively inhibits prolactin secretion. Its ability to normalize prolactin levels and to reduce tumor size has made this agent an effective alternative to surgical therapy for many prolactinomas.[11,12] Bromocriptine is also effective, although to a lesser degree, in reducing GH levels in tumors associated with acromegaly.

With the discovery that GH secretion is physiologically inhibited by somatostatin, the potential therapeutic value of somatostatin in treating GH-secreting tumors was clearly recognized. Somatostatin analogues, which are biologically more stable than native somatostatin, have an evolving role in the management of tumors associated with acromegaly. Although somatostatin analogues have been shown to reduce GH levels, and in some cases effect tumor shrinkage, the consistency and durability of the response is uncertain. Therefore, somatostatin analogues are not currently considered long-term alternatives to surgical therapy. At present, they are best viewed as important adjunctive therapy, reserved for those patients with persistent or recurrent postoperative disease.[11,13]

Radiation Therapy

Radiation therapy has traditionally had a major adjuvant role in the postoperative treatment of pituitary tumors. With the increasing effectiveness of surgical therapy and the increasing feasibility of adjuvant medical therapy, it is becoming increasingly difficult to precisely define the role of radiation in contemporary pituitary tumor management. The goal of radiation therapy is to prevent progression or recurrence of tumor growth. Probably the clearest indication for radiation therapy is the persistence or recurrence of a medically refractory hypersecretory state following surgery. For large nonfunctioning pituitary adenomas, postoperative radiation is also considered in cases of invasive or incompletely resected tumors. Complications of pituitary irradiation include delayed panhypopituitarism, cognitive impairment, optic nerve and temporal lobe radionecrosis, and the possibility of radiation-induced tumors. Conceptual and technical advances in radiation delivery have minimized the frequency of many of these complications. However, delayed panhypopituitarism is still a major concern.

Acromegaly and GH-Secreting Adenomas

Acromegaly is an insidiously progressive, physically disabling systemic affliction having the well-defined metabolic basis of pathologic GH excess.[14] Should this GH excess present at an early age and prior to long bone epiphyseal closure, gigantism is the result. So distinctive is the clinical syndrome that acromegalics and related giants have been the subject of seemingly mythical reference in folklore and legend, as keepers of great strength and power. This was rarely the case, particularly in the later, debilitating stages of the disease when these individuals were relegated to freakish outcasts, often regarded with horror and ridicule.

Most acromegalic patients reach medical attention between the third and fifth decades, although the disease may have been slowly progressive. Focal enlargement of bones and soft tissue is apparent at characteristic body locations. The facial features become classically coarse, with frontal bossing, prognathism, dental malocclusion, and macroglossia. There is broad, spade-like enlargement of hands and feet. Bone density increases, and the hypertrophy of joints and cartilage leads to degenerative joint disease and debilitating spinal stenosis. Peripheral neuropathy in the form of carpal tunnel syndrome and other entrapments produce paresthesias, a common presenting feature. Cardiac enlargement leads to congestive heart failure, which is further complicated by the hypertension seen in these patients. Abnormalities of glucose metabolism are common, ranging from impaired glucose tolerance to insulin resistance and frank diabetes. Finally, depending on the tumor size, local mass effects can produce visual complaints and hypopituitarism.

Suspicion of acromegaly on historical and clinical grounds must be carefully validated with endocrine studies. While elevations of serum GH levels are the hallmark of acromegaly, this finding alone does not conclusively secure a diagnosis of acromegaly. Random elevations of GH occur in a variety of conditions, including diabetes, renal failure, cirrhosis, malnutrition, and stress. The two most sensitive means of confirming a diagnosis of acromegaly are (1) demonstration of a lack of suppression of GH levels following a glucose load, and (2) elevations of somatomedin C levels.[11,14] Somatomedin C, also known as insulin-like growth factor I, is secreted under the influence of GH and is the principal mediator of the clinical effects seen in acromegaly. It is therefore an excellent indicator of active acromegaly for both initial diagnosis and postoperative surveillance of residual or recurrent disease.

An anatomic diagnosis is established with MRI of the head. This will localize all macroadenomas and approximately 90% of small intrasellar tumors. GH levels generally correlate well with the size, invasiveness, and Hardy class of the tumor. With regard to anatomic diagnosis, the rare possibility of extrapituitary causes of acromegaly must always be considered. These include growth hormone-releasing hormone (GHRH)-producing adenomas associated with hypothalamic hamartomas, occasional pancreatic tumors, and carcinoid tumors of the bronchus and intestine. The GHRH produced by these conditions causes hyperplasia of pituitary somatotrophs, with sellar changes mimicking a primary pituitary tumor. Sometimes, the only way these extrapituitary sources of acromegaly can be distinguished is by measuring serum GHRH levels.

Pure GH-producing tumors occur in two forms: the densely granulated GH adenoma and the sparsely granulated GH adenoma. Both occur with equal frequency, but the latter is notorious for its larger size, invasive tendency, and overall more aggressive character.[1] In addition, some GH-secreting tumors may be admixed with neoplastic cellular elements capable of PRL secretion.

Of the three existing treatment modalities (medical, surgical, and radiation therapy), transsphenoidal surgery provides the most satisfactory results and is recommended for virtually all patients with active acromegaly. The other therapeutic options are used adjuvantly. Criteria for successful management or "cure" include removal of tumor mass, resolution of acromegalic signs and symptoms, and restitution of normal GH dynamics. For practical purposes, basal GH levels should be reduced to <5 ng/mL and, following a glucose tolerance test, <2 ng/mL. Normalization of somatomedin C levels occurs over a period of weeks and is probably the single best biochemical and physiologic index of cure. In our surgical series of 360 acromegalics, GH levels decreased significantly in nearly all patients and >90% have shown improvement in acromegalic symptoms. Based on the numerical criteria above, our surgical results indicate that 74% of patients are cured, of whom 7% experienced recurrence during a 10-year follow-up period. The prognostic implications of increasing tumor size and preoperative GH levels are evident in Table 25-3. Radiation therapy is considered for those patients in whom an endocrinologic cure was not achieved surgically, as determined by persistently elevated GH and somatomedin C levels.

Prolactin-Producing Adenomas: "Prolactinomas"

Prolactin-secreting pituitary adenomas are the most common tumors of the pituitary gland, accounting for 30% to 40% of all pituitary tumors encountered in clinical practice. Prolactinomas occur in both sexes, but there are a number of fundamental differences in epidemiology, clinical presentation, and treatment strategies between tumors in men and women. Women are affected almost four times as frequently as men, accounting for 78% of prolactinomas. Prolactinomas usually present in women during the second and third decades, whereas affected males are typically older, in their fourth and fifth decades. Tumors in men are larger and more often invasive, and usually have transgressed sellar confines at the time of diagnosis. Women usually present on an endocrinologic basis with symptoms of amenorrhea and galactorrhea (Forbes-Albright syndrome), as the direct consequence of prolactin excess. Men usually present on a neurologic basis with

Table 25-3. Surgical Results in GH-Producing Adenomas (N = 360)

Tumor Type	Incidence	Postoperative Normalization of GH (Clinical Remission)
Microadenoma	26%	85%
Macroadenoma	50%	65%
Invasive macroadenoma	24%	48%
All tumors, preoperative GH <40 ng/mL		82%
All tumors, preoperative GH >40 ng /mL		35%
Postoperative recurrence (10-year follow-up of 100 cases)	7%	

headache, visual loss, and relative hypopituitarism, features directly attributable to an enlarging sellar mass. As in women, prolactin excess in men produces hypogonadism, but symptoms of impotence and decreased libido are not as conspicuous as the corresponding menstrual disturbances seen in women. This may provide a partial explanation of why tumors in men are so advanced when recognized, while microadenomas are readily detected in women. This explanation is probably not as simple as it seems, especially in the face of a number of longitudinal natural history studies, which suggest that prolactinomas are relatively stable from a growth standpoint; fewer than 8% of microadenomas evolve into macroadenomas.[12] It may be that PRL-producing tumors in men inherently are simply more aggressive.

An endocrine diagnosis is made by confirmation of elevated levels of basal PRL. Other conditions causing hyperprolactinemia (drugs, hypothyroidism, cirrhosis, and renal failure) are usually easily excluded.[11,12] The degree of hyperprolactinemia is a critical determinant of both the nature of the pathologic process and the likelihood of surgical cure. Serum PRL levels are normally <25 ng/mL. As previously discussed, PRL elevations up to 150 ng/mL can be, but are not necessarily, due to a prolactin-secreting tumor. Other nonprolactin-producing pituitary tumors, as well as other structural lesions in the vicinity of the sella, can cause these mild PRL elevations due to the "stalk section effect" (see Table 25-1). PRL levels in excess of 200 ng/mL are very likely prolactinomas, and levels in excess of 1,000 ng/mL are indicative of an invasive prolactinoma.

Once the diagnosis of prolactinoma is established on clinical and endocrinologic grounds, an anatomic diagnosis is obtained with MRI. Macroadenomas will always be identified, as will 90% of microadenomas.[11]

Treatment options for prolactinomas consist of surgical resection, pharmacologic control, and radiation therapy.[11,12] The consistency and efficacy with which bromocriptine normalizes PRL levels, restores reproductive function, and reduces tumor mass adds both dimension and controversy to the relative roles of surgery and medical therapy in the treatment of prolactinomas. Surgical therapy provides the opportunity for both endocrinologic and oncologic *cure*; however, success rates are limited by the size and invasiveness of the tumor. Alternatively, bromocriptine provides for endocrinologic and oncologic *control*. It is effective to some degree in the majority of patients, but often is associated with intolerable side effects and must be taken indefinitely. While some latitude exists in the selection of therapeutic approach, treatment strategies must be individualized, with careful consideration of treatment goals, the size and invasiveness of the tumor, the degree of hyperprolactinemia, and the inclinations of the patient.

Microadenomas, the majority of which occur in women, are usually managed with bromocriptine as primary therapy. It effectively ameliorates the endocrinopathy in most patients and restores ovulation for those desiring fertility. If pregnancy occurs, bromocriptine should be discontinued and resumed following delivery. Although accelerated tumor growth can occur during pregnancy, it rarely occurs in patients with microadenomas. In contrast, patients with PRL-secreting macroadenomas who are receiving bromocriptine have a genuine risk of accelerated tumor growth during pregnancy when therapy is discontinued. Conception in these patients should be withheld until the tumor is definitively treated with surgical resection. Many patients with PRL-secreting microadenomas who desire fertility are also treated surgically. Curative tumor resection and subsequent pregnancy have been achieved in 83% of our patients harboring PRL-secreting microadenomas.

In our clinic, indications for surgical management of PRL-secreting macroadenomas include mass effect (progressive visual loss), apoplexy, bromocriptine resistance, and desire for fertility. "Cure" rates for macroadenomas reach only 53%, which with local invasion is further reduced to 28%. Preoperative PRL levels also serve as a prognostic index of surgical success: tumors with PRL levels <200 ng/mL are most susceptible to surgical "cure" (Table 25-4). In patients with large or invasive tumors, and in those with persistent postoperative hyperprolactinemia, adjunctive therapy with bromocriptine is recommended. Radiation therapy has an adjuvant, though relatively restricted, role in the management of prolactinoma. It is generally recommended for those with recurrent or persistent disease, in whom bromocriptine and surgery fail to control tumor growth or PRL levels.[11,12]

Table 25-4. Surgical Results in PR-Producing Adenomas (N = 737)

Tumor Type	Postoperative Normalization of GH (Clinical Remission)
Microadenoma	74%
Macroadenoma	53%
Invasive macroadenoma	28%
All tumors, preoperative PRL <200 ng/mL	83%
All tumors, preoperative PRL >200 ng/mL	43%

Cushing's Disease and Nelson's Syndrome: Corticotroph Adenomas

Corticotroph adenomas account for 14% of all pituitary tumors. They are hormonally active lesions engaged in the deregulated hypersecretion of ACTH. These tumors result in two clinically distinct, but pathologically related, conditions: Cushing's disease and Nelson's syndrome.

Cushing's Disease

While the term *Cushing's syndrome* is the general description of any iatrogenic or endogenous hypercortisolemic state, *Cushing's disease* refers specifically to a hypercortisolemic state generated in response to a hypothalamic-pituitary disorder of ACTH hypersecretion. When defined etiologically, 80% of noniatrogenic cases of Cushing's syndrome are, in fact, cases of Cushing's disease due to an ACTH-producing pituitary tumor. The remaining causes include cortisol-producing adrenal tumors and ectopic sources of ACTH production (bronchogenic carcinoma, carcinoid tumors, and pancreatic tumors).

Cushing's disease is a serious endocrinopathy, with clinical features that are attributable to endogenous cortisol excess. Women constitute more than 75% of affected patients, with individuals most commonly afflicted between the ages of 30 and 40 years. The classic features include a characteristic change in body habitus with the development of moon facies, centripetal obesity, "buffalo hump," and supraclavicular fat deposition. Skin changes include hirsutism, occasional hyperpigmentation, plethora, and vascular fragility, leading to ecchymoses and purple abdominal striae. Generalized weakness, fatigue, and myopathy are common. Metabolic effects include hypertension, glucose intolerance, and osteoporosis. Menstrual abnormalities, immunosuppression, and psychiatric symptoms also can occur. In its most florid form, the disorder is easily recognizable; however, subtle versions of the condition can occur and may not be immediately obvious. In addition to the genuine hypercortisolemic states listed above, alcoholism, depression, and obesity may mimic some of the features of Cushing's disease, and must be distinguished. In contrast to the other hypersecretory states (hyperprolactinemia, acromegaly), the endocrinopathy of Cushing's disease is life threatening. Untreated, the disease carries a 5-year mortality rate of 50%.[15] For this reason, Cushing's disease is accompanied by certain therapeutic imperatives, which are much more pressing than those occurring in any other hypersecretory state.

Distinguishing Cushing's disease from other hypercortisolemic states is critical, as appropriate therapy for hypercortisolism is contingent on precise identification of the pathologic nature and anatomic site of the causative lesion. In this regard, rigorous endocrine diagnosis is most important. Cushing's disease has the following endocrinologic profile[11]: (1) hypercortisolism, as demonstrated by elevations of serum cortisol and 24-hour urinary free cortisols; (2) loss of diurnal variation in serum cortisol values; (3) moderately elevated ACTH levels; and (4) cortisol suppressibility on high-dose dexamethasone testing, but no suppression on low-dose dexamethasone testing. In many cases, these tests are sufficient to secure an endocrine diagnosis of Cushing's disease, but occasionally atypical results necessitate additional testing. In such circumstances, ACTH measurements of effluent blood in the inferior petrosal sinus can help identify whether a pituitary-hypothalamic source is responsible for ACTH excess, and, if so, where within the pituitary gland the hypersecreting focus is located.[11]

Because the majority of corticotroph adenomas are small microadenomas, anatomic diagnosis is achieved radiologically in only 40% of cases. MRI studies have the highest yield, particularly when gadolinium is used. When pituitary imaging is normal, particularly when endocrine testing is atypical, normal scans of the lungs and adrenals provide indirect evidence of a hypothalamic-pituitary source of excess cortisol production. Nevertheless, even if the causative tumor is radiologically occult, a confirmatory preoperative endocrine diagnosis of Cushing's disease ensures a high measure of confidence that a pituitary adenoma is indeed present and can be selectively identified and removed with transsphenoidal surgery.

Distinguished by ultrastructural morphologic features, corticotroph adenomas are of two pathologic types: densely granulated and sparsely granulated corticotroph adenomas. The former occurs commonly and is well differentiated. The latter is less common, less well differentiated, and notorious for its aggressive and invasive tendencies. ACTH immunopositivity is demonstrated in both tumor types.[1] More than 80% of corticotroph adenomas are microadenomas, often only a few millimeters in size, but usually from

Table 25-5. Surgical Results in Cushing's Disease (N = 260)

Tumor Type	Incidence	Normalization of ACTH (Clinical Remission)	Tumor Recurrence*
Microadenoma	84%	90%	8%
Macroadenoma	16%	66%	18%

*Mean follow-up of 5.3 years.

surrounding normal distinguishable tissue.

The merits of transsphenoidal surgery are particularly well exemplified in the treatment of Cushing's disease. Whether the lesion is visible on imaging studies or is radiologically occult, transsphenoidal exploration of the pituitary gland enables identification and selective resection of the offending microadenoma while preserving normal pituitary function. Based on our series of 260 patients, curative resection can be achieved in >90% of microadenomas and in 65% of macroadenomas and invasive tumors (Table 25-5). Successfully treated patients have an immediate fall in blood cortisol levels and eventual regression of cushingoid features. Recurrence is uncommon, occurring in 8.5% of cases and sometimes many years after successful surgery. In the minority of cases in which surgery fails to achieve an immediate endocrinologic cure, medical therapy, radiation therapy, and bilateral adrenalectomy are all potential options. Medical therapy consists primarily of agents that pharmacologically block adrenal steroidogenesis (mitotane, ketoconazole, and metyrapone). They do reduce cortisol levels, but rarely restore them to normal. Moreover, they are often associated with unpleasant side effects. The delayed therapeutic effect of radiation therapy limits its role in Cushing's disease, although it is used for persistent disease (in conjunction with medical therapy) and in cases of invasive tumors. Bilateral adrenalectomy is immediately effective in ameliorating hypercortisolism and is recommended in patients with persistent and debilitating disease that is unresponsive to other therapies.

Nelson's Syndrome

Nelson's syndrome refers to the clinical condition in which pituitary corticotroph adenomas become manifest following bilateral adrenalectomy for Cushing's disease. Approximately 15% of patients with Cushing's disease so treated will develop Nelson's syndrome. Although these tumors are morphologically identical to tumors responsible for Cushing's disease, they are characteristically much more aggressive, frequently exhibiting unrelenting invasion of neighboring neural, vascular, and bony structures. The enhanced aggressiveness of these tumors has been attributed to loss of negative feedback inhibition consequent to the adrenalectomy. These tumors produce ACTH, but the adrenalectomy prevents the occurrence of hypercortisolemia. Because these tumors also secrete melanocyte-stimulating hormone, patients with Nelson's syndrome are hyperpigmented. The syndrome is easily recognizable, beginning with a history of Cushing's disease in which the pituitary lesion was either unsuspected, undetected, or incompletely resected. Persistent hypercortisolism would subsequently be treated with bilateral adrenalectomy, which effectively ameliorates the hypercortisolemic state. This temporary remission would be followed by aggressive tumor recurrence with manifestations of hyperpigmentation and extrasellar tumor extension (visual loss, cranial nerve palsies, and headache). Serum ACTH levels are elevated, and, depending on the size of the tumor, varying degrees of hypopituitarism will be detected clinically and biochemically.

Therapeutic options for Nelson's syndrome include surgery and irradiation. Because the majority are invasive macroadenomas, these tumors are rarely curable and both surgery and radiation therapy are frequently required for symptomatic control of local disease. Symptomatic resolution of mass effect is usually achieved, but improvements in hyperpigmentation and normalization of ACTH levels occur in only 50% and 25% of patients, respectively. For the occasionally fortunate patient in whom oncologic and endocrinologic cure has been obtained, the recurrence rate of tumors of Nelson's syndrome is approximately 11% in our series.

Glycoprotein-Producing Pituitary Adenomas

Glycoprotein hormone-producing pituitary adenomas are of two major types: gonadotroph adenomas which produce FSH/LH and thyrotroph adenomas which produce TSH. Despite hypersecretion of gonadotropins, gonadotroph adenomas do not produce any recognizable clinical syndrome and are therefore considered among the hormonally inactive pituitary tumors (see below).

TSH-producing adenomas are rare, accounting for approximately 1% of all pituitary tumors. The world literature on the subject consists of less than 100 cases, which emphasizes the relatively limited clinical and pathological experience with this tumor type.[1,11,16,17] Endocrinologically, most patients present with some history of thyroid dysfunction, typically hyperthyroidism, although these tumors can present anywhere along the spectrum of thyroid function, ranging from normal to extremes of hypothyroidism and hyperthyroidism. The most typical scenario includes initial symptoms of hyperthyroidism which, despite unsuppressible TSH elevation, are erroneously attributed to primary thyroid disease. These patients are treated with some form of thyroid ablation, which temporarily ameliorates the hyperthyroid state, only to be followed by accelerated tumor growth and optic nerve compression. It is at this point that a pituitary tumor is correctly recognized as the site of responsible pathology. These tumors are generally macroadenomas at the time of diagnosis and have usually invaded parasellar structures. Their aggressive tendency has been attributed to the typical delay in diagnosis, but also to the loss of feedback inhibition imposed by thyroid ablation.

With the routine availability of sensitive TSH assays, and their increased use to confirm thyrotoxicosis of all causes, most TSH adenomas should now be diagnosed at an earlier stage and inappropriate thyroid ablation occur less frequently. The endocrine diagnosis rests on demonstrating hyperthyroidism in association with inappropriately elevated and unsuppressible TSH elevations. In more than 80% of TSH adenomas, elevations of glycoprotein hormone alpha subunit can also be detected. Co-secretion of other anterior pituitary hormones, particularly GH and PRL, is seen in about 70% of cases.[1,11,16]

Therapy for TSH adenomas is surgical excision.[17] When the diagnosis is established early in the course of the disease, these tumors may be detected at a microadenoma stage, when selective transsphenoidal resection of the tumor should be curative. However, when the diagnosis is delayed, especially in the context of prior thyroid ablation, these tumors are sufficiently large and invasive that cure rates associated with transsphenoidal surgery are reduced to approximately 40%.[17] Adjuvant radiotherapy is usually recommended in such cases of invasive lesions. Pharmacologic therapy in the form of somatostatin analogue has shown some promise in reducing TSH levels, but is generally ineffective in reducing tumor mass.[11]

Nonfunctioning Pituitary Adenomas

Nonfunctioning pituitary adenomas are tumors that do not cause a clinically recognizable endocrinopathy, presenting instead with features of a progressive sellar mass (headache, visual loss, and varying degrees of hypopituitarism). By virtue of their size, they may also produce mild hyperprolactinemia on the basis of the "stalk section effect." Three distinct morphologic entities constitute this nonfunctioning class of pituitary tumors: null cell adenomas, oncocytomas, and gonadotropin-producing adenomas. As mentioned, the last are often functioning tumors, which can liberate gonadotropic hormones (LH and FSH). Because there is no definable endocrinopathy attributable to gonadotropin excess, their presentation is like the genuine nonfunctioning entities and they are therefore discussed here. Collectively, nonfunctioning adenomas account for 25% of all pituitary adenomas, and they can reach such a large size at presentation that their management can be a formidable challenge.

Null cell adenomas and oncocytomas account for 17% and 6% of pituitary adenomas, respectively. Null cell adenomas are so named because they are unassociated with any distinctive morphologic or immunohistochemical marker referable to any one of the five known adenohypophyseal cell types. Oncocytomas are simply null cell adenomas that exhibit intracellular accumulation of large numbers of dilated mitochondria. This is a descriptive term without biological or clinical significance; in practice, both these entities are oncologically equivalent. These tumors typically occur in older patients, and are virtually all large macroadenomas at presentation. It is likely that the majority of these have limited proliferative potential and have been slowly growing for many years before reaching medical attention. Gross invasion of neighboring anatomic structures is present in approximately 40% of these tumors.

Gonadotroph adenomas arise as neoplastic derivatives of normal pituitary gonadotrophs, and account for 3% to 5% of all pituitary adenomas. They most commonly occur in older patients, sometimes in the context of gonadal failure. They are all macroadenomas at presentation and one fifth are locally invasive. Despite the absence of a distinct endocrinopathy, elevations of FSH, the glycoprotein hormone alpha subunit, and rarely LH can be detected.[11] These elevations serve as useful markers for the initial diagnosis and for later postoperative surveillance of residual or recurrent disease.

The diagnosis of nonfunctioning adenoma rests primarily on MRI imaging. As these lesions are usually large, careful consideration must be given to their full extent and their relationships to surrounding neural and vascular structures. These factors are critical in determining optimal surgical access, potential operative hazards, and possibility of cure. Endocrinologic testing is used primarily to exclude a hypersecretory state and to identify the presence and degree of coexisting hypopituitarism. As mentioned, mild elevations of PRL levels are common.

While each of the hyperfunctioning tumors has a pharmacologic option for treatment, none exists for nonfunctioning adenomas. Therapy is therefore primarily surgical, with judicious adjuvant use of irradiation. Despite their size, the majority of nonfunctioning tumors are accessible transsphenoidally. Craniotomy is reserved for the occasional lesion with extreme lateral intracranial extension. Although "total" surgical removal is the intuitive goal for all pituitary tumors, the fact that most nonfunctioning tumors occur in the elderly and are usually slow-growing necessitates that judgment prevail and therapy be individualized. When progressive visual loss occurs in the elderly patient, for example, a radical procedure with attempt at "total" surgical resection may be less prudent than a less radical and less dangerous partial decompression. Guided by these principles, the surgical outcome in our series of more than 600 nonfunctioning tumors have been satisfactory. Visual function improved or was stabilized in 94% of patients, and symptoms of headache and cavernous sinus compression were almost always relieved. Because of their large size and longstanding compression of the normal pituitary, restoration of normal pituitary function, if impaired preoperatively, occurs in only a minority of patients. Therefore, recognition of postoperative pituitary deficiency, followed by adequate hormone replacement therapy, are important components of long-term care. Adjuvant radiation therapy is often recommended in cases of residual or recurrent disease.

Pituitary Carcinoma

Primary carcinoma of the pituitary gland has long been enshrouded in controversy. For some, the entity did not exist, and for those who acknowledged its existence, no consensus could be reached on its definition. Earlier literature suggested that tumors exhibiting local invasion were malignant. However, the observation that up to 85% of benign pituitary tumors show histologic invasiveness has rendered this perspective obsolete.[18,19] The currently accepted operational definition of primary pituitary carcinoma includes those tumors of adenohypophyseal origin that are associated with distant metastases or metastatic dissemination into remote areas of the subarachnoid space.[1] Based on these criteria, there are fewer than 40 cases of genuine pituitary carcinoma described in the world literature.[20]

Unlike most other forms of human cancer, the cytologic hallmarks of malignancy (anaplasia, increased mitotic index, necrosis, and invasiveness) are insufficient to constitute a diagnosis of pituitary carcinoma: these are common features shared by many benign pituitary tumors. Instead, the diagnosis is based on the biological behavior of the tumor rather than on its pathologic characteristics. In this regard, metastatic dissemination occurs most commonly within the CSF axis. The clinical manifestations will depend on the level(s) of the CSF axis affected: intracranial deposits will produce focal motor, cognitive, or cranial nerve findings; spinal lesions will produce paraplegia; and cauda equina metastases will produce polyradiculopathy. Less commonly, extraneural metastases (to the liver, mediastinum, lymph nodes, heart, bone, and kidney) can occur. The mode of systemic spread is presumed to be both hematogenous and lymphatic. The former appears to be a venous phenomenon, presumably beginning with tumor penetration into the cavernous sinus, with subsequent transport to the internal jugular veins via the petrosal sinuses. Although the pituitary gland lacks lymphatic drainage, tumor penetration into the skull base results in access to the rich lymphatics of the latter, providing the necessary conduit for lymphatic dissemination.

Pituitary carcinomas, like their benign counterparts, can be hormonally active or hormonally silent. It is impossible to predict whether any given pituitary tumor harbors metastatic potential. In some patients, the initial clinical course is indistinguishable from that of a benign lesion, except that it is followed by multiple recurrences and eventual dissemination. Alternately, the behavior of other pituitary carcinomas suggests de novo malignancy. Such tumors are biologically malignant from the outset, beginning as locally invasive, unrelentingly progressive, and frequently cytologically atypical tumors, which promptly give way to metastatic dissemination. The preoperative onset of diabetes insipidus is a particularly ominous sign suggesting hypothalamic invasion. This is rarely, if ever, associated with a benign pituitary adenoma. Nevertheless, despite the pattern of initial presentation, no clinical or pathologic parameter has been identified to enable an a priori diagnosis of pituitary carcinoma.

Insofar as most pituitary carcinomas will present unsuspectingly as benign adenomas, their initial management is identical to that of any benign pituitary tumor. Depending on the endocrinologic context, size, and invasiveness of the tumor, surgery, pharmacotherapy, and irradiation may all have temporary effectiveness. When the malignant nature of the pituitary tumor is revealed, as evidenced by CSF or distant metastases, subsequent therapy becomes palliative. Methotrexate and 5-fluorouracil have been used, but due to limited experience and the generally short lifespan of patients with proven pituitary carcinoma, the efficacy of these or other agents is uncertain. It is important to recognize that of the reported cases of pituitary carcinoma, many, if not all, patients have died as a direct consequence of their intracranial disease, and not as the result of secondary systemic dissemination.

Tumors of the Posterior Pituitary

The posterior pituitary is rarely the site of clinically significant primary tumors. Granular cell tumors are the most common primary tumors of the neurohypophysis. Most are only a few millimeters in size and are incidental findings in up to 8% of unselected autopsies. On rare occasion, granular cell tumors can assume sufficient size to cause local compressive symptoms, including visual disturbance and hypopituitarism.[21] Given their posterior lobe origin, diabetes is often a prominent accompanying feature. When symptomatic, granular cell tumors are effectively treated by surgical resection.

Hamartomas and low-grade astrocytomas arising from the infundibular stalk, or extending down from the hypothalamus, are additional rarities constituting the remaining primary neurohypophyseal tumor types. Hamartomas, also known as choristomas or gangliocytomas, may sometimes liberate hypothalamic hormones that produce hyperplasia of adenohypophyseal cells, causing a hypersecretory syndrome such as acromegaly or Cushing's disease. Occasionally, hamartomas are associated with a pituitary adenoma, suggesting the potential inductive effect of excess hypothalamic stimulatory input of the former in the development of the latter. In addition, some hamartomas in this region have been known to release gonadotropin-releasing hormones, which may account for the high frequency of precocious puberty seen with these lesions. Aside from the above-mentioned hypersecretory states which may accompany hamartomas in this region, diabetes insipidus and local compressive symptoms are generally the most common presenting features. When symptomatic, surgical resection aimed at relieving mass effect constitutes appropriate therapy. As implied in their designation, "hamartomas" are generally considered nonneoplastic, and surgical resection is often curative.[22]

Astrocytomas of the infundibulum and posterior lobe, or those descending into the sella from the hypothalamus, third ventricle, or optic nerves, are generally low-grade pilocytic astrocytomas. On the rare occasion when they become symptomatic, surgical debulking is often used to ameliorate mass effect. However, given their critical location and frequently indolent biology, gross total resection is generally not achieved, nor is it advised. Given the complications of radiation therapy in this region of the neuroaxis, postoperative irradiation is generally reserved for tumors with documented progression.

Although primary tumors of the posterior pituitary are rare, metastatic deposits emanating from a variety of systemic and hematopoietic malignancies are not uncommonly featured in the posterior lobe. The predilection of metastatic tumors for the posterior lobe of the pituitary relates to its blood supply. In contrast to the anterior pituitary, which has a somewhat tenuous indirect supply from the portal circulation, the posterior lobe derives its circulation directly from the carotid arterial system. Although the majority of metastatic tumors to this region occur in the context of advanced malignancy, the occasional posterior lobe metastasis may be the first sign of an unrecognized neoplastic process.[23] Of the metastatic cancers, breast is the most common culpable primary tumor, followed by lung and prostate.[24] Hematopoietic malignancies that may present with a posterior lobe deposit include the solitary plasmacytoma (which usually evolves into multiple myeloma), as well as various lymphomas and leukemias. Diabetes insipidus is often an accompanying feature, and its presence in association with a sellar mass should raise the possibility of a metastatic tumor. Additional symptoms include headache, visual field defects, hypopituitarism, and cranial nerve palsies related to cavernous sinus infiltration. With the exception of diabetes insipidus, which is rarely a feature of pituitary adenomas, it is often impossible, in the absence of a known history of malignancy, to distinguish a metastatic tumor to the sella from a pituitary adenoma. Transsphenoidal sellar exploration and decompression will provide the tissue diagnosis and often effect symptomatic improvement, and is therefore the treatment of choice in appropriate patients. Adjuvant radiation therapy is usually required postoperatively. Depending on the responsiveness of the primary tumor and the clinical status of the patient, chemotherapy may also be considered.

References

1. Kovacs K, Horvath E. *Tumors of the Pituitary Gland. Atlas of Tumor Pathology,* Armed Forces Institute of Pathology; 1986: series 2, vol 21;1-262.

2. Thapar K, Kovacs K, Laws ER Jr, Muller PJ. Pituitary adenomas: current concepts in classification, histopathology and molecular biology. *Endocrinologist.* 1993;3:39-57.

3. Burrow GN, Wortzman G, Rewcastle NB, Holgate RC, Kovacs K. Microadenomas of the pituitary and abnormal sellar tomograms in an unselected autopsy series. *N Engl J Med.* 1981;304:156-158.

4. Scheithauer BW, Laws ER Jr, Kovacs K, Horvath E, Randall RV, Carney JA. Pituitary adenomas of the multiple endocrine neoplasia type 1 syndrome. *Semin Diagn Pathol.* 1987;4:205-211.

5. Bystrom C, Larsson C, Blomberg C, et al. Localization of the *MEN1* gene to a small region within chromosome 11q13 by deletion mapping in tumors. *Proc Natl Acad Sci U S A.* 1990;87:1968-1972.

6. Werner S, Bystrom C, Askensten U, et al. Retained constitutional genotype on chromosome 11 in 26 sporadic pituitary adenomas. *J Endocrinol Invest.* 1989;12(Suppl 2):52 (abstract).

7. Herman V, Fagin J, Gonsky R, Kovacs K, Melmed S. Clonal origin of pituitary adenomas. *J Clin Endocrinol Metab.* 1990;71:1427-1433.

8. U SH, Kelly P, Lee WH. Abnormalities of the human growth hormone gene and proto-oncogenes in some human pituitary tumors. *Mol Endocrinol.* 1988;2:85-89.

9. Karga HJ, Alexander JM, Hedley-Whyte ET, Klibanski A, Jameson JL. *Ras* mutations in human pituitary tumors. *J Clin Endocrinol Metab.* 1992;74:914-919.

10. Landis CA, Harsh G, Lyons J, Davis RL, McCormick F, Bourne HR. Clinical characteristics of acromegalic patients whose pituitary tumors contain mutant G_s protein. *J Clin Endocrinol Metab.* 1990;71:1416-1420.

11. Klibanski A, Zervas NT. Diagnosis and management of hormone-secreting pituitary adenomas. *N Engl J Med.* 1991;324:822-831.

12. Molitch ME. Pathologic hyperprolactinemia. *Endocrinol Metab Clin North Am.* 1992;21:877-901.

13. Lamberts SWJ, Reubi JC, Krenning ER. Somatostatin analogs in the treatment of acromegaly. *Endocrinol Metab Clin North Am.* 1992;21:737-752.

14. Melmed S. Acromegaly. *N Engl J Med.* 1990;322:966-977.

15. Boggan JE, Wilson CB. Cushing's disease and Nelson's syndrome. In: Wilkins RH, Rengachary SS, eds. *Neurosurgery.* New York, NY: McGraw-Hill Book Co; 1985:859-863.

16. Gesundheit N, Petrick PA, Nissim M, et al. Thyrotropin-secreting pituitary adenomas: clinical and biochemical heterogeneity. *Ann Intern Med.* 1989;111:827-835.

17. McCutcheon IE, Weintraub BD, Oldfield EH. Surgical treatment of thyrotopin-secreting pituitary adenomas. *J Neurosurg.* 1990;73:674-683.

18. Scheithauer BW, Kovacs KT, Laws ER Jr, Randall RV. Pathology of invasive pituitary adenomas with special reference to functional classification. *J Neurosurg.* 1986; 65:733-744.

19. Selman WR, Laws ER Jr, Scheithauer BW, Carpenter SM. The occurrence of dural invasion in pituitary adenomas. *J Neurosurg.* 1986;64:402-407.

20. Mountcastle RB, Roof BS, Mayfield RK, et al. Pituitary adenocarcinoma in an acromegalic patient: response to bromocriptine and pituitary testing: a review of the literature on 36 cases of pituitary carcinoma. *Am J Med Sci.* 1989;298:109-118.

21. Becker DH, Wilson CB. Symptomatic parasellar granular cell tumors. *Neurosurgery.* 1981;8:173-180.

22. Scheithauer BW, Kovacs K, Randall RV, Horvath E, Okazaki H, Laws ER Jr. Hypothalamic neuronal hamartoma and adenohypophyseal neuronal choristoma: their association with growth hormone adenoma of the pituitary gland. *J Neuropathol Exp Neurol.* 1983;42:648-663.

23. Branch CL Jr, Laws ER Jr. Metastatic tumors of the sellar turcica masquerading as primary pituitary tumors. *J Clin Endocrinol Metab.* 1987;65:469-474.

24. Teears RJ, Silverman EM. Clinicopathologic review of 88 cases of carcinoma metastatic to the pituitary gland. *Cancer.* 1975;36:216-220.

26

MALIGNANT TUMORS OF BONE

Douglas J. Pritchard, MD

Malignant neoplasms of bone are relatively rare, as compared with tumors arising in other organ systems. *Primary* malignant bone tumors appear to arise within or on the surface of the bone, while *secondary* tumors arise elsewhere and metastasize to bone or begin in adjacent soft tissue and subsequently invade bone. This chapter will discuss only malignant tumors that are primary in bone.

Overall, about 1 in 100,000 persons may be expected to develop a primary bone malignancy. In comparison, about 35 times as many people will develop secondary bone malignancies.[1] Some histologic types tend to affect young people, whereas others occur more commonly in older adults. Ewing's sarcoma and osteosarcoma, for example, usually arise in young, growing children or teenagers. Because of this, there has been considerable interest in these tumors, even though they are relatively rare, and considerable research has been done in basic science as well as clinical aspects of these tumors. In addition to age specificity, a number of other key considerations depend on the specific histologic diagnosis. Therefore, each of the more common malignant bone tumors will be considered separately. A discussion of limb salvage procedures concludes the chapter.

Osteosarcoma

Tumor Anatomy

Osteosarcoma may arise in virtually any bone, although about half of all cases occur in the region of the knee, in the metaphysis of either the distal femur or the proximal tibia. It is distinctly rare for osteosarcoma to arise in the small bones of the hand or feet. Indeed, it is rare for this neoplasm to occur distal to the elbow or the ankle.

Epidemiology and Risk Factors

Osteosarcoma tends to occur in individuals younger than 20 years, but may be seen at any age. In some series, there is a secondary peak in incidence among older adults, which reflects the fact that osteosarcoma sometimes arises in patients who have preexisting Paget's disease. This secondary peak is more common in geographic areas with a high incidence of Paget's disease, such as Great Britain. Males are more commonly affected than females, a trait common to almost all malignant neoplasms involving bone.

The etiology of osteosarcoma is not known.[2] However, certain factors, such as radiation, have been found to predispose to the development of this malignancy. The first such tumors of known cause resulted from exposure in the watch industry to the radiation emitted from radium used in dials: watchmakers would lick the tip of the brush they dipped in radium to bring the tip to a fine point. In addition, radiation-induced osteosarcomas may arise following treatment for other conditions, after a lapse of at least four years. Various agents have caused osteosarcoma in experimental animal systems, although the relevance of these experiments to the clinical setting is not known.

A number of genetic abnormalities are now being addressed. It is known, for example, that patients with bilateral retinoblastoma have a chromosomal abnormality, and if these patients survive their retinoblastomas, they often develop osteosarcoma at a later date. It was originally thought that these tumors occurred within the field of radiation for the retinoblastoma, but it is now known that osteosarcoma may arise at any site, even outside the field of radiation therapy.

Natural History

As with almost all sarcomas, there is a great tendency for osteosarcoma to metastasize to the lungs, particularly the peripheral lung fields. Spread to other bones may also occur, but lung metastasis is more common.

Douglas J. Pritchard, MD, Professor of Orthopedic Surgery, Mayo Clinic and Mayo Foundation, Rochester, Minnesota

Rarely, osteosarcoma metastasizes to other sites, such as the heart.

Clinical Presentation and Diagnostic Workup

Most patients with osteosarcoma tend to present with pain, a lump, or sometimes both. About 10% of patients who seek medical treatment have already developed metastasis at the time of the original evaluation.

Initial evaluation of the patient with suspected osteosarcoma should include x-rays of the involved site in two planes. Frequently, these plain x-rays are diagnostic if features characteristic of osteosarcoma are present, such as variable amounts of mineralization that appear as a combination of both lytic and sclerotic areas. The cortical bone often has been penetrated, and there is usually a soft-tissue component of the tumor immediately adjacent to the bone. Reactive new bone may form, particularly at the periphery of these tumors. This combination of destruction of bone and proliferation of new bone is frequently suggestive of the diagnosis of osteosarcoma. Some osteosarcomas appear to be entirely sclerotic or entirely lytic. In virtually every case, a biopsy is necessary to confirm the diagnosis.

Other imaging modalities may be of considerable importance. Magnetic resonance imaging (MRI) appears to be especially useful in establishing the extent of both soft-tissue involvement as well as medullary involvement within the bone. Technetium bone scans may be helpful in showing skip areas within the medullary canal and in ruling out metastatic disease involving other bones of the skeleton. If an osteosarcoma is suspected, it is important to obtain both a chest x-ray and computed tomography (CT) of the lung fields to exclude metastatic disease at the outset and to serve as a baseline for future comparison should positive findings arise on subsequent examinations.

Biopsy of suspected osteosarcoma is particularly important and should be performed only by someone knowledgeable in the management of malignant bone tumors, since placement of the biopsy site may be critical. A poorly placed biopsy may preclude a subsequent limb salvage procedure and create the necessity for amputation.

The histologic diagnosis of osteosarcoma may be difficult. A bone pathologist may need to be consulted to establish the diagnosis. Osteosarcoma is defined as a tumor with malignant osteoid-producing cells.

General Management

Once the diagnosis is established and staging studies have been performed to rule out metastatic disease, treatment may be initiated. Today, most institutions treat osteosarcoma with preoperative chemotherapy for a period of time. Surgery is then required to remove the affected part. In approximately 80% of cases, surgery can be accomplished without having to resort to amputation. Following resection, a variety of reconstructive techniques can restore limb function (Fig 26-1).

Patients need to be followed closely for a number of years following their initial treatment. During the immediate postoperative period, chemotherapy is usually continued for a variable period, after which the patient returns periodically for repeat imaging and staging studies. With this sort of regimen, 70% of patients may be expected to survive long-term. Even patients who develop metastatic disease or who presented initially with metastatic disease may be long-term survivors with aggressive treatment.

Ewing's Sarcoma

Tumor Anatomy

Ewing's sarcoma may affect any bone, although about 60% of tumors arise in the lower extremities and pelvic girdle.

Epidemiology and Risk Factors

Like osteosarcoma, Ewing's sarcoma is a disease of young people. It rarely occurs under the age of 3 or over the age of 25. When a malignant-appearing bone tumor occurs in children younger than 3 years, metastatic neuroblastoma must be considered. Males are more commonly affected than females. There are no known etiologic factors for this neoplasm.

Clinical Presentation and Diagnostic Workup

Pain and swelling are the most common presenting symptoms. Patients also may complain of intermittent fever, which is usually low grade. Pathologic fracture with this disease occasionally occurs, but is unusual.

The evaluation of a patient with suspected Ewing's sarcoma should include plain x-rays as well as routine laboratory screening tests. Patients with Ewing's sarcoma frequently present with mild anemia, mild leukocytosis, and an elevated sedimentation rate. The radiographic appearance is nonspecific, but usually there is evidence of involvement of the tubular portion of a long bone. A mixed or mottled lytic appearance suggests destruction of the cortical bone. Subperiosteal, reactive new-bone formation sometimes gives the characteristic "onionskin" appearance of Ewing's sarcoma. However, this appearance is not always present and, if present, is not always diagnostic.

Other imaging studies, including MRI, frequently show a contiguous soft-tissue mass surrounding the area of bony involvement. The degree of soft-tissue involvement may be underestimated by CT. MRI appears to reflect the extent of the soft-tissue mass

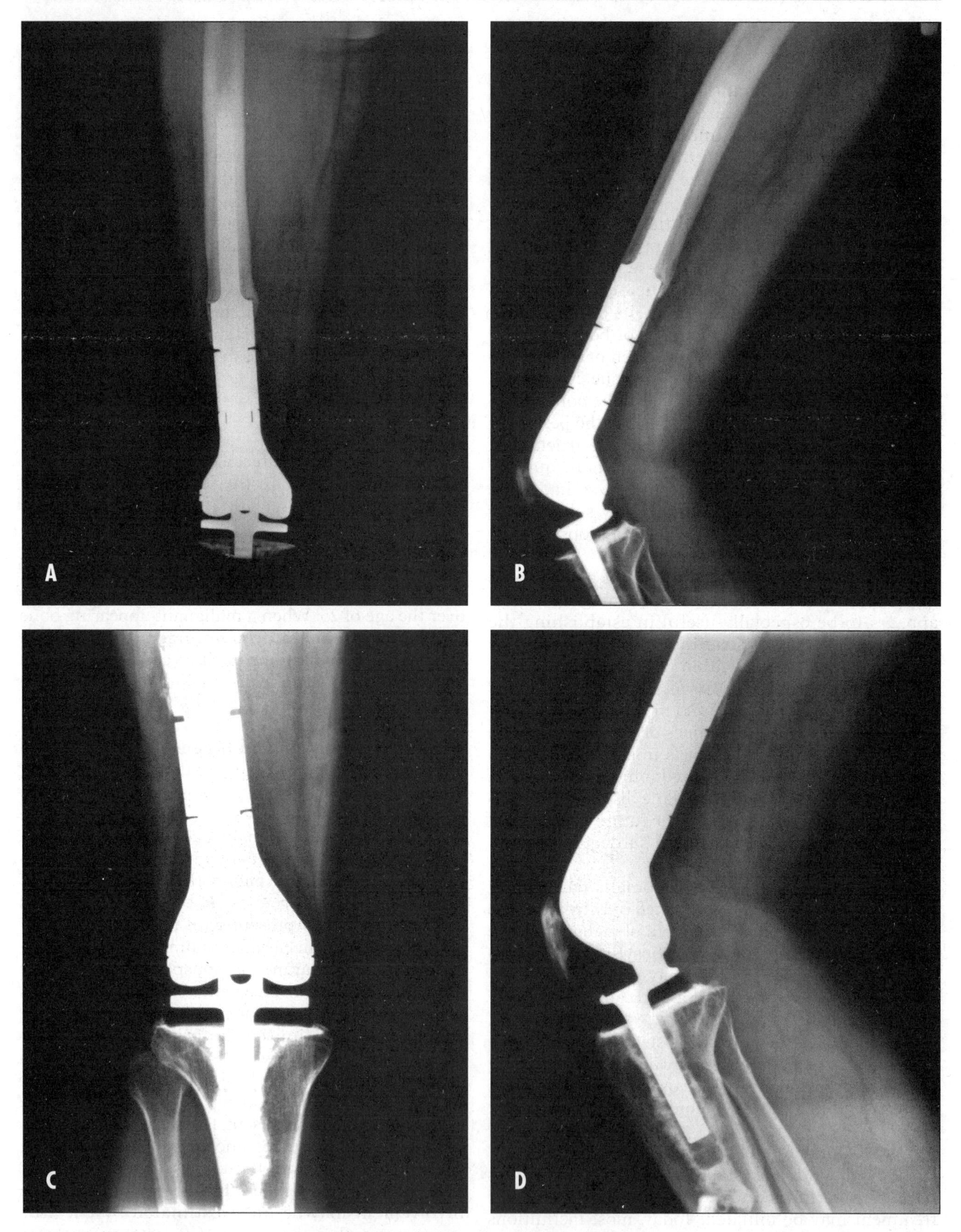

Fig 26-1. "Custom" type modular, rotating-hinge kinematic total-knee replacement following resection for a sarcoma of the distal femur. ***A***: AP view; ***B***: lateral view; ***C***: AP view showing tibial component; ***D***: lateral view showing tibial component.

more accurately. Ewing's sarcoma tends to metastasize to the lungs or other bones; hence, staging studies should include chest x-rays, CT scan of the lungs, and a technetium bone scan of the entire skeleton.

When the tumor is entered, a semi-liquid, almost purulent-appearing material may be encountered. The surgeon may suspect osteomyelitis and obtain cultures, but neglect to obtain histologic samples. If cultures turn out negative, the clinician may realize the need for a histologic examination. It should be noted that in all cases in which biopsy of a suspected bone tumor is performed, material should be submitted for both histology and culture. Ewing's sarcoma is composed of numerous small round cells.

General Management

Once the diagnosis is established, multidrug chemotherapy is initiated. After several courses of induction chemotherapy, management of the primary lesion must be considered. In the past, Ewing's lesions were usually treated by radiation therapy. Today, however, some cases are better suited for surgical resection than radiation therapy (Fig 26-2). After treatment of the primary lesion, the chemotherapy is usually resumed for approximately 1 year.

In the past, patients with Ewing's sarcoma had a dismal prognosis. Only about 10% of patients survived 5 years or longer. Today, however, at least 75% may be expected to survive that long. Patients with this disease require long-term periodic follow-up examinations.[3]

Chondrosarcoma

Tumor Anatomy

Most chondrosarcomas arise de novo within virtually any portion of the skeleton. The predominant site appears to be the region of the triradiate cartilage of the pelvis. It is unusual for chondrosarcoma to arise in the small bones of the hands or feet. Indeed, chondrosarcoma is much more common in the central portions of the skeleton.

Epidemiology and Risk Factors

Chondrosarcoma tends to arise in adults older than 50 years. However, it may occasionally occur even in childhood. Males are more commonly affected than females.

Several predisposing conditions are genetic in origin. Patients with Ollier's disease are predisposed to develop chondrosarcomas. In Ollier's disease, multiple bones may show evidence of enchondromatosis, and there is an element of dysplasia in long bones.

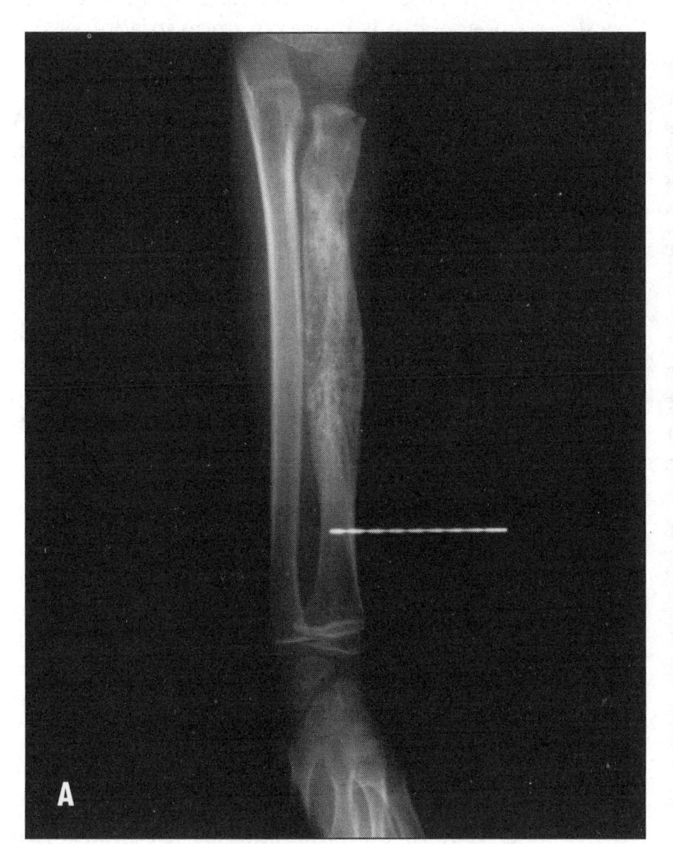

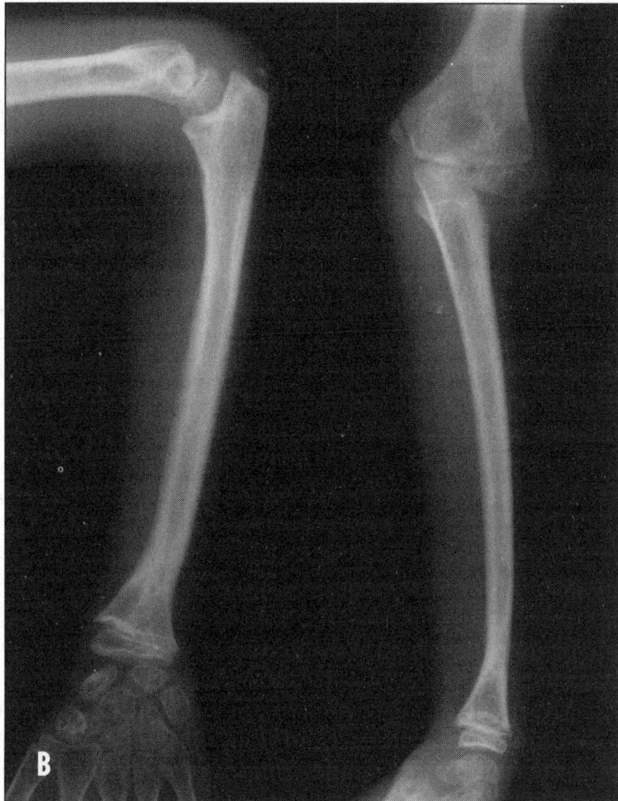

Fig 26-2. Ewing's sarcoma of the radius. ***A***: following preoperative chemotherapy and just prior to resection; ***B***: AP and lateral views of the forearm following resection of the radius and conversion to a one-bone forearm.

Fortunately, Ollier's disease is rare. Patients with an even more infrequent condition, Mafucci's syndrome, have a high incidence of development of chondrosarcoma. This syndrome is the combination of skeletal chondromatosis and various angiomatoid lesions.

Patients with multiple osteochondromas also tend to develop chondrosarcoma in one or more osteochondroma sites. The exact incidence is not known, but is probably <10% of such cases. Patients with solitary osteochondromas, on the other hand, only very rarely develop chondrosarcomas.[4] Patients with any of these conditions who show evidence of an enlarging or changing mass should be suspected for the development of chondrosarcoma.

Clinical Presentation and Diagnostic Workup

Most patients with chondrosarcoma present with a mass or pain or both. Pathologic fractures secondary to this disease are unusual.

The radiographic appearance is sometimes characteristic, since chondrosarcoma is often a slow-growing neoplasm. There may be actual expansion of the cortical bone, a feature rarely seen in other conditions. A spiculed calcification is often seen within the medullary canal, and there may be even larger areas of calcification that have the appearance of popcorn. Erosion of the endosteal surface of bone, or so-called scalloping, also may be prominent. From the plain x-rays, it is sometimes difficult to visualize a tumor in the triradiate cartilage of the pelvis, and the tumor may reach considerable size before its true nature is discovered. Tumors at this site present a differential diagnosis problem since the patient may complain of hip pain and be thought to have osteoarthritis.

The histologic diagnosis of chondrosarcoma is one of the most difficult for the pathologist to consider. The vast majority of chondrosarcomas are low grade, hence difficult to distinguish from their benign cartilage counterparts. High-grade chondrosarcoma is relatively easy to diagnose. Low-grade lesions have a tendency to recur locally, particularly if the tumor is spilled at the time of surgical resection. Even low-grade tumors, however, have the capacity to metastasize; and routine staging studies, including bone scans, chest x-rays, and CT of the lungs, are always indicated.

General Management

At present, chondrosarcoma is managed surgically, with radiation and chemotherapy rarely used in the treatment of the primary lesion. When progression occurs, however, these modalities may be considered and occasionally are effective. The prognosis depends on the histologic grade of the tumor as well as the adequacy of the surgical treatment. Low-grade lesions with an adequate resection have an excellent prognosis.[5]

Unusual Types of Chondrosarcomas

There are several "nonconventional" types of chondrosarcomas. The clear-cell variety tends to involve the epiphyseal areas of long bones and hence may be confused with benign chondrogenic tumors. These tumors are slow-growing. A characteristic histologic feature is the abundant clear cytoplasm of the tumor cells. These tumors may be cured with surgical resection, but complete surgical removal is necessary.[6]

An even more unusual form of chondrosarcoma is the so-called mesenchymal chondrosarcoma, which may arise in either soft tissue or bone. This rare tumor is particularly lethal and requires very aggressive surgical treatment.[7]

Malignant Lymphoma Of Bone

Tumor Anatomy

Malignant lymphomas may affect any bone, but only rarely the small bones of the hands and feet.

Epidemiology and Risk Factors

Lymphoma of bone may present as a primary lesion with no evidence of disseminated disease. Somewhat less than half of all cases of lymphoma involving bone are primary in bone at the outset. Males are more commonly affected than females. Lymphoma may occur at any age, but is more common in adults.

Clinical Presentation and Diagnostic Workup

Most patients complain of pain, swelling, or both. A pathologic fracture may be the presenting symptom.

Roentgenography may show extensive involvement of the affected bone. The appearance is usually a mottled combination of sclerosis and lysis. These findings are nonspecific, and Ewing's sarcoma and osteomyelitis may be in the radiographic differential diagnosis.

The histologic picture is a diffuse pattern of small round cells, which show a mixed-cell infiltrate. With Ewing's sarcoma, the cells all tend to be of the same size and shape, but with lymphoma, there is considerable variation.

General Management

Most patients are treated with combination chemotherapy plus radiation therapy over the bony lesion. The structural integrity of the bone may be threatened and prophylactic internal fixation may be indicated. The prognosis depends on the extent of involvement: with solitary bone involvement, at least 70% of patients may be expected to survive long-term.[8]

Other Malignant Bone Neoplasms

Other rare types of bone malignancy are mentioned briefly.

Parosteal Osteosarcoma

Parosteal osteosarcoma is a relatively low-grade type of sarcoma that tends to occur on the surface of bone, especially on the posterior aspect of the distal femur. Most patients complain of swelling or a mass, which may be present for several years before the patient seeks medical attention. Roentgenographic features are characteristic. The tumor appears to arise on the surface of the bone and tends to encircle the shaft; the periphery of the lesion typically is less mineralized than the base. Medullary bone ordinarily is unaffected except in longstanding or recurrent tumors. Treatment is surgical resection. If the tumor is completely excised, the long-term cure rate is better than 90%. Most authorities agree that chemotherapy is inappropriate in this setting.

Periosteal Osteosarcoma

Periosteal osteosarcoma is another rare tumor arising on the surface of bone.[9] Typically there will be radiating spicules of mineralized tissue, which gives a characteristic roentgenographic picture. Histologically, the lesion is usually a chondroblastic osteosarcoma. By definition, there cannot be medullary bone involvement. This lesion is treated surgically, but the prognosis is not as favorable as with parosteal osteosarcoma. Some feel that chemotherapy is indicated in this setting.

Limb Salvage

The first half of this century saw a number of reports on limb salvage procedures for a variety of malignant bone tumors. In general, these early attempts failed, and the idea of limb salvage was abandoned. By the 1950s, the standard therapy for most malignant bone tumors was dictated by the histologic findings. If the pathologist reported a small round-cell tumor, then the lesion was felt to be amenable to radiation therapy. If, on the other hand, the lesion was felt to be radioresistant, amputation was generally called for. By 1970, approximately 90% of radioresistant malignant bone tumors were being treated by amputation. Today the situation is reversed, and 80% to 90% of radioresistant malignant bone tumors are treated by limb salvage procedures. In addition, many of the radiosensitive tumors previously treated by radiation alone are now being treated by surgery or a combination of surgery and radiation.

The modern era was brought about by a number of factors, not the least of which was better imaging to permit more accurate assessment of the extent of the lesion as well as to enable improved planning for the surgical procedure. The use of neoadjuvant chemotherapy allows time for the manufacture of specialized surgical implants; in addition, surgery is made easier and local control more reliable. Many new and improved surgical procedures are available, and we now have a better understanding of clinicopathologic factors and how they relate to prognosis, which helps in the selection of patients and procedures.

To justify limb salvage, we must be able to provide a functional extremity that is tumor free. Several studies have shown that limb salvage procedures are, in general, safe—that is, patients who undergo limb salvage procedures have local recurrence and overall survival rates that are comparable to those achieved with amputation. The question of functional restoration of the extremity is being studied over time. Some procedures may be expected to fail with time, particularly those involving metallic implants.

Different procedures are currently being assessed by orthopedic oncologists. In general, experts agree that no one procedure is best for every patient, and each situation deserves individual planning. In terms of specific diagnoses, it is probably fair to say that chondrosarcoma is a "surgical" disease with little or no role for adjuvant treatment at present. On the other hand, osteosarcoma is generally treated by both surgery and chemotherapy, whether preoperative, postoperative, or both. Ewing's sarcoma is usually treated by surgery or radiation therapy or, in some instances, both, in conjunction with preoperative and postoperative chemotherapy. Hence, the diagnosis and adjuvant treatment required may influence the extent of surgery required as well as the type of procedure utilized.

Careful preoperative planning and staging is important. It is necessary to define the precise extent of the local disease, which can be done by a number of modalities, including plain films, CT scans, and MRI.

Regarding the type of reconstructive procedure for an individual patient, there are some circumstances in which no reconstruction is necessary. For example, the proximal portion of the fibula can be readily sacrificed, without the need for reconstruction.

A number of prosthetic implants can be utilized, either alone or in conjunction with allografts. Alternatively, an allograft may be used to replace either the end of a long bone or diaphyseal segment of bone.

Many patient factors contribute to determine the particular type of procedure to be utilized. The patient's age is extremely important since future growth should be taken into account in planning for the procedure. If a child has a tumor located near a physeal growth plate, a significant limb discrepancy may result. Fortunately, a number of procedures allow for subsequent equalization of leg lengths.

There are serious potential risks and complication in limb salvage procedures. Two or more operations may be necessary to achieve a stable, functioning limb, and some patients may be better off with an amputation.

References

1. Mirra JM. *Bone tumors: Clinical, Radiographic, and Pathologic Correlations.* Philadelphia, Pa: Lea & Febiger; 1989.

2. Pritchard DJ, Finkel MP, Reilly CA Jr. The etiology of osteosarcoma: a review of current considerations. *Clin Orthop.* 1975;111:14-22.

3. Wilkins RM, Pritchard DJ, Burgert EO Jr, Unni KK. Ewing's sarcoma of bone: experience with 140 patients. *Cancer.* 1986;58:2551-2555.

4. Dahlin DC, Unni KK. *Bone tumors: General Aspects and Data on 8,542 cases.* 4th ed. Springfield, Ill:Thomas;1986.

5. Pritchard DJ, Lunke RJ, Taylor WF, Dahlin DC, Medley BE. Chondrosarcoma: a clinicopathologic and statistical analysis. *Cancer.* 1980;45:149-157.

6. Bjornsson J, Unni KK, Dahlin DC. Clear cell chondrosarcoma of bone: observations in 47 cases. *Am J Surg Pathol.* 1984;8:223-230.

7. Huvos AG, Rosen G, Dabska M, Marcove RC. Mesenchymal chondrosarcoma: a clinicopathologic analysis of 35 patients with emphasis on treatment. *Cancer.* 1983;51:1230-1237.

8. Mendenhall NP, Jones JJ, Kramer BS, et al. The management of primary lymphoma of bone. *Radiother Oncol.* 1987;9:137-145.

9. Ritts GD, Pritchard DJ, Unni KK, et al. Periosteal osteosarcoma. *Clin Orthop.* 1987;219:299-307.

Suggested Readings

Bacci G, Springfield D, Capanna R, et al. Neoadjuvant chemotherapy for osteosarcoma of the extremity. *Clin Orthop.* 1987;224:268-276.

Evans R, Nesbit M, Askin F, et al. Local recurrence, rate and sites of metastases, and time to relapse as a function of treatment regimen, size of primary, and surgical history in 62 patients presenting with nonmetastatic Ewing's sarcoma of the pelvic bones. *Int J Radiat Oncol Biol Phys.* 1985;11:129-136.

Glaubiger DL, Mackuch RW, Schwarz J. Influence of prognostic factors on survival in Ewing's sarcoma. NCI Monograph 1981;56:285-288.

Hall RB, Robinson LH, Malawar MM, Dunham WK. Periosteal osteosarcoma. *Cancer.* 1985;55:165-171.

Han MT, Telander RL, Pairolero PC, et al. Aggressive thoracotomy for pulmonary metastatic osteogenic sarcoma in children and young adolescents. *J Pediatr Surg.* 1981;16:928-933.

Jaffe, N. Chemotherapy for malignant bone tumors. *Orthop Clin North Am.* 1989;20:487-503.

Link MP, Goorin AM, Miser W, et al. The effect of adjuvant chemotherapy on relapse-free survival in patients with osteosarcoma of the extremity. *N Engl J Med.* 1986;314:1600-1606.

Mankin HJ, Gebhardt MC. Advances in the management of bone tumors. *Clin Orthop.* 1985;200:73-84.

Miser JS, Kinsella TJ, Triche TJ, et al. Preliminary results of treatment of Ewing's sarcoma of bone in children and young adults: six months of intensive combined modality therapy without maintenance. *J Clin Oncol.* 1988;6:484-490.

Pritchard DJ. Small round-cell tumors. In: Evarts CM, ed. *Surgery of the Musculoskeletal System.* 2nd ed. New York, NY: Churchill Livingstone; 1990:4853-4893.

Pritchard DJ, Dahlin DC, Dauphine RT, et al. Ewing's sarcoma: a clinicopathologic and statistical analysis of patients surviving five years or longer. *J Bone Joint Surg.* 1975;57A:10-16.

Rosen G. Neoadjuvant chemotherapy for osteogenic sarcoma: a model for the treatment of other highly malignant neoplasms. *Recent Results Cancer Res.* 1986;103:148-157.

Sailer SL, Harmon DC, Mankin HJ, et al. Ewing's sarcoma: surgical resection as a prognosis factor. *Int J Radiat Oncol Biol Phys.* 1988;15:43-52.

27

SOFT TISSUE SARCOMAS

Kevin C. Conlon, MD, Murray F. Brennan, MD

Soft tissue sarcomas constitute a heterogeneous group of malignant tumors that share a common origin in mesenchymal tissue. These tumors are relatively uncommon and provide an extraordinary opportunity for an organized multimodality therapeutic approach.

Incidence and Demographics

Soft tissue sarcomas account for only 1% of all malignant tumors in adults. In 1991 there were approximately 6,000 new cases of soft tissue sarcoma in the United States; the age-adjusted incidence was approximately 2 per 100,000. An estimated 3,300 will die of the disease.[1] Both the incidence and mortality from soft tissue sarcoma in the US appear to be unchanged in recent years. Soft tissue sarcomas have an equal sex distribution, and show no predilection for any particular age group.

At Memorial Sloan-Kettering Cancer Center (MSKCC), a prospective data base for all adult patients (age >16 years) admitted and treated for soft tissue sarcoma was begun in 1982. From July 1, 1982, through May 1, 1992, a total of 1,957 patients with a histologically confirmed diagnosis of soft tissue sarcoma were admitted. Their ages ranged from 16 to 92 years (median, 50 years). There were 1,050 male and 907 female patients (ratio, 1.2:1). Whites comprised 90%; blacks, 6%; and other races, 4%.

The most common sites of initial presentation were the extremities (52%), with 37% in the lower extremity and 15% in the upper extremity (Fig 27-1). Intra-abdominal and retroperitoneal tumors accounted for 14%, visceral tumors for 13%, and truncal tumors for 9%, with thoracic (5%), head and neck (5%), and genitourinary (2%) cancers accounting for the rest.

The histologic types of soft tissue tumors vary. The most common types are liposarcoma (23%), leiomyosarcoma (18%), malignant fibrous histiocytoma (18%), fibrosarcoma (9%), and synovial sarcoma (8%) (Fig 27-2). The histologic subtypes *hemangiosarcoma, lymphangiosarcoma,* and *malignant hemangiopericytoma* are generally classified as vascular soft-tissue sarcomas, accounting for <5% of

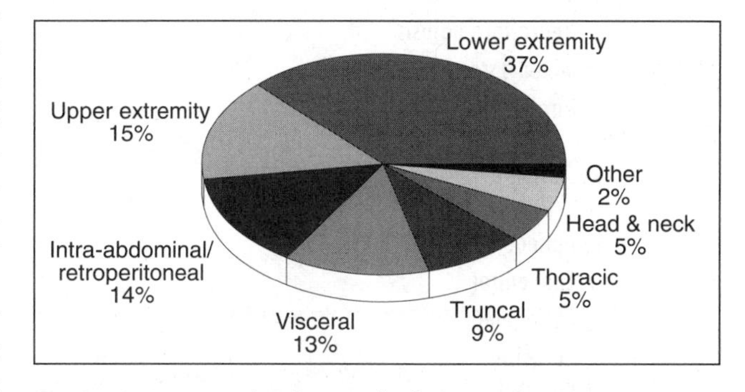

Fig 27-1. Anatomic distribution of soft tissue sarcomas presenting to Memorial Sloan-Kettering Cancer Center between 7/1/82 and 5/1/92 (N = 1,957).

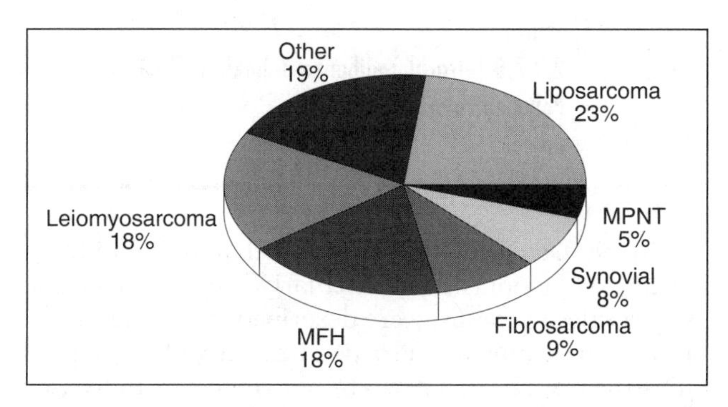

Fig 27-2. Histopathology of soft tissue sarcomas for patients admitted between 7/1/82 and 5/1/92 (N = 1,957). MFH = malignant fibrous histiocytoma, MPNT = malignant peripheral nerve tumor.

Kevin C. Conlon, MD, Attending Surgeon, Memorial Sloan-Kettering Cancer Center, New York, New York

Murray F. Brennan, MD, Chairman, Department of Surgery, Memorial Sloan-Kettering Cancer Center, New York, New York

such tumors in adults. The frequency of a particular histologic type depends on the anatomic location of the tumor. Liposarcomas, malignant fibrous histiocytomas, synovial sarcomas, and fibrosarcomas tend to predominate in the extremities and head and neck. In the retroperitoneum, liposarcomas and leiomyosarcomas are most common. Leiomyosarcomas account for almost all visceral sarcomas. The stomach is the commonest site for leiomyosarcomas (47% to 50%), followed by the small bowel (30% to 35%), colon/rectum (12% to 15%), and esophagus (5%). Malignant fibrous histiocytoma, hemangiopericytoma, and malignant peripheral nerve sheath tumor have also been described, but are very rare.

Etiology

The etiology of soft tissue sarcomas is unknown at present, although many genetic, environmental, and iatrogenic factors have been implicated (Table 27-1).

Table 27-1. Factors Implicated in the Etiology of Soft Tissue Sarcomas

Factors
Genetic
Neurofibromatosis
Mixed sarcoma syndromes
Gardner's syndrome
Radiation exposure
Lymphedema
Congenital
Latrogenic
Parasitic
Surgical
Trauma
Desmoid tumors
Chemical
2,3,7,8-Tetrachlorodibenzo-p-dioxin (TCDD)
Polyvinylchloride
Arsenic

In 1969, a cohort of families with a high incidence of diverse neoplasms, particularly breast cancer and soft tissue sarcomas, were described as having the Li-Fraumeni syndrome. Prospective study of these families over a 12-year period confirmed the increased frequency of neoplasia and suggested an autosomal dominant pattern of inheritance.[2] Recent studies have noted an increased frequency of germ line mutations of the p53 tumor suppressor gene in patients with the Li-Fraumeni syndrome. Mutations of the p53 gene are uncommon in patients with sporadic sarcoma. However, in those with a previous history of malignancy or a strong family history of cancer (but insufficient for the Li-Fraumeni syndrome), germ line mutations of p53 may be more frequent than previously thought. An increased incidence of cancer (of the breast, bone, joint, or soft tissue) in survivors of childhood soft tissue sarcomas and their first-degree relatives has also been noted, suggesting that risk of a second tumor is associated with a family predisposition to cancer.

Familial syndromes, particularly neurofibromatosis (Recklinghausen's disease), have been suggested as predisposing factors. Malignant peripheral nerve sheath tumors develop in 2% to 3% of patients with hereditary neurofibromatosis. Patients with Gardner's syndrome have an increased risk of developing intra-abdominal desmoid tumors (low-grade fibrosarcomas).

Trauma has been implicated in the pathogenesis of soft tissue sarcomas. In the majority of cases, however, it is likely that the trauma merely calls attention to a preexisting mass. Desmoids may be an exception. In a recent review, 8 of 12 abdominal wall desmoids occurred in patients with an antecedent history of trauma or recent pregnancy.[3] This raises the conjecture that abdominal wall desmoids in women may be in some way related to the hormonal milieu. This observation has led to attempts to treat desmoids with estrogen or anti-estrogen therapy.

An association between radiation exposure and the development of soft tissue sarcomas has been recognized for many years. Radiation-associated sarcomas are uncommon, accounting for <3% of all soft tissue sarcomas; they occur most frequently following treatment of breast cancer, lymphoma, or carcinoma of the cervix. There is generally a long latency period (>10 years) between exposure to radiation and development of a sarcoma. However, this delay appears to be age related, with older patients having a shorter latency period. The type (orthovoltage or megavoltage) and dose of the initial radiation may also influence the latency period.

Lymphangiosarcoma has been described in traumatic, idiopathic, congenital, and chronic filarial lymphedema. By increasing the risk of developing lymphedema after mastectomy and axillary lymphadenectomy, radiotherapy may be a contributing factor.

Controversy exists as to the importance of herbicidal exposure in the development of soft tissue sarcomas. Case-control studies from Europe have demonstrated an increased risk of soft tissue sarcomas among farmers and forestry and railroad workers exposed to phenoxyherbicides and chlorophenols. These results are supported by data from an international historical cohort study of 18,910 production workers and sprayers, which demonstrated a nine-fold excess of sarcomas among the sprayers. An increased incidence of soft tissue sarcomas was also seen in a cohort of 1,520 industrial workers exposed for more than one year to 2,3,7,8-tetrachlorodibenzo-p-dioxin (TCDD). However, other studies have failed to substantiate these findings. An analysis of >350,000 Swedish agricultural and forestry workers did not demonstrate an increased risk. A further study of 20,245 Swedish licensed pesticide applicators also failed to confirm the association between herbicidal exposure and soft tissue sarcomas.

The Selected Cancers Cooperative Study Group has performed a population-based, case-control study to assess the risk of soft tissue sarcomas in Vietnam veterans, including those potentially exposed to the herbicide agent orange, which contains dioxin. This study demonstrated no increased risk for the development of sarcomas among any subset of veterans compared with control groups.

Clinical Features and Diagnosis

The majority of patients with extremity lesions present to a physician within a few weeks of discovery of a mass. The mass is usually asymptomatic. However, one third will have a painful swelling as the dominant clinical feature. Pain without a palpable mass is an unusual initial complaint. While many patients report an antecedent history of trauma, the etiologic significance is unclear.

In contrast to extremity sarcomas, clinical presentation of retroperitoneal or visceral sarcomas is usually delayed until the tumor has attained a considerable size. The average duration of symptoms before seeing a physician is approximately 6 months. Patients present with a variety of symptoms, which to an extent depend on the site of the tumor. For retroperitoneal lesions, the most common presenting symptom is abdominal pain, which is often vague and nonspecific. Neurologic symptoms, primarily paresthesias, occur in up to 30% of patients. Significant weight loss is seen in <15%. Early satiety, nausea, and vomiting occur in <40%. Dysphagia, regurgitation, retrosternal chest pain, and weight loss are common presenting complaints of esophageal tumors. Gastric sarcomas frequently present with acute or chronic hemorrhage, dyspeptic symptoms, or the presence of a mass. Abdominal pain, chronic hemorrhage, intestinal obstruction, or perforation occurs more commonly with intestinal tumors. Rectal bleeding and tenesmus are seen with sarcomas of the rectum. Despite the nonspecific nature of these symptoms, they often precipitate radiologic or endoscopic procedures that yield valuable preoperative information.

For extremity lesions, clinical evaluation is directed at determining location, approximate size, and depth (with regard to fascia) of the tumor. Possible bone and neurovascular involvement should be assessed. The status of regional lymph nodes, although infrequently involved, should also be assessed.

Some 50% to 75% of patients with retroperitoneal or visceral sarcoma will have a palpable abdominal mass at presentation. An additional one third of patients will have evidence of increased abdominal girth. The differential diagnosis includes malignant lymphoma, urogenital neoplasms, and extension from adrenal, colonic, pancreatic, or renal tumors. Benign lesions such as hemangiomas, lipomas, lymphangiomas, neuromas, and retroperitoneal cysts account for approximately 12% of retroperitoneal masses. Appropriate preoperative investigations (such as alpha fetoprotein and beta human chorionic gonadotropin, testicular ultrasound for germ cell tumors, and hematologic work-up for lymphomas) can distinguish the majority of these conditions.

Biopsy is a crucial step in the diagnostic algorithm for extremity tumors (Fig 27-3). The method of obtaining tissue is critical (Fig 27-4). Fine needle aspiration rarely establishes a diagnosis of a specific sarcoma type and is grossly inadequate for histopathologic subtyping or assessment of grade. In contrast, a Tru-cut® biopsy,

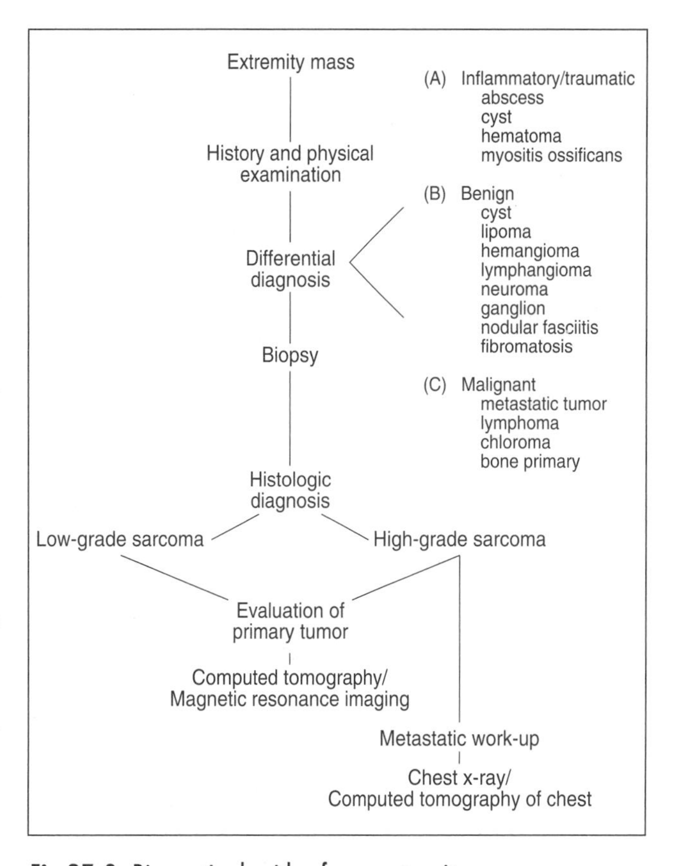

Fig 27-3. Diagnostic algorithm for an extremity mass.

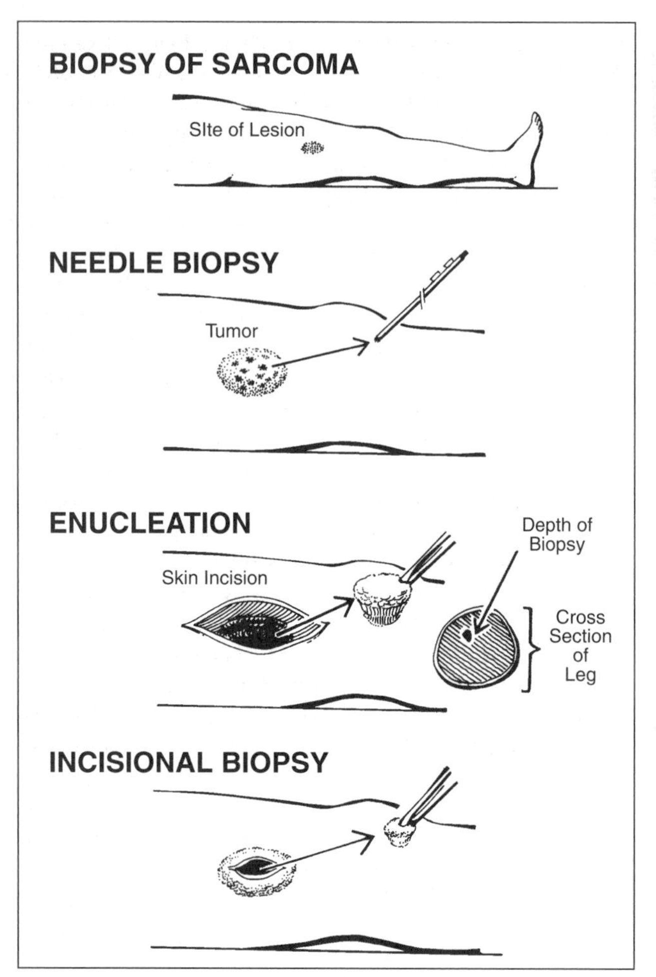

Fig 27-4. Types of biopsy. From Shiu and Brennan.[4]

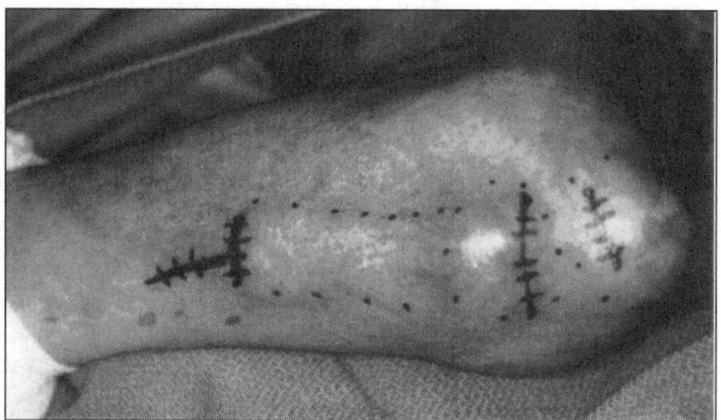

Fig 27-5. Misplaced transverse biopsy incisions. Potentially involved skin is included. Poorly placed incisions and multiple recurrences due to inadequate surgery result in the need for major reconstruction.

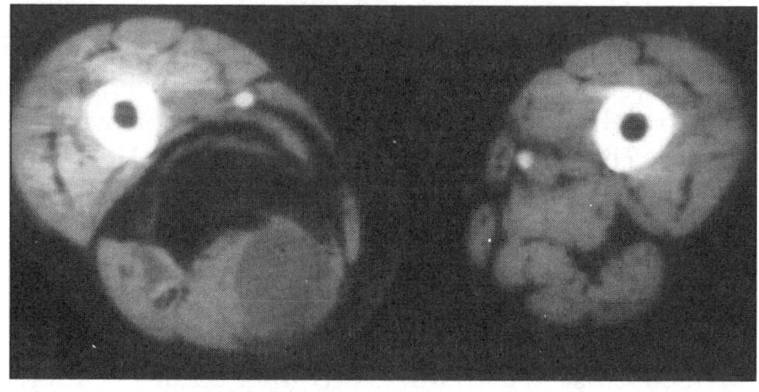

Fig 27-6. CT scan of a large, low-grade myxoid liposarcoma of the posterior thigh in a 69-year-old man.

which yields a core of tissue, is highly sensitive in the diagnosis of soft tissue sarcoma. A well-planned biopsy, with the site selected so as to avoid cystic or necrotic areas of the tumor, allows for adequate tissue sampling. Tumor subtype and grade can be determined accurately from the specimen. Traditionally, an open biopsy has been the procedure of choice. A generous sample of tissue is obtained, allowing an accurate histopathologic diagnosis to be made. Excisional biopsy, or enucleation, is indicated only for small superficial lesions. For larger lesions, this technique disrupts the pseudocapsule and may compromise the subsequent en bloc resection. An incisional biopsy should be performed for the majority of lesions >3 cm in diameter. The placement of the skin incision is important. A misplaced biopsy incision (Fig 27-5) makes definitive excision more difficult. For most extremity lesions, a longitudinal incision is required. No skin flaps should be raised and dissection kept to a minimum. Meticulous hemostasis is important, as wound drainage or tissue hematoma should be avoided. At the time of definitive surgery, the biopsy site should be fully excised in continuity with the tumor. The specimen is sent fresh and sterile to the pathology department. Immunohistochemistry, electron microscopy, and cytogenetic studies can be performed in addition to conventional light microscopy.

In contrast to extremity lesions, preoperative needle biopsy should not be performed for intra-abdominal sarcomas. However, when the tumor is clearly unresectable or an alternate diagnosis such as lymphoma or germ cell neoplasm is suspected, an open biopsy should be performed. Gross tumor spillage should be avoided, so as not to compromise a subsequent resection.

Once the histogenesis and grade are established for extremity sarcomas, a rational radiologic workup can be accomplished. Computed tomography (CT) remains the most popular diagnostic modality for the assessment of the primary lesion. CT enables noninvasive visualization of the tumor and adjacent structures (Fig 27-6). Comparative studies have demonstrated several advantages for magnetic resonance imaging (MRI) over CT. MRI provides imaging

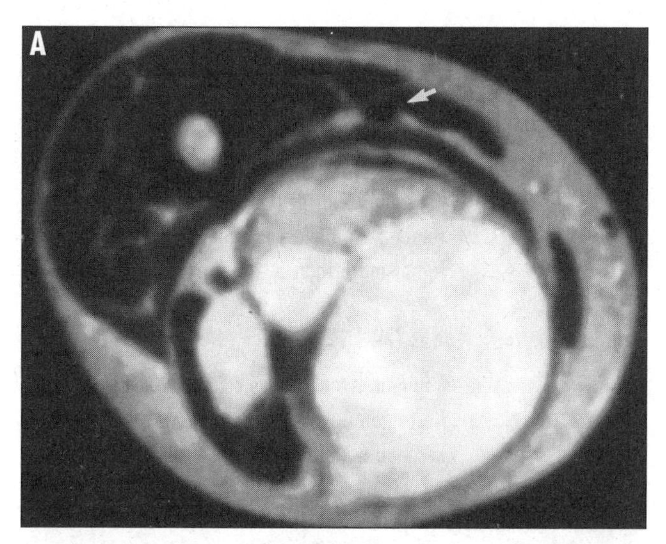

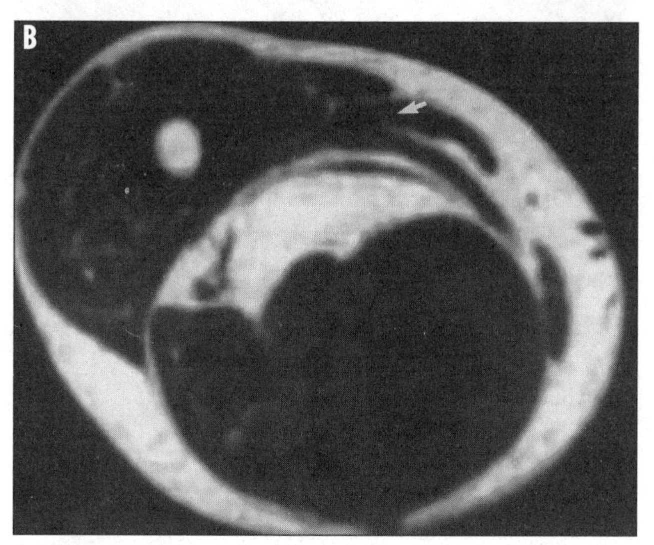

Fig 27-7. T-1 and T-2 weighted magnetic resonance images of the tumor in Fig 27-6. A is T-1; B is T-2. Note the increased signal intensity in the T-1 weighted image and the heterogeneity of the image. The neuromuscular bundle is clearly seen (arrow).

without the use of ionizing radiation or intravenous contrast agents. While both modalities appear equally sensitive in the assessment of tumor size, depth, and relationship to major neurovascular and skeletal structures, the three-dimensional, multiplanar images obtained with MRI appear better at predicting completeness of resection. Currently, MRI is the staging procedure of choice for patients with extremity soft tissue sarcomas at our institution (Fig 27-7).

The extent, size, and anatomic relationships of retroperitoneal and visceral sarcomas can be accurately defined by CT. The presence or absence of hepatic or intraperitoneal metastatic disease can also be assessed. MRI provides coronal, sagittal, and transaxial images of the retroperitoneum, allowing excellent estimation of the configuration, extent, and relationship of the tumor to neurovascular structures and other organs. Recent studies have shown that MRI is superior to CT in delineating tumor, neurovascular, and skeletal relationships. Nonetheless, due to its availability and cost, CT scanning remains the primary diagnostic test in evaluating retroperitoneal tumors. It is our practice to obtain MRI preoperatively when concern exists regarding muscular extension or neurovascular involvement.

Since MRI accurately delineates vascular involvement, angiography is rarely indicated in the preoperative workup. Similarly, as soft tissue sarcomas rarely metastasize to regional nodes, lymphangiography is not indicated.

Nuclear imaging has a limited role in the assessment of sarcomas. Bone scanning has poor specificity and sensitivity in detecting bone invasion and is rarely recommended. Gallium scintigraphy has been demonstrated to have a 96% sensitivity and 87% specificity for detecting malignancy in soft tissue masses.[5] It also can detect occult nonpulmonary metastases. However, it is expensive, provides poor anatomic definition, and does not replace the need for biopsy. Thus, the role for gallium scintigraphy in staging sarcomas is uncertain and unlikely to be of value. Recent studies have suggested that positron emission tomography (PET) may be useful in the assessment of locally recurrent and metastatic disease. However, the cost of the scanner and the requirement for a cyclotron limit this modality to the research setting.

Prior to surgery, a routine chest x-ray should be obtained to exclude metastatic pulmonary disease. Chest CT should be reserved, in general, for patients with abnormalities detected on chest radiographs or patients in whom an extensive and disabling operation is planned.

Histopathology

The pathologic diagnosis and classification of mesenchymal tumors have represented a considerable challenge to the pathologist. Recent advances have enabled a specific histogenesis to be determined for the majority of tumors using a combination of light microscopy, immunohistochemistry, electron microscopy, and chromosomal studies. Advances in immunohistochemistry particularly have contributed to precise identification. Tissue-specific markers help distinguish tumors of myogenic, neurogenic, or epithelial origin. Several soft tissue sarcomas demonstrate specific cytogenic abnormalities that may have diagnostic utility. These include chromosomal translocations in synovial sarcomas (X;18), alveolar rhabdomyosarcoma (2;13), and myxoid liposarcoma (12;16). The absence of specific cytogenic aberrations may also be useful in confirming the diagnosis of some leiomyosarcomas, malignant fibrous histiocytomas, and malignant peripheral nerve sheath tumors.

Histologic grade is the single best prognostic indicator for the development of recurrent disease and eventual outcome. The criteria for histopathologic grading is somewhat subjective. At MSKCC, histopathologic grading is based on a number of parameters, including degree of tissue differentiation, cellularity, amount of stroma, extent of necrosis, vascularity, and mitotic activity (Table 27-2).[6] Tumors are divided into low-grade or high-grade lesions. This simplified system differs from the American Joint Committee on Cancer (AJCC) classification, which also includes two intermediate histologic grades.

Table 27-2. Guidelines to Histologic Grading of Sarcomas

Low-Grade Sarcomas	High-Grade Sarcomas
Good differentiation	Poor differentiation
Hypocellular	Hypercellular
Increased stroma	Minimal stroma
Hypovascular	Hypervascular
Minimal necrosis	Much necrosis
<5 mitoses per 10 HPF*	>5 mitoses per 10 HPF*

*high-power field

From Hajdu et al.[6]

Along with morphologic grade, the estimation of nuclear DNA content and identification of altered gene expression have been shown to have prognostic significance. In high-grade extremity sarcomas, DNA aneuploidy is a negative prognostic factor. Unfavorable clinical outcome has also been predicted by decreased expression of the retinoblastoma susceptibility (Rb) gene, a tumor suppressor gene, in a group of patients with high-grade sarcomas.[7]

Staging

For rational treatment planning, a staging system is required to provide prognostic information on the likelihood of recurrence or metastasis, and to enable meaningful comparison of inter-institutional results. The staging system, proposed by the American Joint Committee on Cancer Staging (AJCC), is based on four variables: histologic grade, tumor size, regional node involvement, and presence of distant metastases (Table 27-3).[8] Of these variables, histologic grade and the presence of metastases are the most important determinant of stage. Stage IV lesions have either lymphatic or distant metastasis. An alternate system

Table 27-3. TNM Staging for Soft Tissue Sarcomas

Primary Tumor (T)

TX	Primary tumor cannot be assessed
T0	No evidence of primary tumor
T1	Tumor 5 cm or less in greatest dimension
T2	Tumor more than 5 cm in greatest dimension

Regional Lymph Nodes (N)

NX	Regional lymph nodes cannot be assessed
N0	No regional lymph node metastasis
N1	Regional lymph node metastasis

Distant Metastasis (M)

MX	Presence of distant metastasis cannot be assessed
M0	No distant metastasis
M1	Distant metastasis

Stage Grouping

Stage IA	G1	T1	N0	M0
Stage IB	G1	T2	N0	M0
Stage IIA	G2	T1	N0	M0
Stage IIB	G2	T2	N0	M0
Stage IIIA	G3,4	T1	N0	M0
Stage IIIB	G3,4	T2	N0	M0
Stage IVA	Any G	Any T	N1	M0
Stage IVB	Any G	Any T	Any N	M1

Histopathologic Grade (G)

GX	Grade cannot be assessed
G1	Well differentiated
G2	Moderately differentiated
G3	Poorly differentiated
G4	Undifferentiated

From American Joint Committee on Cancer.[8]

is currently employed at MSKCC. This system utilizes the depth of tumor invasion, which is a variable excluded in the AJCC system, in addition to tumor size and grade. The relative impact on outcome of each parameter has been determined from a large retrospective analysis. Disease-free survival (Fig 27-8),[9] overall survival, and freedom from distant metastasis are predicted with significant accuracy with use of

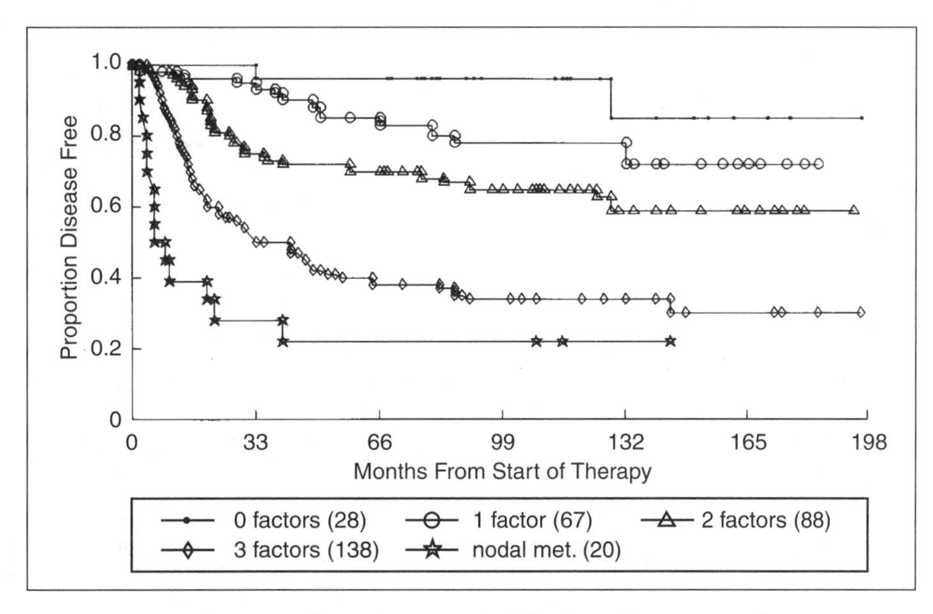

Fig 27-8. Disease-free survival according to number of unfavorable presenting factors. MSKCC experience, 1968-1978; n = 423. Adapted from Gaynor et al.[9]

this system.[9,10] The excellent prognosis (5-year survival rate of >90%) of small, superficial, high-grade sarcomas is evident using this system. In contrast, under the AJCC system, these tumors would be classed as stage III, with an actuarial survival of 29%. It would now seem that grade alone should not determine the categorization of advanced stage if the tumor size is <5 cm.

Prognostic Factors

In an effort to define risk factors for both local recurrence and survival, a retrospective review of 423 patients with an extremity lesion treated at MSKCC between 1968 and 1978 was performed.[10] Of the 196 men and 227 women in the study, 66% presented with a primary tumor and 34% with locally recurrent disease. The lower extremity was the tumor site in 74% of patients, and the upper extremity in 26%. Multivariate analysis identified the following factors associated with an increased risk of local recurrence: age >53 years, presentation with recurrent disease, high histologic grade, limb-sparing surgery, and inadequate surgical margins. Age >53 years, presentation with a painful mass, tumor size >10cm, proximal site, high histologic grade, limb-sparing surgery, and inadequate surgical margins were also independent predictors of poor survival. Embryonal rhabdomyosarcoma, angiosarcoma, and malignant peripheral nerve sheath tumors were unfavorable histologic subtypes for both disease-free and overall survival.

A statistical re-review of this data using Cox models for the rates of tumor mortality, development of distant metastases, local recurrence without metastases, and death following the development of metastases was performed recently.[9] The analysis confirmed the importance of tumor grade, depth, and size with regard to ultimate prognosis. However, the relative prognostic value of each variable changed over time. The effect of histologic grade was initially stronger (in the first 18 months after initial treatment) than either depth or size, with its prognostic value diminishing over time. Grade should, therefore, be given a larger prognostic weight in a staging system based on the risk of early metastatic spread. On the other hand, a clinicopathologic staging system based on ultimate prognosis would give equal emphasis to all three variables.

Prognostic factors were analyzed in 80 patients with primary retroperitoneal soft tissue sarcoma admitted to MSKCC between 1982 and 1988.[11] A complete resection was performed in 62 patients (78%), 16 patients had a partial resection, and 2 underwent biopsy only. Tumors were more likely resectable in women, and least likely resectable if they were midline. Resectability was not associated with age, presentation, or histopathologic features. There was a difference in both disease-free and overall survival rates between patients who underwent a complete resection and those with partially or unresected tumors. This difference was significant only in the subset of patients completely resected with high-grade tumors (Fig 27-9). Tumor size and histopathologic subtype were not prognostic variables. In patients with complete resection, the type of operation, surgical or microscopic margins, and use of adjuvant chemotherapy or radiotherapy were not determinants of survival.

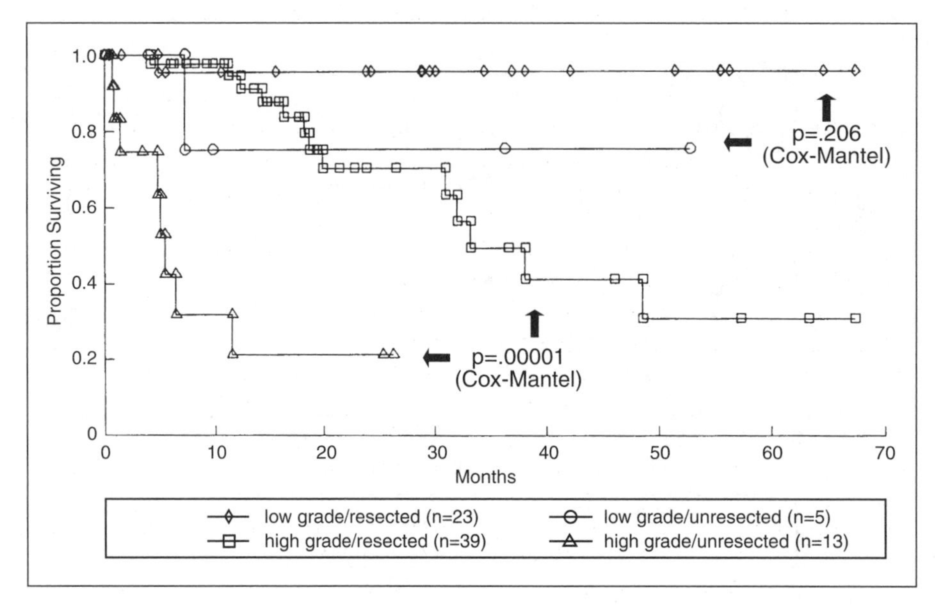

Fig 27-9. Survival in patients with retroperitoneal sarcoma depends on resectability and grade. From Bevilacqua et al.[11]

In a recent review from the MD Anderson Cancer Center of 191 patients with a visceral sarcoma, complete surgical excision without tumor spillage, localized lesions, low histologic grade, and small tumors were found on univariate analysis to be prognostic factors.[12] However, multivariate analysis showed that only the type of surgery was a significant prognostic factor. Patients with a complete resection of localized disease survived a median of 46 months, compared with 21 months for patients with incomplete resections. An overall 5-year survival rate of 65% was reported by MSKCC.[13] Tumor size >5 cm in diameter, extra-intestinal invasion or perforation, and a high histologic grade of malignancy were considered important clinicopathologic factors influencing prognosis. The presence of none, one, two, or three of these factors was associated with 5-year survival rates of 100%, 44%, 31%, and 0%, respectively.

For vascular sarcomas, unlike other sarcomas, histopathologic type or grade, tumor size, and depth of penetration were not significant prognostic variables. Complete excision of all gross disease and the presence of metastasis were the only factors noted to influence survival.[14]

Treatment and Outcome

The management of soft tissue sarcomas has evolved considerably in recent years. Surgery remains the primary treatment modality; however, an increasing number of patients are now receiving adjuvant radiation or chemotherapy.

Extremity Sarcomas: Surgical Therapy

A greater understanding of the biology of soft tissue sarcomas and the development of effective adjuvant therapies have influenced our current approach to surgery. Resection of the tumor with a wide margin of normal tissue remains the primary objective of the surgeon. Traditionally this has been achieved with amputation, resulting in low local recurrence rates. However, limb-sparing procedures now predominate (Fig 27-10). Due to the microscopic infiltration of the tumor beyond the pseudocapsule, marginal excision or enucleation alone is inadequate, resulting in local recurrence in 65% to 90% of cases. Wide-margin excision—ie, the tumor plus 2-3 cm of normal tissue—improves local control, reducing local failure rates to approximately 30%. Using the prognostic factors previously identified, patients at higher risk for local recurrence can be identified. These patients should receive adjuvant therapy. More radical surgery, such as formal compartmental resection, which sacrifices entire muscle groups and often adjacent neurovascular structures, does not obviate the need for adjuvant therapy, and is required only in selected patients.

Extremity Sarcomas: Radiation and Chemotherapy

Early work suggested that soft tissue sarcomas as a group were radioresistant. However, this appears to have been due to inadequate dose administration rather than biologic resistance. Studies published in the early 1980s demonstrated that external beam radiation administrated following conservative surgery

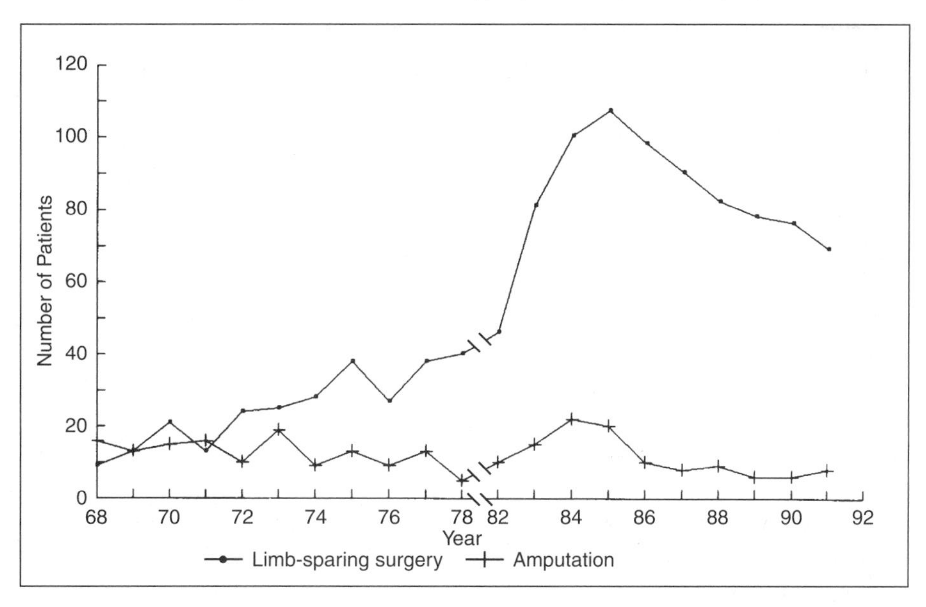

Fig 27-10. Surgical management of extremity soft tissue sarcomas at MSKCC between 1968 and 1991.

(usually wide local excision) reduced local recurrence in irradiated patients compared with non-irradiated controls. A prospective randomized trial from the National Cancer Institute (NCI) in patients with high-grade extremity sarcomas compared amputation to limb-sparing surgery and postoperative radiation therapy.[15] All patients received adjuvant chemotherapy. No difference in 5-year disease-free or overall survival was seen between the two treatment groups. This study supported the concept that limb function could be preserved while maintaining local control by combining a less radical surgical approach with adjuvant radiation therapy. It appears that the benefit of radiation therapy accrues from control of microscopic foci of disease. In a study from the University of California, San Francisco, 3 of 22 patients (14%) with a positive surgical margin who received 5,500 to 7,000 cGy external beam irradiation postoperatively developed a local recurrence. In contrast, 79% of non-irradiated patients with positive margins developed a local recurrence.[16]

Brachytherapy, an alternate method of radiation delivery, has been extensively investigated.[17] It involves either the permanent placement of radioactive sources (eg, iodine 131, gold 98), or the temporary placement of afterloading catheters into the tumor or tumor bed. The catheters are subsequently loaded with radioisotope early in the postoperative period. At our institution the latter technique has been widely utilized with iridium 192 sources. This methodology permits the delivery of high doses of radiation (4,500 to 6,000 cGy) locally to the tumor bed over a short period of time, usually 4-5 days. Reports from our institution have demonstrated its efficacy combined with surgical resection for locally advanced or anatomically unfavorable sarcomas.[18] This method of interstitial irradiation can also be used with surgery in selected patients with recurrent extremity sarcomas who have received prior external beam radiotherapy.

The benefit of chemotherapy in the adjuvant setting is not known at present. The exciting results of systemic chemotherapy obtained in pediatric embryonal rhabdomyosarcoma have not been translated to the adult population to date. In adults, doxorubicin and ifosfamide have been demonstrated to be the most active agents in widely disseminated soft tissue sarcoma. Response rates of 15% to 35% are seen with doxorubicin alone. The majority of studies using single-agent doxorubicin have failed to show an improvement in either disease-free or overall survival in patients receiving postoperative chemotherapy compared with surgery alone. In a trial from the Istituto Ortopedico Rizzoli, improvement in 3-year actuarial disease-free (42% vs 68%, $P<.05$) and overall survival rates (68% vs 86%, $P<.05$) was noted in patients with high-grade extremity lesions receiving postoperative adjuvant doxorubicin.[19] However, this benefit appeared restricted to patients undergoing amputation.

Several prospective randomized trials evaluating combination chemotherapy in patients with extremity soft tissue sarcoma have been reported (Table 27-4). The majority of these studies have included all sites, but subset analyses of the extremity lesions have been performed.

Table 27-4. Combination Adjuvant Chemotherapy for Extremity Soft Tissue Sarcomas: Randomized Trials

Group	Regimen	N	MFU (m)	% Disease-free* Tx	% Disease-free* no-Tx	% Survival* Tx	% Survival* no-Tx
MD Anderson	ACVAd	43	120	54	35	65	36
Mayo Clinic	AVDAd	48	64	88	67	83	63
EORTC	ACVD	233	44	67	52	79	74
NCI	ACMx	67	85	75	54	83	60
	AC	47	53	72	—	75	—

NCI = National Cancer Institute
EORTC = European Organization for Research and Treatment of Cancer
N = number of patients, MFU = median follow-up (months)
* = 5-year, Tx = chemotherapy, no-Tx = no chemotherapy
A = doxorubicin, Ad = actinomycin D,
C = cyclophosphamide, D = dacarbazine (DTIC)
Mtx = high-dose methotrexate, V = vincristine.

Outcome

The actuarial 5-year survival for patients with extremity soft tissue sarcoma treated at our institution is 60% (Fig 27-11). Tumor size and histologic grade affect survival (Figs 27-12 and 27-13). Depth in relation to the muscle fascia is also a significant variable, with deep lesions having a decreased survival ($P<.00001$). Small superficial lesions irrespective of histologic grade are associated with an excellent prognosis, with a 5-year survival of >90%. In contrast, patients with large (>10 cm), proximal, high-grade tumors have a much poorer prognosis, with an estimated 5-year survival of 30% in 1992.

The relationship between local failure and the development of distant metastases is controversial. In an effort to define the effect of radiotherapy on local recurrence, a prospective randomized trial was performed at our institution between 1982 and 1987 to

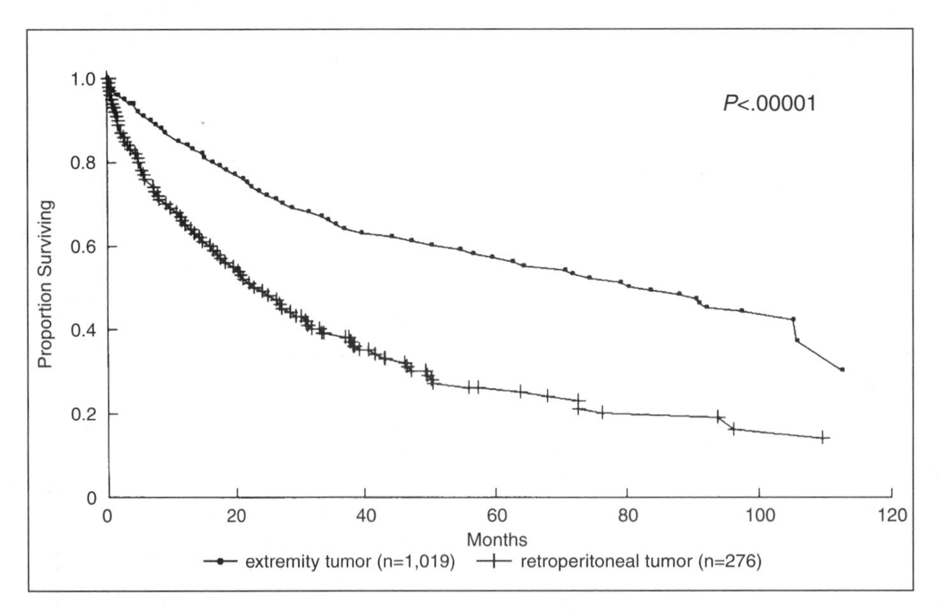

Fig 27-11. Survival by site for soft tissue sarcomas. Patients with a primary tumor of the extremity have a better survival than those with a retroperitoneal tumor ($P<.00001$). Univariate analysis, no other factors considered.

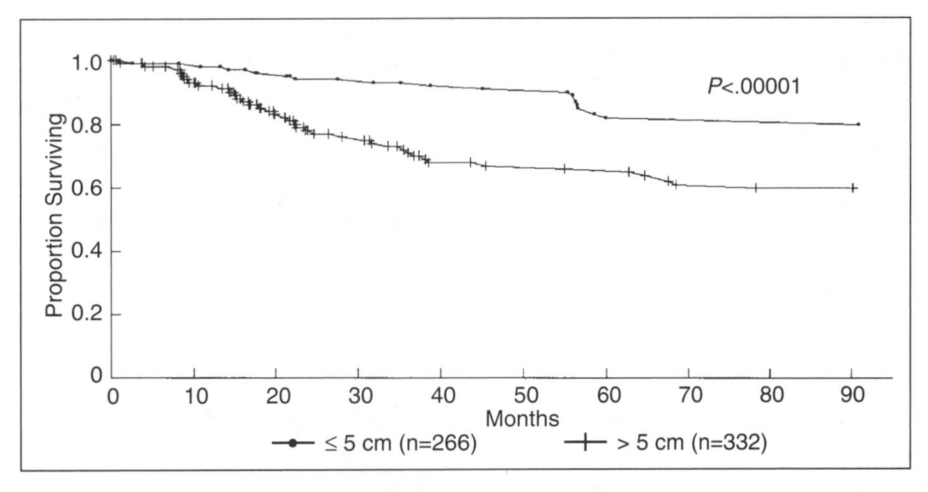

Fig 27-12. Effect of tumor size on overall survival for patients with a primary extremity soft tissue sarcoma (univariate analysis). MSKCC experience, July 1982 - July 1991; follow-up, 1/15/92.

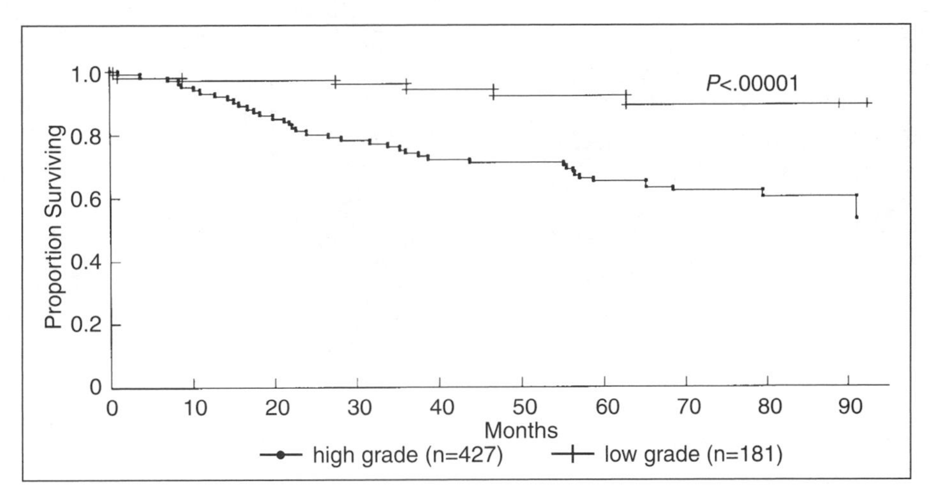

Fig 27-13. Effect of histopathologic grade on overall survival for patients with a primary extremity soft tissue sarcoma (univariate analysis). MSKCC experience, July 1982 - July 1991; follow-up, 1/15/92.

evaluate adjuvant brachytherapy following conservative surgery for extremity soft tissue sarcomas.[20] Patients were stratified according to prognostic criteria, including tumor presentation, size, depth, and histologic grade. A total of 126 patients were randomized to this trial. Brachytherapy (with iridium 192) was administered to 56 patients (44%), while the other 70 received no radiation. Equal numbers of patients in both groups with high-grade lesions received adjuvant doxorubicin chemotherapy. At a median follow-up of 54 months, there was a significant reduction in local recurrence in those receiving brachytherapy. Subset analysis indicated that this effect is due to the impact on local recurrence of high-grade tumors only. The decrease in local recurrence is not accompanied by an improvement in overall survival. This suggests that local recurrence is not a factor in survival.

Distant metastases usually present within 2 years of the initial diagnosis. High-grade sarcomas are at increased risk of distant disease, whereas only 10% to 15% of low-grade extremity sarcomas develop metastases. In a review of 130 patients with localized low-grade lesions treated at MSKCC between 1968 and 1978, 14% developed distant metastases at a median follow-up of 7.5 years.[21] The median time to metastases was 17 months. The lung is the most frequent site of failure regardless of histologic grade of the primary tumor (Fig 27-14). In selected patients, complete resection of pulmonary lesions is worth-

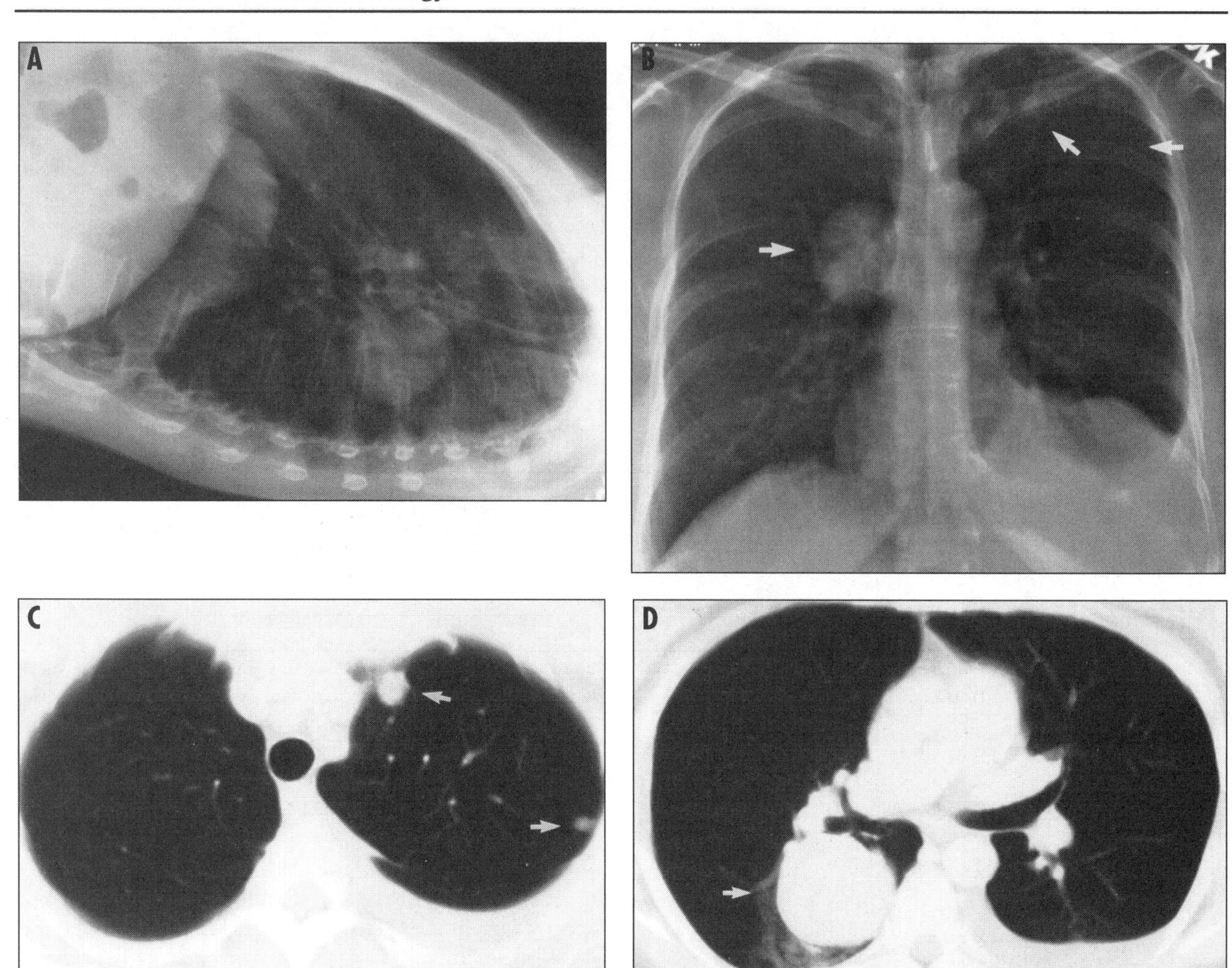

Fig 27-14. Plain radiographs ***A*** and computed tomograms ***B*** of the chest from a 53-year-old woman with recurrent pulmonary metastases (arrow) from a high-grade hemangiopericytoma. The CT scan demonstrates lesions not apparent on the plain radiographs.

while, with long-term disease-free survival being achieved in 25% to 50% of cases. In a recent series from UCLA, 66% of patients were alive after pulmonary metastasectomy at 2 years, compared with <10% survival in patients with unresectable disease.[22] Criteria for resectability include absence of evidence of disease at the primary site, no extrapulmonary metastatic disease, and adequate pulmonary function. Between 1960 and 1983, 208 patients underwent pulmonary resection of metastatic disease at MSKCC.[23] Seventy-two percent had unilateral disease, and 28% bilateral nodules. Wedge or segmental resection accounted for 70% of surgical procedures. Lobectomy was performed in 19%, with pneumonectomy only required in 2%. Depending on the histologic subtype, 5-year survival was 20% and 29%.

Determinants of survival after pulmonary resection include tumor doubling time >20 days, disease-free interval >12 months, and fewer than four nodules on chest CT. Following initial pulmonary metastasectomy, resection of a solitary recurrent metastatic pulmonary nodule can also result in long-term survival. Unfortunately, while selected patients who have curative pulmonary resection can survive over the long term, the overall yield for all patients with pulmonary metastases is low, with <10% of patients being long-term survivors.

Intra-Abdominal Sarcomas: Surgical Treatment

Aggressive surgical extirpation is the mainstay of treatment for primary and recurrent retroperitoneal sarcomas. The aim of surgery should be to completely excise the tumor en bloc with a margin of normal tissue. Extensive local tumor involvement, particularly of the root of the mesentery, vascular invasion, abdominal sarcomatosis, nerve root involvement, and hepatic metastasis are the usual reasons for unresectability. Involvement of adjacent organs is common, and is not, per se, a reason for unresectability. In the most recent series from MSKCC, 83% of patients underwent resection of adjacent organs en bloc with the primary tumor in order to obtain clear margins. The kidney and adrenal gland were the most frequently excised organs (46%), followed by the colon (24%) and pancreas (15%). A major vascular resection occurred in 10% of patients, involving mainly the vena cava or mesenteric vessels. The vena cava can safely be ligated without reconstruction if sufficient collaterals have developed. Because of the possibility of renal or colonic resection, all patients should have their renal status assessed and undergo a complete bowel preparation preoperatively. An extensive lymphadenectomy is not required, as lymphatic involvement occurs in <5% of patients.

The role of palliative resection or "debulking," is controversial. Compared with biopsy alone, no improvement in survival is achieved by partial resection.[24] Partial resection should be reserved for particular cases in which symptomatic palliation can be achieved either by relieving gastrointestinal or urinary obstruction or decreasing the size of an intra-abdominal mass. In these carefully selected cases, prolonged palliation may be obtained with surgery.

Clinical presentation, anatomic site, size, and extent of the tumor determine surgical therapy for visceral sarcomas. For localized gastric lesions, wedge resection of the primary tumor results in overall and disease-free survival rates similar to those achieved with more extensive procedures. Larger gastric lesions may require subtotal or total gastrectomy, with resection of contiguous organs to remove all gross disease. Pancreaticoduodenectomy may be required for sarcomas of the duodenum. Tumors of the small bowel and colon can be excised with a standard segmental resection. Due to the low incidence of nodal metastasis (0% to 15%), a radical mesenteric lymphadenectomy is not required. Small rectal sarcomas can be treated by local excision. Larger lesions may require a low anterior resection, abdominoperineal resection, or total pelvic exenteration to remove all gross disease.

Intra-Abdominal Sarcomas: Radiation and Chemotherapy

Locoregional recurrence in the retroperitoneal space or peritoneum is the predominant pattern of failure following complete surgical resection of retroperitoneal or visceral tumors. Experience with extremity sarcomas suggests that adjuvant radiation therapy could potentially be beneficial at these sites. However, gastrointestinal or neurologic toxicity often limits the delivery of sufficient radiation. As a consequence, the results of radiation therapy have been disappointing. Retrospective studies suggested a benefit for patients treated with postoperative external beam radiation. A prospective randomized trial from the NCI assessed the benefit and morbidity associated with radiotherapy in two groups of patients with resectable retroperitoneal disease.[25] Study participants received either intraoperative radiotherapy (IORT) to 2,000 cGy using high-energy electrons plus low-dose external beam irradiation (3,500 to 4,000 cGy), or standard high-dose postoperative external beam irradiation (5,000 to 5,500 cGy). Morbidity was significant, occurring in 63% of patients, with no difference in frequency between groups. Acute radiation enteritis was more common in the patients receiving high-dose external beam irradiation (60% vs 7%). Four of 15 patients developed delayed peripheral neuropathies after IORT. There was no difference in either disease-free or overall survival rates between the two groups. The 40% overall survival and 20% disease-free survival seen in this trial are similar to results obtained with surgery alone. In a recent series from MSKCC, 11 of 43 patients who underwent complete surgical resection received adjuvant radiotherapy (~4,500 cGy).[24] No benefit in either disease-free or overall survival could be demonstrated in this group compared with non-irradiated patients.

Similar disappointing results have been seen with visceral lesions. Because of the lack of demonstrated efficacy and potential morbidity, routine radiotherapy following complete excision of retroperitoneal or visceral sarcomas cannot be recommended. Radiation therapy for patients with unresectable disease appears to have minimal effect on local control or progression of disease. It should be utilized only in selected cases for symptomatic palliation.

The only published randomized prospective trial evaluating chemotherapy for resectable retroperitoneal sarcomas was from the NCI in 1985.[26] All patients underwent a complete surgical resection plus postoperative radiotherapy with or without adjuvant chemotherapy (doxorubicin, cyclophosphamide, and methotrexate). Despite considerable morbidity, no improvement in survival was noted. Analysis of the MSKCC experience with doxorubicin-based adjuvant chemotherapy has failed to demonstrate any effect of chemotherapy on survival.[12] Current interest lies with high dose-intensity chemotherapy utilizing recombinant human granulocyte-macrophage colony stimulating factors (rhGM-CSF) to ameliorate myelosuppression. Preliminary data from the European Organization for Research and Treatment of Cancer (EORTC) Soft Tissue and Bone Sarcoma Group phase II trial have demonstrated a 50% response rate (complete response rate of 17%) in patients with inoperable soft tissue sarcoma given high-dose doxorubicin and ifosfamide with rhGM-CSF.[27]

Outcome

Between 1982 and 1987, 114 patients were explored for retroperitoneal sarcomas at MSKCC.[24] Sixty-three patients presented with a primary tumor, while 51 had recurrent disease. Complete resection was possible in 65% of primary tumors. A partial resection was performed in 14%, and 21% were unresectable. A complete resection was possible in 51% of patients presenting with recurrent disease. Patients undergoing a complete resection had an actuarial 5-year survival of 74%, compared with 35% after partial resection and 15% for those with unresectable disease. Recent surgical studies confirm the poor outcome associated with partial resection.

In the MSKCC series at 31 months' median follow-up, 49% of patients had developed recurrences, the majority of which were locoregional. The median time to recurrence was 15 months for high-grade tumors and 42 months for low-grade lesions (Fig 27-15). This identifies a time period for careful clinical follow-up. All patients should be evaluated every 2 to 3 months, with a CT or MRI scan obtained at 6-month intervals for 3 to 4 years. Any symptoms suggestive of recurrence should be investigated promptly, as resection of recurrent disease may be associated with prolonged survival. In the MSKCC experience, median survival after complete resection of recurrent tumor was 48 months, compared with 15 months in patients with unresectable disease.

The median interval to recurrence for patients with visceral sarcomas after curative treatment varies from 18 months to 2 years. Intra-abdominal sarcomatosis is the most common cause of death. In patients with distant metastasis, the liver is the most frequent site of disease (>65% of cases). Extra-abdominal disease, while present in up to 30% of patients at death, is an unusual site of first recurrence (<10% of cases). In those who do develop extra-abdominal disease, the lung and bone are the predominant sites. The patterns of failure suggest that the initial postoperative surveillance should concentrate on the abdomen, since extra-abdominal disease appears at a late stage of disease progression.

Specific Soft Tissue Sarcomas

Head and Neck Sarcomas

Soft tissue sarcomas of the head and neck are rare, representing <1% of all malignancies of the head and neck in adults. A primary lesion in the head and neck was found in 5% of adult patients admitted with soft tissue sarcomas to our institution between 1982 and 1991. In contrast, 40% of all pediatric soft tissue sarcomas occur in the head and neck. Neuroblastoma and embryonal rhabdomyosarcoma (orbital and nonorbital) are more common in children, while malignant fibrous histiocytoma, leiomyosarcoma, angiosarcoma, and liposarcoma are more frequent in older patients. A retrospective review of the MSKCC experience between 1950 and 1985 showed that histologic grade, tumor size, presence of positive surgical margins, bone involvement, local recurrence, and metastatic spread were associated with an increased risk of treatment failure and decreased survival. Histologic type also appears to have prognostic value, with angiosarcoma and nonorbital rhabdomyosarcoma predicting poor survival.[28]

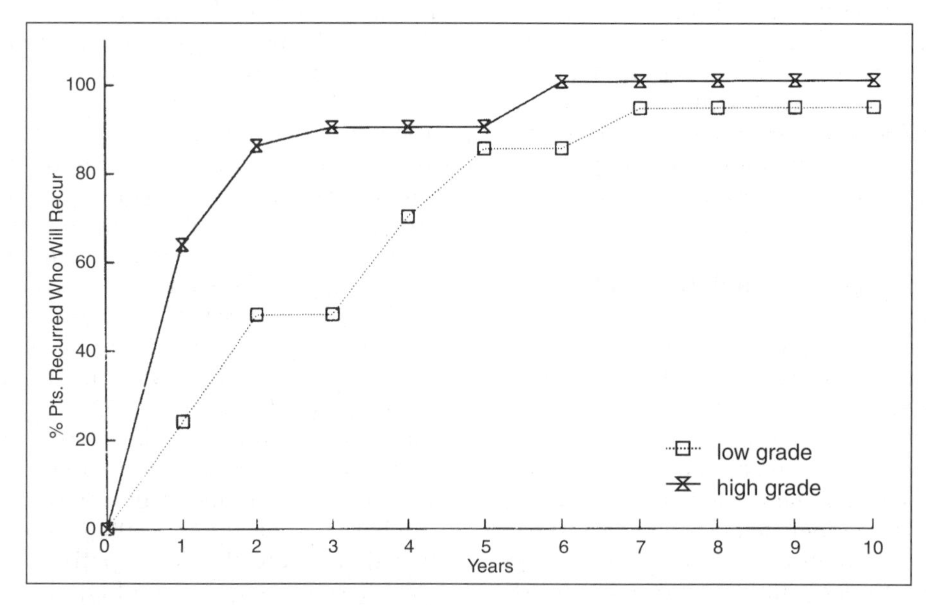

Fig 27-15. Time to recurrence in patients with retroperitoneal sarcomas according to grade. From Jaques et al.[24]

Treatment strategies depend on the age of the patient. In general, a multimodality approach consisting of surgery, chemotherapy, and radiotherapy is utilized in the pediatric age group. The addition of adjuvant chemotherapy to surgery has resulted in an increased overall survival for children with rhabdomyosarcomas. Wide local excision achieving negative surgical margins is the preferred treatment option in adults. A lymphadenectomy is performed only when nodes are clinically suspicious. An elective neck dissection is not required. Radiotherapy should be considered whenever there is doubt as to the adequacy of surgical margins, or when the location of the tumor prevents complete excision. The role of adjuvant chemotherapy has yet to be determined in adults.

Breast Sarcomas

Primary mesenchymal tumors constitute 0.5% to 1% of all primary breast cancers. They should be distinguished from cystosarcoma phyllodes, sarcomatoid carcinoma, and carcinosarcoma. Malignant fibrous histiocytoma, fibrosarcoma, and liposarcoma appear to be the most common histological subtypes.[29] Angiosarcoma appears to occur disproportionally in the breast, compared with other sites. Leiomyosarcoma of the breast is very rare, with only 11 cases reported to date in the literature. Breast sarcomas are usually well circumscribed, large, firm, mobile, and painless. Mammography frequently reveals the mass with well-demarcated edges, in contrast to the usual appearance of breast carcinomas. Diagnosis may be confused with a benign fibroadenoma or cystosarcoma phyllodes.

Because of the rarity of this condition, the prognosis is difficult to determine. Callery reported an actuarial 5-year survival rate of 91% in 25 patients treated at MSKCC between 1949 and 1982.[30] Unlike sarcomas at other sites, tumor size does not appear to be a prognostic determinant.[29] Histologic grade and an infiltrative contour appear to correlate with outcome. A total mastectomy is usually necessary to achieve complete tumor clearance, particularly with angiosarcomas.[29] As sarcomas rarely manifest lymphatic spread, an axillary dissection is not required.[30] Radiation therapy has been recommended when doubt exists as to the adequacy of the surgical margin.[30] However, scant data exist as to its efficacy. The role for adjuvant chemotherapy remains to be determined for mammary sarcomas.

The possible relationship between silicon breast implants and the development of soft tissue sarcomas has generated considerable controversy recently. At present there are no data to support such an association. In our experience, there has been no documented case of a soft tissue sarcoma developing after breast reconstruction with a silicon implant.

References

1. Boring CC, Squires TS, Tong T, Montgomery S. Cancer Statistics, 1994. *CA Cancer J Clin* 1994;44:7-26.

2. Li FP, Fraumeni JF Jr. Prospective study of a family cancer syndrome. *JAMA*. 1982;247:2692-2694.

3. Posner MC, Shiu MH, Newsome JL, Hajdu SI, Gaynor JJ, Brennan MF. The desmoid tumor not a benign disease. *Arch Surg*. 1989;124:191-196.

4. Shiu MH, Brennan MF. Biopsy of soft-tissue sarcoma. In: Shiu MH, Brennan MF, eds. *Surgical Management of Soft-Tissue Sarcomas*. Philadelphia, Pa: Lea & Febiger; 1989: 58-63.

5. Schwartz HS, Jones CK. The efficacy of gallium scintigraphy in detecting malignant soft tissue neoplasms. *Ann Surg*. 1992;215:78-82.

6. Hajdu SI, Shiu MH, Brennan MF. The role of the pathologist in the management of soft tissue sarcomas. *World J Surg*. 1988;12:326-331.

7. Cance WG, Brennan MF, Dudas ME, Huang C-M, Cordon-Cardo C. Altered expression of the retinoblastoma gene product in human sarcomas. *N Engl J Med*. 1990;323:1457-1462.

8. Beahrs OH, Henson DE, Hutter RVP, Kennedy BJ, eds. *American Joint Committee on Cancer Manual for Staging of Cancer*, 4th ed. Philadelphia, Pa: JB Lippincott Co; 1992:131-133.

9. Gaynor JJ, Tan CC, Casper ES, et al. Refinement of clinicopathologic staging for localized soft tissue sarcoma of the extremity: a study of 423 adults. *J Clin Oncol*. 1992;10:1317-1329.

10. Collin CF, Friedrich C, Godbold J, Hajdu S, Brennan MF. Prognostic factors for local recurrence and survival in patients with localized extremity soft tissue sarcoma. *Semin Surg Oncol*. 1988;4:30-37.

11. Bevilacqua RG, Rogatko A, Hajdu SI, Brennan MF. Prognostic factors in primary retroperitoneal soft tissue sarcomas. *Arch Surg*. 1991;126:328-334.

12. Ng E-H, Pollock RE, Munsell MF, Atkinson EN, Romsdahl MM. Prognostic factors influencing survival in gastrointestinal leiomyosarcomas: implications for surgical management and staging. *Ann Surg*. 1992;215:68-77.

13. Karpeh MS Jr, Caldwell C, Gaynor JJ, Hajdu SI, Brennan MF. Vascular soft tissue sarcomas: an analysis of tumor-related mortality. *Arch Surg*. 1991;126:1474-1481.

14. Shiu MH, Farr GH, Egeli RA, Quan SHG, Hajdu SI. Myosarcomas of the small and large intestine: a clinicopathologic study. *J Surg Oncol*. 1983;24:67-72.

15. Rosenberg SA, Tepper J, Glatstein E, et al. The treatment of soft tissue sarcomas of the extremities: prospective randomized evaluations of (1) limb-sparing surgery plus radiation compared with amputation and (2) the role of adjuvant chemotherapy. *Ann Surg*. 1982;196:305-315.

16. Leibel SA, Tranbaugh RF, Wara WM, Beckstead JH, Bovill EG Jr, Phillips TL. Soft tissue sarcomas of the extremities: survival and patterns of failure with conservative surgery and postoperative irradiation compared to surgery alone. *Cancer*. 1982;50:1076-1083.

17. Shiu MH, Hilaris BS, Harrison LB, Brennan MF. Brachytherapy and function-saving resection of soft tissue sarcoma arising in the limb. *Int J Radiat Oncol Biol Phys*. 1991; 21:1485-1492.

18. Zelefsky MJ, Nori D, Shiu MH, Brennan MF. Limb salvage in soft tissue sarcomas involving neurovascular structures using combined surgical resection and brachytherapy. *Int J Radiat Oncol Biol Phys.* 1990;19:913-918.

19. Picci P, Bacci G, Gherlinzoni F, et al. Results of a randomized trial for the treatment of localized soft tissue sarcoma (STS) of the extremities in adult patients. In: Ryan JR, Baker LO, eds. *Recent Concepts in Sarcoma Treatment.* Boston, Mass: Kluwer Academic Publishers; 1988:144-148.

20. Brennan MF, Casper ES, Harrison LB, Shiu MH, Gaynor J, Hajdu SI. The role of multimodality therapy in soft tissue sarcoma. *Ann Surg.* 1991;214:328-338.

21. Donohue JH, Collin C, Friedrich C, Godbold J, Hajdu SI, Brennan MF. Low-grade soft tissue sarcomas of the extremities: analysis of risk factors for metastasis. *Cancer.* 1988;62:184-193.

22. Huth JF, Eilber FR. Patterns of metastatic spread following resection of extremity soft tissue sarcomas and strategies for treatment. *Semin Surg Oncol.* 1988;4:20-26.

23. McCormack PM, Bains MS, Martini N. Surgical management of pulmonary metastases. In: Shiu MH, Brennan MF, eds. *Surgical Management of Soft Tissue Sarcomas.* Philadelphia, Pa: Lea & Febiger; 1989:263-273.

24. Jaques DP, Coit DG, Hajdu SI, Brennan MF. Management of primary and recurrent soft tissue sarcoma of the retroperitoneum. *Ann Surg.* 1990;212:51-59.

25. Kinsella TJ, Sindelar WF, Lack E, Glatstein E, Rosenberg SA. Preliminary results of a randomized study of adjuvant radiation therapy in resectable adult retroperitoneal soft tissue sarcomas. *J Clin Oncol.* 1988;6:18-25.

26. Glenn J, Sindelar WF, Kinsella T, et al. Results of multimodality therapy of resectable soft tissue sarcomas of the retroperitoneum. *Surgery.* 1985;97:316-325.

27. Steward WP, Verweij J, Somers R, et al. High-dose chemotherapy (CT) with two schedules of recombinant human granulocyte-macrophage colony-stimulating factor (rhGM-CSF) in the treatment of advanced adult soft-tissue sarcomas (STS). *Proc Amer Soc Clin Oncol.* 1991;10:349. Abstract.

28. Freedman AM, Reiman HM, Woods JE. Soft tissue sarcomas of the head and neck. *Am J Surg.* 1989;158:367-372.

29. Petrek JA. Other cancers in the breast. In: Harris JR, Hellman S, Henderson IC, Kinne DW, eds. *Breast Diseases.* 2nd ed. Philadelphia, Pa: JB Lippincott Co; 1991;804-809.

30. Callery CD, Rosen PP, Kinne DW. Sarcoma of the breast: a study of 32 patients with reappraisal of classification and therapy. *Ann Surg.* 1985;201:527-532.

28

HODGKIN'S DISEASE AND NON-HODGKIN'S LYMPHOMAS

David S. Rosenthal, MD, and Harmon J. Eyre, MD

The most impressive advances in the treatment of disseminated cancer have been in the management of lymphomas. Indeed, many cases of Hodgkin's disease are now curable. Non-Hodgkin's lymphomas constitute a very large, heterogeneous group of tumors that vary greatly in responsiveness and curability.

The disorders known as malignant lymphomas involve the cells of the lymphatic system and are termed lymphoproliferative disorders, a category that also includes acute and chronic lymphocytic leukemias (ALL and CLL) and Waldenstrom's macroglobulinemia. Although there are similarities between the various lymphomas, they display a wide spectrum of clinical and histologic patterns. The lymphoproliferative disorders may be subclassified not only by morphologic appearance but also by the cell of origin (Table 28-1).

Malignant lymphomas are the fifth most common cancer in the United States, but because of the younger average age of the lymphoma population, they account for more years of potential life lost than many of the more common adult cancers.[1,2]

Because of its characteristic pathology, Hodgkin's disease is considered separately from the other lymphomas. This fact (and the limitations of our knowledge) has led to an unfortunate terminology in which the other lymphoid malignancies are grouped under the term *non-Hodgkin's lymphoma*. Research is active in this area. Malignant lymphomas are being extensively evaluated with immunophenotypes, gene rearrangements, cytogenetic abnormalities, and oncogene activation.

Lymphadenopathy may signify malignant disease, but more commonly enlarged lymph nodes are a secondary phenomenon related to infectious, inflammatory, and other benign disorders. Table 28-2 lists the major causes of lymphadenopathy. A careful history and physical examination are most important in evaluating a patient with enlarged lymph nodes. Infectious nodes are usually soft, tender, <2 cm in diameter, and located in areas that drain common infections; thus, the anterior and posterior cervical nodes of the neck, which drain the ears and throat, are frequently infected. In contrast, malignant nodes are generally firm, hard, or rubbery, fixed to underlying tissue, multiple, nontender, >2 cm in diameter, and located in unusual sites such as the infraclavicular area. When diagnosis is uncertain, histologic examination of an enlarged lymph node is essential.

Hodgkin's Disease

In 1666, a fatal disease was described in which the lymphoid tissues and spleen appeared as a "cluster of grapes." In 1832, Thomas Hodgkin and later Samuel Wilkes described a disease characterized by gradual progressive enlargement of the lymph nodes "beginning usually in the cervical region and spreading throughout the lymphoid tissue of the body, forming nodular growths in the internal organs, resulting in anemia, and usually fatal cachexia."[3] The major features of these cases were (1) slow and relentless growth, the disease sometimes lasting many years, and (2) a characteristic histopathologic pattern (as later elucidated by Reed and Sternberg) that included the distinctive giant cell known as the Reed-Sternberg (RS) cell. Although RS cells occur in other disorders, pathologists now require that this cell be present before establishing a diagnosis of Hodgkin's disease. The RS cell is probably the neoplastic cell, and other cells present are reactive populations of lymphocytes, eosinophils, and plasma cells. The cell of origin of Hodgkin's disease is still not completely defined, but it appears to be from the monocyte-macrophage cell line.[4]

David S. Rosenthal, MD, Director, Henry K. Oliver Professor of Hygiene, Harvard University, University Health Services, Cambridge, Massachusetts

Harmon J. Eyre, MD, Deputy Executive, Vice President for Medical Affairs and Research, American Cancer Society, Atlanta, Georgia

Table 28-1. Classification of Lymphoproliferative Disorders According to B- or T-Cell Markers

B-Cell Disorders	T-Cell Disorders	Cell Type Uncertain
Acute lymphocytic leukemia	Infectious mononucleosis	Hodgkin's disease
Poorly differentiated lymphoma	Mycosis fungoides	Histiocytic lymphoma
Hairy cell leukemia	Sezary syndrome	
Prolymphocytic leukemia	Acute lymphoblastic leukemia (T variant)	
Chronic lymphocytic leukemia	Chronic lymphocytic leukemia (T variant)	
Waldenstrom's macroglobulinemia		
Cold agglutinin disease		
Heavy-chain disease		
Amyloidosis		
Multiple myeloma		

Table 28-2. Major Causes of Lymph Node Enlargement

Infections
- Acute (infectious mononucleosis, toxoplasmosis, cytomegalovirus, generalized dermatitis, common communicable diseases)
- Chronic (syphilis, tuberculosis, sarcoidosis)
- Acquired Immunodeficiency Syndrome (AIDS)

Hypersensitivity reactions and connective tissue diseases
- Serum sickness
- Rheumatoid arthritis
- Systemic lupus erythematosus
- Drug pseudolymphoma (diphenylhydantoin)

Primary lymphoproliferative diseases
- Hodgkin's disease
- Non-Hodgkin's lymphomas
- Leukemia (CLL, ALL, blast crisis of CML)
- Waldenstrom's macroglobulinemia

Endocrine disorders
- Hyperthyroidism
- Hypoadrenocorticism
- Hypopituitarism

Lipidoses

Dermatopathic lymphadenitis

Metastatic cancers
- Breast
- Lung
- Gastrointestinal

Epidemiology

Hodgkin's disease (HD) accounts for approximately 14% of all malignant lymphomas. It occurs in a bimodal age distribution: incidence rates rise sharply after age 10, peak in the late 20s, and then decline until age 45 (Fig 28-1).[5] After age 45, the incidence again increases steadily with age. The histologic pattern and anatomic distribution vary with age. The

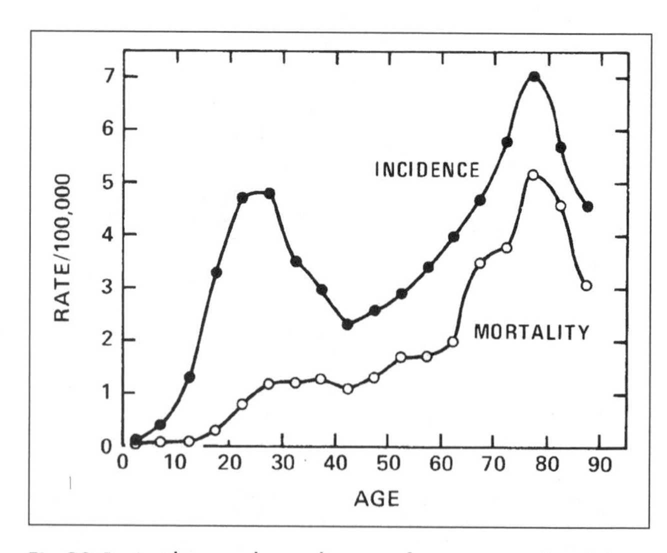

Fig 28-1. Incidence and mortality rates for patients with Hodgkin's disease, as reported by the Surveillance, Epidemiology, and End Results Program of the Biometry Branch of the National Cancer Institute. From Austin-Seymour et al.[5]

nodular sclerosis form of the disease predominates in young adults and the mixed cellularity form is most common in the older age group. At diagnosis, 25% of elderly patients have only subdiaphragmatic disease, compared with <5% of young adult patients. The majority of young patients have mediastinal involvement compared with <25% of elderly patients.[6-8]

Etiology

The clinical manifestations of fever, chills, and leukocytosis, and the histologic similarity to a granulomatous process, have suggested an infectious cause. The epidemiology of Hodgkin's disease implies that the social environment during childhood influences risk of the disease in young adulthood. Exposure to infectious agents appears to be diminished or delayed in persons of higher social class, in more educated individuals, in members of small families, and in older siblings.[9-11]

Epstein-Barr virus (EBV) is a possible etiologic agent, a suggestion supported by an ability to transform lymphocytes, and by the presence of RS-like cells in the lymphoid tissue of patients with infectious mononucleosis. This hypothesis, although supported by an early report of a 3.6-fold increase in the incidence of Hodgkin's disease among persons with a history of infectious mononucleosis, is not supported by other reports, which show a weak association between EBV and HD.[12] The proportion of patients with antibodies to EBV viral capsid antigen is similar to that of controls, but patients with HD consistently have higher titers. These antibody titers have been shown to increase with progressive loss of cell-mediated immunity, as well as after splenectomy and treatment.[13]

Although the question of neoplastic cell lineage remains unresolved, current evidence suggests that the RS cell is derived from the monocyte-macrophage cell line (Fig 28-2). These cells possess Fc and complement receptors and lectin receptors, and express a granulocyte-related differentiation antigen, Leu-M1 (Fig 28-3).[4] RS cells have been shown to have polyclonal immunoglobulins in their cytoplasm, which supports the theory that they retain the phagocytic processes of monocyte-macrophage cell lines.[14] The giant cells cultured in vitro have also been shown to secrete the monokine interleukin-1 into the culture media.[15] This monokine causes proliferation of T lymphocytes and fibroblasts and acts as an endogenous pyrogen[16]; both are common histologic and clinical features of Hodgkin's disease.

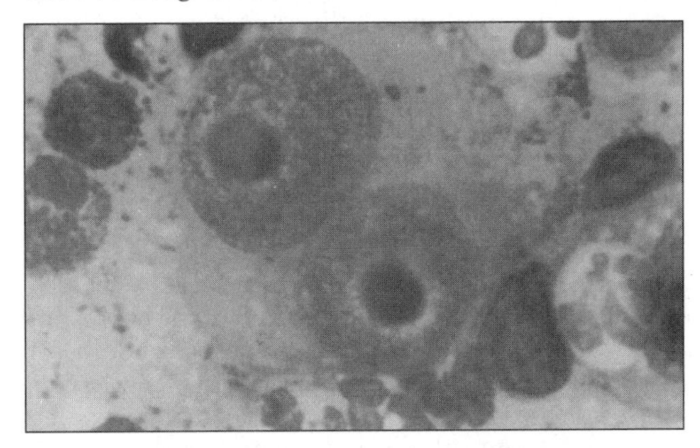

Fig 28-2. Reed-Sternberg cell in bone marrow. (Wright-Giemsa, X 1,000).

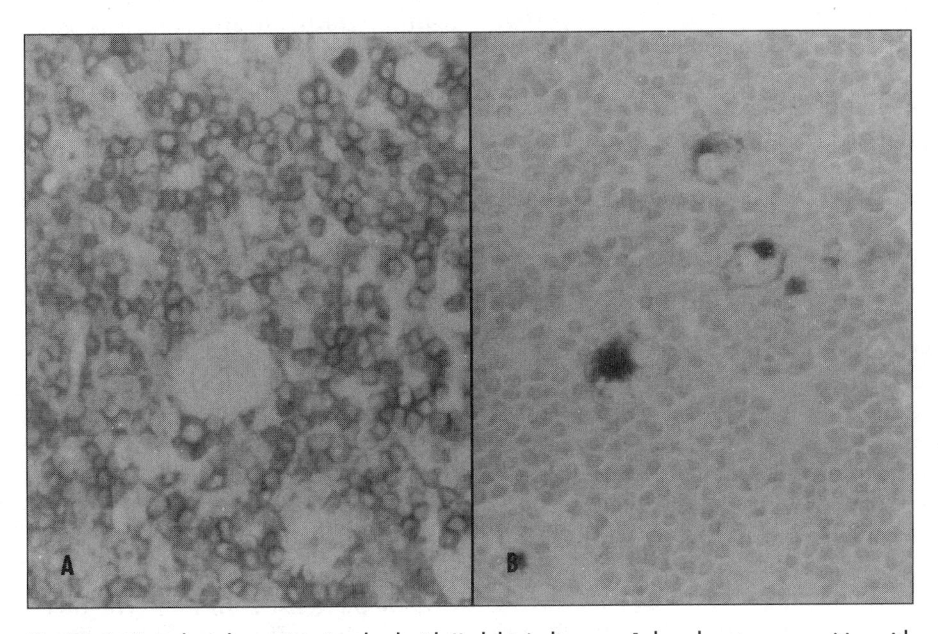

Fig 28-3. Lymph node sections involved with Hodgkin's disease. ***A***, lymphocytes are positive with leukocyte common antigen immunoperoxidase staining, but RS cells are negative. ***B***, Leu-M1 stain is positive in RS cells.

Clinical Presentation and Detection

Typically, HD presents as painless lymphadenopathy in young adults, although there may be associated constitutional symptoms of malaise, fever, night sweats, pruritus, and weight loss. The enlarged lymph node is usually (90%) supradiaphragmatic, and frequently (60% to 80%) in the cervical region. Axillary or mediastinal lymphadenopathy alone is less common. Massive mediastinal lymph nodes may result in symptoms of cough, wheezing, dyspnea, or superior vena cava syndrome. Subdiaphragmatic presentations are uncommon (10%) in young patients, but represent the only site of disease in 25% of elderly patients. Retroperitoneal nodes, the liver, spleen, and bone marrow usually are involved after the disease becomes generalized. Mesenteric lymph nodes are rarely involved, although in advanced cases any organ can be affected.[17]

Unlike the pattern in other lymphoproliferative disorders, Hodgkin's disease usually spreads contiguously from one lymph node region to another. For example, in a patient with early HD there may be involvement of only neck and mediastinal nodes. In advanced disease, diffuse adenopathy, along with involvement of the liver, marrow, lung, or other organs, may be present.

As will be noted, it is customary to speak of the several stages of Hodgkin's disease—and of the process of determining the stage in a given patient's course of disease—as staging. It is the characteristic contiguous nature of the pattern of spread that makes staging important prognostically and therapeutically.

Biopsy

The largest, most central node in an involved group should be removed with the capsule intact. Cervical nodes are preferable to axillary and inguinal nodes since the latter can frequently exhibit reactive changes and not be diagnostic. Needle biopsies yield limited amounts of tissue and often are not helpful for diagnosis. The pathologist should be notified in advance of the surgical procedure to prepare fresh tissue for immunologic and cytogenetic studies prior to freezing or fixing the tissue.

Histologic Classification

The histologic classification currently employed is known as the Rye Conference (1965) system. This classification comprises four major types: lymphocyte predominant, nodular sclerosis, mixed cellularity, and lymphocyte depleted (Table 28-3). The natural history of the disease varies with respect to histologic type. Patients who present with nodular sclerosis and lymphocyte-predominant types generally have a much better prognosis than those with mixed cellularity and lymphocyte-depleted types.

Table 28-3. Histopathologic Classification of Hodgkin's Disease (Rye Classification)

Histology	Relative Frequency (%)
Lymphocyte predominant	5 - 10
Nodular sclerosis	30 - 60
Mixed cellularity	20 - 40
Lymphocyte depleted	5 - 10

Hodgkin's disease is distinguished from other lymphomas by the presence of RS cells, which are large, binucleate cells with vesicular nuclei and prominent eosinophilic nucleoli (Fig 28-2). The RS cells are essential for the diagnosis of Hodgkin's disease, but have been reported in benign conditions such as hyperplastic or inflammatory nodes, mononucleosis, and some viral infections. They also may arise in response to phenytoin therapy. Lymph nodes containing HD show a normal nodal architecture infiltrated diffusely by neutrophils and a variable number of RS cells.

Lymphocyte-Predominant Disease

This type accounts for about 5% to 10% of Hodgkin's disease. Abundant mature lymphocytes diffusely infiltrate the abnormal lymph nodes; RS cells are few in number and difficult to find. The prognosis is excellent, with a 5-year survival rate of approximately 90%.

Nodular Sclerosis

This is the most common type (30% to 60%). Interlacing birefringent bands of collagen that divide the cellular infiltrate into discrete islands produce the lymph node's nodular appearance. Also present is a variant of the classic RS cell, referred to as the lacunar RS cell because of the very faint-staining cytoplasm that appears to be an empty space, or lacuna. Prognosis is good, with a high 5-year survival rate. This disease pattern is most frequently seen in young female adults. At diagnosis, it is most often localized in the cervical nodes and mediastinum.

Mixed Cellularity

This histologic type is the second most common, constituting about 20% - 40% of cases. The nodes contain a pleomorphic infiltrate of eosinophils, normal lymphocytes, and readily identifiable RS cells. Prognosis is slightly less favorable than the first two types with a 5-year survival of all stages of 50% to 60%.

Lymphocyte-Depleted Disease

One of the least common type of Hodgkin's disease, the RS cell predominates and mature lymphocytes are virtually absent in affected lymph nodes. This pattern occurs primarily in older patients and is associated with clinical symptoms and an advanced stage at presentation. The 5-year survival rate is <50%.

Clinical Staging

In addition to histologic type, the prognosis and therapy depend on the extent of disease at the onset. The four clinical stages of Hodgkin's disease are summarized in Table 28-4.[18] The 1971 Ann Arbor symposium on staging in Hodgkin's disease recommended a system using clinical staging (CS) and pathologic staging (PS).[18] In addition, cases are further classified as to the absence (A) or presence (B) of specific symptoms of significant fever, night sweats, and weight loss >10% of body weight.

Systematic clinical staging may include the following evaluations:

- Physical examination with careful attention to all lymph node areas;
- Various routine laboratory studies and chest radiographs;
- Computed tomographic (CT) scans of the abdomen and pelvis, supplying information regarding the liver and abdominal nodes;
- A bipedal lymphangiogram, a procedure in which radiopaque dye is injected into lymphatic channels of the feet with resulting visualization of iliac and para-aortic nodes; and
- Nuclear medicine studies, such as gallium scans.

In some clinics, if CT scans of the abdomen are negative, a staging laparotomy is performed in which the abdomen is explored and suspicious nodes seen on CT or lymphangiogram are removed. Splenectomy is performed, and biopsies are taken of both lobes of the liver and the bone marrow. If operative findings will change the therapeutic plan, then laparotomy is necessary.[19]

Careful and detailed pathologic examination of the spleen can often identify minute areas of Hodgkin's disease (Fig 28-4). Surgical staging may alter the stage in approximately 20% to 30% of patients with clinical stages I and II, which become pathologic stage III or IV. Splenic Hodgkin's disease without evidence of disease elsewhere in the abdomen suggests organ involvement not only by contiguous extension but perhaps also by hematogenous spread. Staging laparotomy alters the patient's stage in one third of cases and, more importantly, may change the plan for therapy.

In the elderly, one must be concerned about the tolerability of general anesthesia and the laparotomy. In one study, 75% of older patients were able to undergo complete staging including laparotomy.[5] It is well

Table 28-4. Stage/Substage Classification of Hodgkin's Disease (Ann Arbor Staging System)

Stage		Substage
Stage I	Single node region	I
	Single extralymphatic; organ/site	I (E)
Stage II	Two or more node regions on same side of diaphragm	II
	Single node region + localized single extralymphatic; organ/site	II (E)
Stage III	Node regions on both sides of diaphragm	III
	+ localized single	III (E)
	extralymphatic organ/site;	III (S)
	spleen, both.	III (ES)
Stage IV	Diffuse involvement extralymphatic organ/site node regions	IV
All stages divided	Without weight loss/fever/sweats	A
	With weight loss/fever/sweats	B

E = extranodal, S = spleen involved.

Adapted from Carbone et al.[18]

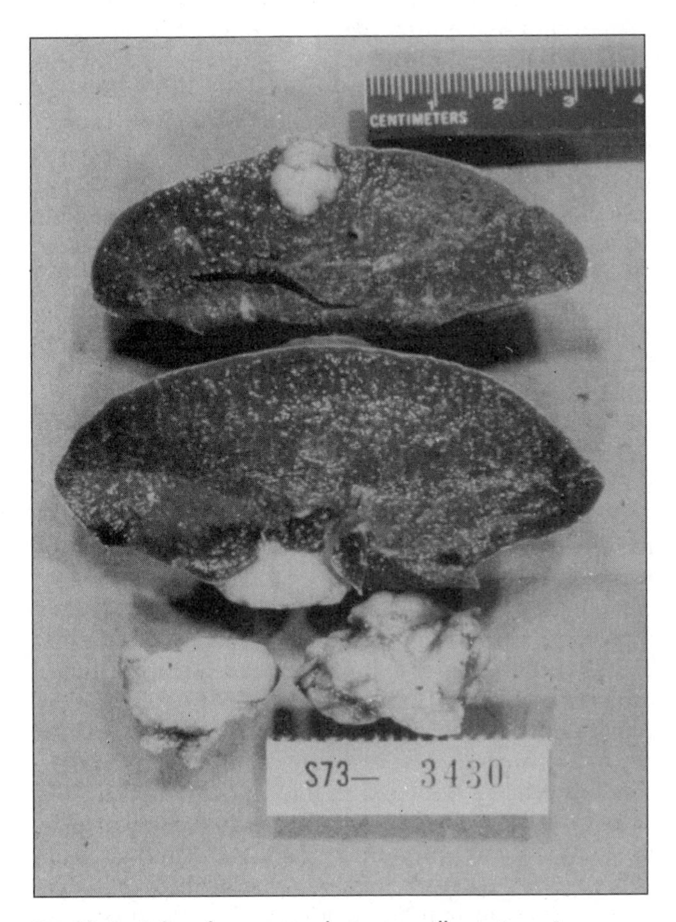

Fig 28-4. Spleen from staging laparotomy illustrating a 1-cm nodule of Hodgkin's disease, which may have been missed by computerized tomography.

recognized that older patients tend to present with more advanced disease. In a prospective study of 39 pathologically staged patients older than 60, 15 (39%) had limited disease (Stage I, II, or IIIA) whereas 24 (62%) had advanced stages, the opposite finding from patients younger than 30 years.[20] With the risk of surgery and the increased prevalence of advanced disease in patients older than 40, it has been suggested that older patients, particularly those with mixed cellularity or lymphocyte-depleted histologic type, may not benefit from laparotomy in determining therapies.[21] These patients may best be treated as if they had widespread disease.

The presence of large mediastinal masses may also preclude the necessity of a staging laparotomy. With masses >30% of the chest wall diameter or the presence of superior vena cava syndrome, curative therapy generally requires systemic chemotherapy with or without radiation therapy. Splenectomy or liver biopsy would not change the primary course of therapy.

Laboratory Studies

There are no pathognomonic hematologic findings in Hodgkin's disease. Leukocytosis with lymphocytopenia is not uncommon. An elevated erythrocyte sedimentation rate (ESR) will correlate with disease activity, and serial ESR studies may be a useful means of following the disease process. Eosinophilia and rarely monocytosis are noted. Other hematologic abnormalities, including leukopenia and thrombocytopenia, usually appear with advanced disease and are secondary to either bone marrow involvement or previous therapy.

Elevated serum alkaline phosphatase levels suggest liver or bone involvement, but may be nonspecific in younger patients. Hypergammaglobulinemia is common in early disease, but immunoglobulin (Ig) levels may decline in advanced disease or during treatment. Elevated serum copper and ceruloplasmin have been reported in active disease.[17]

Patients frequently demonstrate defects in delayed-hypersensitivity reaction and have negative tuberculin reactions even in the presence of active tuberculosis. This defect in cellular immunity is related in part to active suppression of T-lymphocyte function and associated with an increased incidence of infections with unusual organisms, such as *Pneumocystis carinii*, various fungi, and herpes zoster.

Therapy

Therapeutic developments dating from the early 1960s dramatically improved the response rate and survival in Hodgkin's disease. Today, almost 70% of patients with HD are long-term survivors. Success has been attributed primarily to careful staging, an understanding of the pattern of spread, and advances in radiation and chemotherapy.

Management usually consists of treating regions of known disease and the presumed next site of involvement. For example: in a pathologic stage IA patient presenting only with cervical adenopathy, the disease often can be cured by a "mantle" irradiation field plus the contiguous area (ie, the upper abdomen or para-aortic field). In a patient with diffuse adenopathy, above and below the diaphragm, plus fevers and night sweats (stage IIIB), the next potential site of involvement would be extranodal. Therefore, chemotherapy would be the primary therapy.

In general, limited radiation therapy is recommended for early stages of Hodgkin's disease, while chemotherapy with or without irradiation is reserved for advanced stages. Results of such an approach are shown in Table 28-5.

Table 28-5. Five-Year Disease-Free Survival Rates in Hodgkin's Disease

Stage	Therapy	5-Year Disease Free Survival (%)
I, IIA	Intensive radiation therapy	85-95
IB, IIB (rare)	Intensive radiation therapy	80-85
IIIA	Intensive radiation therapy or chemotherapy	60-85
$IIIA_1$	Intensive radiation therapy or chemotherapy	60-85
$IIIA_2$	Chemotherapy ± radiation therapy	60-80
IIIB	Chemotherapy ± radiation therapy	60-80
IVA, IVB	Chemotherapy alone	30-50

Surgery

The primary role of surgery in HD is to obtain tissue for diagnosis or to perform a laparotomy when indicated. An experienced surgical team will decrease operative morbidity and mortality while increasing diagnostic yield.

Therapeutic excision of enlarged nodes (debulking) in early-stage disease is not indicated. Removal of stable residual bulky masses following therapy usually reveals fibrosis.[22]

Radiation Therapy

The concept of intensive, "curative" radiation therapy for Hodgkin's disease was developed by Gilbert and Peters and later by Kaplan and Johnson. Details of therapy and expected results vary according to stage.

Irradiation is curative in most patients with limited

Hodgkin's disease, ie, stages I, II, and some IIIA.[23-25] The addition of chemotherapy to radiation therapy may be indicated in patients with adverse prognostic factors such as B symptoms, bulky disease, and stage III.[19,26,27] Some basic concepts apply to curative radiation therapy for HD: use of megavoltage radiation (linear accelerators), treatment by opposed fields, tumoricidal doses, careful field simulation and verification, and close follow-up of all patients. Treatment should be administered only by a qualified radiation oncologist with full physics and dosimetric facilities. Radiation therapy is usually delivered to three major fields, known as the mantle, para-aortic, and pelvic or inverted Y fields (Fig 28-5). In total nodal radiation therapy, all three fields, which encompass most of the body's lymph node regions are irradiated.

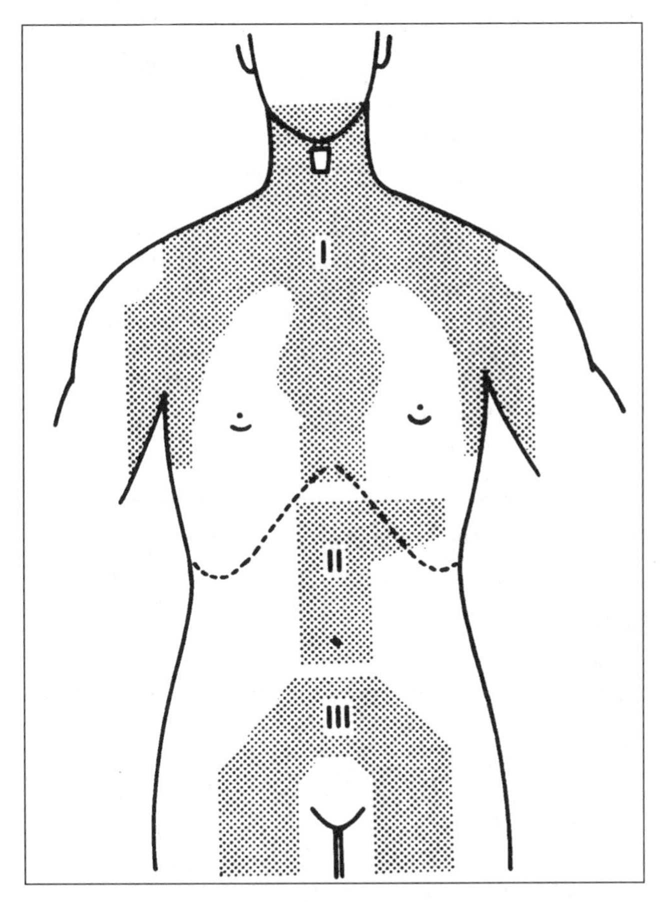

Fig 28-5. Radiation fields in therapy for Hodgkin's disease. Shaded areas represent the three treatment fields. The **mantle field** is the uppermost field (I). Lungs and vocal cords are protected by lead blocks; heart and thyroid are within the field. The **para-aortic field,** or middle field (II), extends from the diaphragm to just above the bifurcation of the aorta. When the spleen has not been removed, this field is extended to include the entire spleen and splenic hilum. The **pelvic** or **inverted Y field** is the lowest field (III). It encompasses the pelvic and inguinal nodes and includes a large area of bone marrow.

The use of extended fields to include the adjacent, clinically negative nodal sites is essential for high cure rates.[28] Extended-field irradiation is based on the contiguity theory of Rosenberg and Kaplan,[29] which suggests that the disease is a monoclonal, unicentric neoplasm that predictably spreads by lymphatics to contiguous node groups. In pathologic stages I and IIA disease, mantle and para-aortic irradiation has become standard therapy and has the advantage of sparing the pelvic bone marrow and reducing exposure of the gonads. Carefully constructed field shapes and blocks (shielding) are used to protect the lungs, heart, spinal cord, larynx, kidneys, gonads, and iliac crest.

The tumoricidal dose level in HD is approximately 40 to 45 Gy, delivered at the rate of 10 Gy/week.[28] Clinically negative adjacent nodal regions can be treated adequately with 35 Gy. The necessary dose of radiation when used in combination with chemotherapy may be lower.

The most efficient treatment of deep-lying tissues requires an opposed-field technique that provides a homogeneous dose distribution throughout the treatment volume and minimizes the chance of radiation damage to adjacent structures. Standard treatment fields employed in patients with Hodgkin's disease use an opposed-field, usually anterior and posterior, technique.

Consolidation irradiation applies to the lower doses (15 to 20 Gy) administered to areas of known disease in advanced stages (IIIB or IV) after a complete response to chemotherapy.[26]

Chemotherapy

Aggressive chemotherapy has also produced long disease-free remissions in advanced Hodgkin's disease. A program developed by DeVita and coworkers, known as MOPP (for the drug combination nitrogen mustard [Mustargen], vincristine [Oncovin], procarbazine, and prednisone) has resulted in complete remissions in 60% to 70% of patients with stages IIIB and IV. However, 5-year disease-free survival was obtained in only 50% of these cases. Recently, other combined chemotherapy programs, employing doxorubicin (Adriamycin), bleomycin, vinblastine, and dacarbazine (the ABVD regimen), have yielded similar results. The duration of therapy is generally 6 to 12 months, or at least 2 months after achievement of complete remission.

Single Chemotherapeutic Agents

Although single chemotherapeutic agents can produce complete and partial responses (CR + PR) in 50% to 70% of patients with HD, the remissions last only a few months and complete responses are unusual (10% to 15%).[30] Single agents can be useful in palliating advanced disease in elderly patients or patients who are heavily pretreated and, due to severe myelosuppression, will not tolerate combination therapy. The use of chemotherapy with a curative intent involves combination, not single-agent, regimens.

Combination Chemotherapy

The MOPP regimen resulted in a high complete response rate and in confirmed durable remissions (Table 28-6).[31,32] The CR rate in 188 patients was 84%, with 66% remaining disease free for >10 years. Patients with no B symptoms and those receiving full doses had a higher CR rate and longer survival. Patients entering complete remission in ≤5 cycles had significantly longer remissions than those requiring ≥6 cycles. Since the introduction of MOPP, investigators have added or substituted other drugs to reduce toxicity and improve results.

The ABVD regimen, a drug combination differing from MOPP in pharmacology and mechanism of action, results in similar CR rates.[33] This regimen has proven to be noncross-resistant with MOPP due to its ability to salvage MOPP failures (59% CR, 13% PR).[34] ABVD produces similar therapeutic results, with a reduced risk of secondary leukemia.[35] Numerous studies have evaluated other second-line salvage therapies.[36] None appears to be clearly superior to or less toxic than ABVD.[37]

Combined Chemotherapy and Radiation Therapy

Specific subsets of patients appear to benefit from combination radiation and chemotherapy. These include patients with large mediastinal masses exceeding one-third the diameter of the thoracic cavity (stage I or II, with so-called massive mediastinum)[38]; patients with stage IIIA disease, with or without bulky sites[39,40]; patients with stage IIIB or IV disease who achieve only a partial remission with chemotherapy that is converted to complete remission with added radiation therapy; and children in whom the use of combination chemotherapy enables reduced doses of radiation, which spare bone growth retardation.[41]

Table 28-6. Chemotherapy for Hodgkin's Disease

MOPP	
Nitrogen mustard (Murstargen)	6 mg/m² days 1 and 8
Vincristine (Oncovin)	1.5 mg/m² days 1 and 8
Prednisone	40 mg/m²/day on days 1-14 (on cycles 1 and 4 only)
Procarbazine	100 mg/m²/day on days 1-14
ABVD	
Doxorubicin (Adriamycin)	25 mg/m² days 1 and 14
Bleomycin	10 mg/m² days 1 and 14
Vinblastine	10 mg/m² days 1 and 14
Dacarbazine	375 mg/m² days 1 and 14

Each regimen is given every 28 days.

Complications of Treatment

Complications of radiation therapy common to patients of all ages include hypothyroidism, pericarditis, and pneumonitis (Table 28-7). Pelvic irradiation can lead to sterility in females and varying degrees of myelosuppression in both sexes. The latter complication varies most with age. Regeneration of marrow activity is quite rapid in patients younger than 20, moderately delayed from ages 20 to 40, and severely delayed from ages 40 to 70. The current recommended dose for Hodgkin's disease is 32 to 40 Gy. Transverse myelitis can occur if the spinal cord is overdosed. To avoid this complication, careful attention should be paid to radiation treatment planning of the gap between two adjacent ports over the cord.

Complications of chemotherapy include myelosuppression, nausea, vomiting, alopecia, paresthesias, pulmonary fibrosis, and rarely cardiomyopathy. Sterility is the rule in males and often occurs in females. There is an increased incidence of second malignancies, usually acute leukemia or non-Hodgkin's lymphoma. The frequency of acute leukemia has approached 5%-7% in patients receiving protracted courses of alkylating agents or chemotherapy combined with total nodal irradiation.

Table 28-7. Complications of Therapy for Hodgkin's Disease

Radiation therapy (RT)
- Myelosuppression
- Hypothyroidism
- Pericarditis
- Pneumonitis

Chemotherapy (CT)
- Nausea, vomiting
- Alopecia (especially with doxorubicin)
- Sterility in males (especially with alkylating agents) and females
- Myelosuppression
- Neuropathy (with vincristine)
- Cardiomyopathy
- Second malignancies, especially acute leukemia.

RT plus CT (combined modality therapy)
- Second malignancies, especially acute leukemia and non-Hodgkin's lymphoma

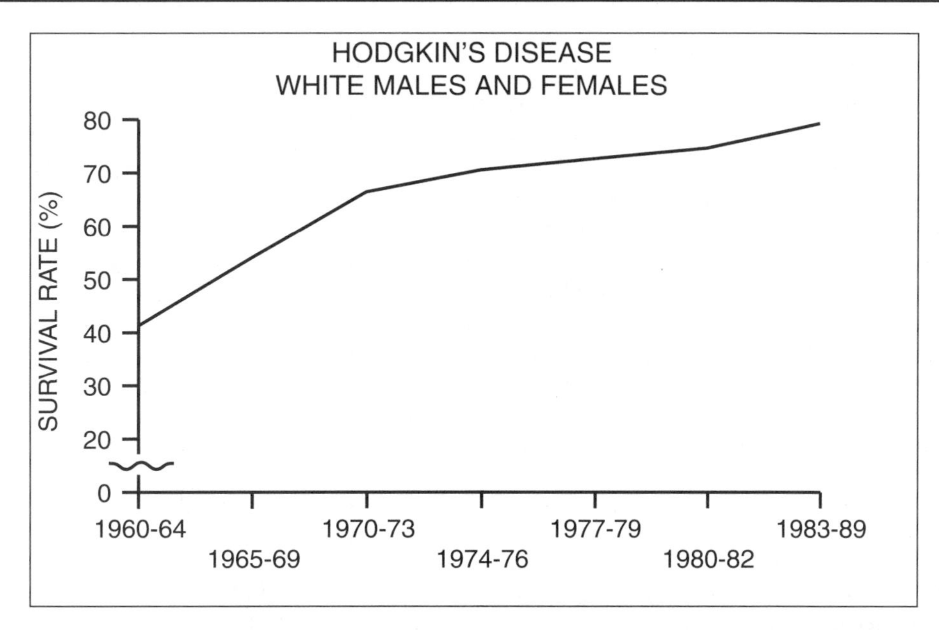

Fig 28-6. Improvements in the 5-year relative survival rate in white males and females with Hodgkin's disease (US 1960-1989).[45]

The Stanford group found a 17.6% cumulative risk (6-fold excess risk) of secondary cancers.[42] The risk of secondary leukemia is greatest in patients older than 40 (20.7% actuarial risk at 7 years).[43] Patients surviving >11 years after treatment appear to be at no increased risk of developing acute leukemia.

Future Directions

The guidelines for treatment selection in HD should be modified depending on the careful evaluation of each individual. Results of therapy have been exciting, with a steady increase in the 5-year relative survival rate (Fig 28-6) and a corresponding decline in the mortality rate (Fig 28-7).

Ongoing studies include noncross-resistant alternating regimens, integrating chemotherapy and radiation therapy, biologic response modifiers, and high-dose chemotherapy with bone marrow transplantation.[44] Further studies are needed to demonstrate the efficacy and toxicity of these modalities.

Non-Hodgkin's Lymphomas

The non-Hodgkin's lymphomas (NHL) are a heterogeneous collection of lymphoid malignancies with some common features and many differences. Unlike Hodgkin's disease, they appear to be multicentric in origin with an early tendency to spread widely. A peripheral blood leukemic phase is not uncommon and there is some evidence that nearly all patients have malignant cells in the blood regardless of the stage of disease.

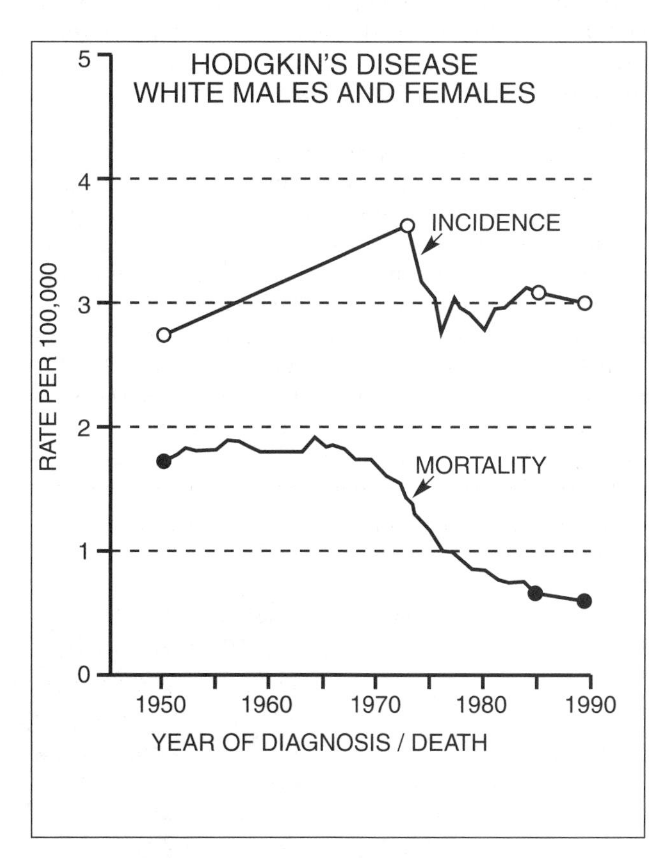

Fig 28-7. Incidence rates per 100,000 population for Hodgkin's disease, age adjusted to 1970, have remained fairly stable. Mortality rates have decreased by more than 50%.

Epidemiology

There is a progressive increase in incidence with age (Fig 28-8).[45] The American Cancer Society estimates that 45,000 new patients with non-Hodgkin's lymphoma was detected in 1994: 25,000 males and 20,000 females. It is estimated that 21,200 deaths occurred.[1] Incidence has increased over 65% since the early 1970s, while mortality rates have not risen as fast. Higher age-adjusted incidence rates are due primarily to increases among older persons. Lower-magnitude increases occur in the 35 to 64 age group, while rates among young adults have not changed substantially.[2] Much of the increase in incidence in the older age group is attributed to a rising incidence of the diffuse large-cell lymphoma histologic subtype.

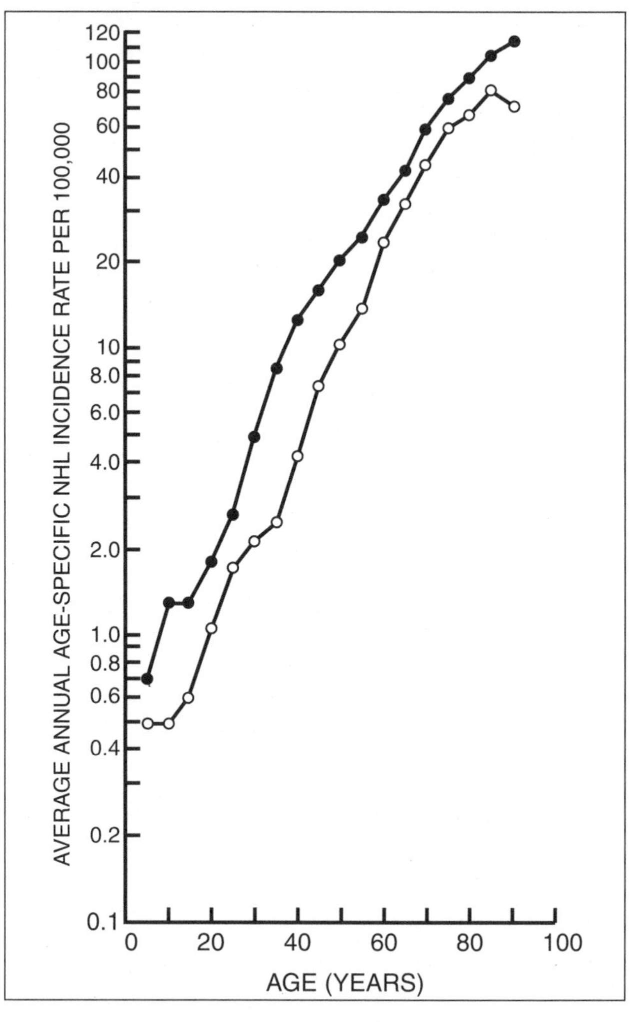

Fig 28-8. Average annual age-specific incidence rates for non-Hodgkin's lymphomas (NHL) per 100,000 population among US white males (closed circles) and white females (open circles).[45]

Etiology

As in Hodgkin's disease, the etiology of most types of non-Hodgkin's lymphoma is unknown. However, several factors suggest possible causal relations. For example, the incidence of non-Hodgkin's lymphomas rises in immunosuppressed patients (eg, patients with acquired immunodeficiency syndrome and renal transplant recipients) and in those with hyperfunctioning immune systems (eg, Sjogren's syndrome). Viruses can cause specific lymphomas. African Burkitt's lymphoma is associated with EBV infection, and an aggressive T-cell leukemia/lymphoma occurring in Japan and Caribbean islands is associated with human T lymphotropic virus type I (HTLV-I) infection. Cytogenetic abnormalities are common, but less consistent than those in the acute leukemias. The exception is Burkitt's lymphoma, which is usually associated with an 8;14 translocation or, in some patients, a variant 8;22 or 8;2 translocation. Interestingly, these translocations all involve the c-*myc* proto-oncogene. About 60% of all non-Hodgkin's lymphomas have a 14q+ marker chromosome. About 35% of nodular B-cell non-Hodgkin's

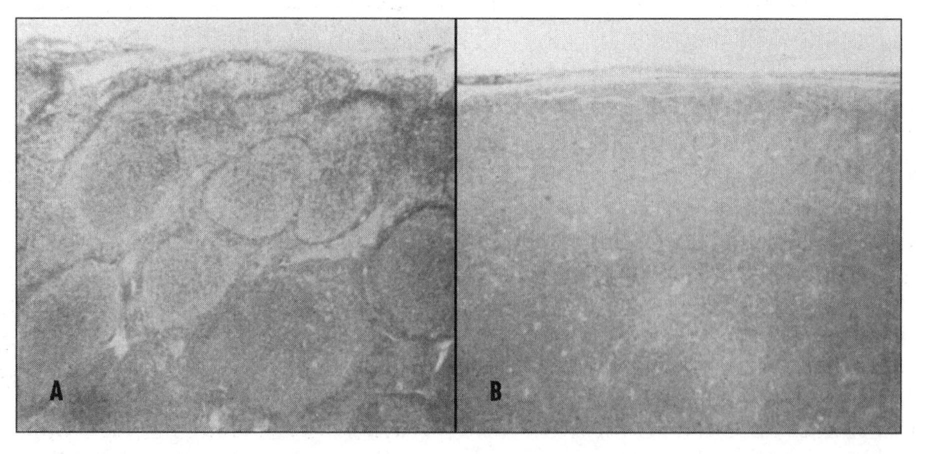

Fig 28-9. Non-Hodgkin's lymphoma. ***A*** shows a follicular, or nodular, histologic pattern; ***B*** shows a diffuse histologic pattern. In general, the follicular architecture portends a more favorable prognosis.

lymphomas have a 14;18 translocation. The significance of these changes is not known. Other cytogenetic studies suggest that non-Hodgkin's lymphomas may be biclonal or multiclonal in origin.

Advances in immunology, particularly in the development of monoclonal antibody technology, have led to the characterization of non-Hodgkin's lymphomas as neoplasms of the immune system. Subclasses of lymphoma are now showing similarities in immunologic phenotype to stages in the normal differentiation of T and B lymphocytes.[46] Molecular genetic analysis has shown that loci involved in the monoclonal cell population for many B-cell lymphomas involve these areas, other specific sites on chromosome 11, and chromosome 18. The T-cell receptor alpha-chain gene locus on chromosome 14 and the T-cell receptor beta-chain locus on chromosome 7 have been involved in translocations. Studies have predicted that specific cytogenetic abnormalities in lymphoma will result in useful prognostic information.[47]

Clinical Presentation and Detection

Most NHL patients are asymptomatic, although 20% may have some constitutional or B symptoms. Often, patients will give a history of "waxing and waning" adenopathy over several months before diagnosis. Presenting signs and symptoms are extremely variable and relate to site and extent of disease. Many patients seek investigation of an enlarged node or abdominal mass. Other cases begin with complaints referable to the alimentary tract, for example, abdominal pain, vomiting, or gastrointestinal bleeding. Systemic manifestations are nonspecific: fever, sweats, and itching are uncommon; weight loss is common. Leukemic transformation of NHL occurs in 10% to 15% of patients.[48] Coombs'-positive autoimmune hemolytic anemia occurs more commonly in NHL than HD.

Central to the diagnosis of all lymphomas is the recognition of lymphadenopathy and the careful histologic evaluation of a lymph node biopsy. As with HD, careful coordination with the pathologist is necessary in order to obtain adequate samples for diagnosis and special studies.

Histologic Classification

Histologic classifications proposed for NHL have included those of Rappaport, Lukes, Kiel, and Lennert. The most widely reported is Rappaport's, on which most of the literature in the US to the mid-1980s is based. In these studies, nodular architecture generally carried a more favorable prognosis than diffuse histology (Fig 28-9). In 1982, a conference held to resolve these differences resulted in the working formulation histologic classification. The Rappaport and working formulation classifications are summarized in Table 28-8. Low-grade lymphomas are predominantly B-cell tumors; intermediate-grade lymphomas include B-cell and some T-cell lymphomas; immunoblastic lymphomas are predominantly B-cell tumors; and the lymphoblastic group usually is composed of T-cell tumors. Burkitt's and non-Burkitt's small noncleaved cell tumors are predominately B-cell tumors. The true histiocytic lymphomas are from the monocyte-macrophage line. Mycosis fungoides has a T-cell origin. Tumors with a good prognosis include all low-grade and some intermediate-grade NHLs. Tumors with a poor prognosis include those in the rapidly progressive high-grade group, particularly diffuse large-cell tumors. Most B-cell tumors are monoclonal and produce either a kappa or lambda light-chain immunoglobulin (usually IgM) molecule.

Table 28-8. Histologic Groups in Non-Hodgkin's Lymphoma

Working Formulation	Rappaport Classification
Low grade	
Small lymphocytic	Well-differentiated lymphocytic lymphoma (WDL)
Follicular small cleaved lymphocytic	Nodular, poorly differentiated lymphocytic lymphoma (NPDL)
Mixed follicular small cleaved cell and large cell	Nodular mixed lymphoma (NM)
Intermediate grade	
Follicular, predominantly large cell	Nodular histiocytic lymphoma (NHL)
Diffuse small cleaved cell	Diffuse, poorly differentiated lymphocytic lymphoma (DPDL)
Diffuse large cell (cleaved or uncleaved)	Diffuse histiocytic lymphoma (DHL)
High grade	
Diffuse large cell immunoblast	Diffuse histiocytic lymphoma (DHL)
B cell	
T cell	
Polymorphic	
Epithelial cell component	
Lymphoblastic	Lymphoblastic lymphoma
Convoluted	
Nonconvoluted	
Small noncleaved	Diffuse undifferentiated lymphoma (DUL)
Burkitt's	
non-Burkitt's	

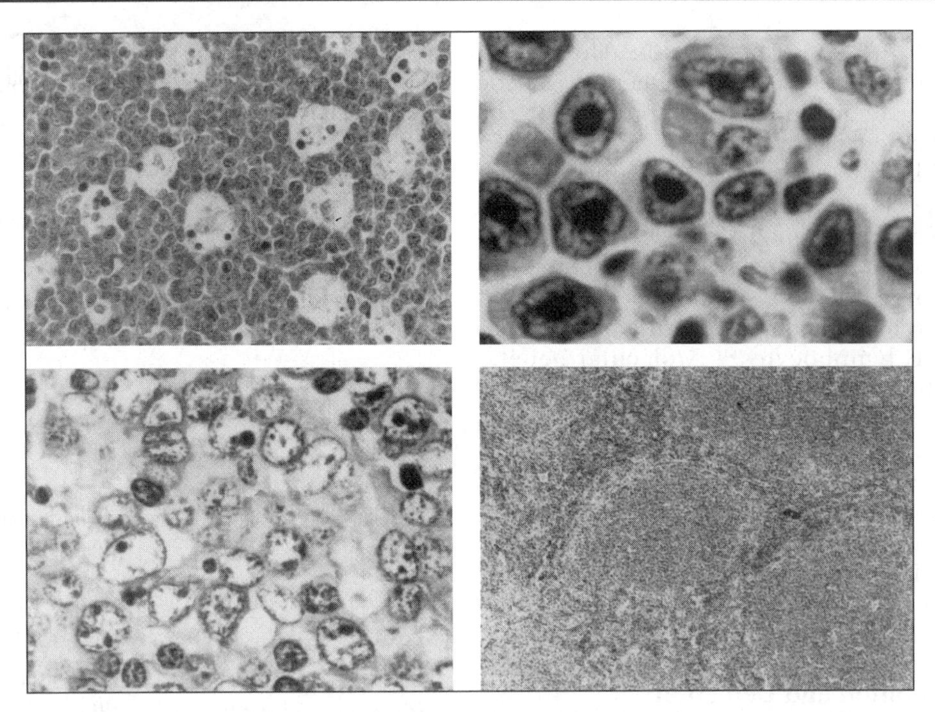

Fig 28-10. *Top left:* follicular small-cleaved cell lymphoma, low-power view. *Top right:* diffuse large-cell lymphoma, high-power view. *Bottom left:* immunoblastic lymphoma, high-power view. *Bottom right:* Burkitt's lymphoma with "starry sky" pattern, low-power view.

The histologic features of the four most common subgroups of NHLs are illustrated in Fig 28-10.

Follicular Small-Cleaved Cell Lymphoma

The vast majority of the neoplastic cells are small, indented lymphocytes with only occasional large cells (Fig 28-11). Mitotic figures are few. Monoclonal populations of these lymphocytes are frequent in the peripheral blood of many patients with follicular lymphomas who do not otherwise have evidence of leukemic changes or elevated lymphocyte counts. The significance of these circulating cells is not yet clear. This is the most common histologic subtype, accounting for approximately 40% of NHL. Patients predominantly present with stages III and IV disease and have a high incidence of bone marrow involvement.

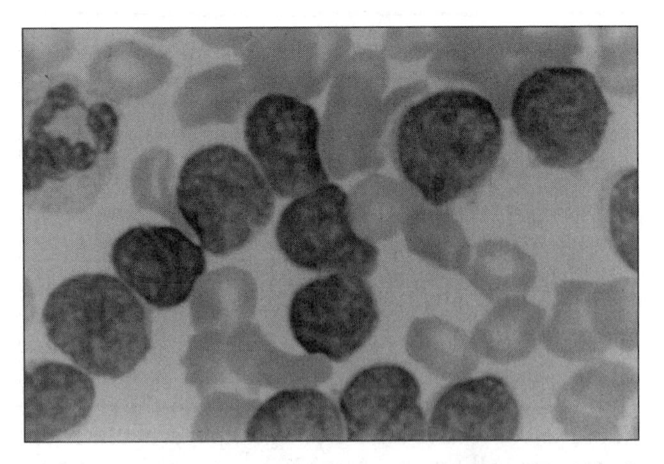

Fig 28-11. Small-cleaved follicular center cells in peripheral blood leukemia phase (Wright-Giemsa, X 1,000). Note the cleavings through the lymphocytes that are otherwise normal sized.

Follicular Mixed Small-Cleaved and Large-Cell Lymphomas

The large cells are more abundant and, in some cases, appear to be mixed with equal numbers of the smaller cells. As with other follicular lymphomas, the lymph node architecture shows distinct nodules usually present throughout the lymph node. However, in mixed cellular lymphomas, more frequent areas of diffuse infiltrate are common. This histologic subtype accounts for 20% to 40% of non-Hodgkin's lymphomas. Marrow involvement is frequent, and most patients have stages III and IV disease at diagnosis.

Diffuse Large-Cell Lymphomas

This subgroup has large lymphocytes with nuclear diameters much greater than a normal lymphocyte. The cells have cytologic features of large noncleaved or large cleaved follicular cells. The cells contain nucleoli and abundant cytoplasm that is slightly amphophilic. Mitoses are more commonly identified in this subgroup. These tumors tend to present frequently in extranodal as well as nodal sites, tend to disseminate rapidly, and involve unusual areas such as the central nervous system, bone, and GI tract.

Immunoblastic Lymphomas

These constitute high-grade neoplasms composed of cells commonly exhibiting a high mitotic rate. Plasmacytoid, clear-cell, and polymorphic subtypes have been proposed. The correlation between morphologic appearance and immunologic subtype is less predictable in these lymphomas.

Clinical Staging

The extent of disease at initial presentation is determined on the basis of history, physical examination, blood studies, bone marrow biopsy, abdominal CT scan, and nuclear medicine scans. Such studies have demonstrated that <15% of patients with NHL are in stage I or II when first seen (compared with 30% to 60% in Hodgkin's disease). Thus, most patients have advanced disease from the onset and staging laparotomy is of no benefit. The same Ann Arbor symposium recommendations used for staging Hodgkin's disease (Table 28-4) are used for staging non-Hodgkin's lymphomas.[18]

The pattern of dissemination in non-Hodgkin's lymphomas is less frequently orderly; there are numerous illustrations of patients with early organ involvement who have minimal adenopathy but extranodal sites (Table 28-9). The prognosis is influenced more by the histologic subtype than by the anatomic extent of disease, as in HD.[49] The clinical characteristics and staging of many patients with NHL evaluated by the working formulation study group are summarized in Table 28-10. There was a high incidence of marrow involvement in stages III and IV patients with low-grade lymphomas and an equal distribution of stages I and II versus stages III and IV with less marrow involvement in the intermediate- and high-grade groups. The survival curves demonstrate the value of histologic subclassification of non-Hodgkin's lymphomas and are helpful with treatment planning (Fig 28-12).

Table 28-9. Extranodal Site Presentations of Non-Hodgkin's Lymphoma

Site	Frequency (%)
Waldeyer's ring	34.4
Gastrointestinal tract	17.2
Skin	11.8
Orbit	5.4
Paranasal sinus	4.8
Bon	4.8
Testis	4.8
Thyroid	4.3
Extradural	4.3
Salivary glands	2.2
Central nervous system	0.5
Other	5.4

The Royal Marsden Hospital, 1962-1972.

Table 28-10. The Relationship Between History, Pathologic Stage and Bone Marrow Involvement at Diagnosis of Non-Hodgkin's Lymphoma

Histology	Stages (%) I	II	III	Bone Marrow Involved
Small lymphocytic	3	8	89	71
Follicular small cleaved cell	8	10	82	51
Diffuse small cleaved cell	9	19	72	62
Diffuse large-cell	16	30	54	10
Large-cell, immunoblastic	23	29	58	2

Treatment

Multidisciplinary Treatment Approach

As with Hodgkin's disease, the non-Hodgkin's lymphomas frequently demand multidisciplinary treatment planning to achieve the most optimal cure rates.[50] Because NHL disseminates early and widely by hematogenous routes rather than through orderly, contiguous node extension,[7,51] radiation therapy is usually considered an adjunct to chemotherapy rather than primary treatment. However, radiation therapy has a role in the management of localized disease.

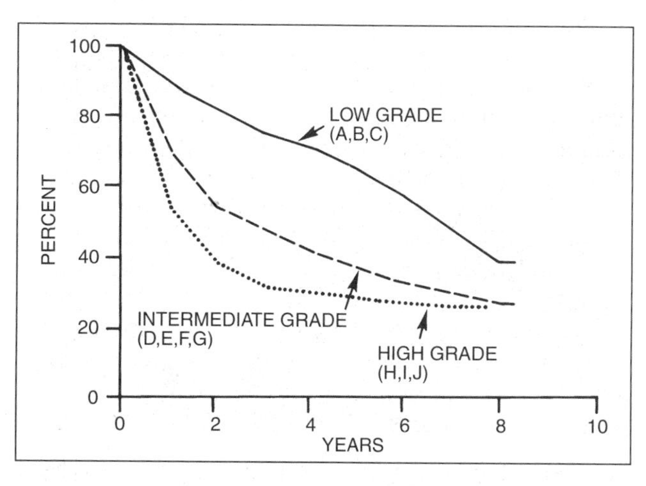

Fig 28-12. Survival of patients with non-Hodgkin's lymphoma classified by the working formulation histologic subgroups.

Surgery

The primary role of surgery is in establishing the diagnosis. In a few circumstances, surgery is a beneficial part of the disease management, for example, in resection of extranodal GI involvement. Localized gastric and small-bowel non-Hodgkin's lymphoma with low-grade histologic patterns may be cured by resection. In addition, GI non-Hodgkin's lymphomas, when treated with chemotherapy or radiation therapy, have a significant risk of perforation or bleeding that can be fatal. To prevent this complication, it is desirable to resect areas of the GI tract involved with the extensive lymphoma.

Radiation Therapy

Before beginning radiation therapy, it is essential to carefully stage NHL patients. The goal of radiation therapy should be to control disease within the confines of the clinically evident disease. Fields utilized in the treatment of HD are often inappropriate for NHL.

The low-grade (favorable) lymphomas are generally highly responsive to irradiation. Local control rates exceeding 90% are achieved with 40 Gy administered to the involved field. Satisfactory control rates are usually achieved with doses in excess of 30 Gy. As indicated in Table 28-10, it is uncommon for favorable-histology lymphomas to be localized at diagnosis; frequently the marrow or other sites are involved.

Long-term follow-up after involved- or extended-field therapy for localized disease (stage I or II low-grade lymphomas) indicates a 10-year survival and freedom from relapse of >50%, especially among younger patients.[52,53] However, late relapses can occur. Studies involving total lymphoid irradiation given alone or combined with chemotherapy, as well as whole-body irradiation, have been used to treat patients with stages III and IV disease. These therapeutic approaches produce a high remission rate, but there is no proof of curative potential in low-grade lymphomas.[54,55]

In contrast to low-grade NHL, more intermediate- and high-grade lymphomas present in localized stages I and II than in disseminated stages III and IV disease (Table 28-10). They also arise much more commonly in extranodal sites such as the GI tract, bone marrow, CNS, and skin. Before the introduction of effective combination chemotherapy, radiation therapy was the standard mode of treatment for patients with stages I and II large-cell lymphomas. The results of several controlled trials demonstrate long-term disease-free survival of >50% for thoroughly studied stage I patients treated with radiation therapy alone.[56,57] Patterns of relapse are less predictable than with Hodgkin's disease, and relapses are more common with systemic disease or other organ involvement. Also, local control rates with radiation therapy are not as predictable as in HD. These features have led to trials combining chemotherapy with radiation therapy for localized NHL.

Radiation therapy is effective for the palliation of symptoms in patients with advanced NHL of low-, intermediate-, and high-grade histology. These situations include relieving superior vena cava obstruction, alleviating spinal cord compression, treating ureter occlusion, and treating painful tumor masses.

Electron beam radiation therapy has been extensively used in the management of patients with early-stage mycosis fungoides. This is an effective palliative modality,[58] because individual tumor nodules are highly responsive.

Chemotherapy

The non-Hodgkin's lymphomas frequently present as disseminated disease and relapse with disseminated involvement following localized radiation therapy. The prime treatment modality is chemotherapy. Useful chemotherapeutic agents are similar to those used in the treatment of HD. The choice of agent or combination is based on histology, stage, and general patient information such as age and performance status.

Low-Grade Histology

Low-grade NHL typically is diagnosed as a systemic disease; approximately 90% of patients demonstrate stage III or IV disease. The peripheral blood is frequently involved with circulating monoclonal lymphoma cells (Fig 28-11). Although generally regarded as indolent diseases, they are progressive and ultimately fatal. Most patients retain a follicular histologic pattern, although some will advance to a high-grade histologic pattern. The natural history of the low-grade lymphomas demonstrates that with minimal therapy, a median survival of 7.5 to 9 years can be expected. Thus, the decision to initiate therapy has to be weighed carefully. The quality of life is usually unimpaired, with long periods of symptom-free survival,[59] and in some series, 25% of asymptomatic patients with low-grade histologic characteristics never require therapy and live a close to normal life with disease.

Treatment with a variety of programs, including single agents, COP, C-MOPP, CHOP, MACOP-B, m-BACOD, and ProMACE-CytaBOM, has been used (Table 28-11). Unfortunately, although there is a high remission rate, the average remission lasts only 2 to 3 years. After subsequent relapses, the remissions induced with second courses of therapy are shorter. Data for all therapies indicate little evidence of curability for stages III and IV disease.[60,61]

Current research questions for this patient population involve the application of aggressive chemotherapy earlier in the course of the disease and biologic response modifiers used in combination with the chemotherapy or during maintenance.[62] Initial results with high-dose chemotherapy followed by

Table 28-11. Combination Chemotherapy for Non-Hodgkin's Lymphomas

COP Regimen

Agent	Dose/Administration Route	Day
Cyclophosphamide	400 mg/m² PO	1-5
	or 700 mg/m² IV	1
Vincristine (Oncovin)	1.4 mg/m² IV	1
Prednisone	100 mg/m² PO	1-5

Repeat cycle every 21 days, usually for ≥6 cycles.

CHOP Regimen

Agent	Dose/Administration Route	Day
Cyclophosphamide	750 mg/m² IV	1
Doxorubicin	50 mg/m² IV	1
Vincristine	1.4 mg/m² IV	1
Prednisone	100 mg PO	1-5

Repeat cycles at 21 to 28 days, usually for ≥6 cycles.

MACOP-B Regimen

Agent	Dose/Administration Route	Week
Methotrexate	400 mg/m² IV (4 h)	2,6,10
Leucovorin	15 mg PO q6h x 6	after Mtx
Doxorubicin	50 mg/m² IV	1,3,5,7,9,11
Cyclophosphamide	350 mg/m² IV	1,3,5,7,9,11
Vincristine	1.4 mg/m² IV	2,4,6,8,10,12
Bleomycin	10 mg/m² IV	4,8,12
Prednisone	75 mg PO day	x 12 wk

m-BACOD Regimen

Agent	Dose/Administration Route	Day
Cyclophosphamide	600 mg/m² IV	1
Doxorubicin	45 mg/m² IV	1
Vincristine	1.0 mg/m² IV	1
Bleomycin	4 mg/m² IV	1
Dexamethasone	6 mg/m² PO	1-5
Methotrexate	200 mg/m² IV	8 and 15
Leucovorin	10 mg/m² PO q6h x 6	after Mtx

Repeat cycles every 21 days for 10 cycles.

Table 28-11 *Continued.* Combination Chemotherapy for Non-Hodgkin's Lymphomas

ProMACE-CytaBOM Regimen

Agent	Dose/Administration Route	Day
Cyclophosphamide	650/mg/m² IV	1
Doxorubicin	25 mg/m² IV	1
Etoposide	120 mg/m² IV	1
Prednisone	60 mg/m² PO	1-14
Cytarabine	300 mg/m² IV	8
Bleomycin	5 mg/m² IV	8
Vincristine	1.4 mg/m² IV	8
Methotrexate	120 mg/m² IV	8
Leucovorin	25mg/m² PO q6h x 4	after Mtx

Repeat cycles every 21 days for ≥6 cycles.

autologous marrow transplantation have been favorable but overall success must be measured by long-term follow-up. Marrow harvested from patients with low-grade NHL is usually involved with lymphoma and is treated in vitro with specific monoclonal antibodies.[63]

Intermediate- and High-Grade Histology

Patients with NHL of unfavorable (intermediate or high-grade) have a much more aggressive disease that results in a rapid downhill course. For these groups, the median survival with minimal treatment ranges from 1 to 2 years. However, this course has been dramatically changed by the introduction of aggressive combination chemotherapy that results in a high percentage of durable, long-term disease-free survival and patients who are cured. For patients with bulky stages II to IV, unfavorable-histology non-Hodgkin's lymphoma, aggressive systemic chemotherapy is the initial treatment of choice. CR rates with a variety of chemotherapeutic regimens vary from 40% to 80%.[64-73] A substantial portion of patients who achieve a complete response, particularly those with diffuse large-cell lymphoma, remain clinically disease free for extended periods and may be cured.

Chemotherapeutic regimens with the best potential to induce prolonged complete remissions are generally high-intensity regimens containing doxorubicin (Adriamycin).[72] The drugs used in combination therapy, frequency of administration, and doses vary con-

Table 28-12. Results of Representative Cooperative Group Treatment

Regimen	No. Patients	No. Responses Evaluable	CR (%)	Toxicity (%) LT	Toxicity (%) Fatal
CHOP	350	350	37-68	10	3
m-BACOD	84	84	65	31	6
ProMACE-CytaBOM	97	83	58	20	5
MACOP-B	72	68	56	28	2

CR=complete response; LT=life threatening

From Miller et al.[75]

siderably among regimens (Table 28-11), and reports primarily of phase II trials give widely different complete response rates and claim superiority of one regimen over another. A high-priority randomized prospective clinical trial of the National Cancer Institute evaluated four combinations: CHOP, m-BACOD, ProMACE-CytaBOM, and MACOP-B.[74] The results of representative Cooperative Group treatment using the four different regimens are given in Table 28-12.[75]

Unfortunately, a significant number of patients with unfavorable-histology NHL either fails to respond or eventually has disease relapse. Prognosis then is uniformly poor, and almost all can be expected to die of progressive lymphoma. Effective salvage

Table 28-13. Prognostic Factors in Non-Hodgkin's Lymphomas

- Performance status
- B symptoms
- More than two extranodal sites
- Mass >10 cm
- Spleen involvement
- Elevated serum LDH
- Stage III/IV
- Effusions

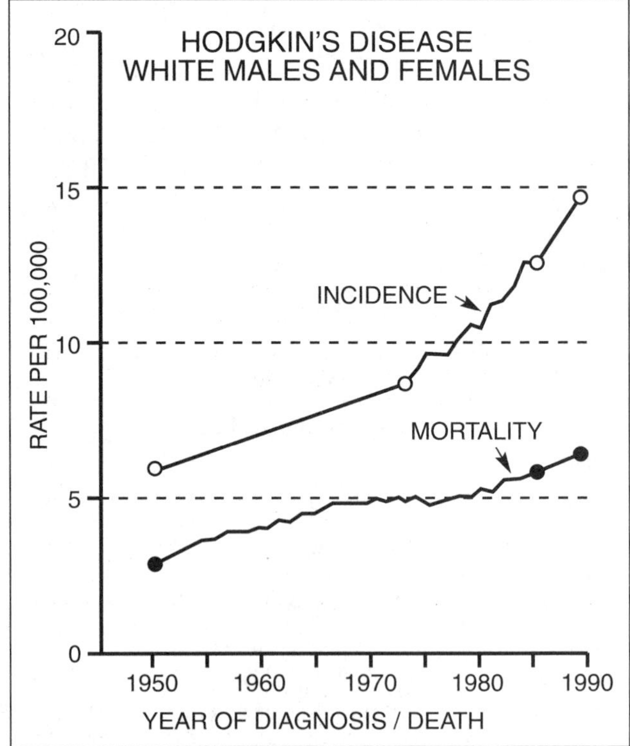

Fig 28-14. Incidence rates per 100,000 population for non-Hodgkin's lymphoma, age adjusted to 1970 have nearly doubled since 1950, as have mortality rates.

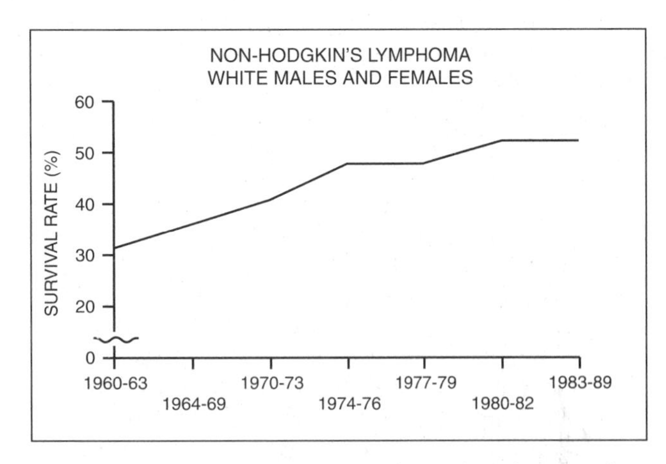

Fig 28-13. Improvements in 5-year relative survival rates in the US (from 31% in 1960 to 52% in 1989).[45]

chemotherapy with a variety of regimens can produce second remissions, but these are rarely of significant duration.[76,77] A number of investigational drugs are being evaluated for their ability to salvage these patients, but the most consistently reported effective salvage therapy for relapsing patients (excluding primary failures) seems to be marrow transplantation. Several centers have reported long-term disease-free survival either using cryopreserved autologous marrow or allogeneic marrow transplantation.[78] The prognostic factors listed in Table 28-13 may help predict poor responses to conventional chemotherapy and select candidates for experimental programs of marrow transplantation.

Summary

Aggressive chemotherapy is the primary therapy for intermediate- and high-grade NHL. Radiation therapy may be used to treat residual disease if limited and localized. Overall treatment results for non-Hodgkin's lymphomas have been steadily improving (Fig 28-13). Improved survival rates, however, are offset by rising incidence rates, which contribute to a slight increase in mortality rates (Fig 28-14).

The non-Hodgkin's lymphomas differ in many ways from Hodgkin's disease. The malignant cell is known in NHL, the frequency of disease is increasing, and there is some evidence for a pathogenetic mechanism. Histologic grading is of much more importance than clinical staging.

The management of malignant lymphomas has taught oncologists many lessons in the cure of malignant disease. Further advances and better control of these diseases will also prove useful in the understanding of other human malignancies.

References

1. Boring CC, Squires TS, Tong T, Montgomery S. Cancer Statistics, 1994. *CA Cancer J Clin* 1994; 44:7-26.

2. Devesa SS, Silverman DT, Young JL Jr, et al. Cancer incidence and mortality trends among whites in the United States, 1947-1984. *J Natl Cancer Inst.* 1987;79:701-770.

3. Hodgkin T. On some morbid appearances of the absorbent glands and spleen. *Med-Clin Tran.* 1832;17:68.

4. Pinkus GS, Thomas P, Said JW. Leu-M1–a marker for Reed-Sternberg cells in Hodgkin's disease: an immunoperoxidase study of paraffin-embedded tissues. *Am J Path.* 1985;119:244-252.

5. Austin-Seymour MM, Hoppe RT, Cox RS, Rosenberg SA, Kaplan HS. Hodgkin's disease in patients over sixty years old. *Ann Intern Med.* 1984;100:13-18.

6. DeVita VT Jr, Jaffe ES, Hellman S. Hodgkin's disease and the non-Hodgkin's lymphomas. In: DeVita VT Jr, Hellman S, Rosenberg SA, eds. *Cancer Principles and Practice of Oncology.* 2nd ed. New York, NY: JB Lippincott Co; 1985: 1623-1709.

7. Rosenberg SA, Kaplan HS, eds. *Malignant Lymphomas: Etiology, Immunology, Pathology, Treatment.* New York, NY: Academic Press; 1982.

8. Cutler SJ, Young JC, eds. Third national cancer survey: incidence data. *Natl Cancer Inst Monographs.* 1975;41: 107-111.

9. Vianna NJ, Polan AK. Immunity in Hodgkin's disease: importance of age at exposure. *Ann Intern Med.* 1978;89: 550-556.

10. Paffenberger RS Jr, Wing AL, Hyde RT. Characteristics in youth indicative of adult-onset Hodgkin's disease. *J Natl Cancer Inst.* 1977;58:1489-1491.

11. Grufferman S, Cole P, Smith PG, Lukes RJ. Hodgkin's disease in siblings. *N Engl J Med.* 1977;296:248-250.

12. Diehl V, Burrichter H, Schaadt M, Fonatsch C, Stein H, Rossbach HC. Hodgkin's disease: the remaining challenge. *Prog Med Virol.* 1984;30:199-203.

13. Hesse J, Levine PH, Ebbesen P, Connelly RR, Mordhurst CH. A case control study on immunity to two Epstein-Barr virus-associated antigens and to herpes simplex virus and adenovirus in a population-based group of patients with Hodgkin's disease in Denmark, 1971-1973. *Int J Cancer.* 1977;19:49-58.

14. Kadin ME, Stites DP, Levy R, Warnke R. Exogenous immunoglobulin in Reed-Sternberg cells in Hodgkin's disease. *N Engl J Med.* 1978;299:1208-1214.

15. Ford RJ, Mehta S, Davis F, Maizel AL. Growth factors in Hodgkin's disease. *Cancer Treat Rep.* 1982;66:633-638.

16. Oppenheim JJ, Stadler BM, Siragnian RP, Mage M, Mathieson B. Lymphokines: their role in lymphocyte responses: properties of interleukin 1. *Fed Proc.* 1982;41: 257-262.

17. Stein RS. Clinical features and clinical evaluation of Hodgkin's disease and the non-Hodgkin's lymphomas. In: Bennett JM, ed. *Lymphomas 1.* Boston, Mass: Marcus Nijhoff; 1981:129-175.

18. Carbone PP, Kaplan HS, Mushoff K, Smithers DW, Tubiana M. Report of the Committee on Hodgkin's Disease Staging Classification. *Cancer Res.* 1971;31:1860-1861.

19. Kaplan HS. *Hodgkin's Disease.* 2nd ed. Cambridge, Mass: Harvard University Press; 1980.

20. Eghbali H, Hoerni-Simon G, deMascarel I, Duran M, Chauvergne J, Hoerni B. Hodgkin's disease in the elderly. *Cancer.* 1984;53:2191-2193.

21. Desforges JF, Rutherford CJ, Piro A. Hodgkin's disease; medical progress. *N Engl J Med.* 1979;301:1212-1222.

22. Chen JL, Osborne BM, Butler JJ. Residual fibrous masses treated in Hodgkin's disease. *Cancer.* 1987;60: 407-413.

23. Cornbleet MA, Vitolo U, Ultmann JE, et al. Pathologic stages IA and IIA Hodgkin's disease: results of treatment with radiotherapy alone (1968-1980). *J Clin Oncol.* 1985;3:758-768.

24. Leslie NT, Mauch PM, Hellman S. Stage IA to IIB supradiaphragmatic Hodgkin's disease: long-term survival and relapse frequency. *Cancer.* 1985;55:2072-2078.

25. Prosnitz LR, Montalva RL, Fisher DB, et al. Treatment of stage IIIA Hodgkin's disease: is radiotherapy alone adequate? *Int J Radiat Oncol Biol Phys.* 1978;4:781-787.

26. Farber LR, Prosnitz LR, Cadman EC, Lutes R, Bertino JR, Fischer DB. Curative potential of combined modality therapy for advanced Hodgkin's disease. *Cancer.* 1980;46:1509-1517.

27. Desser RK, Golomb HM, Ultmann JE, et al. Prognostic

classification of Hodgkin's disease in pathologic stage III, based on anatomic considerations. *Blood.* 1977;49:883-893.

28. Kaplan HS. Hodgkin's disease: unfolding concepts concerning its nature, management and prognosis. *Cancer.* 1980;45:2439-2474.

29. Rosenberg SA, Kaplan HS. Evidence for an orderly progression in the spread of Hodgkin's disease. *Cancer Res.* 1966;26:1225-1230.

30. Coltman CA Jr. Chemotherapy of advanced Hodgkin's disease. *Semin Oncol.* 1980;7:155-173.

31. Longo DL, Young RC, Wesley M, et al. Twenty years of MOPP therapy for Hodgkin's disease. *J Clin Oncol.* 1986;4:1295-1306.

32. DeVita VT Jr, Simon RM, Hubbard SM, et al. Curability of advanced Hodgkin's disease with chemotherapy: long-term follow-up of MOPP-treated patients at the National Cancer Institute. *Ann Intern Med.* 1980;92:587-595.

33. Bonadonna G, Zucali R, Monfardini S, DeLena M, Uslenghi C. Combination therapy of Hodgkin's disease with Adriamycin, bleomycin, vinblastine, and imidazole carboxamide versus MOPP. *Cancer.* 1973;36:252-259.

34. Santoro A, Bonfante V, Bonadonna G. Salvage chemotherapy with ABVD in MOPP-resistant Hodgkin's disease. *Ann Intern Med.* 1982;96:139-143.

35. Santoro A, Bonadonna G, Valagussa P, et al. Long-term results of combined chemotherapy-radiotherapy approach in Hodgkin's disease: superiority of ABVD plus radiotherapy versus MOPP plus radiotherapy. *J Clin Oncol.* 1987;5:27-37.

36. Buzaid AC, Lippman SM, Miller TP. Salvage therapy of advanced Hodgkin's disease. *Am J Med.* 1987;83:523-532.

37. Canellos G, Anderson JR, Propert KJ, et al. Chemotherapy of advanced Hodgkin's disease with MOPP, ABVD or MOPP alternating with ABVD. *N Engl J Med.* 1992;327: 1478-1484.

38. Mauch P, Goodman R, Hellman S. The significance of mediastinal involvement in early stage Hodgkin's disease. *Cancer.* 1978;42:1039-1045.

39. Henkelmann GC, Hagemeister FB, Fuller LM. Two cycles of MOPP and radiotherapy for stage III_1A and III_1B Hodgkin's disease. *J Clin Oncol.* 1988;6:1293-1302.

40. Mauch P, Goffman T, Rosenthal D, et al. Stage IV Hodgkin's disease: improved survival with combined modality therapy as compared with radiation therapy alone. *J Clin Oncol.* 1985;3:1166-1173.

41. Behrendt H, VanBunningen BNFM, Van Leeuwen EF. Treatment of Hodgkin's disease in children with or without radiotherapy. *Cancer.* 1987;59:1870-1873.

42. Tucker MA, Coleman CN, Cox RS, Varghese A, Rosenberg SA. Risk of second cancers after treatment for Hodgkin's disease. *N Engl J Med.* 1988;318:76-81.

43. Coltman CA Jr, Dixon DO. Second malignancies complicating Hodgkin's disease: a Southwest Oncology Group 10-year follow-up. *Cancer Treat Rep.* 1982;66:1023-1033.

44. Linch DC, Winfield D, Goldstone AH, et al. Dose intensification with autologous bone-marrow transplantation in relapsed and resistant Hodgkin's disease: results of a BNLI randomised trial. *Lancet.* 1993;341:1051-1054.

45. Miller BA, Ries LAG, Hankey BF, et al. *SEER Cancer Statistics Review: 1973-1990.* Bethesda, Md: National Cancer Institute; 1993. NIH Pub 93-2789.

46. Foon KA, Schroff RW, Gale RP. Surface markers on leukemia and lymphoma cells: recent advances. *Blood.* 1982; 60:1-19.

47. Rodriguez MA, Pathak S, Trujillo J, et al. Structural abnormalities of chromosome 11q in patients with lymphoma. *Proc Am Assoc Cancer Res.* 1987;23:146. Abstract.

48. Rosenberg SA, Diamond HD, Jaslowitz B. Lymphosarcoma: a review of 1,269 cases. *Medicine.* 1961;40:31-84.

49. Ultmann JE, Jacobs RH. The non-Hodgkin's lymphomas. *CA Cancer J Clin.* 1985;35:66-87.

50. Armitage JO. Treatment of non-Hodgkin's lymphoma. *N Engl J Med.* 1993;328:1023-1030.

51. Vokes EE, Ultmann JE, Golomb HM, et al. Long-term survival of patients with localized diffuse histiocytic lymphoma. *J Clin Oncol.* 1985;3:1309.

52. Paryani SB, Hoppe RT, Cox RS, Colby TV, Rosenberg SA, Kaplan HS. Analysis of non-Hodgkin's lymphomas with nodular and favorable histologies, stages I and II. *Cancer.* 1983;52:2300-2307.

53. Gospodarowicz MK, Bush RS, Brown TC, et al. Prognostic factors in nodular lymphomas: a multivariate analysis based on the Princess Margaret Hospital experience. *Int J Radiat Oncol Biol Phys.* 1981;10:489-497.

54. Glatstein E, Donaldson SS, Rosenberg SA, et al. Combined modality therapy in malignant lymphomas. *Cancer Treat Rep.* 1977;61:1199-1207.

55. Hoppe RT, Kushlan P, Kaplan HS, Rosenberg SA, Brown BW. The treatment of advanced stage favorable histology non-Hodgkin's lymphoma: a preliminary report of a randomized trial comparing single agent chemotherapy, combination chemotherapy, and whole body irradiation. *Blood.* 1981;58:592-598.

56. Hoppe RT. The role of radiation treatment in the management of the non-Hodgkin's lymphomas. *Cancer.* 1985;55:2176-2183.

57. Bush RS, Gospodarowicz M. The place of radiation therapy in the management of localized non-Hodgkin's lymphoma. In: Rosenberg SA, Kaplan HS, eds. *Malignant Lymphomas: Etiology, Immunology, Pathology, Treatment.* New York, NY: Academic Press; 1982:485-502.

58. Hoppe RT, Fuks Z, Bagshaw MA. Radiation therapy in the management of cutaneous T-cell lymphomas. *Cancer Treat Rep.* 1979;63:625-632.

59. Rosenberg SA. Non-Hodgkin's lymphoma: selection of treatment on the basis of histologic type. *N Engl J Med.* 1979;301:924-928.

60. McLaughlin P, Fuller LM. Velasquez WS, et al. Stage III follicular lymphoma: durable remissions with a combined chemotherapy-radiotherapy regimen. *J Clin Oncol.* 1987;5:867-874.

61. Ezdinli EZ, Anderson JR, Melvin F, Glick JH, Davis TE, O'Connell MJ. Moderate versus aggressive chemotherapy of nodular lymphocytic poorly differentiated lymphoma. *J Clin Oncol.* 1985;32:769-775.

62. Young RC, Longo DL, Glatstein E, Ihde CD, Jaffe ES, DeVita VT Jr. The treatment of indolent lymphomas: watchful waiting vs aggressive combined modality treatment. *Semin Hematol.* 1988;25(2, Suppl 2):11-16.

63. Canellos GP, Nadler L, Takvorian T. Autologous bone marrow transplantation in the treatment of malignant lymphoma and Hodgkin's disease. *Semin Hematol.* 1988;25:58-65.

64. DeVita VT Jr, Hubbard SM, Young RC, Longo D. The role of chemotherapy in diffuse aggressive lymphomas. *Semin Hematol.* 1988;25(2, Suppl 2):2-10.

65. Boyd DB, Coleman M, Papish SW, et al. COPBALM III: infusion combination chemotherapy for diffuse large-cell lymphoma. *J Clin Oncol.* 1988;6:425-433.

66. Klimo P, Connors JM. MACOP-B chemotherapy for the treatment of diffuse large-cell lymphoma. *Ann Intern Med.* 1985;102:596-602.

67. Fisher RI, DeVita VT Jr, Hubbard SM, et al. Diffuse aggressive lymphomas: increased survival after alternating flexible sequences of ProMACE and MOPP chemotherapy. *Ann Intern Med.* 1983;98:304-309.

68. Skarin AT, Canellos GP, Rosenthal DS, et al. Improved prognosis of diffuse histiocytic and undifferentiated lymphoma by use of high-dose methotrexate alternating with standard agents (m-BACOD). *J Clin Oncol.* 1983;1:91-98.

69. Freireich EJ, Cabanillas F, Burgess MA, Bodey GP. Sequential chemotherapy and late intensification for malignant lymphomas of aggressive histologic type. *Am J Med.* 1983;74:382-388.

70. Jones SE, Grozea PN, Metz EN, et al. Improved complete remission rates and survival for patients with large-cell lymphoma treated with chemoimmunotherapy: a Southwest Oncology Group study. *Cancer.* 1983;51:1083-1090.

71. Sweet DL, Golomb HM. The treatment of histiocytic lymphoma. *Semin Oncol.* 1980;7:302-309.

72. Jones SE, Grozea PN, Metz EN, et al. Superiority of Adriamycin-containing combination chemotherapy in the treatment of diffuse lymphoma: a Southwest Oncology Group study. *Cancer.* 1979;43:417-425.

73. Coltman CA Jr, Luce JK, McKelvey EM, et al. Chemotherapy of non-Hodgkin's lymphoma: 10 years' experience in the Southwest Oncology Group. *Cancer Treat Rep.* 1977;61:1067-1078.

74. Miller TP, Dahlberg S, Jones SE, et al. ProMACE-CytaBOM is active with acceptable toxicity in patients with unfavorable non-Hodgkin's lymphoma: a Southwest Oncology Group study. *ASCO.* 1987;6:197.

75. Miller TP, Dana BW, Weick JK, et al. Southwest Oncology Group clinical trials for intermediate- and high-grade non-Hodgkin's lymphomas. *Third Int Conference on Malignant Lymphomas.* 1987; Abstract.

76. Cabanillas F, Hagemeister FB, McLaughlin P, et al. Results of MIME salvage regimen for recurrent or refractory lymphoma. *J Clin Oncol.* 1987;5:407-412.

77. Shipp MA, Takvorian RC, Canellos GP. High-dose cytosine arabinoside: active agent in treatment of non-Hodgkin's lymphoma. *Am J Med.* 1984;77:845-850.

78. Applebaum FR, Sullivan KM, Buckner CD, et al. Treatment of malignant lymphoma in 100 patients with chemotherapy, total body irradiation and marrow transplantation. *J Clin Oncol.* 1987;5:1340-1347.

29

MULTIPLE MYELOMA

Glenn J. Bubley, MD, Lowell E. Schnipper, MD

Plasma cell dyscrasia (PCD) is a broad term for a family of clonal neoplastic disorders associated with the overproduction of a monoclonal antibody. The malignant cells in these disorders—plasma cells and plasmacytoid lymphocytes—are the most mature cells of B-lymphocyte origin. B-cell maturation is associated with a programmed rearrangement of DNA sequences in the process of encoding the structure of mature immunoglobulins. This development results in a myriad of plasma cell clones, each making an antibody specific for an almost infinite number of antigens. In PCD, one B-cell clone predominates and results in the production of large quantities of a monoclonal immunoglobulin (Ig).[1]

Multiple myeloma (MM) is the most common malignant PCD, and is characterized by overproduction of monoclonal IgG, IgA, and/or light chains. Waldenstrom's macroglobulinemia (WM), a malignant PCD with a different clinical spectrum from MM, is associated with overproduction of IgM. Occasionally, healthy patients are observed to produce an excess of a monoclonal antibody in the absence of a specific syndrome or symptom complex, and are thus characterized as having a monoclonal gammopathy of undetermined significance (MGUS). Patients in whom the amount of M-protein does not change over time and who remain asymptomatic have a benign monoclonal gammopathy (BMG). Alternatively, MGUS may progress slowly (smoldering myeloma) to become a clinically evident disease associated with progressive overproduction of a monoclonal protein, or M-protein (eg, MM, WM, amyloidosis, or non-Hodgkin's lymphoma). In almost all cases of PCD, an M-protein (usually light chain) can be detected in the serum or urine.[1] In this chapter, the pathophysiology of PCD, each disorder's clinical characteristics, and management are presented.

Antibody Structure

A general model of immunoglobulin structure is shown in Fig 29-1.[2] This monomer is the basic structure of IgG, IgA, IgM, IgD, and IgE. It is made up of identical dimeric units, each composed of a heavy and a light chain bound together by disulfide bridges.[3] Each polypeptide chain contains two general regions: an amino (NH_2)-terminal variable (V) region, and a carboxy ($C0_2H$)-terminal constant (C) region. The antigen recognition site is in the variable region and is composed of terminal heavy- and light-chain components. It is called the fragment antigen binding (Fab) region,[4] and also contains the amino acid sequence that defines the unique antigenic structure of a specific immunoglobulin molecule, termed the idiotype. The other end of the molecule, the Fc region, is responsible for complement activation, cell binding, and placental transport.[4]

Light chains have a single carboxy-terminal domain in contrast to heavy chains, which have three or four constant domains. Both heavy and light chains have one variable domain within which all hypervariable regions (areas of greater amino acid sequence diversity) lie (Fig 29-1); each is made up of approximately 110 amino acids.[3,4]

The major classes of human immunoglobulin—IgG, IgA, IgM, IgE, and IgD—are each defined by a constant heavy chain (C_H) region that is specific for that class. The light chain of the molecule is of two varieties, kappa or lambda. In normal development, B cells progress from producing an IgM molecule to an IgG or IgA by genetic recombination of a segment of

Glenn J. Bubley, MD, Assistant Professor of Medicine, Harvard Medical School, Division of Hematology/Oncology, Beth Israel Hospital, Boston, Massachusetts

Lowell E. Schnipper, MD, Theodore W. and Evelyn G. Berenson Associate Professor of Medicine, Harvard Medical School, Chief, Oncology Division, Beth Israel Hospital, Boston, Massachusetts, of the Charles A. Dana Research Institute, Harvard-Thorndike Laboratory, Department of Medicine of Beth Israel Hospital, Harvard Medical School, Boston, Massachusetts

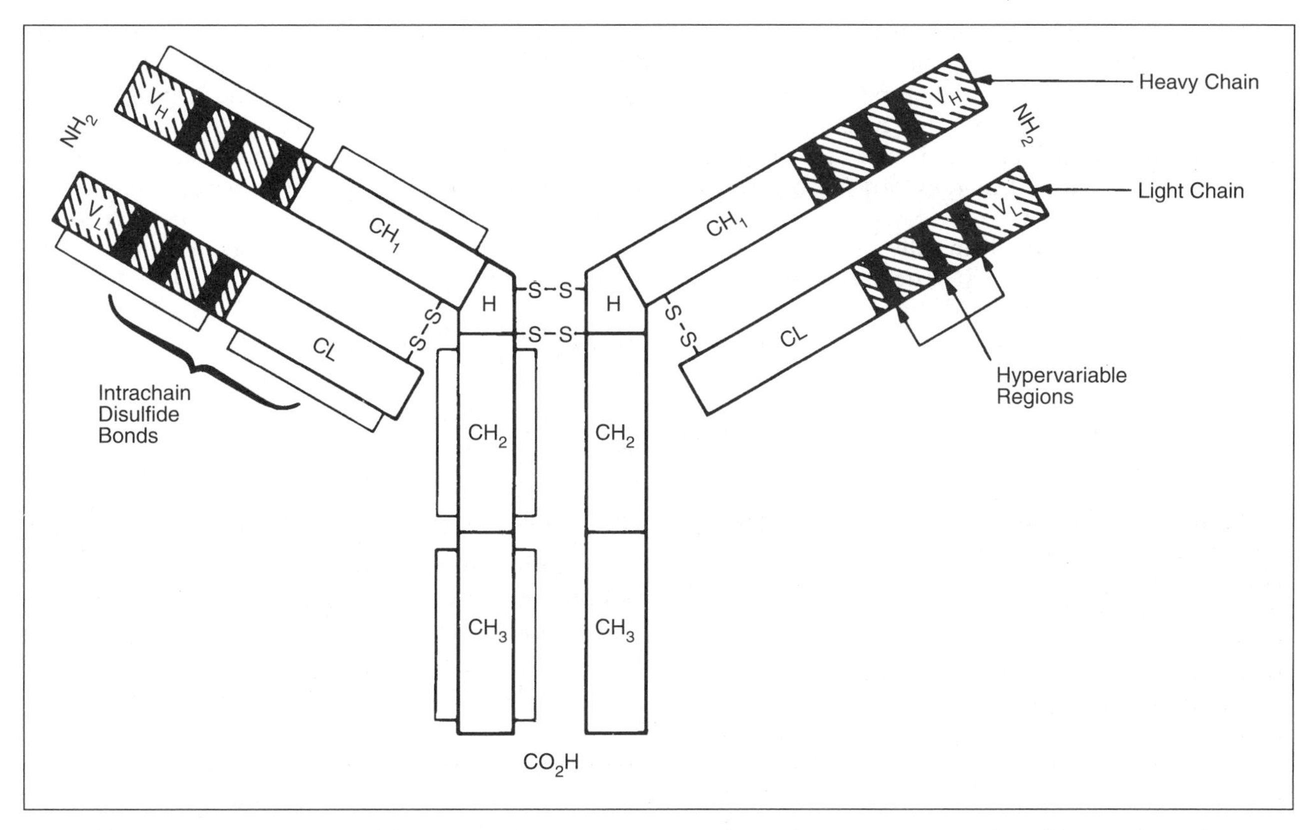

Fig 29-1. Basic structure of immunoglobulin molecule. Each chain consists of variable regions, V_L or V_H, indicated by cross-hatched areas; hypervariable regions (solid black), characterized by minor variations in amino acid sequence; and constant regions (CL or CH). The amino-terminal variable or Fab region is responsible for antigen binding, and the constant carboxy-terminal region (Fc) has separate domains (CH_1, CH_2, or CH_3) responsible for cell or compartment binding. H is the hinge region. From Stamatoyannopoulos et al.[2]

DNA in the C_H region of chromosome 14. A similar process enables a single B-cell clone to produce antibodies of different IgG subclasses that have the same antigenic specificity. Genetic recombination, a process essential to the production of immunoglobulins, is one factor contributing to the amazing diversity of antibody molecules.[4]

During B-cell maturation, the first immunoglobulin produced is IgM; it is also the antibody produced during the primary immune response and is the antibody first produced by infants. The IgM structure is a pentameric ring formed by the attachment of a joining chain to the basic subunits at their Fc portion. These molecules efficiently bind complement and are restricted to the intravascular space. Due to their large size these antibodies are called macroglobulins, and a monoclonal IgM is the M-protein overproduced in WM.

IgG is the major immunoglobulin in serum. It consists of four isotopic subclasses (IgG1-4), within which small differences in the heavy-chain regions account for slightly different biologic properties. For example, IgG1 and IgG3 bind complement and mononuclear cells more effectively than IgG2 and IgG4. IgG1 and IgG3, when overproduced in MM, can be associated

Table 29-1. Frequency of M-Protein Classes Produced by Plasma Cell Neoplasms

	Proportion (%)
M-proteins containing both H and L chains	
1. IgG	52
2. IgA	21
3. IgM	12
4. IgD	2
5. IgE	0.01
M-proteins containing only L chains (κ or λ)	11
M-proteins containing only H chains (γ, α, μ, δ, or ε)	1
≥2 M-proteins	0.5
No M-protein in serum or urine	1

From data on 1,827 patients compiled by Pruzanski and Ogryzlo; adapted from Holland and Frei.[5]

with hyperviscosity due to a propensity to form dimers. They have faster catabolic rates than the other IgG subclasses. IgG is normally produced during the secondary (anamnestic) immune response. It is the only immunoglobulin class that can be transported across the placenta and thereby provide passive immunity to the newborn.[3]

IgA is the chief antibody in saliva, tears, and secretions of the gastrointestinal (GI) and respiratory tracts and serves as the first line of local defense against environmental agents. Its structure includes a secretory component that facilitates transport across the epithelial cell membrane.[3]

IgD and IgE are usually trace proteins in plasma. IgD is thought to act as a cell surface receptor that binds antigen and triggers B-cell proliferation and differentiation.[2] IgE serum levels can be elevated during parasitic infection or in atopic individuals.[3] It binds with high affinity to receptors on basophils and mast cells, and may induce these cells to release vasoactive amines as part of an allergic response.

IgG makes up the largest proportion of immunoglobulins in adult plasma, followed by IgA and IgM.[4] The distribution of these proteins in normal serum has a parallel in the observed distribution of M-protein types in PCDs (Table 29-1).[5] This holds true for the IgG subtypes as well. For example, IgG1 makes up about 65% of the IgG concentration in normal serum and is the M-protein in a comparable percentage of IgG myelomas. These observations suggest that any B-cell clone has an equal chance of evolving into a malignant clone.

B-Lymphocyte Development

The assembly of mature immunoglobulin molecules is the result of several genetic-recombination events that occur at identifiable stages of B-cell development and contribute to generating antibody diversity.[6,7] B-cell ontogeny begins when a lymphoid stem cell is committed to development as a progenitor B cell, and proceeds through developmental steps to become a lymphocyte or a plasma cell (Fig 29-2).[2] In PCD, a malignant B-cell clone producing a monoclonal Ig has undergone a similar pattern of development, although heavy- and light-chain production may be unbalanced.

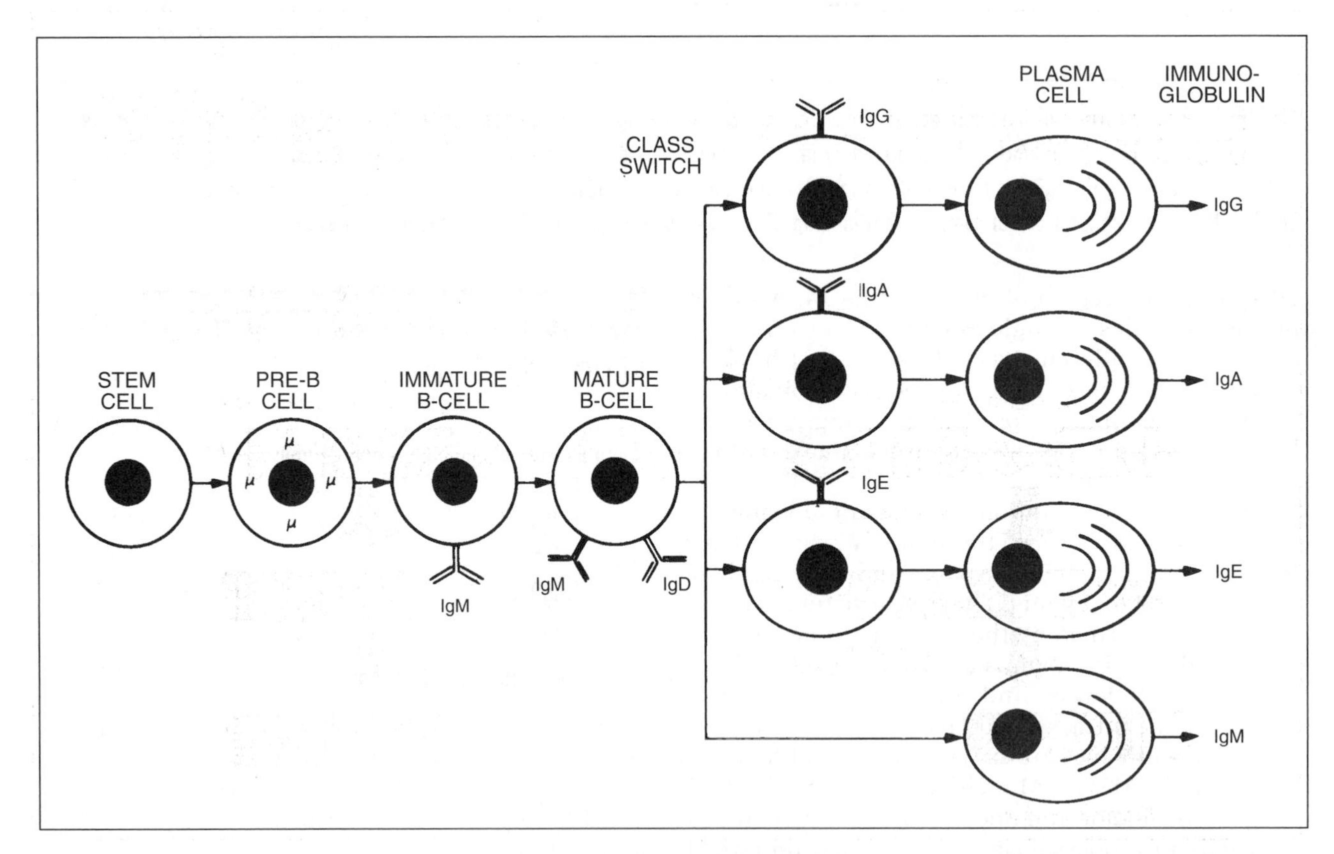

Fig 29-2. Differentiation of B lymphocytes and plasma cells. A pleiotropic stem cell gives rise to the pre-B cell that has acquired the capacity to synthesize heavy chains (μ). The immature B cell can synthesize light chains so that a complete IgM molecule is formed and expressed on the cell surface. Mature B cells express both IgM and IgD on their surfaces. These cells can either mature into IgM-secreting plasmacytoid lymphocytes, or undergo a class switch to express IgG, IgA, or IgE on their surfaces. The latter cells can undergo terminal differentiation into IgG-, IgA-, or IgE-secreting plasma cells. From Stamatoyannopoulos et al.[2]

At least two different gene segments contribute to each constant and variable region of both the heavy and light chains.[6] The DNA segments encoding the heavy-chain gene family are on chromosome 14, kappa light chains are encoded on chromosome 2, and lambda light chains on chromosome 22.

The first step in immunoglobulin production is the heavy-chain rearrangement on chromosome 14 that marks the cell's commitment to B-cell lineage. Initially, one of the 20 or more diverse (D) genes is transposed next to one of six joining (J) region genes on both chromosomes 14. If a DJ rearrangement is completed successfully, then one of at least 50 variable (V) region genes on only one of the chromosomes is translocated (Fig 29-3) to form a continuous VDJ_H complex.[3,6] This genetic complex can encode the entire variable region of the heavy chain.

Transcription into RNA is another mechanism for differential gene expression. When RNA is transcribed from DNA, both coding regions (exons) and noncoding intervening sequences (introns) are transcribed. Splicing is the process by which introns are removed prior to translation. Following removal of introns between the VDJ_H complex and the heavy-chain constant region (Cμ), the IgM heavy-chain can be translated.[3] Splicing, or removal, of different intervening DNA segments can also result in B-cell production of either cytoplasmic or surface IgM, or both (Figs 29-2 and 29-3).

Expression of the heavy or μ chain identifies the pre-B cell phase of development.[7] If a nonproductive rearrangement in the VDJ_H complex occurs on one of the pair of chromosomes 14, then rearrangement activity will shift to the other chromosome. This process, termed allelic exclusion, is repeated during light-chain development and ensures that a B lymphocyte can make only one type of antibody. Cells that do not undergo a functional heavy-chain rearrangement on either chromosome will not initiate light-chain production.

The next step in the gene rearrangement cascade occurs on chromosome 2, which encodes the variable region of the kappa gene. DNA fragments from two separate DNA segments, V and J, undergo a rearrange-

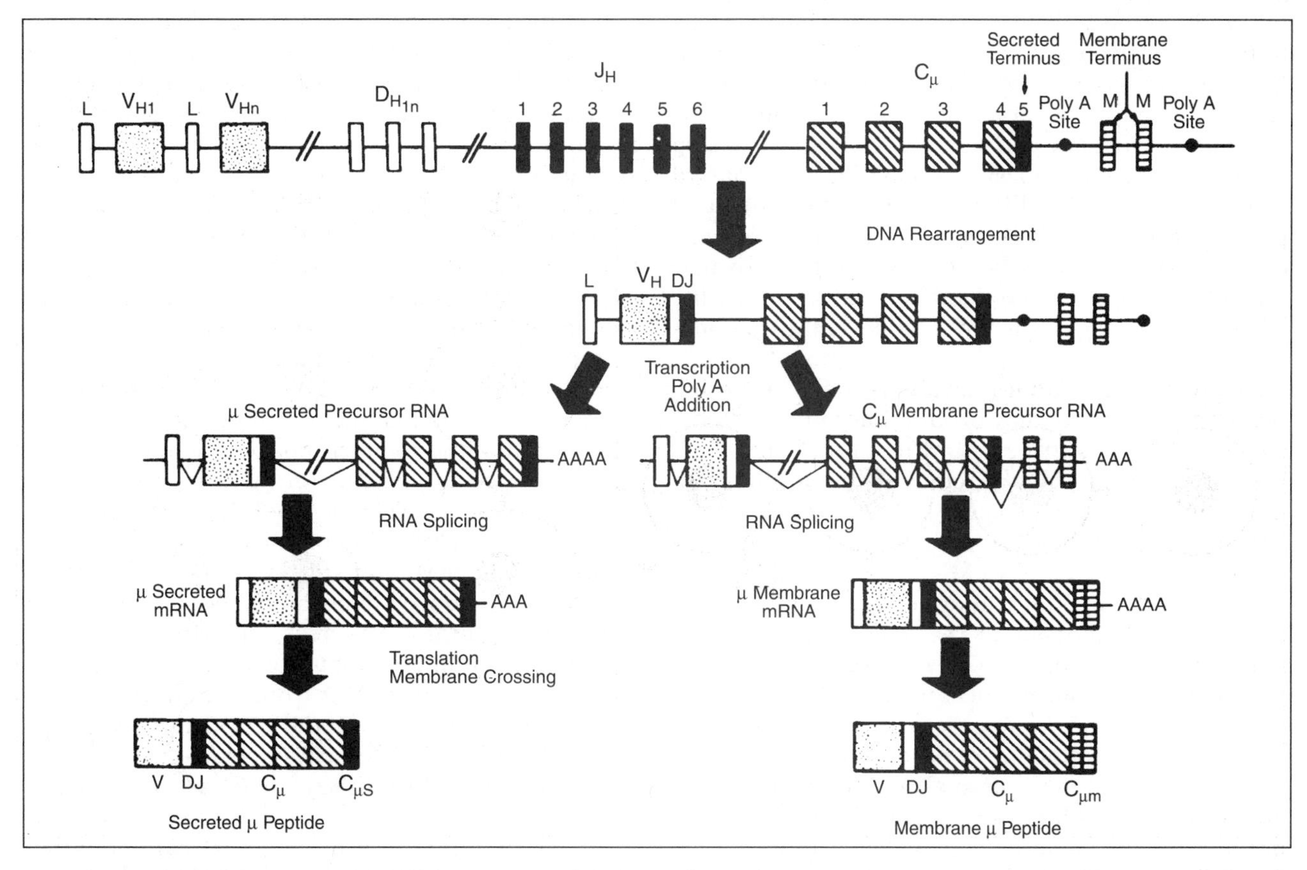

Fig 29-3. Model of the DNA structure and rearrangement of the human heavy-chain gene. The region consists of multiple (300) V_H regions, families of diverse (D_H) segments, six joining (J_H) segments, and a single constant (C) gene made up of a number of domains. Single V_H—D_H—and J_H region gene subsegments are joined at the DNA level. Both secreted and membrane forms of IgM can be derived from a single constant region locus by addition of sites of poly-A residues (adenines added to the end of mRNA) and RNA splicing. From Stamatoyannopoulos et al.[2]

ment to encode the kappa light-chain variable region. If a productive VJ rearrangement does not occur, then rearrangement will shift to the VJ region of the lambda light-chain region on chromosome 22. Successful production of a kappa or lambda light chain allows it to bind to the heavy chain to make a complete IgM monomer. This molecule is then transported to the cell surface, where its expression marks the early stage of B-cell development.[3,6]

The result of multiple genetic rearrangements encoding slight alterations in DNA sequence, especially in the regions joining different segments, is production of millions of different B-cell clones.[6] These enter the circulation from the bone marrow to migrate to the spleen and other lymphoid tissue, where further development depends on antigenic stimulation. If a specific B cell is exposed to an antigen that binds specifically to the variable region of the antibody expressed on its cell surface, the cell will internalize and digest the fragment. The antigen will then be expressed on the surface of the cell with major histocompatibility complex (MHC) class II antigens. This complex can be recognized by helper T cells, which produce factors promoting proliferation and differentiation, allowing the B cell to progress through further stages of development. When antigen-stimulated B cells lose surface IgD and IgM and begin to accumulate cytoplasmic IgG, they become intermediate and mature B cells, the final step prior to maturation into plasma cells (Fig 29-2). Plasma cells are terminally differentiated. The continued production of antibody depends on the continued presence of antigenic stimulation. Following removal of the antigen, antibody production depends on the life span of the plasma cell and the half-life of the immunoglobulin protein.[6]

B lymphocytes in an individual clone can switch from IgM to IgG or IgA production with identical variable-region antigen-binding specificity. This process, termed a class switch, probably results from a deletion on chromosome 14 of DNA between the VDJ complex and the C_H region specific for another Ig class.[2,6]

In general, the proliferation of B cells and production of immunoglobulin in PCD follow the pattern of normal development. In PCD, however, the proliferation of a B-cell clone and its attendant antibody production continue in the absence of an obvious antigenic stimulus. The production of other immunoglobulins may be reduced and the normal antibody responses to antigens may be blunted. Occasionally, the antibody produced in PCD is specific for a known antigen, such as a bacterial or viral surface protein.[8]

Etiology

The etiology of PCD is not completely understood; however, there is now intriguing evidence about a specific factor that may induce growth of a B-cell clone.[9] There is also evidence that the abnormal proliferation of plasma cells may be programmed as early as the pre-B stage of development.[10] In fact, the expression of myeloid, megakaryocytic, and erythroid antigens on the same plasma cell clone has been demonstrated, reinforcing the view that myeloma may originate from an early multipotential progenitor cell.

The role of cytokines in the pathogenesis of PCD is an important area of current research. A number of investigators have shown interleukin-6 (IL-6) to be an important factor promoting the in-vitro growth of myeloma cells.[9,11] This cytokine in the presence of IL-3 may have synergistic effects on the differentiation of B cells to yield a plasma cell clone. IL-6 levels have been reported to be higher in the serum of patients with active myeloma than in those with MGUS or BMG.[12] Exposure of IL-6 receptor expressing human myeloma cell lines to antisense IL-6 mRNA resulted in marked inhibition of proliferation,[13] which suggests that IL-6 may promote growth of myeloma cells through an autocrine loop.

Other cytokines or lymphokines that may be important in the pathogenesis of PCD include tumor necrosis factor and IL-1–beta, both of which have been implicated in the bone destruction prevalent in MM.

To better understand the etiologic factors for PCD, an animal model has been developed in specific strains of mice,[14] in which chronic intraperitoneal injection of an antigenic stimulus such as mineral oil leads to the formation of granulomas, which progress to multiple plasmacytomas with an associated diffuse hypergammaglobulinemia. This progresses to a monoclonal gammopathy, suggesting that a specific clone may outgrow and retard the growth of other B-cell clones. Consistent with this observation in humans is the demonstration that malignant plasma cells release a factor that binds to macrophages and induces these cells to release a soluble factor that suppresses helper B-cell function.[15,16] The release of this factor may contribute to the suppression of normal gamma globulin production in MM, and suggests a possible mechanism of PCD-induced hypogammaglobulinemia.

Chromosomal translocations affecting genes encoding the immunoglobulin loci and the *myc* gene have been detected in DNA from mice having undergone experimentally induced PCD.[14] Translocations of these same genes in man are associated with another B-cell neoplasm, Burkitt's lymphoma.[7] Occasionally, Burkitt's and other non-Hodgkin's lymphomas have been associated with a monoclonal gammopathy.[5] Although specific rearrangements of the *myc* gene have not yet been detected in humans, recently rearrangements 3′ to *myc* have been demonstrated in a minority of cases. Other abnormalities have also been detected on chromosomes 1, 3, 6, 11, 16, and

17.[17,18] These data suggest that PCD, like other human malignancies, results from a multistep progression of genetic changes.

In the mouse plasmacytoma model, host-genetic factors determine susceptibility to malignancy. For instance, only specific strains such as BALB/c and C3H mice develop plasmacytomas following mineral oil instillation.[14] A possible extension to humans is represented by the increased frequency of PCD noted among close relatives of individuals with this disease.[19]

Chronic antigenic stimulation has been implicated in the etiology of PCD. In the mouse model, the mineral oil injected into the peritoneum is not metabolized and serves as a nidus for chronic inflammation. Administration of anti-inflammatory agents such as indomethacin delays the progression of plasmacytomas. In man, a benign monoclonal gammopathy is sometimes preceded by polyclonal hyperglobulinemia in patients with recurrent or chronic inflammatory disorders such as cholecystitis, osteomyelitis, or pyelonephritis.[20] A self-limited or reversible form of PCD can also occur in patients with viral hepatitis or drug hypersensitivity. Monoclonal gammopathies can also be associated with nonlymphoid malignancies,[21] in which case one may speculate that the tumor acts as a chronic antigenic stimulus for a B-cell clone.

A viral etiology has been suggested for PCD. In the mouse model, BALB/c mice infected with a specific RNA virus, MLV-A, have a shorter latency period prior to developing mineral-oil-induced plasmacytomas.[22,23] It has been suggested that the virus may transform B lymphocytes and place them at greater risk for malignant transformation. Although viral particles have been visualized using electron microscopy in mouse plasmacytomas, viruses have not been identified in human myeloma.

Familial factors have been suggested to have a role in the development of the disease and specific environmental exposures may be important, including chemicals used as herbicides[24] and radiation,[25] as demonstrated by the study of atom bomb survivors. Analogous to the animal model of PCD, exposures to chronic antigenic stimulation have been shown to be important in epidemiologic studies in human PCD.[26]

Diagnostic Considerations and Detection of Plasma Cell Dyscrasias

The clinical presentation of MM is characterized by the combination of bone pain (often in the back) and anemia in a middle-aged or elderly patient. It is difficult to specify clinical syndromes typical of MM or other PCD since their presentation is highly variable, depending on the sites of infiltration by neoplastic cells and the biochemical properties of the protein being overproduced. Frequently, patients are asymptomatic and the diagnosis is suggested by detection of an abnormal protein on serum electrophoresis.

The most important means of detecting PCD is electrophoretic measurement of immunoglobulin in both serum and urine. Examination of the urine for immunoglobulin is necessary because many patients with light-chain disease will not have a detectable M-spike in serum.[27] Reliable methods are available for detecting, quantitating, and determining the precise biochemical properties of an M-protein.

Serum protein electrophoresis (SPEP) is a useful screen for detecting M-proteins.[28] Proteins migrating on the basis of their mobility from left to right are: albumin, alpha 1 and alpha 2, beta, and gamma globulin (Fig 29-4).[29] Antibodies are found primarily in the beta and gamma globulin regions. An M-protein detected by SPEP usually appears as a sharp spike, and may represent a complete immunoglobulin or a subunit such as a light chain. In unusual cases, two spikes may appear, possibly indicating a rare biclonal gammopathy. In a polyclonal elevation of Ig, a broad-based band will be demonstrated in the beta-to-gamma region.

Immunoelectrophoresis (IEP), a technique that differentiates proteins on the basis of electrophoretic and immunologic characteristics, is a sensitive method to type and confirm a monoclonal protein observed on SPEP.[30] IEP is generally performed by allowing monoclonal antisera specific for any of the five immunoglobulin heavy-chain types and two light-chain types to diffuse into an electrophoretic gel following electrophoretic separation. At the point where the protein and antisera meet, a precipitin arc is formed that can be quantitated and characterized.

Other techniques such as immunofixation, nephelometry, and radial immunodiffusion are available to quantitate plasma Ig levels. Immunofixation is a sensitive technique that is especially helpful in identifying an IgM spike in WM,[31] and in detecting and quantitating M-spikes in urine.[32]

Dipstick tests of urine are not reliable for detecting urinary light chains because they often identify only albumin. The use of sulfosalicylic acid or Exton's test is valuable for screening a spot urine sample for light chains.[30] If light chains are present, an IEP is performed on a 24-hour collection of concentrated urine, and reacted with anti-κ or anti-λ antibody to determine if the light chain is of monoclonal origin (as in PCD) or a polyclonal broad-based band. As in serum, the amount of M-protein in the urine correlates with plasma cell burden.[33] In some cases, immunofixation will detect a monoclonal urinary light-chain peak in the presence of a large amount of protein, including albumin. This finding raises the possibility of primary amyloidosis or amyloidosis secondary to multiple myeloma.

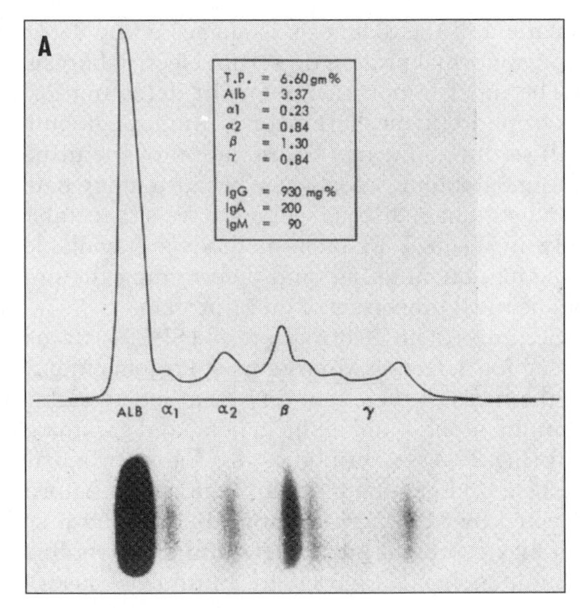

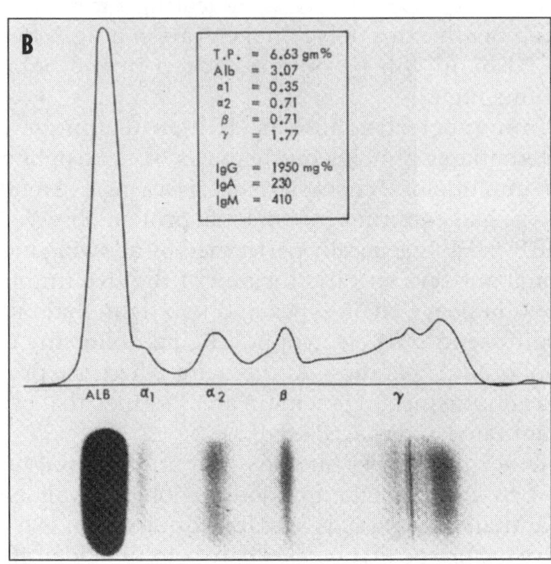

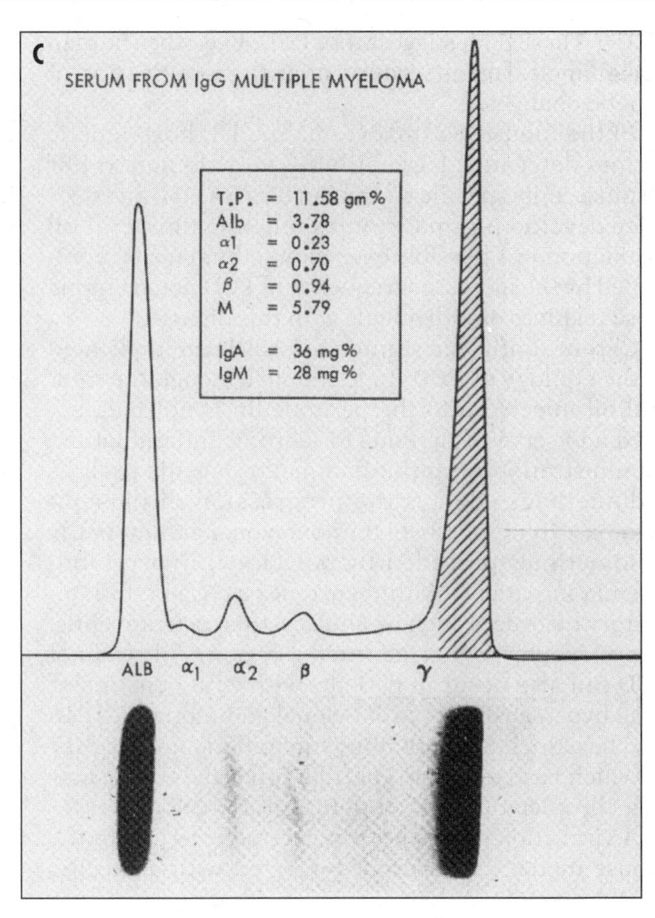

Fig 29-4. Electrophoretic pattern of ***A*** normal human serum, ***B*** hypergammaglobulinemia, and ***C*** IgG multiple myeloma. From Lee et al.[29]

Clinical Aspects of Multiple Myeloma

Multiple myeloma is a malignant neoplasm resulting from monoclonal proliferation of plasma cells. Its clinical consequences result from an increasing tumor cell mass in bone, bone marrow, and extraosseous sites and the production of vast excesses of monoclonal immunoglobulin. The pathophysiologic basis for the clinical sequelae of MM is best understood by thinking of them as the result of an expanding plasma cell mass on the one hand and humoral factors—monoclonal Ig overproduction, osteoclast activating factor (OAF), or other cytokines—on the other (Table 29-2).

The differential diagnosis of PCD includes an abundance of benign and malignant disorders, as shown in Table 29-3. Monoclonal gammopathies are frequent in the elderly, observed in 5% of individuals older than 70 years of age, and are well known in patients with autoimmune diseases.[34] A monoclonal protein, most frequently an IgM, is detected in approximately 5% of patients with B-cell lymphomas.

The appearance of a monoclonal gammopathy may not represent the development of a malignant diathesis, although as many as 11% of patients with BMG will develop MM when followed for 5 years. Monoclonal gammopathies of undetermined significance have been classified into four categories by Kyle[35] in accordance with the outcomes observed in a large group of patients followed because of the presence of an asymptomatic M-component (Table 29-4). Over a 10-year period, the initial levels of monoclonal IgG and hemoglobin had no predictive value for identification of patients who would demonstrate rising M-

Table 29-2. Pathophysiology of Multiple Myeloma

Organ System	Secondary to Cell Proliferation	Serum Protein Abnormalities
Skeletal	1. Isolated plasmacytomas (2%-10% of patients) 2. Widespread lytic lesions or diffuse osteoporosis (more common) 3. Severe bone pain	1. Hypercalcemia—production of osteoclast activating factor (not an immunoglobulin)
Hematologic	1. Bone marrow infiltration or replacement by plasma cells, resulting in: 2. Neutropenia and/or 3. Anemia and/or 4. Thrombocytopenia	1. Anemia: antibody-mediated hemolysis (rare) 2. Bleeding: M-components may specifically interact with clotting factors, or coat platelets leading to defective aggregation; may interfere with fibrin polymerization 3. Hypogammaglobulinemia as a result of plasmacytoma-induced macrophage substance (PIMS) suppression of B-cell function
Renal	1. Hyperuricemia due to plasma cell turnover—uric acid nephropathy 2. Hypercalcemic nephropathy 3. Renal infiltration of plasma cells	1. Myeloma kidney: light-chain nephropathy 2. Amyloidosis 3. Glomerulosclerosis
Nervous system	1. Radiculopathy/cord compression due to skeletal destruction and nerve compression 2. Intracranial plasma cell masses	1. Amyloid infiltration of nerves: neuropathy
General		1. Hyperviscosity syndrome: infrequent in MM, occurs with IgG1, IgG3, or IgA MM, sludging in capillaries due to aggregation of Ig's—purpura, retinal hemorrhage, papilledema, coronary ischemia, CNS symptoms (vertigo, seizures, confusion) 2. Cryoglubulinemia: reversible precipitation of serum protein in the cold—Raynaud's phenomenon, thrombosis, and gangrene in extremities

components that evolve into MM. Most M-proteins were <3 g/dL at diagnosis, only 28% had depression of normal Ig, and urinary light-chain excretion was rare. In Group 1, there was no progression in the magnitude of M-protein in most patients over two decades; the gammopathy was truly benign. In a smaller proportion, the M-component slowly and progressively increased, indicating a gradual clonal expansion, but MM did not develop (Group 2). In Group 4, classical multiple myeloma developed, at a median follow-up of 8 years, and the disease constituted 70% of tumors. The diagnostic criteria for MM is shown in Table 29-5. The remainder of Group 4 individuals developed Waldenstrom's macroglobulinemia or amyloidosis. As a rule, the most consistent sign that an MGUS is evolving into MM is a progressive rise in the level of the paraprotein, which has a rough correlation with the plasma cell mass.[19] Hence, serial measurement of the M-component on at least a yearly basis provides adequate follow-up.

Incidence

MM is an infrequent disease, accounting for 1% of all malignancies in the United States. It is age dependent, with <2% of cases occurring before 40,[36] after which the incidence rises continuously through the eighth decade.[37] The disease is more common in blacks than whites by 2 to 1. This may be due to the higher aver-

Table 29-3. Differential Diagnosis of Monoclonal Gammopathies

A. Neoplasms of immunoglobulin-producing cells
  1. Multiple myeloma (IgG, IgA, IgD, or IgE + free light chain; free light chain alone; rarely [1%], no detectable immunoglobulin abnormality; very rarely biclonal or oligoclonal). Malignancy of plasma cells
  2. Macroglobulinemia (IgM + free light chain). Malignancy of cells apparently transitional between lymphocytes and plasma cells
  3. Heavy-chain diseases (and/or chain or fragment thereof). Malignancies of plasma cells or lymphoid precursors
  4. Primary amyloidosis (IgG, IgA, IgM, or IgD—free light chain; free light chain alone; occasionally no detectable immunoglobulin abnormality). Question: special form of multiple myeloma?

B. Lymphoreticular neoplasms
  Non-Hodgkin's lymphoma, chronic lymphocytic leukemia (often hypogammaglobulinemia; M-component when present often IgM, occasionally IgG). B lymphocytes in these disorders occasionally produce M-component

C. Nonlymphoreticular neoplasms
  Cancer of colon, prostate, breast, stomach, and other sites (no consistent pattern of M-components). Occasionally monoclonal immunoglobulin production is seen in this setting, presumably in reaction to the tumor

D. Diseases with autoimmune features
  1. Mixed cryoglobulinemia (homogeneous IgM acting as anti-IgG)
  2. Hypergammaglobulinemic purpura (homogeneous IgG acting as anti-IgG)
  3. Cold agglutinin disease (predominantly IgM)
  4. Sjogren's disease (IgM)
  5. Lupus and related disorders

E. Disorders of varying and unknown etiology
  Chronic infections, parasitic diseases, cirrhosis of the liver, carcinoid, polycythemia vera, renal tubular acidosis (no consistent pattern of M-components); Gaucher's disease (IgG), pyoderma gangrenosum (IgA), lichen myxedematosus (predominantly IgG). Usually polyclonal, rarely monoclonal reactions are part of the underlying disorder

F. No associated disease
  Monoclonal gammopathy of undetermined significance (MGUS)

Table 29-4. Monoclonal Gammopathies of Undetermined Significance (MGUS)

1.	Monoclonal protein:	IgG <3.5 g/dL IgA ≤ 2.0 g/dL BJ ≤ 1.0 g/24 h
2.	Bone marrow <10% plasma cells	
3.	No bone lesions	
4.	No symptoms	

Table 29-5. Diagnostic Criteria for Multiple Myeloma

Major Criteria
1. Plasmacytoma on tissue biopsy
2. Bone marrow plasmacytosis >30% plasma cells
3. Monoclonal globulin spike on SPEP
   IgG >3.5 g/dL
   IgA >2.0 g/dL
4. κ or light chain >1.0 g/24 h on urine electrophoresis

Minor Criteria
1. Bone marrow plasmacytosis 10% to 30%
2. Monoclonal globulin spike, less than above levels
3. Lytic bone lesions
4. Hypogammaglobulinemia or suppression of antibody production other than monoclonal spike

age Ig levels in blacks, which represent a larger pool of B cells at risk for undergoing neoplastic transformation.[38]

Osseous Disease

The vast majority of patients with MM will develop skeletal manifestations that result from diffuse or focal areas of osteolysis in anatomic relation to an expanding mass of plasma cells. They present with localized areas of bone pain or swelling, or both, in conjunction with marked tenderness. Back pain is particularly common and is occasionally punctuated by episodes of severe, intractable discomfort that may represent a pathologic fracture. Compression fractures of the vertebrae are common and can cause the patient to lose several inches in height.

On x-ray, the most frequent observation is lucent lesions with clearly demarcated borders, the so-called punched-out lesions. There is little osteoblastic activity or periosteal reaction, unlike with most other neoplasms that metastasize to bone. In some patients, bone x-rays demonstrate diffuse osteoporosis; however, if microradiography were performed, it would reveal extensive bone destruction. It is widely acknowledged that bone scintigraphy is considerably less sensitive than routine x-rays in demonstrating bone involvement by MM, presumably due to the minimal osteoblastic activity and hypovascularity associated with this disease.[39] Where clinically indicated, high-resolution computed tomography (CT) often permits visualization of lesions that present early in the course of the illness.[40]

A variant of the skeletal disease associated with MM is solitary osseous myeloma (SOM). These myelomas will present in 3% to 5% of cases of plasma cell neoplasia as pain and tenderness at the site of the bone lesion.[41] Often there is radiologic evidence of bone destruction and accompanying neurologic signs such as nerve root compression causing radiculopathy or spinal cord compression. Many of these patients (75%) do not have a demonstrable M-component; among those that do, it is usually <1.5 g/dL. The detectable paraprotein often disappears following radiation therapy. Unfortunately, 70% of patients develop typical MM within 10 years.

A frequent accompaniment of myelomatous bone involvement is hypercalcemia. Whereas the osseous lesions of MM are secondary to an expanding neoplastic cell mass, elevations in serum calcium have a humoral basis. Myeloma cells secrete OAF, a lymphokine that activates osteoclasts to produce organic acids that demineralize bone.[42,43] Serum calcium is elevated in 30% of presenting patients and rises above normal in another 30% throughout the course of the illness, roughly correlating with a large tumor burden.[44] Hypercalcemia is often precipitated by the enforced bed rest resulting from painful bone lesions, and can be exacerbated by dehydration. Consequently, both bed rest and dehydration are to be avoided if possible.

Hematologic Consequences

The most frequent finding is a normocytic, normochromic anemia, which is often present at the inception of the clinical illness, but which has developed insidiously. Rouleau formation is discernible in the peripheral blood of patients with elevated Ig levels, often in conjunction with a blue background on the smear due to elevated concentrations. The reticulocyte count is typically low, and the erythrosuppression may worsen with disease progression or the initiation of chemotherapy. Leukopenia and thrombocytopenia are frequent, especially as the myeloma cell burden expands in the narrow space, or the patient is exposed to radiation or chemotherapy. Although serious bleeding can often be avoided by platelet transfusions, bleeding will occasionally occur because of nonspecific interactions between the M-component and clotting factors, or defective platelet function secondary to nonspecific coating of platelets by immunoglobulins.[45]

Severe neutropenia is an important contributor to the development of bacterial infection, a predisposition that is enhanced by the hypogammaglobulinemia that is often present. The mechanisms underlying the impairment in humoral immunity are twofold: the increased rate of Ig catabolism, and the production by plasma cells of a factor (PC factor) that stimulates macrophages to produce PIMS (plasmacytoma-induced macrophage substance), which inhibits B-cell function.[46]

Renal Manifestations

Myeloma Cast Nephropathy

Dense tubular casts are a hallmark of MM and are observed in 75% of patients, all of whom are excreting free light chains, or Bence-Jones proteins.[47] The large, hard casts cause compression atrophy of the tubular epithelium. The tubular basement membrane may then rupture and result in interstitial inflammation, subsequent fibrosis, and, ultimately, renal failure. The tubular casts stain positively for Ig light chains, but contain mucoproteins as well. Acute renal failure can be precipitated in patients with MM by acute dehydration, which may occur during preparation for an x-ray study employing iodinated dyes; fever secondary to infection; or hypercalcemia.[48] Dehydration facilitates precipitation of light chains in tubules, which sometimes is compounded by coprecipitation with calcium. Although light-chain nephropathy is an ominous development, acute renal failure arising in this setting is often partially reversible by restoration of renal perfusion and cautious use of loop diuretics.

Glomerular Lesions

Twenty-five percent of patients develop cumulative deposition of the paraprotein in the mesangium that results in glomerulosclerosis. The morphologic pattern is characterized by coarse granular deposits, which stain with antibodies to κ chains and are located at the inner aspect of the glomerular basement membrane. The mechanism by which glomerular damage is produced is not understood.

Another glomerular lesion found in patients with MM is renal amyloid deposits, present in 30% of patients. This material can be found in tubular basement membranes, renal vessels, the interstitium, and glomeruli. The last can be associated with nephrosis in which mixed serum proteins, including albumin, are excreted in the urine, along with light chains.

Renal failure in MM often occurs when dehydration, hypercalcemia, and light-chain excretion are present. Management of acute renal failure that arises in the face of excessive light-chain production may include plasmapheresis to rapidly lower the burden of light chains. The institution of hemodialysis in MM patients with irreversible, profound renal failure is entirely justified if the prospects for systemic control of the disease are favorable. This important management approach has ameliorated the dire consequences otherwise imposed by this complication.

Neurologic Complications

Spinal cord compression is almost always secondary to osseous involvement of ribs or vertebrae in association with an epidural mass. Back pain or radicular pain lasting many months and increasing in severity is a frequent prelude to this severe complication. The importance of prompt diagnosis cannot be overstated, as the appearance of neurologic deficits often progresses to paraplegia within hours or days. Suspicion of cord compression based on new neurologic signs should stimulate the prompt initiation of diagnostic studies to delineate the upper and lower extent of the lesion or lesions. In this particularly challenging clinical situation, nuclear magnetic resonance imaging (MRI) often provides definitive identification of an epidural lesion causing cord compression.

The usual emergency therapy for spinal cord compression is high-dose dexamethasone (Decadron), followed by radiation therapy once the anatomic extent of the lesion is known. Laminectomy is indicated in the circumstance of relapsing cord compression, when radiation is contraindicated, or when an isolated osseous lesion is associated with the neurologic deficit.

Unusual Neurologic Manifestations

Intracranial myeloma is a distinctly rare event that can occur due to extension of a lesion involving the cranium. When myelomatous masses invade the meninges, plasma cells are easily observed in the cere-

Table 29-6. Myeloma Staging System

Stage	Criteria	Measured Myeloma Cell Mass (cells x $10^{12}/m^2$)
I	All of the following: 1. Hemoglobin value >10 g/100 mL 2. Serum calcium value normal (<12 mg/100 mL) 3. On x-ray, normal bone structure (scale 0) or solitary bone plasmacytoma only 4. Low M-component production rates a. IgG value <5 g/100 mL b. IgA value <3 g/100 mL c. Urine light chain M-component on electrophoresis <4 g/24 h	<0.6 (low)
II	Fitting neither stage I nor stage III	>0.6-1.2 (intermediate)
III	One or more of the following: 1. Hemoglobin value 8.5 g/100 mL 2. Serum calcium value >12 mg/100 mL 3. Advanced lytic bone lesions (scale 3) 4. High M-component production rates a. IgG value >7 g/100 mL b. IgA value >5 g/100 mL c. Urine light chain M-component on electrophoresis >12 g/24 h	>1.2 (high)

Subclassification:
A = Relatively normal renal function (serum creatinine value <2.0 mg/100 mL)
B = Abnormal renal function (serum creatinine value >2.0 mg/100 mL)

brospinal fluid (CSF). Immunoelectrophoresis of the CSF will demonstrate the paraprotein. Management consists of detailed analysis of the mass by CT or MRI, followed by surgical decompression or resection, if necessary, and radiotherapy.

Sensorimotor neuropathy occurs in about 1% of myeloma patients, and may precede the onset of illness by years. When it occurs, it is more common in individuals with solitary osseous plasmacytoma, and resembles the syndrome occasionally seen in patients who ultimately develop lung or stomach cancer.[49]

The hyperviscosity syndrome (HVS) is caused by elevated levels of serum proteins with a high intrinsic viscosity, and is usually manifest at serum viscosity levels >4 centipoises (Cp). It is most common in the setting of Waldenstrom's macroglobulinemia, which is characterized by marked overproduction of monoclonal IgM protein. In MM it is associated with overproduction of IgG1 and IgG3 proteins, as the relevant heavy-chain classes within these categories have a propensity to aggregate.[50] HVS is also observed in IgA myeloma, particularly when the M-component exceeds 5 g/dL. The likelihood of these immunoglobulins aggregating is enhanced if the protein is temperature sensitive, such that exposure to cold might precipitate HVS. The clinical picture is characterized by fatigue, headache, sluggish mentation, and visual disturbances. These symptoms can be compounded by vascular effects of sludging, such as myocardial ischemia, and by defects in platelet aggregation. It is important to be alert for the signs of HVS because plasmapheresis can be lifesaving, even in those cases of IgG MM in which the paraprotein is distributed throughout the intravascular and extravascular space (unlike IgM, which is entirely intravascular).

Tumor Kinetics and Staging

The amount of monoclonal immunoglobulin produced in MM closely correlates with the tumor mass of plasma cells. Therefore, serial measurement of the M-protein can be used to assess changes in tumor burden over time or following treatment. M-protein levels reliably serve as a tumor marker that has been useful in providing a model for the growth kinetics of a human malignancy.

Durie, Salmon and Moon developed a method to quantitate tumor burden in MM, defined as total-body myeloma cell number.[51] Their investigation of a large series of MM patients at presentation has led to a staging system that correlates clinical characteristics with total mass of myeloma cells. The latter can be calculated by this formula:

$$\text{Total-body myeloma cell number} = \frac{\text{Total-body M-component synthetic rate}}{\text{M-component synthetic rate per myeloma cell}}$$

The total-body M-component synthetic rate can be calculated from the determination of the M-component serum concentration, the plasma volume, and the predicted catabolic rate for the Ig monoclonal protein in question. The M-component synthetic rate per cell is determined by growing myeloma cells obtained from bone marrow in short-term culture. From quantification of the number of cells in culture and determination of the Ig production rate, the synthetic rate per cell can be calculated.

The total-body myeloma cell burden have been correlated with specific clinical characteristics, and this correlation has led to the identification of three stages of disease (Table 29-6): high cell mass ($>1.2 \times 10^{12}$

Table 29-7. Myeloma Cell Mass and Survival in 160 Patients

Cell Mass Category (cells/m^2)	No. of Patients		Median Survival (months)	p Values
	Alive	Dead		
High				
$>1.2 \times 10^{12}$	38	57	32.6	0.05 0.0002
Intermediate				
$\geq 0.6\text{-}1.2 \times 10^{12}$	20	20	54.5	0.05 0.10
Low				
$<0.6 \times 10^{12}$	16	9	76.5	0.10 0.0002

Adapted from Durie et al.[52]

myeloma cells per m^2)—stage III; intermediate cell mass (0.6-1.2 x 10^{12} per m^2)—stage II; and low cell mass (0.6 x 10^{12} per m^2)—stage I.[41] Important prognostic implications (Table 29-7)[52] are based on these stages, plus the added subclassification for renal failure.[51] Furthermore, the staging system does not require extensive laboratory techniques.

Another important prognostic variable is based on the determination of the number of dividing cells in a population of myeloma cells. This parameter, termed the labeling index (LI), also depends on the ability to grow myeloma cells in short-term culture. It is performed by labeling cells with tritiated thymidine for one hour and counting the number of cells that have taken up the radioactive precursor.[43]

Most patients with MM have an LI of 1% to 5% at presentation. An LI >3% correlates with a poor prognosis, especially if it is associated with a high tumor cell burden. Patients with an LI of <1% have a relatively good prognosis. Patients with MGUS often have an LI of <0.5%.

Measurement of LI has permitted several observations about the kinetics of MM following treatment.[52] Patients who have a high LI respond more rapidly to chemotherapy, but their responses are often of short duration and the disease tends to grow back quickly. Conversely, patients with a low LI take longer to respond to therapy, but have a longer duration of response and survival.

Following effective therapy, the M-component falls until it reaches a plateau. The plateau phase lasts a fixed period of time, even if therapy is continued, until the M-component again starts to increase.[53] In this relapse phase, about two thirds of patients have a higher LI than at presentation, indicating an increasing growth fraction of probably drug-resistant cells.[54] Other relapsing patients can have high tumor masses but a low LI.[55] In these cases, the malignant mass of plasma cells increases in size and the tumor outgrows its blood supply. Growth then slows, resulting in a prolonged doubling time. This pattern of faster growth at smaller tumor volumes is called Gompertzian kinetics and may explain the presumed rapid subclinical growth of MM. Gompertzian kinetics obviously does not apply to all cases of PCD. In MGUS, the growth of plasma cells is halted or slowed at low plasma cell masses.[56] Progression of growth may be controlled by poorly understood host factors.

Another useful prognostic indicator in MM is the measurement of beta-2 microglobulin (β_2M) levels.[57,58] This protein has a structure similar to the constant region of the light chain of the MHC. If renal function is normal, β_2M levels closely reflect tumor load in PCD. The measurement of β_2M is especially useful in patients with light-chain disease or rare nonsecretory myelomas, for which the measurement of M-component levels over time may be problematic or impossible. Some recent observations suggest that in the future thymidine kinase levels may be a useful quantitative marker for disease activity.

Therapy for Multiple Myeloma

Conventional treatment of MM is palliative and fraught with long-term dangers. As a result, observation is appropriate for patients without anemia, bone pain, osteolysis, or renal failure. When therapy is indicated, the mainstay of chemotherapy has been melphalan (M), usually given on an intermittent schedule, eg, 0.25 mg/kg/day for 4 days, in conjunction with prednisone (P), 2 mg/kg/day.[59] The addition of the steroid to melphalan increases the response rate substantially, but it does not have a large effect on survival. Melphalan is well absorbed orally, and can be administered in standard doses to patients with renal failure. Melphalan therapy can be discontinued after the maximal response has been achieved.

Cyclophosphamide is an alkylating agent (AA) that is structurally different from melphalan, is not cross-resistant with it, and can be used when drug resistance to melphalan has developed.[60] It is equally effective in producing remissions in MM, is well tolerated systemically, and can be administered in standard doses to patients with renal failure. Cyclophosphamide is less toxic to thrombopoiesis than other alkylating agents and therefore can be used with greater safety in patients with thrombocytopenia.

The superiority of multiple-drug regimens has not been demonstrated when compared with MP. The VAD regimen, in which vincristine and doxorubicin (Adriamycin) are administered as a continuous infusion along with pulse dexamethasone, is frequently used as primary or salvage treatment. This regimen has a response rate approximately equal to that of MP, and is reported to have the slight advantage of a more rapid response.[61] Combinations of melphalan, cyclophosphamide, BCNU, vincristine, and prednisone, or alternating combinations of subsets of these agents, are effective in inducing remissions, perhaps at faster but not at substantially higher rates than MP. No reproducible survival advantage has been shown with these more intensive regimens, and their additional toxicity and cost raise questions about their utility.

This conclusion has been emphasized in a group of patients at high risk for failure—those with a high LI and elevated β_2M levels. In a recent randomized trial, vincristine, melphalan, cyclophosphamide, and prednisone were alternated with vincristine, carmustine, doxorubicin, and prednisone and compared to the standard MP regimen. The analysis showed no survival advantage, little difference in the time to remission, and no difference in the duration of remission.[62]

A feared long-term consequence of standard therapy for MM is the development of acute leukemia. This secondary neoplasm results from prolonged exposure to AA, and has been reported at a frequency of 20% after 50 months of follow-up.[63] Secondary acute nonlymphocytic leukemia (ANLL) often begins as a myelodysplastic syndrome, demonstrating characteristic karyotypic abnormalities affecting chromosomes 5 and 7. Within several months of onset, the disease progresses to frank acute leukemia, which generally responds poorly to established methods of therapy.

Treatment with interferon has been attempted at different stages of MM. Although one study demonstrated a positive effect of adding alpha interferon to an induction regimen,[64] there is no consensus affirming the value of this approach. Treatment with interferon alfa-2b during the maintenance phase of the disease has, at least in one study, been effective in improving survival.[65] This has yet to be confirmed.

Treatment of Resistant Disease

Approximately 40% of patients are unresponsive to AA at the start of therapy, and virtually all who initially experience tumor regression will ultimately manifest AA resistance. Several salvage regimens have been employed in these patients with variable results. High-dose steroid therapy, with either dexamethasone or prednisone, has demonstrated activity in patients who are either initially or ultimately refractory to alkylating agents.[66] In one study, a 40% response rate was detected following therapy with dexamethasone 40 mg/day for 4 days each week for 8 weeks.[67] The addition of vincristine and doxorubicin as part of the VAD regimen is not likely to improve responses in the resistant patient population, but may allow a reduction in steroid dose and toxicity. An active multidrug regimen based on the continuous infusion of cisplatin combined with etoposide, cytosine arabinoside (ara-C), and dexamethasone is associated with a 40% response rate but considerable toxicity.[68] Other therapies that have some demonstrated activity include hemibody irradiation[69] and beta interferon.[70]

Overexpression of the multiple drug resistance (mdr, p21) gene has been detected in malignant plasma cells from selected previously treated patients who are resistant to chemotherapy.[71] The expression of the MDR phenotype in association with prior treatment with VAD is particularly relevant since vincristine and doxorubicin are extruded by the protein (P-glycoprotein) that is the product of the mdr gene. Treatment of patients who are resistant to VAD with the combination of verapamil, an agent that can partially circumvent the MDR phenotype, and VAD has had limited clinical success.[72] Hopes for an even greater effect on MDR-expressing cells depend on the identification of more effective agents to circumvent the MDR pump. In addition to the presumed relevance of the MDR phenotype to the treatment of MM, it is likely that other factors contributing to drug resistance will be identified.

Bone Marrow Transplantation

MM has been shown to be responsive to dose escalation of the most commonly used first-line agent, melphalan, even in patients resistant to standard doses.[68] These observations suggested that a greater number of complete remissions or a longer duration of response might be achievable by employing high-dose therapy with bone marrow infusion for hematologic support. This has proven to be the case for both autologous and allogeneic transplantation.

Autologous transplantation has been performed in more than 300 patients, most of whom have been reinfused with unpurged marrow. The complete remission rate ranges from 20% to 30%. About one half of patients who achieve a complete remission are disease free after 4 years.[73] Patients with low tumor burdens who are still responsive to chemotherapy derive the greatest benefit. Considering this constraint, the usefulness of this therapeutic option in patients with resistant disease is limited.

Recently, a large trial of allogeneic bone marrow transplantation (BMT) has been reported for MM. In the 90 patients studied, a complete remission rate in excess of 40% was achieved, with a median duration of remission of 48 months. Patients were treated with a combination of total body irradiation (TBI) and high-dose alkylating agents. There was a trend toward better results in patients still responsive to therapy and those with lesser stages of disease, but statistical significance was not reached.[74]

Both forms of transplantation therapy hold promise. Allogeneic therapies are limited by the availability of a compatible donor and the recipient's age. For instance, the median age of patients in the allogeneic BMT trial was 42 years, two decades younger than the median age of patients who receive standard therapy. On the other hand, the benefits of autologous transplantation might be limited by reinfusing myeloma cells, possibly decreasing the duration of response. Autologous BMT is available to an older patient population. Current research is attempting to define effective plasma cell purging techniques to determine its impact on the duration of response.

References

1. Waldenstrom J. *Diagnosis and Treatment of Multiple Myeloma.* New York, NY: Grune and Stratton Inc; 1970.

2. Stamatoyannopoulos G, Nienhuis AW, Leder P, Majerus PW, eds. *The Molecular Basis of Blood Diseases.* Philadelphia, Pa: WB Saunders Co; 1987.

3. Rosen SM, Buxbaum JN, Frangione B. The structure of immunoglobulins and their genes, DNA rearrangement and B cell differentiation, molecular anomalies of some monoclonal immunoglobulins. *Semin Oncol.* 1986;13:260-274.

4. Natvig JB, Kunkel HG. Human immunoglobulins: classes, subclasses, genetic variants, and idiotypes. *Adv Immunol.* 1973;16:1-59.

5. Holland JF, Frei E III, eds. *Cancer Medicine.* Philadelphia, Pa: Lea & Febiger; 1982.

6. Cooper M. B lymphocytes: normal development and function. *N Engl J Med.* 1987;317:1452-1456.

7. Foon K, Todd RF III. Immunologic classification of leukemia and lymphoma. *Blood.* 1986;68:1-31.

8. Seligmann M, Brovet J. Antibody activity of human myeloma globulins. *Semin Hematol.* 1973;10:163-177.

9. Kawano M, Hirano T, Matsuda T, et al. Autocrine generation and requirement of BSF-2/IL-6 for human multiple myelomas. *Nature.* 1988;332:83-85.

10. Pilarski LM, Mant MJ, Ruether BA. Pre-B cells in peripheral blood of multiple myeloma patients. *Blood.* 1985;66:416-422.

11. Hirano T, Taga T, Yasukawa K. Human B-cell differentiation factor defined by an anti-peptide antibody and its possible role in autoantibody production. *Proc Natl Acad Sci U S A.* 1987;84:228-231.

12. Bataille R, Chappard D, Marcelli C, et al. Recruitment of new osteoblasts and osteoclasts is the earliest critical event in the pathogenesis of human multiple myeloma. *J Clin Invest.* 1991;88:62-66.

13. Levy Y, Tsapis A, Brouet JC. Interleukin-6 antisense oligonucleotides inhibit the growth of human myeloma cell lines. *J Clin Invest.* 1991;88:696-699.

14. Potter M. Plasmacytomas in mice. *Semin Oncol.* 1986;13:275-281.

15. Katzmann JA. Myeloma-induced immunosuppression: a multistep mechanism. *J Immunol.* 1978;121:1405-1409.

16. Krakauer RS, Strober W, Waldmann TA. Hypogammaglobulinemia in experimental myeloma: the role of suppressor factors from mononuclear phagocytes. *J Immunol.* 1977;118:1385-1390.

17. Dewald GW, Kyle RA, Hicks GA, Greipp PR. The clinical significance of cytogenetic studies in 100 patients with multiple myeloma, plasma cell leukemia or amyloidosis. *Blood.* 1985;66:380-390.

18. Ferti A, Panani A, Arapakis G, et al. Cytogenetic study in multiple myeloma. *Cancer Genet Cytogenet.* 1984;12:247.

19. Maldonado JE, Kyle RA. Familial myeloma: report of eight families and a study of serum proteins in their relatives. *Am J Med.* 1974;57:875-884.

20. Merlini G, Furhangi M, Osserman EF. Monoclonal immunoglobulins with antibody activity in myeloma, macroglobulinemia, and related plasma cell dyscrasias. *Semin Oncol.* 1986;13:350-365.

21. Zawadski Z, Edwards G. Nonmyelomatous monoclonal immunoglobulinemia. *Prog Clin Immunol.* 1972;1:105-156.

22. Warner N, Potter M, Metcalf D. *Multiple Myeloma and Related Immunoglobulin Producing Neoplasms.* Geneva: Internal Union Against Cancer; 1974. UICC Technical Report Series, vol 13.

23. Potter M, Sklar MD, Rowe WP. Rapid viral induction of plasmacytomas in pristane-primed BALB/c mice. *Science.* 1973;182:592-594.

24. Eriksson M, Karlsson M. Occupational and other environmental factors and multiple myeloma: a population based case-control study. *Br J Ind Med.* 1992;49:95-103.

25. Riedel DA, Pattern LM. The epidemiology of multiple myeloma. *Hematol Oncol Clin North Am.* 1992;6:225-247.

26. Gramenzi A, Buttino I, D'Avanzo B, Negri E, Franceschi S, La Vecchia C. Medical history and the risk of multiple myeloma. *Br J Cancer.* 1991;63:769-772.

27. Kyle R. Multiple myeloma: review of 869 cases. *Mayo Clin Proc.* 1975;50:29-40.

28. Alper CA. Plasma protein measurements as a diagnostic aid. *N Engl J Med.* 1974;291:287-290.

29. Lee GR, Bithell TC, Foerster J, Athens JW, Lukens JN, eds. *Wintrobe's Clinical Hematology.* Philadelphia, Pa: Lea and Febiger; 1993.

30. Kyle RA, Garton JP. Laboratory monitoring of myeloma proteins. *Semin Oncol.* 1986;13:310-317.

31. Ritchie RF, Smith R. Immunofixation, III: application to the study of monoclonal proteins. *Clin Chem.* 1976;22: 1982-1985.

32. Whicher JT, Hawkins L, Higginson J. Clinical applications of immunofixation: a more sensitive technique for the detection of Bence Jones protein. *J Clin Pathol.* 1980;33: 779-780.

33. Cooper DA, Miller AC, Penny R. Biosynthesis of immunoglobulin in human immunoproliferative diseases. II. Comparison of tumor cell mass in multiple myeloma measured by synthetic rate studies with that calculated from clinical staging systems. *Acta Haematol.* 1982;68:224-236.

34. Papadopoulos NM, Elin RJ, Wilson DM. Incidence of gamma-globulin banding in a healthy population by high-resolution electrophoresis. *Clin Chem.* 1982;28:707-708.

35. Kyle R. Monoclonal gammopathy of undetermined significance: natural history in 241 cases. *Am J Med.* 1978; 64:814-826.

36. Hewell GM, Alexanian R. Multiple myeloma in young persons. *Ann Intern Med.* 1976;84:441-443.

37. Turesson I, Zettervall O, Cuzick J, Waldenstrom JG, Velez R. Comparison of trends in the incidence of multiple myeloma in Malmo, Sweden, and other countries, 1950-1979. *N Engl J Med.* 1984;310:421-424.

38. Cutter SJ, Young JL. *Third National Cancer Survey: Incidence Data.* Washington, DC: US. Government Printing Office; 1975. US Dept of Health, Education, and Welfare publication NIH 75-787. National Cancer Institute monograph 41.

39. Frank JW, LeBesque S, Buchanan RB. The value of bone imaging in multiple myeloma. *Eur J Nucl Med.* 1982;7:502.

40. Solomon A, Rahamoni R, Seligsohn U, Ben-Artzi F. Multiple myeloma: early vertebral involvement assessed by computerized tomography. *Skeletal Radiol.* 1984;11:258-261.

41. Conklin R, Alexanian R. Clinical classification of plasma cell myeloma. *Arch Intern Med.* 1975;135:139.

42. Raisz LG, Luben RA, Munds GA, Dietrich JW, Horton JE, Trummel CI. Effect of osteoclast activating factor from human leukocytes on bone metabolism. *J Clin Invest.* 1975;56:408-413.

43. Mundy GR, Raisz LG, Cooper RA, Schehter GP, Salmon SE. Evidence for the secretion of an osteoclast stimulating factor in myeloma. *N Engl J Med.* 1974;291:1041-1046.

44. Bergsagel DE, Griffin KM, Haut A, Stuckey WJ Jr. The treatment of plasma cell myeloma. *Adv Cancer Res.* 1967;10:311-359.

45. Perkins HA, Mackenzie MR, Fudenberg HH. Hemostasis defects in dysproteinemias. *Blood.* 1970;35:695-707.

46. Ullrich S, Zolla-Pazner S. Immunoregulatory circuits in myeloma. *Clin Haematol.* 1982;11:87-111.

47. Hill GS, Morel-Maroger L, Mery JP, Brouet JC, Mignon F. Renal lesions in multiple myeloma: their relationship to associated protein abnormalities. *Am J Kidney Dis.* 1983; 2:423-438.

48. Cohen DJ, Sherman WH, Osserman EF, Appel GB. Acute renal failure in patients with multiple myeloma. *Am J Med.* 1984;76:247-256.

49. Davis LE, Drachman DB. Myeloma neuropathy: successful treatment of two patients and review of cases. *Arch Neurol.* 1972;25:507-511.

50. Hall CG, Abraham GN. Reversible self-association of a human myeloma protein: thermodynamics and relevance to viscosity effects and solubility. *Biochemistry.* 1984;23:5123.

51. Durie BGM, Salmon SE, Moon TE. Pretreatment tumor mass, cell kinetics, and prognosis in multiple myeloma. *Blood.* 1980;55:364-372.

52. Durie BGM, Salmon SE. A Clinical staging system for multiple myeloma correlation of measured myeloma cell mass with presenting clinical features, response to treatment and survival. *Cancer.* 1975;36:842-854.

53. Salmon S. Immunoglobulin synthesis and tumor kinetics of multiple myeloma. *Semin Hematol.* 1973;10:135-144.

54. Drewinko B, Brown BW, Humphrey R, Alexanian R. Effect of chemotherapy on the labelling index of myeloma cells. *Cancer.* 1974;34:526-531.

55. Hobbs JR. Growth rates and responses to treatment in human myelomatosis. *Br J Haematol.* 1969;16:607-617.

56. Kyle R. Monoclonal gammopathy of undetermined significance (MGUS): a review. *Clin Haematol.* 1982;11:123.

57. Bataille R, Maqub M, Grenier J, Donnadio D, Sany J. Serum beta-2-microglobulin in multiple myeloma: relationship to presenting clinical features and clinical status. *Eur J Cancer Clin Oncol.* 1982;18:59-66.

58. Childs J, Crawford S, Norfolk D, O'Quigley J, Scraffe J, Struthers LP. Evaluation of serum B_2-microglobulin as a prognostic indicator in myelomatosis. *Br J Cancer.* 1983; 7:111-114.

59. Alexanian R. Treatment of multiple myeloma. *Acta Haematol.* 1980;63:237-240.

60. Bergsagel DE, Cowan DH, Hasselback R. Plasma cell myeloma: response of melphalan-resistant patients to high-dose intermittent cyclophosphamide. *Can Med Assoc J.* 1972;107:851-855.

61. Alexanian R, Barlogie B, Tucker S. VAD-based regimens as primary treatment for multiple myeloma. *Am J Hematol.* 1990;33:86-89.

62. Boccadoro M, Marmont F, Tribalto M, et al. Multiple myeloma: VCMP/VBAP alternating combination chemotherapy is not superior to melphalan and prednisone even in high-risk patients. *J Clin Oncol.* 1991;9:444-448.

63. Bergsagel DE. Plasma cell neoplasms and acute leukaemia. *Clin Haematol.* 1982;11:221-234.

64. Montuoro A, De Rosa L, De Blasio A, Pacilli L, Petti N, De Laurenzi A. Alpha-2a-interferon/melphalan/prednisone versus melphalan/prednisone in previously untreated patients with multiple myeloma. *Br J Haematol.* 1990;76: 365-368.

65. Mandelli F, Avvisati G, Amadori S, et al. Maintenance treatment with recombinant interferon alfa-2b in patients with multiple myeloma responding to conventional induction chemotherapy. *N Engl J Med.* 1990;322:1430-1434.

66. Norfolk DR, Child JA. Pulsed high dose oral prednisolone in relapsed or refractory multiple myeloma. *Hematol Oncol.* 1989;7:61-68.

67. Friedenberg WR, Kyle RA, Knopse WH, Bennett J, Tsiatis A, Oken M. High-dose dexamethasone for refractory or relapsing multiple myeloma. *Am J Hematol.* 1991;36: 171-175.

68. Barlogie B, Velasquez WS, Alexanian R, Cabanillas F. Etoposide, dexamethasone, cytarabine, and cisplatin in vincristine, doxorubicin and dexamethasone-refractory myeloma. *J Clin Oncol.* 1989;7:1514-1518.

69. Singer CRJ, Tobias JS, Giles F, Rudd GN, Blackman GM, Richards JDM. Hemibody irradiation: an effective second-line therapy in drug-resistant multiple myeloma. *Cancer.* 1989;63:2446-2451.

70. Liberti AM, Cinieri S, Sanatore MG, et al. Phase I-II trial of natural beta interferon in chemoresistant and relapsing multiple myeloma. *Haematologica.* 1990;75:436-442.

71. Dalton WS, Grogan TM, Meltzer PS, et al. Drug-resistance in multiple myeloma and non-Hodgkin's lymphoma: detection of P-glycoprotein and potential circumvention by addition of verapamil to chemotherapy. *J Clin Oncol.* 1989;7:415-424.

72. Salmon SE, Dalton WS, Grogan TM, et al. Multidrug-resistant myeloma: laboratory and clinical effects of verapamil as a chemosensitizer. *Blood.* 1991;78:44-50.

73. Barlogie B, Alexanian R, Dicke K, et al. High-dose chemoradiotherapy and autologous bone marrow transplantation for resistant multiple myeloma. *Blood.* 1987;70: 869-872.

74. Gahrton G, Tura S, Ljungman P, et al. Allogeneic bone marrow transplantation in multiple myeloma. *N Engl J Med.* 1991;325:1267-1273.

30

THE ADULT LEUKEMIAS

A. Jacqueline Mitus, MD, David S. Rosenthal, MD

Leukemia constitutes about 2% of adult cancers. It is a heterogeneous group broadly classified into acute and chronic disorders. While both are clonal diseases of blood-forming elements, the pathophysiologic basis of the two processes is different. *Acute leukemia* is characterized by a block in differentiation resulting in massive accumulation of immature cells, or blasts. In contrast, the defect in *chronic leukemia* leads to unregulated proliferation and hence marked overexpansion of a spectrum of differentiated cells. In general, acute leukemia, unlike the chronic form, is potentially curable by elimination of the neoplastic clone.

Acute and chronic leukemias involve the myeloid elements of the bone marrow—white cells, red cells, and megakaryocytes (acute myelogenous leukemia [AML], chronic myelogenous leukemia [CML])—and cells of the lymphoid lineage (acute lymphoblastic leukemia [ALL], chronic lymphocytic leukemia [CLL]). Malignant cells disrupt normal marrow function and may directly invade the spleen, liver, lymph nodes, central nervous system as well as other organs. Traditional morphologic and histochemical diagnostic criteria have been supplemented by cytogenetic, immunologic, and molecular techniques allowing more precise classification of the disorders. Intensive chemotherapy regimens, invaluable supportive services, and bone marrow transplantation have led to an improved outlook for patients with adult leukemia.

Acute Myelogenous Leukemia

Originally described by Virchow in 1897 as *weisses blood* (white blood), AML (also referred to as acute nonlymphocytic leukemia [ANLL]), gives rise to massive accumulation of immature and undifferentiated cells known as blasts. The ensuing disruption of normal hematopoiesis results in severe and often life-threatening pancytopenia. The French-American-British (FAB) classification established in 1976 organizes AML into eight subgroups based on morphologic, histochemical, and immunologic criteria. Untreated, the disease is fatal within months. With aggressive therapy 70% to 80% of patients will achieve remission (inability to detect residual malignant cells); however, only 25% to 30% of patients will be cured.

Incidence and Epidemiology

The incidence of AML rises sharply with age, increasing from less than 1/100,000 under age 35 to 15/100,000 in individuals over 75.[1] There is no predilection for race or sex.

Etiology

The etiology of AML remains unknown. Aberrant expression of oncogenes and transcription factors form the basis of intense ongoing investigation.[2] One locale of particular interest is the long arm of chromosome 5, where a number of growth factors and growth factor receptors are located (eg, IL-3, GM-CSF, M-CSF receptor c-fms). The cytogenetic abnormality 5q- in myelodysplastic syndromes and AML suggests that deletion of this region may be important in these clonal neoplasms; however, the precise relationship remains speculative.

Perhaps the best characterized molecular disturbance in AML involves the 15;17 translocation of acute promyelocytic leukemia (M3). Empiric trials of the differentiating agent trans retinoic acid (Tretinoin) lead investigators to define the breakpoint on chromosome 17 as arising from the retinoic acid receptor. The breakpoint regions in the PML gene on chromosome 15 have also recently been cloned. Two fusion RNA products result from the reciprocal translocations, both of which may be pathogenetically important. Their role in APL and the mechanism by

A. Jacqueline Mitus, MD, Instructor, Harvard Medical School and Associate Physician, Brigham and Women's Hospital, Boston, Massachusetts

David S. Rosenthal, MD, Harry K. Oliver Professor of Hygiene, Harvard University, Cambridge, Massachusetts

which all trans retinoic acid induces cellular differentiation in this disease is still poorly understood.

Of all the leukemias, AML is most strongly linked to radiation and toxin exposure (Table 30-1). The leukemogenic potential of radiation was recognized decades ago among radiologists; however, the largest experience has been derived from Japanese atomic bomb survivors. A 50-fold risk of AML is reported, peaking at 5 to 7 years but continuing for up to 14 years.[3] Benzene, the best documented chemical leukemogen, was first associated with AML early in this century. A prodromal phase of bone marrow aplasia and cytogenetic abnormalities is characteristic. Chemotherapeutic drugs (usually alkylating agents) have been implicated as causing AML in patients treated for Hodgkin's disease, multiple myeloma, breast, ovarian, and gastrointestinal cancers. Recently, children receiving epipodophyllotoxins (VP-16, VM-26) for acute lymphoblastic leukemia also have been recognized to suffer a higher risk of AML.[4] Unlike other cases of secondary AML, onset is earlier—1 to 4 years following therapy.

Previous bone marrow disorders predispose to AML. Of the myeloproliferative diseases, chronic myelogenous leukemia carries the highest risk (nearly 100%). While only 2% of patients with untreated polycythemia vera develop AML, this number rises steeply for patients given chlorambucil. AML is also a frequent end result of the myelodysplastic syndromes.

Several congenital disorders terminate in AML (Table 30-1). Of these, Down's syndrome is most notable, leading to a 20-fold increased risk of leukemia.

Table 30-1. Pathogenesis of Acute Leukemia

- I. Toxins
  - A. Radiation
  - B. Chemicals: benzene
  - C. Drugs
    1. Alkylating agents: melphalan, cyclophosphamide, chlorambucil, busulfan, thiotepa, CCNU
    2. Chloramphenicol
    3. Phenylbutazone
- II. Congenital Diseases
  - A. Down's syndrome
  - B. Fanconi's anemia
  - C. Klinefelter's syndrome
  - D. Turner's syndrome
  - E. Bloom syndrome
  - F. Wiskott-Aldrich syndrome
- III. Acquired Disorders
  - A. Myeloproliferative
    1. Polycythemia vera
    2. Primary thrombocytosis
    3. Agnogenic myeloid metaplasia
  - B. Myelodysplastic syndromes
  - C. Paroxysmal nocturnal hemoglobinuria (PNH)

Clinical Characteristics

Constitutional symptoms stem from disruption of normal hematopoiesis: fatigue and shortness of breath (anemia), bleeding and easy bruising (thrombocytopenia), and fever with infection (leukopenia). Infiltration of skin (leukemia cutis), gingiva, and other soft tissue occurs in any subtype of AML (approximately 1% to 3%) but is particularly suggestive of the monocytic variants (about 30%). Oropharyngeal complaints are common, leading many patients to first seek attention from their dentist. Involvement of the central nervous system (CNS), suggested by the presence of headache, cranial neuropathy, and unexplained nausea or vomiting, is rare at presentation and poses a greater problem at relapse. When peripheral blast counts exceed 50,000 to 100,000/μL, these large, noncompliant, and "sticky" cells impair normal blood flow and invade perivascular tissue, thus giving rise to leukostasis. Headache, change in mental status, dyspnea, and priapism constitute medical emergencies mandating immediate lowering of the white cell count. Collections of myeloblasts, chloromas, or granulocytic sarcomas can involve any soft tissue and may occur as isolated findings. Inevitable infiltration of the bone marrow results, however, and systemic as well as local therapy is indicated.

Classification

Acute leukemia is defined by the presence of at least 30% blasts in the bone marrow. The FAB classification divides AML into seven groups (M1-M7) based on morphologic, histochemical, and immunologic findings (Fig 30-1—color plate following page 372). Recently, an eighth category—M0—has been proposed.[5] In this latter "minimally differentiated" subtype, diagnosis cannot be made on morphologic grounds but rather on the detection of myeloid-specific surface antigens. This entity should be distinguished from undifferentiated or biophenotypic leukemia (see ALL classification). Table 30-2 summarizes the criteria for recognition of M0-M7 and includes a partial listing of cytogenetic and phenotypic data.

A particularly helpful feature of the FAB system is that it distinguishes subsets of AML of unique clinical and prognostic importance. For example, in acute promyelocytic leukemia (APL or M3), tumor cells are heavily laden with unusual dysplastic granules (Fig 30-1b–color plate following page 372). Rich in procoagulants, release of granular contents often incites fulminant disseminated intravascular coagulation (DIC)

Table 30-2. Classification of AML

FAB	Morphology	Histochemistry	Cytogenetics	Surface Markers	Other
M0	Large, agranular blasts	Peroxidase (-) Sudan black (-)		CD13 or CD 33 (+)	May be confused with ALL (B-cell and T-cell markers [-])
M1	Minimal maturation Scant granules and Auer rods	Peroxidase (+) 3% to 5% cells Sudan black (+) 3% to 5% cells PAS, NSE (-)	t(9;22) + 8 del(5), del(7)	Ia, CD13, CD33 (+) CD14, CD11b (+)	
M2	Greater maturation Granules and Auer rods	Peroxidase (+) Sudan black (+) PAS, NSE (-)	t(8;21) + 8 del(5), del(7)	Ia, CD13, CD33 (+) CD14, CD11b (-)	
M3	Promyelocytes with prominent granules and Auer rods	Peroxidase (++) Sudan black (++) PAS, NSE (+/-)	t(15;17)	CD33, CD13 (+) Ia (-) CD11b (+/-)	DIC common
M4	Myelomonocytic blasts	Peroxidase (+) NSE (+), SE (+)	t(4;11), t(9;11) + 8 del(5), del(7)	CD13, CD11b (+) Ia, CD14 (-)	Increased lysozyme Organ infiltration
M4Eo	Myelomonocytic blasts >5% eosinophils	Esterase and PAS may be (+) in eosinophils	inv(16)		
M5 a	Undifferentiated monoblasts	Peroxidase (-) SE (-), NSE (+)	t(9;11) + 8 del(5), del(7)	CD13, CD11b (+) Ia, CD14 (-)	Increased lysozyme Organ infiltration
b	Differentiated monocytes	Peroxidase (-) SE (-), NSE (+)			
M6	Erythroblasts with dysplasia	PAS coarsely (+)	+ 8 del(5), del(7)	Glycophorin (+)	
M7	Pleomorphic megakaryoblasts	Platelet peroxidase (+) Peroxidase, Sudan black (-) PAS, esterase (+/-)		Factor VIII (+) Gp Ib, IIb/IIIa (+)	Marrow fibrosis common

NSE = Nonspecific esterase: α naphthyl acetate or α naphthyl butyrate esterase
SE = Specific esterase: α naphthyl ASD chloracetate esterase

even before therapy is instituted. The 15;17 translocation is requisite for diagnosis and is invaluable in defining the morphologic microgranular variant of APL. In the latter condition promyelocytes have distinctive folded or bi-lobed nuclei (Fig 30-1c—color plate following page 372) and subtle granulation that can remain undetected until myeloperoxidase staining or electron microscopy is performed. The monocytic forms of AML, M4, and M5 (Fig 30-1d—color plate following page 372) are associated with frequent infiltration of skin and other soft tissues. Monoblasts stain positively for non-specific esterase and may lead to elevated levels of serum and urine lysozyme. Increased eosinophils with scattered basophilic granules suggests the subtype M4Eo. The cytogenetic abnormality inv(16) confirms this diagnosis. Acute megakaryocytic leukemia (M7) is the most difficult form of AML to recognize. Clinically, patients develop sudden pancytopenia and bone marrow fibrosis (hence its alternate name acute myelofibrosis). Bone marrow aspiration is often unsuccessful, yielding a "dry tap." Careful examination of the specimen may reveal small blasts with cytoplasmic blebbing (Fig 30-1f—color plate following page 372). Definitive characterization of these cells as megakaryoblasts, however, rests on histochemical stains (platelet peroxidase reaction) and immunologic markers (surface expression of platelet glycoproteins and Factor VIII).

Table 30-3. Prognostic Factors in AML

Prognostic Factors in AML
Good Prognosis
FAB-M3; t(15;17)
FAB-M4Eo; inv (16)
t (8;21)
t (9;11)
Standard Prognosis
Normal cytogenetics
(+) 8
Poor Prognosis
t(3;3)
t(4;11)
t(9;22)
-5, -7
(+) 21

Laboratory Data

Some degree of anemia, thrombocytopenia, and neutropenia is uniform to all types of AML. Leukocytosis with circulating blasts is usual, although mild pancytopenia may be the only abnormality. "Aleukemia leukemia" is particularly common in APL. Due to rapid cell turnover, hyperuricemia and elevated lactic dehydrogenase (LDH) levels are frequent at onset and are compounded by a variety of other metabolic abnormalities once therapy is initiated, such as tumor lysis syndrome. Coagulation profiles may detect laboratory evidence for DIC before clinical signs have developed and should be monitored frequently.

Prognosis

FAB classification and cytogenetic data help define prognostic subsets of AML (Table 30-3).[6] Patients with M3 [t(15;17)] and M4Eo [inv (16)] are among those with improved survival. In contrast, abnormalities of chromosome 5 and 7 suggest secondary AML arising in the setting of myelodyplasia and portend an unfavorable outcome. Older persons often fare poorly because of decreased drug tolerance and increased toxicity.

Treatment

Initial therapy for AML (induction) is directed at eradication of the leukemic clone and reestablishment of normal hematopoieis. Cytosine arabinoside (ARA-C) and anthracyclines (eg, daunarubicin) form the mainstay of induction regimens and yield response rates of 60% to 80%. Once remission has been achieved (defined as less than 5% myeloblasts in the marrow) additional chemotherapy is required to delay or prevent relapse. Despite many studies, the optimal timing, duration, and dosing of post-remission treatment has not been defined. With chemotherapy alone, only 20% to 30% of patients will be cured of AML. Allogeneic bone marrow transplant (BMT) performed in first remission has improved long-term survival to about 60%.[7] Whether allogeneic BMT should be offered to patients with APL or other subtypes carrying a more favorable prognosis remains unsettled. Because allogeneic BMT is restricted by toxicity and availability of donors, autologous BMT (purged and unpurged) is being investigated. Each is associated with unique advantages and disadvantages (Table 30-4), and ongoing trials may help to define the optimal timing and setting for these treatment modalities.[8]

Approximately 75% of patients achieving complete remission will relapse usually within 2 years of diagnosis. A variety of chemotherapeutic regimens have been used with varied success. Repeated courses of daunarubicin and ARA-C, high-dose ARA-C, etoposide, and mitoxantrone in various combinations as well as single-agent carboplatin and 2-chlorodeoxyadenosine have been reported. In general, remission rates of 25% to 40% are obtained. Only a small percentage of these patients will have long-term survival. Autologous BMT with ex-vivo purging of leukemic cells by chemotherapeutic drugs such as 4-hydroperoxycyclophosphamide (4-HC) is effective at this juncture, yielding long-term relapse-free survival of about 30%.[9]

Recent trials of the oral differentiating agent all trans-retinoic acid have provided exciting and encouraging results in APL. A high proportion of patients will achieve complete remission usually without marrow ablation or induction of DIC.[10] Remission duration, however, is transient and may be associated with severe leukocytosis as well as a clinical syndrome characterized by fever, weight gain, hypotension, hyperbilirubinemia, pulmonary infiltrates, and pleuro-pericardial effusions ("retinoic acid

Table 30-4. Allogeneic vs Autologous Bone Marrow Transplant (BMT)

Allogeneic BMT

Advantages

- Graft vs leukemia effect

Disadvantages

- Age <55
- HLA match required
- Graft vs host disease
- Severe immunosuppression (infection, post-transplant lymphoma)

Autologous BMT

Advantages

- Age <65
- No HLA match required
- No graft vs host disease

Disadvantages

- No graft versus leukemia effect
- Marrow contamination by occult tumor cells
- Prolonged marrow reconstitution

syndrome").[11] Whether the toxicity profile and success rate of retinoic acid will warrant its use as a first-line drug for patients with APL awaits ongoing randomized trials. It should certainly be considered in the relapse setting.

Numerous complications are anticipated during the treatment of AML. Improved supportive measures have proved critical in this regard. Permanent indwelling intravenous catheters, subspecialty nursing services, and increased availability of blood products are central to the success of intensive chemotherapy regimens. Alloimmunization has been decreased by rendering red cells and platelets leukopoor. Prompt recognition and treatment of fever in the neutropenic patient is facilitated by a range of broad-spectrum antibiotics and antifungal drugs. Administration of oral antibiotics during neutropenic nadirs has been shown to reduce the incidence of severe infection while not improving overall survival.

Infiltration of the central nervous system by leukemic cells occurs in about 5% to 10% of all patients with AML during some stage of the disease, most often at the time of marrow relapse. Cranial irradiation and intrathecal administration of ARA-C and/or methotrexate are used to treat leukemic meningitis, although high intravenous dosing of these agents may be equally effective. Prophylactic treatment of the CNS in adults with AML is not generally recommended.

Leukostasis arises when peripheral blast counts exceed 50,000 to 100,000/μL. Altered mental status, dyspnea, retinal hemorrhage, and priapism are felt to arise from arteriolar plugging by leukemia blasts as well as local perivascular tissue infiltration. Cranial irradiation, high doses of rapidly cytolytic drugs (eg, hydroxyurea) and/or leukopheresis are instituted as emergent therapies.

Massive and rapid lysis of leukemic cells can induce acute, life-threatening metabolic derangements including hyperkalemia, hyperuricemia, hyperphosphatemia, hypocalcemia, acidosis, and renal failure, known as the tumor lysis syndrome. Vigorous hydration and administration of allopurinol help circumvent these imbalances.

Serious hemorrhage and less-frequent thrombosis arise from DIC in AML. Management is controversial, but it has been shown that transfusion with plasma, red cells, and platelets is as effective as heparin.

Chronic Myelogenous Leukemia

An early description of CML by Craigie colorfully portrays the cardinal features of this disease: "listlessness...swelling and hardness in the left epigastric region...perspiration at night...blood vessels filled with grumus and clots containing lymph or purulent matter."[12] CML is a clonal myeloproliferative disorder characterized by profound myeloid hyperplasia, splenomegaly, and eventual transformation to acute leukemia, "blast crisis." As the first human malignancy associated with a consistent cytogenetic abnormality, the Philadelphia (Ph) chromosome has provided a model for molecular oncogenesis. Like other chronic leukemias, CML is palliated by standard chemotherapy, and the only potential for cure is afforded by bone marrow transplantation.

Incidence and Epidemiology

CML constitutes about 0.3% of all cancers in the United States and 13% of leukemia in Western countries with an annual incidence of 1.3/100,000.[13] Rates keep rising with age, and males have a rate 1.7 times as high as females.

Etiology

The Ph chromosome is the hallmark of CML. Originally described by Nowell and Hungerford[14] in 1960 as a "minute chromosome," it is now known to represent reciprocal translocation of genetic material between chromosomes 9 and 22, t(9;22) (q34.1;q11.21). Two oncogenes are involved in the formation of the Ph chromosome (Fig 30-2).[15] C-*abl*, located on the long arm of chromosome 9, is juxtaposed to a narrow 5.8 kilobase breakpoint cluster region (bcr) on chromosome 22. Found on chromosome 22, C-*sis* can be reciprocally translocated to chromosome 9 or a variety of other sites. The new fusion gene, bcr-*abl*, results in an

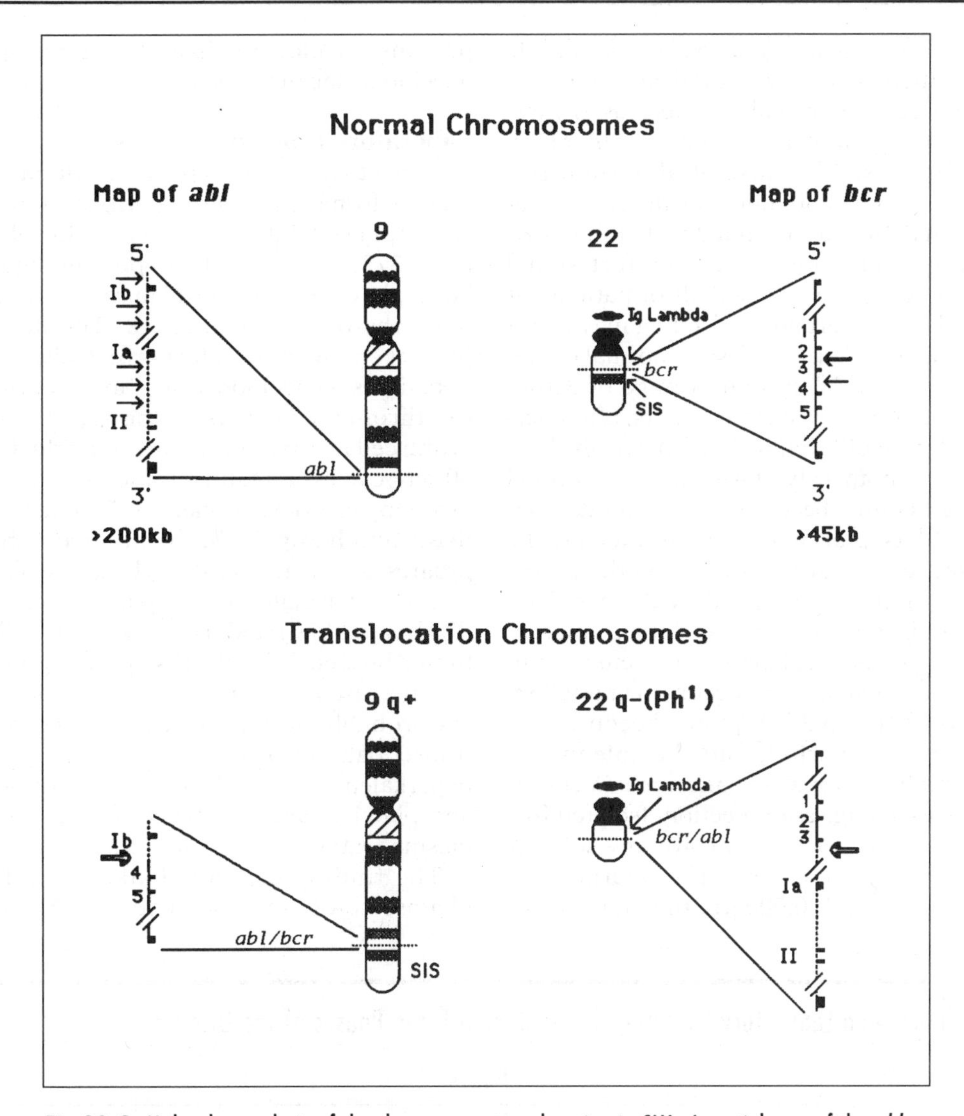

Fig 30-2. Molecular analysis of the chromosome translocation in CML. A partial map of the *abl* proto-oncogene on chromosome 9 (dashed line) and bcr on chromosome 22 (solid line). The exons are indicated by small black squares. The arrows in the upper portion of the figure indicate translocation breakpoints; those in bcr tend to cluster between exons 2 and 3 (heavy arrow), whereas those in *abl* occur anywhere within the 200 kb intron that is 5′ of exon II. The genetic consequences of one translocation are shown in the lower portion. Proto-oncogene *abl* distal to exon Ib is translocated to the Ph chromosome whereas bcr distal to exon 3 is translocated to the 9q+ chromosome, resulting in fusion genes on both translocation partners. Adapted from Rowley.[15]

aberrant 8 kilobase RNA transcript and a p210Kd protein with tyrosine kinase activity. Virtually all cases of CML will show evidence of bcr-*abl* rearrangement, which has become a sine qua non for the disorder. The role of this gene product as well as the importance of the translocated c-*sis* gene remains largely unknown, although undoubtedly central to the pathophysiology of this disease.

Exposure to high doses of radiation promotes evolution of CML with a peak incidence at 7 to 10 years. It comprises one-fifth of leukemias occurring in patients with ankylosing spondylitis treated with radiation and one-quarter of cases arising in Japanese atomic bomb survivors.[3] There has been no demonstrable association with chemotherapeutic drugs or viral agents.

Clinical Characteristics

The course of CML can be divided into three clinical periods: stable or chronic phase, accelerated phase, and an acute phase also known as blast crisis (Table 30-5). Early in the disease, symptoms are mild and non-specific: fatigue, fever, malaise, decreased exercise tolerance, weight loss, and night sweats. Many patients are diagnosed because of abnormalities detected on blood counts obtained for unrelated reasons. Early satiety, left upper quadrant fullness or pain and referred left shoulder discomfort signal splenomegaly noted in about one half of patients at presentation. Thrombosis and/or bleeding may result from impaired platelet function despite normal or elevated platelet number. Within an average of 3 to 4 years, transformation to blast crisis occurs, often heralded by a prodrome of fever, bone pain, weight loss, and increasing splenomegaly. During this accelerated phase, white cell counts become erratic and demonstrate increased basophils and immature forms, the LAP score rises, and additional cytogenetic abnormalities are acquired. Extramedullary disease, lytic bone lesions, and hypercalcemia are other, uncommon, accompaniments. Blast crisis represents evolution to overt acute leukemia and occurs in about 85% of patients. Constitutional symptoms become pronounced during this period, and the spleen can enlarge dramatically. Progressive pancytopenia ensues giving rise to hemorrhage and infection. Isolated foci of tumor cells—chloroma—can involve any soft tissue. Leukostasis may develop if peripheral blast counts exceed 50,000 to 100,000/μL. In a minority of persons, myelofibrosis and massive splenomegaly develop as terminal events.

Laboratory Features

Leukocytosis with a spectrum of early and more mature forms typifies the peripheral blood smear in stable-phase CML (Fig 30-3a—color plate following page 372). Eosinophils, hypogranulated basophils, large platelets, and megakaryocyte fragments complete the observed findings. The hematocrit and platelet count are usually normal, although one-third of patients will demonstrate thrombocytosis. At times the thrombocytosis is pronounced (>100,000/μL). White cell and platelet counts may fluctuate in 30- to 60-day cycles, a feature important to remember in assessing response to therapy. Increasing numbers of blasts and basophils in the peripheral blood suggest progression to accelerated phases or blast crisis (Fig 30-3b—color plate following page 372).

Elevated LDH and uric acid levels reflect the large tumor burden. Vitamin B_{12} and B_{12} binding capacity are increased as in other myeloproliferative disorders probably because of accelerated production of transcobalamin I by mature granulocytes. Pseudohyperkalemia results from in vitro lysis of white cells and platelets and can be confirmed by obtaining a plasma (rather than serum) potassium value.

The finding of a low leukocyte alkaline phosphatase (LAP) score is virtually pathognomonic of

Table 30-5. Clinical and Laboratory Features of CML During Three Phases of the Disease

	Phase		
	Stable	**Accelerated**	**Blast Crisis**
Symptoms*	None/minimal	Moderate	Pronounced
Splenomegaly	Mild	May increase	May be marked
WBC	Elevated	Erratic	High or low
Differential	<1% to 2% blasts on spectrum WBC	Increasing basophils and immaturity†	Circulating blasts often >25%
Hct	Normal	May decrease	Low
Platelets	High/normal	Erratic	Low
LAP score	Low	May increase	Normal
Bone marrow	<10% immature	Increased immaturity	>30% blasts
Cytogenetics	Ph	Ph, additional abnormalities	Ph, additional abnormalities
Median survival	3 to 4 years	6 to 24 months	2 to 4 months

* Fever, bone pain, night sweats, fatigue, weight loss
† Promyelocytes and myeloblasts

stable-phase CML. It is particularly helpful in the evaluation of a patient with leukocytosis; an elevated result suggests a leukemoid reaction, while a depressed value signals CML. During the accelerated phase and blast crisis and during intercurrent infection, the LAP score may normalize.

Morphologic examination of the bone marrow usually adds little, as the diagnosis is suggested by review of the peripheral blood smear in conjunction with physical findings and laboratory data. It is hypercellular with a marked shift in myeloid- to erythroid-ratio (10:1 to 15:1). In the chronic phase, myeloblasts and promyelocytes constitute less than 10% of the leukocyte differential, but as the disease progresses, the proportion of immature cells rises. Blast crises (acute leukemia) assumes a myeloid phenotype (AML) in two thirds of cases and a lymphoid form (acute lymphoblastic leukemia) in one third. Rarely, acute erythrocytic (M6) and acute megakaryocytic (M7) leukemias evolve. The distinction between AML and ALL may be difficult on a morphologic basis alone and is aided by histochemical stains and immunologic markers (Table 30-6).

Table 30-6. Distinguishing AML from ALL

	AML	ALL
Morphology		
Cytoplasm	Lighter blue	Scant rim, dark blue
Nucleoli	Prominent	Subtle
Histochemistry	Myeloperoxidase (+)	PAS (+); TdT (+)
Immunophenotype	Myeloid markers	B-cell, T-cell, CALLA (CD 10)

Prognosis

Chronic myelogenous leukemia is not cured by standard chemotherapy. Median survival in the chronic phase is 3 to 4 years but declines to 6 to 24 months and 8 to 16 weeks for accelerated phase and blast crisis respectively.[16] Overall, the risk of leukemic conversion is about 10% per year. Thus, a small proportion of patients with CML will have prolonged life expectancy. The lymphoid variant of blast crisis carries a somewhat improved outlook: 60% of patients attain a transient remission extending survival to 6 to 8 months.

Treatment

Therapy in chronic phase is palliative, directed simply at control of white blood cell and platelet counts. The most commonly utilized agents hydroxyurea and myeleran are both effective in this regard. Hydroxyurea is generally better tolerated and results in rapid, albeit short-lived, remissions. Myeleran is administered on a pulse rather than daily basis and is thus less cumbersome. However, long-term side effects such as pulmonary fibrosis, Addisonian-like syndrome, xerostomia, and rarely, bone marrow aplasia, render this agent more toxic. Before the introduction of myeleran in the 1950s, splenic irradiation constituted first line therapy. Rarely, it is still employed to control massive or painful splenomegaly. Alpha interferon induces hematologic remission in 70% to 80% of patients with stable phase CML, and it suppresses the number of Ph-positive metaphases in about one half of cases.[17] Less effective in accelerated phase and blast crisis, interferon may play a role in minimal disease states, such as cytogenetic relapse following bone marrow transplantation.

Once blast crisis has evolved, re-establishment of chronic phase is unlikely. Aggressive chemotherapeutic regimens are generally ineffective and highly toxic. The lymphoid variant is more responsive, and temporary remissions can be achieved in about 50% of patients with ALL-directed therapy.

To date, allogeneic BMT affords the only potential cure for CML. It is most successful when performed in the chronic phase, where long-term disease-free survival approaches 50% to 60% (Fig 30-4).[18] Toxicity of transplant remains significant; nearly 20% of patients die within the first 100 days from acute and chronic graft-versus-host disease (GVHD) interstitial pneumonitis and viral infection and failure of engraftment.[19] While diminishing the threat of GVHD, T-cell depletion of the bone marrow significantly increases the risk of leukemic relapse.

Morbidity and mortality of BMT are offset by the potential for long-term survival, and most investigators recommend allogeneic BMT early in chronic phase (within 1 year of diagnosis) for patients under age 55.[19] Increasing experience is being gained with matched unrelated marrow donors. As new immunosuppressive modalities are perfected, this form of BMT may become more widely applied.

Acute Lymphoblastic Leukemia

Acute lymphoblastic leukemia accounts for 78% of childhood leukemia but is uncommon in adults.[13] It is a heterogeneous disorder whose classification rests on both morphologic and immunologic criteria. Remission rates of 60% to 80% and long-term survival of about 40% in adults have been achieved through ad-ministration of prolonged, intensive multidrug chemotherapy regimens and CNS prophylaxis. Prognostic factors that identify high-risk subgroups of ALL help tailor therapy and define a role for allogeneic BMT.

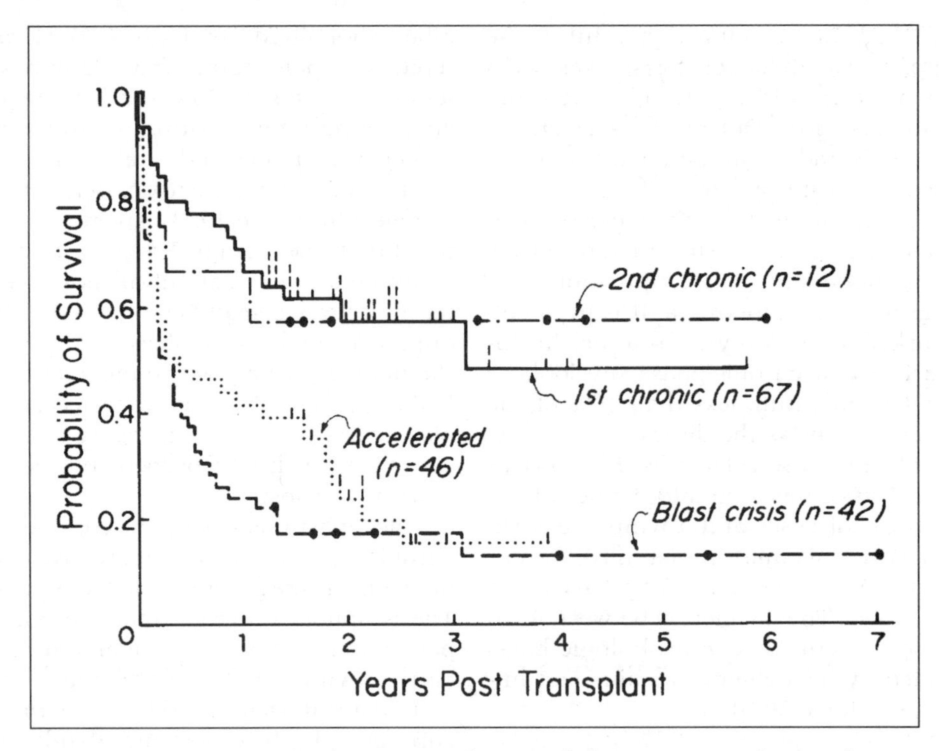

Fig 30-4. Kaplan-Meier product limit estimates for survival after marrow transplantation for patients given allogeneic grafts in the first chronic phase (solid line), second chronic phase (broken line with dots), accelerated phase (dotted line), or blastic phase (broken line). The tick marks and solid circles indicate surviving patients. Adapted from Thomas et al.[18]

Incidence and Epidemiology

ALL comprises about 40% of adult leukemias. A slight male predominance has been noted in the United States, and whites are more frequently affected than blacks.[20]

Etiology

As with other forms of adult leukemia, the etiologic basis of ALL remains unknown. Molecular identification of translocation breakpoints may yield further insights into the pathophysiology of this disease.[2] The best recognized of these is the t(8;14) characteristic of L3 ALL and Burkitt's lymphoma. The oncogene c-*myc* is translocated from chromosome 8 to chromosome 14, where it is strategically positioned adjacent to the heavy chain immunoglobulin locus. How subsequent altered expression of c-*myc* relates to the development and progression of ALL remains largely unknown.

Radiation exposure in Japanese atomic bomb survivors is associated with an increased risk of ALL as are certain congenital disorders including ataxia telangiectasia, Down's syndrome, and Fanconi's anemia. Concurrent development of leukemia in monozygotic twins during early childhood has been noted, suggesting either a shared genetic predisposition or intrauterine exposure.

Clinical Characteristics

Abrupt onset of malaise, fatigue, bony pain, bleeding, and bruising is common. Headache and cranial nerve palsies imply CNS infiltration present in about 10% of patients at onset. Hepatosplenomegaly and lymphadenopathy are frequent in all subtypes, while mediastinal masses and bulky abdominal nodes typify the T-cell and B-cell subtypes respectively.

Classification

ALL is categorized on the basis of both morphologic and immunologic data. The FAB system stratifies this disorder into three groups—L1 through L3. L1, seen most frequently in childhood, is characterized by small, homogenous lymphoblasts with scant cytoplasm, regular nuclei, and indistinct nucleoli (Fig 30-5a–color plate following page 372). L2 lymphoblasts typical of adult ALL are larger and more variable (Fig 30-5b—color plate following page 372). Malignant cells in L3 ALL are morphologically indistinct from Burkitt's lymphoma and tend to be large with vacuolated, deeply basophilic cytoplasm and prominent nucleoli (Fig 30-5c—color plate following page 372).

Immunologic data serve to further classify cell lineage in ALL. The presence of surface immunoglobulin (smIg) defines a mature B-cell phenotype found in

Table 30-7. Classification of Acute Lymphoblastic Leukemia in Adults

Subtype	Clinical Features	Surface Markers	Morphology
T-cell (15% to 20%)	Mediastinal mass CNS involvement	CD2 (Leu 5) (+) CD7 (Leu 9) (+) CD5 (Leu 1) (+)	L1, L2
Pre-B-cell (75% to 80%)		Ia (HLA-DR) (+) 100% CD19 (B4) (+) 95% CALLA (CD10) (+) 75% CD20 (B1) (+) 50% Cytoplasmic m chain (+) 15%	L1, L2
B-cell (2% to 7%)	Abdominal masses CNS involvement Poor prognosis	Surface membrane Ig (smIg) CD20 (+) CD19 (+) Ia (+)	L3

2% to 7% of cases. Initially labeled "null cells" due to their lack of surface markers, the majority of lymphoblasts have been found to express cytoplasmic immunoglobulin and demonstrate immunoglobulin gene rearrangements. This group of early "pre" B cells may also be classified according to the presence of the common acute lymphoblastic leukemia antigen (CALLA). Approximately 20% of lymphoblasts will be derived from T-cell lineage, identified in part by CD2, CD5, CD7. Correlation between morphologic and immunologic findings, while not strict, is presented in Table 30-7.

Biphenotypic Leukemia

Refinement of histochemical, immunologic, and cytogenetic techniques has led to increasingly frequent detection of leukemic blasts that share myeloid and lymphoid features. These so-called biphenotypic leukemias are believed to present "lineage infidelity," co-expressing genes and cell surface markers common to both forms of leukemia. Precise categorization of these processes is controversial (AML with lymphoid markers; ALL with myeloid markers), and at times they are placed under the umbrella of acute undifferentiated leukemia.

Laboratory Data

Circulating lymphoblasts are commonly detected in ALL and accompany anemia, neutropenia, and thrombocytopenia. Lymphoblasts may be difficult to distinguish from myeloblasts (Fig 30-6—color plate following page 372). Histochemistry and immunologic markers have proven invaluable in this regard (Table 30-6). Coarse PAS staining marks 75% of lymphoid blasts, and acid phosphatase serves to identify those of T-cell origin. Particularly helpful is the finding of terminal deoxynucloetidyl transferase (TdT) activity, an enzyme involved in early immunoglobulin and T-cell receptor gene rearrangement.

Cytogenetics are normal in one-third of patients. The Ph t(9;22) is the most frequent anomaly detected (30%) but is distinguished from CML by a unique bcr-*abl* fusion gene and a p190 KD (not p210 KD) protein. The t(8;14) is associated with the L3 (Burkitt's) morphologic subtype and mature B-cell (smIg +) phenotype.

As with other forms of leukemia, elevated levels of uric acid and lactic dehydrogenase reflect large tumor burden. Unlike AML the development of DIC and tumor lysis syndrome are unusual except in the L3 variant, where the latter complication can be profound.

Prognosis

Factors adversely affecting outcome have been defined for childhood ALL, some or all of which can be extrapolated to the adult (Table 30-8). Long-term survival varies from 50% to 60% (favorable) to 20% to 25% (unfavorable). The biphenotypic leukemias carry a particularly poor prognosis, and in these cases therapy should be directed at both the myeloid and lymphoid components of the disease.

Treatment

Treatment programs for adult ALL are based on regimens used in children and differ from therapy for AML in two important respects: prolonged administration of drugs (maintenance) and CNS prophylaxis. Numerous

Table 30-8. Poor Prognosis in ALL

Male sex
Age >9 years or <2 years
WBC >15,000-30,000/mL
Prolonged time to achieve remission (>4 weeks from treatment)
L3-Burkitt's morphology; B-cell phenotype; t(8;14)
t(9;22)
t(4;11)

intensive and complicated protocols have been designed exploiting chemotherapeutic agents of varying toxicities and mechanisms of action. The most active drugs include: anthracyclines, vincristine, prednisone, L-aspariginase, methotrexate, cyclophosphamide, cytosine arabinoside, 6-thioguanine, and 6-mercaptopurine. Combinations of these medications are administered over 2 years. Remission rates of 70% to 90% are reported, but overall survival of only 35% to 50% is expected.[21] CNS prophylaxis follows once the bone marrow has been cleared of lymphoblasts and generally consists of intrathecal methotrexate and/or cytosine arabinoside with cranial irradiation. It has been recognized that patients with the L3 subtype (mature B-cell phenotype, t[8;14]) fare poorly with standard ALL chemotherapy regimens and should be treated with more intensive Burkitt's lymphoma protocols.

Less than one half of patients with ALL will be cured. Allogeneic BMT in first remission remains controversial but should be offered to those with high-risk disease (eg, Ph-positive ALL). When performed in second or subsequent remission, disease-free survival approximates 20% to 30%. Autologous BMT has proven disappointing, complicated by a high rate of leukemic relapse. The role of in vitro purging by monoclonal antibodies or chemotherapeutic drugs remains unproved.

Chronic Lymphocytic Leukemia

Depicted by Dameshek[22] in 1967 as an "accumulation of immunologically incompetent lymphocytes," chronic lymphocytic leukemia (CLL) is an indolent lymphoproliferative disorder characterized by lymphocytosis, lymphadenopathy, and splenomegaly. In the majority of cases (95%) it is a neoplasm of B cells; T-cell CLL represents a somewhat different clinical and laboratory variant (see below). The course of patients with B-cell CLL is highly dependent on stage of disease, with median survival ranging from over 10 years to less than 19 months. The development of autoimmune hemolytic anemia and thrombocytopenia as well as recurrent viral and bacterial infections highlight the profound immunoregulatory deficiencies inherent to this disorder.

Incidence and Epidemiology

CLL is the most common form of adult leukemia and constitutes about 0.9% of all cancers. With an annual incidence of 2.9/100,000, CLL is a disease of the elderly; 90% of cases affect persons over age 50. For reasons that remain unexplained, it is extraordinarily infrequent in the Asian population. Males are affected twice as frequently as females.

Etiology

The cause of CLL remains unknown. It is the only leukemia not associated with radiation or drug exposure. CLL evolves in the setting of immunodeficiency states such as Wiskott-Aldrich syndrome, ataxia telangiectasia, and immunosuppression following organ transplantation, suggesting that altered immune regulatory mechanisms may be of pathophysiologic importance. A notable familial tendency for this disorder has been defined.

Clinical Characteristics

Patients with CLL often present serendipitously with an incidental finding of unexplained lymphocytosis. Fatigue, shortness of breath, night sweats, and bleeding reflect more advanced disease. Recurrent bacterial infections are a major cause of morbidity and mortality. The incidence of viral infections, notably herpes zoster, approaches 20%. An exaggerated response to insect bites (particularly that of mosquitoes) remains unexplained. Despite often extraordinarily high lymphocyte counts (>200,000/μL), signs and symptoms of leukostasis are rare. Lymphadenopathy and splenomegaly are detected in two-thirds of patients at diagnosis.

In 3% to 10% of cases, transformation to an aggressive form of large-cell lymphoma develops (Richter's syndrome).[23] Fever, rapid and disproportional growth of one lymph node group, weight loss, pancytopenia, and abdominal pain serve as warning signs. Involvement of liver, bone, gastrointestinal tract, and other extranodal sites is typical. The prognosis in these cases is extremely poor with only transient responses to intensive chemotherapy. Much less frequent transformation to prolymphocytic leukemia in CLL has also been reported.

Staging

Staging is based on physical findings and laboratory abnormalities. It is most helpful in classifying patients for study purposes but also provides general guidelines of prognosis and indications for therapy. Two classification schemas are widely used, those of Rai and colleagues (Table 30-9)[24] and Binet and colleagues (Table 30-10).[25]

Laboratory Features

CLL is marked by the proliferation of small, mature-

Table 30-9. Rai Classification

Stage	Clinical Features	Median survival (months)
0	Lymphocytosis only (>15,000/mL)	150
I	Lymphocytosis and adenopathy	101
II	Lymphocytosis and hepatomegaly or splenomegaly	71
III	Lymphocytosis and anemia (Hb <11gm)	19
IV	Lymphocytosis and thrombocytopenia (plt <100,000/mL)	19

The *modified* Rai classification further groups stages according to prognosis: stage O (low risk), stages I, II (intermediate risk), stages III, IV (high risk).

appearing lymphocytes (Fig 30-7—color plate following page 372). Occasional variation in size can be observed as well as characteristic "smudge cells." Immunophenotypic data defines the clonal process as of B-cell origin in 95% of cases. Low-intensity surface immunoglobulin (IgM ±IgD) with monotypic light chain expression is noted. Other markers of B-cell lineage include CD19, CD20, CD21, CD23, and CD24. Aberrant expression of a normal T-cell antigen (CD5) remains a distinctive and unexplained feature of CLL cells.

At diagnosis, 35% of patients will present with anemia and 25% with thrombocytopenia. These may result from marrow infiltration or autoimmune destruction. Of interest, the autoantibody appears to be polyclonal in nature. One fifth of patients develop a positive Coomb's (antiglobulin) test, although hemolysis is detected in less than one half of instances. Hypogammaglobulinemia is typical and may be profound. Monoclonal gammopathy is seen in 10%. Elevated levels of LDH and uric acid, reflective of rapid cell turnover, are unusual.

The bone marrow is always affected and may assume one of four morphologic patterns. Diffuse infiltration has been touted to imply a worse prognosis compared to nodular or interstitial involvement. Cytogenetic studies in CLL have been hampered by difficulties in obtaining adequate metaphases for analysis. The most common finding is trisomy 12, accounting for 20% to 60% of karyotypic abnormalities. Lymph node histology is indistinguishable from that of well-differentiated lymphocytic lymphoma.

Prognosis

Prognosis for patients with CLL is determined mainly by clinical stage and is highly variable, ranging from 1 to 2 years to over 10 years. Weight loss, performance status, degree of leukocytosis, elevated LDH, uric acid, and alkaline phosphatase have been identified as additional predictors of adverse outcome perhaps because they reflect increased tumor burden. Lymphocyte doubling time of less than one year has also been associated with poorer prognosis.[26]

Treatment

At the present time, CLL remains incurable, and thus chemotherapy is given with palliative intent. In early-stage patients (Rai stage 0; Binet stage A), treatment with chlorambucil has been shown to afford no survival advantage over observation alone.[27] Systemic symptoms (fever, night sweats, weight loss), bulky adenopathy, progressive pancytopenia, or refractory autoimmune phenomena serve as indications for systemic therapy. Chlorambucil alone is as effective as combination therapy (cyclophosphamide, vincristine, and prednisone) for intermediate-stage patients (Rai stage I, II; Binet stage B).[28] However, it has been proposed, though still not widely accepted, that persons with advanced CLL (stage C or Rai stage III, IV) receive more aggressive regimens such as cyclophosphamide, adriamycin, vincristine, and prednisone (CHOP).[29]

Fludarabine offers an alternative for management of CLL[30]; overall, 56% of previously treated patients will respond to this purine analog. While still generally relegated to the refractory setting, Fludarabine may emerge as an effective front-line therapy. Severe myelosuppression is the most limiting toxicity, and occasional cases of tumor lysis syndrome and pulmonary dysfunction are reported with its use. Patients on Fludarabine acquire significant immunologic defects, further enhancing susceptibility to opportunistic organisms. Patients with advanced-stage, resistant CLL have similar response rates with 2-chlorodeoxyadenosine (2-CDA).

Radiation therapy to sites of bulk disease (lymph nodes and spleen) may be of palliative benefit. Like-

Table 30-10. Binet Classification of CLL

Stage	Clinical Features	Median survival (months)
A	Lymphocytosis and enlargement of ≤3 lymph node groups	108
B	Lymphocytosis and enlargement of >3 lymph node groups	60
C	Lymphocytosis with anemia (Hb <10 g) or thrombocytopenia (platelets <100,000/mL)	24

wise, splenectomy in selective patients can improve blood counts and ameliorate autoimmune hemolysis. Allogeneic BMT is being investigated as a potentially curative option for the young patient but remains completely experimental at this time.

Gammaglobulin replacement in CLL is controversial. While it may diminish the number of bacterial infections, widespread application to all patients has been questioned.[31] Vaccinations against pneumococcus, *H influenza*, and meningococcus are advised. However, live viral vaccinations must be avoided, as they can incite a severe localized necrotizing vasculitis or a potentially fatal systemic illness.

CLL Variants

Prolymphocytic Leukemia

Prolymphocytic leukemia (PLL) was described as a distinct syndrome by Galton[32] in 1974. It is about one tenth as frequent as CLL and occurs somewhat later in life. The majority of cases occur in men. Constitutional symptoms, splenomegaly, and lymphocytosis (100,000 to 500,000/μL) are often pronounced, while lymphadenopathy is minimal. Prolymphocytes are larger than mature lymphocytes with generous amounts of cytoplasm and prominent nucleoli (Fig 30-8—color plate following page 372). Like those found in CLL, they are generally of B-cell origin. However, they are distinguished by intense surface immunoglobulin staining (compared with dim staining in CLL) and absence of the CD5 antigen. Rare T-cell variants have been described. Median survival for PLL is poor (17 weeks to 3 years), and aggressive therapy with anthracycline-based regimens has been advocated.[33] Fludarabine phosphate has also been tried in this disorder.

Hairy Cell Leukemia

Infiltration of the bone marrow and spleen by lymphocytes with unusual hairy projections leads to pancytopenia and splenomegaly in the indolent disorder, hairy cell leukemia (HCL). HCL affects males four times as frequently as females with a median age of onset of about 50 years.

Lymphocytes appear somewhat larger than normal with reniform ("kidney"-shaped) nuclei (Fig 30-9a—color plate following page 372). Fine cytoplasmic projections are particularly evident on phase microscopy. The majority of tumor cells mark with mature B-cell antigens including surface immunoglobulin. They are usually CD25 (IL-2 receptor) positive and CD5 negative. Acid phosphatase staining resistant to treatment with tartrate (TRAP) is a hallmark finding in HCL found in 95% of cases. Infiltration of the spleen occurs in the red pulp distinctive from the usual white pulp involvement of other low-grade lymphoproliferative disorders. While bone marrow aspirates may be unhelpful ("dry taps"), the histologic "fried egg" pattern of the biopsy is often pathognomonic (Fig 30-9b—color plate following page 372).

Patients with HCL develop complications arising from pancytopenia as well as a striking propensity for opportunistic infection and vasculitis. Up to 20% of patients may have prolonged survival without therapeutic intervention. Splenectomy was the traditional first-line approach for this disease but has been largely replaced by treatment with alpha interferon, pentostatin, or 2-chlorodeoxyadenosine (2-CDA). Interferon yields high rates of complete and partial responses (up to 80%), which may be sustained for 12 to 18 months. While patients are unlikely to be cured, they can be palliated by repeated courses of this agent. The adenosine deaminase inhibitor pentostatin (deoxycoformycin) has also been used with success in HCL and may provide a higher number of remissions that are more durable.[34] The most impressive new drug for HCL is 2-CDA. One 7-day infusion can result in permanent eradication of neoplastic lymphocytes from all affected organs.[35] Toxicities are generally mild but include transient leukopenia and immunosuppression (reduction of CD4 counts). Unlike other therapies, 2-CDA offers the potential for cure and thus has become the drug of first choice in this disease.

T-cell Lymphocytosis

T-cell chronic lymphoproliferative disorders have long defied precise categorization. Among the heterogeneous subtypes, T-gamma lymphocytosis and T-cell CLL emerge as two distinct entities.[36] In the former condition a proliferation of large granular lymphocytes (LGL) has given rise to the many pseudonyms for this syndrome (LGL leukemia, T-suppresser cell leukemia). The clinical course is usually benign but is notable for associated autoimmune disease (eg, rheumatoid arthritis), splenomegaly, and neutropenia. Pure red cell aplasia has also been reported. Large granular lymphocytes generally number less than 20,000/μL in the peripheral blood and can be further characterized by surface expression of CD2, CD3, and CD8 and the absence of CD5. While the course of this disease is often indolent and requires no therapy, LGL may progress and prove refractory.

T-cell CLL is distinct from T-gamma lymphocytosis. Lymphadenopathy, lymphocytosis, splenomegaly, and skin involvement are prominent, while neutropenia and anemia are unusual. Morphologically, the cells are similar to their B-cell counterparts and mark with a helper (CD4+) phenotype. Because of the rarity of this disease, its natural history and therapy remain ill defined.

Sezary's syndrome and adult T-cell leukemia-lymphoma both present with a leukemic component that may be difficult to distinguish from CLL. In the former condition (the leukemic phase of mycosis fungoides), infiltration of the skin by malignant T-cells gives rise to a diffuse erythroderm and scaling plaques. Sezary cells have generous cytoplasm, convoluted nuclei, and may demonstrate a characteristic "ring of pearls" pattern (Fig 30-10—color plate following page 372). They are immunologically recognized as helper (CD4+) and CD25 (IL-2-receptor) negative. Topical drugs are effective in the early stages of Sezary's syndrome. However, more advanced disease mandates systemic chemotherapy.

Adult T-cell leukemia-lymphoma is the first human malignancy causally linked to viral infection (HTLV I). Endemic in Japan, southeastern United States, Africa, and the Caribbean, its aggressive course is punctuated by nodular skin infiltrates, lymphadenopathy, hepatosplenomegaly, lytic bone lesions, and hypercalcemia. Circulating malignant cells have markedly convoluted nuclei and deeply basophilic cytoplasm (Fig 30-11—color plate following page 372). Like Sezary cells, these cells are CD4+ but are distinguished by the presence of the IL-2 receptor (CD25). Despite aggressive treatment, the disease is usually fulminant, with a median survival of less than 1 year.

References

1. Sandler DP. Epidemiology of acute myelogenous leukemia. *Semin Oncol.* 1987;14:359-364.

2. Nichols J, Nimer SD. Transcription factors, translocations, and leukemia. *Blood.* 1992;80:2953-2963.

3. Moloney WC. Radiogenic leukemia revisited. *Blood.* 1987;70:905-908.

4. Pui C-H, Ribeiro RC, Hancock ML, et al. Acute myeloid leukemia arising in children treated with epipodophyllotoxins for acute lymphoblastic leukemia. *N Engl J Med.* 1991;325:1682-1687.

5. Bennett JM, Catovsky D, Daniel M-T, et al. Proposal for the recognition of minimally differentiated acute myeloid leukemia (AML-M0). *Br J Hematol.* 1991;78:325-329.

6. Arthur DC, Berger R, Golomb HM, et al. The clinical significance of karyotype in acute myelogenous leukemia. *Cancer Genet Cytogenet.* 1989;40:206-216.

7. Begg CB, McGlave PB, Bennett JM, et al. A critical comparison of allogeneic bone marrow transplantation and conventional chemotherapy as treatment for acute nonlymphocytic leukemia. *J Clin Oncol.* 1984;2:369-378.

8. Mitus AJ, Miller K, Schekein DP, et al. Multicenter trial of allogeneic versus autologous bone marrow transplantation for AML in first remission. *Blood.* 1991;78(suppl 1):268a.

9. Santos GW. Marrow transplantation in acute nonlymphocytic leukemia. *Blood.* 1989;74:901-908.

10. Warrell RP Jr, Frankel SR, Miller WH, et al. Differentiation therapy of acute promyelocytic leukemia with tretinoin (all trans retinoic acid). *N Engl J Med.* 1991; 324:1385-1393.

11. Frankel SR, Eardley A, Lauwers G, et al. The "retinoic acid syndrome." *Ann Intern Med.* 1992;117:292-296.

12. Craigie D. A case of disease of the spleen in which death took place in consequence of the presence of purulent matter in the blood. *Edinburgh Med Surg.* 1845;64:400-413.

13. Miller BA, Ries LAG, Hankey BF, et al. *SEER Cancer Statistics Review 1973-90.* Bethesda, Md: National Cancer Institute; 1993. Dept. of Health and Human Services publication NIH 93-2789.

14. Nowell P. Chromsome studies on normal and leukemic human leukocytes. *J Natl Cancer Inst.* 1960;25:85-93.

15. Rowley JD. Chromosome abnormalities in leukemia. *J Clin Oncol.* 1988;6:198.

16. Champlin RE, Golde DW. Chronic myelogenous leukemia: recent advances. *Blood.* 1985;65:1039-1047.

17. Silver RT. Interferon in the treatment of myeloproliferative diseases. *Semin Hematol.* 1990;27:6-14.

18. Thomas ED, Clift RA, Fefer A, et al. Marrow transplantation for the treatment of chronic myelogenous leukemia. *Ann Intern Med.* 1986;104:155-163.

19. Wagner JE, Zahurak M, Piantadosi S. Bone marrow transplantation of chronic myelogenous leukemia in chronic phase: evaluation of risks and benefits. *J Clin Oncol.* 1992;10:779-790.

20. Pendergrass TW. Epidemiology of acute lymphoblastic leukemia. *Semin Oncol.* 1985;12:80-91.

21. Linker CA, Levitt LJ, O'Donnell M, et al. Treatment of adult acute lymphoblastic leukemia with intensive cyclical chemotherapy: a follow-up report. *Blood.* 1991;78:2814-2822.

22. Dameshek W. Chronic lymphocytic leukemia: an accumulative disease of immunologically incompetent lymphocytes. *Blood.* 1967;29:566-583.

23. Trump DL, Mann RB, Phelps R, et al. Richter's syndrome: diffuse histiocytic lymphoma in patients with chronic lymphocytic leukemia: a report of five cases and review of the literature. *Am J Med.* 1980;68:539-548.

24. Rai KR, Sawitsky A, Cronkite EP, et al. Clinical staging of chronic lymphocytic leukemia. *Blood.* 1975;46:219-234.

25. Binet JL, Auquier A, Dighiero G, et al. A new prognostic classification of chronic lymphocytic leukemia: prognostic significance. *Cancer.* 1981;40:855-864.

26. Montserrat E, Sanchez-Bisono J, Vinolas N, et al. Lymphocyte doubling time in chronic lymphocytic leukemia: analysis of its prognostic significance. *Br J Hematol.* 1986;62:567-575.

27. French cooperative group on chronic lymphocytic leukemia. Effect of chlorambucil and therapeutic decision in initial forms of chronic lymphocytic leukemia (stage A): results of a randomized clinical trial on 612 patients. *Blood.* 1990;75:1414-1421.

28. French cooperative group on chronic lymphocytic leukemia. A randomized clinical trial of chlorambucil versus COP for Stage B chronic lymphocytic leukemia. *Blood.* 1990;75:1422-1425.

29. French cooperative group on chronic lymphocytic leukemia. Effectiveness of "CHOP" regimen in advanced untreated chronic lymphocytic leukemia. *Lancet.* 1986 1:1346-1349.

30. Keating MJ, Kantararijian H, Talpaz M, et al. Fludarabine: a new agent with major activity against chronic lymphocytic leukemia. *Blood.* 1989;74:19-25.

31. Weeks JC, Tierney MR, Weinstein MC. Cost effectiveness of prophylactic intravenous immune globulin in chronic lymphocytic leukemia. *N Engl J Med.* 1991;325:81-86.

32. Galton D. Prolymphocytic leukemia. *Br J Hematol.* 1974;27:7-20.

33. Stone RM. Prolymphocytic leukemia. *Hematol-Oncol Clin N Am.* 1990;4:457-471.

34. Cassileth PA, Cheuvart B, Spiers ASD, et al. Pentostatin induces durable remissions in hairy cell leukemia. *J Clin Oncol.* 1991;9:243-246.

35. Piro LD, Carrera J, Carson DA, et al. Lasting remissions in hairy cell leukemia induced by a single infusion of 2-chlorodeoxyadenosine. *N Engl J Med.* 1990;80:765-769.

36. Berliner N. T-gamma lymphocytosis and T-cell chronic leukemias. *Hematol Oncol Clin N Am.* 1990;4:473-487.

31

CHILDHOOD LEUKEMIAS

Ching-Hon Pui, MD

Leukemia is the most common form of childhood cancer, affecting approximately 2,500 children in the United States each year and accounting for almost one third of all childhood malignancies. Acute lymphoblastic leukemia (ALL) accounts for about 80% of the leukemias in children and acute myeloid (nonlymphoblastic) leukemia (AML) for most of the remainder. The increased precision of diagnostic methods, the development of more effective therapy in controlled clinical trials, and advances in supportive care have substantially improved the outlook for children with leukemia. Today, it is estimated that 70% of children with ALL will be in continuous complete remission 5 years after diagnosis, and most of these children will be cured.[1,2] Progress against AML remains slow, however; even with intensive chemotherapy and bone marrow transplantation, only 30% to 40% of those children can expect to remain in long-term remission.[3,4] Also, the late sequelae of treatment in long-term survivors of leukemia pose new therapeutic problems that are expected to increase as this population grows.

The study of childhood leukemia has yielded benefits that extend beyond improved cure rates. Because of its relatively high incidence, childhood leukemia was one of the first malignant diseases for which large-scale therapeutic trials were conducted and has served as a paradigm for the development of treatment strategies for cancers of all types. Leukemic cells are readily obtained from the blood and bone marrow, and studies of these cells have revealed many of the principles underlying our current knowledge of tumor cell biology.

Ching-Hon Pui, MD, Member, Departments of Hematology-Oncology and Pathology and Laboratory Medicine, Director, Lymphoid Disease Program, St Jude Children's Research Hospital and Professor of Pediatrics, University of Tennessee, Memphis, College of Medicine, Memphis, Tennessee

Morphologic and Cytochemical Classification

Precise classification is essential to understand the pathophysiology of childhood leukemias and to develop more specific methods of therapy. In the broadest terms, leukemias can be classified as acute, chronic, or congenital. The terms *acute* and *chronic* originally referred to survival duration, but with the advent of effective treatment they have taken on new meanings. Acute leukemia now refers to the malignant proliferation of immature (blastic) cells, and chronic leukemia to the proliferation of predominantly more mature (more differentiated) cell types. Unlike leukemia in adults, childhood leukemia is almost always acute. Chronic myeloid leukemia (CML) accounts for approximately 2% of childhood leukemias. Chronic lymphoid leukemia has been reported in only a few children. Congenital or neonatal leukemias are those diagnosed in the first four weeks of life. A related category, myelodysplastic syndrome, is a heterogeneous condition, generally characterized by pancytopenia and bone marrow dysfunction with dysmorphic maturation of the hematopoietic elements, which may evolve into frank acute leukemia.

The acute leukemias are classified as lymphoid or myeloid by their morphologic characteristics on Romanovsky-stained bone marrow smears and by their cytochemical staining properties. In general, lymphoblasts have a smooth, homogeneous nuclear chromatin pattern with indistinct nucleoli and scanty cytoplasm, without granules. Myeloblasts are larger, with abundant granular cytoplasm and one or more distinct nucleoli. However, the only morphologic feature that is diagnostic is the presence of Auer rods, which represent coalescence of azurophilic granules and are pathognomonic for AML. Azurophilic cytoplasmic granules can be identified in blast cells of 10% to 15% of children with ALL. Thus, it is essential to perform cytochemical staining for accurate diagnosis. Although much effort has been devoted to the cytochemistry of leukemia, only a few techniques are routinely necessary—myeloperoxidase, Sudan black B, α-naphthyl acetate esterase, and α-naphthyl butyrate esterase being the prime examples. Myeloperoxidase is positive in all the cells of the granulocytic series, from myeloblasts to granulocytes; weakly positive or negative in cells of the monocytic series; and always negative in lymphoblasts and lymphocytes. Sudan black B positivity usually parallels that of myeloperoxidase. Although Sudan black B positivity has been described in ALL, the staining pattern differs (a few discrete granules compared with the diffuse, intense, coarsely granular appearance of myeloblasts). Monoblasts react with both α-naphthyl butyrate and α-naphthyl acetate esterase, but megakaryoblasts are positive for only the latter stain.

Several attempts have been made to subclassify ALL and AML, but most have been unsuccessful because they were technically difficult to reproduce or lacked meaningful clinical correlation. In 1976, a French-American-British (FAB) cooperative group devised a classification schema based on the morphologic features and cytochemical staining properties of bone marrow blast cells.[5] Over the years, there have been several additions to and refinements in this system (Table 31-1). The FAB system is widely accepted and has been useful in diagnosis, treatment, and data analysis and presentation. Concordance among investigators using the FAB classification is high for AML but not for ALL. Lymphoblastic leukemias are classified as L1, L2, and L3 (Fig 31-1—Color plate following page 372); most childhood ALLs are L1, but the proportion varies according to the series. L3 morphology is clearly distinct and associated with B-cell ALL expressing surface immunoglobulin. However, there is no apparent correlation between the L1 and L2 subtypes and cell surface immunologic markers.

The FAB classification specifies eight major groups of AML: M0 through M7 (Fig 31-2—Color plate following page 372). The diagnosis of M0 leukemia cannot be made on the basis of morphologic or cytochemical tests: blast cells resemble L2 blasts in lacking myeloperoxidase and Sudan black B reactivity, and require confirmation by immunologic techniques (positive myeloid and negative lymphoid markers).[6] The M1 variant is also a poorly differentiated form of AML and is morphologically indistinguishable from L2 ALL, but blast cells are positive for myeloperoxidase. M2 leukemias show differentiation beyond the promyelocyte stage. The M3 group has the largest number of Auer rods (often arranged in bundles or "faggots") of any FAB group. The blasts may be disrupted, leaving Auer rods and granules free in the smears. In the microgranular variant of M3, blast cells have characteristic bilobular nuclei, basophilic hypogranular cytoplasm, multiple Auer rods, and fibril bundles.

In the M4 group, more than 20% of nonerythroid

Table 31-1. Classification of Childhood Leukemias by French-American-British (FAB) Criteria

FAB Designation	% of Total	Prominent Features
ALL		
L1	84	Small blasts with scanty cytoplasm, homogeneous nuclear chromatin, regular nuclear shape, and inconspicuous nucleoli
L2	15	Large blasts with increased cytoplasm, irregular nuclear shape, and prominent nucleoli
L3	1	Large blasts with finely stippled and homogeneous nuclear chromatin, regular nuclear shape, prominent nucleoli, and very deep basophilia of cytoplasm with vacuolation
AML		
M0	2	Minimal myeloid differentiation
M1	18	Poorly differentiated myeloblasts with occasional Auer rods
M2	29	Myeloblastic with differentiation and more prominent Auer rods
M3	8	Promyelocytic with heavy granulation and bundles of Auer rods
M4	16	Myeloblastic and monoblastic differentiation in various proportions
M5	17	Monoblastic
M6	2	Erythroleukemic with bizarre dyserythropoiesis and megaloblastic features
M7	8	Megakaryoblastic with bone marrow fibrosis

bone marrow cells are monoblastic. In some cases of M4 (M4Eo), increased numbers of abnormal eosinophils may contain not only eosinophilic granules but also large basophilic granules and a single unsegmented nucleus. In the M5 subtype, 80% or more of the nonerythroid cells in the bone marrow are monoblasts, promonocytes, or monocytes. There are two subtypes of M5 leukemia: M5a (≥80% of monocytic cells are monoblasts) and M5b (<80% are monoblasts). The presence of spectrin or surface expression of erythroid-associated antigens and dysmyelopoiesis leads to the diagnosis of FAB M6. In M7, the megakaryoblasts have typical cytochemical staining properties (as described before), and are characterized by platelet-associated cell surface antigens (platelet glycoproteins Ib, IIb/IIIa, or factor VIII-related antigen) and, in most cases, platelet peroxidase on electron microscopy. This subtype is often associated with pancytopenia and reticulin fibrosis of bone marrow.

The FAB cooperative group also introduced five categories of myelodysplastic syndromes characterized by defective production of normal hematopoietic cells and dyserythropoiesis with or without dysgranulopoiesis and dysmegakaryopoiesis. These cases are associated with very poor survival and may evolve into AML. Because of their rarity in childhood, these syndromes will not be addressed further.

Epidemiology

In the US, the annual incidence of leukemia in children younger than 15 years is about 4 per 100,000. The ratio of ALL to AML in children is 4 to 1—almost the reverse of that in adults. (The exception is congenital leukemia, which is most often AML.) In ALL, the peak age of occurrence is between 3 and 4 years; no age peak has been observed for AML. Unlike ALL, which usually has a higher incidence among whites than among blacks (1.8 to 1), AML is equally distributed by race. The lower incidence of ALL in black children reflects the absence of the 3- to 4-year age peak observed in white children. Whether this phenomenon reflects differences in genetic susceptibility or environmental factors is unknown. There is no sex-related difference in the incidence of AML, whereas boys are more likely than girls to develop ALL (1.4 to 1), especially during puberty. It is uncertain whether sex hormones play any role in leukemogenesis. There also appear to be geographic differences in the frequency, age distribution, and subtypes of leukemia.

Fraternal twins and siblings of affected children have a twofold to fourfold greater risk of developing leukemia than do unrelated children during the first decade of life. When leukemia occurs in one monozygous twin, the other twin has a 20% chance of developing the disease. The risk for the other twin is nearly 100% if leukemia develops in the index twin before the age of 1 year. The risk diminishes with increasing age at the time of diagnosis. If a twin is diagnosed after age 7, the other twin's risk is the same as that for any sibling. Typically, when the second twin does develop leukemia, this occurs within months of the index twin's diagnosis. Concordant leukemia in monozygotic infant twins may reflect a common prezygotic determinant, shared intrauterine event, or metastasis from one twin to the other. Recent findings of identical leukemia cell genetic abnormalities in monozygous twins with leukemia unequivocally demonstrate that intrauterine metastasis is responsible for the concordant leukemia.

An increased risk of leukemia has been linked to a variety of disorders (Table 31-2). Children with trisomy 21 have a 10- to 30-fold increased risk; acute megakaryoblastic leukemia (M7) predominates in patients younger than 3 years and ALL in the older age group. Autosomal recessive genetic diseases associated with increased chromosomal fragility and predisposition to acute leukemia include Fanconi's anemia, Bloom syndrome, and ataxia-telangiectasia. It is of interest that lymphocytes and leukemic cells of patients with ataxia-telangiectasia frequently have chromosomal rearrangements involving bands 7p13-p14, 7q32-q35, and 14q11 (sites of the T-cell receptor gamma, beta, and alpha/delta genes, respectively) and band 14q32 (site of immunoglobulin heavy-chain gene). The extent to which the associated immunodeficiency contributes to leukemogenesis in patients with ataxia-telangiectasia is unknown. In this regard, children with other constitutional or acquired immunodeficiency diseases are also at increased risk, perhaps due to impaired immune surveillance.

There have been multiple reports of so-called leukemic clusters, that is, a greater than expected

Table 31-2. Congenital Disorders Associated with Increased Risk of Leukemia

Congenital Disorder	Associated Leukemia(s)
Down syndrome	ALL, AML
Fanconi's anemia	AML
Ataxia-telangiectasia	ALL
Bloom syndrome	ALL, AML
von Recklinghausen's neurofibromatosis	AML, juvenile CML
Wiskott-Aldrich syndrome	AML
Congenital X-linked agammaglobulinemia	ALL
Immunoglobulin A deficiency	ALL
Kostmann's infantile agranulocytosis	AML
Variable immunodeficiency	ALL, AML
Shwachman-Diamond syndrome	ALL, AML

number of leukemia cases observed in a given geographic area over a certain period. However, under careful scrutiny, most of these reports have been refuted.

Etiology

Several predisposing or contributing factors have been identified, but the cause of human leukemia remains unknown. Occasional reports of leukemic clusters and the association of Epstein-Barr virus (EBV) with Burkitt's lymphoma suggest a role for infectious agents in human leukemogenesis. The ability to induce leukemia in experimental animals with different strains of retroviruses has led to the search for similar viruses in humans. Human T lymphotropic virus type I (HTLV-I) was the first retrovirus definitively linked to the development of leukemia or lymphoma. The HTLV-I virus is associated with mycosis fungoides and adult T-cell leukemia-lymphoma, a disorder prevalent in the Caribbean basin, southeastern US, and parts of Japan. A related retrovirus, HTLV-II, was subsequently isolated from a patient with hairy cell leukemia. However, attempts to demonstrate the involvement of retrovirus in childhood leukemia have been unsuccessful.

Although exposure to ionizing radiation can cause leukemia, there is little evidence of a leukemogenic effect of natural "background" irradiation. The high prevalence of leukemias in atomic bomb survivors is well recognized. The incidence and type of leukemia varied according to age at exposure, absorbed dose, and perhaps the spectrum of radiation emitted by the bombs. ALL occurred more often in those exposed during childhood, and AML in those who were adults when exposed. The relative risk of acute leukemia was higher in survivors exposed before age 10 years than in adults. There was an increased incidence of CML among Hiroshima survivors but not among those in Nagasaki. This discrepancy has been attributed to the mixture of gamma rays and neutrons emitted by the Hiroshima bomb; the Nagasaki bomb emitted predominantly gamma rays. However, there may have been biologic differences between the inhabitants of the two cities. There was also a linear correlation between the radiation dose and incidence of leukemia in individuals exposed to more than 100 cGy. Bomb survivors exposed in utero have not shown an excess of leukemia, a finding in contrast to studies suggesting an increased risk of leukemia in individuals exposed to diagnostic radiation in utero. An estimated 1% of adult leukemia may result from exposure to diagnostic radiography, but data are not available for childhood leukemia. Whereas therapeutic radiation has been associated with an increased risk of leukemia, the risks from exposure to ionizing radiation from routine emissions of nuclear power plants remain controversial. The data associating leukemia with ultrasound or ultraviolet radiation and with electrical or magnetic field exposure are also inconclusive.

Chemicals have long been suspected to cause leukemia; for example, chronic exposure to benzene results in AML in adults. However, although the percentage of childhood leukemia cases attributable to chemical exposure is unknown, it is thought to be very small. The use of intensified chemotherapy, particularly with alkylating agents, is focusing interest on the association between antineoplastic chemotherapy and leukemogenesis. The leukemias associated with use of alkylating agents are generally AML, characterized by a period of preleukemia, myelodysplasia, and frequent abnormalities involving chromosomes 5, 7, and 17.[7] Other classes of chemotherapeutic agents targeting DNA topoisomerase II, such as epipodophyllotoxins (teniposide and etoposide) and anthracyclines, have been associated recently with the development of secondary AML.[8] These leukemias are characterized by a short latency period, M4 or M5 subtype, and 11q23 or 21q22 chromosomal abnormalities.

With few exceptions, no cause or predisposing factor can be identified in children with leukemia. Some now think that spontaneous mutation may be the major cause of childhood ALL. The target cells for ALL (lymphoid precursor cells) have a high proliferative rate and increased propensity for gene rearrangement during early childhood and are more susceptible to mutation. One mutation or, more likely, sequential mutations arising spontaneously in key regulatory genes in a cell population under proliferative stress could occur often enough to account for most cases of childhood ALL. Research on oncogenes and tumor-suppressing genes promises to increase our understanding of the complex process of leukemogenesis.

Marrow Anatomy and Pathophysiology

Whereas hematopoietic precursors can be identified in a number of tissues, the bone marrow is the only site at which myelopoiesis, erythropoiesis, and lymphopoiesis occur simultaneously. The nutrient artery, the principal source of blood, enters the medullary artery via the nutrient foramen. Tributaries of this vessel feed the cortical capillaries, which in turn join the marrow sinusoids and drain into the central sinus. Hematopoiesis occurs in the intersinusoidal spaces, and maturing blood cells enter the systemic circulation by passing through the endothelial cells and the thin basement membrane on their abluminal side. Thus, bone marrow is a highly compartmentalized organ; its two major compartments are vascular and extravascular (hematopoietic). Hematopoietic cells are closely associated with fixed tissue elements, collectively referred to as stromal cells. Stromal cells, including endothelial cells, reticular cells, fibroblasts, and adipocytes, contribute to the hematopoietic microenvironments that support and regulate blood cell development. Extracellular matrix substances, such as proteoglycans, have recently been implicated in the regulation of hematopoiesis.

The prevailing theory of the pathophysiology of leukemia is that a single mutant hematopoietic progenitor cell, capable of indefinite self-renewal, gives rise to malignant, poorly differentiated hematopoietic precursors. Evidence from several lines of research supports this concept.[9] Similar chromosomal abnormalities found in multiple leukemic blast cells at diagnosis and at relapse support the clonal origin of leukemia. The unicellular development of neoplasia has been demonstrated by findings of a single type of glucose-6-phosphate dehydrogenase (G6PD) in the malignant cells of heterozygous female patients who have a double-enzyme pattern in their normal tissues. Determining the methylation patterns of X-linked restriction fragment length polymorphisms in heterozygous females is another sensitive method of analysis based on the same principle. Detection of immunoglobulin gene and T-cell receptor gene rearrangements by Southern blotting provides an alternative means of demonstrating the clonal origin of leukemia. Finally, demonstration of monoclonal immunoglobulin idiotypes and light-chain types is useful in B-cell malignancies. In fact, differentiated cells in some patients originate from the same leukemic clone.

Most often, leukemia appears to initiate in the bone marrow and spread to other parts of the body. Sometimes, however, leukemia may arise in an extramedullary site and subsequently invade the bone marrow. For example, patients may present with chloroma (granulocytic sarcoma) and no discernible hematologic or marrow abnormalities, yet develop AML months to years later. Further, ALL conceivably originates in the thymus in patients who present with an anterior mediastinal mass and in the intestine in those with an ileocecal tumor. Indeed, many investigators use an arbitrary method to distinguish between lymphoblastic leukemia and lymphoma in these cases: >25% blast cells in bone marrow signifies leukemia and <25% signifies lymphoma. A minimum of 30% blasts is required for the diagnosis of AML.

Leukemic cells divide more slowly and take longer to synthesize DNA than do normal hematopoietic precursors. Despite this seemingly subdued property, leukemic cells accumulate relentlessly in most patients and compete successfully with normal hematopoietic cells. Hematopoiesis may be suppressed by physical displacement of stem cells by leukemic cells or, more likely, by production of inhibitory humoral factors. Leukemia cell-derived inhibitory activity (LIA) and leukemia-associated inhibitor (LAI), which inhibit normal granulocytopoiesis, have been identified in patients with leukemia. Leukemic cells can also suppress stromal cell growth. Because hematopoiesis depends on intact stromal cell function, this suppression might contribute to the development of hematopoietic abnormalities. Finally, because leukemic blast cells from some patients with AML produce biologically active granulocyte-monocyte colony stimulating factor (GM-CSF), the leukemic cell proliferation in at least some cases may be autocrine based.

Failure of normal hematopoiesis leading to anemia, infection, and bleeding is the most serious pathophysiologic consequence of leukemia. In addition, leukemic cells can infiltrate any organ and cause enlargement and dysfunction.

Acute Lymphoblastic Leukemia

Clinical Presentation

The clinical presentation of ALL is variable. Symptoms may appear insidiously or acutely (Table 31-3). Signs and symptoms reflect the degree of bone marrow failure and extent of extramedullary spread. Some patients have life-threatening infections or hemorrhage at diagnosis. In others, the onset of leukemia is asymptomatic and detected only during routine physical examination. Most patients, however, have some history of illness before diagnosis. Their symptoms may have been present for a few days to a few months. Pallor, fatigue, and lethargy are frequent manifestations of anemia. Anorexia is common, but weight loss is usually slight, if at all. A third of patients, especially young children, may present with a limp, painful bone, arthralgia, or refusal to walk. These symptoms may result from leukemic infiltration of the periosteum, bone, or joint or from expansion of the marrow cavity by leukemic cells. Bone marrow necrosis occurs rarely, resulting in severe pain and fever. Almost half of patients have some manifestation of bleeding. Intermittent fever occurs in more than half of patients and is associated with documented infection in at least one fourth. Less common signs and symptoms include headache, vomiting, respiratory distress, oliguria, and anuria.

Physical examination may reveal fever, pallor, petechiae and ecchymoses on the skin or mucous membrane, retinal hemorrhage, enlarged lymph nodes, hepatosplenomegaly, nephromegaly, and bone tenderness. The last, caused by leukemic infiltration or hemorrhage that strips the periosteum, is often observed. Less common presenting features include subcutaneous nodules (leukemia cutis), enlarged salivary glands (Mikulicz's syndrome), painless enlargement of the scrotum (due to testicular leukemia or hydrocele), cranial nerve palsy, leukemic deposits in the retina, papilledema, painful swelling of the joints, and priapism (due to mechanical obstruction of the corpora cavernosa and dorsal veins caused by leukostasis or sacral nerve root involvement). Epidural spinal cord compression may occasionally result in paraparesis or paraplegia, an oncologic emergency requiring immediate treatment. In some patients, infiltration of the tonsils, adenoids, appendix, or mesenteric lymph nodes leads to surgical intervention before leukemia is diagnosed.

Laboratory Features

Initial blood cell counts reveal a wide spectrum of abnormalities. Anemia, abnormal leukocyte and differential counts, and thrombocytopenia are usually present at diagnosis. Very rarely, children have normal blood counts. Leukocyte counts range from 0.1 to 1,600 x 10^9/L (median, 13 x 10^9/L), often with absolute granulocytopenia. Approximately two thirds of patients have leukocyte counts <25 x 10^9/L (Table 31-3). The majority of cells in blood smears are lymphoblasts or lymphocytes. Because the morphology of blast cells in peripheral blood smears may differ from that in bone marrow, the peripheral smears should not be used for definitive diagnosis. Hypereosinophilia, generally reactive, may be present at diagnosis and occasionally will precede the diagnosis of ALL by many months. Several patients, mostly males, have been reported to have ALL with classic t(5;14)(q31;q32) chromosomal abnormalities accompanied by the hypereosinophilia syndrome (hypereosinophilia, pulmonary infiltration, cardiomegaly, and congestive heart failure). Activation of the interleukin-3 gene on chromosome 5 by the enhancer of the immunoglobulin heavy-chain gene on chromosome 14 is thought to play a central role in leukemogenesis and associated eosinophilia in ALL.

Hemoglobin levels range from 2 to 15 g/dL (median, 8 g/dL), and reticulocyte counts are normal or low. Erythrocytes are generally normochromic and normocytic. Platelet counts (median, 50 x 10^9/L) are usually decreased. Coagulopathy, usually mild, can occur in T-cell ALL. Elevated serum uric acid levels are common in patients with large leukemic cell mass, reflecting increased purine metabolism. Patients with massive renal involvement may have increased serum levels of urea, creatinine, and phosphorus. Occasionally, children with T-cell ALL present in acute renal failure. Approximately 0.5% of patients have hypercalcemia at diagnosis, which is attributed to the release of parathyroid hormone-like protein from lymphoblasts and leukemic infiltration of bone and generally resolves rapidly with hydration and chemotherapy. Liver dysfunction, usually mild, from leukemic infiltration occurs in 10% to 20% of children and has no important clinical or prognostic consequence. Urinalysis may reveal microscopic hematuria and the presence of uric acid crystals.

Table 31-3. Presenting Clinical and Laboratory Features in 500 Children with ALL Treated Consecutively at St Jude Children's Research Hospital

Clinical Feature	% of Total	Laboratory Feature	% of Total
Age (y)		Leukocyte count (x 10^9/L)	
≤1	3	<25	65
2-9	72	25-49	9
≥10	25	50-100	9
		>100	17
Male	53		
Race		Hemoglobin (g/dL)	
Black	12	<8	50
Other	88	8-10	18
		>10	32
Symptoms		Platelet count (x 10^9/L)	
Fever	53	<10	15
Malaise	50	10-49	34
Bleeding	38	50-100	21
Bone or joint pain	27	>100	30
Anorexia	19		
Abdominal pain	10		
Lymphadenopathy	35	Immunophenotype	
		Early pre-B	57
		Pre-B	25
		Transitional pre-B	1
		B	2
		T	15
Liver edge below costal margin		Karyotype	
		Hypodiploid	7
1-4 cm	26	Pseudodiploid	42
≥5 cm	35	Hyperdiploid 47-50	15
		Hyperdiploid >50	27
Spleen edge below costal margin		Near triploid/tetraploid	1
		Normal	8
1-4 cm	23		
≥5 cm	34		
Mediastinal mass	10	DNA index ≥ 1.16	20
Central nervous system leukemia	8	Chromosomal translocation	43

Serum immunoglobulin levels are low in approximately a third of patients, reflecting the decreased number and impaired function of normal lymphocytes.

Definitive diagnosis rests on examination of bone marrow, which is usually replaced completely by leukemic lymphoblasts. Fibrosis or tightly packed marrow can lead to difficulties with bone marrow aspiration, necessitating biopsy. A touch preparation of the biopsied tissue can be stained for morphologic diagnosis. A small proportion of patients have bone marrow necrosis, usually in association with severe bone pain and tenderness, a very high serum lactate dehydrogenase level, and fever. Bone marrow scans are sometimes necessary to guide attempts to obtain viable tissue; rarely, a lymph node biopsy is required. The use of magnetic resonance imaging of bone marrow in these patients is being investigated. Although an occasional patient with an aplastic presentation may require multiple procedures before a diagnosis can be made, a marrow aspirate can usually establish the diagnosis of childhood ALL promptly. In children, the usual site for marrow aspiration is the posterior or anterior iliac crest. The use of special histochemical stains, immunophenotyping, and cytogenetic analysis can establish the diagnosis of virtually all childhood ALLs. Molecular studies may help subclassify the disease.

A chest roentgenogram is needed to detect mediastinal nodal enlargement, thymic enlargement, or pleural effusion. Pulmonary infiltrates are occasionally detected and can indicate pneumonia, edema, hemorrhage, or, rarely, leukemic infiltration. Fifty percent of patients have skeletal lesions, including generalized rarification of bones, transverse radiolucent bands in the metaphyses of long bones, periosteal new-bone formation, cortical osteolytic lesions, osteosclerosis, and vertebral collapse. Because these changes have no independent prognostic significance, a skeletal survey is unnecessary unless indicated clinically.

Cerebrospinal fluid should be examined. It contains leukemic blasts in 15% to 20% of patients, regardless of the presence or absence of neurologic manifestations. Concern that this practice may facilitate seeding the central nervous system (CNS) is unfounded. Recent studies indicate that patients with any amount of leukemic blasts identified in the cerebrospinal fluid are at increased risk of subsequent CNS relapse and should receive more intensive CNS treatment.

Immunologic Markers

Differences in expression of surface membrane antigens or cytoplasmic components identify and classify lymphoproliferative diseases by cell origin and stage of differentiation.[10] These studies help establish the diagnosis and determine an effective treatment plan. Virtually all known "differentiation" antigens as well as immunoglobulin and T-cell receptor gene rearrangements lack lineage specificity. The only known exceptions are cytoplasmic CD3 for T cell and cytoplasmic CD22 for B-lineage ALL. Therefore, the classification of leukemia should be based on the pattern of reactivity to a panel of lineage-associated monoclonal antibodies for surface antigens and the presence or absence of cytoplasmic and surface immunoglobulin. Most antigens have been assigned a cluster of differentiation (CD) number in the leukocyte typing conferences.

In general, childhood ALL can be classified as T cell ($CD7^+$ plus $CD5^+$ or $CD2^+$), B cell (positive for sur-

Table 31-4. Comparative Features of 500 Childhood ALL Cases Treated Consecutively at St Jude Children's Research Hospital, According to Immunologic Subclasses

Feature	T Cell	Early Pre-B Cell	Pre-B Cell	Transitional Pre-B Cell	B Cell
Median age (y)	10.3	4.3	4.5	5.0	8.7
Median WBC (x 10^9/L)	110	11.4	13.7	9.7	9
Median LDH (IU/L)	2,043	410	601	Not Done	1,600
% Male	66	49	51	41	75
% Mediastinal mass	62	1	1	0	0
% CD10 (CALLA) positivity	40	95	95	100	47
% Hyperdiploidy	2	38	23	54	0
% Chromosomal translocation	49	45	64	43	100

WBC = white blood count; LDH = lactic dehydrogenase;
CALLA = common acute lymphocytic leukemia antigen.

face immunoglobulin), pre-B (positive for cytoplasmic immunoglobulin), or early pre-B ($CD19^+$, $CD22^+$, $HLA\text{-}DR^+$, $CD7^-$, $CD5^-$, and $CD10^\pm$, and negative for cytoplasmic and surface immunoglobulin).[10] Transitional pre-B ALL, in which lymphoblasts express both cytoplasmic and surface immunoglobulin heavy chains and surrogate light-chain proteins, has been described recently.[10] Male gender, older age, a large leukemic cell mass reflected by a high leukocyte count and elevated serum lactate dehydrogenase level, and a mediastinal mass often characterize T-cell leukemia (Table 31-4). T-cell ALL is further subclassified according to the stage of thymocyte differentiation: early (stage I), intermediate (stage II), and late (stage III). About one third of T-cell cases have late thymocyte stage differentiation; the suggestion in one study that these patients have a poorer prognosis than other T-cell cases remains to be substantiated. Patients with B-cell ALL often present with a massive extramedullary tumor. Their marrow is replaced by blasts with L3 morphology, and more than 90% of cases express cell surface immunoglobulin mu heavy chain. Approximately two thirds of these patients coexpress kappa and the remainder coexpress lambda light chain. B-cell ALL often seems to represent advanced Burkitt's lymphoma in a phase of leukemic evolution. Most ALL cases have been classified as early pre-B. These cases are more likely to have favorable presenting features (eg, age 1 to 9 years and low leukocyte count) and outcome. Children with pre-B ALL have higher serum lactate dehydrogenase levels and are more likely to have unfavorable cytogenetic features than those with early pre-B ALL.[10] Transitional pre-B cases uniformly lack L3 morphology and have a lower presenting leukocyte count, a high prevalence of favorable cytogenetic features, and good clinical outcome. Approximately 94% of children with early pre-B or pre-B ALL and 40% with T-cell ALL express CD10 antigen. Among early pre-B or pre-B cases, CD10-negative patients have greater leukemic cell burden, are more likely to be infants, and have a higher frequency of unfavorable blast cell chromo-somal features. In T-cell cases, lack of CD10 expression is associated with an especially poor clinical outcome.

Cytogenetic and Molecular Genetic Studies

The fundamental changes associated with neoplastic transformation include chromosomal alterations.[11] Clonal cytogenetic abnormalities have been identified in more than 90% of children with ALL. With wider application of improved cytogenetic techniques, recurring structural chromosomal abnormalities will be identified in increasing numbers. Specific chromosomal translocations involving reciprocal exchanges of DNA appear to be the most biologically and clinically significant karyotypic change in human leukemia. Table 31-5 lists some of the more common and better-defined nonrandom translocations.

The most common translocation in childhood ALL is t(1;19), found in 5% to 6% of cases and primarily seen in patients with pre-B ALL. Recent studies reveal that the unfavorable presenting features formerly ascribed to pre-B ALL are closely associated with the t(1;19) subgroup. The 22q- marker, or Philadelphia (Ph) chromosome, results from the balanced translocation t(9;22)(q34;q11). The Ph chromosome is found in leukemic cells of 3% to 5% of children with ALL and in more than 90% of those with CML. Ph^+ ALL and Ph^+ CML differ clinically and molecularly, despite sharing an identical karyotype. Childhood Ph^+ ALL is associated with older age, high leukocyte count, the FAB L2 morphology, CNS involvement at diagnosis, and very poor prognosis.

The most consistently observed association between immunophenotype and chromosomal translocation occurs in B-cell leukemia. B-cell ALL is invariably associated with one of three specific chromosomal translocations: the t(8;14) in approximately 80% of B-cell ALL cases and the t(2;8) or t(8;22) in the remaining patients. Many recurring translocations have been associated with T-cell ALL (Table 31-5). No apparent relationship exists between particular translocations and levels of thymocyte maturation. Among childhood T-cell ALL cases, the t(11;14)(p13;q11) is the most common nonrandom abnormality, occurring in 7%. A normal karyotype is observed in approximately one fourth of T-cell cases; they were reported to have a more favorable outcome than other T-cell ALL patients. The t(4;11) is associated with age <12 months, female sex, hyperleukocytosis, $CD10^-$ early pre-B or pre-B immunophenotype, expression of myeloid-associated antigen CD15, and a very poor prognosis. The dic(9;12) cases are characterized by male gender, low initial leukocyte count, and $CD10^+$ early pre-B or pre-B immunophenotype; none of the roughly two dozen reported cases has relapsed.

Molecular analysis of leukemic lymphoblasts with specific chromosomal rearrangements has identified several genes and their protein products that play important roles in malignant transformation and proliferation. The following general mechanisms are involved: activation of cellular proto-oncogenes by altered transcription, mutation, or gene fusion; induction of gene(s) that prevent programmed cell death (apoptosis); and loss of function of a tumor suppressor gene.[12] The largest class of products implicated in leukemogenesis is the helix-loop-helix (HLH) family of DNA-binding proteins. These proteins apparently control cell growth and differentiation through their transcriptional regulatory functions. The prototypic oncogenic HLH protein is MYC. In B-cell neoplasms, the chromosomal rearrangements consistently bring together the *MYC* proto-oncogene on chromosome 8(q24) and a transcriptionally active gene for the immunoglobulin heavy chain on 14q32, the kappa light chain on 2p11-p12, or the lambda light chain on 22q11, leading to aberrant activation of *MYC*. Similarly, in half of T-cell ALL cases with a translocation, the breakpoints are in regions to which the T-cell receptor genes have been mapped: α-chain at 14q11-q13, β-chain at 7q32-q36, γ-chain at 7p15, and δ-chain

Table 31-5. Common Nonrandom Chromosomal Translocations in Childhood ALL

Immunophenotype and Translocation	Frequency (%)	Involved Gene(s)		Protein Product
Pre-B cell/early pre-B cell /T-cell				
t(9;22)(q34;q11)	3-5	*ABL*	*BCR*	$P185^{BCR\text{-}ABL}$
Pre-B cell/early pre-B cell				
t(1;19)(q23;p13)	5-6	*PBX1*	*E2A*	E2A-PBX1 fusion protein
t(4;11)(q21;q23)	2	*AF4*	*ALL1/MLL*	ALL1-AF4 fusion protein
dic(9;12)(p11-p12;p12)	1	Unknown	Unknown	
t(5;14)(q31;q32)	<1	*IL3*	*IgH*	Interleukin-3
t(11;19)(q23;p13)	<1	*ALL1/MLL*	*ENL*	ALL1-ENL fusion protein
t(9;11)(p21-p22;q23)	<1	*AF9*	*ALL1/MLL*	ALL1-AF9 fusion protein
t(17;19)(q22;p13)	<1	*HLF*	*E2A*	E2A-HLF fusion protein
T-cell				
t(11;14)(p13;q11)	1	*TTG2/Rhom2*	*TCRd*	Zinc-finger protein (rhombotin 2)
t(11;14)(p15;q11)	<1	*TTG1/Rhom1*	*TCRd*	Zinc-finger protein (rhombotin 1)
t(10;14)(q24;q11)	<1	*TCL3/HOX11*	*TCRd*	Homeodomain protein
t(1;14)(p32-p34;q11)	<1	*TCL5/TAL1/SCL*	*TCRd*	Helix-loop-helix protein
t(8;14)(q24;q11)	<1	*MYC*	*TCRad*	Helix-loop-helix zipper protein
t(8;14)(q24;q11)	<1	*PVT1*	*TCRd*	
t(7;9)(q34;q32)	<1	*TCRß*	*TAL2d*	Helix-loop-helix protein
t(7;9)(q34;q34.3)	<1	*TCRß*	*TAN1d*	
t(7;19)(q35;p13)	<1	*TCRß*	*LYL1d*	Helix-loop-helix protein
t(1;7)(p34;q34)	<1	*LCK*	*TCRß*	Tyrosine kinase
B-cell				
t(8;14)(q24;q32.3)	1-2	*MYC*	*IGH*	Helix-loop-helix protein
t(8;22)(q24;q11)	<1	*MYC*	*IgL*	Helix-loop-helix protein
t(2;8)(p11-p12;q24)	<1	*IGK*	*MYC*	Helix-loop-helix protein

ABL = cellular homologue of the Abelson murine leukemia virus oncogene; *BCR* = gene containing the breakpoint cluster region involved in Ph translocation; *PBX1* = pre-B cell transforming gene; *E2A* = gene for Ig enhancer binding proteins E12/E47; *AF4* = *ALL1* fused gene from chromosome 4; *IL3* = interleukin-3; *ALL* = acute lymphoblastic leukemia; *MLL* = myeloid/lymphoid, or *M*ixed-*L*ineage, *L*eukemia; *ENL* = eleven-nineteen leukemia; *AF9* = *ALL1* fused gene from chromosome 9; *HLF* = hepatic leukemia factor; *TCR* = T-cell receptor gene; *TCL* = T-cell leukemia/lymphoma breakpoint regions; *TTG* = T-cell translocation gene; *Rhom* = Rhombotin gene; *HOX* = homeobox gene; *IGH* = Ig heavy-chain gene; *TAL* = T-cell acute leukemia gene; *TAN* = translocation-associated notch homologue; *MYC* = cellular homologue of the transforming sequence of the avian myelocytomatosis virus; *PVT1* = plasmacytoma variant translocation; *LCK* = lymphocyte-specific protein tyrosine kinase; *IGK* = Ig κ light-chain gene; *IGL* = Ig λ light-chain gene; *LYL* = lymphoid leukemia gene.

at 14q11. In T-cell ALL, T-cell receptor genes activate or perturb genes encoded for HLH or other classes of transcriptional proteins in a manner similar to that observed in B-cell neoplasms.

HLH proteins are involved in leukemogenesis by another mechanism. In pre-B ALL, the t(1;19) results in synthesis of a fusion transcript that contains the 5′ sequence of the *E2A* gene, which codes for the HLH protein E12/E47, and 3′ sequences from the homeobox gene *PBX1*. The resulting fusion transcripts have been shown to encode chimeric E2A-PBX1 proteins with transforming potential. Similarly, in most childhood ALLs with the Ph chromosome, the t(9;22) results in fusion of the *BCR* gene on chromosome 22 with the *ABL* gene on chromosome 9, producing a characteristic 7-kb mRNA and a 190-kDa hybrid protein. The fusion protein functions as a constitutively activated tyrosine kinase that can induce malignant transformation of hematopoietic cells.

The product of the human gene *BCL-2* suppresses apoptosis.[13] Overexpression of BCL-2 at critical stages of differentiation may lead to malignant transformation. Indeed, in follicular B-cell non-Hodgkin's lymphoma (NHL) with t(14;18), the translocation juxtaposes the BCL-2 gene on chromosome 18 with the immunoglobulin heavy-chain locus. However, abnormally high levels of BCL-2 protein have also been observed in some cases of NHL and, more recently, in childhood ALL lacking karyotypic and molecular evidence of BCL-2 gene rearrangement. This suggests that other mechanisms may cause inappropriate BCL-2 expression and tumorigenesis.

Tumor suppressor genes have also been implicated in leukemogenesis.[14] Homozygous or hemizygous deletion of the α- and β_1-interferon gene clusters in the 9p22 region has been found in leukemic lymphoblasts; in some cases, the deletions were submicroscopic. Because interferons are known to affect cell proliferation and differentiation, the loss of one or more interferon genes may be related to malignant proliferation in ALL. Deletion, inactivation, or mutation of other tumor suppressor genes (eg, the retinoblastoma gene and the *p53* gene) has also been reported in some cases of ALL.

Cytogenetic and molecular genetic data are also important for the diagnosis and clinical monitoring of leukemia. In cases with equivocal phenotype, cytogenetic findings may be used to classify the disease. For cases with specific chromosomal abnormalities, the polymerase chain reaction (PCR)—a powerful technique that amplifies specific sequences of DNA between two oligonucleotide primers—has been used to monitor minimal residual disease.[15] PCR techniques have been developed to monitor virtually all cases of certain leukemias [eg, t(9;22) and t(1;19) ALL] with characteristic chimeric transcripts. Whether the detection of minimal residual disease by this method can reliably predict clinical relapse remains to be determined in prospective clinical trials.

Prognostic Factors

A more precise estimate of the risk of relapse permits a more accurate assessment of the acceptable therapeutic index. For children with leukemia associated with features that predict a lower risk of relapse, clinical trials can focus on designing therapies that reduce acute toxicities and long-term sequelae, but maintain excellent disease control. For children with higher-risk leukemia, contemporary treatment programs featuring therapy that is more intensive, and hence more toxic, have yielded improved results. Indeed, the "tailoring of therapy" has contributed substantially to the success of modern treatment programs for ALL.

The initial leukemic cell burden, as reflected by the leukocyte count, serum lactate dehydrogenase level, and the degree of organomegaly, is closely linked with treatment outcome.[16] The initial leukocyte count, perhaps the most important prognostic factor, has a linear relationship to the likelihood of disease-free survival. Children with the highest leukocyte counts tend to have the poorest outcome. Age at diagnosis is also a consistently reliable predictor. Patients older than 10 years or younger than 12 months fare much worse than children in the intermediate age group. The extremely poor outcome of infant ALL has recently been shown to be limited to cases with 11q23 chromosomal abnormalities, which correlate with age under 6 months, hyperleukocytosis, and a CD10-negative immunophenotype. Compared with patients between ages 1 and 10, adolescents with ALL are more likely to be male and have a higher leukocyte count, mediastinal mass, and T-cell disease. Their leukemic cells are more likely to have the L2 morphology, CD10 negativity, and unfavorable cytogenetic features. Those older than 16 years have an even worse outcome. Because they are readily available and independently important, leukocyte count and age are universally accepted prognostic factors.

Although black children develop ALL less often than do white children, they are more likely to have a high leukocyte count, mediastinal mass, L2 morphology, CD10 negativity, pre-B phenotype, and pseudodiploidy. Despite these unfavorable prognostic features, their outcome has improved substantially with contemporary treatment. Previous studies showed that girls fare better than boys because of the development of testicular relapse and the higher frequency of T-cell ALL in males. However, modern treatments have improved the prognosis in males.

Among the immunophenotypic subtypes of ALL, early pre-B cases are associated with the most favorable treatment outcome.[10] The generally poorer prognosis of pre-B and T-cell cases are partly explained by larger initial leukemic cell mass and unfavorable leukemic cell cytogenetic features. However, in some small clinical trials, pre-B and T-cell cases fared as well as early pre-B patients. As mentioned earlier, CD10 positivity confers a more favorable prognosis among early pre-B, pre-B, and T-cell cases and is an independent factor in T-cell cases. B-cell ALL cases, once associated with an extremely poor prognosis, now have a long-term survival rate of 80% or higher with the use of extremely intensive but short-term (2 to 6 months) chemotherapy. B-cell ALL with CNS leukemia at diagnosis continues to pose a therapeutic problem.

Chromosomal abnormalities are important prognostic factors in ALL.[11] Hyperdiploid stem lines, with >50 chromosomes per leukemic cell, constitute about 27% of children with ALL and have the most favorable prognosis. This group can be easily identified by flow cytometry analysis of cellular DNA content, an alternative method of establishing leukemic cell ploidy. With improved treatment, the hyperdiploid 47-50 group has apparently been elevated to a risk status comparable with that of the >50 group. Pseudodiploidy (46 chromosomes with structural abnormalities) and hypodiploidy (46 chromosomes) correlate with a poorer outcome. Whether the near-haploid subgroup has a particularly poor outcome among hypodiploid cases remains unknown. Also uncertain, because of the small number of reported cases, is the prognostic significance of near-triploidy or near-tetraploidy. Finally, cases with a Ph chromosome or a t(4;11) have a particularly poor prognosis. Most investigators advocate the use of allogeneic bone marrow transplantation for patients with either abnormality.

The prognostic value of FAB classification in ALL is controversial because of the differences in treatment and classification criteria and the difficulty of reproducing the results of morphologic classification. In studies observing a significant difference, L2 cases fared worse than L1 cases. Other less important presenting features that correlate with poor prognosis include low economic class, presence of mediastinal mass, low serum immunoglobulin levels (especially of IgM), lower platelet counts, larger kidney, lower levels of glucocorticoid receptors in leukemic blast cells, greater pretreatment blast cell proliferative activity, lower periodic acid-Schiff (PAS) positivity in blast cells, and the presence of "hand mirror" cells. Higher levels of serum interleukin-2 receptor and CD8 antigen (the suppressor/cytotoxic T-cell marker) at diagnosis are associated with a poor treatment outcome, suggesting that host immunity may affect the progression of tumors.

Because the prognostic factors in ALL are highly interrelated, multivariate analyses are necessary to identify those with independent significance. Among the clinical features, leukocyte count and age consistently emerge as independent indicators of treatment outcome. Among the biologic features, hyperdiploidy >50 or high leukemic cell DNA content (>1.16 times that of normal cells) is favorable, whereas the Ph chromosome and the t(4;11) are associated with the worst outcome. Improved therapy lessens the usefulness of many determinants of childhood ALL, and prognostic factors should be evaluated in the context of therapy.

Differential Diagnosis

The initial manifestations of ALL are similar to those of several other disorders. The acute onset of petechiae, ecchymoses, and bleeding may suggest idiopathic thrombocytopenia (often associated with a recent viral infection, large platelets in blood smears, and no evidence of anemia). Both ALL and aplastic anemia may present with pancytopenia and complications associated with bone marrow failure. In aplastic anemia, hepatosplenomegaly and lymphadenopathy are unusual, and the skeletal changes associated with leukemia do not occur. Bone marrow aspirations and biopsy usually establish the diagnosis. Distinguishing between the two diseases may be difficult in a child in whom ALL presents with a hypocellular marrow later replaced by lymphoblasts. Childhood infectious mononucleosis and other viral infections, especially those associated with thrombocytopenia or hemolytic anemia, may be confused with leukemia. Atypical lymphocytes and increased viral titers help establish the correct diagnosis. Children with pertussis or parapertussis may have marked lymphocytosis; their leukocyte counts have been as high as 50 x 10^9/L, but the affected cells are mature lymphocytes rather than leukemic lymphoblasts. Bone pain, arthralgia, and occasionally arthritis may mimic juvenile rheumatoid arthritis, rheumatic fever, other collagen-vascular diseases, or osteomyelitis. Some patients with presumed systemic lupus erythematosus actually have ALL. Therefore, to exclude leukemia, bone marrow aspiration should be performed before initiation of steroid treatment for rheumatic diseases. If bone marrow is replaced by metastatic tumor (eg, neuroblastoma, rhabdomyosarcoma, or retinoblastoma), the malignant cells are usually in clumps and a primary tumor can be found.

Therapy

The identification of important prognostic factors and the recognition of ALL as a heterogeneous disease have led to the use of phenotype-specific or risk-directed therapy. B-cell ALL cases are treated separately with protocols featuring short-term intensive chemotherapy (including high-dose methotrexate, high-dose cytarabine, cyclophosphamide, and vincristine). Many protocols using a variety of drug combinations have been developed for non-B-cell ALL and several have yielded a long-term event-free survival rate of 70%. For patients at lower risk of relapse, current treatment programs are based largely on antimetabolites (eg, methotrexate and 6-mercaptopurine) to avoid the long-term sequelae of other chemotherapeutic agents. In general, ALL treatment regimens comprise three main elements: early therapy (remission induction with or without consolidation treatment), subclinical (prophylactic) CNS therapy, and continuation therapy. Because of the diversity of approaches, only the principles of treatment are addressed.

Early Therapy

Inadequate reduction of the initial leukemic cell burden allows regrowth of drug-resistant cells and results in treatment failure. Theoretically, anticancer drugs could cure if early treatments were sufficiently intense to eradicate malignant cells before drug resistance develops. Several studies have shown that the rapidity of leukemic cytoreduction during induction has prognostic significance. Patients with >25% lymphoblasts in their bone marrow after 2 weeks of induction treatment have a significantly poorer treatment outcome than other patients.[2] Indeed, intensive early therapy has been the hallmark of recent successful clinical trials.[1,2]

Most induction regimens include a glucocorticoid (dexamethasone or prednisone), vincristine, and asparaginase. For patients with higher-risk leukemia, additional agents for remission induction (eg, daunorubicin, cyclophosphamide, and high-dose methotrexate) may help. In attempts to further improve treatment results, some investigators use four or more drugs for remission induction, even in lower-risk leukemia. With modern chemotherapy and supportive care, 97% to 98% of children with ALL attain complete remission—ie, the absence of clinical signs and symptoms of disease, the presence of normal blood counts, and a normocellular bone marrow with <5% blasts. Patients theoretically have their leukemic cell burden decreased from 10^{12} or more at diagnosis to fewer than 10^{10} by remission. Induction failure, occurring in no more than 3% of cases, is due to primary drug resistance or toxicity of therapy. Patients who fail to achieve remission at the end of the usual induction period have a short survival, and if remission is eventually achieved, a higher rate of relapse. Consolidation therapy—intensified treatment administered shortly after remission induction—is an integral component of most successful treatment protocols, especially for higher-risk patients. One approach is the use of pulses of an epipodophyllotoxin plus cytarabine and high-dose methotrexate.

Subclinical (Prophylactic) CNS Treatment

The importance of subclinical CNS therapy was first demonstrated by investigators at St Jude Children's Research Hospital in the mid-1960s. Cranial irradiation (24 cGy) plus intrathecal methotrexate on attaining complete remission became the standard treatment in the 1970s. However, concern over its adverse effects has prompted a reappraisal of therapeutic strategies. Newer approaches being studied include lower dose of cranial irradiation (18 Gy) with intrathecal methotrexate; hyperfractionated cranial irradiation (18 Gy) with intrathecal therapy; triple intrathecal therapy with methotrexate, cytarabine, and hydrocortisone; intermediate-dose methotrexate with concomitant intrathecal methotrexate; high-dose methotrexate alone; or periodic intrathecal methotrexate with intensive systemic therapy. In general, CNS irradiation is now reserved for patients who have initial CNS leukemia or who are at high risk of CNS relapse (eg, those with a very high presenting leukocyte count, T-cell ALL cases with a high leukocyte count, and cases with the Ph chromosome).[17] The efficacy of systemic chemotherapy affects that of subclinical CNS therapy.

Continuation Therapy

Whether or not an intensive consolidation regimen is used early in remission, continuation treatment is required. Earlier studies indicated that virtually all patients would otherwise relapse within a few months. Continuation treatment is based largely on daily mercaptopurine and weekly methotrexate. Some studies demonstrated a better treatment response when mercaptopurine was given at bedtime to patients with an empty stomach. Whereas the relative effectiveness of oral versus parenteral methotrexate remains uncertain, the problem of compliance (especially in adolescents) can be at least partly circumvented by the latter route of administration. The addition of intermittent pulses of prednisone and vincristine to continuation treatment comprising mercaptopurine and methotrexate improves the outcome for some patients. For those with higher-risk leukemia, many investigators now recommend more intensive continuation therapies (single agents at an increased dosage, repeated pulses of a multiple drug combination, or rotational combination chemotherapy).

Optimal duration of therapy has not yet been established. Because all drugs induce undesirable toxic effects, chemotherapy cannot be given indefinitely. Prolonged exposure to the same agents may ultimately lead to the emergence of drug-resistant leukemia. Further, the maximum antileukemic effect of any drug combination is most likely reached within a finite period. Early studies indicated no advantage to prolonging treatment beyond 3 years and found that boys require longer treatment duration than girls. Today, discontinuing all therapy in patients in continuous complete remission for 2.5 to 3 years is a common practice. Whether duration of treatment can be shortened for patients receiving more intensive treatment is unknown. Before therapy ends, patients should undergo bone marrow and cerebrospinal fluid examination. Elective testicular biopsy to detect occult leukemia, a previously common practice, is of little value with modern improved treatment. After completion of chemotherapy, children should be evaluated for social, scholastic, and vocational development as well as remission status.

Relapsed ALL

Relapse is the reappearance of leukemia at any site in the body. Although most relapses occur during treatment or within the first 2 years after the end of therapy, initial relapses have been observed as long as 10 years after diagnosis. Anemia, leukocytosis, leukopenia, thrombocytopenia, enlargement of the liver or spleen, bone pain, fever, or a sudden decrease in tolerance to chemotherapy may signal bone marrow relapse.

Bone marrow relapse, the most common form of treatment failure, portends a poor prognosis for most patients. Factors predictive of especially poor prognosis include relapse on therapy, a short initial remission duration, and intensive primary therapy. Although intensified regimens have made it possible to induce second remission in over 90% of patients relapsing on modern therapy, the outlook for long-term survival in this cohort is dim. Prolonged second remission (>3 years) may be obtained with intensive chemotherapy and a second course of subclinical CNS therapy, usually with intrathecal treatment, in approximately 10% of patients who relapse during therapy and in up to one third of those who relapse after therapy has ended.[18] When relapse occurs more than 12 months after elective cessation of therapy, the prospects for inducing and maintaining a new remission are clearly better. Most investigators advocate the use of allogeneic bone marrow transplantation with hyperfractionated total-body irradiation and ablative chemotherapy for patients with bone marrow relapse, especially those suffering an early event.

CNS relapse occurs in 5% to 10% of patients despite subclinical therapy. It may occur alone or with a bone marrow relapse or other extramedullary recurrence (eg, testicular). Some patients have repeated episodes of CNS leukemia while the bone marrow remains in initial remission. Because the cerebrospinal fluid is routinely examined throughout the treatment course and effective subclinical therapy is available, overt meningeal leukemia is uncommon today. It is usually diagnosed when leukemic cells are found on routine examination of cerebrospinal fluid, before symptoms of increased intracranial pressure or cranial nerve involvement develop. Chemotherapy via lumbar puncture or an Ommaya reservoir usually clears leukemic cells from cerebrospinal fluid within a few weeks. However, only cranial or craniospinal irradiation eradicates overt CNS leukemia. Because these patients are at high risk for subsequent bone marrow relapse, intensive systemic chemotherapy is also needed. The outcome of an isolated CNS relapse occurring as the first adverse event depends on the type of initial subclinical CNS therapy administered. Children given intrathecal treatment alone are much more readily salvageable than are those given cranial irradiation.

Leukemic infiltration of the testes presents as painless swelling of one or both gonads. Although testicular relapse may occur during therapy, particularly in patients who had presented with high leukocyte counts or T-cell leukemia, most relapses occur within the first year or so after elective cessation of therapy. Although the disease may be apparent in one testicle only, the other testicle is frequently involved. Because of the overall improved therapy for childhood ALL, the frequency of testicular relapse has decreased substantially. In some studies, only 1% of boys developed an isolated testicular relapse.[2] Children who relapse during continuation therapy tend to have a poor prognosis because of the rapid involvement of bone marrow or other extramedullary sites, whereas those who relapse after completion of therapy are generally treated successfully. Treatment should include local irradiation (24 to 30 Gy) to both testes and systemic combination chemotherapy. Radiation therapy adversely affects testicular function. All patients become sterile and most will require subsequent testosterone replacement therapy.

Leukemic relapse occasionally occurs at other extramedullary sites in patients in hematologic remission. The sites vary widely and include the eye, ovary, bone, tonsil, kidney, mediastinum, and paranasal sinus. As with bone marrow relapse, recurrence during therapy confers a poor prognosis.

Bone Marrow Transplantation

Intensive chemoradiotherapy followed by allogeneic bone marrow transplantation is used with increasing frequency to treat patients with ALL, particularly those who suffer a bone marrow relapse. Recent studies demonstrated long-term survival rates of 10% to 15% in patients who underwent transplantation at relapse and 40% to 50% in those undergoing transplantation in second remission. HLA-identical individuals (usually siblings) served as donors, and preparative therapy comprised hyperfractionated total-body irradiation and marrow ablative chemotherapy. For patients without matched sibling donors, encouraging results have been obtained with transplantation with matched unrelated donors and with family members who are mismatched for only one HLA antigen locus. These methods have largely replaced autologous marrow transplantation, which has a high relapse rate. With better definition of prognostic factors, bone marrow transplantation has also been employed to treat patients with newly diagnosed ALL whose presenting features predict a poor response to chemotherapy [eg, patients with the Ph chromosome or t(4;11) and cases with hyperleukocytosis].

Complications

The most frequent acute complications of antileukemic therapy include nausea and vomiting, stomatitis, diarrhea, alopecia, and bone marrow suppression. Metabolic complications in children with ALL can result from spontaneous or drug-induced leukemic cell lysis and may be life-threatening for patients with a large burden of leukemic cells. The rapid release of blast cell components can cause hyperuricemia, hyperphosphatemia, and hyperkalemia. Some patients develop uric acid nephropathy or nephrocalcinosis. Rarely, urolithiasis with ureteral obstruction occurs after treatment for leukemia. Hydration, administration of allopurinol and aluminum hydroxide or calcium carbonate, and the judicious use of urinary alkalinization may prevent or correct these complications.

Diffuse leukemic infiltration of the kidneys can also lead to renal failure. Vincristine or cyclophosphamide therapy may increase the release of antidiuretic hormones. Hyperglycemia develops in 10% of patients after treatment with prednisone and asparaginase and may require short-term administration of insulin.

Because of the myelosuppressive and immunosuppressive effects of ALL and its chemotherapy, children with this disease are more susceptible to infections than normal, healthy children. The types of infection in immunosuppressed children with leukemia vary with the treatment and stage of the disease. Most early infections are bacterial, manifested by sepsis, pneumonia, cellulitis, and otitis media. *Staphylococcus epidermidis, Escherichia coli, S aureus, Pseudomonas aeruginosa, Klebsiella pneumoniae, Proteus mirabilis,* and *Haemophilus influenzae* are the organisms most often responsible for sepsis. Any febrile patient with severe granulocytopenia should be considered septic and treated with broad-spectrum antibiotics. Granulocyte transfusions may be used for patients with absolute granulocytopenia and documented gram-negative septicemia that has responded poorly to antibiotic treatment.

Because of intensive chemotherapy and prolonged exposure to antibiotics or hydrocortisone, disseminated fungal infections attributable to *Candida* or *Aspergillus* occur more frequently, although the organisms can be difficult to culture from blood. Computed tomography (CT) scans are useful for documenting involvement of visceral organs. Abscesses of the lung, liver, spleen, kidney, paranasal sinus, or skin suggest fungal infection; diagnosis can usually be established by demonstrating the organism in biopsy samples. Amphotericin B is the treatment of choice for suspected or biopsy-proven fungal infections; 5-fluorocytosine and rifampin sometimes potentiate its effect. Fluconazole was recently found effective for the treatment of candidal and cryptococcal infections.

The development of *Pneumocystis carinii* pneumonia during remission of ALL, once a devastating complication, has become rare with routine use of a combination product of trimethoprim and sulfamethoxazole as chemoprophylaxis. Viral infections—particularly those caused by varicella virus, cytomegalovirus, herpes simplex virus, and measles virus—may overwhelm a leukemia patient's immune defenses. Zoster immune globulin given within 96 hours of exposure usually prevents or modifies the clinical manifestations of varicella. Acyclovir is the drug of choice for varicella treatment. Varicella vaccine has been safely administered to children receiving chemotherapy for ALL, with a 90% to 100% seroconversion rate. Nevertheless, a large proportion of patients still receiving chemotherapy lack detectable antibody 18 months after immunization. Other live virus vaccines (poliomyelitis, mumps, measles, and rubella) should not be administered to leukemia patients who receive immunosuppressive therapy. Siblings and other children who have frequent contact with patients should be given inactivated, rather than live, oral poliomyelitis vaccine and can be immunized against measles, mumps, and rubella.

ALL or its treatment can lead to thrombocytopenia. Hemorrhagic manifestations are common in children with this disease but are usually limited to the skin and mucous membranes. Overt bleeding in the CNS, lungs, or gastrointestinal tract is rare but can be life-threatening. Patients with extremely high leukocyte counts at diagnosis are more likely to develop these complications. Coagulopathy attributable to disseminated intravascular coagulation, hepatic dysfunction, or chemotherapy for ALL is usually mild. Cerebral thromboses, peripheral vein thromboses, or both, occur in up to 2% of children after remission induction treatment with prednisone, vincristine, and asparaginase. This complication has been attributed to a drug-induced hypercoagulable state. In general, drugs that can cause impaired platelet function, such as salicylates, should be avoided in patients with leukemia. Irradiation of blood products before transfusion prevents graft-versus-host disease.

With the success of therapy for ALL, much attention has shifted to the late effects of treatment. Subclinical CNS therapy and intensified systemic treatment have been implicated as causative factors in leukoencephalopathy, mineralizing microangiopathy, seizures, and intellectual impairment in some children. Leukemia patients are also at significant risk of developing a second malignancy.[19] Reports of brain tumors developing in these children, especially those irradiated at 5 years of age or younger, are of particular concern. The intensive use of epipodophyllotoxins (teniposide and etoposide) can result in an increase in secondary AML cases.[8] Other late effects include impaired growth; dysfunction of gonads, thyroid, liver, and heart; and aseptic necrosis of the femoral head. Little information is available on the teratogenic and mutagenic effects of antileukemic therapy; however, no evidence exists of increased defects of either kind among children born to parents previously treated for leukemia. In one recent study, increased congenital cardiac defects were reported in children of women who had been treated with dactinomycin, but this drug is not used in the treatment of ALL.

Acute Myeloid (Nonlymphoblastic) Leukemia

Clinical Presentation

The presenting signs and symptoms of AML are similar to those of ALL: fever, pallor, bone or joint pain, fatigue, anorexia, and cutaneous or mucosal bleeding (Table 31-6). Prodromal symptoms last 2 days to 12 months (median, 6 weeks). Patients with transient symptoms usually have fever, bleeding, infection, or gastrointestinal symptoms; those with longer prodromes often present with fatigue and recurrent infection. Unexplained menorrhagia is a common presenting feature in teenage girls. Half the patients have some degree of hepatosplenomegaly. Granulocytic sarcoma (chloroma), consisting of tumorous growth of granulocytic or monocytic precursor cells in the skin or other organs, is also common, especially in infants. Occasionally, it precedes the development of leukemia by a few weeks to as many as 3 years. Some children have presented with ptosis from periorbital chloroma, cauda equina syndrome, or paraparesis from epidural tumor.

Table 31-6. Presenting Features of 328 Children with AML Treated Consecutively at St Jude Children's Research Hospital

Feature	% of Total
Age (y)	
<2	19
2-9	35
>10	46
Male	53
Symptoms	
Fever	30
Bleeding	33
Bone or joint pain	18
Lymphadenopathy	20
Liver edge below costal margin	
1-5 cm	40
>5 cm	13
Spleen edge below costal margin	
1-5 cm	36
>5 cm	13
Chloroma	16
Central nervous system leukemia	20
Leukocyte count (x 10^9/L)	
<25	54
25-49	15
50-100	13
>100	18
Hemoglobin (g/dL)	
<7	21
7-9	55
>10	24
Platelet count (x 10^9/L)	
<10	9
10-49	40
50-100	23
>100	28
Auer rods	46
Coagulopathy	17

Laboratory Features

Presenting leukocyte counts range from 0.8 to 750 x 10^9/L (median, 24 x 10^9/L), platelet counts from 1 to 520 x 10^9/L (median, 58 x 10^9/L), and hemoglobin levels from 2 to 15 g/dL (median, 7 g/dL). Disseminated intravascular coagulation or increased fibrinolytic activity associated with hemorrhagic complications may occur in any subtype of AML but is more common in the promyelocytic (M3), myelomonoblastic (M4), and monoblastic (M5) subtypes. Of the several mechanisms that account for the coagulopathy observed in these patients, the release of thromboplastin from blast cells is probably the most important. CNS leukemia at diagnosis, manifested by leukemic cells in cerebrospinal fluid, occurs in 5% to 20% of patients. Usually asymptomatic, it occasionally presents as cranial nerve palsy or intracerebral chloroma. Infant age group, initial leukocyte counts >25 x 10^9/L, an M4 or M5 leukemia subtype, and an inversion or deletion of chromosome 16q22 are associated with an increased frequency of CNS involvement. A chest x-ray may demonstrate infiltrates caused by pulmonary edema, leukemic infiltration, or pneumonia. Patients with monoblastic or myelomonoblastic leukemia have elevated serum and urine levels of muramidase, a hydrolytic enzyme in the primary granules of myeloblasts or monoblasts causing renal tubular dysfunction with secondary hypokalemia. Although metabolic complications are relatively infrequent in AML, children with very high leukocyte counts (>200 x 10^9/L) may present with lactic acidosis and severe compromise of the CNS, lungs, and kidney secondary to leukostasis. Such patients would benefit from leukapheresis or exchange transfusion.

Although ALL and AML are not easily distinguishable on the basis of presenting features, certain subtypes of AML have distinctive manifestations. Acute promyelocytic leukemia is often associated with disseminated intravascular coagulation and serious hemorrhage. High leukocyte count, gum hypertrophy, skin nodules, and frequent CNS involvement characterize acute monoblastic or myelomonoblastic leukemia.

The definitive diagnosis of AML requires that 30% of cells seen on bone marrow examination be nonlymphoid blasts; the morphology of the blast cells and their cytochemical staining properties are usually adequate for classification. In the occasional difficult case, electron microscopy may demonstrate myeloperoxidase activity in myeloblastic leukemia and platelet peroxidase in megakaryoblastic leukemia. Bone marrow biopsy is sometimes needed to establish the diagnosis of megakaryoblastic leukemia (M7) because of the associated myelofibrosis.

Immunologic Markers

Large numbers of monoclonal antibodies have been developed that recognize determinants expressed on normal and leukemic myeloid cells. However, none of these antibodies is specific for AML. Conversely, the monoclonal antibodies that have identified immunologic subtypes of ALL as well as immunoglobulin and T-cell receptor gene rearrangement are not limited to lymphoid cells. Therefore, detection of immunologic markers is not by itself sufficient for the diagnosis of this disease and is useful only in classifying unusual cases of leukemia and in confirming the AML diagnosis. Moreover, attempts to correlate immunophenotypic data with FAB types have not been entirely successful.

Immunophenotypic studies have disclosed considerable diversity in the expression of surface antigens among AML cells. The more undifferentiated cases tend to express early granulocytic antigens, such as CD33 (MY9) or CD13 (MY7). Several antigens, such as CD14 (MY4) and CD11b (Mo1), correlate with M4 and M5 AML. Leukemic myeloid cells tend to express surface antigens in patterns characteristic of immature normal myeloid cells at various stages of development. This suggests that AML originates in either a multipotent myeloid stem cell (CFU-GEMM) or a more mature committed precursor. Although immunologic classification appears to have some correlation with clinical outcome in adult patients, it has little prognostic significance in children.

Cytogenetic and Molecular Genetic Studies

More than 80% of childhood AML cases are associated with acquired chromosomal abnormalities.[20]

Table 31-7. Common Nonrandom Chromosomal Abnormalities in AML

Abnormality	Frequency (%)	Type of Leukemia	Affected Gene(s)
t(8;21)(q22;q22)	12	Predominantly M2	*AML1, ETO*
inv/del(16)(q22)	12	Predominantly M4 with eosinophilia (M4Eo)	*SMMHC, CBFb*
t(15;17)(q22;q11-q12)	7	M3, M3v	*PML, RARa*
t(9;11)(p21-p22;q23)	7	M5 or secondary AML	*HRX*
-7/del(7q)	5	de novo or secondary AML	
t(1;22)(p13;q13)	2	M7 in infants	
inv (3)(q21;q26) / t(3;3)(q21;q26)	<1	AML with thrombocytosis	*EVI1*
t(9;22)(q34;q11)	<1	M1, M2	*ABL, BCR*
t(6;9)(p23;q34)	<1	M2 or M4 with basophilia	*DEK, CAN*
t(8;16)(p11;p13)	<1	M5 with phagocytosis	
-5/del(5q)	<1	Secondary AML	*IRF1*

Table 31-7 lists the more common, consistent primary abnormalities. The t(8;21), one of the most frequent alterations, is characterized by a high frequency of Auer rods (80%), FAB M1 or M2 morphology, and a high initial remission rate. The inversion or deletion of 16q22 features a strong male predominance, frequent CNS involvement, M4 morphology with bizarre eosinophilia, and longer periods of relapse-free survival. The t(15;17) occurs almost uniformly in cases of M3 AML and its variant form, but has not been reported in other patients. The t(9;11) and other 11q23 structural abnormalities are associated with male predominance, M4 or M5 morphology, frequent coagulation abnormalities, and lower age at presentation (median, younger than 2 years). Monosomy 7 appears in 5% of children with AML, with or without a preleukemic phase. Treatment outcome is extremely poor in this subgroup, for whom bone marrow transplantation should be a prime consideration. M7 leukemia with the t(1;22) is seen in infants with extensive leukemic infiltration of abdominal organs and appears to confer a poor prognosis. The Ph chromosome, t(9;22), is relatively rare in AML. In contrast to CML, cases of AML with this chromosome have a substantial proportion of normal diploid cells at diagnosis, and all Ph-positive cells disappear once remission is induced.

Recent studies have demonstrated that the genes for transcriptional regulatory proteins are frequently involved in chromosomal translocations in AML. In M3 leukemia with the t(15;17), the truncated retinoic acid receptor α *(RARα)* gene at 17q11-q12 is translocated to a locus on chromosome 15, resulting in the expression of the *PML-RARα* fusion transcript. It has been suggested that the chimeric protein may block the function of the normal RARα cellular counterpart. In this regard, it is of interest that retinoid treatment can induce differentiation of the malignant cells and restore normal hematopoiesis.[21] More recently, the t(6;9) associated with a small subset of myeloid leukemias has been demonstrated to fuse two genes, *DEK* and *CAN*, resulting in chimeric protein with a possible role in transcriptional processes. Molecular studies of Ph^+ AML are limited and most of the reported cases have the $P190^{BCR\text{-}ABL}$ fusion protein. The colony-stimulating growth factor (CSF-1) receptors, encoded by the c-*fms* proto-oncogene, have been reported to express aberrantly on blast cells in about 40% of patients with AML. The mechanism of its aberrant expression and its possible link to the abnormal cell growth are under investigation. Similarly, the N-*ras* mutation is common in AML, although its precise role in malignant transformation and proliferation is unclear.

Prognostic Factors

Prognostic factors in AML have not been as clearly defined as they have in ALL. Monocytic leukemia, a young age, a high leukocyte count, a large liver or spleen, coagulopathy, and small megakaryocyte size are presenting clinical features that indicate poor treatment outcome. The cytogenetic subtypes of inv/del(16)(q22) and t(8;21) indicate a somewhat more favorable prognosis, whereas monosomy 7 is associated with a short event-free survival. The drug sensitivity of clonogenic leukemic progenitors in vitro correlates with treatment outcome in some studies. Despite these associations, no factor has had sufficient predictive strength to warrant modifications in therapy. Secondary AML cases induced by chemotherapy (alkylating agents or topoisomerase II inhibitors, such as the epipodophyllotoxins) or radiation[7,8] generally have a dismal treatment outcome with conventional chemotherapy and warrant an alternative treatment approach, such as bone marrow transplantation.

Differential Diagnosis

The considerations that apply to the differential diagnosis of ALL also hold for AML. In addition, the megaloblastic changes in some patients with AML may mimic those related to folic acid or vitamin B_{12} deficiency. Occasionally, AML in children evolves from a preexisting myeloproliferative disorder, or preleukemic syndrome, characterized by a long period of progressive marrow failure. Because of the typically small number of blast cells in marrow aspirates, the diagnosis of malignancy may require demonstration of abnormal karyotype in bone marrow cells.

Therapy

Initial therapy should be directed toward prevention or treatment of life-threatening complications, especially bleeding, infection, and leukostasis. Most investigators would recommend prophylactic platelet transfusion to maintain platelet counts above 10 to 20 x 10^9/L and, in the presence of coagulopathy, fresh frozen plasma transfusion as well. The need for low-dose heparin treatment in patients with M3 or M4 leukemia and disseminated intravascular coagulation is controversial. Broad-spectrum parenteral antibiotics should be given to all febrile, neutropenic patients, half of whom have documented infection. When the leukocyte count exceeds 200 x 10^9/L, fatal intracerebral hemorrhage and respiratory distress from leukostasis can occur in some patients. Leukapheresis (exchange transfusion in infants) or hydroxyurea has been used to reduce large masses of leukemic cells so as to decrease the morbidity and mortality associated with hyperleukocytosis. Although metabolic complications seldom create problems in AML, these patients should be well hydrated and may be given sodium bicarbonate and allopurinol.

Remission Induction

Remission induction should begin as soon as the patient is stable. The few effective antineoplastic agents for AML have narrow therapeutic indices. The most effective remission induction regimens include daunorubicin or doxorubicin and cytarabine, with or without 6-thioguanine. Being less toxic to the gastrointestinal tract, daunorubicin is preferable to doxorubicin during remission induction. All patients, except those with M3 leukemia, must go through a period of bone marrow hypoplasia to achieve remission. Most protocols call for a bone marrow aspiration and biopsy 10 to 14 days after the start of induction, with additional treatment to patients with persistent leukemia. A hypoplastic marrow with <5% blasts often heralds a remission. Patients with M3 leukemia are unique in their ability to achieve remission without experiencing marrow hypoplasia. The leukemic promyelocytes sometimes persist in the marrow for several weeks or longer before eventually disappearing, due in part to leukemic cell maturation. Recently, all-*trans* retinoic acid has been used to induce leukemic cell differentiation and subsequent complete remission in a high proportion (>90%) of adult patients with M3 leukemia without a phase of marrow hypoplasia.[21] In fact, complete remission in some patients was preceded by striking leukocytosis, which then resolved. However, because relapse occurs despite continued all-*trans* retinoic acid treatment, all patients require additional chemotherapy. A national randomized trial using the agent followed by combination chemotherapy is being conducted for children with M3 leukemia.

Approximately 80% to 85% of children with AML attain complete remission. Of the remainder, half acquire drug-resistant blasts and the others succumb to the complications of the disease or its treatment. The intensification of remission induction therapy has led to improved measures of supportive care. Such advances are largely responsible for the higher induction rates now achieved.

Subclinical CNS Treatment

Approximately 10% to 30% of children with AML develop CNS leukemia at diagnosis or relapse. However, no definitive prospective clinical trial has demonstrated the efficacy of preventive CNS treatment in patients without identifiable leukemic cells in cerebrospinal fluid at diagnosis. Perhaps when the duration of hematologic remission improves, the value of CNS prophylaxis may become apparent. While some investigators (eg, the Berlin-Frankfurt-Münster Cooperative Group) choose to use cranial irradiation, most prefer intrathecal treatment. Young patients with M4 or M5 leukemia are at increased risk of CNS relapse and warrant consideration of some form of preventive treatment.

Continuation Therapy

In patients who achieve remission, further cytoreduction by early intensification or consolidation therapy is beneficial. However, the value of continuation therapy in frequent courses of less myelosuppressive treatment over several months or years is unclear. Chemotherapeutic agents commonly used in continuation therapy include doxorubicin or daunorubicin, cytarabine, 6-thioguanine or 6-mercaptopurine, methotrexate, cyclophosphamide, 5-azacytidine, and vincristine. Etoposide and teniposide appear to be more effective for treating M5 leukemia. The addition of nonspecific immunotherapy or early splenectomy has failed to improve treatment outcome. Available chemotherapeutic regimens allow only 30% to 50% of children in first complete remission to remain disease-free over the long term.[3]

Relapsed AML

Several chemotherapeutic regimens have led to a second hematologic remission in about 50% of patients. Recently, 2-chlorodeoxyadenosine has been used to induce second remissions in 50% of children with relapsed AML. Patients who relapse after discontinuation of therapy generally have a longer second remission than those who relapse during therapy. Because very few patients who suffer hematologic relapse survive long-term with chemotherapy alone, they should be treated with bone marrow transplantation. In contrast, CNS relapse in AML does not preclude long-term survival; about a third of these patients will attain a prolonged second remission and cure. Testicular or other extramedullary relapse is extremely rare and is usually followed by a bone marrow relapse. Local irradiation combined with intensive chemotherapy or bone marrow transplantation should be considered for these patients.

Bone Marrow Transplantation

Allogeneic bone marrow transplantation from an HLA-identical donor (most often a sibling) is an alternative therapy for AML. For some patients (eg, those with myelodysplasia or monosomy 7), it is the preferred method of treatment. Several reports indicate that 50% to 60% of children with AML survive after bone marrow transplantation performed soon after they attain complete remission.[4] Despite these promising results, however, controversy continues over the relative efficacy of chemotherapy versus bone marrow transplantation in first remission. Graft versus-host disease and interstitial pneumonia account for most deaths in the transplantation group.

For patients with a hematologic relapse or secondary AML, bone marrow transplantation is clearly the treatment of choice. Some investigators have reported long-term leukemia-free survival in as many as 30% of children transplanted early in second remission. Recurrent leukemia is the major problem of bone marrow transplantation during second remission.

Autologous marrow transplantation, with the patient's own bone marrow harvested during remission, is another promising approach. Because remission marrow is likely to contain leukemic cells, several agents including 5-hydro-peroxycyclophosphamide, mafosfamide (ASTA-Z), and monoclonal antibodies have been used to eliminate residual malignant cells before reinfusion of the bone marrow. However, the need for this purging procedure is controversial. Preliminary results suggest that one third of patients receiving an autologous marrow transplant achieve long-term relapse-free survival. Recently, bone marrow transplantation with family donors mismatched for only a single HLA antigen or with unrelated HLA-identical donors has been attempted with encouraging results.

Complications

Infection is the major cause of death during the first 10 weeks of intensive chemotherapy. Susceptibility to bacterial, fungal, or viral infection arises from granulocytopenia and immunosuppression produced by leukemia and chemotherapy and from the breakdown of anatomic barriers as a result of oral or gastrointestinal mucositis and venous access. Some patients develop typhlitis or necrotizing enterocolitis, a specific syndrome comprising right lower-quadrant abdominal pain with rebound tenderness and distention, vomiting, lower gastrointestinal tract bleeding, fever, and perhaps even septic shock. Typhlitis is most likely caused by neutropenia and mucosal breakdown of the ileocecal area with secondary infection. This complication may be more common in children and in patients treated with doxorubicin rather than daunorubicin. Serious hemorrhagic complications may also occur during induction because of thrombocytopenia and coagulopathy, especially in M3 or M5 leukemia cases. Long-term survivors after marrow transplantation with total-body irradiation have developed endocrine abnormalities that adversely affect growth and development.[22]

Acute Leukemia with Myeloid and Lymphoid Markers

The availability of extensive panels of cytochemical and immunologic tests has enabled identification of blast cells expressing both lymphoid- and myeloid-associated cell surface antigens in as many as 20% of children with acute leukemia. The dual-staining technique discloses simultaneous expression of lymphoid and myeloid characteristics on individual blast cells. This lineage heterogeneity has been variously explained as a reflection of aberrant gene expression, malignant transformation of pluripotent progenitor cells capable of differentiation in either the lymphoid or myeloid pathway, or immortalization of rare progenitor cells coexpressing features of both lineages. Numerous terms have been used to designate these cases, but standard nomenclature is still lacking. No term reflects the heterogeneity that characterizes the entire spectrum of mixed myeloid and lymphoid phenotypes. There is increasing clinical and biologic evidence that distinguishes ALL with myeloid-associated antigens (My^+ALL) from AML with lymphoid-associated antigens (Ly^+AML).[23]

My^+ALL cases have an increased frequency of L2 morphology. Ly^+AML cases are characterized by the M1 or M2 subtype, low levels of myeloperoxidase reactivity, and combined populations of myeloperoxidase-positive large and small blasts generally of hand-mirror morphology. The 11q23 translocations are common in My^+ALL cases, and the 14q32 translocation is often found in both My^+ALL and Ly^+AML cases. Patients with Ly^+AML, after failing on protocols for AML, generally respond to prednisone, vincristine, and L-asparaginase—drugs that are usually reserved for ALL. Although My^+ALL has been associated with a poor outcome, a recent study indicated that, in the context of contemporary intensive multiagent treatment, expression of myeloid-associated antigens on lymphoblasts has no apparent prognostic significance in childhood ALL.[23]

Chronic Myeloid Leukemia

Excessive growth of myeloid cells and their progenitors characterizes chronic myelogenous leukemia, a rare hematologic malignancy that accounts for about 2% of all childhood leukemias. Two types of CML, juvenile and adult (Ph^+), occur in children. Both forms present with an increased number of differentiated myeloid cells in the blood; however, features such as fetal hemoglobin levels and leukocyte alkaline phosphatase activity distinguish between the two types of CML (Table 31-8).

Adult-Type CML

Clinical and Laboratory Features

The presenting signs and symptoms of adult-type CML reflect the excessive accumulation of both mature and immature granulocytic cells. Malaise, abdominal discomfort, bleeding diathesis, and bone and joint pain are the most common presenting features. Leukocytosis found on routine examination occasionally leads to

Table 31-8. Presenting Features of Adult and Juvenile Forms of Chronic Myeloid Leukemia

Feature	Adult CML	Juvenile CML
Median age (y)	14	2
M:F ratio	6:1	2:1
Philadelphia chromosome	Present	Absent
Physical findings		
Skin rash	Unusual	Common
Bleeding	Unusual	Common
Bacterial infection	Unusual	Common
Lymphadenopathy	Unusual	Common with tendency to suppuration
Splenomegaly	Marked	Variable
Laboratory findings		
Leukocyte count >100 x 10^9/L	Common	Unusual
Thrombocytopenia	Unusual	Common
Anemia	Variable	Common
Monocytosis	Unusual	Common
Eosinophilia and basophilia	Common	Unusual
Fetal hemoglobin level	Normal	15%-70%
Erythrocyte I antigen	Normal	Decreased
Decreased leukocyte alkaline phosphatase	Common	Variable
Ineffective erythropoiesis	Absent	Common
Marrow myeloid:erythroid ratio	10:1 to 50:1	2:1 to 5:1
Nature of colony formation	Predominantly	Nearly exclusively monocytic
Urine and serum muramidase	Slightly increased	Markedly increased
Immunologic abnormalities	None	Increased immunoglobulin levels, high frequency of antinuclear and anti-IgG antibodies
Clinical course		
Median survival (y)	4-5	1-2
Blastic phase	Common	Unusual

the diagnosis of CML. Splenomegaly is present in most patients; hepatomegaly and lymphadenopathy are less common. Most patients present with a leukocyte count >100 x 10^9/L and thrombocytosis. Median leukocyte count is approximately 250 x 10^9/L and median platelet count 500 x 10^9/L. The blood smear shows myeloid cells at all stages of differentiation. Leukostasis syndrome, manifested by papilledema, stroke, cerebellar signs, respiratory distress, or priapism, is common. In addition to decreased alkaline phosphatase activity, neutrophils from these patients display many biochemical and functional abnormalities. Bone marrow examination discloses granulocytic hyperplasia, frequently associated with dysplastic eosinophils and basophils. Megakaryocytic hyperplasia or lipid-laden histiocytes that resemble Gaucher's cells or sea-blue histiocytes are found occasionally.

Although CML usually remains stable for several months to years, it eventually transforms to a disorder called blast crisis, which is characterized by the loss of capacity of the leukemic clone to differentiate and results in an increase in immature cells. This phase occurs at a median of about 3 years from the date of diagnosis and may be heralded by a transitional phase of several months of fever, weight loss, basophilia, thrombocytosis or thrombocytopenia, leukocytosis, anemia, splenomegaly, karyotypic evolution, and myelofibrosis. The predominant blast cell may be myeloid (70%) or lymphoid (30%). Myeloid blast crisis is heterogeneous; myeloblastic, erythroid, and megakaryocytic variants all have been observed. In lymphoid crisis, the blasts generally express early pre-B or pre-B phenotype and rarely T-cell markers and may have increased terminal deoxynucleotidyl transferase activity. In some cases, the blasts manifest both lymphoid- and myeloid-associated antigens.

Genetic Features

More than 90% of patients have the Ph chromosome, a shortened chromosome 22 formed by a reciprocal translocation of DNA material between chromosomes 9 and 22, the t(9;22)(q34;q11). The cytogenetic abnormality is limited to hematopoietic cells; bone marrow fibroblasts and other mesenchymal tissues do not appear to be involved. The Ph chromosome usually persists during hematologic remission, although it may decrease in frequency. Even the variant translocations that form in some patients always involve chromosomes 9 and 22. Several consistent secondary chromosome abnormalities, including +Ph, +8, i(17q), +19, and -Y, accompany the accelerated or blastic phase.

The molecular consequence of the Ph chromosome is the translocation of the *ABL* oncogene on chromosome 9 to a 5.8-kb breakpoint cluster region (bcr) on chromosome 22. This region of chromosome 22 is within a gene called *BCR*. This mechanism leads to the formation of a new chimeric transcriptional unit containing genetic information from both the *ABL* and *BCR* genes; the resulting transcript is a newly fused mRNA of about 8.5 kb. The translational product of this hybrid mRNA is a 210-kd phosphoprotein with tyrosine kinase activity, which apparently plays a role in the pathogenesis of CML. Although the Ph chromosomes in acute and chronic leukemia appear similar cytogenetically, they constitute a heterogeneous group at the molecular level.

Pathophysiology

G6PD isoenzyme analyses and cytogenetic studies have shown that CML is a clonal disorder of pluripotent hematopoietic stem cells. A monoclonal pattern of G6PD isoenzyme expression or the Ph chromosome has been identified in granulocytes, monocytes, macrophages, basophils, eosinophils, megakaryocytes, erythrocytes, and their committed progenitors. B lymphocytes also originate from the malignant clone; several reports of T-lymphoblast crisis suggest that the disease may involve a stem cell capable of differentiating to T lymphocytes as well.

The evolution of CML is best explained by a multistep process. An initial transformation event occurs within a multipotential progenitor cell, resulting in a clone of a "premalignant" cell. Subsequent events result in the acquisition of the Ph chromosome, with growth advantage over normal hematopoietic cells. The overproduction of myeloid cells in CML is not caused by a rapid rate of cell division but is attributed to a relative insensitivity to feedback inhibition and the production of humoral factors that suppress normal hematopoietic precursor cells. As the disease progresses, new cytogenetic alterations occur and there is an increasing dissociation between proliferation and differentiation. Eventually, the process terminates in acute leukemia.

Differential Diagnosis

Occasionally, patients with severe infections, congenital heart disease, or metastatic cancer present with a leukemoid reaction. In these disorders, the leukocyte counts are lower than in CML, the differential counts rarely reveal blasts, and leukocyte alkaline phosphatase scores and karyotypes are normal. Some patients with adult-type CML may present in lymphoid blast crisis; in most instances, molecular studies can distinguish these cases from Ph-positive ALL.

Treatment

The major obstacle to successful treatment of CML is the lack of differential drug sensitivity of malignant and normal hematopoietic cells. The median survival of patients with Ph+ CML (about 3 years) has not been altered by chemotherapy. During the chronic phase, busulfan or hydroxyurea controls symptoms or signs by suppressing the growth of malignant cells. Hydroxyurea is sometimes preferred because it is less toxic. Recent clinical trials indicate that recombinant human alpha interferon is effective in inducing hematologic remission in most patients in the chronic phase and in suppressing the Ph chromosome in some patients. Treatment for blast crisis has been disappointing. Although 60% of patients with lymphoid, and 20% with myeloid, blast crisis can achieve remission with chemotherapy, the remissions are generally brief.

Bone marrow transplantation, currently the only treatment capable of eradicating the leukemic clone, has produced the most encouraging results.[24] When transplantation is performed early in the chronic phase, 80% or more of children may become long-term survivors. Treatment results become progressively worse when transplants are performed in the second chronic phase (30% to 50%), accelerated phase (15% to 40%), or blastic phase (10% to 20%). Unrelated-donor bone marrow transplantation can also be effective in the treatment of CML, particularly as the prolonged chronic phase offers an opportunity to search for suitable donors.

Juvenile CML

Juvenile CML occurs during the first few years of life. Common presenting features are skin rashes, prominent lymphadenopathy, bleeding, persistent infections, pulmonary symptoms, fever, and failure to thrive. Patients have various degrees of leukocytosis (generally <100 x 10^9/L), thrombocytopenia, and anemia. Monocytosis in the peripheral blood, bone marrow, or both, is a striking finding. Bone marrow examination reveals myeloid hyperplasia and decreased megakaryocytes. Fetal erythropoiesis, which manifests as increased fetal hemoglobin and fetal-type antigens and enzymes, often characterizes this disease. Leukocytes from the blood and bone marrow in these patients form predominantly monocytic colonies in vitro, in contrast to the myelocytic colony formation in patients with adult-type CML. A recent study suggests that progenitor cells of juvenile CML have increased sensitivity to granulocyte-macrophage colony-stimulating factor.[25] Although different cytogenetic abnormalities appear, the Ph chromosome is not present in these cases. The majority of patients have a normal karyotype. Congenital viral infections or persistent Epstein-Barr virus infection may induce a clinical picture mimicking juvenile CML and should be ruled out.

Children with juvenile CML have a more acute course of disease than those with adult-type CML; their diseases do not respond to busulfan or hydroxyurea. Although cytarabine and mercaptopurine have produced responses in some patients, most survived only 1 to 2 years. Intensive AML-type combination chemotherapy has induced remission in some patients. Bone marrow transplantation is the treatment of choice for patients with a histocompatible donor and has been curative.

Congenital Leukemia

Congenital leukemia is rare. Hyperleukocytosis, hepatosplenomegaly, nodular skin infiltrates, and respiratory distress secondary to pulmonary leukostasis generally mark this form of leukemia.[26] Laboratory findings are similar to those in older children with leukemia. Most newborns with leukemia have the monocytic subtype, although occasional cases of pre-B ALL have been reported as congenital. Congenital leukemia has been associated with Down syndrome, Turner's syndrome, trisomy 9, mosaic monosomy 8, Klippel-Feil syndrome, congenital heart disease, and a variant of Ellis-van Creveld syndrome. A variety of disorders in newborns may mimic leukemia. Leukoerythroblastic reaction from bacterial infection, hypoxia, or hemolytic disease should be considered. The differential diagnosis also includes neuroblastoma as well as intrauterine infection by *Toxoplasma gondii, Treponema pallidum,* rubella virus, herpesvirus, and cytomegalovirus. Treatment outcome in patients with congenital leukemia has been poor. Complete remissions are usually of short duration, and most patients die within a few months. Recently, several newborns with monocytic leukemia responded well to epipodophyllotoxin therapy.

The leukemoid reaction in neonates with Down syndrome or trisomy 21 mosaicism poses a unique problem. This condition usually resolves spontaneously over a matter of weeks or months, but some patients with the presumed leukemoid reaction have developed leukemia. A recent study revealed diffuse liver fibrosis but not bone marrow fibrosis in neonates with Down syndrome and transient leukemoid reaction.[27] It was postulated that the abnormal blasts, generally of megakaryocytic lineage, in these cases are of fetal liver origin and cause liver fibrosis by producing collagen-stimulating cytokines. The transition in the site of hematopoiesis from the liver to the bone marrow after birth could influence proliferation of these blast cells and might induce spontaneous regression. Because neonates with true congenital leukemia cannot be distinguished with certainty from those with leukemoid reaction, judicious supportive care and monitoring for a few weeks is the preferred initial treatment.

References

1. Niemeyer CM, Gelber RD, Tarbell NJ, et al. Low-dose versus high-dose methotrexate during remission induction in childhood acute lymphoblastic leukemia (protocol 81-01 update). *Blood.* 1991;78:2514-2519.

2. Rivera GK, Raimondi SC, Hancock ML, et al. Improved outcome in childhood acute lymphoblastic leukaemia with reinforced early treatment and rotational combination chemotherapy. *Lancet.* 1991;337:61-66.

3. Creutzig U, Ritter J, Zimmerman M, Schellong G. Does cranial irradiation reduce the risk for bone marrow relapse in acute myelogenous leukemia: unexpected results of the childhood acute myelogenous leukemia study BFM-87. *J Clin Oncol.* 1993;11:279-286.

4. Phillips M, Richards S, Chessells J. Acute myeloid leukaemia in childhood: the costs and benefits of intensive treatment. *Br J Haematol.* 1991;77:473-477.

5. Bennett JM, Catovsky D, Daniel M-T, et al. Proposals for the classification of the acute leukaemias: French-American-British (FAB) Co-operative Group. *Br J Haematol.* 1976;33:451-458.

6. Bennett JM, Catovsky D, Daniel M-T, et al. Proposal for the recognition of minimally differentiated acute myeloid leukaemia (AML-M0). *Br J Haematol.* 1991;78:325-329.

7. Rubin CM, Arthur DC, Woods WG, et al. Therapy-related myelodysplastic syndrome and acute myeloid leukemia in children: correlation between chromosomal abnormalities and prior therapy. *Blood.* 1991;78:2982-2988.

8. Pui C-H, Ribeiro RC, Hancock ML, et al. Acute myeloid leukemia in children treated with epipodophyllotoxins for acute lymphoblastic leukemia. *N Engl J Med.* 1991;325:1682-1687.

9. Wainscoat JS, Fey MF. Assessment of clonality in human tumors: a review. *Cancer Res.* 1990;50:1355-1360.

10. Pui C-H, Behm FG, Crist WM. Clinical and biologic relevance of immunologic marker studies in childhood acute lymphoblastic leukemia. *Blood.* 1993;82:342-362.

11. Pui C-H, Crist WM, Look AT. Biology and clinical significance of cytogenetic abnormalities in childhood acute lymphoblastic leukemia. *Blood.* 1990;76:1449-1463.

12. Rabbitts TH. Translocations, master genes, and differences between the origins of acute and chronic leukemias. *Cell.* 1991;67:641-644.

13. Korsmeyer SJ. Bcl-2 initiates a new category of oncogenes: regulators of cell death. *Blood.* 1992;80:879-886.

14. Weinberg RA. Tumor suppressor genes. *Science.* 1991;254:1138-1146.

15. Negrin RS, Blume KG. The use of the polymerase chain reaction for the detection of minimal residual malignant disease. *Blood.* 1991;78:255-258.

16. Pui C-H, Crist WM. High-risk lymphoblastic leukemia in children: prognostic factors and management. *Blood Rev.* 1987;1:25-33.

17. Mahmoud HH, Rivera GK, Hancock ML. Low leukocyte counts with blast cells in cerebrospinal fluid of children with newly diagnosed acute lymphoblastic leukemia. *N Engl J Med.* 1993;329:314-319.

18. Henze G, Fengler R, Hartmann R, et al. Six-year experience with a comprehensive approach to the treatment of recurrent childhood acute lymphoblastic leukemia (ALL-REZ BFM 85): a relapse study of the BFM group. *Blood.* 1991;78:1166-1172.

19. Neglia JP, Meadows AT, Robison LL, et al. Second neoplasms after acute lymphoblastic leukemia in childhood. *N Engl J Med.* 1991;325:1330-1336.

20. Kalwinsky DK, Raimondi SC, Schell MJ, et al. Prognostic importance of cytogenetic subgroups in de novo pediatric acute nonlymphocytic leukemia. *J Clin Oncol.* 1990;8:75-83.

21. Warrell RP Jr, de Thé H, Wang Z-Y, Degos L. Acute promyelocytic leukemia. *N Engl J Med.* 329:177-189.

22. Sanders JE, Pritchard S, Mahoney P, et al. Growth and development following marrow transplantation for leukemia. *Blood.* 1986;68:1129-1135.

23. Pui C-H, Raimondi SC, Head DR, et al. Characterization of childhood acute leukemia with multiple myeloid and lymphoid markers at diagnosis and at relapse. *Blood.* 1991; 78:1327-1337.

24. McGlave P. Bone marrow transplants in chronic myelogenous leukemia: an overview of determinants of survival. *Semin Hematol.* 1990;27(3, suppl 4):23-30.

25. Emanuel PD, Bates LJ, Castleberry RP, Gualtieri RJ, Zuckerman KS. Selective hypersensitivity to granulocyte-macrophage colony-stimulating factor by juvenile chronic myeloid leukemia hematopoietic progenitors. *Blood.* 1991;77:925-929.

26. Weinstein HJ. Congenital leukaemia and the neonatal myeloproliferative disorders associated with Down syndrome. *Clin Haematol.* 1978;7:147-154.

27. Miyauchi J, Ito Y, Kawano T, Tsunematsu Y, Shimizu K. Unusual diffuse liver fibrosis accompanying transient myeloproliferative disorder in Down syndrome: a report of four autopsy cases and proposal of a hypothesis. *Blood.* 1992;80:1521-1527.

32

PEDIATRIC SOLID TUMORS

Neyssa M. Marina, MD, Laura C. Bowman, MD, Ching-Hon Pui, MD, William M. Crist, MD

Although rare in the United States, childhood cancer is the second leading cause of death in persons younger than 15 years. Of the 8,000 children in whom cancer is diagnosed each year, about 19% die despite steady advances in therapy. Childhood neoplasms differ from adult tumors in origin, histologic appearance, prognosis, and responsiveness to therapy. In adults, primary epithelial tumors predominate, and there are many known links to environmental carcinogens. In contrast, childhood neoplasms usually are of mesenchymal origin or involve the hematopoietic and central nervous systems (Table 32-1).[1] In this chapter we describe the most common extracranial childhood solid tumors; brain tumors are discussed in Chapter 24.

Epidemiology

The estimated annual incidence of malignancy in the US in persons younger than 15 years is 142.0 per million whites and 118.0 per million blacks.[1] The highest incidences of childhood cancer are found in Israel and Nigeria, and the lowest in Japan and India.[2] For virtually all childhood cancers except Wilms' tumor, incidence rates exhibit wide geographic variation.[3] Hepatoma is particularly prevalent in the Far East, retinoblastoma in India, neuroblastoma in Western Europe, Burkitt's lymphoma in Uganda, and orbital chloroma in Turkey and Uganda. There are also racial differences within the US; Ewing's sarcoma, testicular cancer, and melanoma are extremely rare in blacks.

Solid tumors of embryonal origin constitute about 40% of childhood malignancies. Neuroblastoma, Wilms' tumor, retinoblastoma, medulloblastoma, central nervous system (CNS) gliomas, and rhabdomyosarcoma all have peak incidences in children younger than 5 years. Other tumors, such as bone sarcomas and the majority of brain tumors, are most often diagnosed during adolescence.[3]

Childhood cancer occurs more often in males than females (1.2:1).[1] Lymphomas have the highest male-to-

Table 32-1. Frequency of Cancers by Race in Children Under Age 15 Years in the US, 1973-1982

Category	Percentage of Total White	Percentage of Total Black
Leukemia	30.9	23.1
Central nervous system	18.9	20.5
Lymphoma	12.7	9.4
Sympathetic nervous system	8.1	8.4
Soft tissue	6.1	7.4
Kidney	6.0	10.6
Bone	4.8	4.6
Retinoblastoma	2.5	4.1
Germ cell tumors	3.1	3.8
Miscellaneous	6.9	8.1
Total	100.0	100.0

Adapted from Miller et al.[1]

Neyssa M. Marina, MD, and Laura C. Bowman, MD, Assistant Members, Department of Hematology-Oncology, St Jude Children's Research Hospital, Memphis, Tennessee, and Assistant Professors of Pediatrics, University of Tennessee, Memphis, College of Medicine, Memphis, Tennessee

Ching-Hon Pui, MD, Member, Department of Hematology-Oncology, St Jude Children's Research Hospital, Memphis, Tennessee and Professor of Pediatrics, University of Tennessee, Memphis, College of Medicine, Memphis, Tennessee

William M. Crist, MD, Member and Chairman, Department of Hematology-Oncology, St Jude Children's Research Hospital, Memphis, Tennessee and Professor of Pediatrics and Chief of Division of Pediatric Hematology-Oncology, University of Tennessee, Memphis, College of Medicine, Memphis, Tennessee

*This work was supported in part by grants CA 23099 and CA 21765 from the National Cancer Institute and by the American Lebanese Syrian Associated Charities (ALSAC).

Table 32-2. Conditions Associated With Increased Risk of Childhood Cancer

Condition	Associated Tumor
Cutaneous syndrome	
Nevoid basal cell carcinoma syndrome	Basal cell carcinoma, medulloblastoma
Familial trichoepithelioma syndrome	Basal cell carcinoma
Tylosis (palmar-plantar keratosis)	Esophageal squamous cell carcinoma
Xeroderma pigmentosum	Basal and squamous cell carcinoma, melanoma
Albinism	Squamous cell carcinoma
Werner syndrome (adult progeria)	Soft tissue sarcomas, carcinoma
Epidermodysplasia verruciformis	Basal and squamous cell carcinoma
Polydysplastic epidermolysis bullosa	Squamous cell carcinoma
Dyskeratosis congenita	Squamous cell carcinoma, mucous membrane carcinomas
Familial atypical mole, malignant melanoma syndrome	Melanoma, breast, colon, leukemia, lymphoma, sarcoma
Neurocutaneous syndrome	
Neurofibromatosis	Brain, pheochromocytoma, neuroblastoma, medullary thyroid carcinoma, Wilms' tumor, leukemia, rhabdomyosarcoma, neurosarcoma
Tuberous sclerosis	Brain
von Hippel-Lindau disease	Brain, pheochromocytoma, hypernephroma
Chromosomal syndrome	
Down syndrome (trisomy 21)	Leukemia
Klinefelter's syndrome (47 XXY)	Breast, leukemia, lymphoma, teratoma
Female XY mosaicism (47 XO/46 XY)	Gonadoblastoma
13q- syndrome	Retinoblastoma
11p-, aniridia-Wilms' tumor syndrome	Wilms' tumor
t(3,8)	Renal cell carcinoma
Bloom syndrome	Leukemia, lymphoma, colon, squamous cell carcinoma
Fanconi's anemia	Leukemia, hepatoma, squamous cell carcinoma
Ataxia-telangiectasia	Leukemia, lymphoma, Hodgkin's disease, brain, gastric, ovarian
Primary immunodeficiency syndrome	
X-linked agammaglobulinemia (Bruton)	Lymphoma, leukemia, brain
X-linked lymphoproliferative disease (Duncan)	Lymphoma
Severe combined immunodeficiency	Lymphoma, leukemia
Wiskott-Aldrich syndrome	Lymphoma, leukemia, brain
IgA deficiency	Lymphoma, leukemia, brain, gastrointestinal
DiGeorge syndrome	Brain, oral squamous cell carcinoma
Common variable immunodeficiency	Lymphoma, gastrointestinal, brain
IgM deficiency	Lymphoma
Gastrointestinal syndrome	
Polyposis coli	Colon
Gardner's syndrome	Colon, soft tissue, bone, thyroid, adrenal
Turcot syndrome	Colon, brain
Peutz-Jeghers syndrome	Gastrointestinal, ovarian, breast
Inflammatory bowel disease	Colorectal

Continued

Table 32-2 *Continued.* Conditions Associated With Increased Risk of Childhood Cancer

Condition	Associated Tumor
Miscellaneous	
Hemihypertrophy	Wilms' tumor, hepatoma, adrenocortical carcinoma
Renal dysplasia	Wilms' tumor
Sporadic aniridia	Wilms' tumor
Beckwith-Wiedemann syndrome	Wilms' tumor, hepatoma, adrenocortical carcinoma
Gonadal dysgenesis	Gonadoblastoma
Cryptorchidism	Testicular
Multiple endocrine adenomatosis type I (Wermer's syndrome)	Schwannoma
Multiple endocrine adenomatosis type II (Sipple's syndrome)	Thyroid carcinoma, pheochromocytoma
Enchondromatosis	Chondrosarcoma
Chediak-Higashi syndrome	Lymphoma
Shwachman syndrome	Leukemia
21-hydroxylase deficiency, congenital adrenal hyperplasia	Adrenocortical, testicular, mesodermal, neurogenic
Galactosemia	Liver
Hereditary tyrosinemia	Liver
Type I glycogen storage	Liver
Hypermethioninemia	Liver
Alpha-1-antitrypsin deficiency	Liver
Familial cholestatic cirrhosis of childhood	Liver

female ratio (2:1), in part because of their association with X-linked immunodeficiency disorders.

Etiology

Prenatal Factors

Maternal cancer is rarely transmitted across the placenta to the fetus, although transplacental transmission of melanoma, lymphoma, and bronchogenic carcinoma has been documented.[4] One study reported that childhood cancers increased almost 50% with prenatal exposure to diagnostic irradiation, but other investigators have been unable to substantiate this finding. Intrauterine irradiation does not appear to have increased the cancer mortality among progeny of survivors of the atomic bomb.[5]

Although the majority of children with cancer have no history of prenatal exposure to known carcinogens, several drugs and chemicals have been implicated as in utero carcinogens. There is a well-established relationship between in utero exposure to diethylstilbestrol (DES) during the first half of pregnancy and subsequent development of clear cell adenocarcinoma of the vagina or cervix.[3] In addition, seminomas have developed in some males exposed to DES in utero. There are associations between the fetal hydantoin syndrome and neuroblastoma, as well as between the fetal alcohol syndrome and hepatoblastoma, neuroblastoma, and adrenocortical carcinoma. The apparent correlation between increased cancer incidence and exposure to certain mutagenic and carcinogenic agents in utero underscores the importance of laboratory tests that screen new drugs for carcinogenicity in humans.

Heredity

Underlying inherited disorders are rare in childhood cancer, but children with certain chromosomal disorders or constitutional syndromes are at increased risk of malignancy (Table 32-2). Many patients have distinctive clinical or laboratory features that bring them to medical attention before the development of an associated malignancy. Genetic forms of cancer share several features: earlier disease onset, higher frequency of multifocal lesions within one organ, bilateral involvement in paired organs, and multiple primary cancers. These observations have led to the hypothesis that malignant transformation occurs after at least two cellular mutational events (the "two hit" model of tumorigenesis). In hereditary cancers, the first (germinal) mutation presumably occurs prezygotically and is present in all somatic cells. Cancer subsequently arises in somatic cells that have undergone a second mutation. In nonhereditary (sporadic) cases, both "hits" presumably occur as chance events in the same somatic cell. This model fits the age pattern and laterality of retinoblastoma and Wilms' tumor, and predicts that about 40% of retinoblastomas and a smaller percentage of Wilms' tumors are heritable. Penetrance is estimated to be 95% for the retinoblastoma gene but is considerably lower for Wilms' tumor.

Rarely, childhood cancer occurs repeatedly within families. These clusters may result from polygenic inheritance, a single-gene defect, exposure to common carcinogens, or a combination of factors. When cancer develops in a child, the risk of cancer in siblings becomes approximately twice that of the general population. If two siblings develop childhood cancer, the risk in other siblings may be even higher. Although tumors are usually of the same type, dissimilar neoplasms have also been reported in young siblings.

There are families in which more than 25% of members develop a malignancy (typically sarcoma, breast cancer, or brain tumor) at some time during their lives. In these patients, the histologic diagnoses may be the same, with tumors developing at a single or multiple sites in the same organ or paired organs, or the histiologic diagnosis may differ within an organ system. Some of these families have been found to have a genetic defect (the Li-Fraumeni syndrome) involving the *p53* tumor suppressor gene previously identified in sporadic malignancies.[6] Individuals with this syndrome carry the *p53* gene in both normal and malignant cells. In families with Li-Fraumeni syndrome, tumors develop years or decades earlier than in the general population, and vertical transmission in consecutive generations is consistent with an autosomal dominant inheritance pattern. Germline mutations of the *p53* gene have recently been found in patients with second malignant neoplasms and in children with sarcoma whose family histories did not indicate Li-Fraumeni syndrome.[7,8]

Environment

Survivors of nuclear warfare, workers exposed to radiation, and patients irradiated for medical reasons have an increased incidence of cancer. The type of radiation, total dose, fraction size, dose rate, and other exposure variables affect cancer induction. The form of cancer and its rate of occurrence are related to patient age at exposure. Depending on the sites irradiated, patients may develop carcinomas of skin, thyroid, breast, and salivary gland; sarcomas of bone and soft tissue; brain tumors; and lymphomas. The latency period between radiation exposure and tumor development ranges from 3 to more than 20 years.[3]

Several inherited syndromes are associated with susceptibility to radiation-induced cancer. Patients with ataxia-telangiectasia are predisposed by a defect in DNA repair to lymphoid malignancies and acute radiation toxicity. Sarcomas may occur after radiotherapy for bilateral retinoblastoma, and patients with nevoid basal cell carcinoma syndrome who receive radiotherapy for medulloblastoma may develop skin cancers. Sun exposure increases the risk of skin cancer globally, but occurrence is rare in young individuals without a genetic predisposition such as xeroderma pigmentosum or another congenital defect in DNA repair.

More than 50 chemical agents and medications have been implicated in human carcinogenesis.[3] Exposure can occur by transplacental passage; contamination of food, water, or air; and medical therapy for benign and malignant conditions. Chemotherapeutic agents associated with second malignancies include the alkylating agents (cyclophosphamide, melphalan, busulfan, nitrosoureas, chlorambucil, nitrogen mustard, procarbazine) and the topoisomerase II inhibitors such as epipodophyllotoxins (teniposide, etoposide)[9] and anthracyclines.

A few human cancers have been associated with specific viral and parasitic pathogens. The most compelling evidence of viral induction of certain childhood cancers is the association between Epstein-Barr virus (EBV) and lymphoproliferative disease, especially in patients with congenital or acquired immunodeficiency. Epidemiologic, serologic, and molecular evidence also links this DNA virus to nasopharyngeal carcinoma (lymphoepithelioma) in children. Prolonged hepatitis B antigenemia has been associated with the development of hepatocellular carcinoma. More recently, non-Hodgkin's lymphoma (NHL), Kaposi's sarcoma, and primary lymphoma of the brain have been noted in children with acquired immunodeficiency syndrome (AIDS).[10] Parasitic agents with carcinogenic potential include *Clonorchis sinensis* and *Schistosoma haematobium*.

Genetics of Oncogenesis

Oncogenes and Tumor Suppressor Genes

Proto-oncogenes comprise a variety of genes whose protein products are involved in normal cellular growth or differentiation.[11] Somatic mutations of these genes or their regulatory elements in specific tissues can convert them into oncogenic alleles. The classic examples of proto-oncogenes with malignant associations are N-*myc* in neuroblastoma and c-*myc* in Burkitt's lymphoma.

The term *anti-oncogene* (tumor suppressor gene) was introduced to describe DNA sequences that restrain or confine cellular proliferation and seem to behave as dominant repressors of cancer.[11] Tumor development requires the loss or inactivation of both alleles. Experimental fusion of normal and cancerous cells suppresses the neoplastic phenotype, suggesting that some cancer cells lack cellular constituents required for the regulation of the normal phenotype.

Tumor suppressor gene abnormalities have been identified in retinoblastoma (RB) and Wilms' tumor in children. Deletion of the two homologous copies of the *RB* gene, which is located in 13q14, is associated with a predisposition to retinoblastoma. Similarly, a deletion at 11p13 is associated with a predisposition to Wilms' tumor. Recessive genetic lesions have also been described in some cases of osteosarcoma (13q14), neuroblastoma (1p32-pter), and embryonal tumors (11p15.5-pter) in patients with Beckwith-Wiedemann syndrome. Recently the genetic defect associated with Li-Fraumeni syndrome has been found to involve *p53,* a tumor suppressor gene previously identified in sporadic malignancies.[6] Delineation of the molecular mechanisms by which oncogenes or tumor suppressor genes cause or control cancer will likely lead to new approaches in diagnosis and therapy.

Cancer Cytogenetics

Childhood solid tumors are technically difficult to characterize cytogenetically, but a growing number of consistent abnormalities have been discovered,[6] which may provide useful diagnostic and prognostic information. There are three main categories of cytogenetic abnormalities. The first is translocation, in which a segment moves from one chromosome to another. Translocation sites are often specific to tumor types. The second is a gain of specific genetic material, either by duplication of all or part of a chromosome(s) or by gene amplification. Gene amplification, demonstrated by extrachromosomal double-minute (DM) chromatin bodies or chromosomally integrated, homogeneous staining regions (HSR), is a common mechanism for oncogene activation and is generally associated with more aggressive disease. Neuroblastoma is the classic example of a human tumor that often shows gene amplification (N-*myc*). The third abnormality involves loss of genetic material from a specific chromosomal band or region that may contain or affect tumor suppressor genes. Deletion of an arm of chromosome 1, commonly found in solid tumors, may confer a cellular growth advantage as part of the multistep process of tumorigenesis.

Principles of Diagnosis

The signs and symptoms of childhood cancer vary with the primary site, tumor type, and extent of disease. They are often subtle or nonspecific, causing delays in diagnosis. Tumors are often discovered by parents or caretakers. Prolonged fever, unexplained pain, or growing masses, especially in association with weight loss, should prompt a complete examination to rule out malignancy.

When cancer is suspected, the immediate goal is to learn the nature and extent of disease. It is always appropriate to search for metastatic disease before deciding to remove a tumor surgically. When metastatic disease is present, a diagnosis can usually be made using less invasive procedures, such as bone marrow aspiration. Because the management of each tumor is distinctive, adequate tissue must be obtained to establish the specific subtype of the cancer. In rare circumstances in which an open biopsy is life threatening, the tumor location coupled with a urine or serum marker can establish the diagnosis, precluding the need for surgery. As a rule, a precise histologic diagnosis by an experienced pediatric pathologist is essential. Comprehensive management also includes biologic studies of tumor tissue to determine the tumor phenotype and cytogenetic and molecular analyses to investigate the mechanism of malignant transformation.

Staging directs therapy for most pediatric solid tumors. Staging systems are based on histologic features, primary site, and extent of disease. The disease stage at diagnosis, as determined by surgery, biochemical studies, and diagnostic imaging techniques, predicts the likelihood of a remission and has an inverse relationship to survival.

Principles of Therapy

Cure of childhood solid tumors requires eradication of both local (gross or microscopic) and systemic disease. The multimodality approach used for most tumors includes surgery, radiation therapy for local control of the primary tumor, and chemotherapy to treat both the local tumor and systemic micrometastases. The combination and timing of the component therapies depend on tumor type and stage. For inaccessible tumors or those that are highly chemosensitive but not radiosensitive, multiagent chemotherapy precedes or replaces definitive surgery, radiation therapy, or the two in combination.

The multidisciplinary treatment plan requires the teamwork of a pediatric oncologist, radiation oncologist, surgeon, pathologist, and radiologist as well as specialized support services (oncology nursing, nutrition, rehabilitation, social work, and psychiatry/psychology). Because of the intensity and complexity of therapy, most children with cancer are treated in pediatric oncology centers or institutions participating in the Pediatric Oncology Group or Children's Cancer Study Group. It is vital that childhood cancer be treated in coordinated clinical trials. This approach ensures use of the most effective treatment available and permits valid assessment of promising new additions or modifications designed to improve cure rates while reducing toxicity.

For most childhood tumors, surgery is the primary

local control method. When feasible, complete excision combined with chemotherapy is the standard treatment for osteosarcoma, soft tissue sarcomas, Wilms' tumor, and germ cell tumors. As cure rates have risen with improved chemotherapy and radiation therapy, surgical approaches for most tumors have been revised with the goal of preserving function.[12] In rare instances, surgery alone is curative (eg, in localized, grossly resected neuroblastoma).

Radiation can cure retinoblastoma and is used as primary or adjunct therapy for some brain tumors (eg, brain stem gliomas and medulloblastomas), Wilms' tumor, rhabdomyosarcoma, and Ewing's sarcoma. The radiotherapy treatment plan is based on the anticipated effects of dosage and timing on the tumor and on normal tissue, as well as interactions with surgery and specific chemotherapeutic agents. A goal of current clinical trials for radiosensitive tumors is to reduce side effects and long-term sequelae by modifying the dosage, field of radiation, or other delivery parameters.

Despite adequate local control with surgery, radiotherapy, or a combination of the two, effective systemic chemotherapy improves the prognoses of children with solid tumors. Specific treatment plans are formulated around three central principles:

1. Expeditious delivery prior to disease progression;

2. Use of multiple drugs with documented efficacy, having either different or synergistic actions and non-overlapping toxicities; and

3. Use of the highest safe dose.

In general, chemotherapy treatment plans are based on combinations proven successful in clinical trials, with the addition of new drugs that have produced responses in relapsed patients. The intensity of therapy and the specific combination of drugs are targeted to both disease histology and stage. While therapeutic doses and effective blood levels are known for most drugs in the medical armamentarium, such studies of chemotherapeutic agents are just beginning. This knowledge is particularly crucial in pediatrics because children have a far greater variation in rates of drug metabolism than do adults. The incorporation of pharmacokinetic studies into contemporary protocols holds promise for ensuring the delivery of effective doses while avoiding unnecessary toxicity.

Chemotherapeutic agents comprise several classes of drugs, including alkylators, antimetabolites, antibiotics, plant alkaloids, and hormones. New active agents are identified by a complex process. They are first screened against tumor cell lines and in animal models. Those with promise are then available for phase I studies in patients with refractory malignancy, in which the maximal tolerated dose (MTD), toxicities, and feasibility of administration are assessed by gradually escalating dosage. After the MTD is determined, phase II studies are conducted in patients with a variety of recurrent tumors. Finally, Phase III trials assess the agent in combination chemotherapy for newly diagnosed cancer.

Another approach has been the use of high-dose chemotherapy followed by autologous bone marrow infusion.[13] Initially the patient's own tumor-free marrow is harvested, and high-dose chemotherapy is given in an attempt to ablate any remaining tumor. The stored marrow is then reinfused to repopulate the bone marrow. This approach has been studied in non-Hodgkin's lymphoma, neuroblastoma, Ewing's sarcoma, Hodgkin's disease and other solid tumors, but its precise role in therapy is not yet defined.

Investigators are exploring the use of biologic response modifiers, such as monoclonal antibodies, interferons, interleukins, and colony-stimulating factors, to treat solid tumors in children. By enhancing host antitumor immune response, interleukin-2 has produced tumor regression in some adults with refractory cancers.[14] Recombinant granulocyte-macrophage or granulocyte colony-stimulating factor may permit intensification of chemotherapy by ameliorating drug-induced bone marrow suppression.[15] These and similar hormones may also prove useful in reducing morbidity and mortality from infections in cancer patients with fever and neutropenia.

Supportive Care

Supportive care is an essential component of therapy for childhood cancer: both the disease and its treatment can cause life-threatening complications. In advanced-stage lymphoid malignancies, expeditious treatment is required to correct severe metabolic derangements such as hyperuricemia, hypocalcemia, hyperphosphatemia, hyperkalemia, and lactic acidosis. Bone marrow function is often suppressed in children with cancer, requiring transfusions of blood products. In these immunosuppressed patients, irradiated blood products are given to prevent graft-versus-host disease. Intravenous broad-spectrum antibiotics are necessary to treat neutropenic patients with fever, who are also at risk for viral and fungal infections. With aggressive use of available antifungal agents, mortality from fungal infections has decreased. However, despite the prophylactic use of amphotericin B in patients with prolonged neutropenia and fever, some fungi are resistant and continue to be of particular concern when the children have received prolonged antibiotic therapy.

Control of chemotherapy-induced nausea and vomiting, proper nutrition, and adequate pain control are also important in the management of childhood cancer. Delivery of therapy has improved dramatically since the development of the indwelling vascular catheter and other venous access devices such as subcutaneous ports. These enable outpatient delivery of antibiotics under close medical supervision without compromising the patient's well-being.

Posttreatment follow-up is necessary. Unfortunately, therapy can produce serious late sequelae such as hormonal deficiency, neurologic dysfunction, hepatic cirrhosis, pulmonary fibrosis, cardiomyopathy, renal dysfunction, and hearing or visual impairment. Physicians should be familiar with drug-induced toxicities. Second malignancies are of particular concern and can occur 10 to 20 years after treatment. Therefore, children who have been treated for cancer should be followed carefully.

Both the patient and family need emotional support. This is especially true of adolescents, because of the physical changes and limitations imposed by treatment. Whenever possible, the child should remain in school and in the usual social settings. Honesty and a positive, hopeful attitude are important in dealing with patients and parents.

Non-Hodgkin's Lymphoma

Non-Hodgkin's lymphoma designates a heterogeneous group of malignant lymphoproliferative disorders that resemble Hodgkin's disease (HD) in clinical presentation, but differ in histology and clinical behavior. Follicular NHL, frequently seen in adults, is rare in children, who typically have diffuse, high-grade neoplasms.

Epidemiology

NHL occurs more frequently than does HD in children, and its incidence increases throughout childhood. Boys are affected two to three times more often than girls. Constitutional and acquired immune system aberrations have been linked to an increased risk of lymphomas. Childhood NHL (most often, B-cell lymphomas) is the neoplasm most commonly associated with inherited immunodeficiencies, including ataxia-telangiectasia, Wiskott-Aldrich syndrome, common variable immunodeficiency, severe combined immunodeficiency, isolated deficiencies of IgA and IgM, X-linked lymphoproliferative syndrome, Bloom syndrome, and other familial immunodeficiency states.[16] The incidence of lymphoma is also increased in immunosuppressed renal transplant recipients. Chronic immunostimulation by an infectious agent may cause uncontrolled proliferation of lymphoid cells in immunodeficient patients, eventually leading to lymphomatous transformation. For example, chronic immunostimulation by malarial parasites in Africa and intestinal parasites in the Middle East may be a factor in triggering NHL.

EBV has been associated with the African type of Burkitt's lymphoma. Tumor cells from these patients usually contain integrated viral DNA and express EBV nuclear antigens; patients have high antibody titers against the virus. Additionally, some cases of T-cell lymphoma and leukemia have been associated with human T-cell lymphotropic virus (HTLV-I).[3] NHL has also been found in patients with human immunodeficiency virus (HIV) infection.[17] Although the exact mechanisms that relate viral infection to the development of NHL are unknown, most cases of childhood NHL have no known predisposing factor.

Pathology and Classification

Most cases of childhood NHL fall into one of three major histologic groups: undifferentiated, or small noncleaved cell; lymphoblastic; and large-cell lymphomas (Table 32-3). All three groups are classified as diffuse high-grade lymphomas in the National Cancer Institute Working Formulation for clinical usage. A small proportion of NHLs have different histomorphologic features—a follicular or diffuse pattern with low- or intermediate-grade cytologic features. Common primary sites include lymph nodes, mediastinum, the ileocecal area, tonsils, adenoids, or Peyer's patches. A minority of cases involve the skin, bone, and other sites. Undifferentiated lymphomas are composed of small, round, noncleaved lymphoid cells that predominantly involve extranodal tissues such as the gastrointestinal tract, retroperitoneal and pelvic viscera, kidneys, gonads, jaws, thyroid gland, and CNS. The tumors invariably are of B-cell origin and typically display monoclonal surface immunoglobulin.

Lymphoblastic lymphomas are composed of small,

Table 32-3. Classification of Childhood Non-Hodgkin's Lymphoma

Histologic Subtype	Approximate Frequency	Immunophenotype
Undifferentiated (small noncleaved cell) Burkitt's Non-Burkitt's	30-40%	B
Lymphoblastic Convoluted Nonconvoluted	30-40%	Usually T, rarely pre-B
Large cell Cleaved cell Noncleaved cell Immunoblastic	20-30%	Usually B, few T, rarely of true histiocytic origin
Others	5-10%	

round, immature cells with scant cytoplasm lacking granules. These cells are indistinguishable morphologically from the blast cells of acute lymphoblastic leukemia. The immunophenotype of most childhood lymphoblastic lymphomas corresponds to that of the cortical thymocytes (T cells), predominantly at the middle or late stage of thymic differentiation. Thymus, lymph nodes, liver, spleen, and bone marrow are commonly involved. A minority of cases demonstrate pre-B-cell phenotype and primary sites generally involve the skin.

Large-cell lymphomas have been inappropriately termed histiocytic. Immunophenotypes are generally those of large transformed lymphocytes or immunoblasts; they are rarely derived from histiocytes. Most large-cell lymphomas are B cell-derived, but a minority have T-cell markers and some are devoid of identifiable surface characteristics.

Genetics

Advances in cytogenetics and molecular biology have helped to further explain the biology of NHL. Three different reciprocal chromosomal translocations have been detected in Burkitt's lymphoma and related B-cell NHL (Table 32-4). In most cases, the distal end of the long arm of chromosome 8 translocates to the long arm of chromosome 14[t(8;14)]. Alternatively, the translocation involves the same region of chromosome 8 and the long arm of chromosome 22 or the short arm of chromosome 2. In these translocations, transcriptional deregulation of the c-*myc* oncogene leads to uncontrolled expression of the gene, an apparently crucial step in malignant transformation.[18]

Table 32-4. Nonrandom Chromosomal Translocations in B-Cell and T-Cell Non-Hodgkin's Lymphoma

Immunophenotype	Karyotype
B cell	t(8;14)(q24.1;q32.3)
	t(8;22)(q24.1;q11)
	t(2;8)(p11-13;q24.1)
T cell	t(11;14)(p13;q11)
	t(11;14)(p15;q11)
	t(10;14)(q24;q11)
	t(1;14)(p32-p34;q11)
	t(8;14)(q24;q11)
	t(7;9)(q34;q32)
	t(7;9)(q34;q34.3)
	t(7;19)(q35;p13)
	t(1;7)(p34;q34)

In T-cell NHL, chromosomal aberrations have been detected in regions that encode polypeptide chains of the T-cell receptor antigen (Table 32-4). Research suggests that genes implicated in malignant cell transformation may be deregulated by the rearrangement of the T-cell receptor gene regions.[19]

Presentation and Diagnosis

In children, NHL can arise at any lymphoid tissue site. Most NHLs grow rapidly, with signs and symptoms typically emerging a few days to a few weeks before diagnosis. Painless, rapidly progressive lymphadenopathy in the head and neck region is a common presenting sign. The axilla or groin may also be primary sites. The nodes are nontender and firm. They are discrete in early phases of growth and later are often confluent. Anterior mediastinal masses may rapidly compress the airway or cause pleural effusion and signs of superior vena cava (SVC) obstruction, a medical emergency.

Gastrointestinal tumors, most commonly involving the distal ileum, appendix, or cecum, may produce symptoms of obstruction or mimic appendicitis. NHL can cause intussusception, and this possibility should be considered in the differential diagnosis of such conditions in children aged 5 or older. NHL is rapidly proliferative, with a high rate of spontaneous cell death and metastasis. As a result, patients frequently present with serious metabolic complications, including elevated serum levels of uric acid, phosphorus, and potassium.

Lymphoma of bone produces local or diffuse pain. Meningeal involvement may cause signs of increased intracranial pressure. Cranial nerve palsies and paraplegia from epidural compression may also be presenting signs. Primary intracerebral lymphoma occasionally develops, especially in immunodeficient patients.

The definitive diagnosis depends on biopsy findings; in general, the least invasive procedure should be used. Patients with massive mediastinal involvement may be poor candidates for surgery because of airway compression and SVC syndrome. Because these patients often have cervical or supraclavicular adenopathy, biopsies of these sites should be obtained under local anesthesia. Normal blood counts do not rule out bone marrow involvement; a bone marrow examination is mandatory before thoracotomy is considered. For patients with pleural effusion, thoracocentesis demonstrating malignant cells is often diagnostic. Similarly, cytologic examination of ascitic fluid or bone marrow may obviate the need for a surgical procedure in patients with massive abdominal lymphoma. If a diagnostic laparotomy is performed, however, an attempt should be made to excise all gross tumor.

A staging workup should precede therapy for NHL

and include a careful physical examination, complete blood count, tests of renal and hepatic function, chest radiograph, abdominal computed tomography (CT), examinations of bone marrow and spinal fluid, and a bone scan to determine the extent of disease. Staging laparotomy and splenectomy are not necessary.

The most common staging system (Murphy's staging) was developed at St Jude Children's Research Hospital, Memphis, Tenn. NHL localized in favorable sites is stage I disease. A single tumor with regional node involvement, a localized primary gastrointestinal tumor, or two tumors on the same side of the diaphragm represent stage II disease. Stage III includes disseminated disease on both sides of the diaphragm, extensive unresectable intra-abdominal disease, and all primary epidural or anterior mediastinal tumors without bone marrow or CNS involvement. Initial CNS or bone marrow involvement (≤25% blast cells) in addition to other tumor sites indicates stage IV.

Treatment and Prognosis

Appropriate treatment varies with the histologic type and disease stage. Surgery can establish the diagnosis by biopsy and can be used to excise localized lymphoma of bowel. Systemic chemotherapy has dramatically improved disease control and survival,[20] and all children, regardless of stage or histologic diagnosis, should receive combination chemotherapy. For the one third of patients with localized disease, excellent cure rates have been achieved with several treatment regimens. Ongoing clinical trials aim at reducing toxicity without compromising outcome. In a recent trial, 6 weeks of intensive therapy with prednisone, vincristine, cyclophosphamide, and doxorubicin followed by 6 months of maintenance therapy with 6-mercaptopurine and methotrexate, without radiation therapy, resulted in a 4-year disease-free survival of 85%.[21] CNS prophylaxis was not required in the absence of lymphoma of the head and neck. Another ongoing study evaluates the need for continuation chemotherapy in these patients.

Principles of therapy for advanced lymphoblastic lymphoma are similar to those for high-risk forms of childhood lymphoblastic leukemia. Current 2-year disease-free survival estimates are 60% to 75%.

Current management of advanced B-cell lymphoma is based on short-term (2 to 6 months) intensive combination chemotherapy. Regimens usually include high-dose cyclophosphamide, high-dose methotrexate, doxorubicin, cytarabine, vincristine, and intensive intrathecal chemoprophylaxis. Three-year survival rates have been reported to exceed 70%.[22]

Appropriate treatment for advanced large-cell lymphoma is less clear. In general, multidrug regimens have yielded 3-year survival rates of almost 70%, with a low risk of primary CNS relapse.

Outcome is extremely poor for patients who relapse while on therapy. However, current trials suggest that allogeneic or autologous bone marrow transplantation can cure a small fraction of patients.

The most reliable prognostic factors in childhood NHL are stage of disease at diagnosis and serum levels of lactic dehydrogenase (LDH). The latter is a reliable indicator of the total burden of malignant cells. Children with CNS involvement at diagnosis have a particularly unfavorable outcome. It has recently been reported that the serum interleukin-2 receptor level has independent prognostic value, even after adjustment for disease stage and LDH level.[23] Serum interleukin-2 receptors may compete for ligands with cellular receptors, suppressing the host antitumor response.

Hodgkin's Disease

Hodgkin's disease is a malignant lymphoma possessing features of a neoplasm, an infectious granulomatous disease, and an immunologic disorder. HD is considered a malignancy because the giant cells have clonal aneuploid karyotypes and produce tumors in athymic mice.[24] Nonmalignant reactions to the tumor cells cause heterogeneous cellular infiltration.

Epidemiology

In the United States, HD is rare in children younger than 5 years, but gradually increases in frequency. In children younger than 15, the annual incidence is 7 per million. The disease has a bimodal age distribution, with peaks between ages 15 and 34 and above age 60. From ages 5 to 11, boys outnumber girls by 3:1. After age 15, the ratio falls to 1.5:1 due to a relative increase in incidence among females at the time of puberty.

Better socioeconomic conditions are associated with later onset in the younger subgroup and a shift of histologic subtypes. In Third World countries and lower socioeconomic groups, peak incidence occurs in the early teens and the mixed-cellularity subtype predominates. Close relatives of patients with HD have a modestly increased risk of developing the disease, and many cases of familial HD have been described. Surveys have found some degree of association between HD and specific human leukocyte antigens (HLA). Neighbor-pairs and occasional clusters have also been reported. Although the cause is not yet established, genetic susceptibility and some environmental agents, including viruses, may influence the development of HD.

Pathology and Classification

HD arises in lymph nodes in 99% of cases. Malignant cells normally occupy less than 1% of involved tissue, a feature that makes their isolation and study difficult. These cells, collectively called Hodgkin's cells, include the classic Reed-Sternberg (RS) cells and their mononuclear variants. Cells resembling RS cells have been reported in infectious mononucleosis, rubeola, and phenytoin-induced pseudolymphomatous adenopathy. Thus, examination by an experienced hematopathologist is essential for accurate diagnosis.

The histologic features may include sparse to abundant neoplastic, inflammatory, reactive, and stromal cells, as well as lymphocytes, collagen, and fibrous tissue. The Rye classification includes four major histologic categories: lymphocyte-predominant, nodular sclerosing, mixed-cellularity, and lymphocyte-depleted HD.

In the lymphocyte-predominant subtype (10% to 20% of patients), almost all cells appear to be mature lymphocytes or a mixture of lymphocytes and benign histiocytes, with only an occasional RS cell. This subtype is associated with low-stage disease and has the best prognosis.

In nodular sclerosing HD (50% of patients), islands of RS cells and associated lymphocytes, eosinophils, and histiocytes are surrounded by fibrotic areas. Clear spaces surround so-called lacunar cells, which are variants of the RS cell. Radiographic evidence of response to therapy may be slow to appear due to the amount of collagen in these lesions, especially in the mediastinum. Nodular sclerosing HD is typically regional, most frequently involving the anterosuperior mediastinum and the scalene, supraclavicular, and lower cervical regions.

Mixed-cellularity HD (30% of patients) is characterized by large numbers of RS cells. Foci of necrosis may be present, and extranodal involvement is common.

Lymphocyte-depleted HD occurs in fewer than 10% of patients. RS cells predominate in the cellular infiltrates of lymph nodes. Associated with advanced disease, this histologic type has a relatively poor prognosis.

The cell of origin in HD is unidentified and controversial. Conflicting studies suggest that the Hodgkin's cell is the neoplastic counterpart of interdigitating reticulum cells,[25] and that it is of lymphoid or phagocytic origin.[26] Others propose that it arises from a primitive stem cell.

Immunology

More than 50% of patients with HD demonstrate defective cell-mediated immunity by impaired reaction to delayed-hypersensitivity skin testing, impaired ability to reject skin homografts, and depressed responses to T-cell mitogens in vitro. The depressed cellular immunity associated with HD has been attributed to intrinsic lymphocyte abnormalities, immunosuppressive factors in serum or plasma, increased suppressor monocyte activity, and increased suppressor T-cell activity.[27] The presence of familial decreased cellular immunity suggests that HD is more likely to develop in hosts with defective immunity. Immunodeficiency is greater in advanced disease, less favorable histologic subtypes, and disease progression or recurrence. Radiation therapy and chemotherapy worsen the impairment, which can persist even in long-term unmaintained remission. The lymphocyte surrounding the RS cells are primarily CD4-positive helper/ inducer cells, and there is a corresponding decrease of these cells in circulating blood. It is unclear whether this is a primary or reactive phenomenon. High serum levels of CD8 antigen, a surface membrane component of suppressor/cytotoxic T cells, have recently been correlated with advanced disease.[28]

Presentation and Diagnosis

More than 90% of patients with HD present with painless, unexplained lymphadenopathy involving cervical (60% to 80%), axillary (6% to 20%), or inguinal nodes (6% to 12%). Nodes, usually firm and discrete, may be noticed by the patient, parents, or caretaker. There is characteristically no regional inflammation to explain the lymphadenopathy. The growth rate of the lymph nodes is variable and they may enlarge or shrink. Signs and symptoms may present a few weeks to many months before diagnosis. Twenty percent to 30% of children present with fatigue, fever, weight loss, night sweats, and pruritus; the likelihood of systemic (or B) symptoms increases with the clinical extent of disease. Fever may be cyclic, continuous, or intermittent. Rarely, classic Pel-Ebstein fever occurs. These 1- to 2-week cycles of high fever are separated by afebrile intervals of similar duration.

The tumor spreads initially to contiguous lymphoid areas and then hematogenously to extranodal organs such as the liver, lung, bone marrow, and CNS. Mediastinal or hilar disease is present in approximately 50% of patients and may cause dyspnea, cough, dysphagia, and SVC compression. Although early liver involvement is associated with intrahepatic biliary obstruction and later involvement with hepatocellular disease, hepatosplenomegaly does not indicate organ involvement. Bone marrow involvement may result in pancytopenia. The tumor can occasionally extend through neural foramina to compress the spinal cord, causing paraparesis or quadriparesis.

Patients with suspected HD should undergo careful clinical and laboratory examination as well as diagnostic imaging to define the extent of disease. Laboratory studies should include a complete blood count, erythrocyte sedimentation rate, and routine liver and renal function tests. Blood counts are normal in localized HD, but progressive disease may be accompanied by neutrophilic leukocytosis, microcytic hypochromic anemia, thrombocytopenia, and lymphopenia. Elevations in sedimentation rate and serum copper or ferritin levels are useful indicators of active disease; they fall to normal levels at remission and are followed to detect early recurrence. Bone marrow biopsy is necessary to determine bone marrow involvement.

Diagnostic imaging is an important staging tool. (Table 32-5 shows the current staging system for HD.[29]) Thoracic CT is crucial for accurate assessment of the extent of disease in the chest and mediastinum. Magnetic resonance imaging (MRI) may provide greater detail of a mediastinal mass. Abdominal-pelvic CT and pedal lymphangiography are complementary in evaluating the extent of disease below the diaphragm. In young children, CT does not clearly show abnormal retroperitoneal lymph nodes. Bipedal lymphangiography does not delineate the celiac nodes but enables visualization of the retroperitoneal nodes. However, patients with massive mediastinal lymphadenopathy or parenchymal pulmonary involvement are at high risk of oil embolism following injection of contrast medium. Skeletal surveys, liver-spleen scans, bone scans, gallium scans, and intravenous pyelography generally have limited utility in staging.

Although the role of staging laparotomy with splenectomy is controversial, it is recommended in patients with clinically localized disease for whom radiotherapy alone is a treatment option. Surgical findings advance the disease staging in one third of children. Preoperative polyvalent pneumococcal vaccine is recommended for patients undergoing splenectomy. A staging laparotomy is not essential for patients receiving combined-modality therapy.

Table 32-5. Staging of Hodgkin's Disease*

Stage	Criteria
I	Involvement of a single lymph node region (I) or of a single extralymphatic organ or site (I_E).
II	Involvement of two or more lymph node regions on the same side of the diaphragm (II) or localized involvement of extralymphatic organ or site and one or more lymph node regions on the same side of the diaphragm (II_E).
III	Involvement of lymph node regions on both sides of the diaphragm (III), which may be accompanied by localized involvement of an extralymphatic organ or site (III_E), by involvement of the spleen (III_S), or both (III_{SE}).**
IV	Diffuse or disseminated involvement of one or more extralymphatic organs or tissues with or without associated lymph node enlargement.

*Each stage can be subdivided into A (no systemic symptoms) or B (systemic symptoms). B symptoms include one of the following: unexplained loss of more than 10% of body weight in the 6 months before admission, unexplained fever with temperatures >38°C, and night sweats.

**Stage III disease has been subdivided into Stage III_1, in which disease is limited to the upper abdomen (spleen; splenic, celiac, or portal nodes), and Stage III_2, which includes all other intra-abdominal nodes (mesenteric, para-aortic, iliac), with or without upper abdominal involvement.

Adapted from Carbone et al.[29]

Treatment and Prognosis

Radiotherapy and chemotherapy are both highly effective in the treatment of HD; however, radiotherapy in children has two major disadvantages. First, staging laparotomy with splenectomy is often necessary to establish the extent of disease and define radiotherapy fields. Second, effective radiation doses disturb musculoskeletal growth. In younger children, extended-field radiation can be unacceptably disfiguring. However, the use of radiation therapy averts the toxicity and late effects of chemotherapy.

The MOPP regimen [mechlorethamine, Oncovin (vincristine), procarbazine, and prednisone] developed at the National Cancer Institute[30] has been the cornerstone of therapy for HD. An alternative, non-cross-resistant four-drug combination, ABVD [Adriamycin (doxorubicin), bleomycin, vinblastine, and dacarbazine] is as effective as MOPP in untreated patients with advanced HD, and produces a 75% complete response rate in patients unresponsive to MOPP.[31] Secondary leukemia and sterility can occur after the MOPP regimen, and cardiopulmonary dysfunction is a potential sequela of the ABVD regimen.

Radiation therapy alone has been traditionally used for stage I or IIA disease; chemotherapy with or without radiation has been used for stage IIB, III, or IV disease. To obviate the need for staging laparotomy and to avert the adverse musculoskeletal effects of more extensive radiotherapy, some studies use combined modalities for clinically low-stage disease. Because local recurrence may follow chemotherapy alone, some investigators give involved-field low-dose radiation to large tumors in advanced disease. The optimal treatment regimen for HD uses the minimum therapy necessary for cure.

Because of the immune defects associated with HD, children are particularly susceptible to a variety of infections, such as herpes zoster and *Pneumocystis carinii* pneumonia. Fever may be the only sign of overwhelming sepsis in children who have been splenectomized. Prompt cultures and antibiotic therapy are mandatory until bacteremia has been ruled out. Physicians should also recognize other potential long-term sequelae of treatment, such as thyroid dysfunction, pericarditis, pulmonary fibrosis, ovarian and testicular failure, growth retardation, and second malignancies.

Progress in the treatment of HD has yielded an initial complete remission rate of more than 90% and a cure rate approaching 80%. Currently, the stage of disease and type of treatment are the most important prognostic factors. The serum interleukin-2 receptor and CD8 antigen levels have important prognostic value and appear to be biologic markers of aggressive disease.[28,32]

Neuroblastoma

Neuroblastoma presents a formidable therapeutic challenge because of its relative frequency and its age-related behavior. This tumor is aggressive in older children, but often pursues a paradoxically benign course in infants and occasionally can regress spontaneously. There is a high incidence of neuroblastoma in situ in infants younger than 3 months. Autopsies performed on infants who died of other causes showed that 0.5% had clusters of primitive neuroblasts in the adrenal gland.[33] The incidence of clinically apparent neuroblastoma is approximately 40-fold less than this figure would indicate. Moreover, autopsies of older children fail to demonstrate either neuroblastoma in situ or active neuroblastoma. Thus, neuroblastoma in situ may represent normal embryonic structures that usually disappear without progression.

Epidemiology

Neuroblastoma is the most common extracranial solid tumor in childhood, accounting for 6% to 8% of all pediatric malignancies; yet it causes 15% of pediatric cancer deaths. Half of all neonatal malignancies and 30% of infant cancers are neuroblastomas; congenital and even fetal neuroblastomas have been described. Approximately 50% of neuroblastomas are diagnosed during the first 2 years of life, and more than two thirds are diagnosed during the first 5 years. It is slightly more common in white children and more frequent in boys. Approximately 50 cases of familial neuroblastoma have been reported. There may be an association between neuroblastoma and neural crest-derived disorders such as neurofibromatosis, pheochromocytoma, tuberous sclerosis, Hirschsprung's disease, and heterochromia of the iris. There is a remarkably low incidence of neuroblastoma in the Burkitt's lymphoma belt of Africa.

Pathology and Classification

Neuroblastoma arises in pluripotent neural crest cells of the sympathetic nervous system. These cells (sympathogonia) may develop into ganglion cells, pheochromocytes, or neurofibrous tissue. Neural crest tumors reflect different stages of differentiation and include neuroblastoma, ganglioneuroblastoma, ganglioneuroma, pheochromocytoma, and neurofibroma. There are reports that neuroblastomas have evolved into ganglioneuroblastomas or ganglioneuromas spontaneously or following chemotherapy or radiation therapy.

Neuroblastoma is one of the "small, blue, round cell" tumors of childhood. It can be difficult to differentiate pathologically from lymphoma, rhabdomyosarcoma, Ewing's sarcoma, and peripheral neuroepithelioma. Aids to diagnosis include clinical presentation, electron microscopy, immunohistochemistry profile (such as desmin, actin, and neuron-specific enolase levels), chromosomal studies showing a deletion of the short arm of chromosome 1, N-*myc* oncogene amplification, elevated urinary catecholamine levels, and the presence of rosette formation or neurofibrils on histologic examinations. In contrast to Ewing's sarcoma and rhabdomyosarcoma, neuroblastomas do not contain glycogen and therefore are negative for periodic acid-Schiff stain. Electron microscopy reveals distinctive peripheral dendritic processes containing longitudinally oriented microtubules and small, spherical, membrane-bound neurosecretory granules with electron-dense cores resulting from cytoplasmic accumulation of catecholamines. Shimada and associates have described a histopathologic classification for neuroblastomas based on the degree of tumor cell differentiation and the stromal tissue organization pattern.[34]

Genetics

Some neuroblastomas are characterized cytogenetically by deletions of the short arm of chromosome 1 (or partial monosomy of the short arm of chromosome 1 in the region 1p32-1pter) and by evidence of gene amplification in the form of DM chromosomes or chromosomal HSRs.[35] One or more genes in the short arm of chromosome 1 may be important to the normal regulation of growth and differentiation in neuroblasts. Deletion or inactivation of this putative neuroblastoma suppressor gene on both chromosomes is associated with malignant transformation. However, deletion of 1p has yet to be identified as a constitutional abnormality predisposing to neuroblastoma.

Extrachromosomal DMs are found in 20% to 30% of primary tumors and almost 50% of neuroblastoma cell lines. HSRs are rarely described in primary neuroblastomas but are found in more than half of established cell lines. Degenerated HSRs may form DMs, which in turn reintegrate into chromosomes in an apparently nonspecific distribution to reform HSRs. Because of its homology to the c-*myc* oncogene, the amplified DNA segment in neuroblastoma cells is designated N-*myc*; its normal location is on chromosome 2. Although the mechanism of amplification is unknown, there is excellent correlation between the presence of DMs or HSRs and N-*myc* amplification, which is associated with advanced disease stage, rapid progression, and poor prognosis.[36] Tumors that have a single copy of N-*myc* per cell at diagnosis rarely, if ever, develop amplification later in the disease course. Thus, tumors with N-*myc* amplification represent a genetically distinct subset of neuroblastomas.

Immunology

Neuroblastoma may elicit both cell-mediated and humoral immune responses. Some patients have been shown to produce specific cytotoxic lymphocytes against neuroblastoma. A relatively favorable prognosis is correlated with a high circulating lymphocyte count, high percentage of lymphoblasts in the bone marrow, and increased lymphoid infiltrates in the tumor itself. Some patients produce antibodies against neuroblastoma-associated antigens. However, immune responses may also interfere with tumor control. Some patients with advanced neuroblastoma appear to have a serum "blocking factor" that inhibits the effect of cytotoxic lymphocytes. Although immuno-therapy has not yet proven beneficial in neuroblastoma, these findings suggest that manipulation of the immune system may offer a future therapeutic advantage.

Presentation and Diagnosis

The signs and symptoms of neuroblastoma consist of localized problems arising from growth of the primary tumor or metastases. Neuroblastoma can originate anywhere in the sympathetic nervous system. The most common primary site is intra-abdominal, in either the adrenal gland (40%) or a paraspinal ganglion (25%). Less frequent primary sites include the thorax (15%), pelvis (5%), and neck (4%). Tumors also may arise in unusual sites, including the nasopharynx (esthesioneuroblastoma), liver, kidney, and intracranial region. In rare cases the primary site is unidentifiable.

A firm abdominal mass that crosses the midline is often the first sign of disease. Large abdominal masses can cause leg edema (venous compression) and hypertension (from stretching of the renal vasculature). Abdominal distention may result from an enlarging primary tumor or from hepatic tumor invasion; extensive liver involvement can cause respiratory distress. Abdominal enlargement may be asymptomatic, but is usually associated with anorexia, malaise, vague abdominal pain, and sometimes diarrhea. Thoracic masses are usually found coincidentally unless their size causes respiratory symptoms. The presence of Horner's syndrome, heterochromia iridis, or aniridia should prompt an evaluation to rule out neuroblastoma. Paraspinal tumors that invade the spinal foramina can cause spinal cord compression with paresis, paralysis, and bladder or bowel dysfunction. This oncologic emergency requires immediate treatment. Skin nodules are seen almost exclusively in infants and are usually nontender, bluish, and mobile.

Eighty percent of children older than 1 year who have neuroblastoma present with disseminated disease; symptoms include pallor, irritability, weakness, limping, and ecchymoses around the eyes. The most common sites of metastasis are the lymph nodes, bone marrow, and bone. Less frequent sites include the liver, skin, and orbit. Some patients present with intractable diarrhea due to tumor secretion of vasoactive intestinal polypeptide, an enterohormone. Rarely, patients present with a cerebellar encephalopathy (opsoclonus-myoclonus syndrome) characterized by progressive ataxia and titubation of the head, myoclonic jerks, chaotic conjugate jerking movements of the eyes, and progressive dementia. Systemic syndromes (diarrhea and opsoclonus-myoclonus) may occur at any stage and do not indicate disseminated disease or a poor prognosis.

An evaluation for suspected neuroblastoma includes a complete blood count, skeletal survey, chest x-ray, bone scan, bone marrow examination, coagulation screen, liver and kidney function tests, and urinary catecholamine determination. For abdominal tumors, CT has replaced intravenous pyelograms, arteriograms, inferior venacavograms, and ultrasonograms. Helpful findings on imaging include stippled calcifications within the tumor (80% of cases), displacement of the kidney with little or no pyelocalyceal distortion, and occasionally hydronephrosis due to ureteral compression. On CT, neuroblastomas generally show mixed solid and cystic components as a result of hemorrhage or necrosis. CT of the head, orbit, chest, and abdomen assists in disease staging. MRI is superior to CT for evaluating epidural spinal cord compression, and may be obtained in conjunction with a metrizamide myelogram. Diagnostic imaging with meta-[^{131}I]-iodobenzylguanidine (MIBG) may be a useful adjunct to other procedures. MIBG is taken up by adrenergic secretory vesicles and undergoes the same cellular processing as norepinephrine. In most patients, MIBG is taken up by the primary tumor and metastases.

Many neuroblastomas are characterized by excessive production and excretion of catecholamines and their metabolites, vanillylmandelic acid (VMA), metanephrine, and homovanillic acid (HVA). A VMA/HVA ratio >1:5 is believed to correlate with a better prognosis, as is a low level of cystathione excretion. Elevated levels of other serum markers (LDH, ferritin, and neuron-specific enolase) are generally associated with more advanced disease and poor outcome.

Table 32-6 describes the most commonly used staging systems.[37] The Evans staging system is based on tumor size and extent, and does not include lymph node status, operability, or completeness of removal. The Pediatric Oncology Group staging system is based partially on clinical and radiologic findings; for localized disease, it is based entirely on surgical and pathologic findings. A new staging system has been proposed that incorporates elements of current systems and standardizes criteria for response to treatment,[38] but it has not been evaluated prospectively. Of special interest is the clinical course of infants with apparently widely disseminated disease (Evans stage IV-S) whose tumors may completely regress even in the absence of systemic therapy. Stage IV-S disease is associated with low serum ferritin levels and generally lacks N-*myc* oncogene amplification. Although investigators have suggested that stage IV-S neuroblastoma is a benign polyclonal proliferative disorder, its clonal and hyperdiploid nature has been demonstrated.[37] Both characteristics are accepted criteria of malignancy.

Table 32-6. Staging Systems for Neuroblastoma

Stage	Criteria
Evans Staging	
I	Tumors confined to the organ or structure of origin.
II	Tumors extending in continuity beyond the origin or structure of origin but not crossing the midline; regional lymph nodes on the ipsilateral side may be involved.
III	Tumors extending in continuity beyond the midline; regional lymph nodes may be involved bilaterally.
IV	Remote disease involving the skeleton, parenchymatous organs, soft tissue, distant lymph node groups.
IV-S	Patients who would otherwise be stage I/II but who have remote disease confined to liver, skin, or bone marrow and who have no radiologic evidence of bone metastases on complete skeletal survey.
Pediatric Oncology Group Staging	
A	Complete gross excision of primary tumor, margins histologically negative or positive. Intracavitary lymph nodes not intimately adherent to and removed with resected tumor must be histologically free of tumor. If primary tumor is in the abdomen (includes pelvis), liver must be free of tumor.
B	Incomplete gross resection of primary tumor. Lymph nodes and liver must be histologically free of tumor as in stage A.
C	Complete or incomplete gross resection of primary tumor. Intracavitary nodes* histologically positive for tumor. Liver histologically free of tumor.
D	Disseminated disease beyond intracavitary nodes.

*Intracavitary nodes are those in the same cavity as the primary tumor.

Adapted from Bowman et al.[37]

Treatment and Prognosis

More than 90% of clinically localized tumors can be cured by excision of the primary tumor mass.[37] The presence of microscopic residual tumor does not affect outcome, and the addition of adjuvant chemotherapy or radiation therapy does not improve the excellent cure rate. The outlook for patients with unresectable localized disease (regardless of age) is also excellent, with a 3-year disease-free survival of more than 80%.[37] For unresectable regional disease, the degree and nature of local extension should be established by regional lymph node and liver biopsies.

The agents most active against neuroblastoma are cyclophosphamide, doxorubicin, cisplatin, teniposide, and etoposide. Experimental treatments include targeted radiotherapy using MIBG or monoclonal antibodies as carriers, bone marrow transplantation, and biologic response modifiers. Phase II trials of MIBG therapy have been conducted, but, owing to the myelotoxicity of the regimen in patients with bone marrow involvement there have been no Phase III trials. High-dose chemotherapy followed by autologous bone marrow rescue may improve the outlook for these patients, but this has not been definitely demonstrated.

The most important prognostic factors in neuroblastoma are the disease stage and patient's age at diagnosis. Children with low-stage disease have a good prognosis, regardless of age.[37] Infants (younger than 1 year at diagnosis) generally do well regardless of stage.[36] In contrast, children older than 1 with advanced disease fare poorly (20% long-term survival), despite the use of very high-dose chemotherapy with autologous bone marrow rescue.[13] Among infants, the DNA index appears to be the most important prognostic factor regardless of disease stage. More than 90% of infants with a DNA index above 1.0 achieve 3-year disease-free survival with relatively nonintensive chemotherapy.[39] Infants with a DNA index of 1.0 have a 3-year disease-free survival of 48% with current therapy.[39] This is the first disease in which a biologic feature (the DNA index) has been used to select therapy.

Because neuroblastoma is highly sensitive to antineoplastic drugs, chemotherapy followed by second-look surgery is preferable to attempts to remove large or invasive tumors at diagnosis. Recent evidence suggests that radiotherapy may benefit patients with regional lymph node involvement. Improved treatment strategies are clearly needed for children older than 1 year with metastatic disease at diagnosis.

Wilms' Tumor

Wilms' tumor, or nephroblastoma, is a malignant embryonal neoplasm of the kidney that occurs most frequently in young children. It was the first childhood cancer in which combined surgery, radiation therapy, and chemotherapy achieved significant cure rates. Treatment programs guided by a surgicopathologic staging system and recognition of prognostically significant histologic subtypes maximize cure rates and minimize toxicity for most patients. The overall cure rate is now more than 80%.[40]

Epidemiology

The incidence of Wilms' tumor is remarkably constant throughout the world and has been used as a standard against which to measure the incidences of other tumors. In the US the annual incidence is 5.0 to 7.8 per million children younger than 15 years. Boys and girls are affected equally. Most children at diagnosis are 1 to 5 years old (median, 3.1 years); 90% of cases occur before age 7. The tumor is rare below the age of 8 months; in these infants most primary renal tumors are benign mesoblastic nephromas. The 5% to 10% of patients who have bilateral disease are significantly younger than those with unilateral tumors.[41] Because some very young patients who present with a single tumor progress to bilateral involvement, the contralateral kidney should be carefully followed in young children for at least 3 to 4 years.[41]

Wilms' tumor occurs in both heritable and sporadic forms. The heritable form develops at an earlier age and is more likely to be bilateral and multicentric. All bilateral and approximately 20% of unilateral cases represent a heritable disease; inheritance is autosomal dominant with incomplete (approximately 40%) penetrance. It is estimated that 8% of the offspring of patients with unilateral, unifocal disease and 20% to 30% of the offspring of those with bilateral or known familial disease will develop Wilms' tumor.

About 15% of patients have associated congenital anomalies, including genitourinary anomalies (5%), hemihypertrophy (2%), and aniridia (1%); these occur more frequently in patients with bilateral disease. Genitourinary anomalies associated with Wilms' tumor include ectopic and solitary kidney, horseshoe kidneys, ureteral duplication, hypospadias, and cryptorchidism. Hemihypertrophy, usually idiopathic, may occur ipsilateral or contralateral to the tumor site and may be present at diagnosis or emerge later. Wilms' tumor has been noted in children and siblings of patients with hemihypertrophy.

Patients with Beckwith-Wiedemann syndrome (omphalocele, macroglossia, and visceromegaly) have a 10% risk of neoplasm; in one report, 6 of 14 neoplasms in these patients were Wilms' tumor. Sporadic bilateral aniridia occurs in 1% of patients with Wilms' tumor, compared with 0.01% of the general population. Children with sporadic aniridia have a 1:3 chance of developing Wilms' tumor and should have frequent examinations with abdominal ultrasonography. Familial aniridia is more common than sporadic aniridia but is rarely associated with Wilms' tumor. Several cases of neurofibromatosis associated with Wilms' tumor have been described.

Pathology and Classification

Most Wilms' tumors contain a mixture of blastemal (undifferentiated spindle cells), epithelial differentiation (tubules), and stromal histologic elements. Abortive glomeruli, smooth and striated muscle, myxomatous tissue, fat, bone, or cartilage may also appear.

Three important histologic variants of Wilms' tumor have been identified by light microscopy: nephroblastomatosis (25%), mesoblastic nephroma (8%), and focal anaplasia (5%).[42] The presence of nephroblastomatosis (foci of persistent blastemal cells, which appear as subcapsular nodules or as sheets of primitive metanephric epithelium) correlates with subsequent development of Wilms' tumor in the remaining renal parenchyma, mandating close surveillance.[42] Mesoblastic nephroma is benign and generally curable by nephrectomy alone. Tumors with focal or diffuse anaplasia (characterized by cellular pleomorphism, nuclear enlargement, hyperchromatism, and the presence of bizarre mitotic figures) are much less responsive to therapy than those with other histologic features.[42] Children with anaplastic Wilms' tumor are generally 1 to 2 years older at diagnosis, are more likely to be black, and experience more frequent local recurrence and pulmonary metastasis. Hyperdiploidy and complex chromosomal rearrangements are characteristic of anaplastic tumors.[43] Clear cell sarcoma of the kidney and malignant rhabdoid tumor, formerly classified as variants of Wilms' tumor, are now considered distinct entities requiring different therapeutic approaches.[42]

Genetics

Several chromosomal anomalies, including 11p-, trisomy 8, trisomy 18, and XX/XY mosaicism, have been associated with Wilms' tumor. Interstitial deletion of chromosome 11 at band p13 (11p13), which is associated with aniridia, ambiguous genitalia, and mental retardation, defines the aniridia-Wilms' tumor association (AWTA). Deletions or rearrangements involving the short arm of chromosome 11, including 11p13, may occur in 30% to 40% of cases.[44] These relationships suggest the existence of a Wilms' tumor suppressor gene in the 11p13 band. In DNA analysis, Wilms' tumor cells from patients with normal constitutional phenotype and genotype have demonstrated loss of genetic material and resultant homozygosity in the 11p region.[45] The chromosomal events leading to

11p homozygosity may constitute the second "hit" in the Knudson model of tumorigenesis.

Presentation and Diagnosis

Eighty-five percent of patients present with an abdominal or flank mass first noticed by a parent or caretaker. Abdominal pain occurs in 40% and is severe enough in about 10% to suggest an acute surgical abdomen. Hypertension, usually mild, is found in 60% to 90% of patients and is often associated with elevated plasma renin levels. About one fourth have fever, sometimes in association with urinary tract infection. Although gross hematuria is rare, about one third of children have microscopic hematuria. Rarer symptoms include weight loss, nausea, vomiting, anorexia, bone pain, dysuria, and polyuria. Metastatic disease is unusual, but when present typically involves the lung and liver.

The laboratory examination of a patient with suspected Wilms' tumor includes a complete blood count, liver and kidney function tests, chest x-rays, and CT of the chest and abdomen. On unenhanced CT, Wilms' tumor appears as a nonhomogeneous mass with areas of low density indicating necrosis. Areas of hemorrhage and small focal calcifications are less common and less prominent than in neuroblastoma. Contrast medium shows a slight tumor enhancement, with sharp demarcation from normal renal parenchyma. CT can be used to establish the intrarenal origin of the tumor, determine the extent of tumor, detect multiple masses, and evaluate the opposite kidney. Abdominal ultrasound can evaluate patency of the inferior vena cava and differentiate solid from cystic masses. Intravenous pyelography is no longer considered essential; if it is performed, characteristic findings include intrarenal distortion of calices and displacement of the urinary collection system; the kidney may not be visible. Chest CT is more sensitive than chest x-ray in detecting metastasis, but about half the lesions found are benign.

Although serum LDH and renin levels may be elevated, neither elevation is sensitive or specific for Wilms' tumor. Certain rare paraneoplastic syndromes may be associated with Wilms' tumor: the neoplasm may produce erythropoietin leading to polycythemia, and secondary hypercalcemia has been reported.

Surgery remains the primary means of diagnosing, staging, and treating Wilms' tumor. It often provides adequate local therapy. The procedure should be performed by an experienced pediatric surgeon or urologist, using a transabdominal approach. Ideally, the tumor-bearing kidney is removed with the capsule intact; the abdominal cavity is then examined thoroughly, with biopsy of adjacent lymph nodes and any suspicious areas in the liver or contralateral kidney. The disease stage is determined by the surgical findings and the pathologist's gross and microscopic findings.

Preoperative chemotherapy or radiotherapy has been advocated as a means of shrinking very large tumors and facilitating surgical removal. However, the use of preoperative therapy is associated with a 6% misdiagnosis rate, changes in histologic pattern, and alteration of eventual stage due to resolution of intra-abdominal metastases. Table 32-7 shows the staging system used by the National Wilms' Tumor Study (NWTS) group.

Treatment and Prognosis

Treatment should begin with transabdominal radical nephrectomy, including abdominal exploration with staging. The transabdominal approach has the advantage of providing adequate exposure, permitting thorough exploration of the abdominal contents and opposite kidney, and allowing a sweeping dissection of the attached renal fossa, thus facilitating removal of the involved kidney and associated lymph nodes. Careful attention to the inferior vena cava and renal vein is required to avoid dislodging any tumor that may be propagating intraluminally. Second-look surgery following chemotherapy or radiotherapy may be useful in patients with a massive unresectable tumor at diagnosis or bilateral tumors. This procedure can either document a complete response or convert a partial response to a complete response by removing residual tumor.

Table 32-7. Clinical Staging of Wilms' Tumor*

Stage	Criteria
I	Tumor limited to the kidney and completely excised.
II	Microscopic residual tumor. Tumor completely excised but penetrates through the capsule into perirenal soft tissues. Local spillage of tumor is confined to the flank.
III	Gross residual tumor confined to the abdomen (lymph node involvement, diffuse peritoneal contamination, peritoneal implants, tumor extends beyond the surgical margins, tumor incompletely excised).
IV	Hematogenous metastases to lung, noncontiguous liver, bone, or brain.
V	Bilateral involvement at diagnosis.

*The patient should be characterized by both disease stage and tumor histology (eg, stage II, unfavorable histology or stage III, favorable histology). Sarcomatous or anaplastic (focal or diffuse) histologic subtypes are unfavorable.

Adapted from D'Angio et al.[40]

Only three chemotherapeutic agents are clearly effective for Wilms' tumor: vincristine, dactinomycin, and doxorubicin. Therapy is traditionally based on the disease stage. Patients with gross total resection (approximately 70%) do not require radiation therapy; vincristine and dactinomycin therapy for 3 to 6 months yields a 2-year disease-free survival of approximately 90%. If there is gross residual disease after surgery, radiotherapy (1,000 cGy) to the tumor bed is necessary, and Adriamycin is added as a third drug. There is a 2-year disease-free survival rate of 83% with this therapy among the 20% of patients with stage III disease.[40] The 9% of patients with metastatic disease (Stage IV) have a 70% two-year disease-free survival with the three drugs plus radiotherapy (1,200 cGy) to all involved sites. Optimal therapy for patients with anaplastic histologic features remains unclear, although the addition of cyclophosphamide may be beneficial.

Treatment of bilateral disease is complicated by the need to preserve functional kidney tissue. Various approaches have been used: nephrectomy of the more involved kidney plus heminephrectomy or biopsy of the other; bilateral heminephrectomy; and bilateral biopsy followed by chemotherapy and second-look surgery. Combined chemotherapy and low-dose radiation therapy (1,200 to 1,500 cGy) have produced a 3-year survival rate of 75%.[41]

Therapy for recurrent disease should be based on the time and site of relapse, tumor histology, and treatment history. A complete reevaluation is recommended. Surgery should be strongly considered to confirm the diagnosis and remove all gross recurrent disease, especially in apparently isolated pulmonary recurrence. Radiation should be considered for all previously unirradiated sites of recurrence. Doxorubicin, cyclophosphamide, or a combination of the two may be given to patients who have not received them previously. Ifosfamide, etoposide, carboplatin, and cisplatin are also useful for recurrent Wilms' tumor. Intensive salvage therapy will produce a 30% 3-year postrelapse survival.[46]

In general, patients under 2 years of age whose tumors weigh <250 g have a favorable prognosis. The most important indicators of poor prognosis are histologic anaplasia and advanced stage. Hyperdiploidy, multiple complex translocations, and multiple tumor cell stem lines also confer a poor prognosis and may reflect genetic instability of tumor cells, which increases the likelihood of drug resistance.[43]

Rhabdomyosarcoma

Rhabdomyosarcoma (RMS) is the most common pediatric soft tissue tumor, representing 5% of childhood malignancies. Although described as a tumor of striated muscle origin, it probably arises from primitive or undifferentiated mesenchyme with the capacity to differentiate into muscle. These tumors can originate virtually anywhere in the body.

Epidemiology

The annual incidence of RMS in the US is 4.4 per million white and 1.3 per million black children younger than 15 years. RMS has a bimodal age distribution with peaks at ages 2 to 6 and 15 to 19. In the younger patient group, primary tumors occur primarily in the head and neck region and genitourinary tract (prostate, bladder, and vagina). Among adolescents, tumors are often seen in the male genitourinary tract, particularly in the testes or paratesticular tissue. The male-to-female ratio is 1.4:1.

RMS has been associated with neurofibromatosis, fetal alcohol syndrome, and Gorlin's (basal cell nevus) syndrome. Relatives of children with RMS have a high frequency of carcinoma of the breast and other sites. Cases of RMS are often found in "cancer families," in which there is a high incidence of sarcoma, brain tumor, and early-onset breast cancer.

Pathology and Classification

RMS is usually associated with extensive necrosis and hemorrhage, and often has ill-defined margins. The characteristic cellular element is the rhabdomyoblast, a primitive skeletal muscle cell with eosinophilic cytoplasm and cross-striations or longitudinal myofibrils. Glycogen granules may be present in the cytoplasm. Rhabdomyoblasts can vary morphologically within individual tumors and have been described as round cells, tadpole cells, spindle cells, spider-web cells, and multinucleated giant cells. Definitive pathologic diagnosis may require additional studies such as immunohistochemistry and electron microscopy. The latter modality reveals cells with eccentric nuclei, abundant mitochondria, and large numbers of thick and thin cytoplasmic filaments that tend to form "Z-bands." The presence of desmin, an intermediate protein, can distinguish RMS from other small, blue, round cell tumors of childhood.[47]

Traditionally, the tumors are classified into four histologic tissue patterns: embryonal, alveolar, pleomorphic, and undifferentiated. The embryonal subtype (50% to 60% of cases) is characterized by a variable number of large acidophilic myoblasts and many primitive round and spindle-shaped cells with little myoblastic differentiation; cross-striations may be found within the cytoplasm. This subtype is most commonly found in the head and neck region and genitourinary tract. Sarcoma botryoides is a polypoid variant of embryonal RMS and usually has a grapelike appearance. The botryoid variant (5% of cases), commonly seen in younger children, usually affects the vagina, uterus, bladder, nasopharynx, and middle ear.

The alveolar subtype (20% of cases) is characterized by a pseudoalveolar growth pattern reminiscent of the alveoli of fetal lung. It occurs more commonly in adolescents, with primary sites in the extremities, trunk, and perineum. It tends to metastasize early, usually to lymph nodes and bone marrow, and is associated with a poor prognosis.[48]

Pleomorphic RMS is rare in children (1% of cases) and almost always arises in the extremities.

About 10% to 20% of patients are considered to have undifferentiated tumor. The first Intergroup Rhabdomyosarcoma Study (IRS-I) included three additional tumor types: sarcoma of undetermined histogenesis and special undifferentiated types 1 and 2 (extraskeletal Ewing's sarcoma).[49]

Genetics

Abnormalities of the short arm of chromosome 3 are found in some rhabdomyosarcomas. The translocation t(2;13)(q35;q14) is found in more than half of the alveolar-type tumors, which are associated with adolescence, metastatic disease at diagnosis, and a poor prognosis, as described above. No specific cytogenetic abnormalities have been consistently identified in the more common embryonal-type histologic pattern. Two cases of RMS have demonstrated a loss of heterozygosity in chromosome 11, suggesting involvement of a tumor suppressor gene in some cases.[50]

Presentation and Diagnosis

Clinical presentation varies with the site of tumor origin, speed of tumor growth, and presence of metastases. The most common presenting feature is a mass, which may be painful. The most common primary sites are the head and neck, including the orbit (37%); genitourinary tract (21%); extremities (20%); retroperitoneum (8%); trunk (7%); gastrointestinal tract (2%); perineum and anus (2%); and intrathoracic area (2%).[49] One percent of patients have disseminated disease, usually involving bone and bone marrow with no identifiable primary site.

Young children with orbital tumor usually present with proptosis, periorbital edema, and ptosis. Tumors of the middle ear are associated with ear pain, chronic otitis media, or hemorrhagic discharge from the ear canal. Tumors of the nasopharynx can present with airway obstruction, local pain, sinusitis, epistaxis, or dysphagia. Parameningeal lesions, such as those in the nasal cavity, paranasal sinuses, nasopharynx, and middle ear, may extend into the middle cranial fossa in 35% of cases and cause cranial nerve paralysis, meningeal symptoms, and signs of brain stem compression.[51]

RMS of the trunk or extremities may appear as an enlarging soft tissue mass, frequently first noticed after trauma and commonly mistaken for a hematoma. Involvement of the genitourinary tract may produce hematuria, recurrent urinary tract infection, incontinence, or obstruction of the lower urinary tract and rectum. Paratesticular tumors usually present as a rapidly growing mass in the scrotum. Vaginal or uterine RMS may present as a grapelike mass bulging through the vaginal orifice.

RMS may spread by local extension or via the venous and lymphatic systems. The most frequent sites of metastasis are the regional lymph nodes, lung, liver, bone marrow, bones, and brain. Regional lymph node involvement is often seen with paratesticular tumors (40%), probably because of the rich lymphatic supply of the testes. By contrast, orbital tumors rarely involve regional lymphatic vessels, which are sparse in this region. Bone invasion is frequent in the orbit and extensive involvement may produce symptomatic hypercalcemia.

Initial studies in patients with suspected RMS should include a complete blood count, liver and kidney function tests, a skeletal survey, bone scan, chest x-ray, bone marrow examination, and other appropriate radiographic studies, depending on the region of origin. CT and MRI are the primary imaging methods for evaluating intracranial extension and bony involvement at the base of the skull. The cerebrospinal fluid should also be examined to rule out meningeal seeding. CT with contrast medium and ultrasonography can help delineate abdominal tumors. These methods are also useful in genitourinary tract tumors, with the addition of a cystourethrogram for patients with bladder tumors. MRI is useful for imaging tumors of the extremities.

The staging system most commonly used in the US (Table 32-8) is based on the extent of local disease and extension, involvement of regional lymph nodes, and presence of distant metastases.[49] A new staging system, also developed by the IRS group for current trials, is based on primary site, tumor size, local invasiveness, and presence of nodal or distant metastases.

Treatment and Prognosis

Total excision of the primary lesion is desirable if it does not result in unacceptable deformity. Irradiation of areas of known residual tumor and systemic multiagent chemotherapy are also indicated. In group I disease, complete local excision is usually followed by chemotherapy. For groups II and III, surgery should be followed by local irradiation and systemic chemotherapy. Patients with group IV disease are treated primarily with systemic chemotherapy. Wide-volume radiation therapy is also given in relatively high doses (4,000 to 5,000 cGy) for 6 weeks. The most effective drugs for RMS, usually given in combination, include vincristine, cyclophosphamide, dactinomycin, and Adriamycin.

The use of combined-modality therapy has substantially improved outcome. However, patients with advanced disease at diagnosis remain a therapeutic challenge (Table 32-8). Survival after relapse is extremely poor regardless of the site of recurrence; only 32% survive 1 year and 17% survive 2 years despite aggressive surgery, radiation therapy, and adjuvant chemotherapy.

The most important prognostic factors in RMS are clinical stage (Table 32-8) and primary site.[49] In general, tumors that produce early symptoms are associated with a better prognosis than those arising in deep, poorly confined areas. The prognosis is good for patients with primary tumors in the orbit or bladder, but intrathoracic or retroperitoneal primary sites are associated with poor outcomes.[49,52] Children with the sarcoma botryoides variant of embryonal RMS have the best survival rates; those with alveolar-type histologic patterns have the worst. Older children have worse prognoses than younger ones, probably due to a greater frequency of alveolar histology and of primary tumors in the extremities.

A current IRS trial is comparing hyperfractionated and conventional radiotherapy in selected patients with residual disease. The study is also evaluating the safety and efficacy of new drug combinations administered before conventional chemotherapy ("therapeutic window") in children with advanced disease and a poor prognosis. A third goal of the trial is to compare the relative efficacy of ifosfamide and cyclophosphamide, given on a randomized basis as part of multimodality therapy.

Osteosarcoma

Osteosarcoma (OS), also known as osteogenic sarcoma, is a malignant tumor of mesenchymal origin that produces malignant osteoid. It is the most common bone tumor in childhood, typically affecting adolescents (median age, 15) and involving the distal portion (metaphysis) of long bones. Because osteosarcoma usually occurs during the second decade of life (when physical appearance is of greatest concern) and because therapy usually involves mutilating surgery, psychologic support is an essential part of treatment.

Epidemiology

The incidence of osteosarcoma appears to correlate with linear bone growth. OS is rare in prepubertal children, but increases in incidence after puberty and peaks between 15 and 19 years of age. It constitutes about 60% of all childhood bone tumors, which occur at an approximate rate of 5.6 cases per million in the US. During the first 13 years of life, the incidence of osteosarcoma is equal in boys and girls. After this age,

Table 32-8. Staging and Outcome of Rhabdomyosarcoma*

Stage	Criteria	Proportion of Patients (%)	8-Year DFS (%)
I	Localized disease, completely resected (regional nodes not involved); Confined to muscle or organ of origin; Contiguous involvement with infiltration outside the muscle or organ of origin, as through fascial planes.	15	74
II	Grossly resected tumor with microscopic residual disease; No evidence of gross residual tumor; no evidence of regional lymph node involvement. Regional disease, completely resected (regional nodes involved or extension of tumor into an adjacent organ); all tumor completely resected with no microscopic residual tumor. Regional disease with involved nodes; grossly resected but with evidence of microscopic residual disease.	25	65
III	Incomplete resection or biopsy with gross residual disease.	41	40
IV	Distant metastatic disease present at diagnosis (lung, liver, bones, bone marrow, brain, or distant muscle and nodes)	19	15

*Based on data from the Intergroup Rhabdomyosarcoma Study—I.

Abbreviations: DFS, disease-free survival.

Adapted from Maurer et al.[49]

the incidence increases in males but not in females, yielding a male-to-female ratio of 1.5:1. The relationship between the adolescent growth spurt and tumor development suggests that a high growth rate increases the risk of somatic mutation, leading to malignant transformation. Indeed, osteosarcoma occurs most commonly in long bones at the metaphyseal ends, the regions most active in growth and reconstruction.

Children with hereditary retinoblastoma have a 500-fold increased risk of developing osteosarcoma. Although these osteosarcomas usually develop in previously irradiated sites, they have arisen in bones outside the irradiated field and at multiple sites. Molecular analysis using DNA markers for chromosome 13 reveals deletion of genetic material at band 13q14 in hereditary retinoblastoma, osteosarcoma associated with retinoblastoma, and sporadic osteosarcoma.[53] A recessive tumor suppressor gene on chromosome 13 may be involved in tumor development. Other conditions associated with osteosarcoma include multiple hereditary exostoses, multiple osteochondromatosis (Ollier's disease), polyostotic fibrous dysplasia, osteogenesis imperfecta, Paget's disease of bone, and exposure to ionizing irradiation. Familial cases of osteosarcoma have occasionally been reported.

Pathology and Classification

Osteosarcoma generally arises within the medullary canal, breaking through the cortex and periosteum to form a soft tissue mass that may reach considerable size. The tumor may also extend along the medullary cavity. In about 20% of cases, tumor deposits develop quite far from the primary tumor.

Histologically, the tumor contains primitive spindle cells that form osteoid. Approximately 75% of cases are considered classic osteosarcoma, which can be subdivided into osteoblastic, fibroblastic, and chondroblastic types depending on the predominant matrix. The remaining 25% comprise several groups with varying features and prognoses. Telangiectatic osteosarcoma is an unusual variant characteristically presenting as a lytic lesion on radiographs, with little evidence of calcification or new-bone formation. Pathologic fractures are common in this variant, which seems to have a particularly poor prognosis. Periosteal osteosarcoma arises from the periosteum and grows outward without cortical invasion. It usually occurs in the proximal metaphysis of the tibia and is more common in adolescents. It tends to be less aggressive and may require only wide resection. Parosteal osteosarcoma is more common in older patients (median age, 30) and most often occurs in the metaphyseal region of the femur. It often surrounds the bone shaft without involvement of the cortex. The tumor's growth is relatively slow, but local recurrence and metastasis can occur. Low-grade intraosseous osteosarcoma is a rare variant confined to the marrow cavity, with a very low metastatic potential. Small-cell osteosarcoma resembles Ewing's sarcoma histologically but produces osteoid. Multifocal sclerosing osteosarcoma, which has a predominant osteoblastic pattern, may appear simultaneously at multiple sites.

Presentation and Diagnosis

The usual presenting symptoms are discomfort, swelling, and pain (often increasing with activity), with or without a soft tissue mass overlying the involved bone. Patients occasionally associate the onset of symptoms with trauma, but trauma has not been shown to cause osteosarcoma. The diagnosis may be delayed if pain is attributed to injury. Any patient with prolonged, unexplained bone pain should undergo appropriate imaging studies to rule out osteosarcoma. Depending on the primary site, the mass may or may not be palpable. Pathologic fractures are uncommon except in telangiectatic osteosarcoma, in which they may occur in up to 30% of patients.

Approximately 60% to 80% of osteosarcomas occur near the knee (distal femur or proximal tibia or fibula); 10% to 15% occur in the proximal humerus. The central axis is involved in fewer than 10% of cases.

The initial workup includes plain radiographs of the involved bone, which in conjunction with symptoms are diagnostic in most cases. Radiographs typically demonstrate permeative destruction of the normal bony trabecular pattern, with indistinct margins. A soft tissue mass is common, and there is usually intense periosteal new-bone formation. The eroded cortex may be traversed by horizontal bone spicules that extend into the surrounding soft tissue mass, resulting in the sunburst sign in 60% of cases. At the tumor margins, a triangular region of periosteal new bone (Codman's triangle) is often present. CT and MRI can reveal the extent of cortical involvement and intramedullary spread, as well as detecting skip lesions and soft tissue extension. These studies are essential for planning surgical treatment. Arteriograms are used to delineate the relationship between the tumor and major vessels in candidates for limb-sparing procedures.

Some 10% to 20% of patients have metastatic disease at diagnosis, most commonly in the lungs. This can be detected by routine chest radiographs or CT. CT is more sensitive but occasionally yields false-positive results. Respiratory symptoms are uncommon unless there is extensive metastatic lung disease. Bone or brain metastases may occur, usually after lung metastases. Bone scan and skeletal survey are indicated to rule out bony metastases. Lymphatic spread occurs in only 3% of patients. At diagnosis, about 60% of patients have increased serum alkaline phosphatase levels, which are associated with an increased likelihood of subsequent pulmonary metastasis.

Treatment and Prognosis

Surgical ablation of the affected bone and surrounding soft tissue is essential for local tumor control. The choice between amputation and limb salvage procedures depends on the age of the patient, anatomic location, extent and size of tumor, soft tissue and neurovascular involvement, surgical expertise, expected function, and the patient's attitude and preference.

Historically, above-the-knee amputation was performed for distal femoral tumors and proximal tibia or fibula tumors, and below-the-knee amputations for distal tibia lesions. Shoulder disarticulation or forequarter amputation was performed for proximal humerus lesions, and hemipelvectomy for tumors of the proximal femoral neck or ilium. The usual practice is to obtain a tumor-free margin of 7 to 10 cm. Following amputation, early rehabilitation of the patient with immediate fitting of a prosthesis is extremely important.

Limb salvage is increasingly favored as an alternative to amputation.[54] Preoperative ("neoadjuvant") chemotherapy, which introduces effective drugs as soon as possible after diagnosis to destroy micrometastases, may shrink the tumor sufficiently so that limb salvage becomes feasible for some patients who would not have been candidates otherwise. In limb-sparing procedures, the tumor-bearing bone is resected en bloc and replaced with a cadaver allograft or a custom-made prosthesis. Complications of the procedure include infections, metal fatigue and breakage, decreased functional activity, and local tumor recurrence. Some patients undergoing this procedure eventually require conventional amputation because of complications. For patients with bony metastases, there is little role for surgery except to relieve pain or resect grossly disfiguring metastatic lesions.

The introduction of adjuvant combination chemotherapy after complete excision of primary lesions of extremities has markedly improved 2-year disease-free survival from 17% to 66%.[55] The agents most active against osteosarcoma are high-dose methotrexate (with leucovorin rescue), doxorubicin, and cisplatin. Ifosfamide has shown substantial antitumor activity in previously treated patients[56] and is currently being incorporated into front-line treatment regimens. Several biologic response modifiers have been tested, including transfer factor and interferons, but none has proven beneficial.

An aggressive surgical approach is warranted for patients who develop lung metastases after multimodality therapy. The number and resectability of pulmonary lesions is a determinant of prognosis. Cure is achieved in up to one third of patients with resectable pulmonary metastases.[57]

Location of the primary lesion and the presence or absence of metastatic or multifocal disease are important prognostic variables for osteosarcoma. The few patients who have axial skeletal osteosarcoma fare poorly because of problems in achieving local control. Metastatic disease at diagnosis also confers a poor prognosis. In general, the farther the primary site is from the axial skeleton, the better the prognosis. Tumor size also appears to be important, with a larger tumor (>15 cm in diameter) conferring a poorer prognosis. Histologically, a relatively good outcome is reported for periosteal, parosteal, and low-grade intraosseous osteosarcomas; the telangiectatic variant is associated with a poor prognosis. Preexisting Paget's disease, radiation-induced malignancy, age under 10 years, male sex, short duration of symptoms, and high alkaline phosphatase levels are also adverse indicators. Osteosarcomas with near-diploid stem lines respond significantly better to adjuvant chemotherapy than do tumors with hyperdiploid lines.[58]

Ewing's Sarcoma

Since the first description of this tumor by James Ewing in 1921, the cell of origin has remained elusive. The tumor is thought to arise from the primitive mesenchyme of the medullary cavity. Extraosseous Ewing's sarcoma is a tumor of similar morphologic features that arises from soft tissue. Ewing's sarcoma involves flat bones in about 40% of reported cases.

Epidemiology

Ewing's sarcoma most commonly occurs in early adolescence, often between the ages of 11 and 15 (median age, 13); 90% of cases are diagnosed before age 30. It represents approximately 1% of childhood cancers and 30% of all primary bone tumors (5.6 cases per million) in children less than 15 years of age. It is more common in males (1.6:1), and is exceedingly rare in American blacks and in native Chinese.[3] Familial cases have been described.

Pathology

The tumors, often soft and friable, consist of undifferentiated small round cells with scant cytoplasm and little or no surrounding stroma. Coagulative necrosis may be prominent, and calcification is rare. The periodic acid-Schiff reaction demonstrates glycogen in 80% of tumor samples. Although electron microscopy discerns no diagnostic feature, it is useful for ruling out other small, blue, round cell tumors of childhood.

Genetics

Cytogenetic analyses of cell lines and fresh tumors have demonstrated a subtle but characteristic chromosomal abnormality, t(11;22)(q24;q12).[59] An apparently identical reciprocal translocation has been described in peripheral neuroepitheliomas (PN) and

Askin tumor, both of which may be closely related to Ewing's sarcoma. Although the c-*sis* oncogene at 22q13 is involved in this translocation, it is not rearranged or activated at the molecular level. It is unknown whether the c-*ets*-1 oncogene, normally located in 11q23-25, is translocated or in any way functionally affected in Ewing's sarcoma.

Presentation and Diagnosis

The usual presenting symptoms are localized pain in the affected bone with subsequent development of swelling, tenderness, and heat. The tumor can be difficult to differentiate from osteomyelitis. Various laboratory abnormalities, such as leukocytosis, anemia, and an elevated sedimentation rate, can suggest infection. When the diagnosis of osteomyelitis is questionable and cultures are negative, Ewing's sarcoma should always be considered.

While the tumor may occur in any bone, it is found most frequently in the midshaft (diaphysis) of long bones. The femur is most frequently involved, followed in descending order by the ilium and pubis, tibia, humerus, fibula, ribs, scapula, hands and feet, vertebra, sacrum, clavicle, skull and facial bones, radius, and ulna.

Up to one third of patients will have evidence of metastatic disease at diagnosis, most commonly in the lungs or bones. Patients with a primary tumor in the proximal extremity or central axis have a higher incidence of metastasis (50%) than those with tumor in the distal extremity (10%). Primary tumors of ribs may be massive and result in respiratory distress. In rare cases (<2%), soft tissue extension of vertebral disease can cause epidural spinal cord compression.

Anemia, leukocytosis with a left shift, elevated erythrocyte sedimentation rate, and increased serum LDH levels may occur in some patients, but are nonspecific findings. The radiographic appearance of Ewing's sarcoma varies, but a diffuse lytic lesion with periosteal reaction and a soft tissue mass are most common. Sclerotic lesions may occur; the so-called onionskin appearance thought to be characteristic of Ewing's sarcoma is seen in only a minority of cases. CT and MRI of the primary lesion define the extent of bone and soft tissue involvement; these techniques are especially important in the pelvic region, where the tumor is often grossly underestimated by usual radiographic imaging. Bone scans show increased uptake at the primary site, and gallium scans are positive in approximately 80% of cases. CT and plain films of the chest, as well as skeletal survey, bone scan, and bone marrow examination, can exclude metastatic disease.

Treatment and Prognosis

With surgery and radiotherapy alone, 5-year disease-free survival was 15% to 20% for patients with Ewing's sarcoma, despite apparent local disease control. The addition of chemotherapy has improved 5-year survival to 35% to 70%.[60,61] Most chemotherapeutic regimens include cyclophosphamide, doxorubicin, vincristine, and dactinomycin. Recently, ifosfamide and etoposide have been found active against Ewing's sarcoma and incorporated into clinical trials.[62] Limiting the volume of radiation appears feasible in small lesions of the extremity; hyperfractionated radiotherapy may be more effective in controlling large localized lesions.[63] For some patients with advanced tumor, autologous bone marrow transplantation and total body irradiation with adjuvant chemotherapy have been successful.[63]

Poor prognostic signs include metastatic disease, primary tumors in the flat bones or proximal extremities, and large tumor size (>8 cm or >100 cc). Treatment of large tumors is often unsuccessful, although recent reports suggest that aggressive surgical resection may be of benefit.[60]

Retinoblastoma

Retinoblastoma arises from primitive neuroectodermal tissue within the nuclear layer of the retina. Histologically, it is similar to neuroblastoma, medulloblastoma, and pineoblastoma, three other malignant neoplasms of neural origin. A so-called trilateral retinoblastoma syndrome has been reported in patients with bilateral retinoblastoma and pineal tumor. Instances of spontaneous regression, multicentric origin, a high frequency of second malignancy, and a pattern of inheritance have been reported in patients with retinoblastoma.

Epidemiology

Retinoblastoma is relatively rare, with an annual incidence of 3.4 per million in the US. About 200 children in the US develop retinoblastoma each year, usually before age 2; 80% of cases are diagnosed before age 3. The mean age at diagnosis is 8 months for bilateral, and 26 months for unilateral, retinoblastoma.

Pathology

Retinoblastoma is an undifferentiated small-cell tumor with deeply staining nuclei and scant cytoplasm. The tumor can also be composed of larger cells that form rosettes around a central cavity. The blood supply is invariably inadequate, and patchy areas of necrosis and degeneration with calcium deposition are characteristic. The tumor may grow into the vitreous cavity (endophytic) or into the subretinal space (exophytic). Tumor fragments may break off from an endophytic tumor and float free in the vitreous body to seed unaffected parts of the retina. Retinoblastoma can grow into the choroid, sclera, optic nerve, or subarachnoid space and seed along the base of the brain and spinal cord. Involvement of periglobal tissue can result in hematogenous spread to bone marrow, bone, lymph nodes, and liver.

Genetics

Retinoblastoma occurs in two forms, sporadic (60% of patients) and inherited. Approximately 30% of patients have bilateral involvement and an inherited predisposition to retinoblastoma. Among these patients, the tumor usually is first diagnosed in one eye and appears in the other eye several months to years later. About 15% of patients with unilateral retinoblastoma also have a genetic predisposition. The incidence rate of the hereditary form is 40%, consistent with an autosomal dominant pattern with 80% penetrance.

Loss of heterozygosity at the retinoblastoma gene (*RB*) locus predisposes to the development of retinoblastoma. Alteration of both copies of *RB* is required to induce malignant growth. Patients with hereditary retinoblastoma have a germline mutation at the *RB* locus; a second somatic mutation is required for the development of neoplasia. Sporadic retinoblastoma arises from two somatic mutations.

Most patients with retinoblastoma have a normal constitutional karyotype. A small number have the 13q- syndrome, characterized by mental retardation, growth failure, characteristic facies, microcephaly, skeletal deformities, congenital heart disease, and eye defects. The long arm of chromosome 13 is deleted in all somatic cells. Fifty percent of patients with this syndrome develop retinoblastoma. The altered *RB* gene in patients with this syndrome also confers an increased risk of other tumors; about 15% of survivors of hereditary retinoblastoma will develop a second malignancy, with a median latent period of 11 years.[64] Most second tumors are osteosarcomas that develop at irradiated and nonirradiated sites, often multifocally.

Presentation and Diagnosis

Sporadic retinoblastomas are rarely diagnosed early, because signs and symptoms are not obvious in the young patient. Only 3% are identified on routine ocular examination. Nonetheless, early diagnosis improves treatment outcome and decreases morbidity. Parents are usually the first to notice an eye abnormality in the child. Cat's eye reflex—a whitish appearance of the pupil—is the most common presenting sign. Strabismus, the next most common sign, can occur early if the tumor develops in the macula. A painful red eye, with or without glaucoma, indicates extensive disease. Limited vision or loss of vision, proptosis, buphthalmos, and increased intracranial pressure are late signs.

All patients should receive meticulous ophthalmoscopic examination under general anesthesia. Ocular conditions that must be differentiated from retinoblastoma include persistent hyperplastic primary vitreous, cysticercus, visceral larva migrans, retrolental fibroplasia, Coat's disease, and bacterial panendophthalmitis. In addition to ophthalmoscopy, staging procedures include orbital ultrasound, CT of the head, and, most recently, MRI. These techniques map the extent of ocular involvement and assess infiltration beyond the globe and into the optic nerve. If advanced disease is suspected, cerebrospinal fluid examination, chest x-ray, skeletal survey, and bone marrow examination may be indicated as well. Calcium is found on high-resolution thin-section CT of the orbit in more than 80% of patients with retinoblastoma. Anterior-chamber paracentesis may identify tumor cells in some cases. CT of the head should be performed to rule out trilateral retinoblastoma syndrome. Table 32-9 shows the staging system most commonly used for retinoblastoma.[65] Clinical staging, usually based on extent of intraocular disease, is designed to predict the potential for ocular preservation rather than survival.

Treatment and Prognosis

Every effort should be made to preserve sight by irradiation, photocoagulation, or cryotherapy. Eyes with extensive retinal destruction or neurovascular glaucoma are enucleated, with an attempt to resect as much of the optic nerve as possible (>10 mm). The orbit should be irradiated if there is regional extraocular extension of the tumor. Reports of newer radiation techniques indicate 90% tumor control for early

Table 32-9. Staging of Retinoblastoma

Stage	Criteria
Group I	Solitary or multiple tumors, <4 disc diameters in size, at or behind the equator.
Group II	Solitary or multiple tumors, 4-10 disc diameters in size, at or behind the equator.
Group III	Any lesion anterior to the equator. Solitary tumors >10 disc diameters, behind the equator.
Group IV	Multiple tumors, some >10 disc diameters; any lesion extending anterior to the ora serrata.
Group V	Massive tumor involving more than half the retina. Vitreous seeding.
Group VI	Residual orbital disease; optic nerve involvement and extrascleral extension (metastatic disease).

Adapted from Bedford et al.[65]

to intermediate disease and 60% for advanced ocular disease.[66] Useful vision is retained in about half the cases; poor vision occurs primarily in cases with macular involvement.[66] Cryotherapy or radioactive plaques may be successful in cases of localized tumors. Cryotherapy is used in conjunction with external-beam irradiation to treat anterior retinal deposits in patients with more advanced disease. If the tumor is advanced or extrabulbar extension has occurred, chemotherapy (cyclophosphamide, doxorbicin, vincristine) should be considered in addition to radiotherapy.

The prognosis depends on tumor size and location and the presence and degree of ocular and extraocular involvement. The cure rate for patients with group I to IV retinoblastoma is more than 90%. Group V patients have a 5-year survival rate of 85%. Once the tumor has extended into the optic nerve, the 5-year survival decreases to about 50%; with extraocular extension, it decreases further to 25%. Cure for widespread metastatic disease is rare despite good response to chemotherapy. Spontaneous regression occurs in 1.8% of patients. Bilateral retinoblastoma carries a significantly higher mortality rate, mostly owing to second malignancies.[67]

Germ Cell Tumor

Germ cell tumors are neoplasms (benign or malignant) originating in primordial germ cells, which may undergo germinomatous or embryonic differentiation. The totipotentiality of germ cells results in a wide array of neoplastic histologic patterns. The migration pattern of the primordial germ cells during embryonic development explains the occurrence of germ cell tumors in midline sites (eg, sacrococcyx, neck, mediastinum, retroperitoneum, pineal gland).

Epidemiology

Germ cell tumors account for 2% to 3% of childhood malignancies. Sacrococcygeal teratoma is the most common solid tumor in newborns, with a higher incidence in females. The incidence of sacrococcygeal, head, and neck tumors peaks between birth and 3 years of age. During puberty there is an increase in incidence of ovarian and testicular tumors. Boys with cryptorchidism have a 50-fold greater risk of developing malignant testicular tumors, which may occur even in the descended testis.

Pathology and Classification

Germ cell tumors that contain a mixture of cell types are generally classified by the most malignant component. Pure germ cell tumors are called germinomas (seminoma and dysgerminoma). Embryonic differentiation may result in embryonal carcinoma or teratoma, and extra-embryonic differentiation in endodermal sinus tumor (yolk sac tumor) or choriocarcinoma. Mixed germ-cell tumors with various histologic types are most commonly observed.[68]

Teratomas contain derivatives of at least two of the three germ layers (ectoderm, endoderm, and mesoderm). Although benign, they may undergo malignant degeneration, most frequently to endodermal sinus tumor. Endodermal sinus tumor, with histologic features resembling the yolk sac, is most frequently found in the ovary, testes, and sacrococcygeal areas. Most commonly, germinoma occurs in the ovary of an early pubertal or adolescent girl, or in the pineal region of an adolescent boy. It is less common in the anterior mediastinum or testis. Embryonal carcinoma, a highly anaplastic tumor that retains the potential to develop along either embryonal or extraembryonal lines, is rare in children. Choriocarcinoma, resembling the chorion layer of the placenta, usually occurs as a nongestational tumor of the pineal region, the anterior mediastinum, or the ovary in early childhood. Gestational choriocarcinoma occurs most commonly in girls aged 15 to 19.

Presentation and Diagnosis

Sacrococcygeal teratoma is usually detected during infancy, frequently at birth. Presenting signs include an external midline sacrococcygeal mass, a pelvic mass, or unilateral gluteal enlargement. Depending on the extent of disease, patients may present with paralysis, constipation, diarrhea, bladder distention, or recurrent urinary tract infections. Associated clinical features include congenital anomalies involving the lower vertebrae, genitourinary system, or anorectum. Testicular tumors usually occur in boys younger than 5 years and present as painless unilateral masses. They are rarely inflamed and a hydrocele is frequently present. Ovarian tumors are usually quite large and may cause pain, nausea, and vomiting. Patients who have ovarian torsion may present with an acute abdomen.

The physical examination can delineate the anatomic extent of the primary tumor, especially a sacrococcygeal tumor. Radiographs of the tumor may show calcification and, in the case of a teratoma, even bone or teeth. All patients should have radiographs, as well as CT scans of the chest, abdomen, and primary site. The most helpful clinical laboratory studies for diagnosis and follow-up are serum biomarkers: alphafetoprotein (AFP) and the beta subunit of human chorionic gonadotropin (hCG). The former is increased in embryonal carcinoma and endodermal sinus tumor; the latter in embryonal carcinoma and choriocarcinoma.[69]

Treatment and Prognosis

Tumors should be completely excised if possible, and the surgical specimen carefully studied for the presence of malignant components, which may occupy only a small proportion of the tumor. Because the incidence of malignancy increases with age, it is imperative to remove the sacrococcygeal tumor as soon as possible.

With current therapy the prognosis for patients with germ cell tumor is excellent, with reports of 80% 5-year survival in most series.[68] Chemotherapeutic regimens consisting of vincristine, actinomycin D (dactinomycin), and cyclophosphamide (VAC) or cisplatin, vinblastine, and bleomycin (PVB) are effective against tumors with a malignant component.[68] The role of radiation therapy in nongerminomatous tumors remains controversial. Traditionally, patients with pure germinomas (radiosensitive) are treated with radiation therapy. However, recent reports suggest that these tumors are chemosensitive, and platinum-based regimens offer the possibility of cure with preserved fertility.[70]

Disease stage is the most important prognostic factor. More than 90% of patients with localized disease reach 5-year survival, in contrast to 50% to 70% of patients with advanced disease.[68] Current studies of the treatment of localized disease are attempting to shorten the duration of therapy to minimize acute and chronic side effects. Patients with advanced disease may benefit from intensification of therapy. Histologically, choriocarcinoma is associated with the worst treatment outcome and germinoma with the best. Infants have a high cure rate, probably because of the age-related incidence of presacral teratomas and localized yolk sac tumors.

Langerhans Cell Histiocytosis

Recognition of the histologic and clinical interrelationships between eosinophilic granuloma, Hand-Schüller-Christian syndrome, and Letterer-Siwe syndrome led to the grouping of all three syndromes under the term *histiocytosis X*. The involved Langerhans cells are dendritic cells derived from the bone marrow, and the disease is now correctly called Langerhans cell histiocytosis. There is some evidence that the disorder reflects an immunologic aberration. Although traditionally treated by oncologists, it is probably not a cancer since it is not monoclonal in origin and does not express cellular atypia.

Epidemiology

This disease is rare (at least 20 times less common than acute leukemia in children) and its exact incidence is unknown. The peak mortality rate occurs in infants, and the reported frequency of disease in siblings or twins suggests the importance of genetic factors.

Pathology

The basic lesion is granulomatous and composed of Langerhans cells with variable numbers of granulocytes and lymphocytes. The Langerhans cells are large and have lobular, folded, and grooved nuclei. They are characterized by the presence of Birbeck granules (intracytoplasmic, rodlike lamellar organelles detected by electron microscopy) and by the presence of antigenic surface markers that react with the monoclonal antibody OKT6/Leu-6.

Presentation and Diagnosis

The clinical manifestations vary with tissue and organ infiltration. Solitary- or multiple-bone involvement (eosinophilic granuloma) occurs in older children, usually in the skull and long bones. Exophthalmos, diabetes insipidus, and membranous bone defects (Hand-Schüller-Christian syndrome) are seen together rarely. Patients may have chronically draining ears, with destruction of the mastoid area or cholesteatomas. The skin may have seborrheic-like lesions. Diabetes insipidus may be present at the time of diagnosis or occur later in the disease course.

Aggressive, often fatal disease (Letterer-Siwe disease) may occur in some patients, particularly children younger than 2 years and those with dysfunctional liver, lungs, or hematopoietic systems. Liver enlargement does not indicate poor prognosis unless accompanied by hypoalbuminemia, hyperbilirubinemia, or edema. Clinical signs such as dyspnea, tachypnea, cyanosis, pneumothorax, and pleural effusion demonstrate pulmonary dysfunction. Hematopoietic dysfunction is characterized by hemoglobin values <100 g/L (not due to iron deficiency or infection), leukocyte count $<4 \times 10^9$/L, or thrombocyte count $<100 \times 10^9$/L. Patients may demonstrate prominent cervical lymphadenopathy, rash resistant to conventional therapy, persistent hepatosplenomegaly, prolonged fever, weight loss, lethargy, diarrhea, and therapy-resistant gingival lesions resembling thrush.

The diagnosis is based on histologic examination of a biopsy specimen, often taken from skin, gingiva, lymph nodes, or skeleton. A biopsy of liver or lung is rarely indicated. A complete excisional biopsy and curettage is both diagnostic and therapeutic for a solitary bone lesion. Complete blood counts, skeletal survey, chest x-ray, and liver function tests should be performed to assess the extent of disease. If indicated, bone marrow biopsy or pulmonary function tests also should be performed.

Treatment and Prognosis

Optimal treatment for multifocal involvement has not been established, but systemic chemotherapy (eg, vinblastine, prednisone, methotrexate) is usually given. Low-dose radiation may be preferred for selected cases, such as single-bone lesions, or used when response to chemotherapy is poor. Good supportive care is essential because of frequent secondary bacterial infection, especially otitis media. A combination of trimethoprim and sulfamethoxazole is recommended for *Pneumocystis carinii* pneumonia prophylaxis in children with extensive disease. Children with diabetes insipidus require vasopressin replacement therapy.

Hematopoietic, hepatic, and pulmonary function are the most important prognostic factors.[71] Younger patients tend to have more widespread disease and thus a poor outcome.

References

1. Miller BA, Ries LAG, Hankey BF, Kosary CL, Harras A, Deresa SS, Edwards BK (eds.). *SEER Cancer Statistics Review: 1973-1990.* National Cancer Institute, NIH Pub. No. 93-2789, 1993.

2. Doll R, Meier C, Waterhouse J. *Cancer Incidence in Five Continents.* New York, NY: Springer-Verlag; 1970, vol 2.

3. Miller RW. Frequency and environmental epidemiology of childhood cancer. In: Pizzo PA, Poplack DG, eds. *Principles and Practice of Pediatric Oncology.* Philadelphia, Pa: JB Lippincott; 1989:3-18.

4. Potter JF, Schoeneman M. Metastasis of maternal cancer to the placenta and fetus. *Cancer.* 1970;25:380-387.

5. Jablon S, Kato H. Childhood cancer in relation to prenatal exposure to atomic-bomb radiation. *Lancet.* 1970; 2:1000-1003.

6. Crist WM, Kun LE. Common solid tumors of childhood. *N Engl J Med.* 1991;324:461-471.

7. Malkin D, Jolly KW, Barbier N, et al. Germline mutations of the p53 tumor-suppressor gene in children and young adults with second malignant neoplasms. *N Engl J Med.* 1992;326:1309-1315.

8. Toguchida J, Yamaguchi T, Dayton SH, et al. Prevalence and spectrum of germline mutations of the p53 gene among patients with sarcoma. *N Engl J Med.* 1992;326:1301-1308.

9. Pui CH, Ribeiro RC, Hancock ML, et al. Acute myeloid leukemia in children treated with epipodophyllotoxins for acute lymphoblastic leukemia. *N Engl J Med.* 1991;325:1682-1687.

10. Kamani N, Kennedy J, Brandsma J. Burkitt lymphoma in a child with human immunodeficiency virus infection. *J* Pediatr. 1988;112:241-244.

11. Friend SH, Dryja TP, Weinberg RA. Oncogenes and tumor-suppressing genes. *N Engl J Med.* 1988;318:618-622.

12. Fleming ID, Eteubanas E, Patterson R, et al. The role of surgical resection when combined with chemotherapy and radiation in the management of pelvic rhabdomyosarcoma. *Ann Surg.* 1984;199:509-514.

13. Graham-Pole J, Casper J, Elfenbein G, et al. High-dose chemoradiotherapy supported by marrow infusions for advanced neuroblastoma: a Pediatric Oncology Group study. *J Clin Oncol.* 1991;9:152-158.

14. Rosenberg SA, Lotze MT, Muul LM, et al. Observations on the systemic administration of autologous lymphokine-activated killer cells and recombinant interleukin-2 to patients with metastatic cancer. *N Engl J Med.* 1985;313: 1485-1492.

15. Furman WL, Fairclough DL, Huhn RD, et al. Therapeutic effects and pharmacokinetics of recombinant human granulocyte-macrophage colony-stimulating factor in childhood cancer patients receiving myelosuppressive chemotherapy. *J Clin Oncol.* 1991;9:1022-1028.

16. Filipovich AH, Spector BD, Kersey J. Immunodeficiency in humans as a risk factor in the development of malignancy. *Prev Med.* 1980;9:252-259.

17. Ziegler JL, Beckstead JA, Volberding PA, et al. Non-Hodgkin's lymphoma in 90 homosexual men: relation to generalized lymphadenopathy and the acquired immunodeficiency syndrome. *N Engl J Med.* 1984;311:565-570.

18. Croce CM, Nowell PC. Molecular basis of human B cell neoplasia. *Blood.* 1985;65:1-7.

19. Mecucci C, Louwagie A, Thomas J, Boogaerts M, van den Berghe H. Cytogenetic studies in T-cell malignancies. *Cancer Genet Cytogenet.* 1988;30:63-71.

20. Murphy SB, Fairclough DL, Hutchinson RE, Berard CW. Non-Hodgkin's lymphoma of childhood: an analysis of the histology, staging, and response to treatment of 338 cases at a single institution. *J Clin Oncol.* 1989;7:186-193.

21. Link MP, Donaldson SS, Berard CW, Shuster JJ, Murphy SB. Results of treatment of childhood localized non-Hodgkin's lymphoma with combination chemotherapy with or without radiotherapy. *N Engl J Med.* 1990;322:1169-1174.

22. Patte C, Philip T, Rodary C, et al. High survival rate in advanced-stage B-cell lymphomas and leukemias without CNS involvement with a short intensive polychemotherapy: results from the French Pediatric Oncology Society of a randomized trial of 216 children. *J Clin Oncol.* 1991;9:123-132.

23. Pui CH, Ip SH, Kung P, et al. High serum interleukin-2 receptor levels are related to advanced disease and a poor outcome in childhood non-Hodgkin's lymphoma. *Blood.* 1987;70:624-628.

24. Kaplan HS. Hodgkin's disease: biology, treatment, prognosis. *Blood.* 1981;57:813-822.

25. Sundeen J, Lipford E, Uppenkamp M, et al. Rearranged antigen receptor genes in Hodgkin's disease. *Blood.* 1987;70: 96-103.

26. Brinker MGL, Poppema S, Buys CHCM, Timens W, Osinga J, Visser L. Clonal immunoglobulin gene rearrangements in tissues involved by Hodgkin's disease. *Blood.* 1987; 70:186-191.

27. Romagnani S, Ferrini PL, Ricci M. The immune derangement in Hodgkin's disease. *Hematol.* 1985;22:41-55.

28. Pui CH, Ip SH, Thompson E, et al. Increased serum CD8 antigen level in childhood Hodgkin's disease relates to advanced stage and poor treatment outcome. *Blood.* 1989;73:209-213.

29. Carbone PP, Kaplan HS, Musshoff K, Smithers DW, Tubiana M. Report of the Committee on Hodgkin's Disease Staging Classification. *Cancer Res.* 1971;31:1860-1861.

30. DeVita VT Jr, Hubbard SM, Moxley JH III. The cure of Hodgkin's disease with drugs. *Adv Intern Med.* 1983;28:277-302.

31. Bonadonna G. Chemotherapy strategies to improve the control of Hodgkin's disease: The Richard and Hinda Rosenthal Foundation Award Lecture. *Cancer Res.* 1982;42:4309-4320.

32. Pui CH, Ip SH, Thompson E, et al. High serum interleukin-2 receptor levels correlate with poor prognosis in children with Hodgkin's disease. *Leukemia.* 1989;3:481-484.

33. Beckwith JB, Perrin EV. In situ neuroblastoma: a contribution to the natural history of neural crest tumors. *Am J Pathol.* 1963;43:1089-1104.

34. Shimada H, Chatten J, Newton WA Jr, et al. Histopathologic prognostic factors in neuroblastic tumors: definition of subtypes of ganglioneuroblastoma and an age-linked classification of neuroblastomas. *J Natl Cancer Inst.* 1984;73:405-416.

35. Brodeur GM, Seeger RC. Gene amplification in human neuroblastomas: basic mechanisms and clinical implications. *Cancer Genet Cytogenet.* 1986;19:101-111.

36. Look AT, Hayes FA, Shuster JJ, et al. Clinical relevance of tumor cell ploidy and N-*myc* gene amplification in childhood neuroblastoma: a Pediatric Oncology Group study. *J Clin Oncol.* 1991;9:581-591.

37. Bowman LC, Hancock ML, Santana VM, et al. Impact of intensified therapy on clinical outcome in infants and children with neuroblastoma: The St. Jude Children's Research Hospital experience, 1962 to 1988. *J Clin Oncol.* 1991;9:1599-1608.

38. Brodeur GM, Seeger RC, Barrett A, et al. International criteria for diagnosis, staging, and response to treatment in patients with neuroblastoma. *J Clin Oncol.* 1988;6:1874-1881.

39. Bowman L, Castleberry R, Altshuster G, et al. Therapy based on DNA index (DI) for infants with unresectable and disseminated neuroblastoma (NB): The Pediatric Oncology Group "better risk" study. *Proc Am Soc Clin Oncol.* 1992;11:365. Abstract.

40. D'Angio GJ, Breslow N, Beckwith JB, et al. Treatment of Wilms' tumor: results of the Third National Wilms' Tumor Study. *Cancer.* 1989;64:349-360.

41. Coppes MJ, de Kraker J, van Dijken PJ, et al. Bilateral Wilms' tumor: long-term survival and some epidemiologic features. *J Clin Oncol.* 1989;7:310-315.

42. Beckwith JB. Wilms' tumor and other renal tumors of childhood: a selective review from the National Wilms' Tumor Study Pathology Center. *Hum Pathol.* 1983;14:481-492.

43. Douglass EC, Look AT, Webber B, et al. Hyperdiploidy and chromosomal rearrangements define the anaplastic variant of Wilms' tumor. *J Clin Oncol.* 1986;4:975-981.

44. Slater RM, de Kraker J, Voute PA, Delemarre JFM. A cytogenetic study of Wilms' tumor. *Cancer Genet Cytogenet.* 1985;14:95-109.

45. Koufos A, Hansen MF, Lampkin BC, et al. Loss of alleles at loci on human chromosome 11 during genesis of Wilms' tumour. *Nature.* 1984;309:170-172.

46. Grundy P, Breslow N, Green DM, Sharples K, Evans A, D'Angio GJ. Prognostic factors for children with recurrent Wilms' tumor: results from the Second and Third National Wilms' Tumor Study. *J Clin Oncol.* 1989;7:638-647.

47. Altmannsberger M, Weber K, Droste R, Osborn M: Desmin is a specific marker for rhabdomyosarcomas of human and rat origin. *Am J Pathol.* 1985;118:85-95.

48. Douglass EC, Valentine M, Etcubanas E, et al. A specific chromosomal abnormality in rhabdomyosarcoma. *Cytogenet Cell Genet.* 1987;45:148-155.

49. Maurer HM, Beltangady M, Gehan EA, et al. The Intergroup Rhabdomyosarcoma Study—I: a final report. *Cancer.* 1988;61:209-220.

50. Koufos A, Hansen MF, Copeland NG, Jenkins NA, Lamphin BC, Cavenee WK. Loss of heterozygosity in three embryonal tumours suggests a common pathogenetic mechanism. *Nature.* 1985;316:330-334.

51. Gasparini M, Lombardi F, Gianni C, Lovati C, Fossati-Bellani F. Childhood rhabdomyosarcoma with meningeal extension: results of combined therapy including central nervous system prophylaxis. *Am J Clin Oncol.* 1983;6:393-398.

52. Crist WM, Raney RB, Tefft M, et al. Soft tissue sarcomas arising in the retroperitoneal space in children: a report from the Intergroup Rhabdomyosarcoma Study (IRS) Committee. *Cancer.* 1985;56:2125-2132.

53. Hansen MF, Koufos A, Gallie BL. Osteosarcoma and retinoblastoma: a shared chromosomal mechanism revealing recessive predisposition. *Proc Natl Acad Sci USA.* 1985; 82:6216-6220.

54. Goorin AM, Perez-Atayde A, Gebhardt M, et al. Weekly high-dose methotrexate and doxorubicin for osteosarcoma: the Dana-Farber Cancer Institute/The Children's Hospital study III. *J Clin Oncol.* 1987;5:1178-1184.

55. Link MP, Goorin AM, Miser AW, et al. The effect of adjuvant chemotherapy on relapse-free survival in patients with osteosarcoma of the extremity. *N Engl J Med.* 1986;314:1600-1606.

56. Pratt CB, Horowitz ME, Meyer WH, et al. Phase II trial of ifosfamide in children with malignant solid tumors. *Cancer Treat Rep.* 1987;71:131-135.

57. Meyer WH, Schell MJ, Kumar APM, et al. Thoracotomy for pulmonary metastatic osteosarcoma: an analysis of prognostic indicators of survival. *Cancer.* 1987;59:374-379.

58. Look AT, Douglass EC, Meyer WH. Clinical importance of near-diploid tumor stem lines in patients with osteosarcoma of an extremity. *N Engl J Med.* 1988;318:1567-1572.

59. Whang-Peng J, Triche TJ, Knutsen T, et al. Cytogenetic characterization of selected small round cell tumors of childhood. *Cancer Genet Cytogenet.* 1986;21:185-208.

60. Jurgens H, Exner U, Gadner H, et al. Multidisciplinary treatment of primary Ewing's sarcoma of bone: a 6-year experience of a European cooperative trial. *Cancer.* 1988; 61:23-32.

61. Kinsella TJ, Miser JS, Waller B, et al. Long-term follow-up of Ewing's sarcoma of bone treated with combined modality therapy. *Int J Radiat Oncol Biol Phys.* 1991;20:389-395.

62. Miser JS, Kinsella TJ, Triche TJ, et al. Ifosfamide with mesna uroprotection and etoposide: an effective regimen in the treatment of recurrent sarcomas and other tumors of children and young adults. *J Clin Oncol.* 1987;5:1191-1198.

63. Marcus RB Jr, Graham-Pole JR, Springfield DS, et al. High-risk Ewing's sarcoma: end-intensification using autologous bone marrow transplantation. *Int J Radiat Oncol Biol Phys.* 1988;15:53-59.

64. Smith LM, Donaldson SS, Egbert PR, Link MP, Bagshaw MA. Aggressive management of second primary tumors in survivors of hereditary retinoblastoma. *Int J Radiat Oncol Biol Phys.* 1989;17:499-505.

65. Bedford MA, Bedotto C, MacFaul PA. Retinoblastoma: a study of 139 cases. *Br J Ophthalmol.* 1971;55:19-27.

66. Schipper J, Tan K, van Peperzeel HA. Treatment of retinoblastoma by precision megavoltage radiation therapy. *Radiother Oncol.* 1985;3:117-132.

67. Abramson DH, Ellsworth RM, Grumbach N, Kitchin FD. Retinoblastoma: survival, age at detection and comparison 1914-1958, 1958-1983. *J Pediatr Ophthalmol Strabismus.* 1985;22:246-250.

68. Marina NM, Fontanesi J, Kun L, et al. Treatment of advanced childhood germ cell cancers: review of the St Jude experience 1979 to 1988. *Cancer.* In press.

69. Kurman RJ, Scardino PT, McIntire KR, Waldmann TA, Javadpour N. Cellular localization of alpha-fetoprotein and human chorionic gonadotropin in germ cell tumors of the testis using an indirect immunoperoxidase technique: a new approach to classification utilizing tumor markers. *Cancer.* 1977;40:2136-2151.

70. Williams SD, Blessing JA, Hatch KD, Homesley HD. Chemotherapy of advanced dysgerminoma: trials of the Gynecologic Oncology Group. *J Clin Oncol.* 1991;9:1950-1955.

71. Berry DH, Gresik MV, Humphrey GB, et al. Natural history of histiocytosis X: a Pediatric Oncology Group study. *Med Pediatr Oncol.* 1986;14:1-5.

33

GYNECOLOGIC CANCER

Hervy E. Averette, MD, Hoa Nguyen, MD

Cervical Cancer

Epidemiology

Cervical cancer accounted for about 4,600 deaths in 1994.[1] A total of 15,000 new cases of invasive cervical cancer is estimated for the same period.[1] Because of Papanicolaou (Pap) smear screening, the lifetime risk of developing cervical cancer has declined in both white and black women (from 1.1% and 2.3%, respectively, in 1975 to 0.8% and 1.4% in 1988-90). Cervical carcinoma is more common in women of low socioeconomic status (Table 33-1).[2] Other risk factors include history of multiple sexual partners, intercourse at young age, and a large number of pregnancies (Table 33-2).[3] Cervical cancer is quite rare in sexually inactive or nulliparous women.

Pathogenesis and Natural History

Human papillomavirus (HPV) infection has been strongly implicated in the pathogenesis of cervical cancer, with the discovery of HPV 16, 18, 31, and 33 in preinvasive and invasive cervical lesions and HPV 6 and 11 in benign condylomatous lesions. In a 2-year follow-up of 513 women, HPV infection regressed in 25%, persisted in 60%, and progressed in 14%.[4] Several oncogenes have been implicated in the natural progression of cervical cancer. The risk of distant

Table 33-1. Ratio of Observed to Expected Cancers by Primary Sites by Ethnic and Income Group, 1988

	Black		White	
Cancer Site	LI	MHI	LI	MHI
Breast	82	87	87	105
Cervix	145	118	104	91
Ovary	82	81	104	102
Uterus	83	75	94	103
Pancreas	143	141	104	95
Lung	106	112	114	99
Other Female	137	113	118	91
Melanoma	12	12	90	105

Expecteds were calculated assuming site distribution was the same for each age group as for the merged data for all groups. Ratio=100 when observed equals expected. LI=low income; MHI=moderate-to-high income. Adapted from Leffall et al.[2]

Table 33-2. Risk Factors for Cervical Carcinoma

Risk Factor	Risk Ratio
Age at first coitus	
<16	16
16-19	3
>19	1
Years from menarche to coitus	
<1	26
1-5	7
6-10	3
>10	1
Number of sexual partners	
>4	3.6
Venereal warts	3.2
Smoking	4.0

Adapted from Morrow and Townsend.[3]

Hervy E. Averette, MD, Professor and Director of Gynecologic Oncology, University of Miami School of Medicine, Miami, Florida

Hoa Nguyen, MD, Assistant Clinical Professor of Gynecologic Oncology, Cleveland Clinic Florida, Ft. Lauderdale, Florida

metastasis has been estimated to increase sixfold with overexpression of c-*myc* oncogene.[5] A relationship has been reported between increased *ras* oncogene expression and nodal metastasis.[6]

Cervical cancer commonly spreads by local extension and lymphatic invasion. Tumor infiltration in the upper vagina, parametria, bladder, and rectum is the most common mode of spread. Early in its course, cervical cancer tends to spread laterally and posteriorly to involve the cardinal and uterosacral ligaments. As the tumor extends to the parametria, one or both ureters may become obstructed. Hydronephrosis and uremia are common end-stage symptoms. Direct extension to the bladder or rectum occurs in advanced cases. Tumor invasion and breakthrough can lead to intraperitoneal spread and small-bowel involvement.

Once lymphovascular invasion occurs, tumor emboli may involve the parametrial, pelvic, or aortic nodes. In advanced cases, left supraclavicular nodes may be involved via the thoracic duct. Lymphatic obstruction may lead to bilateral lymphedema and metastases to the groin and external genitalia. Hematogenous spread can result from direct capillary invasion or through intricate lymphovascular anastomoses.

Clinical Presentation

A majority of women with invasive cervical cancer complain of vaginal bleeding, which may include heavy menses, intermenstrual bleeding, and postcoital bleeding. Pelvic pain, urinary frequency, and hematuria are rare presenting symptoms. Vaginal discharge is more common in adenocarcinoma and may be mistaken for cervicitis. On speculum exam, cervical cancers may appear ulcerative, bleeding, friable, or necrotic. Lesions may involve the fornices or vagina canal. Unilateral or bilateral fixation is a bad sign, indicating pelvic wall involvement. Tumor extension to the bladder or rectum may manifest as fistulae and foul vaginal discharge. Rarely, a patient may present with end-stage symptoms such as uremia, enlarged supraclavicular or inguinal nodes, hepatomegaly, leg swelling, or other distant metastases.

Diagnostic Workup

The minimal requirements for a workup are history, physical examination, chest x-ray, intravenous pyelogram (IVP), cervical biopsy, cystoscopy, and proctosigmoidoscopy. The last five tests plus endocervical curettage should be performed routinely to adequately stage cervical cancer. Computed tomography (CT) scan has become increasingly popular, with several authors suggesting its use in clinical staging. However, Grumbine and colleagues found that CT scans were unreliable in detecting subclinical parametrial disease and nodal metastases <2 cm in diameter.[7] Enlarged lymph nodes should be proven histologically by excisional biopsy or fine-needle aspiration. Magnetic resonance imaging (MRI) has emerged as a new radiologic modality capable of detecting early parametrial and nodal disease. Because of infrequent colon and small bowel involvement, the use of barium enema and upper gastrointestinal (GI) tract series should be restricted to symptomatic patients. Routine bone scan is usually unproductive.

Besides standard blood chemistry tests, patients should be checked for signs of chronic vaginal bleeding and anemia. Elevation of blood urea nitrogen (BUN) and serum creatinine usually means hydroureter and hydronephrosis. Liver function tests should be checked to rule out metastatic disease. Increased values of squamous cell carcinoma antigen (SCC) have been found in 50% to 75% of locally advanced cases.[8] SCC titer appears to correlate well with disease stage, tumor volume, and response to treatment.

Staging System

Clinical Staging

The official staging system for cervical carcinoma is based on clinical assessment (Table 33-3). In a Gynecologic Oncology Group (GOG) study of 320 advanced cervical cancers, lymphangiogram was reported to be a better technique for detecting nodal spread than CT or ultrasound.[9] Optimal staging can be ideally performed under general anesthesia at the time of cystoscopy and proctosigmoidoscopy. Staging should be a collaboration between the surgeon and the radiation oncologist.

Surgical Staging

Studies continue to point out the deficiency of clinical staging. In a study comparing clinical and surgical staging in 282 patients, Averette and colleagues found a discrepancy rate of 38%.[10] Information gained from surgical staging can help to optimize treatment in specific patients; for example, those found to have microscopic aortic disease during surgical staging can be offered extended field radiation. To reduce bowel complications, extraperitoneal staging is currently preferred if postoperative radiotherapy is contemplated.

Pathologic Classification

Most cervical cancers develop from the transformation zone, whereby columnar epithelium undergoes metaplasia to become squamous epithelium. It is generally accepted that squamous cancers of the cervix develop from preexisting dysplastic lesions. Squamous cancer typically presents as an ulcerated and exophytic lesion, while adenocarcinoma presents as an enlarged, barrel-shaped cervix.

Adenocarcinoma of the cervix accounts for 5% to 20% of cervical carcinomas. Epidemiologically, cervical adenocarcinoma affects the same patient popula-

Table 33-3. TNM Staging for Cervix Uteri Carcinoma

Primary Tumor (T)

TNM	FIGO*	Definition
TX	—	Primary tumor cannot be assessed
T0	—	No evidence of primary tumor
Tis	—	Carcinoma in situ
T1	I	Cervical carcinoma confined to the uterus (extension to the corpus should be disregarded)
T1a	IA	Preclinical invasive carcinoma, diagnosed by microscopy only
T1a1	IA1	Minimal microscopic stromal invasion
T1a2	IA2	Tumor with an invasive component 5 mm or less in depth taken from the base of the epithelium and 7 mm or less in horizontal spread
T1b	IB	Tumor larger than T1a2
T2	II	Cervical carcinoma invades beyond the uterus but not to the pelvic wall or to the lower third of the vagina
T2a	IIA	Tumor without parametrial invasion
T2b	IIB	Tumor with parametrial invasion
T3	III	Cervical carcinoma extends to the pelvic wall and/or involves the lower third of the vagina and/or causes hydronephrosis or nonfunctioning kidney
T3a	IIIA	Tumor involves the lower third of the vagina, with no extension to the pelvic wall
T3b	IIIB	Tumor extends to the pelvic wall and/or causes hydronephrosis or a nonfunctioning kidney
T4**	IVA	Tumor invades the mucosa of the bladder or rectum and/or extends beyond the true pelvis
M1	IVB	Distant metastasis

Regional Lymph Nodes (N)

NX	Regional lymph nodes cannot be assessed
N0	No regional lymph node metastasis
N1	Regional lymph node metastasis

*FIGO: Federation Internationale de Gynecologie et d'Obstetrique

**Note: Presence of bullous edema is not sufficient evidence to classify a tumor as T4.

Table 33-3 *Continued.* TNM Staging for Cervix Uteri Carcinoma

Distant Metastasis (M)

TNM	FIGO*	Definition
MX		Presence of distant metastasis cannot be assessed
M0		No distant metastasis
M1	IVB	Distant metastasis

Stage Grouping

AJCC/UICC				FIGO
Stage 0	Tis	N0	M0	
Stage IA	T1a	N0	M0	Stage IA
Stage IB	T1b	N0	M0	Stage IB
Stage IIA	T2a	N0	M0	Stage IIA
Stage IIB	T2b	N0	M0	Stage IIB
Stage IIIA	T3a	N0	M0	Stage IIIA
Stage IIIB	T1	N1	M0	Stage IIIB
	T2	N1	M0	
	T3a	N1	M0	
	T3b	Any N	M0	
Stage IVA	T4	Any N	M0	Stage IVA
Stage IVB	Any T	Any N	M1	Stage IVB

From American Joint Committee on Cancer.[36]

tion as endometrial or ovarian carcinoma. Increased mucous discharge in adenocarcinoma patients can be mistaken for cervicitis or vaginitis. Adenosquamous carcinoma, which represents 5% to 15% of cervical carcinomas, does not differ grossly from cervical adenocarcinoma. Both its glandular and squamous components are usually poorly differentiated. Glassy cell carcinoma is an extremely virulent subtype and may account for <5% of cervical carcinomas. It may develop into invasive cancer and bypass preinvasive stages. Patients often give a history of prior normal Pap smear.

Prognosis

Important prognostic factors include tumor grade, pelvic node involvement, depth of invasion, and lymphovascular space invasion. In general, the more advanced the stage, the poorer the prognosis. From cumulative data, 5-year survival rates were 75% to 90% for stage I, 50% to 70% for stage II, 30% to 35% for stage III, and 10% to 15% for stage IV.[3] Large tumor size is associated with poor survival and increased nodal metastasis. In a study of 100 patients with stage IB cervical cancer, recurrence rates of 7%, 26%, and 57% were associated with primary tumors <2, 2-3, and >3 cm in diameter, respectively.[11] In a GOG study of 732 stage I patients, the 3-year disease-free intervals were 95% for occult lesions, 88% for lesions <3 cm, and 68% for those >3 cm.[12] From the University of Miami experience, 5-year survival rates of 90.7%, 80.5%, and 63.5% were reported for squamous, adenocarcinoma, and adenosquamous cancers, respectively.[13] Thus, adenosquamous cancer appears the most virulent cell type.

In 978 stage IB-IIA patients, median survivals of 7.5 and 3.2 years were reported for well-differentiated (grade 1) and poorly differentiated (grade 3) lesions, respectively.[13] In the GOG study of stage I lesions, 3-year disease-free intervals of 77% and 89% were reported for patients with and without capillary space invasion, as well as disease-free intervals for various stromal invasion: 95% for <5 mm, 86% for 6-10 mm, 75% for 11-15 mm, and 71% for 16-20 mm.[12]

Cervical carcinoma has a tendency to spread to the pelvic and para-aortic lymphatics. In the same GOG study, 3-year disease-free intervals were 86% for those with no lymph node involvement, compared with 74% for those with pelvic node metastasis.[12] In the Miami series, median survival was 5.3 years for stage IB patients with no pelvic and aortic node metastasis, which decreased significantly to 3.2 and 1.3 years, respectively, with pelvic and aortic involvement.[13]

General Management

Treatment recommendations are generally based on the clinical stage of disease. For stage IB-IIA cervical carcinoma, radical hysterectomy with pelvic lymphadenectomy has been established to be as effective as radiation therapy. Surgical therapy is advised for patients with a history of diverticular disease, tubo-ovarian or appendiceal abscess, prior radiation therapy, and pelvic kidney. It is also advised in non-compliant and psychotic patients, in whom rapid treatment is needed. Adjuvant radiotherapy is recommended in radical hysterectomy patients with the following risk factors: microscopic parametrial invasion, large lesions (>4 cm), nodal metastasis, lymphovascular invasion, grade 3 lesions, and surgical margin involvement.[14] Stage IIB-IV cervical carcinoma, or locally advanced disease, is routinely treated by radiotherapy. The literature supports a combination of surgical and radiation therapy for patients with cervical adenocarcinoma. Glassy cell carcinoma appears resistant to conventional treatment and may require combination modalities, such as radical hysterectomy and irradiation for stage IB patients. Patients presenting with distant metastases should be treated with chemotherapy. Currently there is no effective single agent or combination chemotherapeutic regimen for advanced or recurrent cervical cancer. In certain locally advanced cervical cancers, neoadjuvant chemotherapy followed by radical hysterectomy is a viable option.

Surgery

Based on a 25-year experience at one medical center, radical hysterectomy is associated with a 5-year survival of 90.1%.[13] This is consistent with an 89% cumulative 5-year survival based on worldwide experience. Surgical treatment of cervical carcinoma can preserve ovarian function and prevent vaginal stenosis in young women. Hysterectomy patients can avoid the immediate and long-term bladder and bowel complications of radiotherapy. Most surgeons prefer to operate on cervical lesions of <3-4 cm to avoid the increased need of adjuvant radiotherapy with larger lesions.

Radiation Therapy

Postoperative radiation is commonly delivered in fractionation, to a total dose of 4,500-5,000 rads with acceptable toxicity. Even though no survival advantage was shown, radiation therapy appeared to reduce the incidence of pelvic recurrences. About 85% of recurrences had distant metastasis. Hopefully, the results of GOG 92 will help determine the value of adjuvant radiotherapy in high-risk radical hysterectomy patients. Patients with aortic metastasis, in whom 5-year survival is reduced to 20% to 50%, constitute a special management problem.[15] Current treatments include extended field radiation with or without cytotoxic agents as radiosensitizers.

Five-year survival rates in irradiated stage IIB and III patients are 65% and 45%, respectively.[16] Local control of bone or brain metastases can be achieved with palliative radiation.

Chemotherapy

The adjunctive use of short-term chemotherapy, such as hydroxyurea and cisplatin, as radiation sensitizers is ineffective in controlling distant disease. Diverting colostomy is routinely recommended for rectovaginal fistula prior to radiotherapy. However, it is prudent to postpone urinary diversion until after radiotherapy unless the field of radiation includes the perineal area.

Induction chemotherapy has become increasingly popular.[17] Neoadjuvant chemotherapy appears to consolidate local disease and decrease the frequency of regional nodal metastasis. In a large number of patients, tumor reduction may be significant enough to allow safe radical hysterectomy. Response rates from 35% to 85% have been reported with various chemotherapeutic regimens. Further trials are needed in a randomized fashion to fully evaluate neoadjuvant chemotherapy followed by radical hysterectomy.

Complications and Recurrences

Urinary tract fistulae are one of the most serious complications of radical hysterectomy. An overall incidence of 1.4% is based on a 0.8% rate of primary fistulae combined with a 0.6% rate of radiotherapy-associated fistulae. Because of an injured autonomic nerve supply, bladder and rectum dysfunction are the most common complaints after radical hysterectomy. Rarely, prolonged Foley drainage or self-catheterization is required in certain patients who had voiding difficulty prior to surgery. Similarly, denervation of the rectum can lead to constipation. These patients can benefit from laxatives and most are able to overcome this problem within a few months.

Persistent or recurrent cervical cancer is associated with a 5-year survival of <5%. Treatment failure after primary surgical therapy is usually managed by radiation. Most failures occur in advanced cases. About 50% of recurrences are diagnosed in the first year of follow-up, 75% by the second year, and 95% by the fifth year. Thus, follow-up visits should be more frequent during the first 2-3 years. Symptoms of new onset, such as pain and vaginal bleeding or discharge, should be thoroughly investigated.

Because 25% to 50% of cases can be cured with pelvic exenteration, it is important to identify patients with early pelvic recurrence. Pap smear should be routinely obtained since it may be the first sign of an early recurrence. Chest x-ray should be performed annually, or more frequently as indicated. The first evidence of recurrent cancer is frequently a new hydronephrosis. Therefore, IVP should be routinely done 3 and 9 months after definitive therapy. Any suspicion of tumor recurrence should be confirmed by biopsy or needle aspiration.

Systemic cervical carcinoma is rarely curable. Treatment is often palliative and may involve a combination of surgery, radiation, and chemotherapy.

Endometrial Carcinoma

Epidemiology

Endometrial carcinoma is the most common female genital cancer and ranks fourth in prevalence behind breast, lung, and colorectal cancers. About 31,000 new cases and 5,900 deaths associated with this cancer occurred in 1994.[1] Endometrial cancer affects mostly postmenopausal women with a median age of 58 years. However, 25% of cases occur in premenopausal women. The incidence of endometrial cancer varies widely among different ethnic groups and countries (Table 33-4). The risk of uterine cancer over a woman's lifetime is estimated to be 2.7% for whites and 1.6% for blacks.

Obesity, diabetes, hypertension, and nulliparity are common associated conditions of endometrial cancer. Other risk factors include history of chronic anovulation, irregular menses, exogenous estrogen consumption, pelvic irradiation, and late menopause (Table 33-5).[18] The use of unopposed estrogen replacement was thought to account for the dramatic increase in incidence of endometrial cancer in the US between 1970 and 1975.[19] Since then, the addition of progesterone and use of combination estrogen-progestin oral contraceptives appear to protect against endometrial hyperplasia and cancer development. Ingestion of food with high animal fat content has been suggested as a contributing factor of high endometrial cancer rates in Western countries.

Table 33-4. Incidence of Endometrial Carcinoma From 1960 to 1980 (Rate Per 100,000 Women)

	1960	1965	1970	1975	1980
United States					
Alameda County, Calif					
White	–	16.8	33.3	38.5	24.8
Black	–	18.1	13.6	10.5	10.8
New York State	12.0	–	12.7	18.8	16.7
Connecticut	12.8	15.3	17.8	21.3	–
Hawaii					
White	15.6	17.5	28.8	34.8	23.4
Hawaiian	18.1	23.9	31.8	34.6	25.2
Chinese	–	19.5	19.7	28.5	18.7
Japanese	9.8	10.8	15.6	19.4	15.5
Filipino	–	16.2	11.2	14.8	11.0
Puerto Rico	3.0	4.6	6.1	6.3	8.0
Miyagi, Japan	2.0	1.3	1.3	2.0	2.8
Sweden	11.1	12.0	12.1	13.0	13.2
Hamburg, Germany	9.2	–	8.9	10.3	11.3
Cali, Colombia	8.1	6.8	5.1	4.3	6.0

Adapted from Parazzini et al.[19]

Pathogenesis and Natural History

Although estrogen appears to play a pathogenetic role, the exact cause of endometrial carcinoma is still unknown. Certain oncogenes appear to play a role in the genesis and natural progression of endometrial cancer. In a study of 16 primary endometrial cancers, two thirds had overexpression of HER-2/*neu* and c-*myc* oncogenes.[20] Among those with oncogene overexpression, 50% died within 1 year, while all patients with normal expression survived at 31-month follow-up. Using immunocytochemistry, Long et al reported a correlation between tumor grades and expression levels of *ras* oncogene.[21]

Table 33-5. Risk Factors in the Development of Endometrial Carcinoma

Characteristic	Risk Ratio
Obesity >50 lb	10
Unopposed estrogen	9.5
Obesity >30 lb	3
Diabetes	2.8
Late menopause	2.4
Nulliparity	2
Hypertension	1.5

Adapted from Park et al.[18]

Depending on the aggressiveness of tumor biology, invasion of the underlying myometrium may occur early in the course of tumor development. Involvement of the isthmus and cervix can be superficial with gland elements or deep in the stroma. Lymphatic involvement may occur early and varies with tumor grade and site of origin. Lymphatic invasion to the pelvic and aortic areas appears a hallmark of endometrial carcinoma. Endometrial cancers from the lower and middle portions of the uterus usually drain into parametria and the paracervical, hypogastric, and obturator lymph nodes. However, fundal lesions tend to empty into the common iliac and aortic nodes. Invasion of the round ligament can lead to inguinal lymphadenopathy. Peritoneal implants may result from tubal spillage or direct extension.

Clinical Presentation

Ninety percent of patients complain of postmenopausal bleeding or irregular vaginal bleeding. The amount of bleeding does not seem to correlate with disease severity. Unfortunately, many women delay seeking medical attention for vaginal spotting or scant bleeding on an irregular basis. The older the patient, the greater the likelihood of cancer as a cause of postmenopausal bleeding. Patients may also complain of pelvic pain and foul, purulent discharge from pyometria. In advanced cases, endometrial carcinoma may present like ovarian cancer with ascites, pelvic/abdominal mass, and bowel symptoms. Metastases to the vagina and suburethral areas occur with resulting inguinal lymphadenopathy. Hematogenous spread usually involves lung, liver, and bone.

Diagnostic Workup

Currently there is no satisfactory screening procedure for endometrial cancer. Endometrial biopsy and fractional dilation and curettage (D&C), which can reliably and accurately detect endometrial cancer and precursor lesions, are recommended for women with bleeding abnormalities. An endometrial biopsy may miss the representative tissue. If complex endometrial hyperplasia is found on a biopsy specimen, a formal D&C is required to exclude the presence of cancer elsewhere in the cavity. Up to 15% to 25% of patients in whom complex atypical hyperplasia were diagnosed by endometrial biopsy may actually have adenocarcinoma on uterine curettage specimen. A finding of endometrial cells or histiocytes on Pap smears of postmenopausal women is an indication for biopsy. Approximately 2% to 5% of endometrial cancer are diagnosed in the asymptomatic patient during the workup of an abnormal Pap smear. Recently, vaginal sonography and color flow Doppler study have been used to screen for endometrial cancer.

All patients in whom endometrial cancer is suspected should have a complete history, physical examination, fractional D&C, chest x-ray, IVP, cystoscopy, and proctosigmoidoscopy. Additional studies such as ultrasound, CT scan, and MRI may provide useful information such as adnexal involvement, uterine size, degree of myometrial invasion, ascites, and lymphadenopathy.

Endometrial cancer frequently metastasizes to the distal vagina and suburethral areas. Examination of the pelvis should include the external genitalia. The cervix and os should be inspected for signs of tumor extension. Rectovaginal exam should be performed to evaluate the adnexa and parametria for induration and nodularity. The uterus is typically enlarged and softened. Rarely, supraclavicular or inguinal nodes are involved. Routine bone and liver scan are usually nonproductive. Serum CA125 should be drawn in all endometrial cancer patients. Elevated values have been found in 80% of patients with advanced or metastatic lesions and highly correlated with extrauterine disease and deep myometrial invasion.

Staging

Endometrial carcinoma has been staged surgically since 1988 by the International Federation of Gynecology and Obstetrics (FIGO) system (Table 33-6). Several studies have convincingly demonstrated the inadequacy of clinical evaluation.

Pathologic Classification

Endometrial cancer usually develops in the uterine fundus and grows into the endometrial cavity, producing an exophytic lesion (Fig 33-1). It is generally accepted that endometrial hyperplasia results from unopposed estrogen stimulation. While the risk of endometrial cancer is approximately 1% to 3% for simple and complex hyperplasia, complex atypical hyperplasia is considered synonymous with carcinoma in situ. If left untreated, 29% of complex

Table 33-6. TNM Staging for Corpus Uteri Carcinoma

Primary Tumor (T)

TNM	FIGO*	Definition
TX	—	Primary tumor cannot be assessed
T0	—	No evidence of primary tumor
Tis	—	Carcinoma in situ
T1	I	Tumor confined to the corpus uteri
T1a	IA	Tumor limited to the endometrium
T1b	IB	Tumor invades up to or less than one-half of the myometrium
T1c	IC	Tumor invades more than one-half of the myometrium
T2	II	Tumor invades the cervix but not extending beyond the uterus
T2a	IIA	Endocervical glandular involvement only
T2b	IIB	Cervical stromal invasion
T3 and/or **N1**	III	Local and/or regional spread as specified in T3a, b, N1 and FIGO IIIA, B, and C below
T3a	IIIA	Tumor involves the serosa and/or adnexa (direct extension or metastasis) and/or cancer cells in ascites or peritoneal washings
T3b	IIIB	Vaginal involvement (direct extension of metastasis)
N1	IIIC	Metastasis to the pelvic and/or para-aortic lymph nodes
T4**	IVA	Tumor invades the bladder mucosa or the rectum and/or the bowel mucosa
M1	IVB	Distant metastasis (*excluding* metastasis to the vagina, pelvic serosa, or adnexa; *including* metastasis to intra-abdominal lymph nodes other than paraortic, and/or inguinal lymph nodes)

Regional Lymph Nodes (N)

NX	Regional lymph nodes cannot be assessed
N0	No regional lymph node metastasis
N1	Regional lymph node metastasis

*FIGO: Federation Internationale de Gynecologie et d'Obstetrique

**Note: Presence of bullous edema is not sufficient evidence to classify a tumor as T4.

Table 33-6 *Continued.* TNM Staging for Corpus Uteri Carcinoma

Distant Metastasis (M)

TNM	FIGO*	Definition
MX	—	Presence of distant metastasis cannot be assessed
M0	—	No distant metastasis
M1	IVB	Distant metastasis

Stage Grouping

AJCC/UICC				FIGO
Stage 0	Tis	N0	M0	
Stage IA	T1a	N0	M0	Stage IA
Stage IB	T1b	N0	M0	Stage IB
Stage IC	T1c	N0	M0	Stage IC
Stage IIA	T2a	N0	M0	Stage IIA
Stage IIB	T2b	N0	M0	Stage IIB
Stage IIIA	T3a	N0	M0	Stage IIIA
Stage IIIB	T3b	N0	M0	Stage IIIB
Stage IIIC	T1	N1	M0	Stage IIIC
	T2	N1	M0	
	T3a	N1	M0	
	T3b	N1	M0	
Stage IVA	T4	Any N	M0	Stage IVA
Stage IVB	Any T	Any N	M1	Stage IVB

From American Joint Committee on Cancer.[36]

atypical hyperplasia cases would develop into endometrial carcinoma.

The most common histologic type is endometrioid carcinoma, accounting for 75% to 80% of cases. Squamous differentiation occurs in one third to one half of cases. Well-differentiated lesions correspond to adenoacanthoma, and poor differentiation to adenosquamous carcinoma.

Some 10% of endometrial cancers are papillary serous carcinomas, and 4% to 5% are clear cell adenocarcinomas. The former closely resemble serous carcinoma of the ovary and fallopian tube. Histologically, serous tumor is characterized by papillary projections, lined by bizarre cells with scanty cytoplasm, and appears to detach easily. Psammoma bodies and clear cell features are frequently seen. Papillary serous adenocarcinoma tends to be poorly differentiated and highly associated with invasion of the outer half of the myometrium as well as extrauterine spread. Clear cell adenocarcinoma of the endometrium has the same histologic appearance as clear

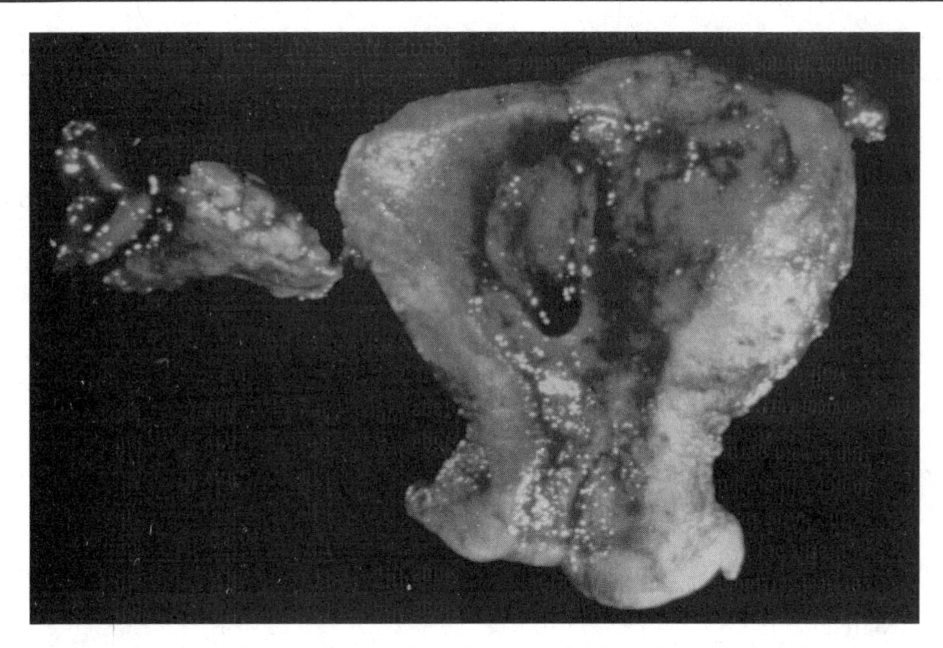

Fig 33-1. Endometrial carcinoma arises from the uterine fundus and grows into a polypoid mass.

cell tumor of the vagina, cervix, and ovary. Histologically, clear cell tumor may assume solid, cystic, tubular, or papillary patterns. Clear cell tumor is characterized by hobnail cells with pink secretions within the gland lumina. These cells produce glycogen and stained positive for PAS. Clear cell adenocarcinoma is an aggressive tumor variant.

Prognostic Factors

Based on GOG studies in women with clinical stage I and II endometrial cancers,[22,23] important risk factors are cell type, tumor grade, depth of myometrial invasion, vascular space invasion, and cervical extension. Among cell types, papillary serous, squamous, undifferentiated, and clear cells are associated with poor outcome. The degree of tumor differentiation was a strong predictor of outcome, with the worst outcome observed in the least differentiated tumors. The GOG study also demonstrated that the incidence of deep myometrial invasion and pelvic and aortic node metastases increased as the tumor became less differentiated.

Depth of myometrial invasion has been consistently shown to be the most important determinant of extrauterine spread, treatment failure, and tumor recurrence. Cervical or isthmic involvement doubled the risk of nodal metastasis and carries a higher relapse rate. When there is evidence of vascular space invasion, the risk of pelvic or aortic node metastasis increases.

Extrauterine risk factors include adnexal involvement, abdominal spread, positive cytologic findings, and pelvic and aortic node metastases. While the incidence of microscopic adnexal metastases is only 6%, its involvement is greatly associated with nodal disease. When there was gross peritoneal disease, the incidence of pelvic and aortic disease climbed to 51% and 23%, respectively. Among cases with positive cytology, the incidences of pelvic and aortic disease were 25% and 19%, respectively. Several investigators have demonstrated a poor outcome for patients with positive cytology.[22,24] Once pelvic node is involved, the risk of aortic disease is 32%.

Studies have confirmed the prognostic value of DNA ploidy in endometrial cancer. Britton observed in 1990 that patients with diploid tumors had a 4-year disease-free interval of 88%, compared with 57% for nondiploid lesions.[25] Diploid cancers are associated with lower relapse rates than aneuploid or tetraploid tumors.

General Management

Standard treatment of endometrial carcinoma is abdominal hysterectomy and bilateral salpingo-oophorectomy. Surgery alone is reserved for patients with little risk of recurrence, such as those with grade 1 or 2 lesions and no myometrial invasion (stage IA G1,2). Adjuvant radiotherapy is recommended for patients with any risk factors. Patients with documented pelvic and/or aortic node metastases should have a CT scan of the chest and abdomen. If lymphadenopathy is found in the thorax or supraclavicular areas, combination chemotherapy is often prescribed since widespread systemic disease is likely. However, patients with limited lymph node disease can be successfully treated with extended field radiotherapy. Advanced endometrial cancer should be managed in the same way as ovarian carcinoma—a combination of surgery, radiation or chemotherapy, and progestin therapy. In medically inoperable patients, radiotherapy alone or high-dose progestin therapy is suggested. Abdominal irradiation should be reserved for optimally debulked cases without extra-abdominal metastasis. In the highly virulent papillary serous carcinoma, careful surgical staging and aggressive therapy are recommended.

Surgery

Surgico-pathologic staging is advised for all medically operable patients with endometrial carcinoma. This phase of the surgery is necessary to identify the high-risk patient who may benefit from adjunctive therapy. Removal of both adnexa is part of the surgical treatment since they may contain microscopic metastases. Furthermore, the ovaries may be the source of estrogen production, which could stimulate residual endometrial carcinoma. Overall 5-year survival in stage I patients treated with primary irradiation is 70% to 80%, compared with 50% in stage II patients.[26]

Radical hysterectomy is restricted to (a) patients with gross cervical involvement (stage II) and contraindications to radiation therapy (history of multiple laparotomies, adnexal mass, tubo-ovarian masses, or diverticular abscess; pelvic kidney); (b) those with cervical cancer who were successfully irradiated and subsequently developed endometrial cancer; and (c) stage II patients who refuse radiotherapy.

Radiotherapy

Radiation therapy can improve local/regional control and serve as an effective adjuvant modality. A recent GOG study reported a local/regional recurrence rate of 34.6% for the surgery-only group, compared with 12.5% for those receiving adjuvant radiotherapy, thus favoring the use of postoperative radiotherapy for high-risk patients.[22] Postoperative pelvic irradiation (4,000-5,000 rads in 6 weeks) is advised for all patients except those with surgical stage IA G1,2 without vascular space invasion.

Vagina cuff implant with a surface dose of 5,000-7,000 rads can reduce cuff recurrence from 12%-15% to 1%-3%. When comparing external beam therapy and vaginal brachytherapy, vaginal implant was clearly superior to pelvis teletherapy in controlling local recurrences. In advanced and recurrent cases, radiation can be used for local control of brain, neck, and bone metastases.

In medically inoperable patients with a small uterus, tandem and ovoid application is probably appropriate. When the uterus is enlarged, Heyman capsules may result in a better cure. In 171 stage I patients treated with Heyman packing, 5-year survival rates of 72% to 76% were reported.[27] High-dose progestin therapy is another alternative in medically inoperable patients. Three months after definitive radiotherapy, a repeat biopsy is recommended to monitor treatment response. In persistent cases, any contraindication to surgery should be reviewed and corrected.

Chemotherapy

Adriamycin has demonstrated some activity in endometrial cancer. The addition of Cytoxan to Adriamycin does not result in improved survival. Cisplatin has modest activity; cisplatin-containing regimens and other combinations have been suggested by many authors, with activity ranging from 30% to 80%. However, most responses were only partial, with median survival commonly <12 months. If a response to chemotherapy is obtained, treatment is continued for 6 to 12 cycles. Serum CA125 may be useful to monitor the disease status if values are elevated. Because of the tendency of endometrial cancer to spread systematically, second-look laparotomy is of limited value.

Hormonal Therapy

Hormonal therapy has been tried for 30 years, with early reports claiming response rates of 20% to 40%. However, a recent GOG study reported a 14% objective response rate with 50 mg of medroxyprogesterone acetate, three times a day orally.[28] Hormonal response correlated well with tumor grade, with response rates of 94%, 15%, and 1.5% for grades 1, 2, and 3, respectively. As side effects of high-dose progestin therapy, many patients reported an improved sense of well-being and enhanced appetite.

Progesterone receptor (PR) levels change with tumor differentiation, with the more differentiated the tumor, the higher the PR. Several authors have demonstrated the independent prognostic value of estrogen receptor (ER) and PR with poor outcome associated with lack of receptors. An overall response rate of 68% has been observed for PR-positive tumors in contrast to 9.9% for PR-negative cancers.[29] Once a beneficial response to hormonal therapy has been determined, progestin therapy should be continued for as long as the disease remains stable or in remission. Occasionally, hormonal response has been observed in patients with known negative receptors.

Follow-up

Careful follow-up is necessary during the first 2-3 years, when approximately 75% of recurrences occur. Routine follow-up should include a detailed history, noting in particular any new complaints, and assessment of the abdominal and pelvic cavities with special attention to the lymph node areas. Vaginal cytology and serum CA125 should be obtained at each visit, in addition to routine blood chemistry studies. Follow-up visits should take place every 2-3 months during the first 3 years and every 6 months thereafter.

Ovarian Carcinomas

Epidemiology

Only 39% of all women with ovarian carcinoma survive for 5 years. This deadly disease accounted for about 13,600 deaths in the US in 1994 as well as some 24,000 new cases.[1] Nearly 60% of ovarian neoplasms are germ cell tumors in children and women younger than 20 years, while epithelial ovarian cancer is predominantly a disease of postmenopausal women. The lifetime risk of a woman developing ovarian cancer is approximately 1.8%. The incidence of this cancer may vary by age and race. As documented by the Surveillance, Epidemiology, and End Results (SEER) study, the rate increases from <1 per 100,000 women aged 20 or younger to 59 per 100,000 in the 75 to 79 age group.[30] In another study, the age-adjusted incidence rate for whites was 12 to 14 per 100,000, compared with 6 to 9 per 100,000 for blacks.[19]

Consistently identified risk factors include a positive family history, few or no children, older age at first marriage, and childbirth (Table 33-7).[31] An association has been shown between ovarian carcinoma and cancers of the endometrium, breast, and colon.

Table 33-7. Relative Risk Associated with Epidemiologic Factors in the Development of Ovarian Carcinoma

Risk Factor	Relative Risk
General population	1.4
Family history	17-50
Nulliparity	4-5
1-2 children	3
Use of talc	3
Obesity	2
Oral contraceptives	0.5

Adapted from Morrow and Townsend.[31]

Pathogenesis and Natural History

There are no known causes of ovarian cancer, but hormones, diet, genetic disposition, and oncogenes may be contributing factors. The protective effects of childbearing have been confirmed by the Ovarian Patient Care Evaluation (PCE) study.[32] To account for this phenomenon, it has been proposed that incessant ovulation may have a role in the development of ovarian carcinoma. Several case-control studies show oral contraceptive use to decrease risk by 30% to 60%.[19,33] Increased dietary intake of fat and coffee is thought to contribute to the high ovarian cancer rates in Western countries. Lynch has reported three familial ovarian cancer syndromes: site-specific ovarian cancer; familial ovarian and breast cancers; and Lynch type II familial cancer syndrome, which predisposes its members to colorectal, endometrial, and ovarian cancers.[34] These syndromes affect younger patients (average age, 48 years) and are associated with poor survival. Genetic transmission follows the pattern of autosomal dominance with variable penetrance. Certain oncogenes may play a role in the genesis or natural progression of ovarian cancer. Overexpression of HER-2/*neu* oncogene, activated *ras* oncogene, and chromosomal abnormalities have been reported in some patients with ovarian cancer, but the significance of these findings has yet to be determined.

Clinical Presentation

Based on the Ovarian PCE study, common symptoms include abdominal pain, abdominal swelling, bloating or dyspepsia, and pelvic pressure.[32] About 50% of those patients presented with ascites or abdominal-pelvic mass. As the tumor grows, patients may complain of abdominal bloating, increased abdominal girth, and weight gain. Advanced disease is associated with anorexia, severe pain, weight loss, nausea, and vomiting. In early stages, pain may be due to stretching of the ovarian capsule, tumor hemorrhage, necrosis, torsion, or rupture. Many patients do not seek medical help until the abdominal mass becomes quite large. The most common physical sign is abdominal distention, which may be difficult to evaluate. Ascites is a strong indication of malignancy; however, a huge ovarian cystic structure can fill the abdomen and elicit fluid waves like ascites. Supraclavicular, inguinal, and axillary areas should be carefully palpated for nodal enlargement. The external genitalia of ovarian cancer patients is usually normal. Speculum examination may reveal a deviated cervix due to extrinsic compression. In the presence of ascites, rectovaginal examination is more informative than abdominal-pelvic exam and may reveal tumor extension.

Diagnostic Workup

The diagnostic workup should be tailored to the patient's age, symptoms, and physical findings. Older patients with persistent unexplained pelvic pain should be laparoscoped to rule out ovarian neoplasm. In childhood and adolescence, torsion of an ovarian tumor may mimic acute appendicitis. Chest x-ray should be routinely ordered to access metastases and pleural effusion. The presence of calcifications on abdominal x-ray suggests a benign pelvic mass. IVP is informative if it shows urinary tract anomalies or ureteral obstruction. Depending on the gastrointestinal symptoms, barium enema and upper GI series may be indicated. Based on findings from the Ovarian PCE study,[32] ultrasound and CT of the abdomen and pelvis should be considered as routine tests in the preoperative assessment of patients suspected of ovarian cancer. These tests can reveal important tumor characteristics such as excrescences, septations, solid components, and ascites; CT is better for evaluating retroperitoneal nodes. The role of MRI is still not well defined. In the absence of cardinal symptoms, bone and liver scans are of little value.

Routine blood chemistry, serum albumin, calcium, magnesium, renal, and liver function tests are essential to complete the evaluation and to help manage the patient postoperatively. When germ cell tumors are suspected, tumor markers such as lactate dehydrogenase (LDH), human chorionic gonadotropin (HCG), and alpha-fetoprotein (AFP) should be routinely ordered. Serum CA125 is a valuable marker for serous ovarian carcinoma; a cutoff value of 35 U/mL is often used because elevated levels are found in 80% to 85% of ovarian cancers but <1% in normal patients.[35]

The risks associated with paracentesis or culdocentesis usually outweigh the benefits. However, paracentesis is sometimes necessary to decompress tense ascites and relieve respiratory distress. Pleural effusion should be tapped to determine cytologic characteristics because results may warrant reclassification to a more advanced stage.

Surgical Staging

Staging of ovarian cancer is based on surgicopathologic findings. The AJCC and FIGO staging systems described in Table 33-8 reflect closely the natural behavior of ovarian cancer biology.[36]

Pathologic Classification

Ovarian neoplasms are classified according to cell of origin, arising from the celomic epithelium (60% to 70% of cases), specialized stroma (5% to 10%), and germ cell layer (or unfertilized ovum) (15% to 20%). The prognosis and management of each of these tumor groups will be discussed separately. Epithelial ovarian neoplasms are derived from the celomic, or mullerian-derived, epithelium of the female genital tract. Coelomic epithelium can give rise to a variety of cell resemblance. For example, serous tumors resemble tubal neoplasms and mucinous tumors correspond to endocervical cancers.

Malignant Epithelial Neoplasms

Epithelial ovarian tumors may be malignant (85% of all ovarian cancers) or borderline. The epithelial component in malignant tumors can usually be classified as serous, mucinous, endometrioid, or clear cell.

The most common ovarian tumor, serous carcinoma tends to grow rapidly with early intraperitoneal spread. Bilateral involvement occurs in 30% of stage I lesions and is the rule in advanced cases. Microscopically, the tumor is solid and cystic with

Table 33-8. TNM Staging for Ovarian Carcinoma

Primary Tumor (T)

TNM	FIGO*	Definition
TX	—	Primary tumor cannot be assessed
T0	—	No evidence of primary tumor
T1	I	Tumor limited to ovaries (one or both)
T1a	IA	Tumor limited to one ovary; capsule intact, no tumor on ovarian surface, no malignant cells in ascites or peritoneal washings
T1b	IB	Tumor limited to both ovaries; capsules intact, no tumor on ovarian surface, no malignant cells in ascites or peritoneal washings
T1c	IC	Tumor limited to one or both ovaries with any of the following: capsule ruptured, tumor on ovarian surface, malignant cells in ascites or peritoneal washings
T2	II	Tumor involves one or both ovaries with pelvic extension
T2a	IIA	Extension and/or implants on the uterus and/or tube(s); no malignant cells in ascites or peritoneal washings
T2b	IIB	Extension to other pelvic tissues; no malignant cells in ascites or peritoneal washings
T2c	IIC	Pelvic extension (2a or 2b) with malignant cells in ascites or peritoneal washings
T3 and/or N1	III	Tumor involves one or both ovaries with microscopically confirmed peritoneal metastasis outside the pelvis and/or regional lymph node metastasis
T3a	IIIA	Microscopic peritoneal metastasis beyond the pelvis
T3b	IIIB	Macroscopic peritoneal metastasis beyond the pelvis 2 cm or less in the greatest dimension
T3c and/or N1	IIIC	Peritoneal metastasis beyond the pelvis more than 2 cm in the greatest dimension and/or regional lymph node metastasis
M1	IV	Distant metastasis (excludes peritoneal metastasis)

Note: Liver capsule metastasis is T3/Stage III; liver parenchymal metastasis, M1/Stage IV. Pleural effusion must have positive cytology for M1/Stage IV.

*FIGO: Federation Internationale de Gynecologie et d'Obstetrique

Continued

Table 33-8 *Continued.* TNM Staging for Ovarian Carcinoma

Regional Lymph Nodes (N)

NX	Regional lymph nodes cannot be assessed
N0	No regional lymph node metastasis
N1	Regional lymph node metastasis

Distant Metastasis (M)

TNM	FIGO	Definition
MX	—	Presence of distant metastasis cannot be assessed
M0	—	No distant metastasis
M1	IV	Distant metastasis (excludes peritoneal metastasis)

Note: The presence of nonmalignant ascites is not classified. The presence of ascites does not affect staging unless malignant cells are present.

pTNM Pathologic Classification
The pT, pN, and pM categories correspond to the T, N, and M categories.

Stage Grouping

AJCC/UICC				FIGO
Stage IA	T1a	N0	M0	Stage IA
Stage IB	T1b	N0	M0	Stage IB
Stage IC	T1c	N0	M0	Stage IC
Stage IIA	T2a	N0	M0	Stage IIA
Stage IIB	T2b	N0	M0	Stage IIB
Stage IIC	T2c	N0	M0	Stage IIC
Stage IIIA	T3a	N0	M0	Stage IIIA
Stage IIIB	T3b	N0	M0	Stage IIIB
Stage IIIC	T3c	N0	M0	Stage IIIC
	Any T	N1	M0	
Stage IV	Any T	Any N	M1	Stage IV

From American Joint Committee on Cancer.[36]

extensive papillary growths and sometimes psammoma bodies.

Mucinous carcinoma tends to be larger than serous tumor and is bilateral in 5% to 10%. Approximately 50% are diagnosed in stage I or II. Grossly, mucinous ovarian carcinoma is multilocular with solid components. The cystic fluid can be watery or gelatinous. Microscopically, these tumors are lined by endocervical or intestinal-type mucous epithelium.

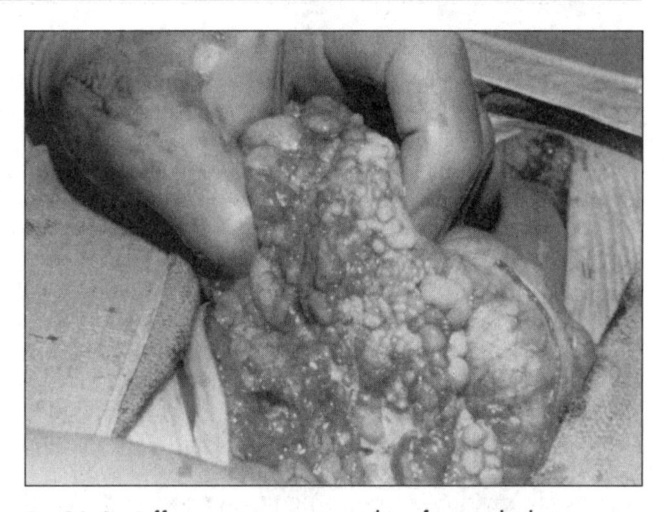

Fig 33-2. Diffuse carcinomatosis resulting from multiple tumor implants.

Endometrioid carcinoma occurs in conjunction with endometrial cancer in 15% to 30% of cases. Endometriosis is found in another 10% of endometrioid cancers. The incidence of bilateralism is about 15% in stage I cases. Microscopically, endometrioid and endometrial carcinomas are indistinguishable.

Clear cell adenocarcinoma is frequently diagnosed in stage I, with a bilateral incidence of 5% to 10%. Endometriosis is found in >25% of cases. In contrast to ovarian endometrioid tumors, endometrial cancer associated with clear cell ovarian carcinoma is more aggressive and less differentiated. Microscopically, clear cell carcinoma is characterized by hobnail cells with clear, glycogen-filled cytoplasm.

Pathophysiology

Ovarian carcinoma can spread via local extension, lymphatic invasion, peritoneal implants, hematogenous metastasis, and transdiaphragmatic passage.

Probably the most common mode of spread is peritoneal implantation. Once the capsule is ruptured, seeding occurs on the surface peritoneum. Multiple tumor implants can develop into diffuse carcinomatosis (Fig 33-2). Averette and colleagues demonstrated the circulatory pathway of peritoneal fluid drainage, which accurately delineated common sites of tumor implantation (Fig 33-3).[37] Preferred sites of tumor implantation include the cul-de-sac, liver surface, and omentum.

Ovarian cancer can invade the lymphatic channels and eventually involve the upper abdomen and beyond. Supraclavicular, inguinal, and axillary node involvement have all been reported. Lymph node metastasis increases from 8% for stage I lesions to 29% for stage III and 53% for stage IV disease. Hematogenous dissemination is common in advanced stages. The presence of distant metastases in advanced disease, such as in the liver or bone, supports the use of systemic therapy.

Several authors have suggested that some ovarian cancers resemble mesothelioma and could conceivably develop simultaneously from peritoneal and ovarian surface epithelium under the same carcinogenic field effect.[38] Primary peritoneal neoplasia is a disease entity that behaves very much like an ovarian carcinoma.

Prognosis

Tumor stage is an important prognostic factor. The Ovarian PCE study revealed worsening 5-year survival rates with advancing stage (89%, 57%, 24%, and 11% for stages I, II, III, and IV, respectively).[32] Cell type appears to have less prognostic value than stage or histologic grade. In the same study, 5-year survival was strongly affected by grade, with rates of 94% for borderline tumors, 74% for grade 1, 45% for grade 2, and 22% to 24% for grade 3 or 4 tumors.[32] Serous and clear cell tumors had the worst overall 5-year survival rates. Friedlander and colleagues observed that early tumors tended to be diploid, while advanced-stage tumors were aneuploid.[39] A median survival of 33 months was reported for diploid tumors, compared with 13 months for aneuploid tumors.

Screening and Prevention

Vaginal ultrasound has been used to screen for ovarian carcinoma in recent years. In a pilot study of 1,000 asymptomatic women aged 40 years and older, an abnormality rate of 3.1% was reported with screening vaginal sonography, of which one ovarian cancer was detected.[40] Because color Doppler flow study may improve the accuracy of vaginal ultrasound, combined use of the two modalities is currently being tested. CA125 is neither specific nor sensitive, and its use as a screening test for ovarian cancer is not supported.

In the Ovarian PCE study, approximately 18.2% of ovarian cancer patients reported a previous hysterectomy in which one or both ovaries were conserved.[32] Thus, prophylactic oophorectomy for women older than 40 years at the time of hysterectomy can significantly reduce the incidence of ovarian carcinoma.

General Management

The management of patients with ovarian carcinoma comprises surgery and adjuvant therapy. The primary goal of surgery is to remove as much cancer tissue as possible without compromising the patient's safety. Other important goals include accurate staging and optimal cytoreduction. Standard procedures include total abdominal hysterectomy, bilateral salpingo-oophorectomy, and omentectomy. Additional procedures, such as sigmoid colectomy and small-bowel resection, may be required to achieve optimal debulking. The aggressiveness of tumor debulking depends on whether resection of abdominal and pelvic disease is safe. For stage I patients, adjuvant radiotherapy but not chemotherapy is recommended; however, melphalan may be effective for high-risk patients with early-stage carcinoma. For advanced ovarian carcinoma, combination chemotherapy may be superior to single-agent therapy. Recently, neoadjuvant chemotherapy followed by interval debulking has been advo-

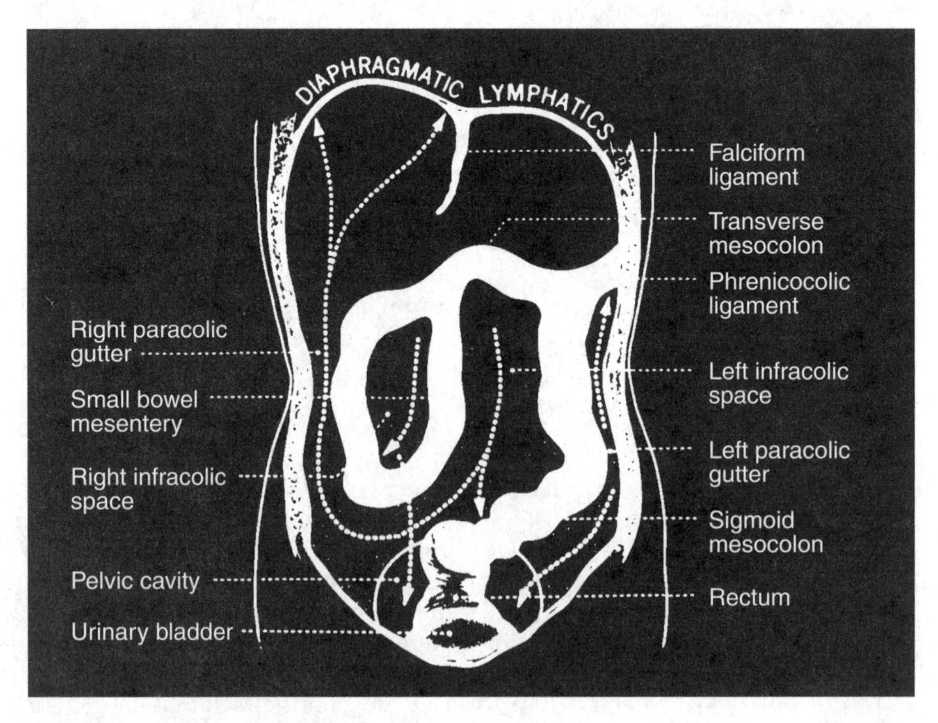

Fig 33-3. Circulation of peritoneal fluid. From Averette et al.[37]

cated for advanced ovarian cancers. After 6 to 12 courses of chemotherapy, second-look laparotomy is indicated to evaluate patients without clinical evidence of disease. Diagnostic tests, including CT, ultrasound, and serum CA 125, have been shown to be ineffective in assessing complete responders. High-dose progestin or tamoxifen may benefit 10% to 15% of patients with recurrent ovarian cancer.

Surgery

Survival has been shown to correlate strongly with residual disease. Aure and coworkers reported improvements in the 5-year survival of stage II patients (from 18% to 55%) and stage III patients (from 8% to 30%) who were optimally resected.[41] Using multivariate analysis, Griffiths found similar survival rates in stage III patients who were optimally debulked to <1.5-cm residual disease and patients who presented with <1.5-cm implants and required no further debulking.[42]

Radiation Therapy

Adjuvant radiotherapy has not been associated with additional benefits in stage I patients.[43,44] The risk of recurrence for stage IA, grade 1 patients was only 4% to 6%, compared with 25% to 29% for stage IA, grade 2 and 3 lesions. Whole abdominal strip radiotherapy was associated with better outcomes than pelvic radiotherapy in terms of relapse rate and 5-year survival in patients with stage I, stage II and III ovarian cancer with optimal debulking.[43] However, serious late complications were found with the strip technique. Thus, whole abdominal radiotherapy with the open field technique may be superior to pelvic radiation in optimally debulked patients. The value of abdominal radiation is still unproven.

Chemotherapy

In 82 stage I patients who received no adjuvant chemotherapy after thorough surgical staging, the recurrence rate was only 2.5% for stage IA and IB, compared with 9.5% for stage IC.[45] In a study of high-risk stage I and II patients, comparable results were reported between melphalan therapy and intraperitoneal P32, with a relapse rate of 12%. However, significant complications were noted in 6% of P32 patients.[46] In a randomized GOG study of stage I patients, postoperative melphalan was associated with better outcomes than pelvic radiation or conservative observation.[44] When Platinol was added to a Cytoxan-Adriamycin combination, the response rate improved from 26% to 51%.[47] GOG investigators reported similar pathologic complete response rates (30% vs 33%) when Adriamycin was deleted from the CAP combination.[48] Because of the potential cardiotoxicity of Adriamycin and the tissue necrosis associated with extravasation, the combination of Cytoxan and Platinol is currently suggested.

Significantly improved rates of successful debulking have been reported in patients treated with 2 to 4 cycles of neoadjuvant chemotherapy, compared with matched controls (77% vs 39%). Overall survival did not differ in the neoadjuvant and control groups. Taxol was reported to have significant activity in advanced ovarian cancers; efficacy is being evaluated in ongoing trials with the NCI and GOG.

Second-Look Operation

The risk of finding cancer at second-look surgery varies inversely with the volume of residual disease after the first debulking, grade, and response to chemotherapy. Long-term survival is rare among patients found at second-look to have residual cancers >2 cm in diameter. Recurrence rates eventually reach 25% to 50% even in patients with negative results at second-look.[49] Among patients with residual microscopic disease, 5-year survival was 70% in those who received additional (3 to 6) courses of chemotherapy.

Based on reports of increased progressive disease and mortality in patients receiving whole abdominal radiation, chemotherapy remains the preferred second-line treatment.

Borderline Epithelial Ovarian Neoplasm

The majority of borderline tumors, which account for 10% to 15% of epithelial ovarian cancers, are diagnosed at stage I. Excellent long-term survival (around 90%) can be expected even in patients with advanced disease or incomplete debulking.

Management

Surgery, including unilateral adnexectomy, continues to be the predominant therapy. The contralateral ovary should be carefully inspected because of the high incidence of bilaterality. If the patient does not desire future fertility, abdominal hysterectomy with bilateral salpingo-oophorectomy is recommended. In advanced cases, complete tumor debulking should be attempted without jeopardizing the patient's life. There is very little evidence to support the use of adjuvant chemotherapy or radiation.

Germ Cell Tumors

Germ cell tumors are the second most common ovarian malignancy, accounting for 15% to 20%. These tumors occur mainly in young women with a median age of 19 years. Malignant germ cell tumors occur in the following order of frequency: dysgerminoma (40%), endodermal sinus tumor (EST), immature teratoma (20%), embryonal carcinoma, and, rarely, choriocarcinoma. Approximately 60% to 75%

of malignant germ cell tumors are found in the early stages.

Up to 75% of dysgerminomas develop in women younger than 35 years; however, 10% are found in prepubertal girls. Dysgerminoma is bilateral in 10% to 20% of cases and tends to spread via the lymphatics. Intersex conditions are predisposing factors. Dysgerminoma is markedly sensitive to irradiation.

EST is the most malignant germ cell tumor, affecting mainly children and women younger than 20 years. Intraperitoneal dissemination appears more frequent than lymphatic spread. This tumor is bilateral in 5% and usually presents as a small component of dysgerminoma, immature teratoma, and choriocarcinoma. Pure EST can rupture and present as hemorrhagic ascites. Microscopically, EST is characterized by a reticular growth pattern with Schiller-Duval bodies and hyaline droplets. Elevated serum AFP can serve as a useful marker.

Immature teratoma is bilateral in <5% of cases. A benign dermoid cyst in the contralateral ovary is present in 10%. Histologically, immature teratoma is characterized by immature tissue from all three germ layers. Typically, these tumors can grow to an average diameter of 18 cm and appear bosselated with solid and cystic components. In addition to stage, grade, and the quantity of malignant tissue, prognosis is influenced by chromosomal abnormality. The finding of immature teratoma at second look usually indicates response to chemotherapy.[50] The majority of pure immature teratomas do not produce hCG or AFP.

Malignancy, most commonly squamous carcinoma, arises in about 1% of benign cystic teratomas. About half of cases are stage IA with a cure rate in the 75% range. Survival is reduced when there's evidence of tumor adhesion, capsular invasion, or rupture.

Approximately 10% to 15% of germ cell tumors are composed of mixed tumors with elevated serum AFP and hCG.

Gonadoblastoma is a small ovarian tumor characterized by germ cells mixing with sex cord elements. Leydig-like cells are commonly present. This tumor is considered premalignant, with up to 50% developing into dysgerminomas. Most gonadoblastomas occur in intersex patients; in those with a Y chromosome, prophylactic gonadectomy is routinely recommended prior to puberty. Genetic abnormality is observed in 90% of cases, with 46XY and 45X/46XY being the most common karyotypes. Ambiguous genitalia is a common feature.

Management

Conservative surgery and chemotherapy can preserve the patient's fertility. Schwartz summarized his 15 years' experience with germ cell tumors and found an 86.4% success rate with primary therapy and an overall survival rate of 92.6%.[51] Unilateral salpingo-oophorectomy, omentectomy, cytology, lymph node samplings, and peritoneal and diaphragmatic biopsies should be performed routinely for accurate staging. Suspicious lesions should be biopsied. Except for grade 1 immature teratoma, all germ cell tumors require adjuvant chemotherapy, with at least 6 cycles of VAC (vincristine, actinomycin D, and cyclophosphamide) in the immediate postoperative period or 3 to 4 cycles of VBP (vinblastine, bleomycin, and Platinol). Management should be dictated by the most malignant element. A second-look operation is advised after 4 to 6 cycles of chemotherapy to help decide whether the latter should be continued. Serial AFP, hCG, and LDH levels can be used to monitor treatment response and disease recurrence. Treatment of early dysgerminomas is unilateral salpingo-oophorectomy. Postoperative adjuvant therapy is not indicated if all biopsy and cytologic findings are negative. Radiotherapy is recommended for patients with pelvic or aortic node metastasis or tumor rupture. Because of the association with intersex and chromosomal anomalies, karyotype analysis should be performed on all patients.

Sex Cord Stromal Neoplasms

Sex cord tumors, which account for 5% of ovarian neoplasms, develop from specialized ovarian stromal tissue with hormone production capability. In general, these tumors are considered benign or of low malignant potential. Because the embryonic gonad is sexually bipotential, its neoplasms can resemble male or female sex cord tumors. Some ovarian stromal tumors resemble adrenal neoplasms. In some tumors, hormonal production is disparate from cell phenotype. For example, a tumor composed of female cell elements can produce androgen. About 15% of stromal tumors are hormonally inactive. Granulosa-theca cell tumors form the majority of sex cord neoplasms. Approximately 50% develop in postmenopausal women, who may have symptoms of excess endogenous estrogen production and such complications as endometrial hyperplasia and endometrial carcinoma. Defeminization or virilization from androgen excess can also occur. Microscopically, granulosa cell tumors can exhibit the microfollicular pattern with Call-Exner bodies. Most of these tumors, which can rupture and present as an acute abdomen, are diagnosed in stage I. Estimated 5- and 10-year survival rates for stage I lesions are 95%, in contrast to 55% and 25% for stages II and III, respectively. Tumor size appears to strongly influence survival.

Thecoma-fibroma tumors consist of theca cells and fibroblasts. When the fibroblast cells dominate, collagen production leads to fibroma. When theca cells are the major component, the tumor is classified as a thecoma. Meigs' syndrome (ovarian fibroma, ascites, and right hydrothorax) is present in only 1 in 150 cases.

Thecomas are estrogen-producing tumors, which may present as postmenopausal bleeding or irregular menses. The risks of endometrial hyperplasia (50%) and endometrial carcinoma (10%) are similar to those of granulosa cell tumors.

Sertoli-Leydig cell tumors constitute <1% of ovarian neoplasms, affecting young women aged 25 to 30 years. Androgen excess leading to defeminization and virilization, as well as excess estrogen, have been reported. As the tumor dedifferentiates, its malignant potential increases. Immature muscle and cartilage may be seen in 90% of poorly differentiated lesions, which carry a high, 50%, recurrence rate.

Both Leydig and hilus cell tumors are composed of the Leydig cells responsible for testosterone production. These tumors are small, unilateral, and yellow to orange. Patients older than 50 years are usually affected. Microscopically, crystals of Reinke are pathognomonic of Leydig cell tumors. Lipid cell tumors are composed of round cells resembling Leydig and adrenocortical cells, with a 20% malignancy rate. These tumors tend to be unilateral and affect younger patients. Although these tumors also produce testosterone, crystals of Reinke are absent.

Management

Primary treatment is conservative surgery—unilateral adnexectomy in young women, and complete removal of the uterus, tubes, and ovaries in postmenopausal women and those without fertility concern. Adjunctive chemotherapy with VAC or VBP is recommended for many patients. Serial measurements of testosterone, dehydroepiandrosterone (DHEA), and estradiol can be used to monitor disease status in hormone-producing tumors.

Fallopian Tube Cancer

Most fallopian tube cancers are metastatic lesions from ovarian or endometrial neoplasms. Primary tubal cancer is the least common gynecologic malignancy, accounting for 0.1% to 0.5%. The mean age at diagnosis is 58 years. Tubal cancer is bilateral in 5% to 30% of cases, with the right and left tubes equally affected. Women of low parity appear to be at higher risk of developing tubal cancer.

Natural History

The ampulla and infundibulum segments appear to be the most common sites of origin. Fallopian tube cancer develops from mucosal epithelium into an exophytic papillary lesion distending the lumen. In early disease, the tumor is confined in an enlarged fusiform tube, which grossly may be mistaken for hydrosalpinx, hematosalpinx, or pyosalpinx. The metastatic pattern of fallopian tube cancer is similar to that of ovarian cancer.[51] Lymphatic spread can manifest early in the disease process.

Clinical Presentation

The classic triad of presenting signs and symptoms consist of abdominal pain, vaginal bleeding or discharge, and adnexal mass. A negative D&C is often found during the workup of postmenopausal bleeding. Early in the disease process, fallopian tube carcinoma tends to cause fimbrial obstruction, which leads to tubal distention and colicky pain. Vaginal discharge can be profuse, watery, and yellow or amber. Even though Pap smear is positive in only 0% to 18% of cases, the finding of cancer cells may be the only sign of an ongoing malignancy. Patients who present with adenocarcinoma on a routine Pap smear should undergo a D&C if colposcopic examination is normal. If the D&C turns out negative, tubal or ovarian carcinomas are likely possibilities.

Surgical Staging

There is no official staging system for tubal cancer. A modified FIGO staging system for ovarian carcinoma is currently the most widely used for tubal malignancy (Table 33-9). The majority of tubal carcinomas are diagnosed in early stages.

Table 33-9. FIGO* Surgical Staging of Fallopian Tube Carcinoma

Stage I	
IA	Tumor limited to one tube
IB	Tumor limited to both tubes
IC	Either IA or IB with ascites or positive washing
Stage II	
IIA	Tumor extension to ovaries or uterus
IIB	Tumor extension to other pelvic tissues
IIC	Either IIA or IIB with ascites or positive washing
Stage III	
IIIA	Microscopic seeding of abdominal cavity
IIIB	Abdominal implants <2 cm in diameter
IIIC	Abdominal implants >2 cm, positive inguinal or retroperitoneal lymph nodes
Stage IV	Parenchymal liver metastasis, distant metastases

*FIGO: Federation Internationale de Gynecologie et d'Obstetrique

Pathologic Classification

Adenocarcinoma of the fallopian tubes typically shares histologic features with ovarian carcinoma. The most common histologic type is papillary serous adenocarcinoma. Rarely, tubal epithelium undergoes squamous metaplasia. The following criteria have been established for the diagnosis of fallopian tube carcinoma: the main tumor must be in the tube and arise from the endosalpinx; the tumor reproduces tubal mucosal pattern with papillary features; if the tumor invades the tubal wall, the transition between benign and malignant epithelium should be present; and both the ovaries and endometrium are either normal or contain less tumor than the tubes.[52,53]

Prognosis

Important prognostic factors include depth of invasion in early disease and disease stage, but not tumor grade. The 5-year survival rate of 91% in patients with mucosal lesions was reduced to 53% and 25% when cancer involves muscularis and serosal layers, respectively.[54] Declining 5-year survival rates of 72%, 38%, 18%, and 0% have been reported for stages I, II, III, and IV, respectively.[55] As with ovarian carcinoma, the success of surgical debulking strongly influences survival.

Management

There is no standard treatment for tubal carcinoma. Most oncologists follow the treatment approach for ovarian carcinoma. Complete surgical staging and optimal cytoreduction is recommended primary treatment.[56,57] Tumor debulking surgery should be carried out as intensely as for ovarian cancer. Chemotherapy, especially cisplatin-based regimens, is routinely advised for patients with extratubal disease or grade 3 lesion. To evaluate the efficacy of chemotherapy, second-look laparotomy is recommended for all cases with stage IIB to IV cases. Radiotherapy may have some role in optimally debulked patients.

Vulvar Malignancies: Squamous Carcinoma

Epidemiology

Squamous carcinoma of the vulva affects mostly older women (median age, 65 years), reflecting an incidence that increases dramatically with age. Risk factors include low socioeconomic status, multiple sexual partners, and regular coffee consumption.[58, 59] Associated factors are a history of vulvar dystrophy, leukoplakia, vulvar or vaginal inflammatory disease, and cervical cancer.[59]

Pathogenesis and Natural History

Several studies have demonstrated a relationship between sexually transmitted diseases and vulvar carcinoma. For example, chronic granulomatous vulvar disease has been observed to increase the risk of vulvar cancer. There is also the possible field-exposure effect of common carcinogens on lower genital tract tissue. Up to 15% of patients with vulvar cancer have invasive or in situ cervical cancer.[59] More recent interest has focused on HPV in the development of vulvar and cervical carcinomas, in particular, HPV 16 and 18 with genital tract squamous cancers. Vulvar dysplasia, which is considered a premalignant lesion, can be found at the periphery of 50% of invasive vulvar cancers. It is currently believed that vulvar carcinoma progresses through a spectrum of intraepithelial neoplasia, to carcinoma in situ and invasive cancer.

Squamous vulvar carcinoma originates in the squamous epithelium of the skin and mucous membrane of the vulva. It tends to grow slowly and may involve the urethra, vagina, perineum, and anal canal. Lymphatic spread is the rule, with drainage toward the mons pubis and then laterally to the groin nodes.[60] The risk of pelvic node metastasis can be substantial when bilateral or three or more ipsilateral groin nodes are involved.[61]

Clinical Presentation and Diagnostic Workup

Vulvar carcinoma commonly appears as a raised, red, pink, or white nodule, with a fleshy, warty, or ulcerated surface (Fig 33-4). About 50% of patients complain of chronic pruritus and a growing mass in their external genitalia. Other complaints are vulvar pain, burning, bleeding, discharge, and dysuria. Early invasive vulvar cancers may be clinically inapparent and can be detected only by punch biopsy. Careful attention should be paid to surrounding external genitalia to detect multifocal lesions. Speculum exam and Pap smear can rule out concurrent disease in the upper genitalia. After identification of the target lesion, it is important to determine lesion size and proximity to the clitorus, urethra, and other structures. The groin nodes should be carefully palpated for evidence of enlargement or fixation. Suspicious lymph nodes should be biopsied or aspirated for cytologic exam.

Staging System

Since 1989, FIGO has approved a surgical staging for vulvar carcinoma (Table 33-10). This system recognizes the inadequacy of clinical palpation and the adverse effect of groin metastasis on survival.

Prognosis

Survival is strongly affected by the disease stage: 5-year survival rates of 91%, 81%, 48%, and 15% have been reported for stages I-IV, respectively.[62] Within each stage, the presence of inguinal metastasis as well as the number of metastatic groin nodes influences survival. For example, with inguinal metastasis, the 5-year survival rate in stages I-II patients declines from 98% to 44%; the decline in stage III patients is from 70% to 27%.[63]

Depth of invasion has been established as a powerful predictor of inguinal metastasis.[64] Other factors that influence the risk of inguinal metastasis include disease stage, size of the primary tumor, clitoral involvement, vascular space invasion, and tumor differentiation (increasing risk with increasing grade).

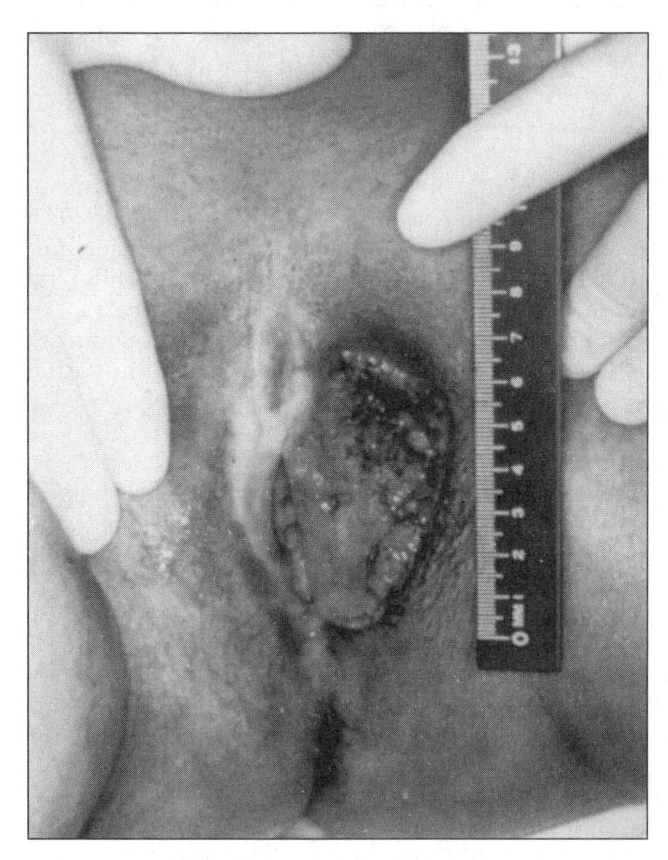

Fig 33-4. Invasive vulvar carcinoma with necrosis and surface ulceration (courtesy of Manuel Penalver, MD)

General Management

Standard therapy for vulvar cancer remains radical vulvectomy and bilateral groin lymphadenectomy. In recent years, more conservative surgery has been advocated to reduce morbidity and long-term sequelae.[65] Therapy may be individualized according to the presence of surgicopathologic risk factors, such as depth of invasion. Small, unifocal, lateralized lesions can be managed by radical hemivulvectomy or radical local excision and ipsilateral groin dissection. Clitoral lesions may best be managed by standard therapy or radiotherapy. Preoperative radiation with or without concurrent chemotherapy can be used to reduce tumor bulk and permit less debilitating surgery. Postoperative radiotherapy is recommended for patients with two or more metastatic groin nodes, and for patients with more than one occult inguinal metastasis. In advanced cancers involving the anorectal canal, vagina, urethra, or bladder, total pelvic exenteration is often necessary to ensure complete resection. Despite high operative morbidity and mortality, a 5-year survival rate of 50% can be expected. Local and groin metastases are usually treated with a combination of surgery and irradiation. Distant metas-

Table 33-10. TNM Staging for Vulvar Carcinoma

Primary Tumor (T)

TX	Primary tumor cannot be assessed
T0	No evidence of primary tumor
Tis	Carcinoma in situ (preinvasive carcinoma)
T1	Tumor confined to the vulva or to the vulva and perineum, 2 cm or less in greatest dimension
T2	Tumor confined to the vulva or to the vulva and perineum, more than 2 cm in greatest dimension
T3	Tumor invades any of the following: lower urethra, vagina, or anus
T4	Tumor invades any of the following: bladder mucosa, upper urethral mucosa, or rectal mucosa, or is fixed to the bone

Regional Lymph Nodes (N)

NX	Regional lymph nodes cannot be assessed
N0	No regional lymph node metastasis
N1	Unilateral regional lymph node metastasis
N2	Bilateral regional lymph node metastasis

Distant Metastasis (M)

MX	Presence of distant metastasis cannot be assessed
M0	No distant metastasis
M1	Distant metastasis (Pelvic lymph node metastasis is M1.)

Stage Grouping

(Correlation of the FIGO, UICC, and AJCC nomenclatures)

AJCC/UICC				FIGO
Stage 0	Tis	N0	M0	
Stage I	T1	N0	M0	Stage I
Stage II	T2	N0	M0	Stage II
Stage III	T1	N1	M0	Stage III
	T2	N1	M0	
	T3	N0	M0	
	T3	N1	M0	
Stage IVA	T1	N2	M0	Stage IVA
	T2	N2	M0	
	T3	N2	M0	
	T4	Any N	M0	
Stage IVB	Any T	Any N	M1	Stage IVB

From American Joint Committee on Cancer.[36]

tases should be treated only with combination chemotherapy.

Surgery

Patients with <1-mm depth of invasion can be managed conservatively with radical local excision without groin dissection because there is virtually no risk of groin metastasis. The posterior half of the vulva and perineum can be spared during excision of a small (<2 cm) anterior vulvar cancer; similarly, the anterior portion can be spared with a posterior lesion. In a recent review, Heaps and colleagues determined that both lateral and deep margins should be at least 1 cm from the tumor.[66] Based on multivariate analysis, free margins of ≥1 cm were the single most important prognostic factor. In this study, patients with free margins of <8 mm had a 48% local recurrence rate regardless of stage. Numerous complications can be expected after radical vulvectomy and groin dissection: wound breakdown and infection, chronic leg edema, groin lymphocysts, lymphangitis, and stress urinary incontinence.

Radiation Therapy

In a randomized GOG study, survival improved significantly among post radical vulvectomy patients treated with pelvic and inguinal irradiation for groin metastasis.[67] Preoperative radiotherapy plus radical vulvectomy have resulted in 65% to 70% success rates, as well as preserved urinary and bowel function in patients with advanced cancer.[68] Chemotherapy has been used in conjunction with radiation as sensitizers; responses in advanced cases have enabled conservative surgery instead of exenteration.

Nonsquamous Vulvar Malignancies

Malignant Melanoma

Malignant melanoma is the second most common malignancy of the vulva, accounting for 5% to 10% of cases. Postmenopausal women with a median age of 57 years are affected. Up to 80% of these melanomas originate in the labia minora and clitoris. Malignant melanoma may develop from preexisting junctional nevus, compound nevus, or de novo. Vulvar melanoma commonly appears as a pigmented, ulcerated growth with an inflammatory margin.

The most common form (66.7% of cases) is superficially spreading melanoma (SSM), which appears as a pigmented flare and has a slow horizontal growth phase prior to invasion. Nodular melanoma (NM) grows vertically at the outset and is commonly found at advanced stages. Mucocutaneous melanoma (MM), which accounts for 10% of vulvar melanomas, has an initial horizontal and radial growth phase prior to invasion. Lentigo malignant melanoma is rarely seen in the vulva. Because most malignant melanomas have an initial horizontal growth phase, all pigmented vulvar lesions should be prophylactically removed.

Vulvar melanoma is staged by tumor thickness (Breslow staging) or depth of invasion (Clark system). Patient survival has been shown to be determined by thickness of invasion, vagina, or urethral involvement, and presence of metastasis.[69] Vulvar melanomas <0.76 mm thick can be treated with wide local excision. For thicker lesions, radical local excision and bilateral groin dissection is preferred because of the risk of groin metastasis. If vaginal, rectal, or urethral mucosa is involved, radical surgery including exenteration should be considered.

Other Vulvar Malignancies

Verrucous carcinoma is usually a locally invasive malignancy that resembles a giant venereal wart. HPV type 6 has been found in verrucous carcinoma. Wide local excision is usually adequate. Radiation is ineffective and may cause the tumor to become aggressive.

Basal cell carcinoma of the vulva is also an indolent, locally invasive cancer that accounts for 2% to 4% of vulvar cancers. It commonly appears on the labia majora as a sessile growth with surface ulceration. Wide excision is the treatment of choice for primary or recurrent lesions.

Vulvar adenocarcinoma develops from the Bartholin's glands. A history of chronic vulvar inflammation or bartholinian abscess is common. Cases tend to be advanced by the time of diagnosis. The carcinoma's deep origin may contribute to a delay in diagnosis and early spread to other pelvic structures. Recommended treatment is radical vulvectomy and bilateral groin lymphadenectomy.

Paget disease is adenocarcinoma in situ of the eccrine or apocrine sweat glands. The typical patient is a white woman aged 65 years who suffers from chronic vulvar pain and pruritus. The lesion can appear red or white, eczematoid, and well demarcated. Paget disease is characterized by large cells with clear cytoplasm clustering near the basement membrane (Fig 33-5). Unlike Paget disease of the breast, only 15% of the vulvar condition is associated with occult adenocarcinoma of the rectum, bladder, urethra, Bartholin's gland, or apocrine gland. Treatment is by wide local excision. Total vulvectomy may be indicated for more extensive lesions. Recurrence can be expected in about one third of cases. Invasion rarely develops; when it does, radical vulvectomy and groin lymphadenectomy are indicated.

Vaginal Malignancies: Squamous Carcinoma

The majority of vaginal carcinomas are metastatic. Primary cancer of the vagina constitutes only 1% to 2% of gynecologic malignancies. The predominant histologic type is squamous cell carcinoma, which makes up 90% of primary vaginal neoplasms.

Epidemiology

Vaginal squamous carcinoma affects mostly postmenopausal women (median age, 62). Generally the disease is diagnosed at an early stage, and the cure rate is high. While one reviewer found no predisposing factors, others have reported an increased risk with low socioeconomic status, history of venereal warts, vaginitis, abnormal Pap smear, hysterectomy, and pessary use.[70,71] About 20% of patients in one study gave a history of prior radiotherapy, mostly for primary cervical cancers.[72]

Squamous carcinoma usually develops in the vaginal mucosa, growing into an exophytic and papillary lesion. It can spread along the vaginal canal, infiltrating the cervix, urethra, or vulva. The most common site of origin (40% to 50% of cases) is the upper vaginal one-third. Distal vaginal involvement can make it difficult to differentiate from primary urethral or vulvar carcinoma. Once vaginal cancer infiltrates submucosal tissue, lymphatic invasion and nodal metastases become likely. Local extension may continue along the paravaginal and parametrial planes and involve the pelvic side walls. Similarly, tumor extension may proceed in the anteroposterior direction and invade the bladder or rectum, resulting in fistulae. Distal vaginal cancers tend to metastasize to inguinal nodes, while tumors from the upper one-third spread directly to pelvic nodes.

Clinical Presentation and Diagnostic Workup

Most patients complain of postmenopausal spotting, bleeding, foul discharge, and pain. A clear plastic speculum is preferred because it allows careful inspection of all vaginal walls. Sometimes, application of Lugol's solution may help delineate lesion sites. Rectovaginal examination is essential to determine submucosal and paravaginal extension or rectal involvement.

Vaginal cancer is detected by routine Pap smear and pelvic examination in only 20% of cases. Besides chest X-ray and IVP, cystoscopy and proctosigmoidoscopy should be routinely performed. CT and MRI can help determine intra-abdominal and retroperitoneal disease. MRI can also distinguish radiation fibrosis from tumor recurrence.

Staging System

Table 33-11 lists the FIGO staging system for vaginal carcinomas.

Prognosis

The most significant prognostic factor is the disease stage: 5-year survival rates of 75%, 55%, 45%, and 30% have been reported for stages I-IV, respectively.[73] Vaginal sarcoma and melanoma tend to have poorer outcomes, with more frequent local recurrences and distant metastases.

Management

Treatment of vaginal carcinoma depends on lesion

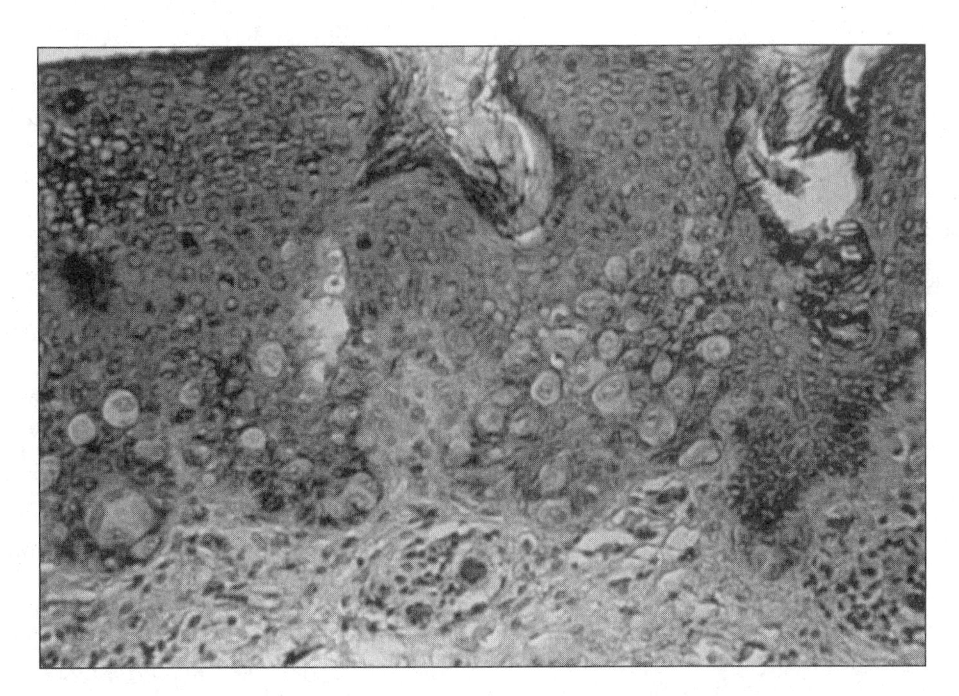

Fig 33-5. Paget disease of the vulva exhibits large epithelial cells with pale cytoplasm and prominent nuclei.

Table 33-11. TNM Staging for Vaginal Carcinoma

Primary Tumor (T)

TNM	FIGO	Definition
TX	—	Primary tumor cannot be assessed
T0	—	No evidence of primary tumor
Tis	0	Carcinoma in situ
T1	I	Tumor confined to the vagina
T2	II	Tumor invades paravaginal tissues but not to the pelvic wall
T3	III	Tumor extends to the pelvic wall
T4*	IVA	Tumor invades the mucosa of the bladder or rectum and/or extends beyond the true pelvis
M1	IVB	Distant metastasis

*Note: The presence of bullous edema is not sufficient evidence to classify a tumor as T4. If the mucosa is not involved, the tumor is Stage III.

Regional Lymph Nodes (N)

NX Regional lymph nodes cannot be assessed
N0 No regional lymph node metastasis

Upper Two-Thirds of the Vagina:

N1 Pelvic lymph node metastasis

Lower One-Third of the Vagina:

N1 Unilateral inguinal lymph node metastasis
N2 Bilateral inguinal lymph node metastasis

Distant Metastasis (M)

TNM	FIGO	Definition
MX	—	Presence of distant metastasis cannot be assessed
M0	—	No distant metastasis
M1	IVB	Distant metastasis

Stage Grouping

AJCC/UICC				FIGO
Stage 0	Tis	N0	M0	
Stage I	T1	N0	M0	Stage I
Stage II	T2	N0	M0	Stage II
Stage III	T1	N1	M0	Stage III
	T2	N1	M0	
	T3	N0	M0	
	T3	N1	M0	
Stage IVA	T1	N2	M0	Stage IVA
	T2	N2	M0	
	T3	N2	M0	
	T4	Any N	M0	
Stage IVB	Any T	Any N	M1	Stage IVB

From American Joint Committee on Cancer.[36]

size and the involvement of adjacent structures. For patients with early lesions and no prior radiotherapy, radiation and surgery offer similar cure rates.[74,75] Radical hysterectomy, pelvic lymphadenectomy, and partial or complete vaginectomy are indicated for early proximal vaginal cancers. Radical vaginectomy or vulvectomy may be required for early lesions in the distal vagina. In selected patients, recurrent vaginal cancers can be treated by total pelvic exenteration.[74]

For advanced (stages II-IV) vaginal lesions, radiotherapy is advised (4,500-5,000 rads to the whole pelvis, followed by 2,500-4,000 rads of intracavitary or interstitial brachytherapy). Because of lymphatic drainage, inguinal areas should be treated for tumors involving the lower third of the vagina. The poor prognosis associated with advanced vaginal cancer suggests that a combination of surgery, radiation, and chemotherapy may prove beneficial.

Nonsquamous Vaginal Malignancies

Adenocarcinoma

Primary adenocarcinoma of the vagina is so rare that the possibility of it being a metastatic lesion should first be ruled out. Adenocarcinomas of the endometrium, ovary, or endocervix are common sites of origin. Occasionally a cancer of the kidney, breast, colon, or pancreas can spread to the vagina. The most frequent histologic type is clear cell carcinoma. The majority of clear cell carcinomas in young women are associated with a history of intrauterine diethylstilbestrol (DES) exposure. Vaginal adenosis has been found in 97% of vaginal and 52% of cervical clear cell carcinomas.

Malignant Melanoma

Vaginal melanoma, which accounts for 3% to 5% of all vaginal cancers, is highly malignant. Junctional activity of epidermal melanocytes is necessary to confirm a primary lesion. The average age at diagnosis is 55 years. Malignant melanoma preferentially develops in the distal third of the vagina and the anterior vaginal wall. Patients may present with vaginal bleeding or discharge. On examination, vaginal lesions may be papillary, polypoid, or pedunculated with ulceration. They may be black, brown, red, or yellow. Vaginal melanoma should be staged by the Breslow system because depth of invasion appears to be the best determinant of survival. Few patients survived more than 5 years. Treatment with local excision or partial vaginectomy and radiation is associated with an 80% recurrence rate. Radical hysterectomy with total vaginectomy or anterior, posterior, or total pelvic exenteration has been advocated for locally advanced disease. Because of a tendency for systemic metastasis, combination chemotherapy will be of value.

Gynecologic Sarcomas

Uterine Sarcomas

Uterine sarcomas comprise 2% to 4% of all uterine cancers and have an incidence of 1.2 to 2.3 cases per 100,000. These sarcomas can develop from myometrial or endometrial tissue and can be divided into three groups: leiomyosarcomas, endometrial stromal sarcomas (ESS), and mixed mesodermal sarcomas. In general, uterine sarcomas tend to be aggressive, with frequent peritoneal, lymphatic, and hematogenous spread. Treatment failures can be expected in 40% to 50% of cases, of which a significant number have distant metastases.[76] The modified FIGO staging system for endometrial cancer is commonly applied to uterine sarcomas (Table 33-12). The value of staging laparotomy and tumor debulking remains controversial for uterine sarcomas.

Table 33-12. FIGO* Staging System for Uterine Sarcoma

Stage	Description
I	Sarcoma confined to uterus
II	Extension to cervix
III	Extension to pelvic structures
IV	Extrapelvic metastases

*FIGO: Federation Internationale de Gynecologie et d'Obstetrique

Leiomyosarcomas (LMS), a homogeneous group, make up 25% of uterine sarcomas. The average patient is 53 years old and complains of postmenopausal bleeding. Uterine enlargement can lead to low abdominal pain, abdominal pressure, constipation, and urinary frequency. Most cases are diagnosed accidentally during surgery for fibroids. The diagnosis requires at least 10 mitoses per 10 high-power fields (hpf) or, if cellular atypism is present, 5 to 9 mitoses per 10 hpf. Five-year survival rates of 50% and 0% have been reported for stages I-II and III-IV, respectively.[77] In addition to stage, mitotic count is a reliable prognostic indicator. Leiomyosarcoma is treated by abdominal hysterectomy and bilateral salpingo-oophorectomy. Once extrauterine, uterine sarcoma tends to be a systemic disease. Radiation may help locoregional control, but does not affect survival outcome. Combination therapy with VAC was associated with a 28% response rate in 14 patients.[78] Even though no cytotoxic regimen has been shown effective, chemotherapy is the only reasonable treatment option.

ESS are pure homologous sarcomas that can be classified into two distinct entities: low-grade tumors (also called endolymphatic stromal myosis) and high-grade tumors. The low-grade ESS tumor occurs mostly in premenopausal women. Uterine curettage may show stromal hyperplasia. The diagnosis can be made intraoperatively by observing characteristic wormlike structures infiltrating the broad ligaments from an enlarged uterus. Histologically, this tumor is characterized by small uniform cells arranged in a whorling pattern around blood vessels. The mitotic count is usually <5 per 10 hpf, with minimal cytologic atypia. Its clinical course is usually indolent with long-term survival to be expected. Because of the tendency to locally invade adjacent pelvic tissues, radical hysterectomy and salpingo-oophorectomy have been recommended as primary treatment for early-stage tumors.[79] Limited data suggest irradiation and chemotherapy to not be valuable. In general, these tumors have high levels of steroid receptors and are hormonally sensitive to progestin therapy.

On the other hand, a high-grade ESS tumor is very aggressive and tends to affect postmenopausal women. The mitotic count is usually >10 per 10 hpf. A majority of these tumors are found to have spread beyond the uterus at the time of diagnosis. A 5-year survival rate of 25% to 50% has been reported for stage I-II disease.[77] Standard treatment for high-grade ESS is total abdominal hysterectomy and bilateral salpingo-oophorectomy. Adjuvant therapy is recommended because of the high recurrence rate. Pelvic irradiation appears useful in controlling local recurrence. Limited data suggest chemotherapy is indicated for advanced disease. Hormone therapy is generally ineffective.

Mixed mesodermal sarcomas mainly affect postmenopausal women (median age, 62 years). This disease shares several epidemiologic risk factors with endometrial carcinomas and affects the same patient groups. An association with pelvic irradiation has been reported, with 9% incidence in 517 cases.[76] Pelvic examination usually reveals an enlarged, soft uterus with tissue protruding from the cervical os. Grossly, the uterine cavity is filled with a polypoid, fungating tumor with hemorrhage and necrosis. Mixed mesodermal sarcomas can have homologous or heterologous components, such as striated muscle, cartilage, and bone. Generally, there is no significant difference in survival between heterologous and homologous sarcomas. Metastases to the lung, abdominal cavity, and retroperitoneal lymph nodes are commonly reported. Standard therapy is total abdominal hysterectomy and bilateral salpingo-oophorectomy. In disease seemingly confined to the pelvis, pelvic radiotherapy is routinely recommended. Currently, there is no effective chemotherapy for advanced or recurrent disease. However, an occasional response has been reported with high-dose progestin therapy.

Vaginal Sarcomas

The most common vaginal sarcoma is rare—sarcoma botryoides, also called embryonal botryoid rhabdomyosarcoma. This tumor occurs almost exclusively in infants and children younger than 5 years. The diagnosis is typically made with the discovery of grapelike tissues protruding at the vaginal introitus. Improvement has been reported with a combination of tumor debulking and adjuvant chemotherapy, with or without pelvic irradiation.

Sarcomas of the Fallopian Tube

Fallopian tube cancer is commonly diagnosed in advanced stages in postmenopausal women. The prognosis is generally poor. Treatment consists of tumor debulking plus chemotherapy with VAC.

Ovarian Sarcomas

The ovary is capable of giving rise to endometrial malignancies from endometrioid adenocarcinoma to sarcomatous tumors (such as endolymphatic stromal myosis, ESS, and adenosarcoma). Mixed mesodermal tumor (MMT) is the most common ovarian sarcoma, affecting postmenopausal women (median age, 60 years). About 50% of MMTs contain heterologous elements. In general, the prognosis is poor even for stage I patients.

Trophoblastic Tumors

Epidemiology

The incidence of molar pregnancy varies from 1:85 to 1:1,700 for different parts of the world. Black Americans appear to be half as likely to have a molar pregnancy as nonblack Americans.[80] A difference in genetic makeup, rather than environmental factors, appears to account for the diverse incidence rates among racial groups: Asian women born and raised in Hawaii share the same incidence as those born in Asia.[80] Hydatidiform mole has a bimodal distribution, with risk ratios of 1.5 and 5.2 for those younger than 20 years and older than 40, respectively.[81] In another study, a 411-fold increased risk was reported in women older than 50 years, compared with a sixfold increase in those younger than 15. The extreme ages of affected patients may reflect a higher incidence of defective gametogenesis at both ends of the reproductive capacity spectrum. The age-related risk is documented for complete mole, but not for partial mole. A history of prior molar gestation confers a 20- to 40-fold increased risk of having another molar gestation. Women with prior miscarriages appear to be at two to three times the normal risk, while childbearing appears to offer some protection.

Pathology and Cytogenetics

Molar pregnancy can be classified as complete or partial moles. Complete hydatidiform mole results when the embryo fails to develop and undergoes hydropic degeneration. Microscopically, the villi appear edematous with trophoblastic hyperplasia and no fetal blood vessels. A partial mole is characterized by hydropic degeneration of the villi and an embryo, which often dies by 9 weeks. Rarely, the fetus survives until the second or third trimester. Hydropic degeneration in a partial mole appears focal and less organized than in a complete mole. Fetal capillaries can be seen, with mild syncytial trophoblastic hyperplasia. Partial mole is associated with a lower frequency of gestational trophoblastic neoplasia (5% versus 15% to 20%).[82] High levels of b-hCG may contribute to ovarian hyperstimulation. Theca-lutein cysts can be detected in one third of molar patients and usually are associated with b-hCG >100,000 mIU/mL.

Karyotyping analysis reveals that approximately 95% of complete moles have a 46,XX composition, and 5% have 46,XY. It has been shown that the 46,XX complete mole results from duplication of a single haploid sperm (23X), while the 46,XY karyotype comes from fertilization with 23X and 23Y sperms. About 80% to 95% of partial moles have a triploid karyotype (two sets of paternal and one set of maternal chromosomes). The triploid fetus rarely survives and develops to term.

Clinical Presentation

Molar gestation commonly presents with vaginal bleeding during the first or second trimester of pregnancy. Patients may complain of passing grapelike tissues. Once this occurs, active vaginal bleeding typically ensues and may lead to hypovolemic shock. Up to 25% to 50% of molar patients have an elevation of total T4 and free T4 values; however, clinical hyperthyroidism is manifested in less than 10%. Additionally, 25% of patients with complete mole present with hyperemesis and preeclampsia.

Diagnostic Workup

The diagnosis of molar gestation should be suspected in any pregnant woman complaining of vaginal bleeding, hyperemesis gravidarum, or toxemia during the second trimester. Commonly, the uterus appears large for gestational age, but no fetal heart tone can be detected. In contrast to a complete mole, patients with a partial mole tend to present with a uterus smaller than date. Preoperative workup includes a complete history and physical examination; chest x-ray; renal, liver, and thyroid function tests; hematologic profiles; urinalysis; and arterial blood gases. The finding of grapelike tissues at the cervical os is almost pathognomonic of molar pregnancy. Currently, pelvic sonogram and serum beta-hCG titers are the only routine diagnostic tests for molar gestation. The former should be performed in all pregnant patients with vaginal bleeding. The classic snowstorm pattern is almost diagnostic. Even in patients passing molar tissue, ultrasound can help identify theca-lutein cysts and twin gestation. Serum beta-hCG levels in excess of the normal pregnancy range (50,000-100,000) provides further evidence of molar pregnancy.

Surgical Management

Most hydatidiform moles can be cured by suction D&C. After completion of the suctioning, sharp curettage is carried out to ensure no residual trophoblastic tissues. The curetting should be thorough, yet gentle to prevent uterine scarring and adhesion. Because of the potential for massive blood loss, rapid fluid resuscitation and blood replacement should be available. Hysterotomy is reserved for patients with a mole and a fetus. Total abdominal hysterectomy is reserved for older patients (>40 years) and those desiring sterilization. Acute pulmonary insufficiency with sudden onset of dyspnea, tachypnea, and cyanosis sometimes occurs from massive trophoblastic emboli, which can be fatal. Human immune globulin (Rhogam) should be administered in patients with nonsensitized Rh-negative to prevent Rh-sensitization problems with future pregnancies. Theca-lutein cysts commonly resolve within three months. In 30% of cases, theca-lutein cysts grow in response to rising hCG titer.

Follow-up

Up to 20% of molar patients develop gestational trophoblastic neoplasia (GTN) and require additional chemotherapy. Serum beta-hCG titers should be followed weekly until it returns to normal (by 60 days in 70% of patients). Pelvic exam is performed at monthly intervals to monitor involution of the uterus and theca-lutein cysts. Once normal, serum beta-hCG is followed monthly for another 6 months. In patients with continued elevated titers, 50% develop invasive mole and 50% choriocarcinoma. Thus, metastatic workup should be initiated in patients with elevated hCG titers at 60 days postevacuation. Metastatic workup is also indicated for those with two consecutively rising titers and those with plateau levels for ≥3 weeks. Diagnostic workup should include a pelvic examination to look for lower genital tract metastases and uterine enlargement; pelvic ultrasound; chest x-ray; and CT of the head, abdomen, and pelvis. In addition to blood chemistry, renal and liver function tests should be routinely ordered. Since pregnancy can delay the diagnosis and treatment of GTN, patients should be placed on oral contraceptives for at least a year.

Gestational Trophoblastic Neoplasia

Invasive mole constitutes 70% to 90% of GTNs, while choriocarcinoma forms the other 10% to 30%. Table 33-13 lists the FIGO staging system for GTN.

Table 33-13. FIGO* Staging System for Gestational Trophoblastic Neoplasia

Stage	Description
I	Confined to uterus
II	Metastasis to pelvis or lower genitalia tract
III	Lung metastasis
IV	Other distant metastases, such as brain or liver

*FIGO: Federation Internationale de Gynecologie et d'Obstetrique

Invasive mole is characterized by hydropic villi and trophoblastic hyperplasia, with deep invasion into the myometrium. The invasive process can penetrate the entire myometrium, rupture, and cause severe intraperitoneal hemorrhage. The diagnosis can be made by pelvic ultrasound, CT, or MRI. Radiologic evidence of intrauterine GTN or distant metastasis coupled with elevated hCG levels should be adequate for implementing chemotherapy. Histologic confirmation is not necessary and may cause bleeding problems.

Approximately 50% of choriocarcinomas develop after a molar gestation, while the other 50% occur after normal pregnancies, abortions, and ectopic gestations. The incidence of choriocarcinoma after a full-term pregnancy has been estimated at 1:20,000 live births. The risk increases ninefold among women older than 40 years. Because vaginal bleeding is frequently attributed to the postpartum period, the diagnosis of choriocarcinoma is usually not made at this time. Those who present with metastatic GTN a few years after the last pregnancy almost invariably have choriocarcinoma. This tumor is highly malignant and characterized by anaplastic proliferation of both syncytiotrophoblasts and cytotrophoblasts without villus formation. The presence of villi indicates an invasive mole rather than choriocarcinoma. Elevation of serum beta-hCG to the million range is highly suggestive of choriocarcinoma.

Choriocarcinoma readily invades blood vessels and spreads hematogenously. Depending on the organs involved, it can masquerade as other diseases and present with hemoptysis, pleuritic chest pain, vaginal bleeding, seizures, neurologic deficit, abdominal pain, hemoperitoneum, anemia, and chronic gastrointestinal bleeding. It is prudent to check beta-hCG level in young women with atypical symptoms.

Management of Nonmetastatic GTN

Seventy-five percent of postmolar GTNs are nonmetastatic.[81] Most cases of nonmetastatic (stage I) GTN can be cured by single-agent chemotherapy with either methotrexate or actinomycin D. If the beta-hCG titer fails to decrease significantly after the first two cycles of therapy, a switch to the other agent is necessary. Once the hCG titer returns to normal, a few additional courses of chemotherapy are generally given to ensure complete resolution. Serum hCG titers should be followed monthly during the first year and every two months during the subsequent year. Hysterectomy is advised for patients who do not respond to chemotherapy or have no desire for fertility. The cure rate for nonmetastatic GTN is close to 100%.

Management of Metastatic GTN

Patients with metastatic (stages II-IV) GTN can be divided into good-prognosis and poor-prognosis groups. The National Institutes of Health have identified the following risk factors: urinary hCG >100,000 IU per 24 hr or serum beta-hCG >40,000 mIU/mL; onset of disease longer than four months since the last pregnancy; brain or liver metastasis; and chemotherapy failure. The World Health Organization (WHO) adapted the Bagshawe scoring system, using nine different criteria.[81] In a recent comparison of the FIGO, NIH, and WHO systems, no system was found superior in identifying high-risk patients.[84] Thus, a careful history and metastatic workup are essential for accurate disease assessment and treatment planning.

In general, good-prognosis metastatic GTN can be treated with single-agent chemotherapy. Approximately 20% of these patients will require combination chemotherapy with MAC (methotrexate, actinomycin D, cyclophosphamide). Morrow and colleagues preferred to treat good-prognosis GTNs initially with the MAC regimen.[81] A five- to tenfold reduction in beta-hCG titer after the first course of chemotherapy usually indicates a good response. If the beta-hCG titer plateaus over two consecutive courses of chemotherapy, drug resistance is likely and a switch to another regimen should be considered.

A majority of patients with poor-prognosis metastatic GTN have choriocarcinoma. These patients commonly have extensive lung, liver, and brain metastases. Standard treatment for high-risk metastatic GTN has been the MAC combination, with cure rates of 50% to 72%.[85] Bagshawe used the CHAMOCA: (Cytoxan, hydroxyurea, actinomycin D, methotrexate, Oncovin, citrovorum factor, Adriamycin) regimen and reported a 75% cure rate.[86] However, in a prospective GOG study, the MAC combination was superior to the Bagshawe regimen in terms of both toxicity and overall survival.[87] A 93% success rate has been reported with an alternating regimen, EMA/CO (etoposide, methotrexate, actinomycin D alternating with Cytoxan, and Oncovin).[88]

Liver metastasis occurs in 5% to 20% of patients with poor-prognosis GTN. It is generally more serious than brain metastasis, with a survival rate of 40%. Currently, there is no optimal therapy for liver metastasis. Radiotherapy has been advocated for the prevention of fatal liver hemorrhage, but is associated with substantial complications. Brain metastasis occurs in 10% of patients with metastatic GTN. Because of the blood-brain barrier, systemic chemotherapy is successful in only 20% of cases. However, a survival rate of 72% has been reported with the EMA/CO regimen in patients with brain metastasis.[89] Whole-brain radiotherapy has been used successfully in combination with chemotherapy,[85,90] with an overall survival of around 50%. Because of the risk of cerebral edema and hemorrhage, dexamethasone should be administered during brain irradiation. Patients who present with neurologic deficit and elevated intracranial pressure may require emergency craniotomy to evacuate the hematoma.

References

1. Boring CC, Squires TS, Tong T, Mongomery S. Cancer Statistics, 1994. *CA Cancer J Clin.* 1994;44:7-26.

2. Leffall LD Jr, Menck HR, Steele GD Jr, Winchester DP. Special populations. In: Steele GD Jr, Winchester DP, Menck HR, Murphy GP, eds. *National Cancer Data Base: Annual Review of Patient Care, 1992.* Atlanta, Ga: American Cancer Society; 1992:48.

3. Morrow CP, Townsend DE. Tumors of the cervix. In: Morrow CP, Townsend DE, eds. *Synopsis of Gynecologic Oncology.* 3rd ed. New York, NY: John Wiley & Sons Inc; 1987:107.

4. Syrjanen K, Mantyjarvi R, Vayrynen M, et al. Evolution of human papillomavirus infections in the uterine cervix during a long-term prospective follow-up. *Applied Pathol.* 1987;5:121-135.

5. Riou GF, Bourhis J, Le MG. The c-*myc* proto-oncogene in invasive carcinomas of the uterine cervix: clinical relevance of overexpression in early stages of the cancer. *Anticancer Res.* 1990;10:1225-1231.

6. Hayashi Y, Hachisuga T, Iwasaka T, et al. Expression of ras oncogene product and EGF receptor in cervical squamous cell carcinomas and its relationship to lymph node involvement. *Gynecol Oncol.* 1991;40:147-151.

7. Grumbine FC, Rosenshein NB, Zerhouni EA, Siegelman SS. Abdominopelvic computed tomography in the preoperative evaluation of early cervical cancer. *Gynecol Oncol.* 1981;12:286-290.

8. Duk JM, de Brujin HWA, Groenier KH, et al. Cancer of the uterine cervix: sensitivity and specificity of serum squamous cell carcinoma antigen determinations. *Gynecol Oncol.* 1990;39:186-194.

9. Heller PB, Malfetano JH, Bundy BN, Barnhill DR, Okagaki T. Clinical-pathologic study of stage IIB, III, and IVA carcinoma of the cervix: extended diagnostic evaluation for paraaortic node metastases: a Gynecologic Oncology Group study. *Gynecol Oncol.* 1990;38:425-430.

10. Averette HE, Donato DM, Lovecchio JL, Sevin BU. Surgical staging of gynecologic malignancies. *Cancer.* 1987;60: 2010-2020.

11. Gauthier P, Gore I, Shingleton HM, Soong S-J, Orr JW Jr, Hatch KD. Identification of histopathologic risk groups in stage IB squamous cell carcinoma of the cervix. *Obstet Gynecol.* 1985;66:569-574.

12. Delgado G, Bundy B, Zaino R, Sevin BU, Creasman WT,

Major F. Prospective surgical-pathological study of disease-free interval in patients with stage IB squamous cell carcinoma of the cervix: A Gynecologic Oncology Group study. *Gynecol Oncol.* 1990;38:353-357.

13. Averette HE, Nguyen HN, Donato D, Penalver M, Sevin BU, Estape R. Radical hysterectomy for invasive cervical cancer: a prospective 25-year experience with the Miami technique. *Cancer.* 1993;71(4):1422-1437.

14. Thomas GM, Dembo AJ. Is there a role for adjuvant pelvic radiotherapy after radical hysterectomy in early stage cervical cancer? *Int J Gynecol Cancer.* 1991;1:1-8.

15. Cunningham MJ, Dunton CJ, Corn B, et al. Extended-field radiation therapy in early-stage cervical carcinoma: survival and complications. *Gynecol Oncol.* 1991;43:51-54.

16. Perez CA, Camel HM, Kuske RR, et al. Radiation therapy alone in the treatment of carcinoma of the uterine cervix: a 20-year experience. *Gynecol Oncol.* 1986;23:127-140.

17. Yordan E. Chemotherapy of cervical carcinoma. In: Deppe G, ed. *Chemotherapy of Gynecologic Cancer.* 2nd ed. New York, NY: Wiley-Liss; 1990:121-153.

18. Park RC, Grigsby PW, Muss HB, Norris HJ. Corpus: epithelial tumors. In: Hoskins WJ, Perez CA, Young RC, eds. *Principles and Practice of Gynecologic Oncology.* Philadelphia, Pa: JB Lippincott;1992:664.

19. Parazzini F, La Vecchia C, Bocciolone L, Franceschi S. Review: the epidemiology of endometrial cancer. *Gynecol Oncol.* 1991;41:1-16.

20. Borst MP, Baker VV, Dixon D, Hatch KD, Shingleton HM, Miller DM. Oncogene alterations in endometrial carcinoma. *Gynecol Oncol.* 1990;38:364-366.

21. Long CA, O'Brien TJ, Sanders MM, Bard DS, Quirk JG Jr. ras oncogene is expressed in adenocarcinoma of the endometrium. *Am J Obstet Gynecol.* 1988;159:1512-1516.

22. Morrow CP, Bundy BN, Kurman RJ, et al. Relationship between surgical-pathological risk factors and outcome in clinical stage I and II carcinoma of the endometrium: a Gynecologic Oncology Group study. *Gynecol. Oncol.* 1991; 40:55-65.

23. Creasman WT, Morrow CP, Bundy BN, Homesley HD, Graham JE, Heller PB. Surgical pathologic spread patterns of endometrial cancer: a Gynecologic Oncology Group study. *Cancer.* 1987;60:2035-2041.

24. Turner DA, Gershenson DM, Atkinson N, Sneige N, Wharton AT. The prognostic significance of peritoneal cytology for stage I endometrial cancer. *Obstet Gynecol.* 1989;74:775-780.

25. Britton LC, Wilson TO, Gaffey TA, Cha SS, Wieand HS, Podratz KC. DNA ploidy in endometrial carcinoma: major objective prognostic factor. *Mayo Clin Proc.* 1990;65:643-650.

26. Varia M, Rosenman J, Halle J, Walton L, Currie J, Fowler W. Primary radiation therapy for medically inoperable patients with endometrial carcinoma, stages I-II. *Int J Radiat Oncol Biol Phys.* 1987;13:11-15.

27. Lehoczky O, Bosze P, Ungar L, Tottossy B. Stage I endometrial carcinoma: treatment of nonoperable patients with intracavitary radiation therapy alone. *Gynecol Oncol.* 1991;43:211-216.

28. Thigpen JT, Blessing J, DiSaia P, Ehrlich C. Treatment of advanced or recurrent endometrial carcinoma with medroxyprogesterone acetate (MPA): a Gynecologic Oncology Group study. *Gynecol Oncol.* 1985;20:250.

29. Deppe G. Chemotherapy for endometrial cancer. In: Deppe G, ed. *Chemotherapy of Gynecologic Cancer.* 2nd ed. New York, NY: Wiley-Liss, 1990:155-174.

30. Miller BA, Ries LAG, Hankey BF, Kosary CL, Harras A, Devesa SS, Edwards BK (eds). *SEER Cancer Statistics Review: 1973-1990.* National Cancer Institute. NIH Pub. No. 93-2789, 1993.

31. Morrow CP, Townsend DE. Tumors of the ovary: general considerations, classification, the adnexal mass. In: Morrow CP, Townsend DE, eds. *Synopsis of Gynecologic Oncology.* 3rd ed. New York, NY: John Wiley & Sons Inc; 1987:233.

32. Averette HE, Hoskins WJ, Nguyen HN, et al. National survey of ovarian carcinoma, I: A Patient Care Evaluation study of the American College of Surgeons. *Cancer.* In press.

33. WHO collaborative study of neoplasia and steroid contraceptives. Epithelial ovarian cancer and combined oral contraceptives. *Int J Epidemiol.* 1989;18:538-545.

34. Lynch HT, Fitzsimmons ML, Conway TA, Bewtra C, Lynch J. Hereditary carcinoma of the ovary and associated cancers: a study of two families. *Gynecol Oncol.* 1990;36:48-55.

35. Einhorn N, Bast RC Jr, Knapp RC, Tjernberg B, Zurawski VR Jr. Preoperative evaluation of serum CA 125 levels in patients with primary epithelial ovarian cancer. *Obstet Gynecol.* 1986;67:414-416.

36. Beahrs OH, Henson DE, Hutter RVP, Kennedy BJ, eds. *American Joint Committee on Cancer Manual for Staging of Cancer.* 4th ed. Philadelphia, Pa: JB Lippincott Co; 1992:155-179.

37. Averette HE, Lovecchio JL, Townsend PA, Sevin BU, Girtanner RE. Retroperitoneal lymphatic involvement by ovarian carcinoma. In: Grundmann E, ed. *Cancer Campaign.* New York, NY: Gustav Fischer; 1983:7:101-109.

38. Genadry R, Poliakoff S, Rotmensch J, Rosenshein NB, Parmley TH, Woodruff JD. Primary, papillary peritoneal neoplasia. *Obstet Gynecol.* 1985;58:730-734.

39. Friedlander ML, Taylor IW, Russell P, Musgrove EA, Hedley DH, Tattersall MHN. Ploidy as a prognostic factor in ovarian cancer. *Int J Gynecol Pathol.* 1983;2:55.

40. van Nagell JR Jr, Higgins RV, Donaldson ES, et al. Transvaginal sonography as a screening method for ovarian cancer: a report of the first 1000 cases screened. *Cancer.* 1990;65:573-577.

41. Aure JC, Hoeg K, Kolstad P. Clinical and histologic studies of ovarian carcinoma: long term follow-up of 990 cases. *Obstet Gynecol.* 1971;37:1.

42. Griffiths CT. Surgical resection of tumor bulk in the primary treatment of ovarian carcinoma. *Natl Cancer Inst Monogr.* 1975;42:101.

43. Dembo AJ, Bush RS, Beale FA, et al. Ovarian carcinoma: improved survival following abdominopelvic irradiation in patients with a completed pelvic operation. *Am J Obstet Gynecol.* 1979;134:793-800.

44. Hreshchyshyn MM, Park RC, Blessing JA, et al. The role of adjuvant therapy in stage I ovarian cancer. *Am J Obstet Gynecol.* 1980;138:139-145.

45. Monga M, Carmichael JA, Shelley WE, et al. Surgery without adjuvant chemotherapy for early epithelial ovarian carcinoma after comprehensive surgical staging. *Gynecol Oncol.* 1991;43:195-197.

46. Young RC, Walton L, Decker D, Major F, Homesley H, Ellenberg S. Early stage ovarian cancer: preliminary results of randomized trials after comprehensive initial staging. *Proc Am Soc Clin Oncol.* 1983. Abstract C-578.

47. Omura G, Blessing JA, Ehrlich CE, et al. A randomized trial of cyclophosphamide and doxorubicin with or without cisplatin in advanced ovarium carcinoma: a Gynecologic Oncology Group study. *Cancer.* 1986;57:1725-1730.

48. Omura GA, Bundy BN, Berek JS, Curry S, Delgado G, Mortel R. Randomized trial of cyclophosphamide plus cisplatin with or without doxorubicin in advanced ovarian carcinoma: a Gynecologic Oncology Group study. *J Clin Oncol.* 1989;7:457-465.

49. Rubin SC, Hoskins WJ, Saigo PE, et al. Prognostic factors for recurrence following negative second-look laparotomy in ovarian cancer patients treated with platinum-based chemotherapy. *Gynecol Oncol.* 1991;42:137-141.

50. Nielsen SNJ, Scheithauer BW, Gaffey TA. Gliomatosis peritonei. *Cancer.* 1985;56:2499-2503.

51. Podratz KC, Podczaski ES, Gaffey TA, O'Brien PC, Schray MF, Malkasian GD Jr. Primary carcinoma of the fallopian tube. *Am J Obstet Gynecol.* 1986;154:1319-1326.

52. Hu CY, Taymor ML, Hertig AT. Primary carcinoma of the fallopian tube. *Am J Obstet Gynecol.* 1950;59:58

53. Yoonessi M. Carcinoma of the fallopian tube. *Obstet Gynecol Surv.* 1979;34:257-270.

54. Peters WA III, Andersen WA, Hopkins MP, Kumar NB, Morley GW. Prognostic features of carcinoma of the fallopian tube. *Obstet Gynecol.* 1988;71:757-762.

55. Denham JW, Maclennan KA. The management of primary carcinoma of the fallopian tube: experience of 40 cases. *Cancer.* 1984;53:166-172.

56. Harrison CR, Averette HE, Jarrell MA, Penalver MA. Donato D, Sevin BU. Carcinoma of the fallopian tube: clinical management. *Gynecol Oncol.* 1989;32:357-359.

57. Barakat RR, Rubin SC, Saigo PE, et al. Cisplatin-based combination chemotherapy in carcinoma of the fallopian tube. *Gynecol Oncol.* 1991;42:156-160.

58. Peters RK, Mack TM, Bernstein L. Parallels in the epidemiology of selected anogenital carcinomas. *J Natl Cancer Inst.* 1984;72:609-615.

59. Mabuchi K, Bross DS, Kessler II. Epidemiology of cancer of the vulva: a case-control study. *Cancer.* 1985;55:1843-1848.

60. Iversen T, Aas M. Lymph drainage from the vulva. *Gynecol Oncol.* 1983;16:179-189.

61. Hacker NF, Berek JS. Vulvar cancer. In: Haskell CM, ed. *Cancer Treatment.* 3rd ed. Philadelphia, Pa: WB Saunders; 1990:351-361.

62. Morrow CP, Townsend DE. Tumors of the vulva. In: Morrow CP, Townsend DE, eds. *Synopsis of Gynecologic Oncology.* 3rd ed. New York, NY: John Wiley & Sons, Inc; 1987:68-77.

63. Morley GW. Infiltrative carcinoma of the vulva: results of surgical treatment. *Am J Obstet Gynecol.* 1976;124:874-888.

64. Rutledge FN, Mitchell MF, Munsell MF, et al. Prognostic indicators for invasive carcinoma of the vulva. *Gynecol Oncol.* 1991;42:239-244.

65. Thomas GM, Dembo AJ, Bryson SCP, Osborne R, Depetrillo AD. Changing concepts in the management of vulvar cancer. *Gynecol Oncol.* 1991;42:9-21.

66. Heaps JM, Fu YS, Montz FJ, Hacker NF, Berek JS. Surgical-pathologic variables predictive of local recurrence in squamous cell carcinoma of the vulva. *Gynecol Oncol.* 1990;38:309-314.

67. Homesley HD, Bundy BN, Sedlis A, Adcock L. Radiation therapy versus pelvic node resection for carcinoma of the vulva with positive groin nodes. *Obstet Gynecol.* 1986;68:733-740.

68. Boronow RC, Hickman BT, Reagan MT, Smith A, Steadham RE. Combined therapy as an alternative to exenteration for locally invasive vulvovaginal cancer, II: results, complications, and dosimetric and surgical considerations. *Am J Clin Oncol.* 1987;10:171-181.

69. Jaramillo BA, Ganjei P, Averette HE, Sevin BU, Lovecchio JL. Malignant melanoma of the vulva. *Obstet Gynecol.* 1985;66:398-401.

70. Herbst AL, Green TH, Ulfelder H. Primary carcinoma of the vagina. *Am J Obstet Gynecol.* 1970;106:210.

71. Brinton LA, Nasca PC, Mallin K, et al. Case-control study of in situ and invasive carcinoma of the vagina. *Gynecol Oncol.* 1990;38:49-54.

72. Pride GL, Schultz AE, Chuprevich TW, Buchler DA. Primary invasive squamous carcinoma of the vagina. *Obstet Gynecol.* 1979;53:218-225.

73. Perez CA, Gersell DJ, Hoskins WJ, McGuire WP. Vagina. In: Hoskins WJ, Perez CA, Young RC, eds. *Principles and Practice of Gynecologic Oncology.* Philadelphia, Pa: JB Lippincott Co; 1992:567-590.

74. Al-Kurdi M, Monaghan JM. Thirty-two years experience in the management of primary tumours of the vagina. *Br J Obstet Gynaecol.* 1981;88:1145-1150.

75. Rubin SC, Young J, Mikuta JJ. Squamous carcinoma of the vagina: treatment, complications, and long-term follow-up. *Gynecol Oncol.* 1985;20:346-353.

76. Hannigan E, Curtin JP, Silverberg SG, Thigpen JT, Spanos WJ. Corpus: mesenchymal tumors. In: Hoskins WJ, Perez CA, Young RC, eds. *Principles and Practice of Gynecologic Oncology.* Philadelphia, Pa: JB Lippincott; 1992:696-708.

77. Morrow CP, Townsend DE. Tumors of the vagina. In: Morrow CP, Townsend DE, eds. *Synopsis of Gynecologic Oncology.* 3rd ed. New York, NY: John Wiley & Sons, Inc; 1987:211-219.

78. Hannigan EV, Freedman RS, Elder KW, Rutledge FN. Treatment of advanced uterine sarcoma with vincristine, actinomycin D, and cyclophosphamide. *Gynecol Oncol.* 1983;15:224-229.

79. Krieger PD, Gusberg SB. Endolymphatic stromal myosis: a grade I endometrial sarcoma. *Gynecol Oncol.* 1973;1:299-313.

80. Matsuura J, Chiu D, Jacobs PA, Szulman AE. Complete hydatidiform mole in Hawaii: an epidemiological study. *Am J Obstet Gynecol.* 1982;89:258.

81. Morrow CP, Townsend DE. Tumors of the placental trophoblast. In: Morrow CP, Townsend DE, eds. *Synopsis of Gynecologic Oncology.* 3rd ed. New York, NY: John Wiley & Sons, Inc; 1987;367-377.

82. Berkowitz RS, Goldstein DP, Bernstein MR. Natural history of partial molar pregnancy. *Obstet Gynecol.* 1985;66:677-681.

83. Vejerslev LO, Dueholm M, Nielsen FH. Hydatidiform mole: cytogenetic marker analysis in twin gestation. *Am J Obstet Gynecol.* 1986;155:614-617.

84. Dubuc-Lissoir J, Sweizig S, Schlaerth JB, Morrow CP. Metastatic gestational trophoblastic disease: a comparison of prognostic classification systems. *Gynecol Oncol.* 1992;45:40-45.

85. Lurain RL, Brewer JI. Treatment of high-risk gestational trophoblastic disease with methotrexate, actinomycin D, and cyclophosphamide chemotherapy. *Obstet Gynecol.* 1985;65:830.

86. Bagshawe KD. Treatment of high-risk choriocarcinoma. *J Reprod Med.* 1984;29:813-820.

87. Curry SL, Blessing JA, DiSaia PJ, et al. A prospective randomized comparison of methotrexate, dactinomycin and chlorambucil versus methotrexate, dactinomycin, cyclophosphamide, doxorubicin, melphalan, hydroxyurea, and vincristine in poor-prognosis metastatic gestational trophoblastic disease: a Gynecologic Oncology Group study. *Obstet Gynecol.* 1989;73:357.

88. Newlands ES, Bagshawe KD, Begent RHJ, Rustin GJS, Holden L, Dent J. Developments in chemotherapy for medium- and high-risk patients with gestational trophoblastic tumours (1979-1984). *Br J Obstet Gynaecol.* 1986;93:63-69.

89. Rustin GJS, Newlands ES, Begent RHJ, Dent J, Bagshawe KD. Weekly alternating etoposide, methotrexate, and actinomycin/vincristine and cyclophosphamide chemotherapy for the treatment of CNS metastases of choriocarcinoma. *J Clin Oncol.* 1989;7:900-903.

90. Yordan EL, Schlaerth J, Gaddis O, Morrow CP. Radiation therapy in the management of gestational choriocarcinoma metastatic to the central nervous system. *Obstet Gynecol.* 1987;69:627-630.

34

NUTRITION AND THE CANCER PATIENT

John M. Daly, MD, and Michael Shinkwin, MD

Progressive weight loss and nutritional depletion are common among cancer patients.[1] The importance of malnutrition as a major source of morbidity and mortality is widely appreciated. Furthermore, antineoplastic therapy modalities can exert a varying impact on the host's nutritional status, adding to the cachectic state caused by the tumor and leading to a more profound nutritional depletion and increased morbidity.[2] Malnourished cancer patients should be identified prior to initiation of antineoplastic treatment, and efforts should be made to improve their nutritional status. This chapter outlines the causes of cancer cachexia, the impact of antitumor therapy on nutrition, the nutritional assessment of the cancer patient, and the provision of optimal nutritional support for each patient.

Cancer Cachexia

The term "cancer cachexia" describes a group of symptoms and signs that encompass inanition, anorexia, weakness, tissue wasting, and organ dysfunction. Cachexia, common in patients with advanced metastatic disease, also occurs in patients with localized disease. DeWys and colleagues[1] noted substantial weight loss in 40% of patients with breast cancer and in 80% of patients with gastric or pancreatic carcinoma. The relationship of cachexia to tumor burden, disease stage, and cell type is inconsistent, and no single theory satisfactorily explains the cachectic state. A variety of etiologic factors can occur simultaneously or sequentially to produce cachexia.

John M. Daly, MD, Lewis Atterbury Stimson Professor and Chairman, Department of Surgery, Cornell University Medical School and Surgeon-in-Chief, New York Hospital, New York, New York

Michael Shinkwin, MD, Fellow in Surgical Oncology, University of Pennsylvania School of Medicine, Philadelphia, Pennsylvania

Diminished Nutrient Intake

Anorexia accompanies most neoplasms to some extent and is a major contributing factor in the development of the cachectic state. Often, loss of appetite is an important symptom of an underlying neoplasm. Several physiologic derangements have been cited as possible reasons for anorexia. Abnormalities in taste perception such as reduced threshold for sweet, sour, and salty flavors have been demonstrated. DeWys and Walters[3] have shown that a reduced taste sensitivity for sucrose and urea is associated with reduced caloric intake; the reduced oral threshold for urea correlates with an aversion to red meat. In contrast, others have noted increased taste sensitivity in cancer patients. Deficiencies in zinc and other trace elements may contribute to altered taste sensation. Patients with hepatic metastases accompanied by some degree of hepatic insufficiency may develop anorexia and nausea as a result of difficulty in clearing lactate produced by anaerobic tumor metabolism of glucose. Substances released by the tumor or by the host's monocytes (cachectin) may act on the feeding center in the hypothalamus and cause anorexia. Recent studies have demonstrated the presence of cachectin in the plasma of tumor-bearing rodents that correlated with the onset of anorexia.

Many studies have been conducted to elucidate the specific metabolic processes that affect nutrient intake in cancer patients. Results of parabiosis studies performed by Lucke and colleagues[4] indicate the presence of a humoral factor that produces in the nontumor-bearing rat characteristics of the tumor-bearing state. Theologides[5] proposed that tumor peptides acting through neuroendocrine cells and neuroreceptors alter metabolic pathways. Nakahara[6] described a "toxohormone" capable of mimicking the cancerous state when injected into normal animals. Toxohormone is a 75,000 d protein identified in several tumors such as melanoma and carcinoma; it leads to increased lipolysis and immunosuppression. Experiments in which rats were given cachectin intraperitoneally for 5 days show that cachectin causes decreased dietary intake with a corresponding decline in host weight. Rats given cachectin for 10 days developed tolerance to cachectin after 5 days.[7] When subsequently inoculated with tumor, these rats survived for a significantly longer period than control animals not pretreated with cachectin. This result strengthens the evidence that endogenously produced cachectin may mediate the development of cachexia in the tumor-bearing host. Krause and coworkers[8] postulated that abnormalities in the central nervous system's metabolism of serotonin may be responsible for the cancer-associated anorexia.

The local effect of the tumor may lead to reduced food intake, especially when the tumor arises from or impinges on the alimentary tract. Patients with cancer of the oral cavity, the pharynx, or the esophagus may have reduced intake because of the odynophagia or dysphagia due to partial or complete obstruction. Patients with gastric cancer often have reduced gastric capacity or partial gastric outlet obstruction leading to nausea, vomiting, and an early feeling of fullness. Intestinal tumors can cause partial obstruction or blind-loop syndrome and interfere with nutrient absorption. Pancreatic carcinomas frequently lead to exocrine enzyme deficiencies, bile salt unavailability, and malabsorption syndromes.

Psychologic factors such as depression, grief, or anxiety resulting from the disease or its treatment may lead to poor appetite, abnormal eating behavior, and learned food aversions, and thus to a diminished or unbalanced dietary intake.

Abnormalities of Substrate Metabolism

Extensive changes in energy, carbohydrate, lipid, and protein metabolism have been demonstrated in patients with malignant disease.[9,10] Increased energy expenditure and inefficient energy utilization are frequently cited causes of malnutrition in tumor-bearing hosts. The normal response to diminished food intake is a reduction in basal metabolic rate (BMR); the BMR or resting energy expenditure is basically the sum of all the energy-requiring processes of vegetative function and accounts for 75% of total energy expenditure in normal individuals.

There have been many studies of the energy requirements of cancer patients. Young[11] reviewed a number of them and could not conclude that resting metabolism is consistently elevated in cancer patients, although the data did show increased resting energy expenditure in leukemia and lymphoma patients. One study demonstrated that increases in resting metabolic rate paralleled advancing disease and reduced nutrient intake. Shike and colleagues[12] demonstrated in a group of patients with small-cell lung carcinoma that basal energy expenditure was elevated. Responders to chemotherapy had a significant decrease in basal energy expenditure, while nonresponders exhibited no change. In 1983, Knox and colleagues[13] measured energy expenditure in 200 malnourished cancer patients by indirect calorimetry. Patients considered normal were also studied and exhibited resting energy expenditure levels within 10% of the value predicted by the Harris-Benedict equation. Only 41% of cancer patients had a normal resting energy expenditure (REE), while decreased and increased REE was observed in 33% and 26% of patients respectively (Fig 34-1). Similarly, Heber and colleagues[14] found no clear evidence of hypermetabolism in noncachectic lung cancer patients. They argued that since malnourished patients normally decrease BMR as an adaptation to starvation, even normal predicted metabolic rates are inappropriately elevated in malnourished cancer patients. Shaw, Humberstone, and Wolfe[15] argued that the alteration in metabolic rate depends on the type of tumor. They demonstrate an elevated rate of energy expenditure in sarcoma-bearing patients associated with increased Cori cycle activity, glucose turnover, reduced glucose oxidation, and increased protein catabolism. Others have shown an elevation in resting energy expenditure with lymphomas, lung cancer, and head and neck cancers. Buzby and coworkers[16] showed a reduction in metabolic rate associated with pancreatic cancer. Patients with lower gastrointestinal (GI) neoplasms tend to be metabolically similar to normal volunteers, whereas upper GI tumors result in an elevated metabolic rate.

Inefficient energy utilization by the tumor-bearing host was studied by Holroyde and Reichard,[17] who reported increased Cori cycle activity in patients with malignancy. This futile cycle, in which glucose is converted to lactic acid and subsequently reconverted to glucose by hepatocytes, is an energy-wasting process. The highest level of Cori cycle activity was observed in patients with the greatest energy expenditure and weight loss. Young[11] has suggested that increased rates of protein turnover also result in significant energy losses due to the failure of normal adaptation to starvation. During the first 2 days of fasting, endogenous glycogen stores of muscle and the liver are depleted. Glucose utilization by the brain and erythrocytes continues, resulting in the breakdown of protein for gluconeogenesis. In noncancer patients, muscle protein breakdown is gradually replaced by fat fuel metabolism in which fatty acids are converted to ketone bodies. These are used for energy by peripheral tissues and eventually up to 95% of energy utilization by the brain; this results in decreased glucose utilization with secondary sparing of muscle protein. In cancer patients, these adaptive mechanisms do not occur, resulting in increased glucose production and protein catabolism.

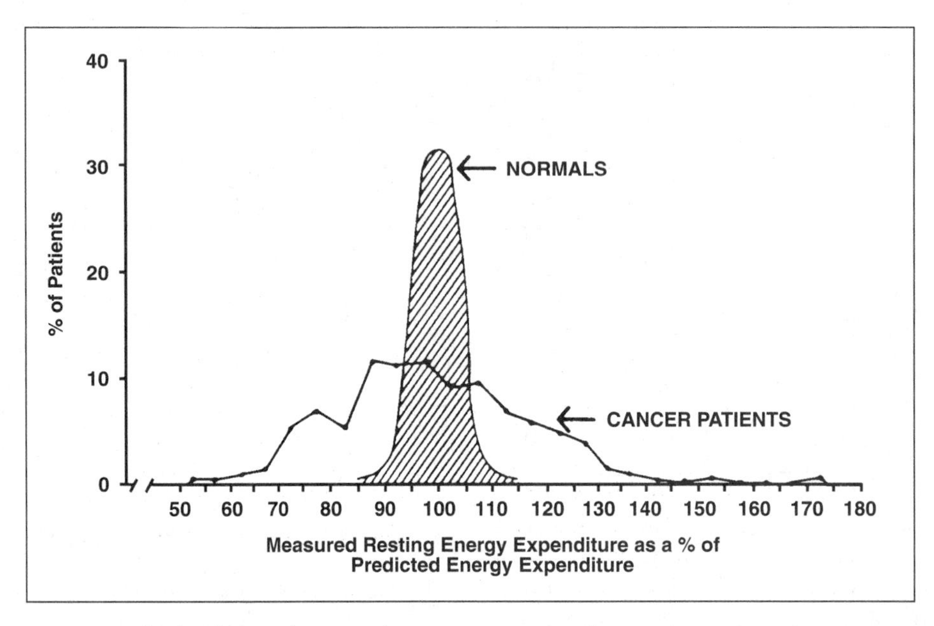

Fig 34-1. The distribution of measured resting energy expenditure in "normals" and in 200 cancer patients. From Knox et al.[13]

Although cancer patients have normal levels of circulating insulin and glucose, they have impaired insulin sensitivity. Glucose intolerance is documented by hyperglycemia and delayed clearance of blood glucose in cancer patients after oral or intravenous glucose administration. Glucose intolerance is due in part to decreased tissue sensitivity to insulin, but may also involve an attenuated secretory response to glucose. Cancer patients also exhibit increased gluconeogenesis from alanine and lactate. Using carbon 14 (^{14}C) labeled alanine, Waterhouse and colleagues[18] found that the apparent increase in gluconeogenesis from alanine reflected a very rapid glucose turnover. Feedback control of glucose production may be impaired because gluconeogenesis and Cori cycle activity are not inhibited by glucose administration in the cancer patient.

Alterations in lipid metabolism in cancer patients include changes in body composition and increased lipid mobilization.[19] Decreases in total body fat are common among these patients and are most likely related to insulin deficiency. Increased oxidation of fatty acids also occurs. Glycerol and fatty acids, the byproducts of lipolysis, serve as substrates for gluconeogenesis and energy production. Waterhouse[20] found that fatty acids are the major substrates in patients with progressive malignant disease. Increased plasma clearance of endogenous fat stores and exogenously administered fat emulsions in cancer patients have been demonstrated in both fasting and fed states. Patients with malignancy fail to suppress lipolysis after glucose administration and continue to oxidize fatty acids.

Several abnormalities of protein metabolism occur in cancer patients, including host nitrogen depletion, decreased muscle protein synthesis, and the occurrence of abnormal plasma aminograms. Nitrogen balance is negative in 30% to 100% of patients with progressive malignancy. Amino acid trapping by tumor cells has been demonstrated clinically and experimentally. In a study of sarcoma-bearing limbs, Norton and colleagues[21] found that affected limbs released less than 50% of the amount of amino acids released from tumor-free limbs. Evidence obtained with whole body protein studies using nitrogen 15 (^{15}N) labeled glycine indicates that cancer patients have increased protein turnover, a circumstance that contributes to increased energy expenditure.

Also associated with cachexia are changes in body composition such as increased extracellular fluid and total body sodium and decreased intracellular fluid and total body potassium. Cohn and others,[22] using prompt gamma-neutron activation to evaluate total body nitrogen and a whole body counter to measure potassium 40 (^{40}K), found that total body potassium was diminished out of proportion to total body nitrogen. On the basis of this finding, they concluded that endogenous nutrient losses in cancer patients were predominantly in the skeletal muscle compartment, since muscle comprises 45% of total body nitrogen and 85% of total body potassium. A recent study, using ^{40}K and a whole body counter, measured body cell mass (BCM) in relation to body weight in normal volunteers, anorexia nervosa patients, and cancer patients. In the normal volunteers, body cell mass tended to decrease with increasing age as an absolute value and as a percentage of total body weight. In anorexia nervosa patients, there was a significant depletion of BCM, but with relative sparing of the BCM when expressed as a percentage of total body weight. This reflects the normal adaptation to starvation when fat utilization predominates and endogenous protein is spared. In cancer patients, there was a significant degree of weight loss accompanied by a proportional decline in BCM, indicating that protein is depleted to the same extent as fat stores.[23]

The Impact of Antitumor Therapy on Nutrition

Antineoplastic therapy invariably affects the host, either by mechanical and physiologic alterations due to surgery or at the cellular level with chemotherapy or radiation therapy.[2] The effects of therapy may add to the cachexia of malignancy and leave the patient with a more severe nutritional deficiency.

Surgical therapy is the primary treatment modality of many cancers, particularly those of the GI tract. The immediate metabolic response to surgery in patients with cancer is similar to that of patients who have surgery for benign disease: increased nitrogen losses and energy requirements. However, because cancer patients tend to have significant weight loss prior to surgery, their ability to cope with stress is impaired, resulting in increased morbidity and mortality.[16] The physical insult, the associated pain, and the emotional response to surgery set off an integrated endocrine and metabolic reaction designed to maintain body functions. There is an increased output of catecholamines, glucagon, and cortisol that results in hypermetabolism, weight loss, negative nitrogen balance, and retention of sodium and water. As well as the general response to injury, surgery of the oropharynx and GI tract have specific nutritional sequelae depending on the site (Table 34-1).

Cancer chemotherapy may profoundly alter the host's nutritional state. The effects may be direct (by interfering with host cell metabolism or DNA synthesis and cellular replication), or indirect (by producing nausea, vomiting, changes in taste sensation, and learned food aversions). Most agents have the ability to stimulate the chemoreceptor trigger zone, resulting in nausea and vomiting. The rapid cell turnover in the alimentary tract mucosa makes it especially vulnerable to chemotherapy, resulting in stomatitis, ulceration, and decreased absorptive capacity. These effects result, in turn, in decreased intake and absorption of nutrients and further predispose the cancer patient to malnutrition. The bone marrow is another organ with a high cell turnover; toxicity is manifested by anemia, leukopenia, and thrombocytopenia. Neutropenia is, in turn, associated with an increased risk of sepsis.

Radiation therapy may affect the host's nutritional state by its effects on the GI tract. The severity of the injury is related to the dose of radiation and the volume of tissue treated. The effects of radiation therapy are classified as early or late. Early effects are transient and are manifested by diarrhea, bleeding, nausea, vomiting, weight loss, mucositis, xerostomia, alterations in taste, and food aversions. Late effects include intestinal strictures, fistulae, and malabsorption.

Table 34-1. Nutritional Consequences of Radical Operative Resection

Organs Resected	Nutritional Sequelae
Oral cavity and pharynx	Dependency on tube feedings
Thoracic esophagus	Gastric stasis (secondary to vagotomy) Fat malabsorption Gastrostomy feedings in patients without reconstruction
Stomach	Dumping syndrome Fat malabsorption Anemia
Small intestine	
Duodenum	Pancreatobiliary deficiency with fat malabsorption
Jejunum	Decrease in efficiency of absorption (general)
Ileum	Vitamin B_{12} and bile salt absorption
Massive (>75%)	Fat malabsorption and diarrhea Vitamin B_{12} malabsorption Gastric hypersecretion
Colon (total or subtotal)	Water and electrolyte loss

From Lawrence.[52]

Consequences of Malnutrition in the Cancer Patient

The clinical relevance of severe malnutrition has been demonstrated by increased morbidity and mortality and poor treatment tolerance in malnourished tumor-bearing individuals. In 1932, after reviewing 500 autopsy reports on cancer patients, Warren[24] found that malnutrition was a major factor contributing to their deaths. The protein-calorie malnutrition produced by the cancer-bearing state leads not only to obvious weight loss, but also to visceral and somatic protein depletion that compromises enzymatic, structural, and mechanical functions. Impairment of immunocompetence and increased susceptibility to infection frequently result. The effect on immune function may be further exacerbated by chemotherapy. Moreover, poor wound healing, increased wound infections, prolonged postoperative ileus, and longer hospital stays have all been linked to poor nutritional status in cancer patients. Meguid and coworkers[25] demonstrated that in patients undergoing colorectal cancer operations, the return to adequate oral food intake was significantly delayed in those patients classified as malnourished based on preoperative assessment. In this study, the morbidity and mortality in malnourished patients was 52% and 12% respectively, compared with 31% and 6% in well-nourished patients.

In animal studies, severe protein restriction depresses both humoral and cellular immune responses. In 1978, Daly, Copeland, and Dudrick[26] demonstrated that only 30% of tumor-bearing rats had a delayed hypersensitivity response to intradermal purified protein derivative after 2 weeks on an oral protein-free diet. Protein repletion with 7 days of total parenteral nutrition (TPN) or oral *ad libitum* feeding restored the response in 91% and 78% of rats, respectively. Only 17% of animals who remained on protein-free diets for the following 7 days showed a delayed hypersensitivity response. Law, Dudrick, and Abdou[27] found reduced titers of antibodies, IgM-producing cells, reduced lymphocyte response to mitogens, and decreased delayed hypersensitivity in rats after 6 weeks on protein-free nutrition.

In human studies, there is evidence for increased morbidity and mortality with depressed immunocompetence. In addition, it has been documented that nutritional therapy reverses anergy. In a group of 161 cancer patients undergoing nutritional support, 32 were anergic prior to therapy. In 27 of these patients anergy was reversed, and three of this group died. Of the five patients who remained anergic, all died. Daly, Dudrick, and Copeland[28] documented that 51% of anergic patients undergoing cancer treatment had restoration of skin test reactivity in response to intravenous hyperalimentation.

Effects of Preoperative Nutrition Support

Since its advent in the late 1960s, TPN has gained wide acceptance as an important route of nutrient administration. Recognition of the prevalence and consequences of malnutrition in the tumor-bearing host has fostered the development of TPN in these patients. More recently, however, routine use of TPN has been the subject of critical debate. In particular, controversy exists regarding the role of preoperative TPN in relation to perioperative morbidity, duration of hospital stay, and health care costs. There have been at least 30 studies to date, both retrospective and prospective, examining the role of perioperative TPN. The majority of these studies consistently demonstrate improved nutritional status in TPN-treated patients, including weight gain, improved serum albumin levels, and positive nitrogen balance. Most of these studies also have substantial defects, lacking adequate sample size, proper design, randomization, and statistical analysis. Failure of studies to date to demonstrate a significant reduction in postoperative complications and mortality in parenterally fed patients has led to conflicts regarding the use of TPN.

As shown in Table 34-2, retrospective analyses include four major studies in surgical patients. Three of these studies demonstrated improved clinical outcome. In an analysis of 244 esophageal cancer patients, Daly and colleagues[29] demonstrated a significant

Table 34-2. Preoperative Total Parenteral Nutrition in Cancer Patients (Retrospective)

Author	No. of Patients	Pre-operative TPN	Nutritional eligibility criteria defined	Complication rate	Mortality rate
Daly (1980)	160	14		na	na
Mullen (1980)	150	7	Yes	Yes	Yes
Smale (1981)	159	6-7	Yes	Yes	Yes
Bristar (1984)	64	25.4	Yes	No	No

na = not assessed

Adapted from Redmond et al.[53]

decrease in major complications in patients who received 5 or more days of TPN preoperatively compared with both concurrent and historical controls (Fig 34-2). In two other studies, preoperative TPN significantly reduced complications in patients deemed to be high risk by their prognostic nutritional index. An increased risk of pulmonary complications and longer hospital stay was shown in patients receiving TPN, but length of preoperative TPN was not documented. More TPN patients underwent operative resection than did controls. Retrospective data must be cautiously interpreted, and design defects identified in these studies include lack of appropriate randomization and inadequate sample size.

Sixteen randomized, prospective trials (Table 34-3), including some presented in abstract form only, have evaluated the effects of preoperative TPN on clinical outcome in cancer patients. In 1979, Heatley and colleagues[30] studied 74 gastric cancer patients who either received TPN for 7 to 10 days or served as controls. TPN patients had fewer wound infections and lost less body weight. Mueller and colleagues[31] studied 125 patients with GI cancer who were randomized to receive 10 days of preoperative TPN (n=66), or standard diet (n=59). Postoperative major morbidity and mortality were significantly lower in the TPN group. In an extension of their work, the authors published the results of a large trial in 1986 that included three groups: (1) control (regular hospital diet only), (2) TPN (amino acids/glucose), and (3) TPN (amino acids/glucose/lipid emulsion). The duration of preoperative TPN was 10 days. Acute and constitutive proteins and cellular and humoral immune parameters were assessed, as well as postoperative morbidity and mortality. Significant differences were noted for weight gain, increased protein and immune parameters, and major complications and mortality between group 2 and controls. However, group 3 was abandoned when a significantly higher mortality rate was noted during the study.

More recently, Starker and colleagues[32] and Bellantone and colleagues[33] have examined the role of preoperative TPN. Both studies included patients with benign and malignant disease. In the first study, 59 malnourished patients were divided into three groups based on initial response to TPN. Patients received intravenous feeding for a period ranging from 5 days to 6 weeks. The authors noted a high morbidity and mortality in those patients who remained hypoalbuminemic after 1 week of TPN. Their data suggest that a prolonged period of TPN decreased postoperative complications in this group of patients. Bellantone's study also randomized malnourished patients to TPN vs control treatment groups. Total parenteral nutrition decreased the incidence of septic complications ($p<.05$) compared with results in control patients.

Foschi and colleagues[34] studied the effects of TPN in 64 jaundiced patients treated preoperatively

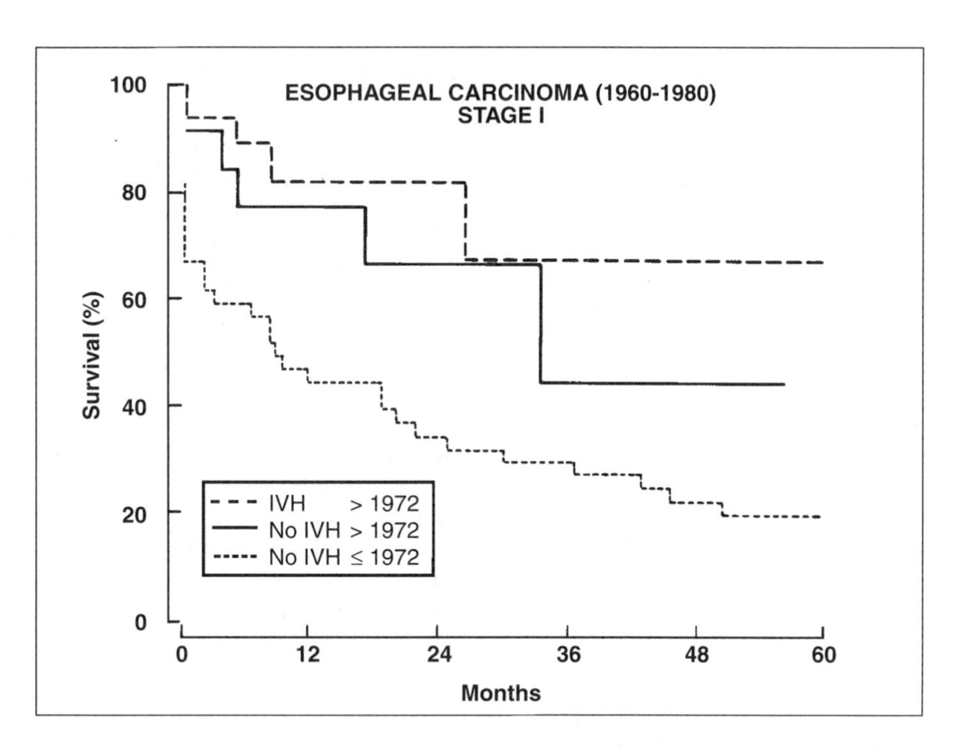

Fig 34-2. Five-year survival curves for patients with stage I esophageal cancer show a significant improvement in survival with TPN over concurrent non-TPN patients treated from 1960 to 1972. Adapted from Daly et al.[29]

Table 34-3. Prospective Randomized Trials of Preoperative Total Parenteral Nutrition in Surgical Patients

Author	No. of Patients	Preoperative TPN Duration(d)	Complication Rate TPN vs Control (%)	Mortality Rate TPN vs Control (%)
Hotler (1977)	56	3	13 vs 19	7 vs 8
Heatley (1979)	74	7-10	28 vs 25	15 vs 22
Holter (1976)	26	2	16 vs 18	ND
Moghissi (1977)	15	5-7	30 vs 50	ND
Preshaw	47	1	33 vs 17	ND
Simms (1980)	40	7-10	ND	0 vs 10
Lim (1981)	19	21-28	30 vs 50	10 vs 20
Schildt (1981)	15	14	39 vs 57	0 vs 0
Thompson (1981)	41	5-14	17 vs 11 vs 10	0 vs 0 vs 0
Sako (1981)	69	8-32	50 vs 56	50 vs 25
Mueller (1982)	125	10	11 vs 19*	3 vs 11*
Burt (1982)	18	14	ND	ND
Jenson (1982)	20	2	Sig in TPN*	ND
Starker (1986)	59	5-42	12.5 vs 45†	0 vs 10†
Foschi (1986)	64	20	18 vs 47	3.5 vs 12.5
Bellantone (1988)	100	7	5.3 vs 22	5.3 vs 6.6

ND = not determined.

*Sig in TPN = significant in TPN group

†Number of control patients vs those patients who received prolonged TPN.

Adapted from Redmond et al.[53]

with percutaneous transhepatic biliary drainage. They hypothesized that the operative risks in jaundiced patients were related to malnutrition, and in the study 20% were malnourished. Patients receiving TPN and/or enteral nutrition had significantly lower morbidity and mortality after surgery than control patients.

Recently, the results of a carefully designed prospective trial have become available. Four hundred fifty-nine patients were studied: 231 received TPN, and 228 served as controls. Mortality rates were similar for both groups, but a slightly higher incidence of pneumonia and wound infection was noted in the TPN group. There was also a higher incidence of septic complications associated with TPN administration at 30 and 90 days. In a subgroup of patients with severe malnutrition measured by subjective global assessment and nutritional index, preoperative TPN was beneficial.

In summary, trials of perioperative TPN have demonstrated improved nutritional status as reflected in body weight, serum proteins, immune function, and nitrogen balance. Effects on clinical outcome remain less well defined. To date, only a few studies of perioperative TPN have demonstrated a significant reduction in postoperative complications and reduced mortality. Failure to demonstrate improved outcome with TPN in other trials may accurately reflect the limited value of TPN. However, because of design defects in these studies, including defects in statistical design, inappropriate patient selection, and treatment regimens, and inadequate definition of endpoint criteria, the role of TPN remains undefined in the mild-to-moderately malnourished. However, in severely malnourished patients, a subgroup that usually includes cancer patients, preoperative TPN appears to have a beneficial role.

A narrow margin of therapeutic safety exists for chemotherapeutic drugs and adequate levels of radiation therapy; cachexia may reduce the therapeutic index of those modalities. Animal studies indicate that protein depletion increases the toxicity and lethality of chemotherapy. Furthermore, TPN or increased dietary protein reduces toxicity in animals, compared to regular or protein-depleted diets. In the 1970s, clinical reviews correlated malnutrition with a poor prognosis in patients with metastatic disease receiving chemotherapy. This suggested that nutritional support should increase therapeutic benefit, and many trials using TPN as adjunctive therapy were initiated. In 1986, Chlebowski[35] reviewed recent randomized trials and found no clear evidence that TPN alleviates chemotherapy-related toxicity or enhances the tumor response in people (Table 34-4). Although randomized trials have failed to demonstrate an adjunctive role for TPN or a reduction in side effects, nutritional therapy is an important supportive measure. It may permit some patients, who are not otherwise candidates for treatment due to inanition, to undergo continuing chemotherapy and, potentially, achieve disease-remission.

Some researchers have demonstrated reduced mortality and increased response rates in patients receiving extensive radiation therapy with adjunctive TPN compared to patients not receiving nutritional support. However, these studies were carried out in small groups of patients. Donaldson[36] reviewed these and other prospective trials in 1984 and failed to show that adequate nutritional support reduced the complication rates or improved local cancer control and survival. This suggests that TPN or enteral feeding is an important support measure in patients undergoing a planned course of radiation therapy but does not sensitize the tumor to irradiation or prevent GI side effects.

Effect of Malnutrition and Nutritional Support On Tumor Growth

Severe protein-calorie malnutrition inhibits tumor development and retards tumor growth in the experimental animal, but these apparent benefits are countered by loss of host body weight and impaired immune function. Malnourished animals that undergo nutritional repletion orally or with TPN may have a significant increase in tumor growth. Stimulation of tumor growth does not appear to be selective, as evidenced by constant tumor weight-to-host ratios

Table 34-4. Randomized Trials of TPN Addition to Chemotherapy in Patients With Cancer

Tumor Type	Patients Entered	Summary Results	Reference
Lung Cancer			
Small-cell	119	More febrile episodes (p 0.001) on TPN	Clamon et al. 1985
	49	No difference in outcome	Valdievieso et al. 1981
	19	No difference in outcome	Serrou et al. 1982
Non-small cell	26	Less myelosuppression on TPN	Issel et al. 1978
	65	*Decreased survival on TPN	Jordan et al. 1981
	31	No difference in outcome	Moghissi et al. 1977
	27	No difference in outcome	Lanzotti et al. 1980
Colon	45	*Decreased survival (p 0.03) on TPN	Nixon et al. 1981
Lymphoma	42	No difference in outcome	Popp et al. 1983
Testicular	30	Trend to more infections (p 0.07) on TPN	Samuels et al. 1981
Sarcoma	27	*Increased relapse (p 0.01) in patients on TPN made NED	Shamberger et al. 1984
Acute leukemia	24	No difference in outcome	Coquin et al. 1981
	21	More rapid bone marrow recovery on TPN	Hays et al. 1983
Pediatric malignancies	19	No difference in outcome	Van Eys et al. 1980

*Trials suggesting adverse effect of TPN addition to chemotherapy. NED = no evidence of disease.
From Chlebowski.[35]

in nutritionally depleted and repleted animals. Thus, it is of great concern in the clinical setting that nutritional support may promote tumor growth.

One of the most extensive clinical studies on nutritional support is that of Copeland and colleagues.[37] After following over 1,500 patients with cancer, they observed no increase in tumor growth attributable to nutritional support. Nixon and others[38] in 1981 noted no direct clinical or biochemical evidence of tumor stimulation with TPN in patients with metastatic colon cancer, although they did note that survival duration was less in the patients given TPN. Tumor protein synthesis, as determined by [^{15}N] glycine metabolism, shows no differences in patients on TPN from those fed orally, despite a substantial increase in protein and calorie intake in the TPN group. To date, numerous retrospective and prospective studies in humans have shown no enhanced tumor growth in response to increased nutritional intake. The issue is complicated by the fact that most patients studied were having antitumor treatment during their nutritional support. Also, the changes may be difficult to assess precisely by clinical or radiologic methods. Malnutrition may affect tumor growth by impairing the host's antitumor immune response. In animal studies, the effects of nutritional repletion appear to vary specifically with tumor immunogenicity and the host's immune response. In animals that do not develop an immune response to the tumor, nutritional repletion results in enhanced tumor growth.[39] Conversely, nutritional repletion in animals with an immunogenic tumor results in diminished tumor growth. Although increased nutritional intake may stimulate tumor growth in animal studies, it may decrease toxicity of chemotherapy without decreasing the response and lead to prolonged survival after treatment.

Nutritional Management of the Cancer Patient

Nutritional support for cancer patients is time-consuming, costly, and has its own inherent complications. There is no doubt that in malnourished patients, nutritional support can restore body composition and substrate metabolism towards normal. It also reduces the morbidity and mortality associated with major surgery. Nutritional therapy has also allowed the administration of more intensive antineoplastic therapy or radical surgery to patients who might otherwise have been considered unacceptable candidates. Thus, it is important to assess cancer patients accurately prior to treatment in order to identify those who may benefit from nutritional intervention. The object of nutritional assessment is to characterize the type and degree of malnutrition and relate these factors to the risk of morbidity and mortality.

The decision to nutritionally support a cancer patient requires decisions about the route and duration of administration and the formulation of the quantity and quality of nutrients.

Nutritional Assessment

The patient's history and physical examination may indicate the need for nutritional support. Once malnutrition is diagnosed, more precise measurements of nutritional status may be carried out. The patient's history allows for estimates of the rate and extent of weight loss and the quantity and quality of nutritional intake. Recent weight loss of more than 10% of body weight (over a period of 3 months) signifies substantial protein-calorie malnutrition. In Western society, where obesity is more the norm than the exception, the percent loss of body weight may be more relevant than comparison with ideal body weight standards. In 1936, Studley[40] showed a strong correlation between preoperative weight loss and postoperative complications in 50 patients undergoing gastric surgery. The patient's history may also provide information regarding special diets; problems with taste, chewing, or swallowing; food allergies; medicine and alcohol intake; and learned food aversions. Physical examination may reveal dry, scaly, atrophic skin; muscle wasting; pitting edema; and loss of muscle strength. A thorough history and physical examination by an experienced clinician is the simplest, and perhaps the best, method of nutritional assessment.

As an initial test, serum albumin can give important information. Values <3.4 g/dL are associated with increased morbidity and mortality following therapy. Less than 3 g/dL indicates significant visceral protein depletion. Albumin having a half-life of 20 days changes slowly in response to additional stress, such as antineoplastic therapy, or in response to nutritional support. Serum prealbumin, retinal binding globulin, and transferrin, with half-lives of 0.5, 2, and 8 days respectively, may be more useful under these circumstances. Alterations in serum levels of these proteins may occur with varying levels of hydration, and it is not uncommon for serum albumin to fall initially when patients are on TPN. This decrease reflects increased hydration rather than a worsening malnourished state.

The degree of visceral protein depletion is also reflected by impaired cell-mediated immunity evaluated by determining recall antigen skin testing and by total lymphocyte count. Loss of immunocompetence is not a sensitive indicator because weight loss usually exceeds 10% before anergy develops. Therefore, anergy with malnutrition indicates a significant visceral protein depletion leading to higher morbidity and mortality in hospitalized patients. Anergy has been associated with decreased serum albumin and transferrin levels. Delayed hypersensitivity is tested by the administration of subdermal injections of five antigens (purified protein derivative, candida, trichophytin, mumps skin test antigen, and streptokinose-streptodornase). A positive reaction with each antigen is defined as induration >5 mm diameter at 24 hours after injection. A normal delayed hypersensitivity response is defined as two or more positive reactions. Anergy is defined as no reaction, and one reaction is relative anergy.

Anthropometric measurements are noninvasive methods of determining body compartments and relate to measurements of age- and sex-matched normal populations. Skinfold thicknesses measured over the triceps, scapular area, iliac crest, and thigh provide an estimate of subcutaneous and total body fat, since 50% of total body fat is in the subcutaneous layer. Midarm muscle circumference, calculated as arm circumference, is measured at a point midway between the tip of the shoulder and the olecranon, minus .314 mm triceps skinfold thickness. This is measured on the nondominant arm and reflects lean body mass, which makes up most of the body's protein. Creatinine-height index, defined as 24-hour creatinine urinary excretion divided by the expected 24-hour excretion of creatinine by a normal adult of the same height, provides another measurement of muscle protein mass in patients with normal renal function. Substantial protein-calorie malnutrition would be defined as a level less than 75% of standard. Skeletal muscle mass may also be determined using a whole body counter to detect [^{40}K], which is present in small amounts, primarily intracellularly in skeletal muscle. From this value, total body potassium, a reasonable estimate of lean body mass, can be calculated.

Nutritional measurements have proved accurate in population surveys but have varying sensitivity and lack specificity. For example, anergy can occur due to exogenous steroid administration, inhalation anesthetics, trauma, radiation therapy, or sepsis; anthropometric measurements may increase with edema; and changes in serum albumin levels may result from alterations in hydration. Thus, the value of nutritional measurements lies in supporting the clinical diagnosis of malnutrition. With each individual patient, these measurements can help define the nutritional status and allow objective assessment of the efficacy of nutritional therapy (Table 34-5).

While the initial clinical assessment and blood tests select nutritionally depleted patients, complete nutritional assessment provides an estimate of body composition and quantifies the magnitude of malnutrition. This may be helpful in determining which patients may benefit from maintenance or anabolic nutritional therapy. These measurements have also been used individually or in various combinations as predictors of surgical risk, in order to select specifically those patients who would benefit from nutritional support. Examples are serum albumin, serum transferrin,[41] delayed hypersensitivity skin tests, and total lymphocyte count.[42] Clinical judgment also plays a role in such assessments.[43]

Table 34-5. Summary of Nutritional Assessment

Measurement	Body Compartment
Recent weight loss	Total body mass
Skinfold thickness over triceps, scapula, iliac crest	Total body fat
Midarm muscle circumference	Lean body mass
Creatinine height index	
Serum albumin, transferrin, retinal binding globulin, and prealbumin	Visceral protein
Total lymphocyte count	Immune competence
Delayed hypersensitivity to common skin antigens	

The key issue is whether there is a correlation between the risk of complications and the degree of malnutrition. Mullen and his coworkers developed an index of risk based on some nutritional parameters for patients undergoing surgery. The resulting formula was termed the prognostic nutritional index (PNI):

$$PNI=158\%-16.6(ALB)-0.78(TSF)-0.2(TFN)-5.8(DH)$$

(ALB = albumin [g/dL]; TSF = triceps skinfold thickness [mm]; TFN = transferrin [mg/dL]; DH = delayed hypersensitivity to any of 3 recall antigens graded from 0 to 2 where 0 is no reaction, 1 is a reaction <5 mm in diameter, and 2 is a reaction >5 mm in diameter at 24 hours after injection.)

A PNI <30% (low risk) was associated with an 11.7% complication rate and a mortality of 2%. A PNI >60% (high risk) was associated with an 81% complication rate and a mortality of 59%. In general, a PNI >40% is regarded as an indication for nutritional support. Cancer patients with a PNI >40% have been shown to have a significant decrease in postoperative mortality and morbidity if given total parenteral nutrition.

A simple, practical definition of significant malnutrition that can be applied clinically includes recent unexpected (ie, not due to dieting) weight loss of 10% or more of body weight, a serum albumin <3.4 g/dL, and a serum transferrin <190 mg/dL (normal range 210 to 375 mg/dL). Any combination of two of these criteria is an indication for nutritional support. The efficiency of PNI for patient selection was assessed for cancer surgery in 1981. Based on the PNI, patients were allocated to high risk (PNI>40%) or low risk (PNI<40%) groups. Within each group patients were assigned to TPN or no nutritional support. In the low-risk group there was no operative mortality and similar complication rates in TPN and no-TPN groups. In the high-risk category patients without nutritional support had a complication rate of 66% and a mortality rate of 40%, while in the TPN group the results were 31% and 15%, respectively. This study indicated that an adequate period of TPN is effective in reducing mortality and morbidity in cancer patients undergoing major surgery. The PNI, which is a nutritional composite representing fat stores, visceral protein, and immunocompetence, provides the clinician with an accurate and objective measure of risk for each individual.

Designing Nutritional Support

Route of Administration

In the presence of a normal GI tract, enteral feeding is preferred because it is more physiologic, less expensive, and has fewer complications associated with it than does parenteral feeding. Animal experiments indicate that adequate caloric and protein intake lead to the same benefits in terms of weight gain and serum albumin levels, irrespective of whether the route of administration is enteral or intravenous. A recent study of surgical patients compared those on enteral feeding to patients not receiving nutritional support. Sixty-seven patients were given a protein hydrolysate solution containing 14,700 to 16,800 J/day by nasogastric feeding tube; 43 patients received no treatment. Results showed highly significant advantages with enteral nutritional support in terms of body weight, serum albumin, nitrogen balance, immunocompetence, morbidity, and mortality. An earlier study of 24 esophageal cancer patients compared preoperative enteral feeding per gastrostomy with TPN. Weight gain was greater in the TPN group; the percentage gain in serum albumin was similar in both groups. In a study of nonsurgical cancer patients randomized to TPN, jejunostomy feeding, or normal oral diet, the TPN and enterally fed groups appeared to stabilize nutritionally; no significant differences could be found between the enteral and parenteral groups of patients.[44] Overall, these studies indicate that enteral and parenteral methods are equally efficacious in supplying nutritional requirements, although if rapid repletion is required, intravenous methods are preferable.

In some patients adequate intake may be achieved orally with aggressive dietary counseling; the normal diet can be supplemented with preparations containing high calorie content, amino acids, vitamins, and minerals. However, the presence of anorexia or upper GI cancers such as oropharyngeal or esophageal neoplasms may necessitate enteral tube feeding to achieve adequate nutritional intake.

For enteral feeding, nasogastric or nasoduodenal tubes, feeding gastrostomy, or jejunostomy routes provide access to the GI tract. Nasogastric tube feeding is the method most commonly used. Recent refinements in design have resulted in smaller-bore (6F to 8F) and more pliable tubes made from silicone or polyurethane. These are available weighted or with a stylet to facilitate passage of the tip. They can be left in place for 4 to 6 weeks with fewer complications (such as mucosal irritation, erosions, and sinusitis) than with the large-bore, less pliable nasogastric tubes. A large number of commercially prepared formulas are available that are homogenous and sterile, flow easily through small-bore tubes, and require little preparation.

If it is anticipated that the duration of enteral feeding will be longer than 6 weeks, gastrostomy or jejunostomy feeding should be considered. Large-bore gastrostomy tubes allow easy administration of bolus feeding but require surgical insertion using local or general anesthesia. Endoscopic techniques permit insertion of smaller percutaneous gastrostomy tubes using a local anesthetic and sedation. A jejunostomy tube is recommended when there is a proximal GI obstruction or fistula. The jejunostomy tube is associated with less stomal leakage, skin erosion, nausea, vomiting, and bloating compared with gastrostomy feeding. The conventional feeding tubes are made of rubber or latex; needle insertion of small-bore polyurethane catheters has become popular. Small-bore jejunostomy feeding requires a continuous flow pump to avoid clogging of the tube. The main disadvantage of jejunostomy feeding is diarrhea. Administration of hyperosmolar solutions within the small intestine results in diffusion of water into the lumen. To reduce the incidence of diarrhea, jejunal feeding should commence with small volumes (25 to 30 mL/h) of full-strength formula with a gradual increase in volume over 3 to 5 days, depending on the patient's tolerance. If diarrhea persists, antiperistaltic agents may be administered in the feeding formula. Gastric feeding allows the stomach to dilute hyperosmolar solutions and reduces the incidence of diarrhea, but it carries the risk of regurgitation and pulmonary aspiration and is contraindicated in the presence of gastric outlet obstruction, obtundation, or laryngeal incompetence.

The candidate for TPN is a malnourished patient who cannot be renourished enterally and who is potentially responsive to antineoplastic therapy. Total parenteral nutrition should also be given to patients with severe protein-calorie malnutrition (PNI>40%), who would be considered for treatment if their nutritional status improved. In these patients, severe visceral protein depletion may decrease the absorptive capacity of the intestine and delay the administration of treatment if enteral feeding methods are used. Total parenteral nutrition is also indicated in patients who, as a result of their treatment, are unable to maintain their nutritional status by oral or enteral feeding. To administer sufficient calories and amino acids intravenously, it is necessary to use hypertonic solutions, administered through a high-flow vein to prevent chemical endothelial phlebitis and thrombosis. The standard approach is central venous access using percutaneous, infraclavicular subclavian vein catheterization. In patients with emphysema, the risk of pneumothorax is high, and access through the internal jugular vein is preferred, though it may be less comfortable.

Nutritional Requirements

In normal individuals, calorie and nitrogen requirements can be calculated based on age, gender, height, and weight. Ideally, caloric requirement should be calculated for each patient by adjusting the calculated or measured REE for the level of physical activity and the degree of stress (Table 34-6). Indirect calorimetry is a more precise measurement of REE in each patient. Calorie requirements can be conveniently calculated using the Harris-Benedict equation:

For women:

REE (kcal/d) = 655 + 9.6W + 1.7H – 4.7A

For men:

REE (kcal/d) = 66 + 13.7W + 5.0H – 6.8A

(W = weight [kg]; H = height [cm]; A = age [years].)

Table 34-6. Determination of Energy Requirements

1. Resting energy expenditure; Harris-Benedict equation/indirect calorimetry	
2. Stress factors:	
Starvation	0.85
Elective surgery	1.0-1.2
Major sepsis	1.4-1.8
Fever	1.0 + 0.13 per degree C
Peritonitis	1.2-1.5
Cancer	1.1-1.45
3. Activity factor:	
Confined to bed	1.2
Mobile	1.3
4. Total energy expenditure = REE x stress x activity	

Adapted from Shanbhogue et al.[54]

Nonprotein caloric intake in excess of 130% of the REE is necessary for positive energy balance and repletion of fat stores. Dempsey, Hurwitz, and Mullen[45] found that increasing energy intake beyond 115% of REE did not improve nitrogen balance. Several studies have shown that provision of excessive caloric intake, especially in the form of hypertonic dextrose, leads to lipogenesis when the glycogen stores are repleted and results in impaired hepatic function. Using both fat and carbohydrate for nonprotein calories minimizes the complications of administering excessive glucose calories alone. Most organs use fat and carbohydrate for energy; the central nervous system, red blood cells, and the renal medulla preferentially metabolize glucose. Providing all the required calories as glucose results in simpler preparation and efficient utilization by all tissues; it spares the use of amino acids for gluconeogenesis. Hypertonic glucose solutions may result in high blood glucose levels leading to loss of glucose in the urine, resulting in an osmotic diuresis with electrolyte loss and tissue dehydration. Coadministration of insulin improves glucose uptake and utilization. High serum insulin levels, whether the result of exogenous administration or stimulated by high glucose levels, inhibit lipolysis and promote fat deposition, decreasing the availability of fat as an energy source. Glucose provides 4 kcal/g, and utilization is optimal when it is given at rates of 4 mg/kg/min to 5 mg/kg/min. Administration at rates in excess of 7 mg/kg/min does not further increase glucose oxidation rates. Glycogenolysis is stimulated, and excess glucose is converted to glycerol and fatty acids leading to fat deposition in the liver. Insulin has an anabolic effect on skeletal muscle, increasing uptake and decreasing release of amino acids that may bias protein repletion in favor of muscle protein at the expense of visceral protein. The provision of a liquid source of calories helps to overcome these problems. When plasma levels of fatty acids are elevated, they become the main source of energy for peripheral tissues, sparing glucose for tissues that preferentially metabolize it. In addition, using glucose alone as a caloric source results in an increase in carbon dioxide (CO_2) production, since glucose is oxidized with a respiratory quotient (RQ) of 1.0. Fat, on the other hand, has an RQ of 0.7 and fat oxidation produces less CO_2. Conversion of glucose to lipid is associated with an RQ of 8.0 and a substantial rise in CO_2 production. This requires the patient to increase minute ventilation to cope with rising CO_2 production and may cause respiratory distress with acidosis in patients with chronic obstructive airways disease. This is evidenced clinically by the fact that patients are more easily weaned off mechanical ventilators if they are receiving lipid in their diet or TPN solution.

Fat is usually given as lipid emulsions mainly made up of long-chain fatty acids with a caloric value of 9 kcal/g. Large quantities of long-chain fatty acids may impair neutrophil and reticuloendothelial macrophage function and reduce bacterial clearance. Thus, long-chain fatty acids should be limited to a maximum of 1.5 g/kg/day. Medium-chain triglycerides are available and do not impair macrophage function. They do not contain essential fatty acids, and thus a mixture of long- and medium-chain triglycerides is commonly used.

Administration of amino acids and calories adds to the circulating pool of amino acids supplying the liver with substrates for protein synthesis and reduces protein catabolism for energy production. In the malnourished patient, pyruvate is converted to alanine in skeletal muscle, receiving an amino group from one of the branched-chain amino acids (BCAA), leucine, isoleucine, and valine. In the liver, alanine is deaminated to pyruvate and converted to glucose. The administration of BCAA has been advocated to improve nitrogen balance in hypercatabolic patients. However, because of high costs, the use of these solutions is not warranted.

In addition to protein and calorie requirements, minerals, trace elements, and vitamins must be supplied. The clinical course of the patient should be monitored closely. Each day the patient's temperature, weight, glucose excretion, fluid and electrolyte balance, and physical findings should be reviewed. Serum urea, calcium, and phosphorus; and electrolyte concentrations, liver function, and blood glucose should be measured two or three times weekly to assess the effects of nutritional therapy on the patient. As part of the initial assessment, serum trace elements can be measured so that specific deficits can be corrected.

Numerous standard commercial solutions are available for TPN, some of which may be combined to provide the total daily nutrient requirements for each patient. The solutions can be combined into large bags containing up to three liters that can be changed once each day. This reduces the risk of contaminating the central venous line and is more convenient for the nursing staff. Mixing is carried out in the pharmacy under sterile conditions within a laminar flow hood. Standard amino acid TPN solutions are comprised of 500 cc 8.5% amino acids of which 30% to 50% are essential amino acids. Table 34-7 shows the composition of three typical standard amino acid solutions. These solutions are available at 10% concentrations for protein-depleted patients such as cancer cachexia patients. Solutions varying from 3% to 14% amino acids are available depending on the patients' needs. For renal failure patients, a 3% to 5% solution mainly made up of essential amino acids is usually used. Some of the amino acids, such as glutamine, degenerate in solution and are not included. In the future, glutamine should be added because it is an important amino acid for the maintenance of GI mucosal integrity.

Nonprotein calories can be given as glucose or lipid. A combination of fat and carbohydrate minimizes the complications of excessive administration of glucose calories. Fat emulsions also provide essential fatty acids. Intravenous fat emulsions are usually prepared from soybean or sunflower oils and are rich in polyunsaturated fatty acids. They are usually prepared as a 10% or 20% emulsion using egg phospholipid as the emulsifier and providing 1.1 kcal/mL or 2.2 kcal/mL, respectively. The commercially available emulsions are similar in composition and are therapeutically equivalent.

Glucose is usually administered as dextrose, a polymer of glucose, which yields 3.4 kcal/g. Solutions are available from 5% to 70% concentrations but a 50% solution is most commonly used.

Table 34-7. Composition of 8.5% Amino Acid Solutions

Amino Acids (g/L)	Freamine III	Aminosyn	Travasol
Essential			
Leucine	7.7	8.1	5.3
Isoleucine	5.9	6.2	4.1
Valine	5.6	6.8	3.9
Phenylalanine	4.8	3.8	5.3
Methionine	4.5	3.4	4.9
Lysine	6.2	6.2	4.9
Histidine	2.4	2.6	3.7
Threonine	3.4	4.6	3.6
Tryptophan	1.3	1.5	1.5
Non-Essential			
Alanine	6.0	11.0	17.6
Glycine	11.9	11.0	17.6
Arginine	8.1	8.5	8.8
Proline	11.2	7.5	3.6
Tyrosine	0	0.4	0.3
Serine	5.0	3.7	0
Cysteine	0.2	0	0
Glutamic Acid	0	0	0
Aspartic Acid	0	0	0

Nutritional and metabolic support includes electrolytes, vitamins, and trace elements. Daily intravenous requirements of minerals are as follows:

Sodium 60-140 mEq
Potassium 60-100 mEq
Chloride 60-120 mEq
Magnesium 8-10 mEq
Calcium 200-400 mg
Iron 1-2 mg

These must be provided daily, but the amounts administered must constantly be re-evaluated in light of existing deficits or abnormal losses.

Parenteral vitamin requirements for maintenance and repletion are poorly defined. The standard approach is to give the recommended daily allowance (RDA) of each vitamin as set down by the Food and

Drug Administration (Table 34-8). Dempsey and colleagues[46] determined the prevalence of abnormal vitamin levels in adult hospitalized patients prior to receiving TPN and found abnormally low levels in 42% of the patients. Standard parenteral vitamin therapy resulted in marginal improvement. A higher repletion dose resulted in significant improvement in vitamins A and C and pyridoxine. Commercially available multivitamin products contain more than the RDA, and the addition of one vial to the TPN solution each day is recommended. Vitamin K is not available in multivitamin preparations because vitamin K therapy is not required by all patients, such as those on anti-coagulants. Vitamin K is available as a separate parenteral injection as phytonadione. The recommended dosage is 10 mg once a week. Trace elements are also available commercially for TPN regimens, and the daily requirements of zinc, copper, manganese, selenium, and chromium can be added to the TPN solution. These elements and others are also available individually and can be added for specific deficiencies. All the above can be added together in a 3-liter bag. Heparin (8,000 to 10,000 units) is added to reduce the incidence of subclavian vein thrombosis. More water may be added to make up the daily fluid requirements. Initially the solution is given at 40 mL/h to 50 mL/h; the rate is gradually increased over 2 or 3 days until the full daily requirements are tolerated. Insulin can be added to the solution as required and six hourly blood sugars checked until they are stable. Suggested daily TPN regimen for an adult cancer patient is given in Table 34-9.

Table 34-8. Food and Drug Administration Recommended Daily Allowance of Vitamins

Vitamin	RDA
A (IU)	4,000-5,000
D (IU)	400
E (IU)	12-15
C (mg)	45
B_1 (mg)	1.0-1.5
B_2 (mg)	1.1-1.8
B_6 (mg)	1.6-2.0
B_{12} (μg)	3
Folate (μg)	400
Niacin (mg)	12-30
Pantothenic acid (mg)	5-10
Biotin (μg)	150-300

Table 34-9. Suggested Daily TPN Regimen for an Adult Cancer Patient

Protein-calorie		kcal
700 mL 50% dextrose		1,190
400 mL 20% lipid emulsion		880
1,000 mL 10% amino acid solution		400
Total calories		2,470
Total calorie: protein nitrogen ratio		154:1
Total volume		2,100 mL
Additives		
Electrolytes	Sodium chloride	60-140 mEq/d
	Potassium chloride	60-100 mEq/d
	Magnesium sulfate	8-10 mEq/d
	Calcium gluconate	9 mEq/d
	Potassium phosphate	30-45 mEq/d
Trace minerals	Copper	
	Zinc	
	Manganese	1 vial/d
	Chromium	
	Selenium	
Iron		1 mg/d
Multivitamin preparation		one vial/d
Vitamin K_1		10 mg/once weekly
Heparin		8,000 u/day
Glutamic acid		4 g/d

Nutrition and Immunity

Immunosuppression is a common finding in the cancer patient. Malignancy, malnutrition, surgery, anesthesia, blood transfusions, chemotherapy, and radiation treatment have all been found to depress the immune system. Patients with cancer show depression of both cellular and humoral immune functions. Classically, T-cell proliferative responses to both mitogen and alloantigen are reduced with increasing tumor burden. Patients with advanced disease often lack a delayed-type hypersensitivity reaction to skin-recall antigens (anergy). Anergy is clearly predictive of increased sepsis and mortality in patients undergoing major surgery.

In analyzing anergy, defects in T-cell activation have been found to be the primary abnormality in the delayed hypersensitivity response. When removed from "anergic environment" and cultured in vitro with recall antigen, however, T cells proliferate normally. These activated T cells then can elicit the delayed-type hypersensitivity response when reinjected into the patient. Cytotoxic T lymphocytes isolated from patients with breast, lung, and colon carcinomas as well as from sarcomas demonstrate decreased cytotoxicity to autologous tumor. Natural killer cells, the body's putative first line against cancer, are also less active when isolated from tumor-bearing animals and patients.

In addition to the immunosuppression that occurs in the presence of malignancy, surgical therapy intended to eradicate tumors may promote metastatic tumor growth. Patients undergoing diverting colostomy followed by colectomy for cancer have been shown to do less well than those treated by one operation. Controlled experiments in animal models corroborate enhancement of tumor growth, but mechanisms remain obscure. Functionally, T cells show depressed responses to mitogen or alloantigen. Although blood transfusions are often unavoidable in oncologic surgery, they may adversely affect outcome in the cancer patient. Perioperative blood transfusion has been associated with significantly poorer prognosis in patients with breast carcinoma, colon cancer, non-small cell lung cancer, and sarcoma. The mechanisms involved are complex and multifactorial, but multiple blood transfusions depress the immune response manifested in vitro by poor T-cell proliferative indices and decreased effector cell response to various lymphokines.

Certain nutrient substrates may have a major role in the nutritional support of the cancer patient. Specific amino acids, RNA ω-3 fatty acids, and trace metals such as zinc have all been shown to affect host immune function.

Arginine is a semi-essential dibasic amino acid that is a component of the urea cycle. It is converted by the enzyme arginase into ornithine and urea. Arginine has potent secretagogue effects on several endocrine and neuroendocrine glands. Administration of arginine induces the secretion of growth hormone, prolactin, insulin, glucagon, insulin-like factor-1, pancreatic polypeptide, somatostatin, and catecholamines. In laboratory studies, arginine supplementation has thymotropic properties and enhances the responsiveness of thymic lymphocytes to mitogens in normal and traumatized animals. Arginine enhances cellular immunity, as evidenced by improved delayed-type hypersensitivity responses and improved bacterial containment and survival in animal burn models. Arginine has also been demonstrated to have antitumor effects in both chemically and virally induced and transplanted solid tumor models. Studies from our laboratory have demonstrated beneficial effects of supplemental arginine in the tumor-bearing host by noting increased Concanavalin A (con-A) mitogenic responses and IL-2 production by host splenocytes and increased host reactivity against tumor antigens in the tumor-bearing group.[47] Supplemental arginine significantly retarded the growth of C1300 neuroblastoma in protein-depleted mice and prolonged median host survival. These effects were dependent on tumor antigenicity.

Few clinical studies have examined the role of oral or intravenous supplemental arginine in humans. In healthy volunteers, supplemental dietary arginine increased peripheral blood lymphocyte mitogenic response to con-A and phytohemagglutinin (PHA). Our group investigated the effects of supplemental arginine in cancer patients undergoing major surgery.[48] Thirty patients were randomized to receive either supplemental arginine (25 g/d) or isonitrogenous L-glycine (43 g/d) as part of the graduated enteral diet for 7 days after surgery. Supplemental arginine significantly increased mean mitogenic responses to con-A and PHA on postoperative days four and seven compared to postoperative day one. No differences were found in the glycine-treated group. Mean CD4+ phenotype levels on postoperative day seven were also significantly increased compared to the glycine group. Mean plasma levels of somatomedin-C were also significantly increased on day seven in the arginine group compared with the glycine group.

RNA has been demonstrated to be essential for the continued maturation of T cells in animal models. Absence of RNA from the diet results in depressed cell-mediated immune function, decreased survival after *Staphylococcus aureus* injection, and diminished rejection of allografts. Fatty acids in the diet affect levels of arachidonic and eicosapentaenoic acid, resulting in changes in prostaglandin synthesis. Increased intake of ω-3 fatty acids has been reported to improve immunologic function by decreasing prostaglandin E_2 production after major injury. Animal studies by Alexander and coworkers have demonstrated improved response to infectious challenges in animals supplemented with ω-3 fatty acids. Recent studies in cancer patients undergoing major upper GI surgery demonstrated a significant reduction in postoperative infections, wound complications, and hospital length of stay in patients receiving arginine, RNA, and ω-3 fatty acids compared with patients receiving a standard diet.[49]

Specific Nutritional Manipulation of Host and Tumor

Visceral protein and lean body mass depletion result in a worse prognosis than does fat depletion. This is to be expected, since proteins are the constituents of enzymes, hormones, immunoglobulins, and the contractile elements of muscle tissue. Using standard nutritional support, weight can be maintained or gained during repletion. This may not, however, represent true anabolism in most patients. Animal evidence suggests that increases in body weight in response to TPN are due to excess water and increased lipid stores. Most prospective studies using TPN have failed to detect a therapeutic benefit to the host in terms of prolonged survival or in tumor response to chemotherapy or radiation therapy. For nutritional therapy to be maximally effective, the aim should be to increase host protein while inhibiting—or at least not stimulating—tumor growth, as animal studies suggest.

In simple chronic starvation, the body adapts by relying on fat as its main energy source. Free fatty acids are used in muscle and liver metabolism for energy, and excess free fatty acids are converted to ketones by the liver to be used as an energy source in other tissues. In these tissues, the ketones are reconverted to acetyl coenzyme A and enter the Krebs cycle. This spares glucose utilization, the need for gluconeogenesis, and reduces nitrogen output. In the cancer cachectic state, these adaptive mechanisms are not effective, and this results in continuous protein catabolism. Exogenously administered ketones have been given to normal humans as an external energy source; they produce a fall in urinary nitrogen excretion, reflecting protein conservation. A number of tumors specifically metabolize glucose, and the administration of a lipid source of energy may reduce the substrate available to the tumor. Another approach is to use the nutrient-induced phase of tumor stimulation to enhance the effect of therapy. Torosian and coworkers[50] have shown in animals that the percentage of cells in the S-phase increases significantly 2 hours after the commencement of TPN. This may enhance tumor response to cycle-specific chemotherapy.

An alternative approach to shifting nutritional balance in favor of the host is to reduce tumor metabolism by blocking the utilization of a substrate necessary for tumor growth. It has been noted that some animal and human tumors metabolize large amounts of glutamine. Increased activity of enzymes that utilize glutamine for the production of purines and pyrimidines in a variety of rodent tumors has also been shown. Acivicin is a potent inhibitor of this enzyme system, and recent work has shown that acivicin reduces tumor growth in rats fed regular rat chow or on TPN.[51] In addition, the TPN resulted in a significant gain in body weight in these animals. Thus, the specific nutritional requirements of tumors may be used as a weapon against tumor growth while the host benefits from TPN.

Tumor growth may be altered by dietary immunomodulation. Dietary supplementation with arginine demonstrated an inhibition of tumor growth in mice bearing C1300 neuroblastoma. This was associated with augmented specific antitumor immune response.[47]

Conclusion

Frequently, cancer patients are malnourished at the time of diagnosis. These patients develop anorexia and reduced nutritional intake. Specific abnormalities in substrate metabolism and energy expenditure have been detected in patients and in tumor-bearing animals. Protein catabolism, increased lipolysis, and glucose availability help to create a milieu favorable to tumor growth at the host's expense. There is evidence that the tumor can control these changes through neurohumoral mechanisms. There is little doubt that malnutrition associated with cancer has a negative prognostic effect and can contribute directly to the patient's death. It can also increase postoperative morbidity and decrease tumor response and patient tolerance to all modalities of treatment.

Nutritional therapy is an important supportive measure for the patient undergoing antineoplastic treatment. It increases the patient's well-being and may permit the administration of more intensive therapies. There is no conclusive evidence that adequate nutritional support preferentially feeds the tumor and results in increased tumor growth in humans. There is good evidence that effective nutritional repletion can reduce the postoperative complication and mortality rates after surgery. Weight gain is possible, and immune status may be improved, but definite improvement in tumor response rates and patient survival following chemotherapy or radiotherapy remains unproven. In the future, more specific manipulation of substrates and hormones administered to the host may improve the results.

References

1. DeWys WD, Begg C, Lavin PT, et al. Prognostic effect of weight loss prior to chemotherapy in cancer patients. *Am J Med.* 1980;69:491-497.

2. McAnena OJ, Daly JM. Impact of antitumor therapy on nutrition. *Surg Clin North Am.* 1986;66(6):1213-1228.

3. DeWys WD, Walters K. Abnormalities of taste sensation in cancer patients. *Cancer.* 1975;36:1888-1896.

4. Lucke B, Borwick M, Zeckwer I. Liver catalase activity in parabiotic rats with one partner tumor bearing. *J Natl Cancer Inst.* 1952;13:681-686.

5. Theologides A. Pathogenesis of cachexia in cancer. *Cancer.* 1972;29:484-488.

6. Nakahara W. A chemical basis for tumor host relations. *J Natl Cancer Inst.* 1960;24:77-86.

7. Stovroff MC, Norton JA. Cachectin: a mediator of cancer cachexia. *Surg Forum.* 1987;413-415.

8. Krause R, Humphreys C, von Meyenfeldt M, et al. A central mechanism for anorexia in cancer: a hypothesis. *Cancer Treat Rep.* 1981;65(suppl 5):15-21.

9. Brennan MF. Uncomplicated starvation versus cancer cachexia. *Cancer Res.* 1977;37:2359-2364.

10. Brennan MF. Total parenteral nutrition in the cancer patient. *N Engl J Med.* 1981;305:375-381.

11. Young VR. Energy metabolism and requirements in the cancer patient. *Cancer Res.* 1977;37:2336-2347.

12. Shike M, Russel D, Detsky A, et al. Changes in body composition in patients with small-cell lung cancer: the effect of TPN as an adjunct to chemotherapy. *Ann Intern Med.* 1984;101:303-309.

13. Knox LS, Crosby LO, Feurer ID, et al. Energy expenditure in malnourished cancer patients. *Ann Surg.* 1983; 197:152-162.

14. Heber D, Chlebowski RT, Ishibashi DE, et al. Abnormalities in glucose and protein metabolism in noncachectic lung cancer patients. *Cancer Res.* 1982;42:4815-4819.

15. Shaw JM, Humberstone DM, Wolfe RR. Energy and protein metabolism in sarcoma patients. *Ann Surg.* 1988;207:283-289.

16. Buzby GP, Muller JL, Matthews DC. Prognostic nutritional index in gastrointestinal surgery. *Am J Surg.* 1980;139:160-167.

17. Holroyde CP, Reichard A. Carbohydrate metabolism in cancer cachexia. *Cancer Treat Rep.* 1981;65(suppl):55-59.

18. Waterhouse C, Jeanpretre N, Keilson J. Gluconeogenesis from alanine in patients with progressive malignant disease. *Cancer Res.* 1979;39:1968-1972.

19. Lundholm K, Edstron S, Ekman L, et al. Metabolism in peripheral tissues in cancer patients. *Cancer Treat Rep.* 1981;65(suppl):79-83.

20. Waterhouse C. Nutritional disorders in neoplastic diseases. *J Chron Dis.* 1963;16:637-644.

21. Norton JA, Stein TP, Brennan MF. Whole body protein synthesis and turnover in normal and malnourished patients with and without known cancer. *Ann Surg.* 1981;194: 123-128.

22. Cohn SH, Gartenhaus W, Sawitsky A, et al. Compartmental body composition of cancer patients by measurement of total body nitrogen, potassium, and water. *Metabolism.* 1980;30:222-229.

23. Moley JF, Aamodt R, Rumble W, et al. Body cell mass in cancer bearing and anorexic patients. *J Parenteral Enteral Nutr.* 1987;11:219-222.

24. Warren S. The immediate cause of death in cancer. *Am J Med Sci.* 1932;184:610-615.

25. Meguid MM, Mughal MM, Debonis D, et al. Influence of nutritional status on the resumption of adequate food intake in patients recovering from colorectal cancer operation. *Surg Clin North Am.* 1986;66(6):1167-1176.

26. Daly JM, Copeland EM, Dudrick SJ. Effect of intravenous nutrition on tumor growth and host immunocompetence in malnourished animals. *Surgery.* 1978;84:655-658.

27. Law DK, Dudrick SJ, Abdou NI. The effects of protein-calorie malnutrition on immunocompetence of the surgical patient. *Surg Gynecol Obstet.* 1974;139:257-266.

28. Daly JM, Dudrick SJ, Copeland EM. Intravenous hyperalimentation: effect on delayed cutaneous hypersensitivity in cancer patients. *Ann Surg.* 1980;192:587-592.

29. Daly JM, Massar E, Giacco G, et al. Parenteral nutrition in esophageal cancer patients. *Ann Surg.* 1982;196:203-208.

30. Heatley RV, Williams RHP, Lewis MH. Preoperative intravenous feeding: A controlled trial. *Postrad Med J.* 1979;42:541-545.

31. Mueller JM, Keller HW, Brenner U, et al. Indications and effects of preoperative parenteral nutrition. *World J Surg.* 1986;10:53-63.

32. Starker PM, LaSala PA, Askanazi J, et al. The influence of preoperative total parenteral nutrition upon morbidity and mortality. *Surg Gynecol Obstet.* 1986;162:569-574.

33. Bellantone R, Doglietto G, Bossola M, et al. Preoperative parenteral nutrition of malnourished surgical patients. *Acta Chir Scand.* 1988;22:249-251.

34. Foschi D, Cavagna G, Callioni F, et al. Hyperalimentation of jaundiced patients on percutaneous transhepatic biliary drainage. *Br J Surg.* 1986;73:716-719.

35. Chlebowski RT. Effect of nutritional support on the outcome of antineoplastic therapy, *Clin Oncol.* 1986;5:365-379.

36. Donaldson SS. Nutritional support as an adjunct to radiation therapy. *J Parenteral Enteral Nutr.* 1984;8:302-309.

37. Copeland EM, Daly JM, Ota DM, et al. Nutrition, cancer, and intravenous hyperalimentation. *Cancer.* 1979;43: 2108-2116.

38. Nixon DW, Moffitt S, Lawson DH, et al. Total parenteral nutrition as an adjunct to chemotherapy of metastatic colorectal cancer. *Cancer Treat Rep.* 1981;65(suppl):121-128.

39. Karpeh MS, Kehne JA, Choi SH et al. Tumor immunogenicity, nutritional repletion, and cancer. *Surgery.* 1987; 102:283-290.

40. Studley HO. Percentage of weight loss: a basic indicator of surgical risk in patients with chronic peptic ulcer. *JAMA.* 1936;106:458-460.

41. Mullen JL, Buzby GP, Waldman TG, et al. Prediction of operative morbidity and mortality by preoperative nutritional assessment. *Surg Forum.* 1979;30:80-82.

42. Grant JP, Custer PB, Thurlow J. Current techniques of nutritional assessment. *Surg Clin North Am.* 1981;61: 437-463.

43. Baker JP, Detsky AS, Wesson DE, et al. Nutritional assessment: a comparison of clinical judgment and objective measurements. *N Engl J Med.* 1982;306:969-972.

44. Burt ME, Stein TP, Brennan MF. A controlled randomized trial evaluating the effects of enteral and parenteral nutrition on protein metabolism in cancer-bearing man. *J Surg Res.* 1983;34:303-314.

45. Dempsey DT, Hurwitz S, Mullen JL. Selective repletion of fat and/or protein stores. *J Parenteral Enteral Nutr.* 1985;9:117.

46. Dempsey DT, Mullen JL, Rombeau JL, et al. Treatment effects of parenteral vitamins in total parenteral nutrition patients. *J Parenteral Enteral Nutr.* 1987;11:229-237.

47. Reynolds JV, Zhang S, Thom AK, et al. Arginine, protein malnutrition and cancer. *J Surg Res.* 1988;45:513-522.

48. Daly JM, Reynolds JV, Thom AK, et al. Immune and metabolic effects of arginine in surgical patients. *Ann Surg.* 1988;208:512.

49. Daly JM, Lieberman MD, Goldfine J, et al. Enteral nutrition with supplemental arginine, RNA and omega-3 fatty acids in postoperative patients: Immunologic, metabolic and clinical outcome. *Surgery.* 1992;112:56-67.

50. Torosian MH, Tsou KC, Daly JM, et al. Alteration of tumor cell kinetics by pulse total parenteral nutrition. *Cancer.* 1984;53:1409-1415.

51. Chance WT, Cao L, Nelson JL, et al. Acivicin reduces tumor growth during TPN. *Surgery.* 1987;102:386-394.

52. Lawrence W Jr. Nutritional consequences of surgical resection of the gastrointestinal tract for cancer. *Cancer Res.* 1977;37:2379-2386.

53. Redmond HP, Daly JM. Preoperative nutritional therapy in cancer patients is beneficial. In: Simmons R, ed. *Debates in Clinical Surgery.* vol 2. St. Louis, Mo: Mosby Year Book, Inc; 1991.

54. Shanbhogue LK, Chwals WJ, Weintraub M, et al. Parenteral nutrition in the surgical cancer patient. *Br J Surg.* 1987;74:172-180.

35

ONCOLOGIC EMERGENCIES

John H. Glick, MD, Donna Glover, MD

Advances in therapy and supportive care have led to an increase in oncologic emergencies as the survival of cancer patients improved. Before initiation of treatment, several factors must be considered in evaluating an oncologic emergency (Table 35-1).

Aggressive treatment is indicated if a histologic diagnosis of malignancy has not been established or if the patient has a good prognosis with surgery, radiotherapy, or chemotherapy. If there is a chance for cure or prolonged palliation, radical treatment plans may be indicated. However, in advanced malignancies, the primary goal is often palliation and relief of symptoms, even if the patient has a limited life expectancy. Restoring functional status will frequently lead to improved quality of life. If the oncologic emergency is directly due to the malignant process, the general approach is to treat the underlying malignancy if there is effective therapy. Treatment should be initiated promptly to prevent complications and permanent disability. However, for terminal cancer patients, withholding treatment and controlling pain may be the most appropriate decision.

This chapter will review the pathophysiology, clinical presentation, diagnostic evaluation, and therapy for common oncologic emergencies.

Pericardial Effusions and Neoplastic Cardiac Tamponade

At autopsy, up to 20% of cancer patients have cardiac or pericardial metastases.[1-4] Cancers of the lung or esophagus grow by direct extension into the pericardium, while distant primary malignancies metastasize to the pericardium hematogenously. Carcinomas of the lung and breast, lymphoma, leukemia, melanoma, gastrointestinal (GI) cancers, and sarcomas are the most common primary tumors associated with malignant pericardial effusions.[2,3]

Pathophysiology

Tamponade usually occurs because of cardiac compression from large malignant pericardial effusions,

Table 35-1. Management Factors in the Evaluation and Treatment of an Oncologic Emergency

Symptoms and Signs

1. Are the symptoms and signs due to the tumor or to complications of treatment?
2. How quickly are the symptoms of the oncologic emergency progressing?

Natural History of the Primary Tumor

1. Is there a previous diagnosis of malignancy?
2. What is the disease-free interval between the diagnosis of the primary tumor and onset of the emergency?
3. Has the emergency developed in the setting of terminal disease?

Efficacy of Available Treatment

1. No prior therapy versus extensive pretreatment
2. Should treatment be directed at the underlying malignancy and/or the urgent complications?
3. Will the patient's general medical condition influence the ability to administer effective treatment?

Treatment and Goals

1. Potential for cure
2. Is prompt palliation required to prevent further debilitation?
3. What is the risk versus benefit ratio of treatment?
4. Should treatment be withheld if there is a minimal chance of response to available antitumor therapies?

John H. Glick, MD, Director, Cancer Center, Hospital of the University of Pennsylvania, Philadelphia, Pennsylvania

Donna Glover, MD, Chief of Hematology and Oncology, Department of Medicine, Presbyterian Medical Center, Philadelphia, Pennsylvania

although encasement of the heart by tumor or postirradiation pericarditis can mimic tamponade.[5,6] With cardiac tamponade, signs of circulatory collapse appear suddenly, even though the effusion or constriction may have developed gradually.[5] The severity of tamponade depends on the rate of pericardial fluid accumulation and the volume of accumulated fluid. Pericardial fluid accumulation may stretch the pericardium but not impair cardiac contractility. However, if the pericardium is surrounded by tumor or radiation fibrosis, a small effusion may produce significant cardiac compression.[6,7] Elevated pericardial pressures reduce ventricular expansion and diastolic filling. As stroke volume falls, hypotension and compensatory tachycardia occur, along with equalization and elevation of mean left atrial, pulmonary arterial and venous, right atrial, and vena caval pressures. Tachycardia and peripheral vasoconstriction develop in an attempt to maintain arterial pressure, increase blood volume, and improve venous return.[5,7]

Clinical Presentation

In a large autopsy series, fewer than 30% of patients with malignant pericardial effusion had symptoms of pericarditis. In most patients, the diagnosis of pericardial tumor is not made before death.[2,4] With tamponade or pericardial constriction, patients may complain of dyspnea, cough, and retrosternal chest pain relieved by leaning forward. When cardiac output falls, decreased cerebral blood, peripheral cyanosis, decreased systolic and pulse pressures, and pulsus paradoxus occur.[4] Occasionally, patients with large effusions develop hoarseness, hiccups, nausea, vomiting, and epigastric pain. Physical examination may reveal engorged neck veins, distant heart sounds, edema, ascites, hepatosplenomegaly, and hepatojugular reflex.[4]

Diagnostic Evaluation

More than half of patients with pericardial effusion have cardiac enlargement, mediastinal widening, or hilar adenopathy that can be seen on chest x-ray. As the fluid accumulates, the mediastinum shortens and widens, the normal arcuate borders are lost, and the cardiac silhouette becomes globular.[5,8,9] Electrocardiographic (ECG) abnormalities are often nonspecific. With pericarditis, the ECG may show low QRS voltage in the limb leads, sinus tachycardia, ST elevations, and T-wave changes.[5,10] Electrical alternans may occur with tamponade, but is not a reliable diagnostic parameter.[11] Echocardiography, the most specific and most sensitive noninvasive test, should be performed immediately if the diagnosis is suspected.[7,12,13] With posterior effusions, two distinct echoes are seen: from the effusion and from the posterior heart border. The space between these echoes indicates the size of the effusion or thickness of the pericardium.[8,13] Inconclusive physical examination and noninvasive studies warrant performing a right ventricular catheterization to diagnose pericardial tamponade or constriction.[12,14]

Pericardiocentesis should be performed for both diagnostic and therapeutic purposes. The fluid is analyzed for cell count, cytology, and appropriate cultures. The cytology is usually positive in patients with metastatic carcinoma, but is frequently inconclusive with lymphoma and mesothelioma.[3,4,15,16] If a histologic diagnosis is important and pericardial fluid cytologic findings are negative, a pericardial biopsy is performed, either under local anesthesia with a subxiphoid approach or under general anesthesia with an anterior thoracotomy. The latter procedure is more sensitive since more tissue can be obtained, but is associated with morbidity and mortality.[17,18]

Therapy

A significant decrease in cardiac output warrants emergency pericardiocentesis before initiation of definitive local therapy to prevent recurrent tamponade. Emergency pericardiocentesis should be performed when the patient develops: (1) cyanosis, dyspnea, shock, or impaired consciousness; (2) pulsus paradoxus >50% of the pulse pressure; (3) decrease of >20 mm Hg in pulse pressure; or (4) peripheral venous pressures >13 mm Hg.[5,18] Oxygen should be administered, but positive-pressure breathing is contraindicated because of impaired venous return from increased intrapericardial and intrapleural pressures.[5] If emergency pericardiocentesis cannot be performed immediately, cardiac contractility and filling can be improved with isoproterenol and volume expansion.[4]

Tamponade will recur within 24 to 48 hours unless promptly treated to prevent pericardial fluid reaccumulation. Therapeutic options depend on the sensitivity of the primary tumor to specific modalities; prior treatment; and life expectancy. Pericardial windows, sclerosing agents, radiotherapy, effective systemic antineoplastic drugs, and pericardiectomy have produced excellent long-term palliation in selected series. These treatments are difficult to compare since responses are not based on objective criteria. The duration of response and survival are influenced by the extent of metastatic disease, and the degree of response to concurrent systemic hormonal therapy or chemotherapy.[3,4,17-21]

Tamponade can be controlled by pericardial catheter drainage and sclerosis. An indwelling pericardial catheter is left in place until pericardial drainage stops. Tetracycline 500 to 1,000 mg is then instilled through the pericardial cannula and flushed with normal saline. The procedure is repeated every 2 to 3 days until there is no fluid drainage in the preceding 24 hours.[20,21] The inflammatory response and fibrosis from intrapericardial tetracycline obliterate the space between the parietal and visceral pericardium and prevents fluid formation.

Recent reports have shown effective pericardial sclerosis with a single instillation of bleomycin (30 or 60 mg) through the catheter. Bleomycin is instilled after evacuation of pericardial fluid for 24 hours. The tube is clamped for 10 minutes and then withdrawn. In a recent study,[22] no major side effects were noted, except for one transient elevation in temperature, which resolved in <12 hours. Bleomycin may have certain advantages over tetracycline, such as fewer side effects, especially less pain. Severe fibrosis was not reported after local instillation, nor was there fibrous thickening of the pericardium at autopsy. None of the patients died from pericardial tamponade.[22]

Palliation may also be obtained with pleural-pericardial windows. Under local anesthesia, inferior pericardiotomy provides immediate relief of cardiac compression and tissue for histologic diagnosis, with complication rates of 2%.[17] Symptoms of tamponade recur in <5% of patients. A thoracotomy may be required if the heart is encased with tumor, or additional tissue is required for diagnostic purposes.[18]

Although radiotherapy has been reported to control most malignant pericardial effusions, the radiosensitivity of the tumor will determine the response and duration of palliation. Radiation doses are given in 1.5 to 2 Gy fractions to a total dose of 25 to 30 Gy. Patients with lymphoma or leukemia may respond to lower doses (eg 15 to 20 Gy over 2 weeks).

Pericardiectomy is warranted if radiation-induced pericardial disease is not controlled with conservative medical management. However, it is contraindicated in the presence of extensive pericardial tumor. With extensive pericardial metastases, life expectancy is short and surgical morbidity and mortality rates with pericardiectomy are high.[4]

After the patient is clinically stable, systemic therapy should be administered if effective regimens are available. If a rapid chemotherapeutic response can be obtained (eg in lymphoma or small-cell lung cancer), the patient may be treated with pericardial drainage and systemic chemotherapy.[4]

Data suggest that cytotoxic therapy may be effective in chemotherapy-sensitive tumors such as lymphoma, leukemia, and breast cancer. Patients with lymphoma who have not received first-line therapy responded well to combination chemotherapy for pericardial effusion. In one series of three patients with malignant pericardial effusion due to breast cancer,[23] control of effusion was achieved with single pericardiocentesis followed by systemic chemotherapy. No other local therapy was necessary. Similar results have been observed in patients with effusion due to acute leukemia.

Superior Vena Cava Syndrome

Etiology and Pathophysiology

The superior vena cava (SVC) is easily compressed by adjacent expanding masses.[4] Obstruction produces pleural effusions and facial, arm, and tracheal edema. With severe SVC obstruction, brain edema and impaired cardiac filling may produce alterations in consciousness and focal neurologic signs. Symptoms depend on the extent and rapidity of SVC compression. Table 35-2 lists the signs and symptoms of SVC syndrome.[24] If the SVC is gradually compressed and collateral circulation develops, symptoms may be indolent and subtle.[24]

Most cases of SVC syndrome are caused by malignant mediastinal tumors.[25-27] More than 75% of malignant SVC obstructions are secondary to small-cell or squamous cell lung cancer;[25-28] 10% to 15% are secondary to mediastinal lymphomas, most often diffuse large-cell subtypes.[29] Less than 15% have benign causes, such as tuberculosis and aneurysm.[24,27,30,31] The most common nonmalignant cause of SVC obstruction is thrombus in central venous catheters.[27]

Table 35-2. Symptoms and Signs of Superior Vena Cava Syndrome

Finding	Number	Percent
Thoracic vein distention	56	67
Neck vein distention	49	59
Edema of face	47	56
Tachypnea	34	40
Plethora of face	16	19
Cyanosis	13	15
Edema of upper extremities	8	9.5
Paralyzed true vocal cord	3	3.5
Horner's syndrome	2	2.3
Total no. of patients	84	

Adapted from Perez et al.[24]

Diagnostic Evaluation

It is easy to diagnose SVC obstruction if facial edema, venous engorgement, and impaired consciousness are present. However, if SVC obstruction develops slowly, venography or radionuclide scans may be necessary to confirm the diagnosis. Angiographic or radionucleotide studies also help to localize the site of obstruction and plan radiation portals.[31,32] Computed tomographic (CT) scans of the chest with intravenous contrast or magnetic resonance imaging (MRI) scans provide excellent anatomic detail and help to define radiation portals.[27]

Most patients with SVC syndrome do not present with histologic diagnosis of malignancy.[24,25] The least invasive techniques should be employed to establish the diagnosis by biopsy or cytology. Sputum cytology, bronchoscopy with brushings and washings, and biopsy of palpable adenopathy provide the correct diagnosis in 70% of cases.[24] If small-cell lung cancer or lymphoma is suspected, bone marrow aspirates or biopsies may confirm the diagnosis. Fine needle biopsy of mediastinal masses under CT guidance may provide sufficient tissue for a cytologic diagnosis.[33] If necessary, invasive diagnostic procedures (eg thoracotomy or mediastinoscopy) can be performed safely if the trachea is not obstructed.[26,27] In the past, invasive procedures were postponed until after initiation of radiotherapy, to prevent complications from bleeding or airway compromise. However, delaying diagnostic procedures several days after radiotherapy may yield only necrotic tissue.[25,26]

Therapy

Only a small percentage of patients with rapid onset of SVC obstruction are at risk for life-threatening complications.[26,27] Emergency treatment is indicated when there is brain edema, decreased cardiac output, or upper airway edema. Most patients with malignant SVC obstruction are treated with radiotherapy, initially given in high daily fractions (4 Gy for 3 days), followed by 1.5 to 2 Gy daily to a total dose of 30 to 50 Gy. The radiation dose depends on the tumor size, radioresponsiveness, and probability of achieving a response with systemic therapy.[24,26,28] The radiation portal should include a 2-cm margin around the tumor. In patients with locally advanced nonsmall-cell lung cancer and no distant metastases, the mediastinal, hilar, and supraclavicular lymph nodes and any adjacent parenchymal lesions should be irradiated. Mantle irradiation may be preferable to mediastinal irradiation in selected cases of Hodgkin's disease or malignant lymphoma.[24,28] During irradiation, patients improve clinically before objective signs of tumor shrinkage are evident on chest x-ray.[28] Radiation palliates SVC obstruction in 70% of patients with lung carcinoma and in >95% with lymphoma.[28]

In a review of 125 patients with SVC syndrome due to malignancies, radiotherapy at high initial doses (3 to 4 Gy daily for three fractions) provided symptomatic relief in <2 weeks in 70% of patients.[34] When irradiation at conventional doses (2 Gy daily, five weekly fractions) was used, 56% of patients respond. A combination of radiation and chemotherapy did not improve overall response. However, this would be difficult to assess, depending on the tumor types treated. SVC syndrome recurred in 13% of patients. The most common complaint is dysphagia.

Radiation therapy is effective in most cases of SVC syndrome due to malignancy. However, when signs and symptoms are not relieved, one must suspect a persistent tumor outside the treatment portals. Invasive diagnostic procedures such as contrast venography should be performed to establish the cause of treatment failure.[35] This would enable the clinician to modify treatment and achieve a higher complete response rate. A superior venacavogram, radionucleotide venacavogram, or angiogram may reveal almost complete obstruction of the superior or inferior vena cava, if this diagnosis is suspected because of pedal edema.

Chemotherapy may be preferable to radiation for patients with disseminated disease if a prompt response is anticipated. For example, small-cell anaplastic carcinoma and lymphoma respond to radiation,[24] but may be more sensitive to systemic chemotherapy.[29,36,37] Sclerosing agents given to patients with SVC syndrome should not be injected into dilated arm veins. Anticoagulation may help relieve venous obstruction by preventing thrombus formation. Although anticoagulated patients improve more rapidly and have shorter hospitalizations, there is no difference in overall survival.[38,39] Generally, the risks of hemorrhage associated with antithrombotic therapy outweigh the temporary benefit if the venous obstruction is due to tumor rather than clot. Corticosteroids decrease edema associated with inflammatory reactions following tumor necrosis from irradiation. If clinical signs of venous obstruction progress shortly after initiation of radiotherapy, steroids are administered for 3 to 7 days. When SVC obstruction is due to thrombus around a central venous catheter, patients may be treated with antifibrinolytics or anticoagulants. Surgical removal of the catheter may be required.[27]

Spinal Cord Compression

Etiology and Pathophysiology

Spinal cord compression is always an emergency, especially when neurologic deterioration is rapid. Once the patient becomes paraplegic, there is little chance of regaining function. The most common tumors associated with spinal cord compression are carcinomas of the breast, lung, and prostate; multiple myeloma; and lymphoma.[40-42] At autopsy, >5% of patients with metastatic disease have epidural tumors,[42] which generally arise within the vertebral body and grow along the epidural space anterior to the spinal cord.[43] Patients with paraspinal tumors (eg, lymphoma) may develop epidural metastases when the neoplasm grows through the intervertebral foramina from adjacent nodes. Spinal cord and nerve root compression can occur secondary to epidural tumor or vertebral collapse from destructive osseous metastases. Permanent neurologic dysfunction may occur if vascular compromise produces prolonged ischemia or hemorrhage.[40,43]

Clinical Presentation

More than 95% of patients with spinal cord compression complain of progressive central or radicular back pain. The pain is often aggravated by recumbency, weight bearing, coughing, sneezing, or the Valsalva maneuver, and is relieved by sitting.[41] The earliest neurologic symptoms are sensory changes, including numbness, paresthesias, and coldness. The incidence of motor dysfunction has decreased due to earlier diagnosis and treatment. Although bladder and bowel dysfunction are rarely the first signs of cord compression, metastases to the cauda equina typically produce impaired urethral, vaginal, and rectal sensation; bladder dysfunction; saddle anesthesia; and decreased sensation in the lumbosacral dermatomes.[40,41,43] The level of cord compression may be determined by pain elicited by straight leg raising, neck flexion, or vertebral percussion. The upper limit of the sensory level is often one or two vertebral bodies below the site of compression. Decreased rectal tone and perineal sensation are often observed when there is autonomic dysfunction. Deep tendon reflexes may be brisk with cord compression and diminished with nerve root compression.[40,42]

Symptoms and signs indicating spinal cord compression may be due to a number of noncompressive causes, including paraneoplastic syndromes, carcinomatous myopathy or neuropathy, radiation myelopathy, herpes zoster, subacute myelopathy, pain from a pelvic or long bone metastasis, anterior spinal artery occlusion, retroperitoneal tumor, or the toxicity of cytotoxic drugs. Nonmalignant diseases such as herniated disks, osteoporotic vertebral fractures, and intraspinal abscess can also cause cord compression in the cancer patient. The cause of neurologic symptoms is generally evaluated by plain film myelography, MRI, and CT scans.

Diagnostic Evaluation

Rodichok and colleagues initiated a prospective clinical trial designed to diagnose spinal cord compression before irreversible neurologic damage occurred. In his series, more than 90% of patients with epidural tumor had radiographic evidence of vertebral metastases (eg, vertebral collapse, osteolytic lesions, pedicle erosion, or a paraspinal mass).[44] However, in another series, 15% of cancer patients with vertebral compression had only benign disease on CT scan of the spine. There was a high correlation between posterior cortical bone discontinuity and the presence of epidural tumor.[45] Myelograms revealed epidural metastases in 81% of patients with roentgenographic abnormalities. However, only 14% of patients with negative bone films had positive myelograms regardless of neurologic deficits. Although bone scans were more sensitive in detecting early osseous metastases, up to 30% of abnormalities on bone scan may be due to benign disease; they are less accurate in predicting spinal cord compression.[44]

The accuracy of MRI in detecting metastatic compression of the spinal cord or cauda equina has been compared with other findings—at myelography, surgery, clinical follow-up, and autopsy. MRI has a sensitivity of 93%, specificity of 97%, and overall accuracy of 95%.[46] The SIRs of 41 metastatic and 15 posttraumatic collapsed vertebrae were calculated in one study. All benign and only one malignant compression fracture had SIRs greater than 0.8.

MRI offers advantages over myelography in that no uncomfortable positions or contrast injections are required. In addition, it can demonstrate multiple sites of epidural metastasis, which may not be obvious on the initial myelogram unless special attention was paid. The detection of cord displacement, however, becomes less certain and more subjective when the spine is scoliotic. The use of a surface coil may improve image detail.

The disadvantages of MRI include the necessity to lie still in one position. Many patients with severe central back pain cannot maintain a position for long periods.

Therapy

All patients with suspected cord compression should have emergency myelography or an MRI scan of the spine. These studies are necessary to determine the proximal and distal extent of the epidural defect as well as whether there is more than one area of cord or nerve root compression. If a complete block is found on myelogram, a cisternal or lateral cervical puncture is required if the upper limit of the block cannot be defined by air injection following lumbar Pantopaque™ myelography.[47] If there is not a complete block, cerebrospinal fluid (CSF) can be obtained safely. The CSF is then sent for glucose, protein, cell count, cytology, and appropriate stains and cultures, if infection is suspected.[40] If a complete block is demonstrated, no more than 1 cc of CSF should be removed. In place of a myelogram, either an MRI scan or metrizamide CAT scan may delineate the subarachnoid space and define the area of block. MRI or CAT scans of the spine, spinal canal, vertebral foramina, and paravertebral soft tissues may also identify abnormalities not seen on plain film or myelography.

When spinal cord compression is suspected, the radiation oncologist and neurosurgeon should be consulted immediately. Treatment decisions must be based on the radiosensitivity of the tumor, compression, rate of neurologic deterioration, and prior radiotherapy. Radiotherapy is the primary treatment for most patients with epidural metastases and once the diagnosis of cord compression is confirmed, emergency radiotherapy should be given. Radiation portals include the entire area of block and two vertebral bodies above and below the block. Radiation doses range from 30 to 40 Gy administered over 2 to 3 weeks. Radioresponsive tumors (eg, lymphoma and multiple myeloma) have a higher chance of neurologic recovery with radiotherapy than radioresistant tumors (eg, melanoma).[40-42,48] More than half of patients with rapid neurologic deterioration improve with radiotherapy.[41] However, the prognosis for patients with autonomic dysfunction or paraplegia is poor despite surgery or radiotherapy.[42,49,50]

Laminectomy provides prompt decompression of the spinal cord and nerve roots. However, with a posterior laminectomy, it is extremely difficult to remove the tumor, since most epidural metastases arise in the vertebral bodies anterior to the spinal cord. Because the tumor cannot be removed surgically, postoperative radiotherapy is given to decrease residual tumor, relieve pain, and improve functional status. Most ambulatory patients have improved neurologic function after surgical decompression, but those with severe preoperative neurologic deficits rarely benefit from surgery.[41,42,50] Surgery is generally contraindicated when there are multiple areas of cord compression.

A recent review suggests that patients with vertebral collapse rarely benefit from surgical laminectomy due to an increased risk of major neurologic deterioration by at least one grade.[51] The higher risk is probably due to the presence of a destructive lesion in the anterior spinal column, which results in further instability with posterior laminectomy. In most cases, laminectomy is contraindicated in the presence of a collapsed vertebral body. Radiation therapy should not affect spinal stability, but there is no evidence that it improves neurologic results. The most logical approach may be to use an anterior surgical approach to the spine (either transthoracic or thoracoabdominal) which will enable immediate spinal stabilization and early mobilization.

If there is no prior histologic diagnosis of malignancy or if infection or epidural hematoma must be ruled out, a laminectomy is indicated. High cervical cord lesions can cause death from respiratory paralysis unless surgical decompression is accomplished. If surgery is not viable, the patient's neck should be stabilized in a halo. When neurologic signs progress over 48 to 72 hours despite high-dose steroids and radiotherapy, emergency decompression should be attempted although results are generally poor when there is rapid neurologic progression. After a long interval subsequent to radiotherapy for spinal cord compression, surgery may be beneficial when the epidural tumor recurs.

Corticosteroids may promptly reduce peritumoral edema and improve neurologic function.[41] Prior to emergency diagnostic procedures, patients with neurologic symptoms from possible cord compression should receive dexamethasone 10 mg. Generally, dexamethasone (4 to 10 mg every 6 hours) is continued during radiation therapy, then tapered. Steroids initially improve neurologic function, but it is not clear that they affect the ultimate outcome. The side effects of high-dose glucocorticoids (Table 35-3) must be considered before these drugs are prescribed.

Table 35-3. Side Effects of Corticosteroids

Life-Threatening Side Effects
1. Diabetes
2. Proximal muscle weakness
3. Increased risk of infection
4. Edema
5. Peptic ulcer disease
6. Psychosis
7. Adrenal suppression

Bothersome, Cosmetic Side Effects
1. Weight gain
2. Striae
3. Moon facies
4. Acne

Rare Side Effects
1. Hiccups
2. Insomnia
3. Pseudorheumatoid arthritis

Chemotherapy rarely has a major therapeutic role in spinal cord compression. However, if the malignancy is sensitive to chemotherapy, the regimen can be administered concurrently with or soon after radiotherapy or surgery is complete.

Although the management of spinal cord compression due to multiple myeloma usually involves radiation, with or without decompressive surgery, chemotherapy may play a role in patients who have had prior radiation. In one series,[51] six myeloma patients became ambulatory with melphalan and prednisone alone. Three of the patients had total paraplegia, and two had moderate paresis. The duration of symptoms in four patients ranged from 2 weeks to 2 months. Three patients had loss of bladder control. The time to full ambulation ranged from 2 weeks to 8 months.[52,53]

Although hormonal therapy or chemotherapy should not be the mainstay of treatment for oncology patients who have not had prior radiation therapy or surgery, systemic therapy may play a role in certain tumor types. Spinal cord compression due to lymphoma, malignant thymoma, or seminoma has been reported to respond to glucocorticoids alone, but it is not known whether this is due to reduction of edema or a direct antitumor effect. Neurologic recovery in patients with lymphoma and cord compression has been observed with single-agent chemotherapy. Paraplegia due to prostate carcinoma has been found to respond to hormonal manipulation without radiation treatment.

Obstructive Uropathy

Etiology

Obstructive uropathy is frequently associated with intra-abdominal, retroperitoneal, and pelvic malignancies. The diagnostic and therapeutic approach depends on whether the site of obstruction is the bladder neck or ureter. Bladder outlet obstruction is often secondary to cancer of the prostate, cervix, or bladder, or to benign prostatic hypertrophy. Ureteral blockage is due to para-aortic malignancies such as lymphoma, sarcoma, and nodal metastasis from carcinoma of the cervix, bladder, prostate, rectum, or ovary.[54-56]

Most cancer patients have obstructive nephropathy due to tumor, but benign conditions must be considered in the differential diagnosis. Chronic hypercalcemia, hyperuricemia, and urinary tract infection predispose patients to renal calculi. Ureteral strictures are delayed complications of surgery and radiotherapy. Following retroperitoneal surgery, abscesses or hematomas can cause ureteral obstruction. The primary cause of acute hyperuricemic nephropathy is uric acid deposition in the renal tubules. However, ureteral obstruction from uric acid calculi has been reported in association with myeloproliferative disorders.[55,57] Bladder outlet obstruction may be secondary to clots, urethral strictures from radiation fibrosis, or cyclophosphamide cystitis. Patients with locally advanced bladder cancer or with metastasis to the brain, spinal cord, or sacral roots may have impaired bladder emptying. Voiding problems may be secondary to medications that alter the central or autonomic nervous system.[58,59] Whatever the cause of obstruction, pathologic changes in the dilated structures proximal to the site of obstruction ultimately culminate in renal failure and death.[59] The initial staging evaluation for patients with locally advanced pelvic or retroperitoneal malignancies should include studies to ensure patency of the urinary tract.

Clinical Presentation

Oliguria is a common problem in cancer patients who are ill. Obstruction should be suspected when patients complain of urinary tract infections. Unfortunately, ureteral obstruction often goes undiagnosed until renal failure results in obtundation, seizures, volume overload, and anuria.[55,58,61] Ureteral obstruction and neurogenic bladders are recognized earlier than ureteral blockage. Impaired bladder emptying causes symptoms of hesitancy, urgency, nocturia, frequency, and decreased force of urinary stream.[55,58-61] Partial kidney obstruction should be suspected when polyuria alternates with oliguria. Physical examination may reveal an enlarged prostate or bladder, or a pelvic, flank, or renal mass. Decreased anal sphincter tone or diminished bulbocavernosus reflexes should suggest a neurogenic bladder.[58]

Diagnostic Evaluation

The diagnosis of obstructive uropathy can be readily made on intravenous pyelography (IVP), renal ultrasound, renal radionuclide scans, or CT. However, an IVP will rarely delineate adequately the renal pelvis and ureters in patients with rising creatinine levels (≥3 mg/dL). Negative findings on renal ultrasound do not rule out an obstruction. The bladder must be catheterized to exclude urethral obstruction. Routine serum chemistry studies, including creatinine, electrolytes, blood urea nitrogen (BUN), calcium, phosphorus, uric acid, and hematologic profiles, should be monitored frequently. Pyuria and bacteriuria suggest an accompanying obstruction that requires immediate drainage and parenteral antibiotics.

The site of obstruction must be identified prior to planning appropriate therapy. Hydronephrosis usually is confirmed by renal ultrasonography, since the risks of contrast-induced nephrotoxicity are high and poor renal function can result in inadequate IVP images. Renal ultrasound can demonstrate pelvic or retroperitoneal masses, ureteral dilatation, and calculi.[61] Unless the patient is allergic to contrast dye or has severe renal dysfunction, intravenous urograms will define the site of blockage in 80% of cases of acute urinary obstruction. However, a dilated collecting system does not always imply obstruction. These selected cases may require a repeat injection of contrast or a radionuclide scan after hydration and intravenous diuretics. CT is more expensive and less specific, but can help differentiate hydronephrosis from renal cysts and identify obstructing masses.[62]

The most reliable means of ruling out renal obstruction are cystoscopy and bilateral retrograde pyelography. However, the latter is contraindicated in cases of infection. If obstruction is proven, a stent can be placed to relieve an obstruction. Stents should be rechecked to avoid reobstruction and reinfection.

Percutaneous antegrade pyelography has the advantage of both diagnosing and relieving obstruction without the risks of anesthesia. Under ultrasonic guidance, a catheter is inserted in the dilated renal pelvis. Urine is aspirated and sent for analysis and culture. To localize the site of obstruction, contrast is injected through the catheter. Once the site is determined, an attempt is made to advance the catheter through the obstruction to restore internal ureteral drainage. If internal drainage is ineffective, external drainage can be achieved via the percutaneous catheter until indwelling ureteral stents are placed with cystoscopy and retrograde pyelography.[63]

Urodynamic and urethrocystography are helpful in differentiating bladder dysfunction secondary to neuromuscular or mechanical causes. Generally, transurethral or suprapubic cystoscopy is required to determine the cause of bladder outlet obstruction. The ureteral orifices must be visualized and urinary flow confirmed from each orifice. Appropriate biopsies and cytologic samples should be obtained.[58]

Therapy

Lower urinary tract obstruction can be relieved temporarily by an indwelling urethral catheter, suprapubic cystostomy, or cutaneous vesicostomy. If bladder outlet obstruction cannot be promptly correctly, suprapubic cystostomy is preferable to an indwelling urethral catheter. The former is more comfortable, associated with a lower risk of infections, and avoids prostatic swelling. For partially denervated bladders, parasympathomimetic drugs (eg, bethanechol) can improve bladder contraction and prevent overflow incontinence. Low-pressure incontinence can be treated with adrenergic agonists (eg, ephedrine). Anticholinergics (eg, propantheline bromide) are prescribed for patients with uninhibited or reflex neurogenic bladders.[58] Generally, prostatic obstruction is corrected by transurethral resection. Obstructive symptoms from advanced prostate cancer also can be relieved by orchiectomy, hormonal therapy, and radiation. However, if transurethral resection is not performed, temporary urinary diversion is required since maximal benefit from hormonal manipulation or radiation is often delayed for a few weeks.[54,64-66]

Radiation therapy or chemotherapy may effectively relieve obstruction if the tumor is responsive to the treatment modality.[67-69] Dosages should be adjusted for renal insufficiency, and nephrotoxic drugs (eg, cisplatin and methotrexate) should be avoided. Cyclophosphamide and ifosfamide should not be given, since the uroepithelium can be damaged severely after prolonged exposure to the active urinary metabolites of these drugs. After the obstruction is relieved, intravenous or oral fluids administered for a few days can compensate for the postobstructive diuresis.

Infection, hyperkalemia, and acidosis must be treated promptly. Unless obstruction is relieved promptly, permanent renal damage will result. The decision to relieve an obstructing lesion must be carefully considered in terminally ill patients, because patient survival, but not comfort, may be prolonged.

Airway Obstruction

Etiology

Tracheal or endobronchial tumors that cause significant airway obstruction must be treated promptly to prevent postobstructive pneumonia, respiratory distress, and irreversible lung collapse.

Lung cancer is the primary cause of bronchial obstruction. At diagnosis, partial or complete bronchial obstruction is present on chest x-ray in 53% of patients with squamous cell carcinoma; in 25% with adenocarcinoma; in 33% with large-cell anaplastic carcinoma; and in 38% with small-cell carcinoma.[70] Endobronchial tumor is seen in 70% of lung cancer patients at thoracotomy. Endobronchial lesions are found in the main stem and lobular bronchi in 20% and 50% of cases, respectively.[71]

In contrast to primary bronchogenic carcinomas, significant endobronchial metastatic lesions are rare. Only 2% of cancer patients have significant endobronchial metastases. However, if patients with microscopic endobronchial disease are included, the incidence of endobronchial metastasis ranges from 25% to 50%.[71-74] The most common malignancies metastasizing to the bronchial tree are carcinomas of the breast, colon, and kidney; sarcoma; melanoma; and ovarian cancer.[74,75]

Tracheal obstruction is often secondary to benign conditions such as tracheal stenosis, tracheomalacia, and edema from infection or recent irradiation.[69] Patients with cancer of the head and neck usually have elective tracheostomies prior to developing upper airway obstruction.[68]

Clinical Presentation

Bronchial and tracheal obstructions are often difficult to differentiate on physical examination. Presenting symptoms include dyspnea, orthopnea, cough, wheezing, stridor, hoarseness, and hemoptysis. Symptoms of bacterial postobstructive pneumonia may be found with complete obstruction. High-pitched breathing or stridor is usually associated with laryngeal or tracheal obstruction. Wheezing and rhonchi may be audible or palpable over a partially obstructed airway. If the bronchus is significantly obstructed, the trachea will deviate toward the obstructed side. Most patients are asymptomatic until at least 75% of the lumen is occluded.[68,75]

Diagnostic Evaluation

Lateral neck radiographs with soft tissue technique provide the best view of the upper third of the trachea, but tracheal narrowing may be seen on routine chest x-ray or bilateral oblique views. Prior to initiation of treatment, overpenetrated tracheal films, tomography, and barium swallow should be obtained to evaluate tracheal narrowing.[76] If radiologic studies are not definitive, upper airway obstruction can be confirmed with flow-volume loops using an 80% helium/20% oxygen mixture. Tracheostomy and directed biopsies are usually needed to obtain a definitive histologic diagnosis.

With bronchial obstruction, chest x-rays may reveal atelectasis or segmental consolidation. Cultures should be obtained if fever or other signs of postobstructive pneumonitis are present. A definitive diagnosis is made with fiberoptic bronchoscopy, biopsy, and brushing.[74,76]

Therapy

Significant upper airway obstruction requires immediate treatment to prevent respiratory failure and death. A low tracheostomy should be performed if the obstruction is in the hypopharynx, larynx, or upper third of the trachea. A long tracheostomy tube may be inserted after tracheal dilatation if the lower trachea is obstructed.[68] Once the airway is secured, most patients are treated with emergency radiotherapy. High-dose corticosteroids (eg, dexamethasone 10 to 16 mg a day) are often administered to reduce edema during the initial days of radiation treatment. Patients with a neoplasm sensitive to chemotherapy, such as small-cell anaplastic lung cancer or lymphoma, may respond more promptly to combination chemotherapy.[77]

Patients with tracheal tumors should be considered for surgical resection and reconstruction in the absence of evidence of extratracheal metastasis.[68,69,77] When nonsmall-cell lung cancer obstructs a major bronchus, surgical resection is rarely curative.[71] Curative radiotherapy for an obstructing non-small-cell lung cancer may be problematic: Obstructing pneumonitis makes it difficult initially to plan radiation portals. As atelectasis resolves, the portal should be reduced. Patients with endobronchial obstruction from small-cell lung cancer may respond promptly to combination chemotherapy or radiotherapy. If an endobronchial lesion regrows in the irradiated field, palliation may be achieved with laser therapy, iridium seed implantation, or cryosurgery.[77]

Brain Metastases

Emergency measures are indicated when patients present with signs of increased intracranial pressure, herniation, or hemorrhage due to brain metastases. Even when patients have more gradual neurologic deterioration, prompt treatment is warranted to prevent permanent neurologic damage. The incidence of brain metastasis has increased among patients with cancer of the breast, bladder, or lung because of prolonged survival with combination chemotherapy. Most chemotherapeutic regimens penetrate the blood-brain barrier poorly, and brain metastases may develop without disease progression outside the central nervous system (CNS).[77,78] The most common malignancies metastasizing to the brain are cancers of the lung and breast and melanoma. In patients with small-cell lung cancer, 10% have brain metastases at presentation and 80% of those who survive 2 years develop brain metastases unless the cranium is irradiated prophylactically.[79,80] Up to one third of patients with metastatic breast cancer show CNS involvement at autopsy.[81]

Most neurologic deficits in cancer patients are secondary to CNS metastases, but benign conditions must be excluded. Elderly patients may develop neurologic signs due to metabolic disturbances, cerebrovascular thrombosis, or hemorrhage. Meningitis and brain abscesses occur with increased frequency in immunosuppressed patients. When neurologic deficits recur long after high-dose whole-brain radiotherapy, it may be difficult to differentiate brain necrosis from recurrent metastatic disease.[77]

Pathophysiology and Clinical Presentation

More than 60% of patients with brain metastasis will have multiple lesions at autopsy,[82] with lesions occurring predominantly in the cerebrum. Signs and symptoms depend on the location of the lesion, the extent of brain edema, and the intracranial pressure. Extensive edema surrounding the brain metastasis or ventricular obstruction by tumor results in increased intracranial pressure, with the characteristic symptoms of decreased mental status, vomiting, nausea, and headache. Headache is usually present before arising from bed and improves within an hour of arising. Engorged retinal veins lead to papilledema, which results in blurred vision.[77,83] Seizures occur more frequently among patients with increased intracranial pressure, melanoma, or carcinomatous meningitis.[77,83]

There are three types of cerebral herniations. Uncal herniation presents with lateral, rapidly expanding supratentorial masses. The temporal lobe is displayed and compresses the ipsilateral third cranial nerve, ipsilateral posterior cerebral artery, and upper brain stem. Patients present with headache, vomiting, unilateral pupillary dilatation, rapid loss of consciousness, and decerebrate posturing. Central herniation occurs with multifocal supratentorial mass lesions, expanding unifocal mass lesions in the frontal or parietal areas, and hydrocephalus. These patients generally present with headache, progressive drowsiness, small reactive pupils, periodic Cheyne-Stokes respirations, and bilateral extensor plantar responses. Subsequently, these patients develop hyperventilation, disconjugate gaze, pupillary fixation, and abnormal motor postures. Tonsillar herniation occurs with large posterior fossa masses. These patients have signs of direct brain-stem compression and acute hydrocephalus with headache, vomiting, hiccups, nuchal rigidity, rapid loss of consciousness, deviation of the eyes, irregular respirations, and hypertension.

A variety of metastatic and nonmetastatic diseases cause seizures in patients with malignancy; brain metastases are the most common cause.

Diagnostic Evaluation

MRI and CAT scans are the safest and most accurate tests available. When the latter is performed, with or without contrast, most lesions >1 cm are detected. MRI scans are more sensitive and do not require contrast, but usually are more expensive. MRI scans will determine the lesion size, number, and location, as well as whether there is significant edema, hemorrhage, shift of midline structures, or ventricular dilatation.[77,83] Skull films may be helpful in the rare patient with increased intracranial pressure due to a skull metastasis that either occludes the sagittal sinus or produces focal neurologic signs because of extrinsic compression of the underlying brain. Angiograms may be necessary to determine the tumor's blood supply if surgery is planned.[77,83]

Intraoperative fine needle aspiration biopsy (FNAB) of the brain performed through either a burr hole or a craniotomy is useful in determining the type of neoplasm. Stained smears can be evaluated immediately to assess the adequacy of the specimen and, in most cases, provide a rapid preliminary diagnosis. The cytologic preparation demonstrates superior cellular detail, without the artifactual distortion seen on frozen section preparations. FNAB uses only a small amount of tissue, saving residual tissue for permanent section. Special studies including electron microscopy and immunohistochemistry may be particularly valuable in patients with deep-seated lesions in whom biopsy would cause severe neurologic complications.[85]

In patients with seizures, laboratory studies should be performed for serum glucose, BUN, electrolytes, calcium, magnesium, liver function, complete blood counts and differentials, cultures, arterial blood gases, and coagulation profiles. A CAT or MRI scan of the brain and lumbar puncture may also be done.

Therapy

When patients have signs of increased intracranial pressure or rapid neurologic deterioration, high-dose corticosteroids (dexamethasone 10 mg qid) and emergency radiotherapy are indicated. If intracranial pressure does not decrease promptly, mannitol is given as a 50-g intravenous bolus or a 20% infusion.

Patients presenting with acute deterioration from increased intracranial pressure and possible herniation should be managed acutely with the following measures:

- Maintain the airway; intubate comatose patients and lower the PCO_2 to 25 to 30 mm Hg.
- Administer mannitol in 25- to 100-g intravenous boluses using a 20% solution.
- Administer dexamethasone intravenously at a dose of 100 mg as soon as possible, followed by 25 mg qid.
- Perform emergency CAT or MRI scan.
- If feasible, perform surgical decompression.

Hyperventilation will produce cerebral vasoconstriction and decreased brain blood volume and intracranial pressure. Mannitol will reduce brain water content, brain volume, and intracranial pressure. Steroids will take a few hours to produce their desired effect.

If steroids, mannitol, and radiation fail to lower the intracranial pressure, an emergency neurosurgical procedure should be performed. A ventricular needle or Scott cannula may be inserted through a burr hole. Ventriculoperitoneal shunts are indicated if there is significant ventricular obstruction.[77]

Although steroids initially may benefit 60% to 75% of patients, without radiotherapy or surgical resection patients will rarely survive more than a few weeks. Table 35-4 lists the possible mechanisms by which steroids may reduce brain edema. Symptoms may improve within 4 hours following steroids or may improve gradually over several days. Dexamethasone is recommended because of its minimal salt-retaining properties.[82] If there are not signs of increased intracranial pressure, the initial daily regimen of dexamethasone is 16 mg in divided doses. If there is not clinical improvement, higher doses (up to 100 mg daily) may be required for several days.[77,82,83] Common practice has been to continue steroids during radiation therapy because of the fear of radiation-induced edema exacerbating symptoms or herniation.[82] After several days of irradiation, the steroid dose may have to be increased temporarily. Although steroids improve neurologic deficits more quickly, they do not improve the response rate to radiation or patient survival, unless there is significantly increased intracranial pressure.[77,83,84] Anticonvulsants are not prescribed unless there is a history of seizures or increased intracranial pressure. When phenytoin and corticosteroids are used concurrently, doses may have to be increased because of increased drug metabolism.[83]

Radiation therapy provides prompt palliation for most patients with brain metastases. The indications for surgical consultation are listed in Table 35-5. Surgical resection may be indicated if the diagnosis of brain metastasis is uncertain, particularly in patients without a history of malignant disease. Patients with a solitary brain metastasis but no other systemic metastasis may be candidates for surgery if resection would not produce neurologic defects. Emergency neurosurgical consultation is indicated for patients with increased intracranial pressure from cerebellar

Table 35-4. Possible Mechanisms by Which Corticosteroids Reduce Brain Edema

Decreased Edema Production
1. Decreased tumor capillary permeability
2. Anti-inflammatory effects by reducing oxygen free radical damage
3. Alteration of sodium and water transport across endothelial cells
4. Antitumor effects

Increased Edema Reabsorption
1. Decreased CSF production in choroid plexus
2. Improved pressure gradient for edema fluid to pass from extravascular space into CSF

Table 35-5. Possible Indications for Neurosurgical Intervention or Consultation for Brain Metastases

1. Uncertain diagnosis of brain metastases
2. Solitary metastasis with small chance of postoperative neurologic deficit
3. Increased intracranial pressure from cerebellar or temporal lobe lesion
4. Ventricular obstruction
5. Radioresistant tumors
6. Long interval between diagnosis of primary tumor and brain metastasis
7. Rapid neurologic deterioration despite osmotic therapy and radiation

or temporal lobe lesions or ventricular obstruction. There is debate over whether surgery or radiation is preferred for patients with (1) a solitary brain metastasis and a long interval between the initial primary malignancy and the brain metastasis; (2) slow-growing radioresistant tumors; or (3) rapid neurologic deterioration despite mannitol and steroids.[83,86] Mortality rates with surgical resection range from 10% to 30%. Patients with poor performance status, cardiopulmonary insufficiency, or increased intracranial pressure are at highest surgical risk. Prognostic factors that predict a long survival after surgery for solitary brain metastasis include minor preoperative neurologic deficits, a long interval between diagnosis of the primary neoplasm and the brain metastasis, total resection of the brain metastasis, and postoperative radiotherapy.[86]

Patients with brain metastases from metastatic melanoma appear to have improved survival after surgery. In one series the mean survival after radiation therapy was 14 weeks in 66 patients with brain metastasis. Survival was improved (median, 36 weeks) only in patients who underwent subtotal or total resection of a solitary brain metastasis prior to radiation therapy.[87]

Almost all patients with brain metastases receive cranial irradiation, and because most patients have multiple metastases at autopsy, the whole brain is irradiated.[77,83,88] Most patients receive 30 Gy over 2 weeks or 40 Gy over 3 weeks.[77,84] More than 69% of patients show improvement in neurologic deficits. Neurologic signs resolve entirely in 32% to 66% of patients after radiotherapy. However, 30% to 50% die from recurrent brain metastases. Although patients may benefit from additional brain radiation, they must be warned of the risk of brain necrosis.[77,82,86]

In ambulatory patients with brain metastases as the only site of disease, a higher total dose of 4,500 to 5,000 cGy is recommended, with 1,500 to 2,000 cGy given as a boost to the localized metastatic sites in the brain. Retreatment is possible, particularly in patients responsive to previous radiation who had received <4,000 cGy over 3 to 4 weeks.

Carcinomatous Meningitis

Etiology and Clinical Presentation

Carcinomatous meningitis is increasing in frequency because of improved survival due to systemic antineoplastic therapies and increased awareness of this problem among oncologists. At autopsy, 4% of patients have leptomeningeal spread, most commonly associated with lymphoma, leukemia, cancers of the breast and lung, and melanoma.[81,83,89,90] Because most chemotherapeutic drugs fail to penetrate the blood-brain barrier, carcinomatous meningitis develops frequently in patients without signs of progressive systemic diseases outside the CNS.[91]

At autopsy, the brain and spinal cord may be covered by a sheet of malignant cells, or the spinal and cranial nerve roots may have multifocal metastases. The malignant cells tend to settle in the basal cisterns, where they interfere with CSF flow and absorption, leading to obstructive hydrocephalus.[89]

Carcinomatous meningitis should be suspected when neurologic signs indicate that more than one structural area of the nervous system is affected. Clinical symptoms depend on the extent of tumor involving the brain, cranial nerves, or spinal cord. Occasionally, neurologic symptoms may be subtle and exist for several weeks prior to diagnosis. Headache may be associated with nausea and vomiting, and mental status changes, lethargy, and decreased memory are frequent. The most common cranial nerve deficits cause diplopia, visual blurring, hearing loss, and facial numbness. More than 70% of patients have neurologic signs due to spinal cord or nerve root involvement; symptoms of spinal cord compression may be present.[81,83,89]

Diagnostic Evaluation

The diagnosis of carcinomatous meningitis is established by cytologic examination. At least 5 mL of CSF should be sent for cytology, although repeated lumbar punctures may be required to confirm the diagnosis. In retrospective series, malignant cells were seen in the first, second, and third CSF samples in 42% to 66%, 60% to 87%, and 68% to 96% of cases, respectively. With obstruction of normal CSF pathways, patients may have repeatedly negative lumbar CSF cytologies, while cytologies of cisternal or ventricular fluid are positive.[89,92,93] More than 50% of patients with carcinomatous meningitis have one or more of the following CSF abnormalities: opening pressure >160 mm of water, increased white cell count, a reactive lymphocytosis, elevated CSF protein, and decreased glucose.[89,93]

CT scans may reveal contrast enhancement in the meninges and periventricular area; hydrocephalus; or brain metastases, which are present in 20% of patients.[89] Emergency myelograms or MRI scans of the spine should be performed in patients with symptoms or signs of metastasis to the spinal cord or cauda equina.

If CSF cytologies are repeatedly negative and neoplastic meningitis is strongly suspected, CAT scan, myelography, CSF markers, or MRI may be useful. Brain scans may show hydrocephalus; contrast enhancement of the basal cisterns, cortical foci, or tentorium; obliteration of the basal cistern or cortical sulci; or multiple small cortical nodules. Irregular filling of the spinal arachnoid space due to thickening and nodularity of nerve roots may be seen on myelography. Gadolinium-enhanced MRI may be more sensitive than the above studies. Flow cytometry of CSF may identify a monoclonal lymphocytic infiltrate in leukemic or lymphomatous meningitis.

Therapy

Treatment for carcinomatous meningitis consists of intrathecal chemotherapy and radiation therapy to the areas of the neuroaxis responsible for the neurologic deficits. Without treatment, patients will die within 4 to 6 weeks. Therapeutic drug levels generally are not achieved in the CSF with parenteral chemotherapy. Intraventricular chemotherapy via an Ommaya reservoir is preferable to lumbar injections, which may distribute drug only to epidural or subdural spaces. Even when the drug reaches the subarachnoid space, therapeutic levels are rarely reached in the ventricles. Intraventricular injections via the Ommaya are less painful than lumbar punctures and allow drug concentrations to follow the normal pathways for CSF flow.[90,93] Compared with retrospective series in which drugs were given by lumbar puncture, it appears that with intraventricular therapy and radiation therapy, responses are higher and longer in duration. In Wasserstrom's series,[89] more than 60% of patients with leptomeningeal metastases from breast cancer, 100% with lymphoma, 50% with lung cancer, and 40% with melanoma improved or stabilized with therapy; median survival was 5.8 months (range, 1 to 29 months).

Ommaya reservoirs can be placed with <2% morbidity and no mortality. If intracranial pressure is increased, an Ommaya reservoir can be placed and connected to a ventricular peritoneal shunt. The shunt has an on-off valve that allows it to be closed off for about 4 hours after intraventricular drug administration.[89]

The most frequently used intrathecal drugs are methotrexate, thiotepa, and cytosine arabinoside; recommended doses are listed in Table 35-6. Leucovorin (10 mg every 6 hours for 6 doses) will reduce systemic side effects associated with methotrexate. Since methotrexate does not cross the blood-brain barrier, the antitumor efficacy in the CSF will be unaffected.

Table 35-6. Dosage Regimens for Treatment of Carcinomatous Meningitis

Drug	Lumbar Puncture Injection (mg)	Intraventricular Ommaya Injection (mg)
Methotrexate	12-15	10-12
Cytosine arabinoside	45	30-45
Thiotepa	15	10

Methotrexate and thiotepa are usually administered for solid tumors associated with carcinomatous meningitis. Cytosine arabinoside alone or with methotrexate is used in leukemic and lymphomatous meningitis. Intrathecal therapy is given twice a week until symptoms improve or stabilize and the cytology becomes negative. Intrathecal therapy may then be given weekly, and gradually spaced out to monthly injections if cytologic findings are persistently negative.[81,89]

Whole-brain and brain-stem radiation are beneficial in the presence of cerebral or cranial nerve abnormalities. When spinal cord or nerve root signs are present, myelograms or MRI scans of the spine are required to plan radiation portals. Radiation doses are usually 30 Gy over 2 weeks.

Lymphomatous and leukemic meningitis are more responsive to intrathecal therapy and may also respond to high-dose systemic methotrexate with leucovorin rescue. Because of the high incidence of leptomeningeal involvement, patients with acute lymphocytic leukemia, acute lymphoblastic lymphoma, and Burkitt's lymphoma receive prophylactic intrathecal chemotherapy via lumbar puncture and whole-brain irradiation after a complete remission.

Metabolic Emergencies

Hypercalcemia

The most frequent metabolic emergency in oncology is hypercalcemia, which develops when the rate of calcium mobilization from bone exceeds the renal threshold for calcium excretion. Neoplastic disease is the leading cause of hypercalcemia among inpatients.[94-96] The most common tumors associated with hypercalcemia are carcinomas of the breast and lung, hypernephroma, multiple myeloma, squamous cell carcinoma of the head and neck and esophagus, and thyroid cancer.[95] Parathyroid carcinoma is rare, associated with intractable hypercalcemia due to elevated parathyroid hormone (PTH) levels.

Although more than 80% of patients with hypercalcemia have osseous metastases, the extent of bony disease does not correlate with the level of hypercalcemia.[95] During the course of their disease, about 40% to 50% of patients with breast carcinoma metastatic to the bone will develop hypercalcemia. While hypercalcemia generally suggests disease progression, these patients develop hypercalcemia associated with hormonal therapy. Estrogen and antiestrogens stimulate breast cancer cells to produce osteolytic prostaglandins and to increase bone resorption.[97] Within several days of initiating hormonal therapy for metastatic breast cancer, the calcium level may rise and the bone pain increase. This tumor flare in response to hormonal therapy usually predicts an excellent antitumor response. However, the hormonal therapy must be temporarily withdrawn and the hypercalcemia corrected before the drug is reinstituted.

In the majority of patients with bone metastases, direct neoplastic bone resorption is not felt to be the cause of hypercalcemia. It is now known that malignant cells in the bone produce various growth factors that activate osteoclast precursors to destroy surrounding bone. Many of these growth factors and cytokines will also inhibit osteoblast activity to allow the tumor to grow into the space destroyed by the osteoclast. Twenty percent of solid tumors associated with hypercalcemia have no evidence of osseous spread. In these cases, investigators have found humoral substances secreted by tumor cells, such as parathyroid-related peptide and osteolytic cytokines and growth factors. In multiple myeloma, hypercalcemia occurs because of production of osteoclast activating factors (cytokines including interleukin I, lymphotoxin) by the abnormal plasma cells, rather than from a direct neoplastic bone effect.

These factors stimulate osteoclast activity and proliferation and often inhibit new-bone formation. Although osseous metastases are frequently surrounded by a zone of osteoclasts, it is now clear that hypercalcemia results from release of osteolytic substances from the malignant cells.

Patients with squamous cell carcinoma of the head and neck, lung, and esophagus may develop a clinical syndrome suggestive of hyperparathyroidism due to ectopic secretion of a parathyroid-related peptide. In association with hypercalcemia, patients develop hypophosphatemia, increased urinary cyclic adenosine monophosphate (AMP) activity, and elevations in bone alkaline phosphatase.[95] Although it is clear that parathyroid carcinoma cells produce excessive PTH, recent data suggest that ectopic PTH production in other tumor types is really due to a structurally similar parathyroid hormone related peptide. Except in parathyroid carcinoma, extractable PTH is not found in neoplastic tissue. Most cases of hypercalcemia which were presumed to be secondary to ectopic PTH production are now felt to be due to ectopic secretion of PTH-like substances that bind to PTH receptors. In contrast to hypercalcemia due to hyperparathyroidism, these patients have impaired production of 1,25-dihydroxy vitamin D, decreased new-bone formation, and no evidence of renal bicarbonate wasting.[97]

Osteoclast activating factors cause bone reabsorption and secondary hypercalcemia in multiple myeloma and lymphoma.[98,99] However, despite the potent in vitro osteolytic activity of these cytokines, patients with elevated levels do not always develop hypercalcemia unless there is renal dysfunction.[97] Patients with lymphoma due to the human T-cell lymphotrophic virus (HTLV) present with severe hypercalcemia due to ectopic production of several osteotrophic factors (osteoclast activating factor, colony-stimulating factor, gamma interferon, and an active vitamin D metabolite).[97]

Clinical Presentation and Diagnostic Evaluation

Hypercalcemia is rarely a presenting sign of malignancy, except in patients with parathyroid carcinoma, HTLV-1 T-cell lymphomas, or multiple myeloma. Most hypercalcemic patients present with nonspecific symptoms of fatigue, anorexia, nausea, polyuria, polydipsia, and constipation. Neurologic symptoms of hypercalcemia begin with vague muscle weakness, lethargy, apathy, and hyporeflexia. Without treatment, symptoms progress to profound alterations in mental status, psychotic behavior, seizures, coma, and ultimately death. Patients with prolonged hypercalcemia eventually develop permanent renal tubular abnormalities with renal tubular acidosis, glucosuria, aminoaciduria, and hyperphosphaturia.[96] Sudden death from cardiac arrhythmias may occur when the serum calcium rises acutely.[95,98] Except for those with parathyroid cancer, hypercalcemic cancer patients rarely survive to develop signs of chronic hypercalcemia.

All hypercalcemic patients should have serial measurements of serum calcium, phosphate, alkaline phosphatase, electrolytes, BUN, and creatinine.

Elevated immunoreactive PTH levels in association with hypophosphatemia may suggest ectopic hormone production. In malnourished patients with low albumin levels, the ionized calcium value may help to determine therapy, since symptoms of hypercalcemia correlate with elevation in ionized but not protein-bound calcium. Patients with multiple myeloma may have elevated serum calcium levels secondary to abnormal calcium binding to paraproteins without an elevation in ionized calcium, while malnourished patients with hypoalbuminemia may have symptoms of hypercalcemia with normal serum calcium levels. The ECG often reveals shortening of the QT interval, widening of the T wave, bradycardia, and PR prolongation.[95]

Therapy

The cause of hypercalcemia, severity of associated clinical signs, and chances of response to antitumor treatment must be considered in selecting the most appropriate therapy. Mild hypercalcemia is frequently corrected with intravenous hydration alone. If effective antitumor therapy is available, the serum calcium level will gradually decline as the tumor regresses. However, most hypercalcemic cancer patients require additional hypocalcemic therapy until an antitumor response is achieved. Calcium balance can be corrected by directly decreasing bone reabsorption, promoting urinary calcium excretion, and decreasing oral calcium intake. Patients should be mobilized to avoid osteolysis. Constipation should be corrected, and medications such as thiazide diuretics and vitamins A and D that may elevate calcium levels should never be used.[95]

All hypercalcemic patients are dehydrated because of polyuria from renal tubular dysfunction. Intravenous hydration with normal saline will increase urinary calcium excretion, since the urinary clearance rates for calcium parallel sodium excretion.[95] When hypercalcemia is life threatening, aggressive hydration (eg, 250 to 300 mL/h) and intravenous furosemide should be administered to decrease reabsorption of calcium.[95]

Corticosteroids, which block bone reabsorption due to certain cytokines, have been effective hypocalcemic agents in multiple myeloma, lymphoma, breast cancer, and leukemia. High-dose steroids also may have hypocalcemic effects by increasing urinary calcium excretion, inhibiting vitamin D metabolism, and decreasing calcium absorption; long-term steroid use produces a negative calcium balance in bone.[95,97] High doses of corticosteroids are generally required for several days before an effective hypocalcemic response is seen. Most patients require prednisone 40 to 100 mg daily.[95]

Most hypercalcemic patients are treated with the diphosphonates etidronate and pamidronate. Pamidronate can be given at a dose of 60 to 90 mg either over 2 to 4 hours or as a 24-hour infusion. Responses are seen within 24 to 48 hours. Pamidronate 90 mg has the longest duration of activity. Gallium nitrate also has been used, but requires five daily doses and has a potential for renal toxicity. Diphosphonates inhibit osteoclast activity; pamidronate has less effect on osteoblasts, while etidronate can also inhibit new-bone formation. Mithramycin is rarely used now that diphosphonates are available. Mithramycin is a chemotherapeutic agent that decreases bone reabsorption by reducing osteoclast number and activity.[99] Mithramycin is a sclerosing agent and must be given as a bolus through a freshly started intravenous line. Low doses will control hypercalcemia, but repeated use may lead to side effects such as thrombocytopenia, coagulopathy, hypertension, liver function abnormalities, and nephrotoxicity.[95,96,99,100]

When hypercalcemia occurs following hormonal therapy for metastatic breast cancer, patients should be treated with hydration, steroids, and if necessary mithramycin. If the hypercalcemia is severe, hormonal therapy should be discontinued immediately. Once the calcium level normalizes, the hormone can be restarted at lower doses and gradually increased. When the hypercalcemia is mild, hormone therapy frequently can be continued without undue risk while the patient is managed with hydration.[95]

Calcitonin promptly inhibits bone reabsorption, causing a fall in serum calcium within hours of administration.[95,101] Although there is a prompt hypocalcemic response, tachyphylaxis develops unless glucocorticoid therapy is given concomitantly. For some reason, a secondary response will occasionally occur within 48 hours of reinstitution of calcitonin after the latter had been discontinued due to a rise in serum calcium. Calcitonin is given in daily intravenous doses (3 to 6 Medical Research Council [MCR] units/kg), or twice-daily intramuscular or subcutaneous injections (100 to 400 MRC units/kg).[95,102] Calcitonin is rarely employed except in emergency situations requiring rapid decreases in calcium.

Most patients are effectively managed with hydration, mobilization, effective antitumor therapy, and diphosphonates. If effective antitumor therapy is not available, patients must be maintained on hypocalcemic therapy indefinitely and serum calcium should be monitored at least twice a week.

Uric Acid Nephropathy

Uric acid nephropathy is usually associated with malignancies that have an increased rate of cell turnover. While this condition can be spontaneous, it most frequently is reported as a complication of cytotoxic therapy that produces a rapid antitumor response. With rapid cell death, increased uric acid production results in hyperuricemia and uric acid crystal deposition in the urinary tract.[55,57] Hyperuricemia and associated renal uric acid deposition occur most commonly with the tumor lysis syndrome, which is often associated with Burkitt's lymphoma. Most episodes of uric acid nephropathy are associated with effective cytotoxic chemotherapy or radiation therapy, but spontaneous hyperuricemic nephropathy has been reported occasionally in patients with lymphoma and leukemia.[57] Untreated leukemic patients have increased uric acid excretion. The degree and incidence of hyperuricemia correlates with the cytologic type of leukemia, rather than the degree of white count elevation. For example, uric acid excretion is typically higher in "aleukemic" acute myelocytic leukemia than in chronic lymphocytic leukemia.[55,95]

Uric acid stones are seen in fewer than 10% of patients in recent series and occur most often in patients with chronic hyperuricemia, such as those with chronic myeloproliferative syndromes.[57,95]

The incidence and severity of hyperuricemic nephropathy have decreased with prophylactic treatment with allopurinol, vigorous hydration, and alkalinization of the urine. In earlier studies, mortality rates ranged from 47% to 100%. However, with current aggressive medical therapy, most patients regain normal renal function within a few days of treatment, after the serum uric acid level falls below 10 mg/dL.[57]

Clinical Presentation and Diagnostic Evaluation

Patients rarely develop ureteral obstruction, so flank pain and gross hematuria are uncommon.[57] The most common presentation is signs of uremia, including nausea, vomiting, lethargy, and oliguria. Early treatment affords an excellent chance of rapidly reversing renal dysfunction.[57,95] It is often difficult to differentiate acute uric acid nephropathy from other causes of renal failure with secondary hyperuricemia. In acute uric acid nephropathy, the mean serum uric acid level at presentation is 20.1 mg/dL (range 9.2 to 92 mg/dL).[57,95]

If flank pain or gross hematuria occurs, a renal ultrasound should be performed to exclude ureteral obstruction. Hyperuricemia increases the incidence of dye-induced renal dysfunction, so intravenous contrast should be avoided. In the tumor lysis syndrome, hyperphosphatemia and hypocalcemia often occur out of proportion to the degree of renal insufficiency.[57] Serial blood studies for electrolytes, BUN, creatinine, calcium, phosphorus, and uric acid should be obtained. Urinalysis will be helpful if uric acid crystals are seen, but their absence does not exclude the diagnosis since crystalluria and hematuria occur only in the acute phase.[57] Kelton has demonstrated that a ratio of urinary uric acid to creatinine of >1 is relatively specific for hyperuricemic nephropathy.[95]

Therapy

The primary goal of therapy should be prevention of hyperuricemia. Patients at high risk should be treated with allopurinol, vigorous hydration, and urinary alkalinization for at least 48 hours prior to cytotoxic therapy. Drugs that block tubular reabsorption of uric acid (such as aspirin, probenecid, and thiazide diuretics) as well as radiographic contrast should be avoided. Prior to chemotherapy, the serum uric acid level should be normal, the urine pH >7, and intravenous hydration given to ensure a urine volume of >3 L/day.[55,57,95] To alkalinize the urine, intravenous sodium bicarbonate, 100 mEq/m^2, should be given daily. When the urinary pH is >7.5, uric acid solubility is maximal and it is unnecessary to produce significant metabolic alkalosis, which may complicate the clinical situation.[57,103] Serum potassium and magnesium levels should be monitored closely and allopurinol administered in doses ranging from 300 to 800 mg/day to decrease uric production by competitively inhibiting xanthine oxidase.[55,57,103] Although high xanthine levels might precipitate xanthine stones, this has not been reported in patients treated for hyperuricemic nephropathy.[95] Prophylactic colchicine is not required when allopurinol is administered, because patients rarely develop acute gouty arthritis.

If oliguria or anuria develops, ureteral obstruction must be excluded by renal ultrasound or antegrade or retrograde pyelography; nephrotoxic contrast must be avoided. Once ureteral obstruction is excluded, mannitol or high-dose furosemide should be given in an attempt to restore urine flow. A Foley catheter should be inserted to measure urine output accurately. If diuresis does not occur promptly within a few hours, emergency hemodialysis is necessary to reverse uric acid obstruction of the renal tubules.[57]

A hollow-fiber kidney apparatus will decrease serum uric acid levels more rapidly than peritoneal or coil hemodialysis.[55,95] With hemodialysis, all patients in Kjellstrand's series had rapid normalization of renal function and a prompt diuresis when the serum uric acid level decreased below 10 to 20 mg/dL. Within 6 hours of hemodialysis, uric acid levels generally fall by 50%. Most patients will require 6 days of dialysis before hyperuricemia resolves and renal function returns to normal values.[57]

In patients undergoing dialysis, a low calcium dialysate should be used to prevent calcium phosphate precipitation, which theoretically would increase nephrotoxicity. Aluminum hydroxide antacids may help to decrease GI phosphate absorption.[57] If hemodialysis cannot be done, uric acid clearance can be improved by adding albumin to the peritoneal dialysis. Albumin will increase uric acid protein binding and removal. Alkalinizing the dialysate to a neutral pH with sodium bicarbonate will also enhance uric acid clearance.[104] Fortunately, with aggressive measures for prevention and treatment, acute uric acid nephropathy is now associated with extremely low morbidity and mortality rates.[57,95]

Hyponatremia

Only 1% to 2% of patients with malignancy develop the syndrome of inappropriate antidiuretic hormone secretion (SIADH). Despite a low plasma osmolality, the urine is inappropriately concentrated with a high sodium level. This situation can also occur in renal disease, hypothyroidism, and adrenal insufficiency, which should be included in the differential diagnosis of SIADH.[105-107] Most patients are asymptomatic unless the serum sodium concentration falls abruptly.[95]

Ectopic antidiuretic hormone (ADH) secretion has been confirmed only in patients with bronchogenic carcinoma. Small-cell anaplastic carcinoma of the lung is the most common malignancy associated with SIADH.[95] At presentation, more than 50% of patients with small-cell lung cancer may develop hyponatremia following a water load, but fewer than 15% of patients develop clinically significant hyponatremia.[95,108] Case reports of SIADH have also been published involving patients with cancers of the prostate, adrenal cortex, esophagus, pancreas, colon, head and neck; carcinoid; thymoma; lymphoma; and mesothelioma.[95,107]

Since ectopic ADH production is rarely seen except in patients with small-cell carcinoma, SIADH is more frequently associated with pulmonary or CNS metastases. Inappropriate ADH secretion can also occur with medications such as morphine, vincristine, and cyclophosphamide.[105,106] With advanced malignancy, patients may also develop hyponatremia due to a "reset osmostat," in which mildly depressed serum sodium levels are corrected with effective antitumor therapy. Kern and associates reported SIADH secretion with pituitary prolactinomas,[109] which are not associated with detectable arginine vasopressin levels. In this setting, bromocriptine induces both tumor regression and correction of hyponatremia.

Adrenal insufficiency resulting from withdrawal of corticosteroids or metastases to the adrenal or pituitary glands may cause mild hyponatremia. In severe liver disease, heart failure, or acute renal insufficiency, patients may develop dilutional hyponatremia.[105,106] Vomiting diarrhea, ascites, or diuretics may precipitate hyponatremia.[14] Patients with plasma cell dyscrasias may have artifactual hyponatremia. Electrolytes should be followed when patients are treated with high-dose cisplatin with mannitol diuresis.[95,110]

Pathophysiology

With increased ADH secretion, excessive water is reabsorbed in the collecting ducts. This leads to increased distal sodium delivery by producing a mild increase in intravascular volume. Volume expansion also increases renal perfusion, decreases proximal tubular reabsorption of sodium, and decreases aldosterone effect.[110] Ectopic ADH secretion has been measured in patients with small-cell lung carcinoma.[111] In other conditions associated with increased ADH secretion, there is excessive production of ADH by the posterior pituitary.[95]

Dilutional hyponatremia occurs in volume-overloaded states secondary to cardiac, hepatic, or renal dysfunction. Although total body sodium and water content is increased, the circulating plasma volume is reduced. With impaired renal perfusion, there is greater reabsorption of water in the collecting duct and increased ADH secretion, resulting in a dilutional hyponatremic state.[105] With dehydration, total body salt and water content is generally decreased, leading to reduced renal perfusion and increased ADH secretion. Diuretics, interstitial renal disease, and mineralocortocoid deficiency are also associated with excessive renal sodium losses. Pseudohyponatremia is associated with elevated parathyroid levels in patients with plasma cell dyscrasias. Since the plasma sodium concentration is measured as the sodium concentration per unit of plasma, with elevated paraprotein levels, the percentage of water in plasma is decreased.[105] With mannitol infusion or hyperglycemia, an osmotic gradient increases water movement into the extravascular spaces, resulting in hyponatremia.[95]

Clinical Presentation

With mild hyponatremia, patients may complain of anorexia, nausea, myalgias, and subtle neurologic symptoms. When hyponatremia develops rapidly or sodium falls below 115 mg/dL, patients frequently have alterations in mental status ranging from lethargy to confusion and coma. Seizures and psychotic behavior have also been reported. With profound hyponatremia, alterations in mental status, pathologic reflexes, papilledema, and rarely focal neurologic signs may be found on physical examination.[106,107] The cause of hyponatremia must be determined before appropriate therapy can be initiated. If pseudohyponatremia due to hyperproteinemia, hyperlipidemia, or hyperglycemia is suspected, serum protein electrophoresis, lipids, and glucose levels should be checked. Medication records should be reviewed since chemotherapeutic agents (such as vincristine or cyclophosphamide), mannitol, morphine diuretics, and abrupt steroid withdrawal may contribute to hyponatremia.[95]

A careful history, physical examination, and review of patient's intake and output will help to determine whether the patient is volume expanded, dehydrated, or euvolemic. Serum and urine electrolytes, osmolality, and creatinine should be measured. With SIADH,

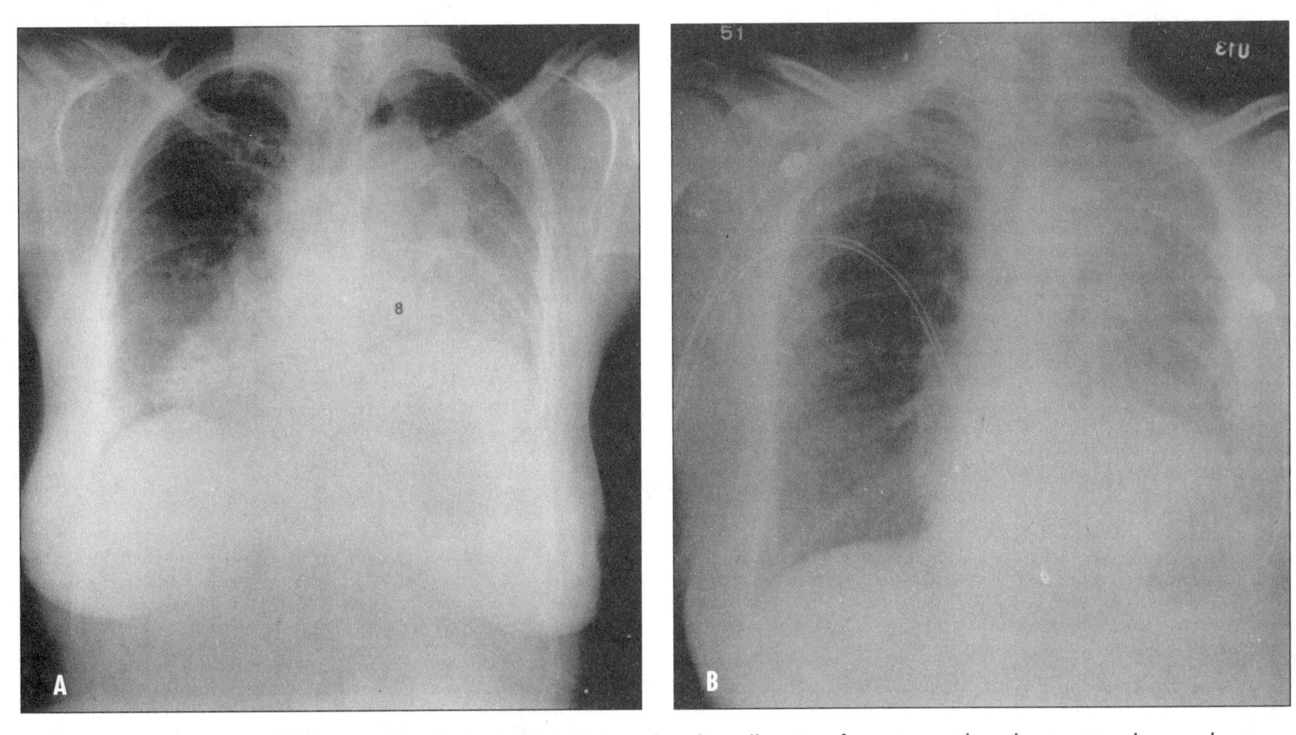

Fig 35-1. Treatment of pericardial tamponade. ***A*** shows the enlarged cardiac silhouette of a patient with cardiac tamponade secondary to metastatic lung carcinoma. In ***B***, a pericardial catheter is placed for draining of the effusion and institution of tetracycline. ***C*** *(below left)* shows a chest film obtained after sclerosis was complete and the catheter removed.

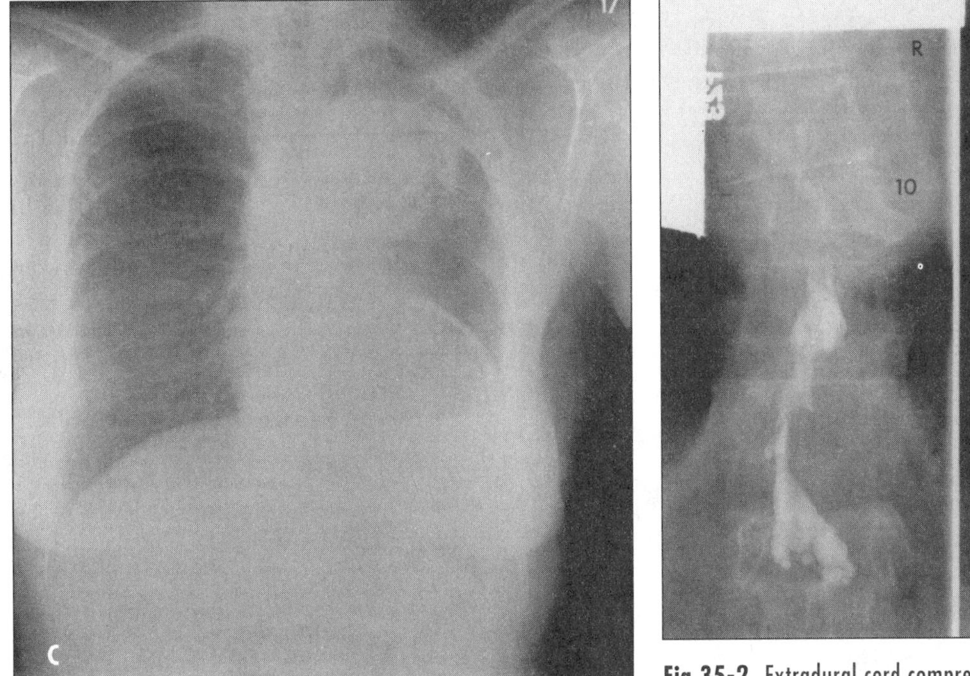

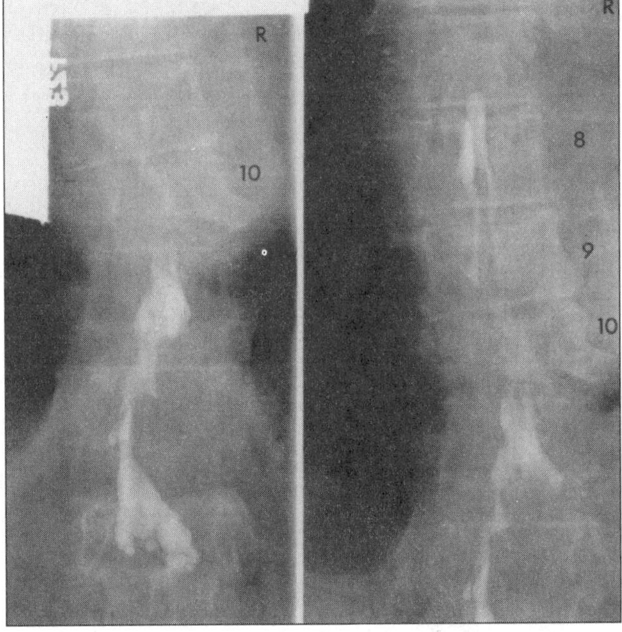

Fig 35-2. Extradural cord compression (complete block demonstrated) secondary to metastatic breast carcinoma.

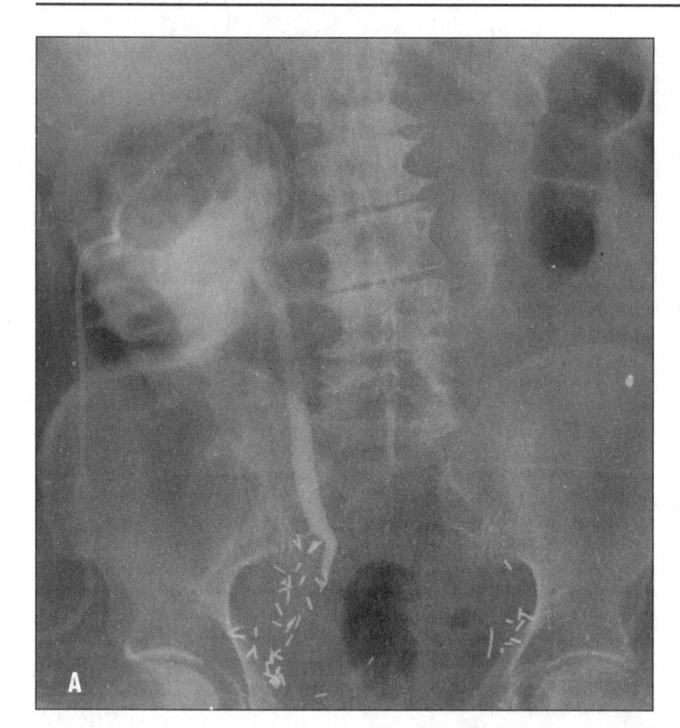

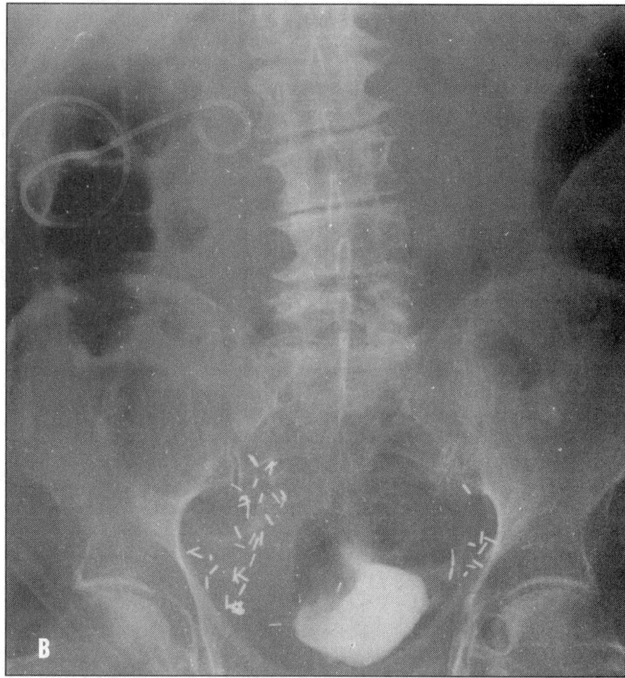

Fig 35-3. Ureteral obstruction secondary to locally advanced transitional cell carcinoma of the bladder. *A* shows a percutaneous catheter placed into the distended right renal pelvis and contrast injected; *B*, delayed film demonstrating the bladder tumor.

there is inappropriate sodium concentration in the urine for the level of hyponatremia. The urine osmolality is greater than plasma osmolality, but is never maximally dilute. With SIADH, BUN is usually low from volume expansion. Hypouricemia and hypophosphatemia may result from decreased proximal tubular reabsorption.[95,105,106] Thyroid and adrenal dysfunction should be ruled out if laboratory studies suggest SIADH. Chest x-ray and CT scans of the brain may reveal pulmonary or neurologic disorders associated with excessive ADH production.

Therapy

Ideally, treatment should correct the cause of hyponatremia. SIADH will resolve when the underlying cause of excessive ADH hormone production is removed. Following effective combination chemotherapy for small-cell lung cancer, serum sodium will rise to normal levels. Corticosteroids and radiotherapy may alleviate SIADH due to brain metastasis. In cases of induced SIADH, serum sodium will return to normal once the offending agent is discontinued.[95] If the cause of excessive ADH secretion cannot be corrected, initial therapy is water restriction. If free water intake is restricted to 500 to 1,000 cc per day, the negative free water balance will correct the hyponatremia within 7 to 10 days.[95,105-107] If water restriction is ineffective, demeclocycline may correct the hyponatremia by decreasing stimulus of ADH for free water reabsorption in the collecting ducts.[105,106,108,112] Demeclocycline produces a dose-dependent, reversible nephrogenic diabetes insipidus.[105,112,114]

Within 3 to 4 days of initiating treatment with demeclocycline, serum sodium increases, on average, from 121 to >130 mEq/L despite liberal fluid intake.[107] The only side effect of demeclocycline is reversible nephrotoxicity.[95,107] Renal dysfunction develops in fewer than half of patients and is generally mild. Most patients who experience nephrotoxicity are taking either higher doses of demeclocycline or other nephrotoxic drugs. Demeclocycline is excreted in the urine and bile; patients with renal or hepatic dysfunction should either avoid this drug or take lower doses.[95,107,112] The usual initial dose of demeclocycline is 600 mg/day.[115] If hyponatremia persists, doses may increase to 1,200 mg/day. Demeclocycline is administered in doses, divided two or three times a day.[95]

Patients with coma or seizures from SIADH should receive 3% hypertonic saline or isotonic saline with intravenous furosemide 1 mg/kg.[95] In volume-expanded patients, hyponatremia will resolve if the associated cardiac, renal, or liver dysfunction is corrected. Dehydrated hyponatremic patients are managed with intravenous isotonic saline solutions.[105,106]

Hypoglycemia

Fasting hypoglycemia occurs with insulinomas and, rarely, with other islet cell tumors of the pancreas. Hypoglycemia is also associated with large, bulky, slow-growing mesenchymal malignancies, including fibrosarcomas, mesotheliomas, and spindle-cell sarcomas.[95,116-118]

Normally, glucose homeostasis is maintained by appropriate hormonal regulation of gluconeogenesis and glycogenolysis in patients with adequate caloric intake.[95] Tumor-induced hypoglycemia may be caused by secretion of insulin or an insulinlike substance, increased glucose utilization by the tumor, or altered regulatory mechanisms. Although insulin levels are elevated in hypoglycemia from islet cell cancers, increased insulin secretion has not been observed with other neoplasms.[95,117] Increased levels of substances with insulinlike activity—referred to as nonsuppressible insulinlike activity (NSILA)—have been measured in serum samples from patients with hypoglycemia and nonislet cell malignancies. Only 5% to 10% of the insulinlike activity can be neutralized with anti-insulin antibodies. NSILA appear to be combinations of somatomedins A and C, high-molecular-weight glycoproteins, and low-molecular-weight growth factors, and have the growth-promoting and metabolic effects of insulin. However, the growth-promoting effects of the low molecular weight substances are 54% greater than insulin's effects, while their metabolic effects are only 1% to 2% as potent. The high molecular weight substances have minimal growth-promoting capabilities but maintain their metabolic effects.[95]

Elevated levels of low-molecular-weight NSILA have been demonstrated in patients with nonislet cell tumors, causing hypoglycemia by both radioreceptor and bioassay techniques. Elevated levels of these substances have been observed in patients with hemangiopericytomas, hepatomas, pheochromocytomas, adrenocortical carcinomas, and large mesenchymal tumors. Low to normal levels of NSILA have been measured in patients with hypoglycemia in association with leukemia, lymphoma, or gastrointestinal primary tumors.[95,117] The majority of hypoglycemic patients with fibrosarcomas will have elevated levels of high-molecular-weight NSILA.[95] When glucose levels decline rapidly in the normal patient, counterregulatory mechanisms should increase secretion of adrenocorticotropic hormone, glucocorticoids, growth hormone, and glucagon. However, in patients with tumor-induced hypoglycemia, the fall in glucose is usually not rapid enough to produce increased hormone levels.[117]

Cancer patients have reduced rates of hepatic gluconeogenesis-reduced glycogen breakdown following epinephrine or glucagon, and decreased hepatic glycogen stores.[95] These date suggest that impaired glucose homeostasis may contribute to tumor-induced hypoglycemia. In the past, increased glucose utilization by the tumor was thought to be a cause of hypoglycemia. However, increased glycogen breakdown and gluconeogenesis should compensate for increased glycolysis. Before assuming that the metabolic abnormality is caused by the malignancy, more common causes of hypoglycemia (ie, exogenous insulin use, oral diabetic agents, adrenal failure, pituitary insufficiency, ethanol abuse, or malnutrition) should be excluded.[95]

Most patients complain of excessive fatigue, weakness, dizziness, and confusion. Rarely are there symptoms suggestive of reactive hypoglycemia. Symptoms tend to occur after fasting in the early morning or late afternoon. If the blood sugar remains depressed below 40 mg/dL, seizures may result.

Fasting and late-afternoon glucose levels are helpful in making the diagnosis. Patients with insulinoma will have increased insulin levels with fasting glucose levels below 50 mg/dL, while patients with nonislet cell tumors will have normal to low insulin levels during periods of hypoglycemia.[95,117] Leukemic patients with high leukocyte counts may have artifactual hypoglycemia when blood remains in collection tubes for prolonged periods.[95]

Insulinomas have elevated ratios of proinsulin to insulin, with malignant tumors producing higher proinsulin levels. If technically feasible, insulinlike plasma factors should be measured by bioassay or radioreceptor technique.[95]

Hypoglycemia is corrected rapidly with intravenous injections of 50% dextrose, which should be followed by a continuous infusion of 10% dextrose. Insulinomas are frequently cured by surgery, while the rare patient with an inoperable insulinoma can be managed with chemotherapy or diazoxide.[95]

If effective antitumor therapy is available for nonislet cell tumors associated with hypoglycemia, the metabolic abnormalities should resolve with tumor regression. Following surgical resection of fibrosarcomas, hypoglycemia will resolve. Effective chemotherapeutic regimens for mesotheliomas have also corrected hypoglycemia.[117] To prevent nocturnal hypoglycemia, patients should be awakened from sleep for meals and have frequent between-meal and bedtime snacks. Occasionally, corticosteroids may provide temporary relief. Patients have also benefited from intermittent subcutaneous or long-acting intramuscular glucagon injections.[95]

Summary

As antitumor therapy becomes more effective and less toxic, it is imperative to recognize potentially life-threatening or permanently disabling complications that may be prevented or reversed by prompt action. Accurate diagnosis and treatment of oncologic emergencies can improve quality of life and prolong survival, allowing more patients to receive an adequate trail of definitive therapy designed to eradicate or effectively palliate their malignant disease.

References

1. Goudie RB. Secondary tumours of the heart and pericardium. *Br Heart J.* 1955;17:183-188.

2. Thurber DL, Edwards JE, Achor RWP. Secondary malignant tumors of the pericardium. *Circulation.* 1962;26:228-241.

3. Martini N, Bains MS, Beattie EJ Jr. Indications for pleurectomy in malignant effusion. *Cancer.* 1975;35:734-738.

4. Theologides A. Neoplastic cardiac tamponade. *Semin Oncol.* 1978;5:181-192.

5. Spodick DH. Acute cardiac tamponade: pathologic physiologic, diagnosis, and management. *Prog Cardiovasc Dis.* 1967;10:64-96.

6. Applefeld MM, Slawson RG, Hall-Craigs M, Green DC, Singleton RT, Wiernik PH. Delayed pericardial disease after radiotherapy. *Am J Cardio.* 1981;47:210-213.

7. Pories WJ, Gaudiani VA. Cardiac tamponade. *Surg Clin North Am.* 1975;55:573-589.

8. Hancock EW. Constrictive pericarditis: clinical clues to diagnosis. *JAMA.* 1975;232:176-177.

9. Martin N, Ruckdeschel JC, Chang P, Byhardt R, Bouchard RJ, Wiernik PH. Radiation-related pericarditis. *Am J Cardiol.* 1975;35:216-220.

10. Niarchos AP. Electrical alternans in cardiac tamponade. *Thorax.* 1975;30:228-233.

11. Lawrence LT, Cronin JR. Electrical alternans and pericardial tamponade. *Arch Intern Med.* 1963;112:415-418.

12. Morris AL. Echo evaluation of tamponade. *Circulation.* 1976;53:746-747.

13. Millman A, Meller J, Motro M, et al. Pericardial tumor or fibrosis mimicking pericardial effusion by echocardiography. *Ann Intern Med.* 1977;86:434-436.

14. Hudson REB. Diseases of the pericardium. In: Hurst JW, Logue RB, Schlant RC, Wenger NK, eds. *The Heart.* 4th ed. New York, NY: McGraw-Hill Information Services Co; 1978.

15. Krikorian JG, Hancock EW. Percardiocentesis. *Am J Med.* 1978;65:808-814.

16. Zipf RE Jr, Johnston WW. The role of cytolgy in the evaluation of pericardial effusions. *Chest.* 1972;62:593-596.

17. Hankins, JR, Satterfield JR, Aisner J, Wiernik PH, McLaughlin JS. Pericardial window for malignant pericardial effusion. *Ann Thorac Surg.* 1980;30:465-471.

18. Hill GJ II, Cohen BI. Pleural pericardial window for palliation of cardiac tamponade due to cancer. *Cancer.* 1970;26:81-93.

19. Lajos TZ, Black HE, Copper RG, Wanka J. Pericardial decompression. *Ann Thorac Surg.* 1975;19:47-53.

20. Davis S, Sharma SM, Blumberg ED, Kim CS. Intrapericardial tetracycline for the management of cardiac tamponade secondary to malignant pericardial effusion. *N Engl J Med.* 1978;299:1113-1114.

21. Rubinson RM, Bolooki H. Intrapleural tetracycline for control of malignant pleural effusion: a preliminary report. *South Med J.* 1972;65:847-849.

22. Van Belle SJP, Volckaert A, Taeymans Y, Spapen H, Block P. Treatment of malignant pericardial tamponade with sclerosis induced by instillation of bleomycin. *Int J Cardio.* 1987;16:155-160.

23. Buzaid AC, Garewal HS, Greenberg BR. Managing malignant pericardial effusions. *West J Med.* 1989;150:174-179.

24. Perez CA, Presant CA, Van Amburg AL III. Management of superior vena cava syndrome. *Semin Oncol.* 1978;5:123-134.

25. Shimm DS, Logue GL, Rigsby LC. Evaluating the superior vena cava syndrome. *JAMA.* 1981;245:951-953.

26. Ahmann FR. A reassessment of the clinical implications of the superior vena caval syndrome. *J Clin Oncol.* 1984;2:961-969.

27. Sculier JP, Feld R. Superior vena cava obstruction syndrome: recommendations for management. *Cancer Treat Rev.* 1985;12:209-218.

28. Davenport D, Ferree C, Blake D, Raben M. Radiation therapy in treatment of superior vena caval obstruction. *Cancer.* 1978;42:2600-2603.

29. Kane RC, Cohen MH, Broder LE, Bull MI. Superior vena caval obstruction due to small-cell anaplastic lung carcinoma: response to chemotherapy. *JAMA.* 1976;235:1717-1718.

30. Schraufnagel DE, Hill R, Leech JA, Pare JAP. Superior vana caval obstruction: is it a medical emergency? *Am J Med.* 1981;70:1169-1174.

31. Van Houtte P, Fruhling J. Radionuclide venography in the evaluation of superior vena caval syndrome. *Clin Nucl Med.* 1981;6:177-183.

32. Gollub S, Hirose T, Klauber J. Scintigraphic sequelae of superior vena cava obstruction. *Clin Nucl Med.* 1980;5:89-93.

33. Barek L, Lautin R, Ledor S, Ledor K, Franklin B. Role of CT in the assessment of superior vena cava obstruction. *J Comput Tomogr.* 1982;6:121-126.

34. Armstrong BA, Perez CA, Simpson JR, Hederman MA. Role of irradiation in the management of superior vena cava syndrome. *Int J Radiat Oncol Biol Phys.* 1987;13:531-539.

35. Kumar PP, Good RR. Need for invasive diagnostic procedures in the management of superior vena cava syndrome. *J Natl Med Assoc.* 1989;81:41-47.

36. Perez-Soler R, McLaughlin P, Velasquez WS, et al. Clinical features and results of management of superior vena cava syndrome secondary to lymphoma. *J Clin Oncol.* 1984;2:260-266.

37. Miller JB, Variakojis D, Bitran JD, et al. Diffuse histiocytic lymphoma with sclerosis: a clinicopathologic entity frequently causing superior vena caval obstruction. *Cancer.* 1981;47:748-756.

38. Salsali M, Cliffton EE. Superior vena caval obstruction with carcinoma of the lung. *Surg Gynecol Obstet.* 1965;121:783-788.

39. Ghosh BC, Cliffton EE. Malignant tumors with superior vena cava obstruction. *N Y State J Med.* 1973;73:283-289.

40. Rodriguez M, Dinapoli RP. Spinal cord compression with special reference to metastatic epidural tumors. *Mayo Clin Proc.* 1980;55:442-448.

41. Gilbert HA. Kagan AR, Nussbaum H, et al. Evaluation of radiation therapy for bone metastases: pain relief and quality of life. *Am J Roentgenol.* 1977;129:1095-1096.

42. Posner JB. Management of central nervous system metastases. *Semin Oncol.* 1977;4:81-91.

43. Bruckman JE, Bloomer WD. Management of spinal cord compression. *Semin Oncol.* 1978;5:135-140.

44. Rodichok LD, Harper GR, Ruckdeschel JC, et al. Early diagnosis of spinal epidural metastases. *Am J Med.* 1981;70:1181-1188.

45. Redmond J III, Friedl KE, Cornett P, Stone M, O'Rourke T, George CB. Clinical usefulness of an algorithm for the early diagnosis of spinal metastatic disease. *J Clin Oncol.* 1988;6:154-157.

46. Li KC, Poon PY. Sensitivity and specificity of MRI in detecting malignant spinal cord compression and in distinguishing malignant from benign compression fractures of vertebrae. *Magn Reson Imaging.* 1988;6:547-556.

47. Katz PB, Lee Y, Wallace S, and Ray RD. Myelography of spinal block from epidural tumor: a new approach. *Am J Radiol.* 1981;136:945-947.

48. Rubin P, Mayer E, Poulter C. Extradural spinal cord decompression by tumor. Part I: High daily dose experience without laminectomy. *Radiology.* 1969;93:1248-1260.

49. Wild WO, Parker RW. Metastatic epidural tumor of the spine: a study of 45 cases. *Arch Surg.* 1963;87:137-142.

50. White WA, Patterson RH Jr, Bergland RM. Role of surgery in the treatment of spinal cord compression by metastatic neoplasm. *Cancer.* 1971;27:558-561.

51. Findlay GFG. The role of vertebral body collapse in the management of malignant spinal cord compression. *J Neurol Neursurg Psychiatry.* 1987;50:151-154.

52. Sinoff CL, Blumsohn A. Spinal cord compression in myelomatosis: response to chemotherapy alone. *Eur J Cancer Clin Oncol.* 1989;25:197-200.

53. Greenberg HS, Kim JH, Posner JB. Epidural spinal cord compression from metastatic tumor: results from a new treatment protocol. *Ann Neurol.* 1980;8:361-366.

54. Michigan S, Catalona WJ. Ureteral obstruction from prostatic carcinoma: response to endocrine and radiation therapy. *J Urol.* 1977;118:733-738.

55. Garnick MB, Mayer RJ. Acute renal failure associated with neoplastic disease and its treatment. *Semin Oncol.* 1978;5:156-165.

56. Williams G, Peet TND. Bilateral ureteral obstruction due to malignant lymphoma. *Urology.* 1976;7:649-651.

57. Kjellstrand CM, Campbell DC II, von Hartitzsch B, Buselmeier TJ. Hyperuricemic acture renal failure. *Arch Intern Med.* 1974;133:349-359.

58. Herwig KR. Management of urinary incontinence and retention in the patient with advanced cancer. *JAMA.* 1980;244:2203-2204.

59. Gutmann FD, Boxer RJ. Pathophysiology and management of urinary tract obstruction. In Rieselbach RE, Garnick MB, eds. *Cancer and the Kidney.* Philadelphia, Pa: Lea & Febiger;1982:594-624.

60. Pillay VKG, Dunea G. Clinical aspects of obstructive uropathy. *Med Clin North Am.* 1971;55:1417-1427.

61. Russell JM, Resnick MI. Ultrasound in urology. *Urol Clin North Am.* 1979;6:445-468.

62. McClennan BL, Fair WF. CT scanning in urology. *Urol Clin North Am.* 1979;6:343-374.

63. Hepperlen TW, Mardis HK, Kammandel H. Self-retained internal ureteral stents: a new approach. *J Urol.* 1978;119:731-734.

64. Kraus PA, Lytton B, Weiss RM, Prosnitz LR. Radiation therapy for local palliative treatment of prostatic cancer. *J Urol.* 1972;108:612-614.

65. Megalli MR, Gursel EO, Demirag H, Veenema RJ, Guttman R. External radiography in ureteral obstruction secondary to locally invasive prostatic cancer. *Urology.* 1974;3:562-564.

66. Green N, Melbye RW, George FW III, Morrow J. Radiation therapy of inoperable localized prostatic carcinoma: an assessment of tumor response and complications. *J Urol.* 1974;111:662-664.

67. Kopelson G, Munzenrider JE, Kelley RM, Shipley WU. Radiation therapy for ureteral metastases from breast carcinoma. *Cancer.* 1981;47:1976-1979.

68. Sise JG, Crichlow RW. Obstruction due to malignant tumors. *Semin Oncol.* 1978;5:213-224.

69. Grillo HC. Obstructive lesions of the trachea. Ann *Otol Rhinol Laryngol.* 1973;82:770-777.

70. Miller WE. Roentgenographic manifestations of lung cancer. In: Straus MJ, ed. *Lung Cancer: Clinical Diagnosis and Treatment.* New York, NY: Grune & Stratton; 1977.

71. Brewer LA III. Patterns of survival in lung cancer. *Chest.* 1977;71:644-650.

72. Rosenblatt MB, Lisa JR, Trinidad S. Pitfalls in the clinical and histologic diagnosis of bronchogenic carcinoma. *Dis Chest.* 1966;40:297-404.

73. Braman SS, Whitcomb ME. Endobronchial metastasis. *Arch Intern Med.* 1975;135:543-547.

74. Baumgartner WA, Mark JBD. Metastatic malignancies from distant sites to the tracheobronchial tree. *J Thorac Cardiovasc Surg.* 1980;79:499-503.

75. Fitzgerald RH Jr. Endobronchial metastases. *South Med J.* 1977;70:440-441.

76. Weber AL, Grillo HC. Tracheal tumors: a radiological, clinical and pathological evaluation of 84 cases. *Radiol Clin North Am.* 1978;16:227-246.

77. Glover DJ, Glick JH. Metabolic oncologic emergencies. *CA Cancer J Physicians.* 1987;37:302-320.

78. Shapiro WR, Chernik NL, Posner JB. Necrotizing encephalopathy following intraventricular instillation of methotrexate. *Arch Neurol.* 1973;28:96-102.

79. Bunn PA Jr, Schein PS, Banks PM, DeVita VT Jr. Central nervous system complications in patients with diffuse histiocytic and undifferentiated lymphoma: leukemia revisited. *Blood.* 1976;47:3-10.

80. Nugent JL, Bunn PA Jr, Matthews MJ, et al. CNS metastases in small cell bronchogenic carcinoma: increasing frequency and changing pattern with lengthening survival. *Cancer.* 1979;44:1885-1893.

81. Yap HY, Yap BS, Tashima CK, DiStefano A, Blumenschein GR. Meningeal carcinomatosis in breast cancer. *Cancer.* 1978;42:283-286.

82. Weissman DE. Glucocorticoid treatment for brain metastases and epidural spinal cord compression: a review. *J Clin Oncol.* 1988;6:543-551.

83. Posner JB, Howeison J, Cvitkovic E. Disappearing spinal cord compression: oncologic effect of corticosteroids (and other chemotherapeutic agents) on epidural metastases. *Ann Neurol.* 1977;2:409-413.

84. Kramer S, Hendrickson F, Zelen M. Therapeutic trials in the management of metastatic brain tumors by different time/dose fractionation schemes of radiation therapy. *Nat Cancer Inst Monogr.* 1977;46:213-221.

85. Silverman JF. Cytopathology of fine-needle aspiration biopsy of the brain and spinal cord. *Diagn Cytopathol.* 1986;2:312-319.

86. Winston KR, Walsh JW, Fischer EG. Results of operative treatment of intracranial metastatic tumors. *Cancer.* 1980;45:2639-2645.

87. Rate WR, Solin LJ, Turrisi AT. Palliative radiation therapy for metastatic melanoma: brain metastasis, bone metastasis and spinal cord compression. *Int J Radiat Oncol Biol Phys.* 1988;15:859-864.

88. Shehata WM, Hendrickson FR, Hindo WA. Rapid fractionation technique and re-treatment of cerebral metastases by irradiation. *Cancer.* 1974;34:257-261.

89. Wasserstrom WR, Glass JP, Posner JB. Diagnosis and treatment of leptomeningeal metastases from solid tumors: experience with 90 patients. *Cancer.* 1982;49:759-772.

90. Bunn P, Rosen S, Aisner J, et al. Carcinomatous leptomeningitis in patients with small-cell lung cancer: a frequent, treatable complication. *Proc Am Assoc Cancer Res ASCO.* 1981;231:641 (abstr C-39).

91. Shapiro WR, Posner JB, Ushio Y, Chernik NL, Young DF. Treatment of meningeal neoplasms. *Cancer Treat Rep.* 1977;61:733-743.

92. Kirkwood JM, Bankole DO. Carcinomatous meningitis at Yale, 1970-1980. *Proc Am Assoc Cancer Res ASCO.* 1981;22:633.

93. Olson ME, Chernik NL, Posner JB. Infiltration of the leptomeninges by systemic cancer: a clinical and pathologic study. *Arch Neurol.* 1974;30:122-137.

94. Besarab A, Caro JF. Mechanisms of hypercalcemia in malignancy. *Cancer.* 1978;41:2276-2285.

95. Glover DJ, Glick JH. Oncologic emergencies and special complications. In: Calabresi P, Schein PS, Rosenberg SA, eds. *Medical Oncology: Basic Principles and Clinical Management of Cancer.* New York, NY:MacMillan Publishing Co;1985:1261-1326.

96. Mazzaferri EL, O'Dorisio TM, LoBuglio AF. Treatment of hypercalcemia associated with malignancy. *Semin Oncol.* 1978;5:141-153.

97. Mundy GR. Pathogenesis of ypercalcaemia of malignancy. *Clin Endocrinol* (Oxf). 1985;23:705-714.

98. Besarab A, Caro JF. Mechanisms of hypercalcemia in malignancy. *Cancer.* 1978;41:2276-2285.

99. Elias EG, Evans JT. Hypercalcemic crisis in neoplastic diseases: management of mithramycin. *Surgery.* 1972;71:615-635.

100. Perlia CP, Gubisch NJ, Wolter J, Edelberg D, Dederick MM, Taylor SG III. Mithramycin treatment of hypercalcemia. *Cancer.* 1970;25:389-394.

101. Binstock ML, Mundy GR. Effect of calcitonin and glucocorticoids in combination on the hypercalcemia of malignancy. *Ann Intern Med.* 1980;93:269-272.

102. Body JJ. Cancer hypercalcemia: recent advances in understanding and treatment. *Eur J Cancer Clin Oncol.* 1984;20:865-869.

103. Seyberth HW, Segra GV, Morgan JL, Sweetman BJ, Potts JT Jr, Oates JA. Prostaglandins as mediators of hypercalcemia associated with certain types of cancer. *N Engl J Med.* 1975;293:1278-1283.

104. Knochel JP, Mason AD. Effect of alkalinization on peritoneal diffusion of uric acid. *Am J Physiol.* 1966;210:1160-1164.

105. DeFronzo RA, Thier SO. Pathophysiologic approach to hyponatremia. *Arch Intern Med.* 1980;140:897-902.

106. Goldberg M. Hyponatremia. *Med Clin North Am.* 1981;65:251-269.

107. Trump DL. Serious hyponatremia in patients with cancer: management with demeclocycline. *Cancer.* 1981; 47:2908-2912.

108. Lockton JA, Thatcher N. A retrospective study of 32 patients with small-cell bronchogenic carcinoma and inappropriate secretion of antidiuretic hormone. *Clin Radiol.* 1986;37:47-50.

109. Kerne PA, Robbins RJ, Bichet D, Berl T, Verbalis JG. Syndrome of inappropriate antidiuresis in the absence of arginine vasopressin. *J Clin Endocrinol Metab.* 1986;62:148-152.

110. Brereton HD, Halushka PV, Alexander RW, Mason DM, Keiser HR, DeVita VT Jr. Indomethacin-responsive hypercalcemia in a patient with renal-cell adenocarcinoma. *N Engl J Med.* 1974;291:83-85.

111. Spencer HW, Yarger WE, Robinson RE. Alterations of renal function during dietary-induced hyperuricemia in the rat. *Kidney Int.* 1976;9:489-500.

112. Skrabanek P, Powell D. Ectopic insulin and Occam's razor: reappraisal of the riddle of tumour hypoglycaemia. *Clin Endocrinol* (Oxf). 1978;9:141-154.

113. Geheb M, Cox M. Renal effects of demeclocycline. *JAMA.* 1980;243:2519-2520.

114. Forrest JN Jr, Cox M, Hong C, Morrison G, Bia M, Singer I. Superiority of demeclocycline over lithium in the treatment of chronic syndrome of inappropriate secretion of antidiuretic hormone. *N Engl J Med.* 1978;298:173-177.

115. Koff SA, Thrall JH, Keyes JW Jr. Diuretic radionuclide urography: a non-invasive method for evaluating nephroureteral dilatation. *J Urol.* 1979;122:451-454.

116. Anderson N, Lokich JJ. Messenchymal tumors associated with hypoglycemia: case report and review of the literature. *Cancer.* 1979;44:785-790.

117. Kahn CR. The riddle of tumour hypoglycaemia revisited. *Clin Endocrinol Metab.* 1980;9:335-360.

118. Smitz S, Legros JJ, Franchimont P, Le Maire M. High molecular weight vasopression: detection of a large amount in the plasma of a patient. *Clin Endocrinol* (Oxf). 1985;23:379-384.

36

AIDS-RELATED CANCER

Tony W. Cheung, MD, FACP, Frederick P. Siegal, MD, FACP

In early 1981, cases of Kaposi's sarcoma (KS) and *Pneumocystis carinii* pneumonia (PCP) developing in previously healthy young men of homosexual or bisexual orientation were first reported.[1-3] The etiologic agent of this disease is a new retrovirus of the lentivirus group, human immunodeficiency virus type I (HIV-I, or simply HIV).[4-6] This syndrome, now known as acquired immunodeficiency syndrome (AIDS), results from a virally-induced, progressive depletion of cell-mediated immunity. The resulting immunologic deficiency predisposes the host to a variety of opportunistic infection and unusual neoplasms, especially KS and aggressive lymphomas.

In addition, in transforming T-cell tropic retrovirus distantly related to HIV, the human T-cell leukemia viruses type I (HTLV-I) and type II (HTLV-II) have now been shown to be causally linked to adult T-cell leukemia-lymphoma (ATLL)[7] and, possibly, to some cases of hairy-cell leukemia, respectively.[8] These retroviruses can also predispose to immune deficiency, but they are principally recognized to immortalize and transform some of the cells they infect, leading after a long incubation to characteristic lymphoid tumors.

The appearance of certain neoplasms among patients with AIDS resembles closely the previously observed association of neoplastic processes with other states of immunodeficiency (Table 36-1). The pattern of neoplasms is sufficiently stereotyped to provide information about the role of the immune system in the containment of neoplasms in general. These patients do not seem to develop the common tumors of the breast, lung, and colon in increased frequency; instead, they are plagued with a limited group of neoplastic diseases: a variety of monoclonal non-Hodgkin's lymphomas (NHL), polyclonal lymphoid tumors including some limited to the central nervous system (CNS), Hodgkin's disease (HD), Kaposi's sarcoma, and squamous carcinomas of the skin.[9,10] This peculiar disease spectrum appears to be associated with a viral role in tumor induction. In particular, human herpesviruses (including Epstein-Barr virus [EBV], herpes simplex, possibly human herpes virus type 6) and human papillomaviruses have been implicated. In the special case of common, variable immunodeficiency (acquired hypogammaglobulinemia) there is an additional unexplained increased incidence of colon and stomach cancers.

Kaposi's Sarcoma

In 1872 Moritz Kohn Kaposi, a Hungarian dermatologist, identified the sarcoma that bears his name as an "idiopathic multiple pigmented sarcoma of the

Table 36-1. Examples of Immune Deficiency Disorders With Increased Risk for Neoplasia

Primary Immunodeficiency States
- Congenital or genetically determined
  - severe, combined immune deficiency
  - X-linked agammaglobulinemia
- Acquired
  - common, variable immunodeficiency
  - syndrome of thymoma with immune deficiency
- Iatrogenic immunosuppression
  - organ transplant recipients

Secondary Immunodeficiency States
- Chronic lymphocytic leukemia

Adapted from Penn[9] and Spector et al.[10]

Tony W. Cheung, MD, FACP, Assistant Professor, Department of Medicine, Mount Sinai School of Medicine, New York, New York

Frederick P. Siegal, MD, FACP, Professor of Medicine, Albert Einstein College of Medicine, Bronx, New York and Head, Section of Hematology Research, Division of Hematology-Oncology, Long Island Jewish Medical Center, New Hyde Park, New York

skin."[11] From that time until the recent epidemic, classic KS remained a rare and unusual tumor often found in men with preexisting immune suppression (Table 36-2). Most cases were seen in elderly men of Italian or eastern European Jewish ancestry.

Epidemiology and Etiology

Kaposi's sarcoma has been widespread among both children and older people in sub-Saharan Africa. In children, the disease tends to involve lymph nodes and occurs at a male-to-female ratio of about 1:1; among African adults, the male-to-female ratio is about 11:1. In 1950, 43 cases of KS were reported from South Africa.[12] Since then, increasing numbers of KS have been reported in central Africa.[13]

Two distinct clinical forms have been identified. An indolent variety is characterized by cutaneous plaque and nodular lesions. This benign type is similar in

Table 36-2. Clinical Classification of Kaposi's Sarcoma

	AGE	RISK GROUPS	CHARACTERISTICS	COURSE
Classic	50-80	Older men of Jewish and Italian origin M:F = 12:1	Skin lesions confined to lower extremities: later can spread cutaneously and to visceral organs	Indolent: survival 10-15 years
African				
Nodular	25-40	Young black men Central Africa M:F = 13:1	Localized nodular lesions, rarely involving bone and lymph nodes	Indolent
Florid	25-40		Fungating exophytic skin lesion, often involving bone (38%), but rarely lymph nodes	Locally aggressive
Infiltrative	25-40		Diffuse skin infiltration always involving bone, but rarely lymph nodes	Locally aggressive
Lymphadenopathic	2-13	Children	Generalized lymphadenopathy (5%), rarely involving the skin	Rapidly progressive: survival 3 years
Immunosuppressive Therapy-Related		Renal transplant patient or patients with autoimmune disease on immunosuppressive therapy M:F = 3:1	May be localized to skin or widespread with systemic involvement	Can be indolent or rapidly progressive. Tumor may regress when immunosuppressive therapy is discontinued.
AIDS-KS	19-64	HIV-infected patients, primarily homosexual men; few Haitians; IV drug abusers	Commonly presents with generalized mucocutaneous lesions often involving lymph nodes and visceral organs.	Variable; without OI,* 80% survival at 2 years; <20% survival if associated with OI

*OI = opportunistic infection

behavior to the classic (western European) type in its clinical pattern and is associated with a long survival. A more aggressive form of KS has been observed in young black Africans. If not treated appropriately, this type of tumor can kill the patient within a year. The aggressive form is subdivided morphologically into florid, infiltrative, and generalized lymphadenopathic types. The most aggressive "florid" lesions grow into fungating and exophytic masses and often invade the subcutaneous and surrounding tissues, including the underlying bone. Both the localized (indolent) and aggressive forms occur mostly in young male adults between the ages of 25 and 40.

Kaposi's sarcoma has also been a known complication of iatrogenically induced or late-onset idiopathic (primary) immunodeficiencies associated with spindle-cell thymoma. Interestingly, it occurs in the same ethnic groups as does classic KS, but at an earlier age, and tends to regress as a result of reduction or cessation in immunosuppressive treatment.[14] Kaposi's sarcoma has also been reported to develop after the use of immunosuppressive agents in the treatment of various autoimmune disease, such as rheumatoid arthritis.

Histopathology and Pathogenesis

Kaposi's sarcoma is a vascular tumor arising from the mid-dermis. It consists of interweaving bands of spindle cells and irregular slit-like vascular channels embedded in reticular and collagen fibers, infiltrations with mononuclear cells, and plasma cells. There are extravasated erythrocytes along with erythrophagocytosis and hemosiderin deposition.

There are many controversies regarding the cellular origin of KS. Some phenotypic markers strongly suggest that KS arises from lymphatic endothelial cells[15]: positive for histochemical marker HLA-DR (Ia), 5'-nucleotidase, and lectin binding protein Ulex europaeus I; weakly positive for factor VIII-related antigen and monoclonal antibody EN-4.[16] However, further studies carried out chiefly by Folkman and coworkers indicated that the AIDS-KS cells also have specific markers of vascular smooth muscle cells (synthesis and expression of smooth muscle alpha-actin).[17] Taken together, these results suggest a possible vascular origin of these cells. Nevertheless, these spindle cells are not identical to vascular smooth muscle cells, but may represent an earlier precursor of undifferentiated smooth muscle cells. Therefore, AIDS-KS cells may originally derive from a pluripotent mesenchymal cell that then differentiates into a smooth muscle-like form.

Detailed studies of long-term culture of Kaposi's sarcoma-derived cell lines[16] demonstrate that these cells express a variety of potent biologic activities including 1) growth-promoting activities for KS spindle cells, normal endothelial cells, fibroblasts, and some other mesenchymal cell types; 2) neoangiogenic activity; 3) induction of a tumor histologically similar to KS, when the cells are inoculated subcutaneously into nude mice; 4) chemotactic and chemoinvasive activities for KS spindle cells, normal endothelial cells, and fibroblasts[18]; 5) interleukin-1 (IL-1) and granulocyte-macrophage colony stimulating factor (GM-CSF)-like activities. In addition, these cells express high levels of mRNA for IL-IB and basic fibroblast growth factor (bFGF).

Both bFGF and IL-1B have been demonstrated to exert significant effects on KS cells, mesenchymal cells, and immune cells.[19] Kaposi's sarcoma cells proliferate in response to the mitogenic effects of recombinant IL-1B, platelet-derived growth factor (PDGF) and transforming growth factor α and ß (TGF-α,ß), whereas smooth muscle cells respond to acidic and bFGF, IL-1 and PDGF.[19] These observations indicate that KS cells produce cytokines that could support both their own growth (autocrine) and the growth of other cells (paracrine), and that these cytokines may play a role in the pathogenesis of AIDS-associated KS.[20]

Recently, by inserting the *tat* gene into the genome of transgenic mice, skin lesions histologically similar to early KS developed in most male mice, and only their skin expressed the *tat* gene mRNA. The fact that KS-like lesions developed only in male mice is consistent with the general clinical prevalence of KS for males and implies a possible hormonal influence in the development of this tumor. Interestingly, *tat* gene mRNA was not found in tumor cells. This suggests that the *tat* gene product (*tat* protein), released by nearby or perhaps distant cells, is able to affect the growth of KS-like tumor.[21]

Epidemiologically, AIDS-associated KS occurs almost exclusively in homosexual men. Homosexual men with AIDS-associated KS, compared with a group of "healthy" homosexual controls, had a much higher rate of passive (receptive) anal intercourse associated with rectal deposition of the sexual partner's semen, as well as higher frequencies of traumatic sexual practices such as "fisting," which would allow entry of infectious agents and exposure to the partner's allo-antigens.[22] It is possible that this practice sets the stage in some way for the pathogenesis of KS.

A recently proposed hypothetical model for the pathogenesis of AIDS-associated KS (Fig 36-1) assimilates much of our current knowledge of this disease.[19]

Kaposi's Sarcoma Associated With AIDS

Epidemiology and Immunogenic Data

The form of KS associated with the AIDS outbreak is sometimes referred to as epidemic KS or AIDS/KS.

Approximately 96% of all cases of epidemic KS in the United States have been diagnosed in homosexual or bisexual men. The patients range in age from 19 to 64 years, with a mean age of 37.7.[23] Very rarely, KS occurs in people with AIDS who are not homosexual or bisexual males. Only about 3% of all reportedly heterosexual intravenous drug abusers with AIDS and about 9% of Haitian AIDS patients develop this form of KS.[23,24] The reason for this striking difference is still unclear. The observation of KS developing in some homosexual men who apparently are not HIV-infected could suggest that another transmissible agent, most common among homosexual males or selectively transmitted via anal intercourse, is involved in the induction of KS.

The majority of AIDS/KS patients are male. However, rare cases of females with AIDS/KS have been reported. Preliminary data showed that these patients may have a higher incidence of visceral involvement and more aggressive disease.[25,26]

Early expression of AIDS/KS has been linked to the major histocompatibility cell-surface antigen, HLA-Dr5, among patients seen in New York City.[27,28] A significantly higher percentage of companions of homosexual men studied early in the epidemic expressed this antigen than did a normal control population; Dr5 was about three-fold more frequent among the men with KS. Dr5 was found with progressively less frequency in successive cohorts of affected men as the epidemic progressed, until in the most recently studied cohorts, the presence of the antigen was found to be less common than in the general population. This observation suggests that genetic factors play an important role in clinical expression of KS. A number of other studies failed to find as significant an association with Dr5, but they may have begun later than did the New York investigations.

Clinical Expression

Kaposi's sarcoma usually presents on the skin as one or more painless red, purplish, or brown patches, plaques, or nodules (Table 36-2). Except for the African form, the classical KS lesions are localized mainly to one or both lower extremities. The classic disease commonly runs a relatively benign and indolent course for 10 or more years with slow enlarge-

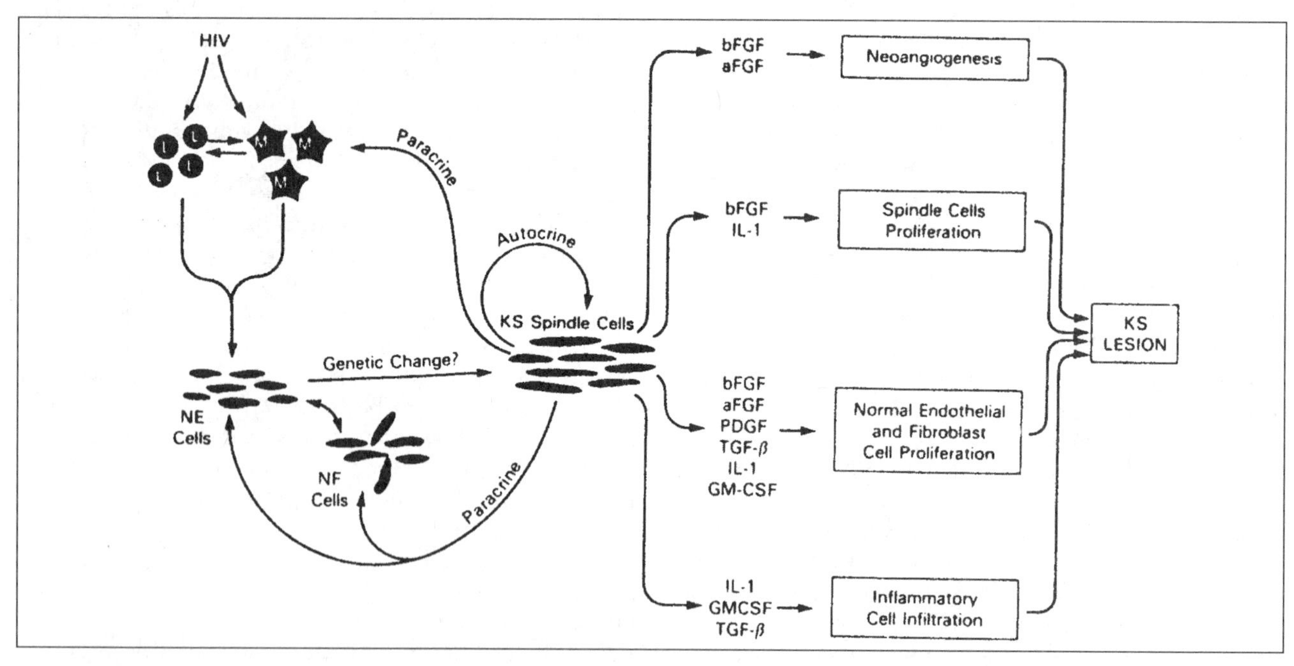

Fig 36-1. A model for the pathogenesis of Kaposi's sarcoma lesion in AIDS patients. NE = normal endothelial cells; NF = normal fibroblasts; L = lymphocytes; M = monocyte-macrophages. HIV-infected cells (L and M) release viral and/or cellular factor(s) capable of stimulating activation and proliferation of a particular cell type of mesenchymal origin. These cells (endothelial cells?) then acquire the peculiar spindle-shaped morphology characteristic of KS cells. The KS cells, in turn, begin to produce and release several cytokines that maintain and amplify the cellular response via autocrine and paracrine pathways. Paracrine activation of normal cells (NE, NF, L, and M) leads to fibroblast proliferation, neoangiogenesis, and inflammatory cell infiltration. These phenomena, together with the spindle cell proliferation, could underlie the typical histologic changes observed in early KS lesions. Later, interactions between cells of the immune system, NE, and NF could amplify cell activation and cytokine production. If the initial stimulus persists, a vicious cycle could be established which, under certain circumstances (eg, specific genetics changes), would lead to tumor transformation. From: Ensoli et al.[19]

ment and local spread of the original lesion, and gradual development of additional tumors and progressive edema, most likely related to obstruction of the normal lymphatic channels by tumor. Patients usually die from causes unrelated to KS. In contrast, the clinical manifestations and extent of dissemination seen in patients with underlying immune deficiency, including AIDS, tend to relate to the degree of immune compromise, the genetics of the host, and factors that are largely unknown.

The earliest presentation of AIDS/KS is often characterized by multifocal, widespread lesions. Sometimes multiple lesions appear suddenly over the body surface. The skin, oral mucosa, lymph nodes, and visceral organs such as the submucosa of the gastrointestinal (GI) tract, lung, liver, and spleen may be affected, sometimes in the absence of skin involvement. Because of its simultaneous development at multiple sites, the disease is generally not considered to be metastatic from a primary focus, but arises independently as a polyclonal disorder. No evidence for a clonal population of neoplastic cells has been reported in KS.

The sites of disease at presentation are much more varied in AIDS/KS than in classical KS. Widespread involvement is relatively common; the skin of the face, extremities, and torso are commonly affected, as are the mucous membranes of the oral cavity, especially the palate. Sixty-one percent of patients have generalized lymphadenopathy at the time of the first examination; in at least some of these, the adenopathy will reflect the reactive lymphadenopathy of early HIV infection (progressive, generalized lymphadenopathy—PGL), rather than nodal KS. In 45% of the patients in one study, KS lesions were found in one or more sites along the GI tract.

Systemic manifestations of AIDS may be present simultaneously, or even precede the appearance of the tumor lesions by several months. These manifestations include persistent or intermittent fever, weight loss, diarrhea, malaise, and fatigue[29] and usually develop in the context of severe cellular immune deficiency, probably reflecting the presence of unrecognized opportunistic infections.

Untreated, almost all patients with KS develop progressive disease. A few localized or isolated mucocutaneous lesions can progress to more numerous and generalized skin, lymph node, and GI tract involvement. The development of pleuropulmonary KS is an ominous sign, usually leading to death within a median of 2 months.[30]

The natural history of KS is highly variable and is closely linked to the degree of coexisting cellular immune deficiency. In one study, patients with epidemic KS who never developed an opportunistic infection had an actuarial survival of 80% at 28 months from diagnosis, as compared to less than 20% survival in those who had an opportunistic infection at some time during the course of their illness.[29] The occurrence of opportunistic infection indicates a coexistent severe immune deficit.

Leukopenia (including lymphopenia) and mild anemia are laboratory abnormalities found commonly in HIV infection. These abnormalities usually reflect the stage of the viral infection at which KS develops. Thrombocytopenia, presented as immune thrombocytopenic purpura (ITP), occurs sometimes as a further complication of the syndrome, but there is no evidence for a selective association of this complication of HIV infection with KS.[31]

Kaposi's sarcoma can develop in persons at risk at almost any stage of HIV infection. Even though KS in an HIV-seropositive person is definitive for AIDS by the surveillance definition of the Centers for Disease Control (CDC), certain individuals fitting this definition through biopsy of skin lesions can remain well—apparently for many years—evidently because the factors that open the door to KS expression do not invariably include clinically significant immune deficiency. There is, however, in AIDS/KS a significant relationship between the absolute numbers of circulating T-helper (CD4) lymphocytes and outcome, both with respect to the development of advancing KS and towards susceptibility to opportunistic infections. There is also a statistical correlation between the number of T-helper lymphocytes and the number of granulocytes and erythrocytes.[32,33] Hematocrit and the number of T-helper lymphocytes are useful independent prognostic factors in this disease (Table 36-3).[34]

Staging

Since KS is a multicentric neoplasm, a TNM classification does not apply. However, certain clinical features can identify different presentations and prognostic indicators of KS and the overall clinical course.

A recent multivariate analysis of nine variables

Table 36-3. Indicators of Poor Prognosis of AIDS-Related Kaposi's Sarcoma

- Visceral involvement
- Prior or coexistent opportunistic infection
- Systemic symptoms (fever, night sweats, weight loss ≥10% of baseline body weight, and unexplained diarrhea)
- Low number of circulating T-helper (CD4) lymphocytes (<250/mm³)
- Low T-helper to T-suppressor (CD4:CD8) ratio (<0.2)
- Low hematocrit[37]
- Presence of serum acid labile alpha-interferon[38]

in 212 patients showed three variables to be significant: a CD4 count below 300 cells/mm^3, "B" symptoms (unexplained fever, night sweats, more than 10% involuntary weight loss, or diarrhea persisting more than 2 weeks), and a history of opportunistic infection.[35] A staging system based on these three variables that identifies four distinct prognostic groups has been proposed (Table 36-4). Another staging classification, recommended by the AIDS Clinical Trials Group (ACTG), uses three parameters to divide patients into good- and poor-risk groups: extent of tumor, immune status, and presence of systemic illness (Table 36-5).[36] Prospective clinical trials will be useful to evaluate the benefits of these staging systems.

Table 36-4. Chachouas' Staging Classification of AIDS-Associated Kaposi's Sarcoma

Stage	Variable
I	No OI,* no B symptoms, CD4 >300
II	No OI, no B symptoms, CD4 <300
III	No OI, B symptoms
IV	OI

*OI = opportunistic infection

Modified from Chachoua.[35]

Therapy for AIDS-Related Kaposi's Sarcoma

Therapeutic interventions in most neoplasms are based on the extent of disease (Table 36-6). In AIDS/KS, this approach is often not practical or straightforward, as the more extensive disease is frequently associated with severe immunodeficiency or myelosuppression, both of which limit tolerance for therapy. Patients with only a few cutaneous KS lesions may simply be observed or treated on protocol with experimental agents, exploring the role of antiretroviral drugs or biologic response modifiers.

Radiation Therapy

Kaposi's sarcoma tumors are generally very radiosensitive. Excellent palliation can be obtained with doses not much higher than 20 Gy. Good cosmetic results can be obtained, especially in patients with lymphedema. However, an increased risk of toxicity, especially severe mucositis, has been noted.[39] The use of radiation with limited potential for tissue penetration (eg, electron beam, which affects tissues no deeper than 1.5 cm below the surface) appears to be a satisfactory and relatively nontoxic approach to dermal KS.[40]

Table 36-5. ACTG* Kaposi's Sarcoma Staging Classification

	Good Risk (0) (All of the Following)	Poor Risk (1) (Any of the Following)
Tumor **(T)**	Confined to skin and/or lymph nodes and/or minimal oral disease†	Tumor-associated edema or ulceration Extensive oral KS Gastrointestinal KS KS in other nonnodal viscera
Immune system **(I)**	CD4 cells $\geq 200/\mu L$	CD4 cells $<200/\mu L$
Systemic illness **(S)**	No history of OI‡ and/or thrush No B symptoms§ Performance status ≥70 (Karnofsky)	History of OI and/or thrush B symptoms present Performance status <70 Other HIV-related illness (eg, neurological disease, lymphoma)

*ACTG = AIDS Clinical Trial Group

†Minimal oral disease is nonnodular KS confined to the palate.

‡OI = opportunistic infection

§B symptoms are unexplained fever, night sweats, >10% involuntary weight loss, or diarrhea persisting more than 2 weeks.

From Krown et al.[36]

Biologic Response Modifiers

Among the biologic response modifiers, recombinant alpha-interferon (IFN-α) has been studied most extensively. Alpha-interferon has been evaluated either at low dose (1 million to 3 million units/m^2) or higher doses (20 million to 36 million units/m^2), given intramuscularly three times weekly.[35,36,41-43] The response rates vary from 13% to 42%, with major responses occurring most frequently in patients receiving higher doses and in those who have had better residual cellular immunity, limited disease and/or absence of other AIDS-related infectious complications.[41]

Clinical trials have demonstrated that features associated with poor response to interferon are a history of opportunistic infections, systemic B symptoms, and anemia. The most important laboratory parameter that predicts responsiveness is the number of CD4+ lymphocytes. Patients with CD4+ counts greater than 600 cells/mm^3 have response rates greater than 80%. Patients with CD4+ counts below 200 cells/mm^3 are unlikely to have a response.[45,46]

The combination of IFN-α and zidovudine has been shown to result in synergistic suppression of HIV replication in vitro, and studies have been conducted to evaluate this combination in AIDS/KS. In two early reports, the maximum tolerated dose combinations were 18 million units of IFN-α daily and 100 mg of zidovudine every 4 hours.[35,47] The dose-limiting toxic effects were anemia and neutropenia for zidovudine and hepatotoxicity for IFN-α. Tumor response rates were higher than expected given the relative low dose of IFN-α used, suggesting antitumor synergy.

Chemotherapy

In the classic and African forms of KS, vinblastine has been the most commonly used chemotherapeutic agent. A response rate as high as 95% has been reported.[48] In AIDS/KS, chemotherapy has presented major problems because of the patients' often severe neutropenia and advanced immune deficits; thus, regimens should be tailored to this special problem, using agents that are relatively marrow-sparing. Vinblastine used alone, or alternating with vincristine, produces objective responses in over one-quarter of patients.[44,49] Other active single agents include etoposide (VP-16), bleomycin, and methotrexate.[50] Adriamycin appears to be one of the most effective agents; it can be used in combination with less myelosuppressive agents such as bleomycin, vincristine, or vinblastine.

Tumor response rates over 80% were initially reported with multidrug regimens; for example, a combination of doxorubicin, bleomycin, vinblastine, and dacarbazine (ABVD) was used early in the out-

Table 36-6. Therapy Guidelines for AIDS/Kaposi's Sarcoma

Disease Characteristics	First Option	Second Option
Minimal Tumor Extent* and Slow Rate of Progression		
Favorable prognostic factors	Observation	Experimental immunomodulators and/or antiviral drugs; vinblastine/vincristine Local therapy with the above agents
Unfavorable factors†	Vinblastine, vincristine, or experimental immunomodulators and/or antiviral drugs; investigational drugs	Observation
Extensive Disease, Rapid Growth		
Favorable prognostic factors	VP-16, Adriamycin, vinca alkaloids	Immunomodulators
Unfavorable factors	VP-16, Adriamycin	Vinca alkaloids or experimental chemotherapy
Locally-Symptomatic Lesions		
Lymphedema or painful necrotic lesions	Radiation therapy	Excision, cryotherapy, electrodesiccation

*25 cutaneous lesions, no known visceral involvement

†See Table 36-3.

Adapted from Volberding.[54]

break.[2] Preliminary results showed that a protocol including vincristine, bleomycin, and doxorubicin achieved superior response rates and duration of response than doxorubicin alone.[51] Unfortunately, the majority of responses to chemotherapy (whether with a single agent or in a combination regimen yielding a high initial response rate) have been relatively short-lived, and long-term disease-free survival is rare.[52]

Regimens with significant myelosuppression should be used with greater caution, because the already increased risk of opportunistic infections in this patient population may be compounded by leukopenia. However, the recent use of hematopoietic growth factors such as G-CSF or GM-CSF concomitantly with chemotherapy may lead to further protection against opportunistic infections and prolonged survival. In clinical practice, chemotherapy should probably be reserved for patients with extensive, visceral, edema-producing or rapidly progressive disease (Table 36-6). Under other conditions, the role of chemotherapy is undefined and patients should be encouraged to participate in ongoing clinical trials or be observed until disease progresses.

Local Treatment

The local treatment of AIDS/KS is important for the control of pain, edema, improvement of function, and the improvement of cosmetic appearance. Various modalities, such as excision, electrodesiccation, currettage, and local radiation therapy, have been found to be relatively safe and effective. Cryotherapy is also commonly used, although there is often residual brown pigmentation and, in darker skinned individuals, cosmetically unacceptable hypo- and hyperpigmentation. Local treatment with low dose vinblastine has resulted in a complete response in 13% and a partial response in 78%.[53] The side-effects are mainly local pain (100%) and skin irritation (90%).

Malignant Lymphoma Associated with AIDS

Epidemiology

In June 1985, the surveillance-definition criteria of AIDS were expanded to include individuals who have high-grade B-cell lymphomas with positive serologic or virologic evidence of infection with HIV.[55] Prior to that time, epidemiologic data had suggested that there was a statistical increase in the incidence of non-Hodgkin's lymphoma (NHL) among intravenous drug abusers[56,57] and among "never-married men."[58] Although the overall incidence of lymphoma was inordinately high in this population group, the most significant increase was in the category of high-grade B-cell disease (Burkitt's lymphoma and immunoblastic sarcoma).

AIDS-related lymphomas have now been reported in all populations at risk for HIV infection, including intravenous drug abusers and hemophiliacs; however, most cases reported to date have occurred in homosexual men.[59] The clinical or pathologic aspects of this disease or their response to therapy and survival among the AIDS risk groups are quite similar.[60,61]

Analyses of recent epidemiologic trends suggest that patients with HIV infection are experiencing somewhat improved survival and a later development of AIDS as a result of advances in antiretroviral and antimicrobial prophylactic therapies.[62,63] Recently, Pluda and colleagues examined the incidence of AIDS/NHL in a cohort of 55 patients who had received zidovudine as antiretroviral therapy for an extended period. Based on this population, he estimated by the Kaplan-Meier method the probability of developing lymphoma to be 28.6% within 30 months of initiating antiretroviral therapy and 46.4% within 36 months of beginning such therapy.[64] This study implied that the longer survival with severe immunodeficiency afforded by antiretroviral agents may lead to an increase in the incidence of lymphoma in patients with HIV infection.

In a similar way, the NCI Multicenter Hemophilia Cohort Study has also shown an exponential rise in lymphoma cases with increasing duration of HIV infection.[65] Although the greatest absolute risk of lymphoma was in the oldest age group, the relative increase compared with general population rates was 38-fold in subjects 10 to 39 years old and 12-fold in older subjects ($p < 0.05$).

Pathogenesis of AIDS-Related Lymphoma

The role of EBV in the pathogenesis of AIDS-related lymphoma has been discussed for some time, based on observations made in various animal systems and in the settings of immunosuppression. Recent work by Birx and colleagues[66] who described defective regulation of EBV infection in patients with AIDS has given much credence to the role of the EBV in lymphomagenesis. In this setting, EBV-immune T cells, which normally suppress EBV-induced B-cell activation, conversely enhanced B-cell activation. Ernberg and colleagues[67] subsequently described the presence of EBV genome within lymphoma cell DNA in a patient with HIV infection. Hamilton and colleagues, using in situ hybridization techniques, detected EBV genome in eight of 16 lymphomas.[68] Further, Shibata and colleagues demonstrated an increased likelihood of progression to lymphoma in a group of HIV-infected men in whom B cells derived from enlarged reactive lymph nodes were found by the polymerase chain reaction to contain EBV DNA. The presence of EBV genome within lymphoma DNA was also demonstrated in approximately 40% of patients with AIDS-related lymphoma.[69] Of great interest, Epstein-Barr virus Early Region proteins have been demonstrated in 100% of primary CNS lymphoma.[70]

Cytogenetic studies of AIDS-related Burkitts' lymphoma have shown a high frequency of t(8;14) and t(8;22) translocations. These associated chromosomal abnormalities occurred as frequently as in ordinary Burkitt's lymphoma. However, an unusual trisomy was observed in three of 13 AIDS-related Burkitt's lymphoma cases.[71]

Rearrangements of the c-*myc* oncogene (located at chromosome 8) has also been frequently described, occurring in 12 of 16 cases reputed by Subar and colleagues.[72] Recent work by Lawrence and colleagues demonstrated that HIV infection of already immortalized EBV-positive B-cell line can lead to upregulation of c-*myc* transcripts and EBV.[73]

Like most neoplasia, the pathogenesis of AIDS-related lymphoma is a multi-step process, and a model of lymphomagenesis can be postulated based on the above data. With underlying immunosuppression by HIV, current or prior EBV infection may be activated, with resultant ongoing B-cell proliferation. Human immunodeficiency virus may promote ongoing B-cell activation and proliferation either directly or via production of certain cytokines such as interleukin-6 from HIV-infected cell, resulting in a state of ongoing B-cell proliferation.[74] An accidental chromosomal abnormality could occur leading to immunoglobulin gene rearrangements and the selection of several clones with potential growth advantage. With further chromosomal aberrations leading to c-*myc* translocation, a single clone may subsequently be selected, leading to a monoclonal B-cell malignancy.

However, the above model is opened to challenge in light of a very recent finding from McGrath's group, which showed that the most prevalent genotype of AIDS-associated lymphoma was polyclonal, EBV-negative tumors with no evidence of c-*myc* rearrangement (14 of 40 or 35%). Monoclonal, EBV-positive tumors with no evidence of c-*myc* rearrangement comprised the second most prevalent class (10 of 40 or 25%); monoclonal, EBV-negative tumors with c-*myc* rearrangement were the third most prevalent class (7 of 40 or 18%) and polyclonal, EBV-positive were observed only in a small subset (3 of 40 or 8%) of specimens analyzed.[75] Further studies will be needed to confirm this data.

Histology

Approximately 60% to 80% of patients with AIDS-related lymphoma have had B-cell tumors of high-grade pathologic types.[75,76] Histologically, these are usually small, noncleaved lymphomas, either Burkitt's lymphoma or Burkitt-like, and immunoblastic lymphoma (immunoblastic sarcoma). Intermediate-grade lymphomas (diffuse large cell) were also reported in a smaller percentage of patients.[76] In addition, cases of more clinically indolent low-grade lymphoma have been noted in HIV-positive patients,[39] as have other lymphoproliferative malignancies including multiple myeloma, plasmacytoma, and B-cell acute lymphocytic leukemia (Burkitt's lymphoma, L-3).

Clinical Expression

Although high-grade lymphoma may be the first manifestation of AIDS, a sizable number of these patients have already had another AIDS-defining illness (47%), opportunistic infection (25%), or KS (11%) by the time the lymphoma is expressed.[76] Many patients have developed an AIDS-related lymphoma in the setting of previously recognized AIDS-related complex, or out of a background of persistent, generalized lymphadenopathy (PGL).

AIDS-Related Central Nervous System Lymphoma

Lymphoma of the central nervous system (CNS) has been considered an illness definitive for AIDS since the beginning of the epidemic. Central nervous system lymphoma, previously well-described in other states of acquired or congenital immune deficiency, is often recognized to be an opportunistic complication in the immunocompromised host.[77]

AIDS-related CNS lymphoma usually occurs relatively late in the course of HIV infection with 75% having a history of AIDS-defining illness. Histologically, the tumors are usually of the immunoblastic or large-cell type, as opposed to the Burkitt sub-type.[70,78] The most common presenting features include headache, cranial nerve palsies, other focal neurologic deficits, or a seizure disorder. Altered mental status or a personality change may coexist with neurologic deficits or may be the only initial manifestation of disease.[79,80]

Clinically, lymphoma most often has to be differentiated from CNS toxoplasmosis or brain abscess. On radiographic evaluation by computed tomography (CT), most patients have definite space-occupying lesions, which are isodense or hyperdense prior to the administration of contrast media, with varying degrees of edema and mass effect. With double contrast studies, most lesions appear as homogeneous or heterogeneous contrast-enhancing masses. The ring-enhancing mass lesions are very similar to those seen in CNS toxoplasmosis. However, patients with toxoplasmosis are more likely to have multiple, smaller CNS lesions on CT scans (mean 1.5 cm, range 1 to 4 cm); they also generally have serologic evidence for prior infection with the organism. Those with primary CNS lymphoma tend to present with fewer, larger lesions (mean 4.5 cm, range 3 to 5 cm).[81] Nevertheless, a definitive diagnosis of lymphoma can only be made by brain biopsy. Lacking this, a trial of empirical therapy for toxoplasmosis, especially in the presence of a positive serologic test for *Toxoplasma gondii*, may be justified.

Whole brain radiotherapy, with corticosteroids, is the standard treatment for CNS lymphoma. Approximately 50% of patients do not respond to such treatment; their median survival is less than 6 months. For the responders, the duration of remission is usually brief.[80] The role of chemotherapy has yet to be defined, but in people with CNS lymphoma without HIV infection, the use of drugs capable of crossing the blood-brain barrier (eg, methotrexate, Ara-C) appears to provide some survival advantage. In rare cases of polyclonal B-cell lymphoproliferative brain disease, treatment with acyclovir has been reported to be helpful. The causes of death may be lymphoma or multiple opportunistic infections occurring in the brain, as well as systemic sites.

Systemic AIDS-Related Lymphoma

The pattern of lymphoma expression often differs from that of the nodes usually involved in PGL. In the latter condition, axillary and inguinal/femoral nodes are preferentially involved, while epitrochlear, retroperitoneal, and intrathoracic nodes are usually spared. Biopsies in PGL usually reveal polyclonal hyperplasia with germinal center activities.[82] Lymphomatous nodes can also appear at these sites, but clinical clues to a malignant transformation include the development of rapidly enlarging, tender nodes; nodes at sites other than those common to PGL; or an extranodal mass with local symptoms, including intestinal obstruction. In addition to benign reactive adenopathy and lymphoma, such nodes can also harbor mycobacteria and other opportunistic pathogens.

Sixty percent to 70% of patents with AIDS-related lymphoma first present with systemic B symptoms, including fever, night sweats, and/or weight loss. Occasionally, some patients can present with a peripheral neurologic syndrome.[83] In the experience of the group at the University of Southern California (USC) with 82 cases, 54 (66%) presented with stage IV disease, while 17 (21%) had stage IE, involving a single extranodal site; a total of 87% presented with extranodal disease.[84] The sites of extranodal disease are variable. Central nervous system involvement is seen in approximately 30% of those with systemic disease; bone marrow (25%), liver (12%), and GI tract (26%) are also commonly involved. Unusual sites of disease (eg, heart, adrenals, rectum, small intestine) have been reported.[80-87]

Therapy

Presently, the therapy of choice in AIDS-related NHL is undefined; the therapy should be tailored to the specific situation. Patients usually have high-grade, advanced disease that requires intensive multiagent chemotherapy. However, because of underlying HIV-induced immunosuppression, the use of multiagent chemotherapy may lead to even greater risk of immune compromise and opportunistic infection.[88] It is also apparent that CNS prophylaxis must be administered, since about 40% of these patients have had documented CNS lymphoma at some time during the course of illness. Furthermore, in an autopsy series from USC, eight of 12 (66%) patients with systemic lymphoma were found to have involvement of the brain, which had been suspected clinically in only three.

Various chemotherapeutic regimens have been tried without significant success. At USC, a prospective study using a modified combination chemotherapeutic regimen, M-BACOD (methotrexate, bleomycin, Adriamycin (doxorubicin), cyclophosphamide, vincristine, and dexamethasone) was superior to a novel, intensive regimen that included high-dose cytosine arabinoside and high-dose methotrexate.[88]

A group of 26 patients was treated with a variety of standard chemotherapeutic regimens, and another group of 38 was treated with a regimen consisting of cyclophosphamide, vincristine, methotrexate, etoposide, and cytosine arabinoside (COMET-A).[89] Although patients treated with COMET-A had a slightly higher complete response rate (58% vs 46%), they had a significantly shorter median survival (5.2 months) than those treated with standard chemotherapy (11.3 months), and 28% developed opportunistic infections from which they died. In addition, patients receiving the higher doses of cyclophosphamide had significantly shorter median survival. These data support the earlier suggestion that more aggressive chemotherapy regimens may result in shorter survival.[88]

Levine and colleagues used a low-dose modification of the M-BACOD regimen in a prospective multi-institutional trial sponsored by the ACTG. A complete remission rate of 46% was achieved in 35 patients (overall response rate of 51%).[90] Responses were also seen in patients with poor prognostic indications and were durable. With the use of intrathecal cytosine arabinoside, CNS relapse appeared to be prevented. This study again suggests less intensive regimens may produce the same as or better results than the standard dosage with less incidence of opportunistic infection.

In an attempt to define the role of hematopoietic growth factors, Kaplan and colleagues reported a phase III trial that used different schedules of rGM-CSF along with the CHOP regimen.[91] In the third week after chemotherapy, there was a significant increase in p24 antigen in patients given rGM-CSF, suggesting stimulation of HIV replication. The clinical outcome of this HIV stimulation could not be determined, and the clinical significance of this finding remains unclear.

To ascertain the precise role of chemotherapeutic dose intensity and the concomitant use of hematopoietic growth factors, the ACTG has now embarked on a Phase III trial in which patients are stratified by prognostic indicators and randomly assigned to receive either the low-dose M-BACOD regimen or standard dose M-BACOD with rGM-CSF.

Hodgkin's Disease

Presently, there is no definitive epidemiologic proof that HD, on the basis of increased frequency, is part of the spectrum of opportunistic diseases comprising AIDS. However, it is apparent that patients who are HIV-positive may present with HD, perhaps because the age-related frequencies of these two diseases of the lymphoid system tend to overlap. Hodgkin's disease is, additionally, a disorder known to appear in increased frequency among the immunocompromised. Patients with HD and concurrent HIV infection more often present with systemic B symptoms and extensive stage III or stage IV disease than do other patients without HIV infection.

Further, unusual disease sites including skin and bone marrow may be seen.[92-94] Such individuals also tolerate chemotherapy poorly; significant neutropenia and opportunistic infections can develop during their treatment.[95] While complete remission rates may be similar to those for other patient groups, the median survival of HIV-positive patients has been shorter than usually expected.

Other Malignancies in HIV-Infected Individuals

Anal Intraepithelial Neoplasia

In 1986, Frazer first reported a study of 61 homosexual men by means of anal Papanicolaou (PAP) smear and HPV analysis.[96] Cytologic dysplasia with concomitant HPV infection was noted in 40%, while another 40% had evidence of HPV infection without dysplasia. With the rise of anal carcinoma in New York City, Beckman and colleagues noted a correlation between prior HPV infection and subsequent development of anal carcinoma. The HPV types most commonly associated with anal cancer have included types 16, 18, 31, 33, and 35.[97]

Recently, Palefsky and colleagues reported an interesting relationship between HIV infection and the development of anal intraepithelial neoplasia. A group of 97 homosexual men with symptomatic HIV infection and without anal symptoms were studied by anal cytology. Abnormal anal cytologic findings were detected in 39% and consisted of anal intraepithelial neoplasia in 15%, atypical cytology in 20%, and condyloma in 4%.[98]

Cervical Intraepithelial Neoplasia

In view of the above findings the association of HIV infection with cervical squamous intraepithelial lesions (SIL) and HPV infection of the cervix was prospectively investigated in 132 women attending a methadone clinic.[99,100] Evidence for HPV infection was detected in 67% of symptomatic HIV-positive women, 31% of asymptomatic HIV-positive women, and 27% of HIV-negative women. Human papillomavirus was more strongly associated with SIL in HIV-positive women than in HIV-negative women. In women who were not infected with HPV, no association was found between HIV and SIL. The findings of this investigation suggest that HIV-induced immunosuppression may predispose to HPV-mediated cervical cytologic abnormalities.

The characteristics of cervical disease were assessed in women with known HIV status attending a medical center for evaluation of abnormal Pap smears.[101] Colposcopic evaluations of 77 patients suggested that cervical intraepithelial neoplasia (CIN) was more severe and extensive in 25 HIV-positive women than in 52 HIV-negative women. Among the HIV-positive women, CIN was a higher grade and was more likely to involve multifocal or extensive cervical lesions, multiple sites of the lower genital tract, and the perianal area. These investigators also reported that seropositive patients with advanced stages of cervical cancer had poorer outcomes after therapy and more aggressive disease than seronegative patients with similar stages.

The long-term consequences of anal dysplastic changes and even intraepithelial neoplasia remain to be clarified. However, the model of HPV infection, long-term cervical dysplasia, CIN and the subsequent development of invasive cancer may serve as an opportunity for the study of carcinogenesis and cancer prevention.

Miscellaneous Malignancies in HIV-Infected Individuals

Patients who have undergone organ transplantation, with subsequent use of long-term immunosuppressive agents to prevent graft rejection, are at increased risk for development of viral lymphomas; KS; squamous cell carcinomas of the cervix, vulva, anus, and skin; basal cell carcinomas of the skin ; and lip cancers.[102-104] This may be due to the breakdown of normal immune or surveillance factors as well as the presence of various oncogenic viruses.

Although KS and high-grade lymphoma have already been linked epidemiologically with AIDS, the other cancers that have been noted in organ transplant recipients have not yet increased statistically in association with the HIV epidemic. In addition to HD and squamous cell carcinoma of the anus and cervix, head and neck carcinoma and basal cell carcinoma have been reported to occur in HIV-infected individuals. It is possible that such associations will become established in future years.

Anecdotally, single-case reports of adenosquamous carcinoma of the lung,[105] adenocarcinoma of the colon and pancreas,[106] and cloacagenic carcinoma[107] have been described in HIV-infected individuals. An increased incidence of testicular carcinoma has also been described in young homosexual men.[108] The significance of these reports is unclear.

Other Retroviruses

In addition to HIV, there is very strong evidence that other related retroviruses can play an important role in the induction of neoplastic diseases. In general, these agents have transmission routes similar to that of HIV and would therefore be expected to be present in HIV-infected individuals at a higher rate than in the general population.

Human T-Cell Leukemia Virus Type I

Human T-cell leukemia virus type I is the primary etiologic agent of ATLL.[108] This retrovirus selectively infects and sometimes transforms and immortalizes the CD4+ T cell, leading to expression of receptors for IL2 and substantial IL2 production by the transformed cells. It has been hypothesized that an autocrine interaction of IL2 and IL2 receptors on the transformed cells provides them with a survival advantage, leading to lymphoproliferation that becomes monoclonal.

Adult T-cell leukemia-lymphoma was first described in 1977 and has been studied in detail in endemic areas in southern Japan.[109] The HTLV-I and its resulting disease were also found to be endemic in the West Indies and in Africa; it is also seen sporadically worldwide, including cases in Israel, the Pacific basin, and the southeastern US, where people of African descent are most often affected.

As many as 5% of persons infected with HTLV-I have developed ATLL. Patients characteristically present with leukemia, lymphadenopathy, and hepatosplenomegaly. They also have skin lesions showing leukemic infiltration with the morphologically typical leukemic cells of ATLL. This cell is a mature T-lymphocyte with a lobulated nucleus and is usually of the CD4+ (helper) T-cell phenotype. Some of the earlier cases of ATLL were considered variants of Sezary syndrome. The disease is usually aggressive and leads to death in several months. In addition, HTLV-I infection is associated with a myelopathy known as tropical spastic paraparesis.

Recently, cases of asymptomatic HTLV-I infection, with ATLL, and of coinfection with HIV and HTLV-I have been described among intravenous drug abusers in New York City.[110,111] In addition, one case of CD8+ (suppressor phenotype) monoclonal lymphoproliferative disease has been described in a patient with coinfection by HIV and HTLV-I. In this unique situation, the lymphoproliferative disorder apparently involved the CD8 cell as the target for transformation and immortalization by HTLV-I, in a setting in which CD4+ cells had been depleted. This combination may have represented an unusual opportunistic neoplasm of AIDS.[112]

Chemotherapy for ATLL has been generally disappointing, although combinations including pentostatin (deoxycoformycin) have shown somewhat encouraging results.[113]

Human T-Cell Leukemia Virus Type II

Human T-cell leukemia virus type II has primarily been associated with intravenous drug abusers and their sexual partners in the US. The role of HTLV-II in human leukemogenesis has not been clear. However, HTLV-II was first isolated from a cell line derived from the spleen of a patient with hairy-cell leukemia.[8] Recently, HTLV-II was also isolated in a patient with T-cell prolymphocytic leukemia.[114] The initiation of volunteer blood-donor screening for HTLV infection in November, 1988, resulted in the identification of approximately 2,000 seropositive units of blood donated each year. Of these, at least half were infected with HTLV-II.

Overview

The management of AIDS-associated neoplasms is difficult and complex. Care of the underlying disease with antiviral agents, appropriate prophylactic antimicrobial therapy, hematopoietic growth factors, patient education, and prompt recognition and intervention at the time of intercurrent opportunistic complications are essential, although this obvious principle is sometimes forgotten in the face of the administration of already complex chemotherapeutic protocols. The recent advances in our understanding of these neoplasms open new avenues in treating these diseases. Physicians managing persons infected with HIV can, to an extent, practice preventive medicine via surveillance for these neoplasms: compulsive history-taking; careful and repeated examinations of lymphoid tissue, the entire skin surface, and the oral cavity; and the performance of frequent Pap smears.

References

1. Siegal FP, Lopez C, Hammer GS, et al. Severe acquired immunodeficiency in male homosexuals, manifested by chronic perianal ulcerative herpes simplex lesions. *N Engl J Med.* 1981;305:1439-1444.,

2. Hymes K, Cheung T, Greene JB, et al. Kaposi's sarcoma in homosexual men. *Lancet.* 1981;II:598-600.

3. Gottlieb MS, Schroff R, Schanker HM, et al. *Pneumocystis carinii* pneumonia and mucosal candidiasis in previously healthy homosexual men: evidence of a new acquired cellular immunodeficiency. *N Engl J Med.* 1981;305:1425-1431

4. Siegal FP. Immune deficiency of AIDS. In: Wormser GP, Stahl RE, Bottone EJ, eds. *Acquired Immune Deficiency Syndrome.* Park Ridge, NJ: Noyes Publications;1987:304-330.

5. Barre-Sinoussi F, Chermann JC, Rey F, et al. Isolation of T-lymphotropic retrovirus from a patient at risk for acquired immunodeficiency syndrome (AIDS). *Science.* 1983;220:868-871.

6. Gallo RC, Sarin PS, Gelmann EP, et al. Isolation of human T-cell leukemia virus in acquired immune deficiency syndrome (AIDS). *Science.* 1983;220-865-867.

7. Poiesz BJ, Ruscetti FW, Gazdar AF, et al. Detection and isolation of type C retrovirus particles from fresh and cultured lymphocytes of a patient with cutaneous T-cell lymphoma. *Proc Natl Acad Sci (USA).* 1980;77:7415-7419.

8. Kalyanaraman VS, Sarngadharan MG, Robert-Guroff M, et al. A new subtype of human T-cell leukemia virus (HTLV-II) associated with a T-cell variant of hairy cell leukemia. *Science.* 1982;218:571-573.

9. Penn I. Immunosuppression and malignant disease. In: Towmey JJ, Good RA, eds. *Immunopathogenesis of Lymphatic Neoplasm. Comprehensive Immunology.* New York, NY: Plenum Press; 1978:4:223-237.

10. Spector BD, Perry GS III, Good RA, et al. Immunodeficiency diseases and malignancies. In: Towmey JJ, Good RA, ed. *Immunopathogenesis of Lymphatic Neoplasm. Comprehensive Immunology.* New York, NY: Plenum Press; 1978;4:203-222.

11. Kaposi M. Idiopathigches multiples pigment sarcom der Haut. *Arch Dematol Syphil (Berlin).* 1872;4:265-273.

12. Ackerman LV, Murray JF. *Symposium on Kaposi's sarcoma.* Basel: S. Karger; 1963.

13. Taylor JF, Templeton AC, Vogel CL, et al. Kaposi's sarcoma in Uganda: a clinicopathologic study. *Int J Cancer.* 1971;8:122-135.

14. Myers BD, Kessler E, Levi D, et al. Kaposi's sarcoma in kidney transplant recipients. *Arch Intern Med.* 1974;133:307-311.

15. Beckstead JH, Wood GS, Fletcher V. Evidence for the origin of Kaposi's sarcoma from lymphatic endothelium. *Am J Pathol.* 1985;119:294-300.

16. Salahuddin SZ, Nakamura S, Biberfeld, et al. Angiographic properties of Kaposi's sarcoma derived cells after long-term culture in vitro. *Science.* 1988;242:430-433.

17. Weich HA, Salahuddin SZ, Gill P, et al. AIDS-associated Kaposi's sarcoma-derived cells in long-term culture express and synthesize smooth muscle alpha-actin. *Am J Path.* 1991;139(6):1251-1258.

18. Thompson EW, Nakamura S, Shima TP, et al. Supernatants of AIDS-related Kaposi's sarcoma cells include endothelial cell chemotaxis and invasiveness. *Cancer Res.* 1991;51:2670-2676.

19. Ensoli B, Salahuddin SZ, Gallo RC. AIDS-associated Kaposi's sarcoma: a molecular model for its pathogenesis. *Cancer Cells.* 1989;1:93-96.

20. Ensoli B, Nakamura S, Salahuddin SZ, et al. AIDS-Kaposi's sarcoma-derived cells express cytokines and autocrine and paracrine growth effects. *Science.* 1989;243:223-226.

21. Vogel J, Hinrichs SH, Reynolds RK, et al. The HIV tat gene induces dermal lesions resembling Kaposi's sarcoma in transgenie mice. *Nature.* 1988;335:606-611.

22. Darrow WW, Jaffe HW, Curran JW. Passive anal intercourse as a risk factor for AIDS in homosexual men. *Lancet.* 1983;2:160.

23. Centers for Disease Control Update. Acquired immunodeficiency syndrome—United States. *MMWR.* 1986;35:757-765.

24. Pitchenik AE, Fischl MA, Dickinson GM, et al. Opportunistic infectious and Kaposi's sarcoma among Haitians: evidence of a new acquired immunodeficiency state. *Ann Intern Med.* 1983;98:277-284.

25. Cheung TW, Siegal FP. Kaposi's sarcoma in women with AIDS (abstr). The Fifth International Conference on AIDS. 1989 M.B.P. 297.

26. Desmond-Hellmann SD, Mbidde EK, Kizito A, et al. The epidemiology and clinical features of Kaposi's sarcoma in African women with HIV infection (Abstr). The Sixth International Conference on AIDS. 1990 S.B. 508.

27. Pollack MS, Safai B, Dupont B. HLA-Dr5 and Dr-2 are susceptibility factors for acquired immunodeficiency syndrome with Kaposi's sarcoma in different ethnic subpopulations. *Dis Markers.* 1983;1:135-139.

28. Rubenstein P, de Cordoba S, Oestricher R, et al. Immunogenetics and predisposition to Kaposi's sarcoma. In: Groopman J, ed. *Acquired Immune Deficiency Syndrome.* New York, NY: Alan R. Liss; 1984:309-318.

29. Friedman-Kien AE, et al. Disseminated Kaposi-like sarcoma syndrome in young homosexual men. *J Am Acad Dermatol.* 1981;5:468-471.

30. Meduri GU, Stover DE, Lee M, et al. Pulmonary Kaposi's sarcoma in the acquired immune deficiency syndrome. *Am J Med.* 1986;81:11-18.

31. Morris L, Distenfeld A, Amorosi E, et al. Autoimmune thrombocytopenic purpura in homosexual men. *Ann Intern Med.* 1982;96:714-717.

32. Tayler J, Afrasiabi R, Fahey JL, et al. Prognostic significant classification of immune changes in AIDS with Kaposi's sarcoma. *Blood.* 1986;67:666-671.

33. Mitsuyasu RT, Glaspy I, Taylor JM, et al. Heterogeneity of epidemic Kaposi's sarcoma: implications for therapy. *Cancer.* 1986;57(suppl 8):1657-1661.

34. Stahl RE, Friedman-Kien A, Dubin R, et al. Immunologic abnormalities in homosexual men: relationship to Kaposi's sarcoma. *Am J Med.* 1982;73:171-178.

35. Chachoua A, Krigel R, Lafleu F, et al. Prognostic factors and staging classifications of patients with epidemic Kaposi's sarcoma. *J Clin Oncol.* 1989;7:774-780.

36. Krown SE, Metroka C, Wernz JC, et al. Kaposi's sarcoma in the acquired immune deficiency syndrome: proposal for a uniform evaluation, response, and staging criteria. *J Clin Oncol.* 1989;7:1201-1207.

37. Volberding PA, Kaslow K, Billie M, et al. Prognostic factors in staging Kaposi's sarcoma in the acquired immune deficiency syndrome (Abstr). *Proc Am Soc Clin Oncol.* 1984;3:51.

38. Vadhan-Rai S, Wong G, Gnecco C, et al. Immunologic variables as predictors of prognosis in patients with Kaposi's sarcoma and the acquired immunodeficiency syndrome. *Cancer Res.* 1986;46:417-425.

39. Chak LY, Gill PS, Levine A, et al. Radiation therapy for

acquired immunodeficiency syndrome-related Kaposi's sarcoma. *J Clin Oncol.* 1988;6:863-867.

40. Nobler MP, Leddy ME, Huh SH. The impact of palliative irradiation on the management of patients with acquired immune deficiency syndrome. *J Clin Oncol.* 1987;5:107-112.

41. Groopman JE, Gottlieb MS, Goodman J, et al. Recombinant alpha-2 interferon therapy for Kaposi's sarcoma in the acquired immunodeficiency syndrome. *Ann Intern Med.* 1984;100:671-676.

42. Krown SE, Real FX, Vadhan-Raj S, et al. Kaposi's sarcoma and the acquired immune deficiency syndrome. *Cancer.* 1986;57:1662-1665.

43. Abrams DI, Volberding PA. Alpha-interferon therapy of AIDS-associated Kaposi's sarcoma. *Semin Oncol.* 1987;14(suppl 2):43-47.

44. Volberding PA, Abrams DI, Conant M, et al. Vinblastine Therapy for Kaposi's sarcoma in the acquired immunodeficiency syndrome. *Ann Intern Med.* 1985;103:335-338.

45. Volberding PA, Mitsuyasu RT, Golando JP, et al. Treatment of Kaposi's sarcoma with interferon alpha-2b (intron A). *Cancer.* 1987;59:620-625.

46. Krown SE, Gold JWM, Niedzwiecki D, et al. Interferon-α with zidovudine safety, tolerance, and clinical and virologic effects in patients with Kaposi's sarcoma associated with the acquired immunodeficiency syndrome (AIDS). *Ann Intern Med.* 1990;112:812-821.

47. DeWit R, Danner SA, Bakker JM, et al. Combined zidovudine and interferon-alpha treatment in patients with AIDS-associated Kaposi's sarcoma. *J Intern Med.* 1991;229:35-40.

48. Klein E, Schwartz RA, Loar Y, et al. Treatment of Kaposi's sarcoma with vinblastine. *Cancer.* 1980;45:427-431.

49. Kaplan MH, Volberding P, Abrams D. Treatment of Kaposi's sarcoma in acquired immunodeficiency syndrome with an alternating vincristine-vinblastine regimen. *Cancer Treat Rep.* 1986;70:1121-1122.

50. Laubenstein LJ, Krigel RL, Odajank CM, et al. Treatment of epidemic Kaposi's sarcoma (EKS) with etoposide or a combination of doxorubicin, bleomycin, and vinblastine. *J Clin Oncol.* 2:1115-1120.

51. Gill PS, Krailo M, Slater L, et al. Randomized trial of ABV (Adriamycin, bleomycin, vincristine) vs. A in advanced Kaposi's sarcoma (KS): preliminary results (Abstr). *Proc Am Soc Clin Oncol.* 1988;7:3.

52. Gelmann EP, Longo D, Lane HC, et al. Combination chemotherapy of disseminated Kaposi's sarcoma inpatients with the acquired immune deficiency syndrome. *Am J Med.* 1987;82:456-462.

53. Newman SB. Treatment of epidemic Kaposi's sarcoma (KS) with intralesional vinblastin injection (IL-VBL). *Proc Am Soc Clin Oncol.* 1988;7:A19.

54. Volberding PA. The role of chemotherapy for epidemic Kaposi's sarcoma. *Semin Oncol.* 1987;14(Suppl 3):23-26.

55. Centers for Disease Control. Revision of the case definition of acquired immunodeficiency syndrome for national reporting — United States. *Ann Intern Med.* 1985;103:402-403.

56. Cheung TW, Silber R. Malignant lymphoma among drug addicts (Abstr). *Proc Am Soc Oncol.* 1982;1:4.

57. Ahmed T, Wormser GP, Stahl RE, et al. Malignant lymphomas in a population at risk for acquired immune deficiency syndrome. *Cancer.* 1987;60:719-723.

58. Ross RK, Dworsky RL, Paganini-Hill A, et al. Non-Hodgkin's lymphomas in never-married men in Los Angeles. *Br J Cancer.* 1985;52:785-787.

59. Levine AM, Gill PS, Meyer PR, et al. Retrovirus and malignant lymphoma in homosexual men. *JAMA.* 1985;254:1921-1925.

60. Levine AM, Meyer PR, Begandy MK, et al. Development of B-cell lymphoma in homosexual men: clinical and immunologic findings. *Ann Inter Med.* 1984;100:7-13.

61. Monfardini S, Vaccher E, Tirelli U. AIDS-associated non-Hodgkin's lymphoma in Italy: intravenous drug users versus homosexual men. *Ann Oncol.* 1990;1:203-211.

62. Lemp GF, Payne SF, Neal D, et al. Survival trends for patients with AIDS. *JAMA.* 1990;263:402-406.

63. Gail MH, Rosenberg PS, Goedert JJ. Therapy may explain recent deficits in AIDS incidence. *J Acquir Immune Defic Synd.* 1990;3:296-306.

64. Pluda JM, Yarchoan R, Jaffe ES, et al. Development of lymphoma in a cohort of patients with severe human immunodeficiency virus (HIV) infection on long-term antiretroviral therapy. *Ann Intern Med.* 1990;113:276-282.

65. Rabkin CS, Hilgartner MW, Hedberg KW, et al. Incidence of lymphomas and other cancers in HIV-infected and HIV-uninfected patients with hemophilia. *JAMA.* 1992;267:1090-1094.

66. Birx DL, Redfield RR, Tosato G. Defective regulation of Epstein-Barr virus infection in patients with acquired immunodeficiency syndrome (AIDS) or AIDS-related disorders. *N Engl J Med.* 1986;314:874-879.

67. Ernberg I, Bjorkholm M, Zech L, et al. An EBV genome carrying pre-B cell leukemia in a homosexual man with characteristics karyotype and EBV-specific immunity. *J Clin Oncol.* 1986;4:1481-1488.

68. Hamilton-Dutort S, Pallensen G, Karkov J, et al. Identification of EBV-DNA in tumor cells of AIDS-related lymphomas by in situ hybridization (letter). *Lancet.* 1989;1:554.

69. Shibata D, Weiss LM, Nathwani BN, et al. Epstein-Barr virus in benign lymph node biopsies from individuals infected with the human immunodeficiency virus is associated with the concurrent or subsequent development of non-Hodgkin's lymphoma. *Blood.* 1991;77:1527-1533.

70. MacMahon EM, Glass JD, Hayward SD, et al. Epstein-Barr virus in AIDS-related primary central nervous system lymphoma. *Lancet.* 1991;338:969-973.

71. Bernheim A, Berger R. Cytogenetic studies of Burkitt's lymphoma-leukemia in patients with acquired immunodeficiency syndrome. *Cancer Genet Cytogenet.* 1988;32:67-74.

72. Subar M, Neri A, Inghirami G, et al. Frequent c-*myc* oncogene activation and infrequent presence of Epstein-Barr virus genome in AIDS-associated lymphoma. *Blood.* 1988;72:667-671.

73. Laurence J, Astrin A. Human immunodeficiency virus induction of malignant transformation in human B lymphocytes. *Proc Natl Acad Sci (USA).* 1991;7635-7639.

74. Nakajima K, Martinez-Maza O, Hirano T, et al. Induction of Il-6 (B-cell stimulatory factor-2/IFN-beta 2) production by human immunodeficiency virus. *J Immunol.* 1989;142:531-536.

75. Shiramizu B, Herndie B, Meeker T, et al. Molecular and immunophenotype characterization of AIDS-associated, Epstein-Barr virus-negative, polyclonal lymphoma. *J Clin Oncol.* 1992; 10:383-389.

76. Ziegler JL, Beckstead JA, Volberding PA, et al. Non-Hodgkin's lymphoma in 90 homosexual men: relationship to generalized lymphadenopathy and acquired immunodeficiency syndrome (AIDS). *N Engl J Med.* 1984;311:565-570.

77. Frizzera G, Rosai J, Dehner LP, et al. Lymphoreticular disorders in primary immunodeficiency: new findings based on an up-to-date histologic classification of 35 cases. *Cancer.* 1980;46:692-699.

78. Raphael J, Gentihomme O, Tulliez M, et al. Histopathologic features of high-grade non-Hodgkin's lymphomas in acquired immunodeficiency syndrome. *Arch Pathol Lab Med.* 1991;115:15-20.

79. Gill PS, Levine AM, Meyer PR, et al. Primary central nervous system lymphoma in homosexual men: clinical, immunologic and pathologic features. *Am J Med.* 1985;78:742-748.

80. So YT, Beckstead JH, David RL. Primary central nervous system lymphoma in acquired immune deficiency syndrome: a clinical and pathological study. *Ann Neurol.* 1986;20:566-572.

81. Gill PS, Graham RA, Boswell W, et al. A comparison of imaging, clinical, and pathologic aspects of space occupying lesions within the brain in patients with acquired immune deficiency syndrome. *Am J Physiol Imaging.* 1986;1:134-141.

82. Poon TP, Matoso IM, Datta B. Ultrastructural study of a primary central lymphoma in acquired immunodeficiency syndrome. *NY Med Quar.* 1988;1:65-68.

83. Gold JE, Jimenez E, Zalusky R. Human immunodeficiency virus-related lymphoreticular malignancies and peripheral neurologic disease. *Cancer.* 1988;61:2318-2324.

84. Levine AM. Reactive and neoplastic lymphoproliferative disorders and other miscellaneous cancers associated with HIV infection. In: De Vita VT, Hellman S, Rosenberg SA. *AIDS PA.* Philadelphia, Pa: JB Lippincott Co; 1988:263-276.

85. Constantino A, West TE, Gupta M, et al. Primary cardiac lymphoma in a patient with acquired immune deficiency syndrome. *Cancer.* 1987;60:2801-2805.

86. Ioachim HL, Weinstein MA, Robbins RD, et al. Primary anorectal lymphoma: a new manifestation of acquired immune deficiency syndrome (AIDS). *Cancer.* 1987;60:1449-1453.

87. Estrin HM, Farhi DC, Ament AA, et al. Ileoscopic diagnosis of malignant lymphoma of the small bowel in acquired immunodeficiency syndrome. *Gastrointest Endosc.* 1987;33:390-391.

88. Gill PS, Levine AM, Krailo M, et al. AIDS-related malignant lymphoma: results of prospective treatment trials. *J Clin Oncol.* 1987;5:1322-1328.

89. Kaplan LD, Abrams DI, Feigal E, et al. AIDS-associated non-Hodgkin's lymphoma in San Francisco. *JAMA.* 1989;261:719-724.

90. Levine AM, Wernz JC, Kaplan L, et al. Low-dose chemotherapy with central nervous system prophylaxis and zidovudine maintenance in AIDS-related lymphoma. *JAMA.* 1991;266:84-88.

91. Kaplan LD, Kahn JO, Crowe S, et al. Clinical and virologic effects of recombinant human granulocyte-macrophage colony-stimulating factor in patients receiving chemotherapy for human immunodeficiency virus-associated non-Hodgkin's lymphoma: results of a randomized trial. *J Clin Oncol.* 1991;9:929-940.

92. Scheib RG, Siegal RS. Atypical Hodgkin's disease and the acquired immunodeficiency syndrome (letter). *Ann Intern Med.* 1985;102:68-70.

93. Schoeppel SL, Hoppe RT, Dorfman FT, et al. Hodgkin's disease in homosexual men with generalized lymphadenopathy. *Ann Intern Med.* 1985;102:68-70.

94. Subar M, Chamulak G, Dalla-Favera R, et al. Clinical and pathologic characteristics of AIDS-associated Hodgkin's disease (Abstr). *Blood.* 1986;68:135a.

95. Bear DM, Anderson ET, Wilkinson LS. Acquired immune deficiency syndrome in homosexual men with Hodgkin's disease. *Am J Med.* 1986;80:738-740.

96. Frazer IH, Crapper RM, Medley G, et al. Association between anorectal dysplasia, human papillomavirus and human immunodeficiency virus infection in homosexual men. *Lancet.* 1986;2:657.

97. Beckman AM, Daling JR, Sherman KJ, et al. Human papillomavirus infection and anal cancer. *Int J Cancer.* 1989;43:1042.

98. Palefsky JM, Gonzales J, Greenblatt RM, et al. Anal intraepithelial neoplasia and anal papillomavirus infection among homosexual males with group IV HIV disease. *JAMA.* 1990;263:2911-2916.

99. Feingold AR, Vermund SH, Burk RD, et al. Cervical cytologic abnormalities and papillomavirus in women infected with human immunodeficiency virus. *J Acquir Immune Defic Syndr.* 1990;3:896-903.

100. Vermund S, Kelley KF, Burk RD, et al. Risk of human papillomavirus (HPV) and cervical squamous dysplasia (SIL) highest among women with advanced HIV disease (Abstract). VI International Conference on AIDS. Vol. 3. San Francisco, June,1990:215.

101. Maiman M, Fruchter RG, Serur E, et al. Human immunodeficiency virus infection and cervical neoplasia. *Gynecol Oncol.* 1990;38:377-382.

102. Li FP, Osborn D, Cronin CM. Anorectal squamous carcinoma in two homosexual men. *Lancet.* 1982;II:391.

103. Daling JR, Weiss NS, Klopfenstein LL, et al. Correlation of homosexual behavior and the incidence of anal cancer. *JAMA.* 1982;247:1988-1990.

104. Sitz KV, Keppen M, Johnson DF. Metastatic basal cell carcinoma in acquired immunodeficiency syndrome-related complex. *JAMA.* 1987;257:340-343.

105. Irwin LE, Begandy MK, Moore TM. Adenosquamous carcinoma of the acquired immunodeficiency syndrome. *Ann Intern Med.* 1984;100:158.

106. Kaplan MH, Susin M, Pahwa SG, et al. Neoplastic complications of HTLV-III infection: lymphomas and solid tumor. *Am J Med.* 1987;82:389-396.

107. Cooper HS, Patchefsky AS, Marks G. Cloacagenic carcinoma of the anorectum in homosexual men: an observation of four cases. *Dis Colon Rectum.* 1979;22:557-558.

108. Logothetis CJ, Newell GY, Samuels ML. Testicular cancer in homosexual men with cellular immune deficiency: report of two cases. *J Urol.* 1985;133:484-486.

109. Uchiyama T, Yodoi J, Sagawa K, et al. Adult T-cell leukemia: clinical and hematologic features of 16 cases. *Blood.* 1977;50:481-492.

110. Dosik H, Denic S, Patel N, et al. Adult T-cell leukemia-lymphoma in Brooklyn. *JAMA.* 1988;259:2255-2257.

111. Robert-Guroff M, Weiss SH, Giron JA, et al. Prevalence of antibodies to HTLV-I, II, and III in intravenous drug abusers from an AIDS endemic region. *JAMA.* 1986;255:3133-3137.

112. Sohn CC, Blayne DW, Misset JL, et al. Leukopenic chronic T-cell leukemia mimicking hairy-cell leukemia: association with human retroviruses. *Blood.* 1986;67:949-956.

113. Daenen S, Rojer RA, Smit JW, et al. Successful chemotherapy with deoxycoformycin in adult T-cell lymphoma-leukemia. *Br J Hematol.* 1984;58:723-727.

114. Cervantes J, Hussain S, Jensen F, et al. T-prolymphocytic leukemia associated with human T-cell lymphotropic virus II. *Clin Res.* 1986;34:454A.

37

REHABILITATION AND SUPPORTIVE CARE OF THE CANCER PATIENT

Robert J. McKenna, Sr, MD, David Wellisch, PhD, and Fawzy I. Fawzy, MD

In the United States today, 54% of cancer patients can look forward to being cured. More than 8 million Americans are alive today with a history of cancer, 5 million of them 5 years or more after their diagnosis. Most people, however, are skeptical about the efficacy of cancer treatment, in part because they are not aware of recent medical advances and in part because they have known people whose cancers have not been cured. People with limited educational and financial resources may not obtain competent medical care for their cancer—or may not seek it. Others use unproven methods that promise a cure without complications.

Quality of Life—The Heart of Rehabilitation

Today's advanced cancer therapies must be accompanied by supportive care in order to maintain quality of life. Many physicians tend to concentrate on the scientific application of modern cancer knowledge and forget that emotional and psychosocial support are also essential. Without this support, such treatment may result in failure to obtain maximum rehabilitation. Physicians must always be aware that their patients are people with individual goals, dreams, hopes, and concerns. The oncologist's role is not only to provide the best quality cancer treatment, but also to consider the disease's impact on each patient's lifestyle and to aid the patient in returning to a normal or near-normal life.

Simply asking the question "How does the patient feel?" is not a valid means of assessing a cancer patient's quality of life. The physician must assess symptoms, side effects of treatment, physical functioning, psychologic distress, social interaction, sexuality, self-image, and satisfaction with care. Moreover, these issues are not static, but change with the stage of the cancer, the passage of time, and the complications and morbidity associated with the disease process. Thus, no simple or single instrument can measure quality of life.

The matrix shown in Figure 37-1 is a good expression of this aspect of care. Four dimensions are listed: physical side effects, which may be both general and a result of treatment; functional status, both personal and social; psychological morbidity, expressed in both distress and depression; and coping and/or satisfaction in work or social relationships.

Yancik and Yates[1] emphasize that the care of the cancer patient must encompass not only the illness but also the social and psychological needs of the patient. They suggest that the use of toxic drugs, high dosages, and even some surgery and hospitalizations might be prevented if physicians treating cancer were better able to predict and monitor the course of the disease as it affects the patient's quality of life.

Cancer Rehabilitation

Goals

Almost all patients who have been treated for cancer need some measure of rehabilitation, since more than half of all cancer patients can now expect to live at least 5 years after they have been diagnosed with cancer, and many live a normal lifespan. Even for those who are not so fortunate, rehabilitation is an integral part of good, comprehensive care.

In 1972, the National Cancer Institute identified four objectives for cancer rehabilitation: psychological support at the time of diagnosis; optimal physical functioning after treatment; vocational counseling, when indicated; and—the ultimate goal of cancer

Robert J. McKenna, Sr, MD, Clinical Professor of Surgery, Los Angeles County Medical Center, University of Southern California Medical School, Los Angeles, California

David Wellisch, PhD, Professor, Department of Psychiatry and Behavioral Sciences, UCLA School of Medicine, Los Angeles, California

Fawzy I. Fawzy, MD, Professor and Associate Chair, Department of Psychiatry and Biobehavioral Sciences, UCLA School of Medicine, Los Angeles, California

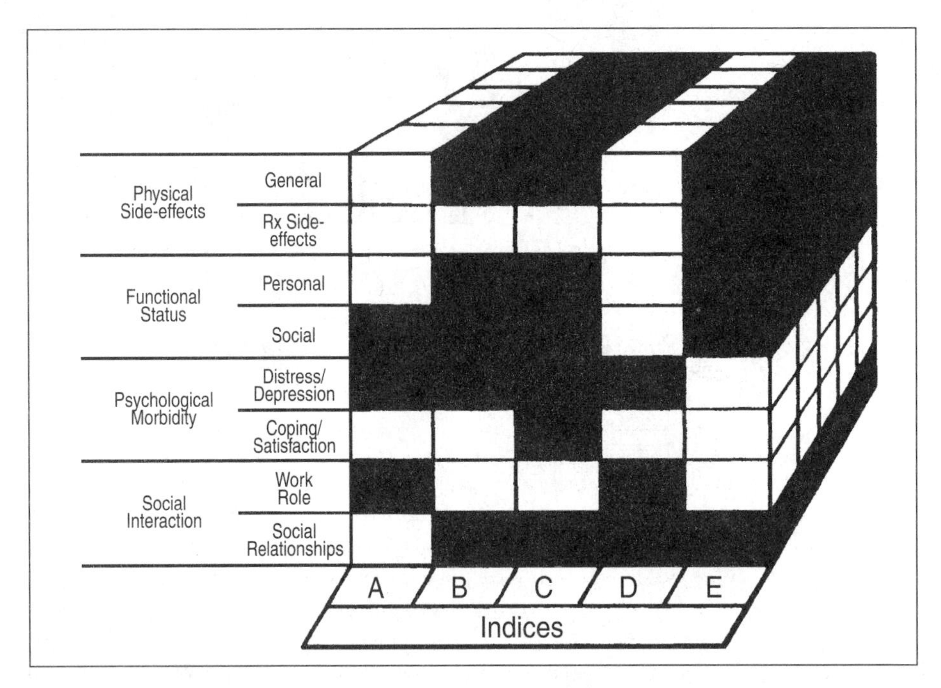

Fig 37-1. Quality-of-life matrix includes dimensions of physical side effects, functional status, psychological morbidity, and social interaction. From Yancik and Yates.[1]

treatment and control—optimal social functioning. In its broadest sense, the goal of cancer rehabilitation is to enable patients to achieve as normal and full a life as possible.

The Rehabilitation Team

Rehabilitation is a team effort focusing on the whole person rather than on a site-specific cancer, although the site is an important factor and will necessarily direct the emphasis of the rehabilitation plan. The physician directing the treatment team should be the one closest to the patient—either the primary physician, the oncologist, or another responsible physician, such as the surgeon, radiotherapist, or psychiatrist. The support team may include oncology nurses, a psychologist or other mental health professional, a physiatrist, a physical therapist, a speech therapist, an occupational therapist, a social worker, home care nurses, clergy, and lay volunteers. The rehabilitation effort may also include ongoing counseling, hospice services, and other long- or short-term programs of supportive care. Not every patient needs the team's services because patients' requirements, desires, and personal resources vary. However, the physician should be alert to any need for services, particularly when the cancer has not been cured.

Although effective rehabilitation has recently become more available and less expensive, many patients still encounter difficulties in securing it. Physicians may be more familiar with diagnosis and treatment than with rehabilitation; community hospitals may lack the full complement of personnel for a team approach; social workers may be unaware of specific appropriate resources; and, in general, the readaptation needs of the cancer patient may be poorly understood. Effective coordination of services is essential for maximum rehabilitation. However, state and federal agencies are of little help. They traditionally assign a low priority to cancer patients because cancer patients in the past have had such low survival rates. They have been slow in responding to the greatly improved outlook for cancer patients.

Interventions

The rehabilitation goals must be realistic and individualized for each patient. They depend on the patient's functional abilities and the stage of the disease. Interventions may be preventive, restorative, supportive, or palliative.

Preventive interventions lessen the impact of an anticipated disability through patient training and education (eg, teaching a woman about to undergo a mastectomy the exercises she will need to perform after the operation to prevent swelling and loss of arm function). *Restorative* procedures aim to restore, as closely as possible, the patient's physical integrity (eg, breast reconstruction following mastectomy). *Supportive* rehabilitation interventions may be provided for the patient who has a disabling condition as a result of the cancer and its treatment, who can learn to cope with that condition, and who retains control over many or most of the activities of daily living (eg, teaching esophageal speech to a patient who has had a total laryngectomy). *Palliative* interventions provide comfort, assistance in everyday functioning, and emotional support in those cases where cancer is advanced and recovery is not expected.

Patient Profile

The most fortunate patients—the majority—are those with an early stage of cancer, who can be treated successfully. They have minimal disability and are likely to have a normal lifespan free of cancer recurrence. These patients live with the fear that their cancer may recur.

A second group includes people who have curable cancer from an anatomic standpoint, who have a total response to treatment, and who have an interval of time free from cancer before experiencing a recurrence, either locally or at a distant site. Some individuals in this group can be cured by further treatment and have a normal lifespan. Others fail to respond and develop progressive disease and eventually die. Crises occur at all stages in the course of their treatment. These patients need major psychological support that emphasizes the hope that the treatment side effects will be short-lived.

Patients in a third group are those treated for cancer and cured, only to develop a second (or a third or fourth) cancer. Some of these later cancers are related to the lifestyle that caused the first (eg, tobacco-induced cancers in the oral cavity, larynx, and lung, or alcohol-induced cancers in the oral cavity). Other second cancers are bilateral disease in the breast, which occurs in up to 20% of women over a 30-year follow-up, and multicentric disease in the colon, which develops frequently during the follow-up after the first cancer. Patients in this group are strong candidates for curative treatment and often tolerate their later cancer well. They are seasoned fighters in the battle against their malignancy and are some of the best participants in volunteer programs to help others with newly diagnosed cancer. This group will probably increase in size as more people are cured of their first cancer and as they live longer.

Patients in the last group present incurable disease at the onset and require palliative and supportive therapy to correct the complications caused by their cancer. It is often difficult for these individuals to accept their diagnosis. Such patients should always be offered worthwhile treatment modalities if there is a high probability of response. The aim should be to help the patient live a normal life as long as possible at reasonable cost. Discomfort can usually be reduced and suffering minimized. Multidisciplinary care is especially appropriate for patients in this group.

Treating the Individual

Each cancer site presents a unique problem related to the function of the anatomy, including physiologic and cosmetic changes. The problems of a woman who loses a breast will differ from those of a man who loses his rectum. Skin cancer is rarely a significant problem unless it is very advanced; it is easily treated with minimal cost and often without hospitalization. In contrast, cancer of the pancreas is almost never curable, has a fairly rapid progression, and is often associated with severe nutritional problems and pain. The experiences of the vast majority of people with cancer fall somewhere between these extremes.

The need for individualization, both in treatment and in support systems, cannot be overemphasized. Some guidelines to follow include:

1. The patient has the right to accept or refuse offered treatment. (If the patient is a child, the parents should have this right.)

2. The patient should be respected in his or her desire to discuss their illness with others.

3. The rehabilitation team should help remove the stigma of cancer as a "dread disease" by encouraging optimism when appropriate.

4. The patient should be treated as an individual rather than as someone with cancer.

The Psychosocial Impact of Cancer and Cancer Treatment

Understanding the Meaning of Cancer to the Patient

Patients with cancer experience the disease's impact in many different ways and at many different times. Nevertheless, as a group they share some common, important concerns: the threatened loss of life; the threat posed by the disease to the patient's relationships with others; fears about loss of independence, job, and career; and concern about the integrity of their body and its functions. These fears, centering first on the threat to life itself and then on the quality of life, constitute the basic meaning of cancer for the patient. A patient's age and the extent to which the disease threatens life goals and activities modify that meaning. To an older person, cancer may predominantly mean becoming a burden to others in the course of a serious illness; for a younger patient, the disease threatens career, sexuality, and family life. Older individuals may display greater depression, while younger ones may show more anger and be less cooperative as an expression of their anger. At any age, disruption of function, even when temporary, becomes disturbing if it involves valued life activities or forces a change in goals.

Each individual's reactions to his or her cancer and treatment should be viewed as a sequence of related events. The sequence begins with the first appearance of symptoms. It continues through the realization that the diagnosis is cancer, to treatment, convalescence, and cure—or recurrence and death. Predicting a patient's reactions is very difficult and requires considerable knowledge of the individual's basic behavior patterns and of his or her ability to develop compensatory patterns.

Patients' behavior and emotions are usually appropriate to their view of what is happening and are designed to minimize or repair the damage of events. For example, delay in seeking help may be the patient's way of averting injury. Many who suspect cancer procrastinate in seeking care, maintaining that their symptoms are not real. They deny their symptoms to avoid the anxiety that acknowledging them would produce. People most likely to delay seeking help are those whose attitudes toward cancer are characterized by shame, guilt, or extreme fear; the elderly; those with a family history of cancer; those who are uneducated or have a language barrier; and those who have no personal physician.

Some patients interpret their illness as a sign of personal weakness or failure. Others believe that their stressful lives caused their disease, or that it is a punishment for some past wrongdoing. Such feelings may be compounded by friends' and families' uneasiness in dealing with cancer, leading to increased isolation of the patient.

Stress

In a paper written in 1951 that has become a classic in the cancer literature, Arthur Sutherland[2] emphasized that a cancer patient is a person under a special and severe form of stress: the threat of a disabling disease, mutilation or loss by surgery of an important body part, or death. Stress caused by cancer can disrupt important patterns of adaptation, defined by Sutherland as the beliefs and behavior designed to bring the individual's physical and emotional needs into harmony with the demands of the environment. When such patterns are threatened, much anxiety is generated, and patients may believe that they are unable to meet environmental demands or fulfill their emotional needs. A loss of self-esteem commonly results.

In a 1979 study conducted by the California Division of the American Cancer Society,[3] the time period immediately following diagnosis was reported as the highest period of stress for 30.5% of patients. The period of hospitalization and initial treatment was the most upsetting for 16.7%; 11.1% reported release from the hospital as the most stressful. Some who had coped well with stress during the diagnosis and treatment phases experienced a delayed reaction 6 months or more after the end of treatment. They expressed this reaction by depression or heavy drinking.

Stress is also due to the uncertain outcome after cancer treatment. The person who has had cancer is a life-long patient, subject to the continuing threat of recurrence, to complications of the treatment, and to sequelae from altered anatomy and physiology. Some individuals are unable to overcome concern about their illness and remain physically and psychologically uncomfortable whenever the disease is discussed, even when treatment has been successful. Others are afraid to return to their normal activities and withdraw to their home environments.

The Patient's Treatment Concerns

The average patient knows little about radiation therapy before the treatment is recommended, and almost all patients have strong preconceived notions, some of which are erroneous. For example, many patients believe that radiation treatment will cause hair loss over their entire body, even though only one area is being treated. They are understandably apprehensive about nausea, skin effects, loss of energy and appetite, and, depending on the site treated, may be concerned about dysphagia, cough, diarrhea, urinary frequency, or other problems. In addition to these fears, the coldness of the radiation room often conveys feelings of isolation, even of danger, and the sight of others who are much sicker than they leads to an expectation that the treatment will be very hard to bear.

Most patients are extremely fearful of chemotherapy. They associate the drugs with major side effects such as nausea, vomiting, diarrhea, and harm to the hemopoietic and immune systems. Many assume that it is never helpful or curative because they have known patients whose chemotherapy has not cured their cancer. Simply approaching the facility where the medications will be administered induces anticipatory nausea in many patients. Anxiety due to the disease process combined with anxiety about the treatment often causes patients to fail to complete treatment as planned. The lay public frequently advises the cancer patient that chemotherapy is dangerous and that alternative treatments that have less toxicity and a guaranteed cure are available for the asking.

Although surgery cures more cancer than any other modality of treatment, patients often look for an alternative in order to avoid disfigurement. Many associate cancer surgery with the word "radical," despite the fact that most procedures are far less radical than in the past. Those patients who believe that surgeons are all-powerful and that all cancers can be totally removed with surgery are equally misguided.

Depression

Two great myths about cancer and depression are in desperate need of debunking. The first is that all cancer patients are depressed. Numerous studies have shown that not all cancer patients are depressed, and those that are, exhibit widely varying degrees of depression. The second myth is that cancer patients should be depressed, and therefore, treatment is unnecessary. The ramifications of untreated depression in cancer patients range from lack of treatment compliance to suicide. Depression in cancer patients can and should be treated. An understanding of what is meant by "depression," how to assess it, and how to treat it are essential to the comprehensive care of many cancer patients.

Depression involves feelings of sadness, grief, hopelessness, and helplessness. Some level of sadness and grief are normal responses to cancer diagnosis and treatment. It is the degree of these feelings and their manifestations that distinguish between normal adaptation and normal depression. This is not a dichotomy but rather a continuum ranging from sadness to depressed mood in reaction to diagnosis and treatment (ie, adjustment disorder with depressed mood) to major depression.

Approximately 6% of the general population[4] suffers from major depression. Therefore, approximately 6% of cancer patients may be assumed to have a preexisting disorder that predisposes them to greater levels of depression during their course of cancer. However, the trauma generated by cancer diagnosis and treatment may manifest itself by depression in those not so pre-disposed.

Numerous studies have been done[5] to determine the actual incidence of depression in cancer patients. Differing methodologies, including lack of predefined diagnostic criteria and the use of patients with different diagnoses, prognoses, and stage of disease, have resulted in reports of depression from 4.5% to 58% of cancer patients.

Derogatis and colleagues[6] found that 47% of 215 patients from three centers met the criteria for a psychiatric disorder. However, only 13% of these patients actually had a major affective disorder (ie, depression). Sixty-eight percent had an adjustment disorder with a depressed or anxious mood. Eight percent of the remaining patients with psychiatric disorder had organic mental disorder, 7% had personality disorder, and 4% had anxiety disorder.

Taking all of these studies into account, it is now generally assumed that at least 25% of all cancer patients will meet criteria for adjustment disorder with depressed mood or major depression.[7] Interestingly, studies have shown that cancer patients are no more likely to suffer from depression than other equally seriously ill medical patients.[7]

Several factors have been identified that may significantly increase a patient's vulnerability to depression. These include a history of depression in either the patient or the family, a history of alcoholism, advanced cancer, or cancers at any stage that have an exceptionally poor prognosis such as pancreatic cancer.[8] In addition, patients with poorly controlled pain are highly likely to be depressed.[9] Many cancer patients who are suicidal may be so due to severe uncontrolled pain (or the anticipation of such agonizing pain) and may actually be helped psychologically simply by treating their pain effectively. Further, a common side effect of some cancer treatment drugs (eg, vinblastine, vincristine, procarbazine) as well as other commonly prescribed medicines (eg, steroids/hormones, certain hypertensive medications, and barbiturates) is depression.[9,10] Finally, some researchers now believe that some cancers themselves may secrete or cause the secretion of substances that cause depression.

Not surprisingly, physical status appears to have the strongest correlation to clinical depression.[11] Depression in physically healthy people is usually manifested in symptoms of loss of appetite, weight, energy, interest in sex, and psychomotor skills, as well as inability to sleep. Since all of these symptoms may also occur as a result of cancer and/or its treatment, the diagnosis of depression in this population has to rely more on reports of the severity of the depressed mood, feelings of hopelessness, helplessness, and guilt, low self-esteem, loss of interest(s), concentration problems, as well as suicidal ideation.[12]

All cancer patients should be treated in an emotionally supportive manner by all of the health professionals with whom they interact. Providing patients with information and support continuously throughout the course of their cancer may go a long way towards preventing the development of adjustment disorder and/or major depression. However, should such conditions develop, a combination of relatively short-term psychotherapy and pharmacologic therapy should prove effective in most cases. In a very few cases electroconvulsive therapy (ECT) may be effective.[5] The psychological care of depressed cancer patients should be managed by a competent psychiatrist who is familiar with the many aspects of cancer as well as the various forms of therapy that are available and compatible with cancer treatment. Good communication between the cancer team and the psychiatrist is essential.

Psychological Impact on the Family

Serious illness in one family member causes stress in all. Children are particularly vulnerable, and their anxieties may be expressed in ways that are not obviously related to the illness in the family.

Children of Cancer Patients

Children of cancer patients can be profoundly affected by the parental experiences with diagnosis and treatment of cancer. Children often believe that they are the cause of their parent's cancer.[13] This emerges from the naturally ambivalent feelings of children toward their parents ("I love you/I hate you"). Such feelings are accentuated during a parent's illness, the child being fearful and loving as well as irritated, disappointed, and angry. The treating physician can help the parents reassure the children that they had no responsibility for causing the cancer.

In a large-scale study of children of cancer patients, the children's problems were found to have been minimized by the overwhelmed parents during the illness, and the children were essentially invisible to the medical staff. These children were noted to have increased symptoms of vegetative disturbance (sleep disorders, eating disorders, mood/affect disorders), school problems, and acting-out/behavioral disturbances during the parental illness.[14] The physician can intervene in this situation during the rehabilitation period by asking the parents how the child is coping and adapting, listening for target symptoms in children, and if those target symptoms are noted, referring the family for professional mental health intervention. Table 37-1 lists the symptoms in pre-adolescents and adolescents and identifies the potential need for referral and absolute need for referral to a psychologist or psychiatrist.

Another common problem for children of cancer patients is role reversal, where the parent turns to the child, or more likely to the adolescent, for support and comfort.[15,16] Role reversal impedes the normal development of the adolescent toward appropriately separating from the parents and developing love interests outside the family. The physician can identify such a pattern and intervene to reinforce appropriate roles for children and encourage normal separations. Parents who are over-dependent on their young children can be referred for professional psychological help or possibly to a support group where adult-to-adult support is obtainable.

Daughters of breast cancer patients who are genetically at risk may overly identify with their sick parent. A recent study showed several variables to define daughters of breast cancer patients at highest emotional risk.[17] These variables included daughters who were adolescent at the time of her mother's diagnosis, daughters whose mothers were terminally ill or who died of breast cancer, or daughters whose mothers were overly dependent on the child for support. In these cases the daughter became the "mother's mother" emotionally. The physician should refer such a family to a child guidance department or clinic. Without professional intervention, these children may suffer sexual dysfunction, unresolved grief, and severe breast-focused anxiety.

Spousal Relationships

When the relationship between spouses has been strong, patients can expect continuing sympathy and support. A weak marriage may be disrupted by anxiety that seems intolerable, but some marriages become stronger under the stress of a spouse's cancer. When a child has cancer, stress on the parents results in a greater than 50% probability that the marriage will dissolve.

A significant number of cancer patients (47 out of 567 in this study) reported sexual problems with their partners. Fear and misunderstanding often lead to impotence, frigidity, or loss of libido. When a partner has gynecologic cancer, fear of contagion can make sexual relations very difficult. Abdominal perineal resection with a colostomy is associated with a high incidence of impotence. In other cases, there may be

Table 37-1. Behaviors of Children of Cancer Patients Indicating Need for Psychological Intervention

Developmental Phase	Behavior or Concern
Pre-Adolescence	Potential Need for Referral
	Sudden learning problems
	Distractibility
	Episodes of sadness
	Sleep problems
	Appetite problem
	Some withdrawal from peers/playing
	Absolute Need for Referral
	Cruelty to animals
	Fire setting
	Stealing
	Loss of toilet training (if previously established)
	Refusal to go to school
	Chronic sleep problems
	Chronic eating disorder (anorexia, obesity)
	Sudden aggression toward peers
	Serious withdrawal
	Somatic identification with sick parent
	Suicidal ideation
Adolescence	Potential Need for Referral
	Same as pre-adolescent
	Absolute Need for Referral
	Stealing
	Drug abuse
	Promiscuity
	Running away episodes
	Persistent somatic identification with sick parent
	Suicidal ideation
	Chronic sleep, eating, grooming problems
	Rage reactions

an actual sexual deficit caused by either the tumor or its treatment. Many patients are reluctant to discuss sexual problems with their physicians, but the sooner such problems are identified and addressed, the better the chance for resolution.

Other marital problems that commonly result from cancer include anger engendered by the diagnosis, financial burdens, neglect by the spouse, drinking or gambling or frequent absences on the part of the spouse, and the fear of contagion.

Effect of Cancer on Other Relationships

A patient who is without spouse or family usually has a greater need for supportive care than one with family support. Family members can be of great help to the patient in adjusting psychologically to diagnosis, treatment, and disability, and in ensuring compliance with treatment. A supportive family can also do much to prevent the seeking of multiple second opinions and unproven treatments. However, the presence of family members does not in itself mean that the patient is not isolated; some patients choose not to "burden" others with their fears and concerns, some find it very difficult to talk to anyone about their illness.

In the American Cancer Society study,[3] 23.2% (N=810) of patients and 35.2% of families reported that patients' roles in the household changed as a result of their cancer. The changes reported most frequently were: a diminished role as a homemaker (119); loss of the role of breadwinner, either partially or entirely (94); inability to fill the role of companion, usually to a spouse (76); and a diminution of the parenting role (35). Adverse effects on household roles were more common in the lower than in the higher income groups.

Friends can provide a cancer patient with much needed emotional support. Unfortunately, they sometimes abandon the patient, perhaps because they fear contagion, or because they assume that a bad lifestyle led to the illness, or because their own sense of security is threatened by the disease.

Sexual Problems in Cancer Rehabilitation

Human sexuality is usually impacted by the diagnosis and treatments of cancer. The main concept for the physician in rehabilitation is that sexual feelings and function can resume after treatment. Sometimes these feelings and functions return in different behavioral patterns, and often barriers must be removed to allow this area of human nature to be expressed.

Tumor sites in men that are associated with sexual dysfunction include prostate cancer, penile cancer, and testicular cancer. Without rehabilitation approximately 85% to 90% of men with prostate cancer suffer erectile impotence secondary to surgery or radiation—this is due to nerve trauma and fibrosis of the pelvic vasculature.[18] Studies have shown younger men treated for testicular cancer can have distress after treatment related to retrograde ejaculation, decreased pleasure with orgasm, and increased rates of erectile dysfunction.[19]

Parallel tumor sites for women include breast, cervical, ovarian, and vulvar cancers. Impaired sexual response for a large number of breast cancer patients usually occurs several months after surgery rather than at the time of surgery.[20]

Another important issue in sexual rehabilitation is the reluctance of patients to discuss treatment-related sexual problems with their physician. A study of cervical cancer patients showed that while 80% desired more information from their doctors, 75% said they were reluctant to raise the issue.[21] It is the responsibility of the physician to ask the patient about sexual functioning after treatment.

Special issues must be addressed in sexual rehabilitation of the young or single patient. Young patients often lack basic information about sexuality. The single patient is burdened by facing dating and mate selection while often feeling like "damaged goods" because they have been treated for cancer. These patients frequently have lowered self-esteem after treatment leading to withdrawal from dating and sex. They are afraid to tell dates about their cancer and its effects on sensuality and body image.[22]

The physician in post-treatment evaluation needs to assess six basic areas in sexual rehabilitation. These include (1) chief complaint; (2) sexual status—what is the nature of sexual functioning?; (3) medical status including cancer treatment status; (4) psychiatric status looking for clinical depression and anxiety; (5) family and psychosexual history—are these new or old problems? and (6) in couples, relationship assessment—how has the patient's partner responded to the cancer and its treatments?[23]

The following are guidelines for the physician in sexual rehabilitation after cancer treatment:

1. Take a complete sexual history including the quality of the patient's sexual activity. Avoidance of this topic by the rehabilitation team is the chief obstacle toward satisfactory sexual functioning.

2. Include the partner in sessions whenever possible.

3. Convey a positive message—some form of sexual expression is always possible. Offer information, reassurance, support, and hope.

4. Perform a thorough work-up to diagnose any associated medical or treatment-related conditions impeding sexual functioning.

5. Counsel with simple, direct suggestions.

6. Refer to a sex therapist for persistent sexual problems.[22]

Several medications that are used during or after cancer treatment may affect sexual response. These include: hormones, antihypertensives, antidepressants, narcotics, diuretics, and adrenergic-receptor blockers. If the patient is experiencing drug-related sexual dysfunction, the treating oncologist should be consulted to determine if the offending drug can be eliminated or the dosage lowered.

Physician-Patient Communication and Support

Cancer forces major changes in normal functioning and brings with it a wide variety of psychological problems and problems in living. Mobility and physical functioning are reduced; work and family roles are altered; needs for emotional and social support increase. Patients experience fear, uncertainty about the future, loss of self-esteem, high stress levels, disability, and pain. Good communication between patient and physician will bring such problems to light. In such cases this communication helps to reduce fears and anxiety, assist the patient in completing treatment, counter feelings of isolation, and correct misconceptions. Poor physician-patient communication, on the other hand, gives rise to anxiety, leading to poor compliance and often resulting in incomplete or inadequate treatment. The physician who is not sensitive to the patient's increasing anxiety may lose the patient's trust and hope. Such a patient may, in desperation, seek help from unproven treatments. The physician should not hesitate to call on the other medical and paramedical personnel who make up the treatment team for assistance.

Most patients will benefit psychologically by having an accurate conceptual framework with which to understand their cancer and assist them in making decisions about their treatment. Patient education is basically the responsibility of the physician, whether specialist or primary care physician. The primary care physician often has the advantage of a relationship with the patient and family that spans a number of years and a knowledge of their emotional strengths and weaknesses, as well as their other medical problems.

Patients should be told the truth about their condition, realistically but optimistically. Few patients are better off not knowing the facts or being deceived or knowing less than the full truth. Lies are invariably exposed, and the patient who has been lied to will be unable to give the physician the trust that is essential for maximum cooperation. Frank, open discussion is mandatory. Such discussions should be conducted with patience and understanding; explanations should be clear, and patients should be given as much (or as little) honest medical information as they desire. An essential part of good management rests with the physician's availability to answer questions at any time during the course of the illness.

There should be no discrepancy between the facts presented to the patient and those given to the family. The best way to accomplish this is to provide information to the family and patient together. Families sometimes claim that patients should be protected from the truth because they "won't be able to handle it." However, in such situations it is usually the family members who cannot deal with the facts.

It is characteristic of supportive families to encourage and maintain close communication with both the patient and the doctor about the disease and therapy. Many physicians support this process by including a family member—or other person significant to the patient—in all their discussions with the patient about his or her illness. This approach encourages further discussion in the physician's absence, eliminates suspicion of secrets, and makes misunderstandings less likely.

Presenting the diagnosis requires sensitivity and some knowledge of the patient's ability to handle stress. It may be useful to use the word "tumor" initially, saving "cancer" for later in the discussion or for a later meeting. Often only a portion of the information given at the first meeting is absorbed because of the emotional upheaval created by the diagnosis and the feared outcome. Patients need help in understanding the implications of the diagnosis and in dealing with fear.

For most patients, cancer treatment is a new experience. Unless plans and procedures are explained as often as necessary, fear and anxiety will increase for both the patient and the family. Nurses and technicians should reinforce educational efforts daily. Support mechanisms are essential throughout the course of treatment to control side effects, maintain nutritional status, and preserve hope. Under no circumstances should technicians or laboratory personnel make remarks that could be interpreted to mean that the patient's situation is hopeless.

A period of emotional turmoil generally follows patients' acceptance of their diagnosis. Anxiety, depression, insomnia, lack of appetite, and poor concentration should be expected; patients may also be unable to carry out the activities of daily living. Many patients express anger at what has happened to them and ask "Why me?" In most cases these problems gradually ease as treatment plans are developed and the patient gains confidence that there may be a solution to the threat of an aggressor disease.

Counseling focusing on issues of self-respect and self-image may be indicated when patients believe that their illnesses are caused by a weakness in their own characters. Depression should be treated in order to minimize sequelae such as drinking or feelings of general tiredness. Serious emotional deterioration is unusual, but an earlier psychiatric disturbance may be reactivated.

The majority of people cope with cancer fairly well, but at least 20% of hospitalized patients have significant emotional distress. A battery of psychological tests is not necessary to determine which patients might be expected to have difficulty handling illness-associated crises. Careful attention to what the patient says and a review of his or her past medical experiences will often give clues to anticipated problems. Psychological disturbances in patients undergoing cancer treatment include depression, anxiety, and central nervous system dysfunction. Some disturbances are due to analgesic agents, steroids, or chemotherapy agents that cause electrolyte imbalance, hypercalcemia, or altered brain function.

Some patients require mild antianxiety medications to help them through crises. The severely depressed or extremely anxious patient may need psychiatric care, especially from a professional skilled in the problems of cancer patients.

Oncology nurses today are also often skilled in giving psychological and emotional support to the patient, and are in an excellent position to alleviate families' anxieties. Counseling by a volunteer from a support group is especially useful to those patients who must make major physical and emotional adjustments to their illness. A patient with a *stoma*, for example, often finds that talking with an ostomate allays many apprehensions.

Follow-up of the Treated Cancer Patient

Good physician-patient communication is as essential in the follow-up period as in the initial treatment phase. Continued follow-up and monitoring for recurrence should be mandatory because those patients with a history of the disease are the people most commonly affected by it in the form of a second or third cancer. Moreover, delayed effects of radiation therapy and chemotherapy often become apparent in the follow-up period, and dysfunction may occur after surgical treatment and require surgical intervention.

All patients are anxious when coming for checkups, and many experience significant anxiety about recurrence for years after they have been cured, despite freedom from any sign of the disease. Living with uncertainty is one of the most troublesome psychological problems associated with cancer; adaptation requires flexible adjustment to day-to-day changes and emotional fluctuations. Patients need the physician's constant reassurance that the disease is controlled or cured, in order to go on with their lives.

Terminal Stage

When a patient has advanced progressive cancer and has failed to respond to definitive local and systemic treatment, it is unlikely that further traditional therapy will be of benefit. The physician must then tell the patient and the family that attempts at heroic treatment are unwise and that the goal should now be relief of distressing symptoms.

Communication with patient and family must be maintained through the final stages of the illness. Some patients wish to be told when death is near, some do not, and some know without being told. Physicians and members of the support team can greatly aid a patient's psychological adaptation to approaching death.

The physician should raise the question of resuscitation with the patient and family ahead of any imminent need. A decision not to resuscitate must be based on the patient's beliefs and value systems. A living will may provide pertinent evidence of the wishes of a patient who is no longer competent; if such a document does not exist, the decision remains with the patient's family or surrogate. Resuscitation should never be withheld simply because a patient has a terminal illness.

Some physicians find it very difficult to continue to treat a terminally ill patient; abandonment is not uncommon. This may be because physicians' training prepares them poorly for the supportive role that they must provide cancer patients.

Financial Concerns for the Patient

Cancer care continues to be ever more costly, notwithstanding an increasing trend toward early discharge from the hospital and outpatient treatment. Patients often experience major economic stress due to the cost of treatment, loss of earning power, and physical or emotional disability.

More than 16% of patients sampled in the California study[3] felt less secure financially as a result of their illness. There was a correlation between the proportion with financial concerns and income. When family income was less than $15,000 a year, it was often difficult to meet the needs of the household. Pre-illness lifestyles could not be maintained, and dependents were affected in 13% of the patients sampled. This was more common in lower income and younger age groups.

Health insurance is a significant factor in reducing cancer's financial impact. Of those in this study, only 40% reported that all hospital and medical costs were covered by insurance.

Among those who were employed at the time of this study, almost 20% were apprehensive that their cancer would adversely affect fringe benefits. Others reported that their disease effectively locked them into their current jobs.

A Patient's Right to Employment

Patients with cancer should have the same opportunity for employment befitting their skills, training, and experience as an individual with no cancer history. They should not have to accept jobs that they would not have considered before their illness solely because of a cancer history. Hiring, promotion, and treatment in the workplace should depend on ability and qualifications and should not be affected by a history of cancer.

Those cancer patients who return to work usually have adapted to treatment and disability. They often have stronger support systems than those who cannot continue working.

Sections 503 and 504 of the Federal Rehabilitation Act of 1973 provide that employment discrimination is illegal, but many workers are not covered by this act. Forty-seven states have statutes related to the employment of people with various illnesses; some of these statutes are cancer specific. It is unfortunate that a cancer patient's ability to continue employment or to gain new employment without discrimination must so often depend on legislation.[24]

Employment Discrimination

Cancer survivors have experienced discrimination in the workplace because cancer is often perceived as a fatal disease. Employers are also reluctant to take a chance on a cancer survivor because they may believe that cancer survivors will not be able to do their job and because of the increasing costs of fringe benefits, including health insurance. While employment discrimination continues to exist, it is less frequent than in the past, primarily because of public education.

Legally, the cancer patient can now rely on new legislation to overcome employment discrimination. The Americans with Disabilities Act (ADA) became effective on July 26, 1992, and could be a milestone in overcoming employment discrimination against cancer survivors. The ADA expands the protection of sections 503 and 504 of the Federal Rehabilitation Act of 1973 by including *all* employers with 25 employees or more. As of July 26, 1994 businesses with 15 to 24 employees must follow these employment provisions.

Under the ADA, all cancer survivors are considered legally "disabled." The ADA is a federal civil rights law that requires that disabled people be given the same chances and opportunities as the able-bodied. The law provides that employers cannot discriminate against persons with a disability in any phase of employment—hiring, training, job assignment, classification, promotion, transfer, benefits, leave of absence, layoff, or termination. The ADA is *not* an affirmative action statute—there are no quotas or goals for hiring the disabled.

The ADA applies to any qualified individual with a disability who can perform the essential functions of the job regardless of whether the job applicant needs a reasonable accommodation from the employer. Most important for cancer survivors, the ADA protects an individual with a record of impairment. Every cancer survivor has a record of substantial impairment, so this law applies to them for the rest of their lives. The ADA protects cancer survivors whether the cancer is cured, controlled, or in remission.

The cancer patient cannot be asked and does not have to disclose any disability that would affect job performance. There need be no explanation of gaps in the employment history.

When a disabled person applies for a job, he or she should be aware of their rights under the law. If a test is part of the job application, the applicant is allowed to ask for a reasonable accommodation because of the disability.

Eight agencies will enforce the ADA. The four most important for the cancer patient are: the Equal Employment Opportunity Commission (1-800-669-4000), the Department of Justice (1-800-347-4283), the Department of Health and Human Services (1-800-368-1019), and the Department of Education (1-800-572-5580).

Legal action against employment discrimination seems to be more frequent each year and is increasingly successful.

Supportive Services

Supportive services are those that assist patients and their families in handling the many emotional, physical, and practical problems that follow the diagnosis and treatment of cancer. Supportive and referral services are usually offered initially as the patient is being admitted to the hospital for the first course of treatment. At this time it is possible to start defining concerns and setting a course of action.

In the California study,[3] supportive and referral services were rated "somewhat inadequate" to "grossly inadequate." Of those surveyed, 27% received literature about cancer and its treatment; 22% met with other cancer patients; 20% received visits from volunteers who themselves had cancer; 14% had visits from social workers; 12% had the services of a psychologist or psychiatrist. Only 9% of family members received psychological help. One fourth of the patients used no support service due to lack of knowledge of the service or rejection of the service offered. An overwhelming majority of patients stated that services, if available, could have been used at the time of diagnosis and treatment. Patients and families agreed that support to family members from medical personnel in times of crisis would be desirable.

The service most often reported as necessary (22% of the patients) was daily home assistance. This need was seen as a continuing one, although with time it became less important. Whether this type of assistance was available was not related to ability to pay. Other service needs were marital or family counseling (1% to 3%); psychological counseling (5% to 10%); nursing care (4% to 7%); child care (2.5%); a live-in homemaker (1% to 5%); financial aid (4% to 6%);

transportation (1.6%); financial planning (2.3%); and yard work or repairs (1% to 2%). Ranges are included in the above figures because additional assistance is usually acute at the time of diagnosis and early treatment, decreasing thereafter. The need for financial assistance, however, does not decrease with time.

Hotlines for information and services are provided by the American Cancer Society (1-800-ACS-2345), the cancer information services of the Comprehensive Cancer Centers (1-800-FOR-CANCER), and community agencies. The questions received by the University of California at Los Angeles cancer hotline indicating the type and relative frequency of the psychosocial concerns of cancer patients and their families are listed in Table 37-2.

Table 37-2. Relative Frequency of Psychosocial Concerns (N = 1,071)

Rank	Concerns	Frequency	%
1	Referral to support group	210	19.6
2	Anxiety/fear associated with illness	190	17.7
3	Family problems associated with illness	133	12.4
4	Patient-physician relationships	110	10.3
5	Sadness/depression associated with illness	105	9.8
6	Financial demands of illness	91	8.5
7	Death-related feelings, thoughts	82	7.6
8	Unproven methods/compliance	63	5.9
9	Coping with treatment and side effects	63	5.9
10	Referral to professional psychotherapy	56	5.2

Personal written communication, 1989, Helene Brown, UCLA Cancer Center, Office of Cancer Communication.

Support Groups for Cancer Patients

The emotional support offered by specialized groups can be especially helpful to cancer patients. Many different types of support groups are available to cancer patients. The goals of these groups are fourfold: (1) decrease the patient's sense of alienation by talking to others in a similar situation, (2) reduce anxiety about the treatments, (3) assist in clarifying misperceptions and misinformation, and (4) lessen feelings of isolation, helplessness, and neglect by others.[25] Support groups are designed to help the patient feel less helpless and hopeless, and perhaps take more responsibility for planning and/or complying with medical regimens. The public is aware of the many therapeutic interventions for cancer patients, and with the popularity of some approaches (such as hypnosis and guided imagery), patients may often specifically request such services. The four most common forms of intervention groups are education, behavioral training (ie, stress management), problem-solving and coping skills, and psychological support. In addition, self-help groups have expanded and grown tremendously in the past decade.

Education

Educational intervention groups provide information about the disease and about health-enhancing behaviors such as diet and exercise. Educational information is especially important during the diagnosis and treatment phase of cancer, when patients generally have a lot of unanswered questions and concerns. In general, education alone is often insufficient to change attitudes or improve coping skills.[26] However, education coupled with counseling has been shown to decrease depression, hostility, and anxiety.[27]

Behavioral Training

Behavioral training groups consist of stress management and relaxation training such as hypnosis, deep muscle relaxation, and guided imagery. Patients are taught relaxation techniques to help reduce their anxiety and stress levels. Chemotherapy patients have used behavioral training to help decrease the side-effects from the drug treatments. In fact, relaxation training and hypnosis have been described as effective in reducing nausea, emotional distress, and physiologic arousal following chemotherapy.[28,29]

Problem-Solving and Coping Skills

Teaching patients how to effectively cope with the stress and anxiety associated with the diagnosis and treatment of cancer is a very important component of the support group process. The Omega Project at the Harvard Medical School originally developed problem-solving interventions for cancer patients. The Omega Project found that highly distressed patients used fewer coping strategies, employed less effective ones, had more problems and concerns, and achieved poor resolutions when attempting to solve critical illness-related concerns.[30,31] An important aim of the coping skills component is to increase the patient's awareness of what Weisman[32] termed the key ingredients of good coping: optimism (the expectation of positive change), practicality (learning that options and alternatives are seldom completely exhausted), flexibility (changing strategies to reflect the changing nature of perceived problems), and resourcefulness (developing the ability to obtain additional information and support to strengthen coping).

Psychological Support

Support groups provide psychological support on two levels—from the professional group leader(s) and from the group members themselves. There is some evidence to suggest that social support groups are associated with better psychosocial adjustment to illness.[27,33-38] Professional group leaders can help patients cope with their cancer by being aware of the many behavioral, cognitive, emotional, and social issues faced by patients at each disease stage, allowing each patient to communicate openly about his or her own issues and fears, listening to these concerns, assuring the patient that his or her feelings are normal, sharing information about the successful coping efforts of other patients, and referring patients to a psychologist or psychiatrist for intensive therapy if other interventions fail to provide sufficient help.[39]

Self-Help Groups

The endurance of self-help groups as a phenomenon highlights the powerful healing nature of these groups. Self-help groups can be defined as groups of patients and/or family members who meet and exchange common experiences, provide mutual help and support, share in the collective group spirit, exchange information, and develop coping mechanisms for constructive action toward shared goals.[40] These groups are led by a group facilitator who is not a mental health professional.

Being part of a group of people with similar stresses has great healing potential. Sharing common experiences creates a special atmosphere of understanding and caring. Group members are encouraged to express feelings and viewpoints and to help each other cope. In addition, these groups serve as a safe environment in which to adjust to the lifestyle changes caused by cancer.

Home Care

Cost-containment issues have limited hospitalization time and have made it essential that home care assume a greater role in the management of the cancer patient. Creative coordination of home care and outpatient care can result in a significant decrease in the amount of time a patient is disabled, in an earlier return to work, and a better quality of life. The first 3 months following hospital discharge are a critical period during which problems tend to be most severe, but in many cases good home care can prevent rehospitalization.

In a randomized trial to evaluate home nursing care for patients with progressive lung cancer,[41] patients cared for by oncology nurses, rather than those who had regular home care nurses or office nurses, showed better control of symptoms and reduced rehospitalization. Reasons for rehospitalization included bleeding and infection, further treatment, palliation, and diagnostic workups. A major finding in this study was that a large number of complications and rehospitalizations occur over a 6-month period.

Parenteral nutrition, pain control, performance of activities of daily living, and physical therapy can be provided by many home health care services, without jeopardizing rehabilitation. Unfortunately, in many communities such facilities are grossly lacking.

Successful management of cancer requires significant cooperation between health providers and patients' families. Most families can participate in home health care when provided with basic knowledge and some monitoring of their services. Difficulties arise, however, when a patient's spouse is elderly and other family members are not readily available.

Provision for transportation to treatment facilities goes hand-in-hand with home health care. Frequently a patient is rehospitalized when medical care is not available at home and the family is unable to provide transportation to the treatment facility or outpatient service.

Hospice

Hospice is an integral part of the broad spectrum of cancer care. It is defined as an integrated program of appropriate hospital and home care for the patient with a limited life expectancy (usually the eligibility guideline is 6 months or less). The usual goal is to help the patient live as fully as possible for whatever time remains, but not to perform heroic, uncomfortable, or meaningless treatments or procedures. A high degree of skilled professional services is required to provide symptom control. The program provides a physician-directed, nurse-coordinated, interdisciplinary approach to patient care, 24 hours per day, 7 days per week. Medicare will reimburse for hospice care for people over 65 years of age.

Hospice is not necessary for every dying person, but it is an option. Whether or not it is appropriate and acceptable depends largely on the patient's lifestyle, beliefs, and value systems.[42] However, acceptance of hospice services is generally high among seriously ill patients. One of the accomplishments of hospice should be to increase the number of patients who die at home rather than in the hospital, which is now 70% of all Americans.

Approximately 1,500 programs[43] in the US are designated as hospices. Some are free-standing units; others are hospice units within general hospitals; others are consultation teams within medical centers; still others are community-based home care programs. The concept is care, not location.

Much research remains to be done to determine the true role and effectiveness of hospice facilities. One study conducted at the hospice connected with the UCLA Medical Center was reported by Rainey and colleagues.[44] In this study, 115 patients were being treated for cancer, and 74% of them were outpatients at the time. The study showed that there was considerable interest in hospice services among these patients, although almost all expressed a desire to continue their involvement with their personal physicians during the period of hospice care. Their priorities for services are listed in Table 37-3. It is interesting to note that bereavement care, which is an integral part of most hospice programs, was ranked last in importance by the patients.

Because specialization usually leads to improved outcomes, hospice programs can be important in three major areas: better pain control, better psychological support for the patient/family matrix, and improved nursing and supportive services. The hospice milieu gives the family a respite from direct care that allows them to emotionally re-group and take the patient home again if they choose. If the family becomes "burned-out," this can create depression in the patient or other family members, possibly leading to suicide. The use of the team approach including physicians, nurses, and mental health personnel in a hospice can prevent burn-out because it provides a wider base of support than exists in the home-based and confined family.

Table 37-3. Patient Priorities for Hospice Services

Rank	Service
1	Medical control of symptoms
2	Home nursing care
3	Psychological counseling
4	Nutrition evaluation
5	Respite care
6	Spiritual guidance
7	Home support services
8	Legal and financial advice
9	Occupational, physical, and speech therapy
10	Bereavement care

Bereavement

The rehabilitation aspect of hospice is mainly for the family that survives the death. The key issue is bereavement resolution for the survivors. It is estimated that between 5% to 9% of the US population is bereaved annually.[45] How well family members work through their feelings will help determine their long-term mental health. Morbidity and mortality of family members are also affected by death of a loved one. Increases may be seen in psychological distress; physical symptoms, use of health services; and self-medication for distress (alcohol, tobacco, drugs). Mortality is higher in men than in women aged 55 to 74. In women, mortality is the same for those widowed or married. For both women and men, mortality is higher for those living alone, higher moving to a nursing home, but not elevated in the first year after the death occurred.[46]

Role of the Physician

The responsibilities of the physician include identification of the best program and the best patient-family-program match. Some families are so dysfunctional or overwhelmed that they need a break, and the patient should be placed in a hospital facility. Others do very well with a visiting team model. The physician should find out if the program screens patients and families or accepts all referrals. The treating physician should decide whether to continue to care for the patient if it is an option in the program and whether or not the program can realistically fulfill the patient's needs and improve his care.[47]

In summary, the physician should decide whether the hospice experience will facilitate a more peaceful and resolved death than the patient would otherwise have. This is one of the primary goals of cancer care. The physician's responsibility toward the family is helping them feel they did the best possible job of supporting their family member through the dying process. The better they feel about the job they did, the less psychological trauma and scarring remains in the period of bereavement and thereafter. Thus, hospice becomes a potentially powerful tool for reducing post-cancer psychiatric morbidity for the family.

Pastoral Care

Robert Hudnut[48] once described organized religion in America as a "sleeping giant—a collection of individuals who might do a great deal of good in the world if only they would wake up." The involvement of organized religion in cancer care began about 20 years ago when the American Cancer Society started professional education programs for the clergy and produced its first training program. Clergy, as a group, need more education about cancer if they are to have a truly effective role in supportive care.

According to the Reverend Mark Peterson,[49] who works with patients in the Bayfront Medical Center, St. Petersburg, Florida, there are four reasons why cancer facilities and organized religion should work together. First, when people are sick, the goals of medicine and religion are much the same: cure, comfort, and care. Second, although many patients do not practice their religion before or after their hospitalization, once admitted to the hospital they generally become more concerned with spiritual matters. Third, all health care has a moral and ethical dimension. Finally, community religious groups could serve as a valuable resource for practical aid in every community in America.

Volunteer Support Groups

Volunteer support groups aiding in cancer patient rehabilitation fall into two general categories. One has as its primary focus helping cancer patients with the difficult periods of adjustment during and after treatment. The oldest group in this category is the International Association of Laryngectomies, founded in 1952. Its activities include the development of educational materials, assisting patients with speech therapy, and pre- and postoperative counseling. Another group with a similar focus is the Reach to Recovery program of the American Cancer Society. Volunteers in the program are women who have had a mastectomy and have been trained to help others receiving such treatment. Other support groups of this kind are ostomy clubs and the Leukemia Society of America (patients and family members). Volunteers can offer a patient the kind of support that comes only from personal experience with cancer at a specific site.

A second category focuses on broad issues of coping with cancer. Support groups include the American Cancer Society programs I Can Cope and CanSurMount; Make Today Count, another nationwide program for those who have experienced cancer, either themselves or in their families; and Candlelighters, a support organization of parents whose children have had cancer. Additional organizations that offer support programs for cancer patients include the American Red Cross, the Salvation Army, and the YMCA/YWCA.

Some Problems in Palliation

Nutrition

Cancer cachexia is characterized by anorexia, weight loss, early satiety, and asthenia. The common association of weight loss and cancer is the effect of a number of factors including anorexia, primary involvement of the gastrointestinal tract, infection, and tumor growth. A significant loss of taste and an aversion to meat are seen in many patients. Cachexia results in a decrease in caloric intake; depletion of essential nutrients; a decrease in protein, fat, carbohydrate, mineral, and vitamin metabolism; and possibly a tumor-host competition for nutrients.[50]

Not all cancer patients have good nutritional status prior to their diagnosis. For example, patients with oral or esophageal cancer are frequently heavy drinkers; excessive alcohol consumption, if associated with an inadequate food intake, predisposes to significant nutritional deficiencies. Therapy may have to be delayed in patients with a compromised nutritional status.

It is generally agreed that nutrition through the alimentary canal is preferable to intravenous feeding. Numerous commercially available enteral products can supplement or replace a patient's oral diet.

Dietitians can be extremely helpful in evaluating patients' food likes and dislikes and their ethnic preferences, as well as in recognizing the special problems that individuals have with cancer at certain sites. The use of a blender to liquefy an ordinary select diet is valuable for the person with dysphagia. The patient with a bowel obstruction is not a suitable candidate for an oral diet and will need intravenous alimentation.

Total parenteral nutrition (TPN), using central venous access, can create an anabolic state in patients who are incapable of adequate oral food intake, or who have significantly deficient absorption ability from the GI tract. Although expensive, TPN is indispensable in a number of situations, including extreme cachexia and prolonged nausea and vomiting, or where there are alimentary tract fistulas or significant complications from radiation therapy or chemotherapy.

The potential risks of IV hyperalimentation are subclavian vein thrombosis, thrombophlebitis, and sepsis. The risk of these complications may be decreased to about 2% when hyperalimentation is undertaken by a skilled cancer care team.

Pain

For the patient with cancer, pain is the most feared complication of the disease process. However, when current knowledge is applied, pain can be controlled or even eliminated. Fear contributes greatly to the perception of pain; hypnosis, behavioral training, biofeedback, and relaxation training may be useful in such cases.

The goal of pain therapy for patients receiving active treatment is to provide relief sufficient for the tolerance of the necessary diagnostic and therapeutic approaches. In cases of advanced cancer, pain control should be sufficient to allow patients to function at a level of their choosing, or to die relatively free of pain. The oncologist must understand the physiology, pharmacology, and psychology of pain perception; must constantly monitor the effectiveness of treatment; and must change the pain medication as necessary.

The type of pain encountered in the cancer patient varies. Acute cancer pain may be related to the presence of the disease and the therapy that is given. Chronic pain may be associated with progression of the disease or with treatment. Some patients have preexistent chronic pain on which the cancer-related pain is superimposed. Many of those dying of cancer have pain that is controllable, but physicians and nurses may be reluctant to provide drugs in the dosages sufficient to give relief. In cancer patients with a past history of drug addiction, the problem of pain relief is a double one.

Non-narcotic analgesics are the first-line agents for the management of mild-to-moderate cancer pain. Where there is severe pain, these drugs serve to potentiate the effects of narcotic analgesics. Adjuvant analgesic drugs constitute a third group of medications and include several different categories: anticonvulsant drugs, phenothiazines, butyrophenones, tricyclic antidepressants, antihistamines, amphetamines, and steroids.

Some useful guidelines for the use of narcotic analgesics in cancer pain management are:[51]

1. Start with a specific drug, and know its pharmacology.

2. Adjust the route of administration to the patient's needs.

3. Administer the analgesic on a regular basis after initial titration of the dose.

4. Use drug combinations to provide additive analgesic effect.

5. Avoid drug combinations that increase sedation without enhancing analgesia.

6. Anticipate and treat side effects such as sedation, respiratory depression, nausea, vomiting, and constipation.

7. Watch for the development of tolerance; if it develops, switch to an alternative narcotic analgesic.

8. Prevent acute withdrawal.

9. Anticipate and manage complications such as overdose or seizures.

The use of intravenous morphine delivered either as a continual drip or by a patient-administered bolus has increased in the past 15 years. A major barrier to the use of continual infusions in the past was fear that drug addiction would result. However, this is not a serious problem for those who have severe cancer pain and do not have a tendency toward addiction.

Regional blocks were utilized extensively in the past but have gone into disfavor because fewer physicians feel comfortable with, or have had sufficient training in, nerve block administration. There is still a place for this approach. Neurosurgical approaches are also used, but infrequently.

Venous Access

Cancer patients require frequent monitoring of hematologic toxicity, transfusions, and IV alimentation. Venous access is a problem when there is repeated venesection, and the placement of a central line is becoming routine for all people with cancer who need continued therapy. Two choices exist: the standard percutaneous transneedle catheter bedside insertion, or the surgical placement of a tunnelled catheter such as a Broviac, Hickman, or Groshong. These latter catheters seem to be less irritating and appear to have fewer complications. They are mandatory if the venous access is expected to be needed for more than a month's time. Nursing care for these catheters has become routine, and patients can easily be taught to manage them.

Infection

Infection is a major cause of morbidity and mortality among oncologic patients and complicates all forms of treatment. The presence of infection may delay definitive tumor management.

Infection may be associated with diagnostic procedures and antitumor therapy, as well as with the tumor itself. Many cancer patients are immunocompromised, either because of their disease or because of its treatment. The multimodal treatment of cancer may render such patients vulnerable to opportunistic organisms. Nutritional deficits, although not a cause of infection, are often associated with it and influence its outcome. Infections can offset the significant gains that are being made in patient survival.

Gram-negative bacteria are the most significant and common cause of infection in cancer patients. Organisms such as *Pseudomonas* sp, *Bacteroides* sp, *E Coli*, *Klebsiella* sp, and *Proteus* sp are frequently found to be responsible for infections in the lung, alimentary tract, and skin. Fungal infections are commonly caused by *Candida albicans*, *Aspergillus* sp, and *Cryptococcus* sp. Herpesviruses cause a large number of infections, and *Pneumocystis carinii*, a common protozoal parasite, is increasingly responsible for pulmonary infections in leukemia patients and those with AIDS.

Cultures with sensitivity should be done to determine which antibiotic to use to treat infection. While waiting for the cultures to be reported, a combination of carbenicillin and gentamicin should be given. This is considered to be the most effective treatment available at present. Amphotericin B is the most commonly used drug in the treatment of fungal infections. Isolation techniques are indicated when the patient is immunosuppressed.

In about one fourth of the febrile episodes that occur in people with leukopenia, a septicemia is diagnosed on blood culture. Usually the organisms responsible are gram-negative bacilli or other major pathogens, but in some institutions gram-positive bacteria surpass gram-negative bacteria as the most frequent aerobic isolate. Mortality from septicemia generally runs from 20% to 40% but can be much higher when multiple microbial sepsis is present.

Although many patients with venous-access catheters have fever, only rarely does such a catheter need to be removed, providing the appropriate treatment is instituted after blood cultures have established the offending organism.

Unexplained fever is present in about 50% of granulocytopenic patients. Empirical antibiotic therapy is mandatory in the absence of positive blood cultures.

Infection occurs most commonly when the host is compromised due to the cancer treatment. More than 80% of the organisms arise from the patient's endogenous microbial flora, and nearly half of these organisms are acquired during hospitalization. Because many of the organisms for infection require a human vector, hand washing remains the most important preventive procedure. Isolation techniques offer very little protection against newly acquired infection. Total protective environments may be useful in special situations such as bone marrow transplantation.

Much remains to be learned about prevention as well as treatment for some of the more exotic infections that develop in the immunocompromised patient. Members of the oncology team need to consult with an infectious disease specialist about the management of these complex issues.

Blood Products

Blood replacement is more often used in cancer therapy than in the treatment of any other medical condition. Patients with cancer may have anemia because of a depressed marrow production, nutritional deficiencies, cytotoxic chemotherapy, radiation therapy sepsis, chronic illness, or increased red cell destruction such as in hypersplenism. Blood loss may be acute or chronic, due to bleeding from a tumor's raw surface.

The signs and symptoms of anemia include malaise and increased fatigue, tachycardia, dyspnea, or headache. These indications are nonspecific and should not be ascribed to anemia unless other possible causes have been excluded. When deciding whether to transfuse a patient, the total medical picture must be taken into account; in general, the hemoglobin level should be kept at 10g/100c, using packed red cells as necessary in order to maintain adequate oxygenation.

Platelet therapy is used when there is a risk of spontaneous hemorrhage, a risk that is significant when counts drop below 20,000/mm^3. Spontaneous intracranial hemorrhage increases substantially when platelet counts of 10,000/mm^3 or less are present.

Nausea and Vomiting

Nausea and vomiting may be complications of any cancer treatment, whether it is surgery, radiation, or chemotherapy. Prophylactic therapy for vomiting is much more effective than after-the-fact treatment. The physiology of vomiting is now well understood, as is the pharmacology of the numerous drugs that are used for the prevention and treatment of nausea and vomiting. Oral therapy, suppository administration, or intermittent IV therapy can be used in selected patients. The phenothiazines are effective as antiemetic drugs; the dosage must be individualized in each patient, depending on the response. The newest group of antiemetic agents include metoclopramide (Reglan) and ondansetron (Zofran).

Care of the Professional Caregiver

The most serious complication of being a caregiver for cancer patients is burnout. Burnout is a reaction to chronic, job-related stress. It is an emotional state that may be accompanied by a number of physical and behavioral changes. Individuals experiencing burnout have greater rates of divorce, suicide, job turnover, drug and alcohol abuse, caffeine and nicotine addictions, and shorter life expectancy.[52] Patients are in danger of receiving poor quality care and even potentially life-threatening care from a burned-out health care worker. A number of authors have described burnout, but the transactional model is perhaps the most useful (Table 37-4).[53]

Stage I of this process occurs when an individual perceives specific demands as taxing or exceeding his or her resources.[54] Such demands and resources may come from external factors such as the environment, relationships, community, goals, or achievements. There are also internal demands such as self-concept, identity, roles, lifestyle, and developmental issues, as well as beliefs and assumptions.[54] A demand and a resource could be identical depending on the individual and the situation. For instance, one person who has a large family may perceive it to be a demand, since he or she has the financial responsibility to care for it. Another person (or even the same person at another time) might see the same large family as a significant resource in terms of emotional support. There are initial, short-term physical and emotional responses to this appraisal of demand/resource imbalance. Feelings of tension and anxiety as well as fatigue and exhaustion are common at this time.

Stage II involves coping attempts to re-establish a balance between demands and resources. If a balance is not achieved, either because coping behaviors were not instituted or they failed, then burnout occurs.

In *Stage III*, a number of maladaptive coping mechanisms are seen. Along with these are common physical and emotional responses to burnout. The number of these symptoms necessary for a diagnosis of burnout has yet to be determined, but the presence of several of them should be a warning signal of possible burnout. The most serious of these is depression with suicidal ideation. While it is true that major depression may occur without burnout, the depressive illness will decrease the ability of the caregiver to cope with the demands of professional responsibili-

Table 37-4. Model of Burnout

Stage I

Appraisal of External and Internal Demands vs Resources

Demands		BALANCE		Resources
Environment Relationships Community Goals Achievements	←	B A L A N C E	→	Self-Concept Identity Roles Lifestyles Development Beliefs/Assumptions

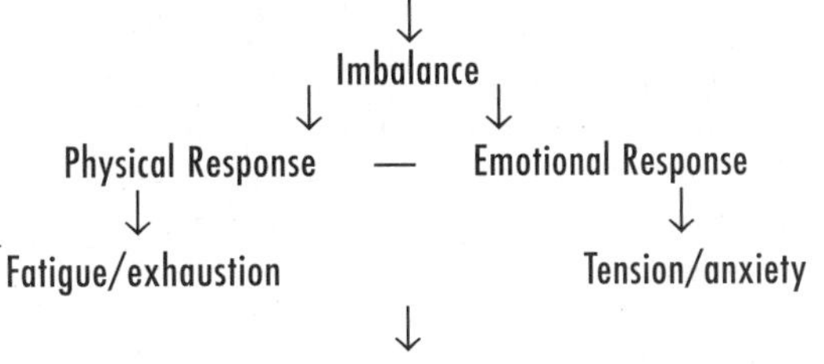

↓

Stage II

Coping Attempts to Re-establish Balance

Unsuccessful	Successful
	(a) Balance restored (b) Responses resolved

↓

Stage III

Burnout

Maladaptive Coping Mechanisms	Adaptive Coping Mechanisms
Cynicism, negativism	Learn and apply principles of stress management
Withdrawal/isolation from coworkers/patients	Participate in support groups (staff support, patient care conferences, patients' family support groups)
Altered work patterns (clock-watching, arrive late/leave early, absenteeism)	Seek appropriate substance abuse treatment
Family conflicts	Seek appropriate family therapy
Uncontrollable crying	
Excessive death watch	
Substance abuse (drugs, alcohol, caffeine, nicotine)	
↓	↓
Responses	(a) Balance restored (b) Responses resolved

Physical	Emotional
Chronic fatigue	Hopelessness
Sleep disorders	Powerlessness
GI disorders	Guilt
Headaches	Detachment
	Depression

ties. If the depressed mood is the reaction to the burnout, it is equally dangerous and threatening to the individual's life and future.

Physician Burnout

Physicians become familiar with the stresses leading to burnout as early as medical school. They may go on to experience "house officer stress syndrome,"[55] at which time they experience episodic cognitive impairment, chronic anger, pervasive cynicism, and family discord. More severe symptoms are major depression, suicidal ideation, and substance abuse. Once in practice, many are disillusioned because instead of the ideal life they envisioned, more stressors await (eg, large numbers of demanding patients, endless paper work, threats of malpractice suits, and a rapid increase in information to learn). A major source of stress for oncology physicians is the daily confrontation with sickness and death. Although much can now be offered to cancer patients, there are always some who will die despite the best efforts of the medical team. Sometimes the morbidity associated with treatment may seriously impair quality of life, forcing both the patient and physician to deal with some serious ethical issues such as when and how much to treat. Physicians are thus forced to face their own mortality and the purpose and meaning of life.

Nurse Burnout

Nurses also experience a great deal of stress that can lead to burnout. Large numbers of patients and meager ancillary support leaves little time for meal and rest breaks, let alone reflective moments or some of the more satisfying aspects of nursing such as patient teaching and support. Many nurses also have to contend with working rotating shifts, holidays, and double shifts due to understaffing. A low sense of authority, involvement, peer cohesion, daily accomplishment, and/or task orientation can also contribute to dissatisfaction and burnout. There is often major conflict between ideas of "good nursing" taught in school and the real world. Nurses, like physicians, are confronted with sickness and death on a regular basis. The nature of the work often involves unpleasant tasks. Recovery for many patients is uncertain and for others, incomplete. Cancer nurses frequently get to know their patients and their families well during the course of treatment. When a patient dies, the nurse must handle her own grief as well as that of the family.[56]

Interventions for Physicians and Nurses

Physicians must learn to recognize that their own expectations are often their greatest source of stress.[57] They must recognize that they are not immune to the same difficulties and psychological problems as others who are involved in high-stress jobs. Many medical schools are now addressing these issues, and some programs have even appeared for physicians in practice. The first and most important aspect of these programs is that they teach physicians that it is acceptable and even desirable to ask for help. The goals of these programs are to provide practitioners with effective ways to cope with stress and to prevent burnout. If burnout has already occurred, it must be handled in a helpful, rather than a punitive, way.[58]

Both physicians and nurses have to learn the principles of stress management. The first of these is awareness. Each individual must determine his or her own personal sources of stress as well as their physical, cognitive, and behavioral responses to acute and chronic stress. Once this awareness has occurred, it is possible to begin to manage the stress. This can be done through problem solving to eliminate or alter the stressors. Altering the cognitive appraisal of the importance of stressors can also be effective. Finally, lowering the physiologic response to stressors via techniques such as progressive muscle relaxation, meditation, yoga, or tai chi can be very helpful.

Focusing on the positive aspects of care of the cancer patient and minimizing those that are stressful are the aims of any intervention.[59] These include giving good care, seeing patients get well, working with families, teaching, and performing stimulating and challenging tasks. Using some creative problem solving can often eliminate or modify some stressors such as poor staffing patterns, noise, and congestion. "Breathing time" away from the work to allow for the restoration of internal resources is a necessary balance between work and rest/play and is essential.

For both doctors and nurses, a team approach (including physicians, nurses, and other health care personnel) and patient care conferences helps to facilitate clear communication about treatment plans and allows opportunity for some creative brainstorming to help solve problems. Feelings as well as ideas need to be voiced. Responsibilities can be shared and emotional support provided.

Continuing education can increase knowledge and a sense of mastery in many areas as well as providing time away from direct patient care.

Both doctors and nurses need to encourage hospital administrations to understand the problems being faced by the staff and to support creative ways of handling those stressors. Ongoing communication is essential. Recognition and rewards for work well done should occur frequently. Opportunities for continuing education should be provided.

It is important to note that burnout can be prevented by psychological and/or social interventions. However, even in the best of all worlds, burnout can and will occur. Supervisors and co-workers need to be alert to this phenomenon and ensure that those who are showing signs and symptoms of burnout receive the understanding, compassion, and professional psychological care that they deserve and that is essential to their recovery. Anyone could be next!

Summary

There are 1.2 million new patients with cancer each year in the US, and there is significant variability in the quality of care they receive. Cancer teams may render good or poor therapy, depending on their medical knowledge and experience, whether the care is multidisciplinary, and whether cancer therapy is the team's full-time activity. Excellent cancer care is a team effort that includes not only the scientific application of medical knowledge but supportive, compassionate care for the individual patient. Patients know that cancer can recur and that it can be fatal; they seek a quality of life comparable to that which existed before their diagnosis. Few can adapt to the stresses of treatment without good communication with a compassionate physician and the cancer team. Too often, cancer care is rendered impersonally, but supportive care that recognizes the patient's fears and dreams, hopes and worries, helps the patient to better tolerate the illness and its treatment.

References

1. Yancik R, Yates JW. Quality of life assessment of cancer patients: conceptual and methodological challenges and constraints. *Cancer Bull.* 1986;38:217-222.

2. Sutherland AS. Psychological impact of cancer and its therapy. In Holleb AI, Randers-Pehrson MB, eds. *Classics in Oncology.* Atlanta, Ga: American Cancer Society; 1987:449-461.

3. American Cancer Society California Division. Report on the social, economic, and psychological needs of patients in California: major findings and implications. 1979.

4. Locke BZ, Regier DA. Prevalence of selected mental disorders. In: Taub CA, Barrett SA, eds. *Mental Health in the United States 1985.* Rockville, Md: National Institutes of Mental Health; 1985:1-6.

5. Massie MJ. Depression. In: Holland JC, Rowland JH, eds. *Handbook of Psychooncology.* New York, NY; Oxford University Press Inc; 1989:283-290.

6. Derogatis LR, Morrow GR, Fetting J, et al. The prevalence of psychiatric disorders in cancer patients. *JAMA.* 1983;249:751-757.

7. Massie MJ, Holland JC. Depression and the cancer patient. *J Clin Psychiatry.* 1990;51:12-19.

8. Holland JC, Korzun AH, Tross S, et al. Comparative psychiatric disturbance in pancreatic and gastric cancer. *Am J Psychiatry.* 1986;143:982-986.

9. Massie MJ, Holland JC. The cancer patient with pain: psychiatric complications and their management. *Med Clin North Am.* 1987;71:143-148.

10. U.S. Department of Health and Human Services. National Institutes of Health. *Chemotherapy and You: A Guide to Self-Help During Treatment.* Nov. 1990:55.

11. Buckberg J, Penman D, Holland JC. Depression in the hospitalized patient. *Psychosom Med.* 1984;46:199-212.

12. Petty F, Noyes R. Depression secondary to cancer. *Biol Psychiatry.* 1981;16:1203-1217.

13. Rait D, Lederberg M. The Family of the Cancer Patient. In: Holland JC, Rowland JH, eds. *Handbook of Psychooncology.* New York, NY: Oxford University Press Inc; 1989:585-597.

14. Cancer Care, Inc and National Cancer Foundation. Listen to the children: a study of the impact on the mental health of children of a parent's catastrophic illness. New York, NY: Cancer Care Inc; 1977.

15. Nir Y, Pynoos R, Holland J. Cancer in a parent: the impact on mother and child. *Gen Hosp Psychiatry.* 1981;3:331-342.

16. Wellisch D. Adolescent acting-out when a parent has cancer. *Int J Family Therapy.* 1979:230-241.

17. Wellisch D, Gritz E, Schain W, et al. Psychological functioning of daughters of breast cancer patients. II: characterizing the distressed daughters of the breast cancer patients. *Psychosomatics.* 1992;33(2):171-179.

18. Stroudmire A, Techman T, Graham S. Sexual assessment of the urologic oncology patient. *Psychosomatics.* 1985;26:405-410.

19. Sohover L, Von Eschenbach A. Sexual and marital counseling with men treated for testicular cancer. *J Sex Marital Ther.* 1984;10:29-40.

20. Maguire G, Lee G, Bevington C, et al. Psychiatric problems in the first year after mastectomy. *Br Med J.* 1978;1:963-965.

21. Vincent C, Vincent F, Greiss C, Linton E. Some marital-sexual concomitants of cancer of the cervix. *South Med J.* 1975:68;552-558.

22. Auchincloss S. Sexual dysfunction in cancer patients: issues in evaluation and treatment. In: Holland JC, Rowland JH, eds. *Handbook of Psychooncology.* New York, NY: Oxford University Press Inc; 1989:383-413.

23. Kaplan H. *The Evaluation of Sexual Disorders.* New York, NY: Brunner/Mazel Inc; 1983.

24. McKenna RJ, Toghia N. Maximizing the productive activities of the cancer patient: policy issues in work and illness. In: Borofsky I, ed. *The Cancer Patient.* New York, NY: Praeger Publishers; 1989.

25. Holland J. The current concepts and challenges in psychosocial oncology. In: Holland J, ed. *Current Concepts in Psychosocial Oncology: Syllabus of Postgraduate Course.* New York, NY: Memorial Sloan-Kettering Cancer Center; 1982.

26. Zimbardo P, Ebbeson EB. *Influencing Attitudes and Changing Behavior.* Reading, Mass: Addison-Wesley Publishing Co Inc; 1970.

27. Gordon WA, Freidenbergs L, Diller L, et al. Efficacy of psychosocial intervention with cancer patients. *J Consult Clin Psychol.* 1980;48:743-759.

28. Burish TG, Lyles JN. Effectiveness of relaxation training in reducing adverse reactions to cancer chemotherapy. *J Behav Med.* 1981;4:65-78.

29. Burish TG, Snyder SL, Jenkins RA. Preparing patients for cancer chemotherapy: effect of coping preparation and relaxation interventions. *J Consult Clin Psychol.* 1991;59(4):518-525.

30. Weisman AD, Worden JW, Sobel HJ. *Psychosocial screening and intervention with cancer patients.* (Project Omega, Grant No. CA–797). Boston, Mass: Harvard Medical School, Massachusetts General Hospital, 1980.

31. Sobel HJ, Worden JW. *Helping Cancer Patients Cope: Practitioner's Manual.* New York, NY: The Guilford Press; 1982.

32. Weisman AD. *Coping With Cancer.* New York, NY: McGraw-Hill Inc; 1979.

33. Spiegel D, Bloom JR, Yalom ID. Group support for metastatic cancer patients: a randomized prospective outcome study. *Arch Gen Psychiatry.* 1981;38:527-533.

34. Fawzy FI, Cousins N, Fawzy NW, et al. A structured psychiatric intervention for cancer patients: 1. Changes over time in methods of coping and affective disturbance. *Arch Gen Psychiatry.* 1990;47:720-725.

35. Fawzy FI, Wellish D, Yager J. Psychiatric liaison to the bone-marrow transplant project. In: Hollingsworth CE, Pasnau RO, eds. *The Family in Mourning.* Philadelphia, Pa: Grune & Stratton Inc; 1977:181-189.

36. Spiegel D, Bloom JR. Pain in metastatic breast cancer. *Cancer.* 1983;52:341-345.

37. Bloom JR. Social support systems and cancer: a conceptual view. In: Cohen J, Cullen J, Martin RL, eds. *Psychosocial Aspects of Cancer.* New York, NY: Raven Press; 1982.

38. Cunningham AJ, Tocco EK. A randomized trial of group psychoeducational therapy for cancer patients. *Patient Education and Counseling.* 1989;14:101-114.

39. Meyerowitz BE, Heinrich RL, Schag CAC. Helping patients cope with cancer. *Oncology.* 1989;3(11):120-129.

40. American Cancer Society. *Guidelines on Self-Help and Mutual Support Groups.* Atlanta, Ga: American Cancer Society; 1988:3.

41. McCorkle R. Complications of early discharge from the hospital. In: *Proceedings of the Fifth National Conference on Human Values in Cancer.* San Francisco, Calif: American Cancer Society; 1987:67-74.

42. Jacob GA. Hospice: what it is not. *CA.* 1984;34:191-201.

43. Magno J. Management of terminal disease: the hospice concept of care. *Henry Ford Hospital Medical Journal.* 1991;39(2):74-76.

44. Rainey LC, Crane LA, Breslow DM, Ganz PA. Cancer patients' attitudes toward hospice services. *CA.* 1984;34:191-201.

45. Frost N, Clayton P. Bereavement and psychiatric hospitalization. *Arch Gen Psychiatry.* 1977;34:1172-1175.

46. Hesing K, Szklo M. Mortality after bereavement. *Am J Epidemiology.* 1981;114:41-52.

47. Torrens P. Hospice programs. In: Haskell C, ed. *Cancer Treatment.* 2nd ed. Philadelphia, Pa: WB Saunders Co; 1985:963-970.

48. Hudnut R. *The Sleeping Giant.* New York, NY: Harper & Row Publishers Inc; 1971:127.

49. Peterson MB. The potential of the clergy in cancer rehabilitation programs. In: *Proceedings of the Fifth National Conference on Human Values in Cancer.* San Francisco, Calif: American Cancer Society; 1987:122-128.

50. Ota DM, Kleman G, Diamond K. Practical considerations in the nutritional management of the cancer patient. *Curr Probs Cancer.* 1986;10:347-398.

51. Foley KM. The treatment of pain in the patient with cancer. *CA.* 1986;36:194-212.

52. Schneider J. Self care: challenges and rewards for hospice professionals. *Hospice Journal.* 1987;121-146.

53. Fawzy FI, Fawzy NW, Pasnau RO. Burnout in the health professions. In: Judd FK, et al, eds. *Handbook of Studies on General Hospital Psychiatry.* New York, NY: Elsevier Science Publishing Co Inc BV (Biomedical Division); 1991:121-130.

54. Lazarus RS, Folkman S. The coping process: an alternative to traditional formulation. In: Lazarus RS, Folkman S, eds. *Stress, Appraisal, and Coping.* New York, NY: Springer Publishing Co Inc; 1984:141-180.

55. Small G. House officer stress syndrome. *Psychosomatics.* 1981;22:860-864.

56. Fawzy FI, Wellish DK, Pasnau RO, Leibowitz B. Preventing nurse burnout: a challenge for liaison psychiatry. *Gen Hosp Psychiatry.* 1983;5:141-149.

57. Trubo R. Burnout. *Medical World News—Psychiatry Edition.* 1984;3:18-32.

58. Caldwell T, Weiner MF. Stress and coping in ICU nursing 1. A review. *Gen Hosp Psychiatry.* 1981;3:119-127.

59. Coombs RH, Fawzy FI. The impaired-physician syndrome: a developmental perspective. In: Scott J, Hawk J, eds. *Heal Thyself.* New York, NY: Brunner/Mazel Inc; 1986:44-559.

38

EFFECTIVE TREATMENT OF PAIN IN THE CANCER PATIENT

C. Stratton Hill, Jr, MD

The title of this chapter suggests that there is also an ineffective treatment of pain in the cancer patient. "Ineffective" treatment implies that the patient is treated but does not experience satisfactory relief of pain. Without pursuing the semantics further, it is well established that in a significant percentage of cancer patients, pain is inadequately treated, causing needless suffering.[1-3] After observing three episodes of undertreatment of pain in members of his own family over a 25-year period, Dr. Jerome H. Jaffe, a renowned teacher and researcher in the field of opioid pharmacology, asked, "How can it be that after 25 years we have made so little progress in teaching our students and colleagues about the management of pain?"[4]

Indeed, progress in improving pain treatment has been inordinately slow even though knowledge about all aspects of pain and its treatment has increased over the 25 years referred to by Dr. Jaffe. The number of medical organizations dedicated to disseminating such information has increased significantly. Nevertheless, neither organizations like the International Association for the Study of Pain nor state cancer pain initiatives, which have provided information about the effective methods of pain control, have made a strong impact on pain treatment practices.

The slow pace leads one to conclude that providing adequate pain relief for cancer patients is a complex issue. Merely giving healthcare providers current information on drugs that relieve pain and interventional pain-relieving techniques is inadequate to effect improvement. The problem is multifactorial and involves cultural and societal barriers to the appropriate and adequate use of opioids (narcotics), knowledge deficits about pain treatment among healthcare providers, and a fear of possible disciplinary action by healthcare licensing boards and of criminal prosecution by drug enforcement agencies.[5]

C. Stratton Hill, Jr, MD, Professor of Medicine, The University of Texas, MD Anderson Cancer Center, Houston, Texas

Evidence exists that inadequate pain relief concerns society as a quality-of-life issue.[6] For patients with chronic painful medical conditions, pain relief is a major factor in determining an acceptable quality of life. As the percentage of the population living into older age increases, more individuals become vulnerable to painful conditions. The rise of a "book of recipes" on how to commit suicide[7] to the top of a leading national best-seller list (faster than any other "how to" book in the history of the list) can be interpreted as a manifestation of societal concern, and indeed impatience, with what is perceived to be a lack of availability of adequate pain relief, resulting in the need to "take matters into one's own hands." Further testimony of society's concern is seen in attempts to legalize physician-assisted suicide in two states (California and Washington) and the passage in 1994 of such legislation in Oregon.

Because traditional educational efforts have not produced the desired result of improving pain treatment, the approach to presenting material in this chapter represents a departure from the usual encyclopedic inclusion of all possible causes of pain in cancer patients and the possible methods of treatment. Instead, an attempt has been made to discuss barriers and pitfalls that prevent *effective* pain relief at points in the patient's evaluation when they usually arise. This may create a "stream of consciousness" style of presentation—eg, a point about treatment may be made during a discussion of the physical examination—but hopefully this approach will be helpful rather than distracting, and provide guidance in developing a comprehensive treatment plan. Factual information will also be presented on the causes of pain, assessing pain and relating it to these causes, recognizable pain syndromes, and strategies to treat pain, plus a discussion of when to seek consultation.

An important goal is to provide the tools to make every physician responsible for the care of cancer patients a "pain treatment expert," in the sense that most patients experiencing pain can be *effectively* treated with the modalities available to all physicians. The emphasis will therefore be on the proper use of analgesic drugs. Most patients do not require sophisticated pain treatment modalities that have to be administered by specially trained personnel. However, because of the multitude of factors contributing to the chronic pain experience, support from other healthcare personnel is desirable. The practitioner can utilize only available resources, but in most communities some type of "team," embracing nurses, pharmacists, social workers, and clergy, can be assembled to address some or all of the factors involved in the patient's pain.

Causes of Pain in the Cancer Patient

A knowledge of the causes of pain is essential at the time of the initial interview for the physician to direct the interview to uncover important clues as to cause. For that reason, the causes of pain are elucidated before a discussion of evaluation of the report of pain.

Pain in cancer patients can be attributed to: 1) tumor impingement on, or invasion of, pain-sensitive structures; 2) any type of treatment for the tumor, but particularly treatments that damage the nervous system; 3) changes in body structure as a result of tumor effects that cause muscle imbalance or other changes that result in mechanical skeletal stresses; and 4) acute and/or chronic medical conditions and acute surgical conditions unrelated to the malignant disease.

Damage to Nerves: Neuropathic Versus Nociceptive Pain

One must be alert to the particular type of pain associated with damage to the nervous system, more commonly the peripheral nervous system. Cancer patients may experience nerve damage either by direct tumor effect or as a result of tumor treatment. Direct tumor effect is usually obvious by observing tumor progression. This commonly occurs with tumor involvement of the brachial and lumbar plexuses. Cancer treatment of all types is more aggressive now than in the past. Consequently, there is greater potential for injury to the peripheral nervous system. Injury, when used in this context, is subtle, not dramatic as the term *injury* often implies. A peripheral nerve can be injured merely by being cut, as in surgery. "Injury" also may occur in the course of usual and acceptable treatment (external-beam or other types of irradiation, neurotoxic chemotherapy, and biological therapy) and does not imply negligence. That some patients (fortunately a small number) develop neuropathic pain as a result of treatment cannot be explained. As far as can be determined, treatment for the primary neoplastic condition is identical in patients who subsequently experience neuropathic pain and in those who do not develop such pain.

Neuropathic pain can occur anywhere in the body. Several recognizable syndromes present with some regularity; two associated with surgery are post-mastectomy and postthoracotomy syndromes. Peripheral neuropathies are the most frequent postchemotherapy syndromes. Any nerve can be affected, but the sensory cutaneous nerves of the soles of the feet are frequently involved, causing a persistent, burning pain. Radiation effects on the brachial and lumbosacral plexuses account for most neuropathic pain following radiotherapy; pain is also experienced by some patients in whom relatively large anatomic areas are irradiated. Graft-versus-host disease is a painful condition associated with biological therapy.

Some or all of the painful sensations may be extremely intense, and the patient totally unable to function. Sleep is interfered with, and interpersonal relationships may be strained. A host of negative emotional states is likely to ensue, and the end result is severe depression.

The history taker may find that patients experiencing the strange painful sensations associated with neuropathic pain are often reluctant to reveal them for fear they will be considered "crazy" or histrionic. They may begin to doubt the validity of their own observations and fear that they are "losing their minds." These feelings are compounded when a patient obtains only partial pain relief with commonly prescribed analgesics, including strong opioids, which is usually the case.

Another frequent negative experience is skepticism by healthcare providers, who may be unfamiliar with this type of pain, who may openly express surprise and doubt about the report of only partial pain relief even with strong opioids. This reinforces a patient's fears of mental instability, especially if a healthcare provider overtly or by innuendo accuses the patient of being a drug abuser or manipulating the caregiver to obtain drugs for subsequent sale on the street. Tension may enter the relationship, further adding to the patient's feeling of helplessness.

Neuropathic pain is characterized by the features listed in Table 38-1. Two important diagnostic features obtained from the patient's history and physical examination are a delay in pain onset after damage to the nervous system and the absence of an obvious ongoing cause for the pain. A classic example of these two features is postmastectomy syndrome. After undergoing a mastectomy, a patient may suffer postoperative (nociceptive) pain but recover completely, resume activities of daily living, and even return to work. After a variable time, many of the features described in Table 38-1 occur. On physical examination, nothing is visible but the mastectomy scar, which is healing or has healed normally, essentially leaving no evidence of an obvious pain-producing process. Allodynia and hyperalgesia are usually present.

Various terms (including *neurogenic* and *deafferentation*) have been used to describe this type of pain, but Fields suggests the term *neuropathic pain* as the most appropriate because it implies only that the pain is due to functional abnormalities of the nervous system.[8]

Nociceptive pain may be defined as a state of continuous stimulation of nociceptors by a noxious stimulus; removal of the stimulus will relieve the pain. Nociceptive pain is usually associated with overt tissue damage and is the most commonly encountered type of pain. A common example of nociceptive pain is acute postoperative pain and acute pain associated with trauma.

Distinguishing nociceptive from neuropathic pain is of increasing importance because the incidence of the latter appears to be increasing in cancer patients and, if treatment is to be successful, treatment must be tailored to each type.

The outcome of treatment for neuropathic pain is problematic. There is probably no other painful experience in which the actual participation of the physician and his or her staff is essential to obtaining an acceptable (though often incomplete) level of pain control. The first task is to assure patients that the symptoms reported—ie, the strangeness of the pain they are experiencing—are believed and help them develop a realistic set of expectations about results. They must be aware that treatment results will not be dramatic. Patience is the watchword. In addition to analgesics, medications recommended for this type of pain include antidepressants, anticonvulsants, and antiarrhythmic drugs. They must be taken continually despite the fact that little immediate relief of pain is evident and minor undesirable side effects occur. A schema for treatment is presented in Fig 38-1.

Analgesic drugs are highly effective in relieving nociceptive pain. In contrast, neuropathic pain is characteristically not satisfactorily relieved by common nonnarcotic analgesics or by weak or strong narcotic analgesics. Since most patients with pain of any type are treated with opioids given orally, the failure of patients with neuropathic pain to obtain relief is often attributed to the oral route of administration. Unfortunately, other routes of drug administration, including the spinal route, fail to improve responsiveness to opioids.[9,10]

Table 38-1. Clinical Features of Neuropathic Pain

- Delay in onset of pain, ranging from days to months after the event that produced nerve damage (eg, surgery, radiation, chemotherapy, biological therapy)
- Absence on examination of painful area of an ongoing tissue-damaging process that would be considered painful (eg, pain in a mastectomy site that appears to be healed)
- Sensations that the patient considers painful, but also abnormal, unfamiliar, unpleasant, "strange," or "weird," and that the physician may consider histrionic
  - Typical painful and/or unpleasant sensations are burning, pressure, twisting or torque-like sensations, stabbing, knife-like sensations, and shooting electrical sensations
  - Sensations may be paroxysmal and their duration varies; also, sensations may alternate in the same general area
- Stimuli that are not usually painful (eg, touch) may now produce pain in the affected area that patient indicates
- Pronounced summation and after-reaction with repetitive stimuli
- Pain in an area of numbness
- Relief with nonopioid and opioid analgesics that is usually less than relief seen with these agents in nociceptive pain (use of coanalgesics is highly desirable)

Pain Associated With Tumor Impingement or Invasion

In cancer patients, pain is most often caused by the presence or effects of the tumor itself. Therefore, a meticulous initial and ongoing effort should be made to demonstrate the presence of tumor. Early detection of recurrent tumor offers the best opportunity for effective treatment of both the pain and the tumor. However, one should never simply assume that pain is caused by the tumor without appropriate investigation even though pain often precedes the examiner's ability to demonstrate objectively the tumor's presence by either physical examination or sophisticated imaging techniques. Treatment decisions based on an erroneous assumption about etiology can be detrimental to the patient. While efforts to demonstrate the presence of the tumor or other potential causes of the pain are continuing, symptomatic treatment of the pain should be started. Analgesics that are strong enough or that are appropriate for the specific cause of the pain should be administered.

Some tumors characteristically metastasize to certain areas of the body; eg, breast and prostate cancer metastasize to bone. However, regardless of the tumor type, pain in any area of the body of a cancer patient should be investigated to rule out metastasis. Pain in the head and neck area requires the early use of sophisticated imaging techniques because plain radiographs are often not discriminative enough to detect tumor invasion or bone destruction. Computed

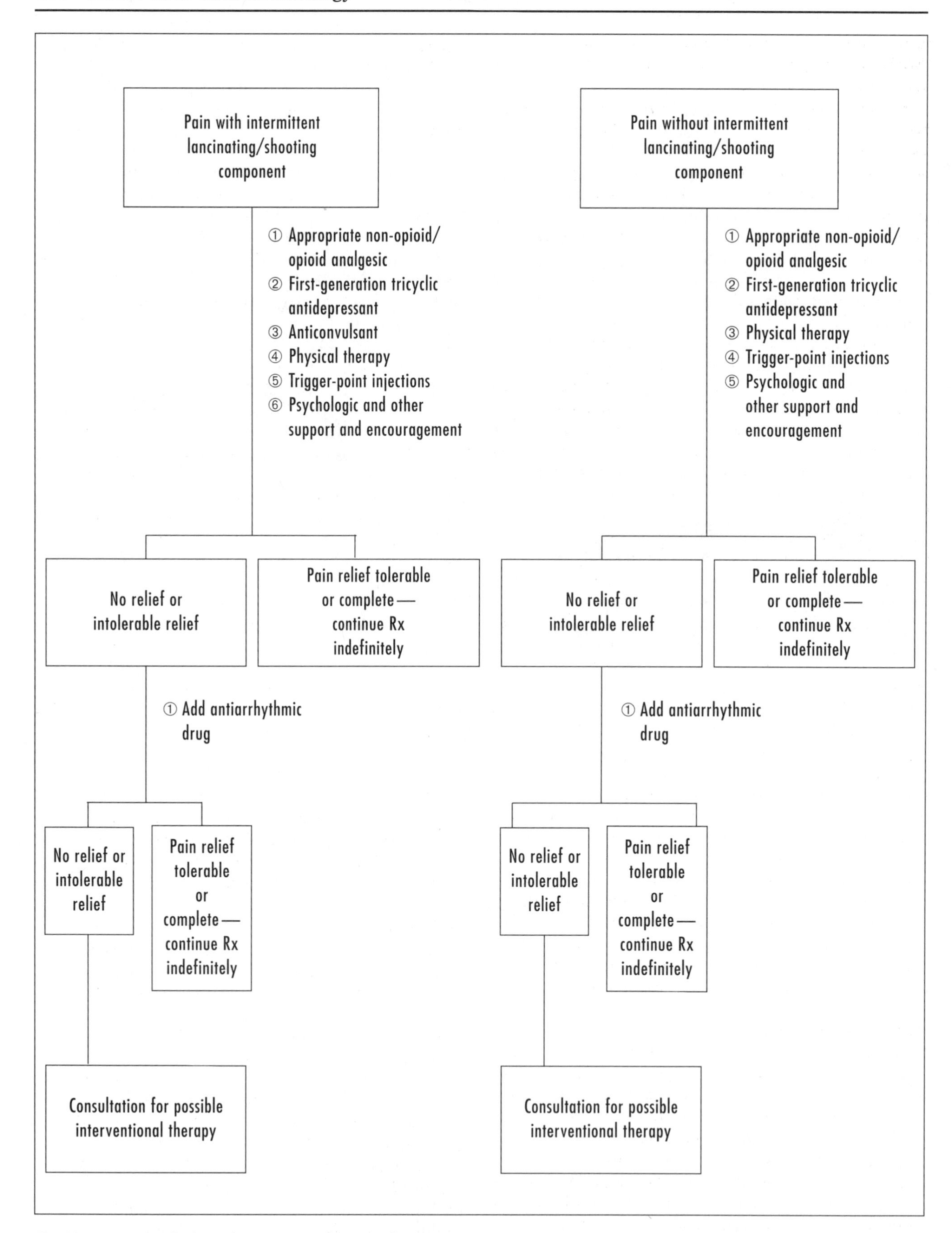

Fig 38-1. Suggested schema for treatment of neuropathic pain.

tomography (CT) and magnetic resonance imaging (MRI) are the procedures of choice for demonstrating lesions in this area.

Back pain is commonly observed in cancer patients because many tumors metastasize to vertebral bodies and other spinal structures. Two conditions deserve particular mention: epidural metastatic disease and spasm of paravertebral and other back muscles. If epidural metastatic disease goes undetected, it most likely will ultimately cause paralysis from spinal cord compression. Epidural spinal cord compression should be considered in the differential diagnosis of back pain in cancer patients. Its presence should be considered a medical emergency. Early diagnosis and prompt treatment can prevent paralysis in most cases. Vertebral body metastases, with or without subsequent partial or complete collapse of the vertebrae, are a frequent cause of spasm of the paravertebral and other back muscles, which produces moderate to severe pain. Pain caused by vertebral body invasion, in the absence of vertebral collapse, muscle imbalance, and associated muscle spasm, is nociceptive and more likely to be controlled by an analgesic than pain caused by muscle spasm. Physical therapy is usually more effective for controlling the latter. A common cause of failure to control back pain caused by muscle spasm is an overreliance on analgesic and muscle relaxant drugs in lieu of physical therapy modalities.

Tumor invasion of individual nerves or plexuses and invasion of pain-sensitive structures in soft tissue are other common causes of pain related to direct tumor involvement. The character of the pain will vary depending on the structure involved. As mentioned earlier, invasion of nerves with subsequent nerve damage produces neuropathic pain. Damage to axons and myelin sheaths has been suggested as a mechanism for this type of pain.[11] Another characteristic of tumor involvement of these structures is motor weakness.

Abdominal visceral pain is caused by tumor obstruction of hollow organs, tumor invasion of pain-sensitive soft tissue, and peritoneal irritation. Tumor obstruction can be partial or complete and may require surgical intervention. Characteristically, pain caused by tumor invasion of pain-sensitive soft tissue or the peritoneum is diffuse and poorly localized.

Pain Associated With Cancer Treatment

Regardless of the therapeutic modality, patients expect pain, discomfort, and other distressing symptoms during active cancer treatment and for a variable period after treatment. These symptoms are also expected to gradually diminish during healing until they disappear. In most cases, if no complications supervene, this is what happens. In a minority of patients, however, pain may either persist or develop following a pain-free interval of variable length despite apparent healing of the damaged tissue. This minority is the subpopulation of pain patients who are suffering from neuropathic pain. However, in all situations in which pain is thought to be due to treatment, the possibility of recurrent tumor must be ruled out.

Pain Associated With Structural Body Changes

Tumor invasion of vertebral bodies may cause pain in two ways: direct involvement of a vertebra activates local nociceptors, and collapse of the vertebra as a result of tumor invasion often causes change in body structure, particularly muscle imbalance, which causes paravertebral and other muscle spasms. Sustained spasm produces pain in the involved muscle and secondary tenderness in the surrounding muscles.

Scoliosis following surgery for thoracic tumors causes muscle imbalance and can be painful. Such pain usually occurs only in the upright position—an incident pain—and for that reason is difficult to treat. Doses of opioids sufficient to relieve pain when the patient is upright are frequently excessive when the patient lies down. Exercises designed to strengthen compensatory muscles may be helpful in controlling this type of pain.

Pain From Causes Other Than Cancer or Its Treatment

Cancer patients may suffer from painful chronic medical illnesses acquired before or after the diagnosis of cancer. Therapy for these conditions is the same as if the patient never had cancer, unless such therapy causes complications or interferes with the cancer treatment.

Acute painful surgical conditions that occur in cancer patients can be unrelated to the neoplasm or may be a complication of tumor progression or its treatment.

A list of common causes of pain and specific pain syndromes in cancer patients is presented in Table 38-2.

Assessing the Report of Pain

Assessment of pain involves two components: 1) the initial assessment and 2) persistent, frequent reassessments as long as the pain persists. In the initial assessment, one determines the pain's location(s), onset, characteristics (eg, quality, radiation), possible clues to its cause, intensity, dynamics (eg, static, progressive), and influence on the patient's psychosocial function and activities of daily living. In addition, the contributing influence of previous therapy; the kind and effectiveness of previous pain treatment (whether nonpharmacologic or pharmacologic); whether the patient has discovered methods to modulate the pain (by lying down or standing up); and whether it is "incident pain" (ie, pain associated with a specific

Table 38-2. Common Causes of Pain and Specific Pain Syndromes in Cancer Patients

A. Pain Syndromes Associated With Direct Tumor Involvement
  1. Tumor infiltration of bone
    a. Base-of-skull syndromes
      1) Jugular foramen metastases
      2) Clivus metastases
      3) Sphenoid sinus metastases
    b. Vertebral body syndromes
      1) C2 metastases
      2) C7-T1 metastases
      3) L1 metastases
    c. Sacral syndromes
  2. Tumor infiltration of nerve
    a. Peripheral nerve
      1) Peripheral neuropathy
    b. Plexus
      1) Brachial plexopathy
      2) Lumbar plexopathy
      3) Sacral plexopathy
    c. Root
      1) Leptomeningeal metastases
    d. Spinal cord
      1) Epidural spinal cord compression

B. Pain Syndromes Associated With Cancer Therapy
  1. Postsurgery syndromes
    a. Postthoracotomy syndrome
    b. Postmastectomy syndrome
    c. Postradical neck syndrome
    d. Phantom limb syndrome
  2. Postchemotherapy syndromes
    a. Peripheral neuropathy
    b. Aseptic necrosis of the femoral head
    c. Steroid pseudorheumatism
    d. Postherpetic neuralgia
  3. Postradiation syndromes
    a. Radiation fibrosis of the brachial and lumbar plexus
    b. Radiation myelopathy
    c. Radiation-induced second primary tumors
    d. Radiation necrosis of bone

C. Pain Syndromes Not Associated With Cancer or Cancer Therapy
  1. Cervical and lumbar osteoarthritis
  2. Thoracic and abdominal aneurysms
  3. Diabetic neuropathy

incident, such as weight bearing or movement) are assessed.

The assessment is done primarily by taking a thorough history. However, pain parameters can also be evaluated by tools such as scales to measure pain intensity (Fig 38-2).[12] These scales also can be used in reassessment.

Occasionally, during the initial assessment of a pain report in a patient who appears healthy and is not suspected of having cancer, cancer is found. Unless the pain in such a patient is unequivocally proven to be due to the cancer, investigation of the pain complaint should not stop with diagnosing either primary or metastatic cancer because many cancers in the early stages are not painful. The pain may have another cause. Patients with pain unrelated to their cancer should have treatment appropriate for the specific cause of the pain.

The assessment should contain, at a minimum, the following information, but each interview must be tailored to the individual clinical situation.

Location of Pain

Identifying the location(s) of pain will help to discern, among other things, whether the pain is related to the cancer, whether it is related to the primary tumor or its metastases, and whether it is of radicular or musculoskeletal origin or is referred.

Onset of Pain

Determining the onset of pain will identify whether the pain is cancer related and was the presenting symptom that prompted the patient to seek medical advice, or was an unrelated preexisting symptom. If it was the presenting symptom of the cancer, subsequent pain episodes will almost invariably be interpreted by the patient as being a harbinger of tumor recurrence or progression. However, it cannot be assumed that the pain experienced by a cancer patient is inevitably caused by the cancer.

Because of its prevalence in the general population, preexisting back pain, due to a variety of traumatic and other causes, is common in patients who subsequently develop cancer. If a successful program for treatment of this pain exists, it should be continued. However, these patients may subsequently develop back pain or pain in other parts of the body due to their cancer. Separate treatments for the two types of pain are necessary for optimum pain relief.

Pain Characteristics

Descriptors are important in determining the type of pain (Fig 38-3).[13] Some descriptors for neuropathic pain are distinct from those for nociceptive pain. The two types of pain may coexist, and thus descriptors for both types may be used by a patient. Because treatment is different for each type, it is important to be alert to descriptors identifying each type.

Special Clues to Etiology

Obviously, pain in the region of a primary tumor or metastatic lesion is considered, *prima facie*, to be due to the tumor. Other clues to etiology from the history include tumor treatments—such as surgery, radiotherapy, chemotherapy, and biological response modifiers—that may cause nerve damage and therefore neuropathic pain. Thus, all previous cancer treatments are potentially chronic pain producers. Evidence of other medical conditions that produce pain, such as the various arthritides, diabetic neuropathy, and herpes zoster, will help establish a differential pain diagnosis.

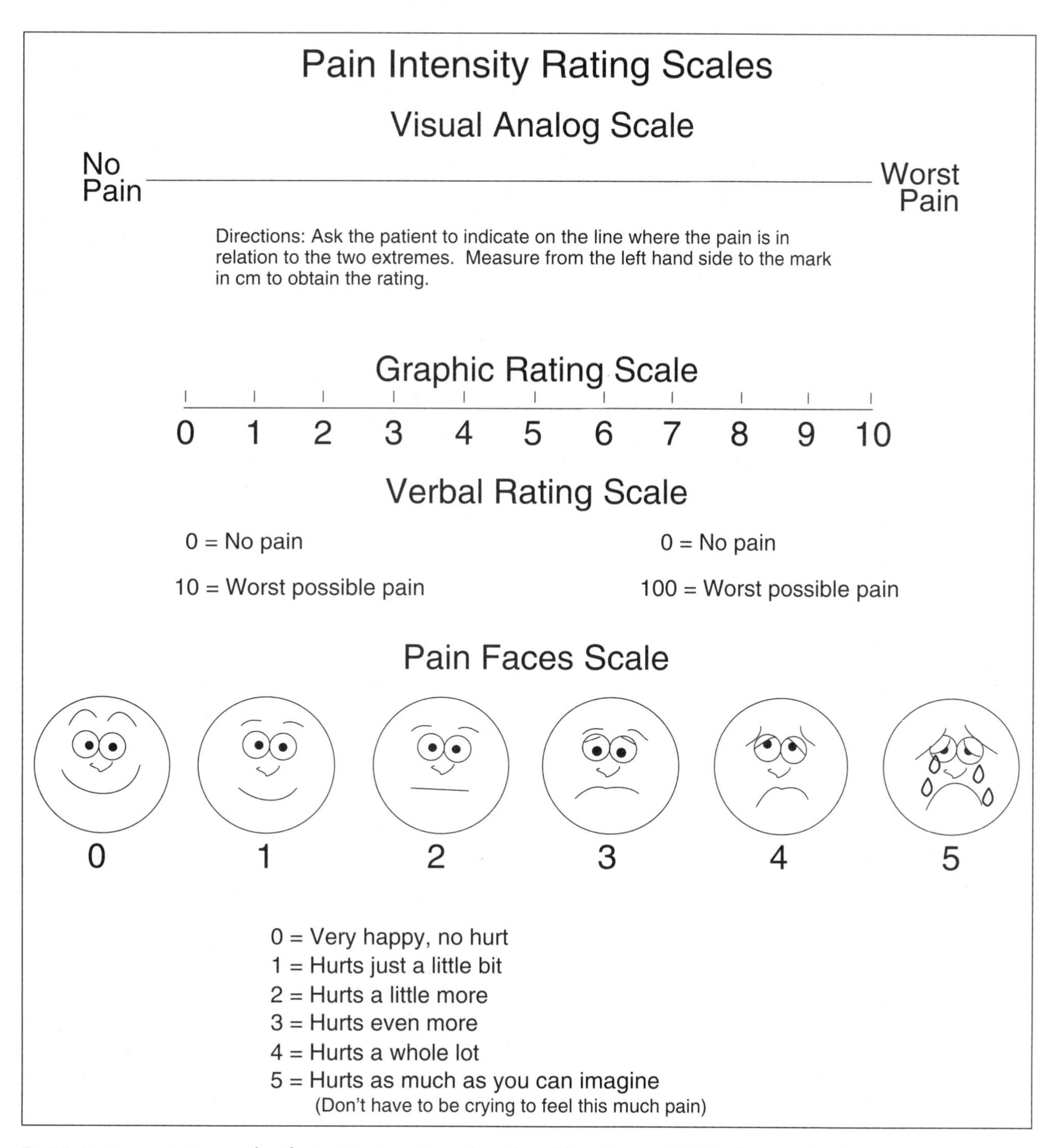

Fig 38-2. Representative samples of pain intensity rating scales. Adapted from Wong and Whaley,[12] reprinted with permission.

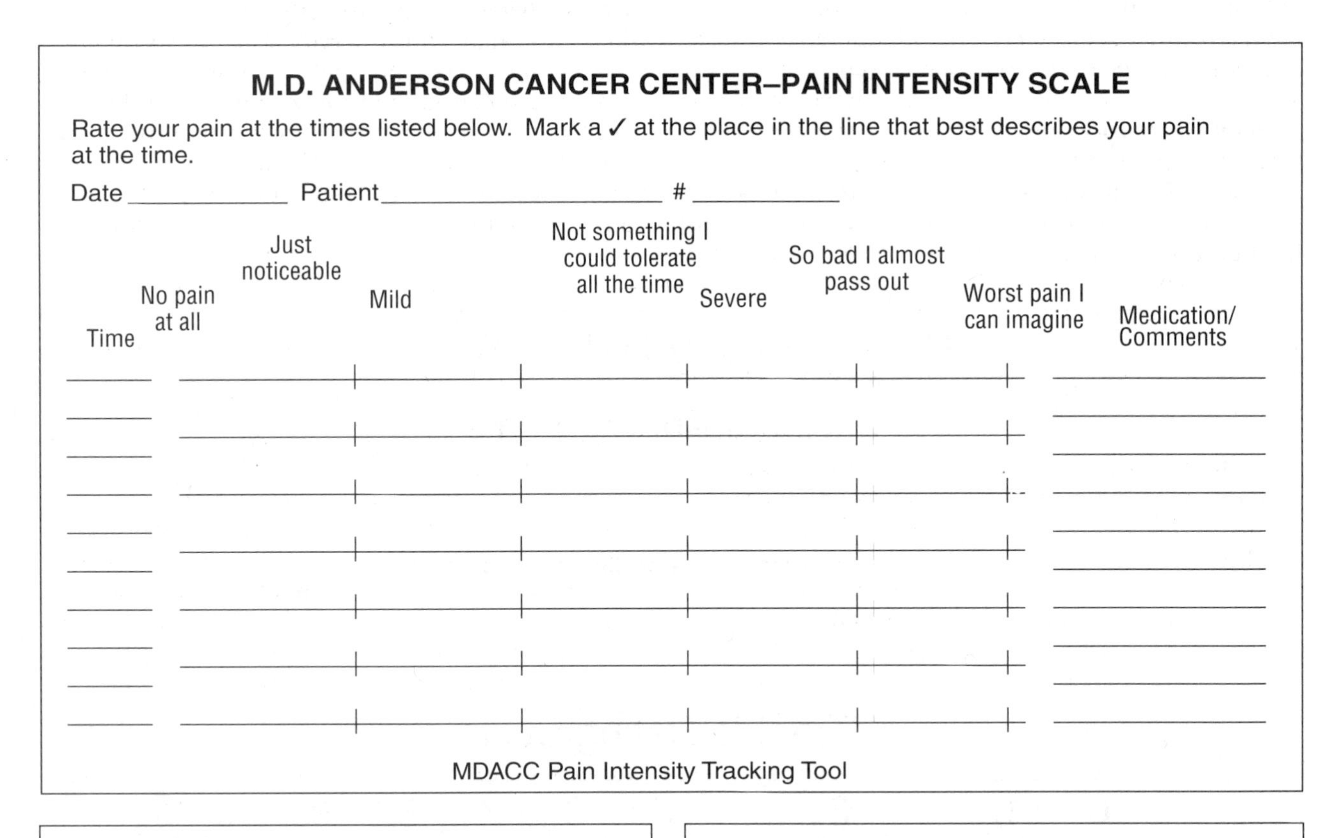

M.D. ANDERSON CANCER CENTER–PAIN INTENSITY SCALE

Rate your pain at the times listed below. Mark a ✓ at the place in the line that best describes your pain at the time.

Date ____________ Patient ______________________ # __________

Time	No pain at all	Just noticeable	Mild	Not something I could tolerate all the time	Severe	So bad I almost pass out	Worst pain I can imagine	Medication/ Comments

MDACC Pain Intensity Tracking Tool

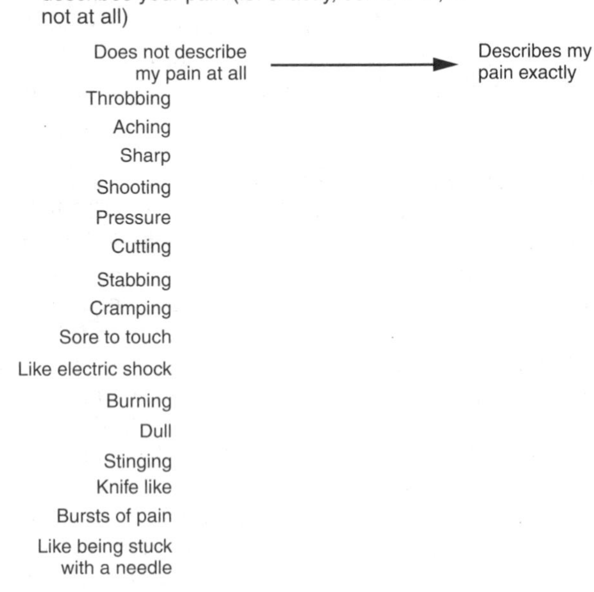

PAIN CHARACTERISTICS

For each word or phrase below, mark a ✓ on the corresponding line at the place that best shows how well that word or phrase describes your pain. Please make a mark on the line for each word or phrase that describes the degree to which it describes your pain (ie: exactly, somewhat, or not at all)

Does not describe my pain at all ⟶ Describes my pain exactly

Throbbing
Aching
Sharp
Shooting
Pressure
Cutting
Stabbing
Cramping
Sore to touch
Like electric shock
Burning
Dull
Stinging
Knife like
Bursts of pain
Like being stuck with a needle

PAIN DISRUPTIVENESS

For each phrase listed below, mark a ✓ at the place on the corresponding line that best shows how well that phrase describes the effects of your pain on your daily activities. Be sure to make a mark for each phrase indicating the degree to which it describes your pain (ie: not at all, somewhat, or exactly)

Does not describe my pain at all ⟶ Describes my pain exactly

Makes me want to give up
My pain is all I can think about
All I can do is lie in bed
Can't do the things I feel I need to
Can't go out
Makes me irritable
Can't do what I enjoy
Keeps me awake
Unable to eat
Makes me tired
Annoys me, but I can distract myself and go on

Fig 38-3. Descriptors of pain. Adapted from Nemni.[13]

Intensity

Intensity is frequently the only characteristic of the pain assessed by the healthcare provider. A crude measure of intensity can be obtained by having the patient rate it using a simple verbal scale of 0 to 10, with 0 being no pain and 10 being the worst pain the patient can imagine. However, these scales are useful only in following the course of pain in the *same* individual. Changes in intensity of pain are meaningful. Inexorable progression of intensity most often signals progression of the cancer, whereas lessening of intensity means either control of the cancer or adequate pain relief. Pain intensity may start as mild and progress in crescendo fashion to severe. Alternatively, it may be severe at onset. An accurate evaluation is important because treatment should be tailored to the intensity of pain at presentation (strong narcotics for severe pain at onset and nonnarcotics or weak narcotics for mild pain at onset).

Influence on Psychosocial Function and Activities of Daily Living

Chronic pain spawns a variety of negative emotions that frequently culminate in clinical depression, which can produce profound changes in interpersonal relationships. When present, these effects of chronic pain must be recognized and treated appropriately if the desired outcome of adequate pain relief and return to normal, or near-normal, lifestyle, including interpersonal relationships, is to be achieved.

Effect of Previous Treatment

It is important to know not only whether previous treatment for the tumor is the cause of the pain but also what prior treatments have been used and whether they were effective. If treatment with analgesics failed to relieve the pain, one must determine whether the problem was failure to use an analgesic strong enough to match the intensity of pain, an inadequate or untolerated dose, or the patient is suffering from neuropathic pain.

Patient's Capacity to Modulate Pain

Patients can, on occasion, modulate pain by their own efforts. They may use biofeedback, guided imagery, relaxation, or self-hypnosis as primary or adjuvant treatment modalities.

The patient's ability to modulate pain is often a clue in diagnosing "incident" pain, ie, pain a patient experiences only if he or she engages in a specific activity (such as sitting or moving) and when not engaging in this activity is either entirely free of pain or the pain is greatly reduced in severity. Incident pain is difficult to treat when an opioid is required because during the pain-free intervals the patient is often oversedated by the opioid.

Reliability of the Pain Report

Many factors can influence the reliability of the pain report. Pain is a subjective complaint. One must rely on and believe the patient's report of pain; however, the intactness of the cognitive powers of the patient and his or her memory must be factored in. Age, central nervous system (CNS) disease, systemic disease, metabolic derangements, and effect of treatment on the body in general, and the CNS in particular, can influence the mental status of the patient.

Loss of memory is an especially serious problem when one is attempting to evaluate the effect of pain treatment from one day to the next. It is usually impossible for a patient with defective memory to remember the intensity or other characteristics of the pain from the day before. Confusion based on organic or metabolic impediments should be differentiated from attempts to manipulate healthcare providers to obtain drugs for mood-altering purposes and from temporary confusion resulting from opioid administration. A neuropsychologic mental status examination should be done in patients giving inconsistent answers about their experience of pain and those having apparent trouble with memory.

Reassessment

All components of the initial assessment are likely to be components of the reassessment. Pain is an ever-changing, dynamic process and treatment must constantly be evaluated to determine its effectiveness. Therefore, treating pain is not easy. It requires constant surveillance and decision making. The frequency of reassessment varies from hourly to only when a change in the patient's symptoms occurs. Nurses, other healthcare providers, family members, and friends are important allies in reassessing the effectiveness of treatment and thereby helping the physician make treatment decisions.

Interpreting the Assessment

After examining the patient's report of pain in light of knowledge of the causes of pain, it is likely that a reasonable preliminary diagnosis about its cause and tentative treatment plan can be made. A meticulously obtained history provides the physician with sufficient information about the characteristics of the pain and how it is affecting the patient to better enable him or her to focus on specific elements of the physical examination and select appropriate laboratory and imaging studies. The location of the pain, whether it radiates, whether it preceded the diagnosis of cancer, its intensity and dynamics, how it impacts the patient and his or her family, and the effectiveness of previous and current treatment can be established on the basis of the history alone. The history also affords clues about the etiology of the pain and whether it is nociceptive or neuropathic in nature. The physical examination should elaborate and expand on information gained from integrating knowledge of the causes of pain with its historical features.

Physical Examination*

Quality medical practice requires that all patients have a thorough physical examination. In addition to completing a standard complete physical examination, the physician should use information gained from the history to guide the examiner to focus on the local examination of the painful area, skin, and musculoskeletal and nervous systems. Maneuvers that stress the area under examination and reproduce the pain are also important to identify the pain source.

Local Examination

Each painful area should be carefully examined for physical changes, such as swelling and inflammation, that contribute to the pain experience. Muscle tenderness and spasm may account for pain. If the cause of these findings is not apparent from the physical examination, appropriate diagnostic studies should be ordered. Pain may vary with positional changes; eg, pain present when the patient is sitting may completely disappear with lying down, or vice versa. Abdominal pain should be carefully evaluated. The abdomen is a frequent site of intermittent acute painful disorders secondary to obstruction by either tumor or adhesions from previous surgery or radiotherapy. Neuropathic pain secondary to previous therapy of any type also may be located in this area. Because outward or ongoing evidence of a pain-producing process is frequently absent, patients complaining of neuropathic abdominal pain often have difficulty convincing the physician that pain actually exists. Bladder, bowel, and vaginal spasms and a distressful "bearing down" sensation deep in the pelvis and rectal area are frequent sequelae of radiotherapy for pelvic lesions. These are visceral forms of neuropathic pain. Because these symptoms frequently are episodic or may be constant with irregular episodes of exacerbation, complete pain control is usually not possible.

Skin

When examining the skin, the examiner may find allodynia, hyperalgesia, dysesthesia, hypalgesia, numbness, cellulitis, neuritis, neuropathy, edema, heat, ulceration, direct tumor invasion, trophic changes, and various dermatologic eruptions. Some of these findings lend support for the diagnosis of neuropathic pain. They also help determine a complete treatment plan, eg, antibiotic therapy to relieve the pain of cellulitis and local treatment to relieve ulcer pain, in addition to systemic analgesic drugs.

Musculoskeletal System

There may be both joint and muscle signs and symptoms, and changes in these structures may affect the overall structural integrity of the skeleton. The function of major muscle groups should be tested. Muscle spasm, atrophy, tenderness (perhaps "secondary" hyperalgesia), a hypersensitive focal area or site in muscle or connective tissue (trigger point), and muscle imbalance secondary to previous surgery may be present. A careful examination in search of clues to the pathogenesis is important. Joint swelling and tenderness may indicate an acute or chronic process, related or unrelated to the malignant process. So-called paraneoplastic syndromes frequently involve the nervous and musculoskeletal systems. Limitation of motion of a joint, such as the shoulder, may cause a painful adhesive capsulitis (frozen shoulder), which is not infrequently seen in patients who limit motion in the shoulder following breast and thoracic surgery. Physical therapy modalities are frequently more effective than drug treatment for long-term improvement. However, analgesics and muscle relaxants may be necessary to facilitate the physical therapy.

Nervous System

The nervous system is one of the most frequently affected systems in cancer patients, and warrants particular attention during examination. At a minimum, all sensory and motor deficits should be identified. Specific neurologic deficits can help locate obscure metastatic deposits in difficult-to-identify locations. As mentioned previously, special attention should be given to back pain to identify leptomeningeal disease and the possibility of spinal cord compression. Preventing spinal cord compression, with its subsequent likelihood of paralysis, can significantly enhance the patient's quality of life. Spinal cord compression requires immediate treatment with corticosteroids, which reduce swelling, thus relieving pain, and may provide interim protection against permanent damage to neurologic structures until definitive measures, such as radiation and surgery, can be initiated. Careful neurologic examination can differentiate peripheral from central causes of pain. This determination is important in directing treatment.

Laboratory and Imaging Studies

Perhaps the two most important diagnostic tests in patients with pain are computed tomography and magnetic resonance imaging. Both are noninvasive and provide relatively detailed images of normal and abnormal anatomic structures. Nervous system structures are better visualized on MRI, which is particu-

*See glossary for definition of terms used in this section.

larly useful for detecting early spinal cord compression. Positron emission tomography can demonstrate specific metabolic and functional CNS changes, but is still an investigational tool.

In selected cases, testing of muscle and peripheral nerves by electromyography and nerve conduction studies is useful. Electroencephalography is useful in evaluating patients with suspected seizure disorders and metabolic derangements of the brain. Psychologic testing may be helpful in identifying brain metastases and assessing higher integrative functioning; this is useful in evaluating the validity of patients' responses to questions and the state of their memory and can provide a clue to their ability to comply with instructions.

Blood chemistry tests that reflect the functioning capacity of the major organ systems are important for determining how the organs are likely to metabolize analgesics and other drugs used to treat pain and other distressing symptoms. Proper dosing of analgesics will depend on this information. The kidney and liver are the two most important organs involved in analgesic metabolism.

Developing a Treatment Plan

To treat pain due to a primary or metastatic tumor, the first treatment consideration for both tumor control and pain relief is treatment directed at the neoplastic process. Treatments designed to remove, or otherwise ablate, the tumor—surgery, radiotherapy, chemotherapy, and biological response modifiers—should be selected depending on their effectiveness alone or in combination. However, it is necessary to concurrently provide pain relief with appropriate analgesics, whether nonopioids or strong opioids, until the antitumor treatment relieves the pain.

The emphasis in this chapter, however, is on the 60% to 90% of cancer patients in whom the cause of pain cannot be removed or who cannot be treated effectively by pain pathway blockade (nerve blocks) or neurosurgical techniques. Nor are they candidates for alternative or adjunctive forms of therapy used alone. These patients must rely on the use of strong systemic opioids.[14] The reliance on strong opioids makes this group of patients the most likely to experience inadequate pain relief. They fall into the following categories[5]:

- Patients who require opioids in "unusual" doses (doses considered "high") over protracted periods to treat pain;
- Patients with predominantly neuropathic pain, or pain only partially responsive to narcotics, who are treated solely with opioids;
- Patients whose pain can be relieved by opioids but in whom no anatomic, physiologic, or pathologic cause of pain can be demonstrated by either physical examination or diagnostic techniques, and who therefore are denied access to opioids; and
- Patients with cancer pain who concomitantly abuse drugs, those who previously abused drugs, and those who fit the "profile" of a drug abuser.

In contrast, the patient in whom the cause of pain can be removed or who responds to nonpharmacologic treatment modalities such as nerve blocks, physical therapy, hypnosis, relaxation, or guided imagery or is a candidate for anesthetic or neurosurgical techniques is unlikely to suffer unrelieved pain because there is no reluctance to apply these modalities.

The goal of education in pain control is to make every physician involved in the daily care of patients a "pain expert." To accomplish this, the proper use of systemic analgesic drugs must be mastered. Fortunately, most pain in cancer patients is of nociceptive origin and can be adequately relieved by the means readily available to the majority of physicians and other healthcare providers. Specialized pain-relieving techniques, which are needed in only a selected, relatively small percentage of patients, will continue to be carried out in hospitals and pain treatment centers.

"Analgesic Ladder" Approach

The World Health Organization (WHO) recommends an "analgesic ladder" approach to pain treatment (Fig 38-4).[15] Patients whose pain starts off as mild and progresses to severe in a crescendo fashion are treated stepwise using increasingly stronger analgesics, which may or may not be combined with a nonsteroidal anti-inflammatory drug (NSAID) and/or various adjuvant or coanalgesic drugs. For mild pain, a nonopioid analgesic, such as acetaminophen, aspirin, or another NSAID, can be used along with an adjuvant drug such as an antidepressant or another appropriate psychoactive drug. For moderate pain, a weak opioid alone or in combination with acetaminophen, aspirin, or another NSAID is recommended, again adding an adjuvant drug such as an antidepressant or another appropriate psychoactive drug. For severe pain, a strong opioid should be used along with the same psychoactive adjuvant drugs used to treat mild and moderate pain. The minimum opioid dose employed for any degree of pain intensity should be that which is adequate to relieve the pain. The so-called usual or recommended doses found in standard references are merely recommended starting doses and frequently must be exceeded to provide optimum relief.

One must keep in mind that the analgesic ladder can be accessed initially on any rung. Pain may not progress in severity in a crescendo fashion. At the outset, it may be severe and require initial treatment with a strong opioid. Assessing the intensity of the pain, as described by the patient, is essential to selecting the proper analgesic at the onset of pain to achieve optimum relief.

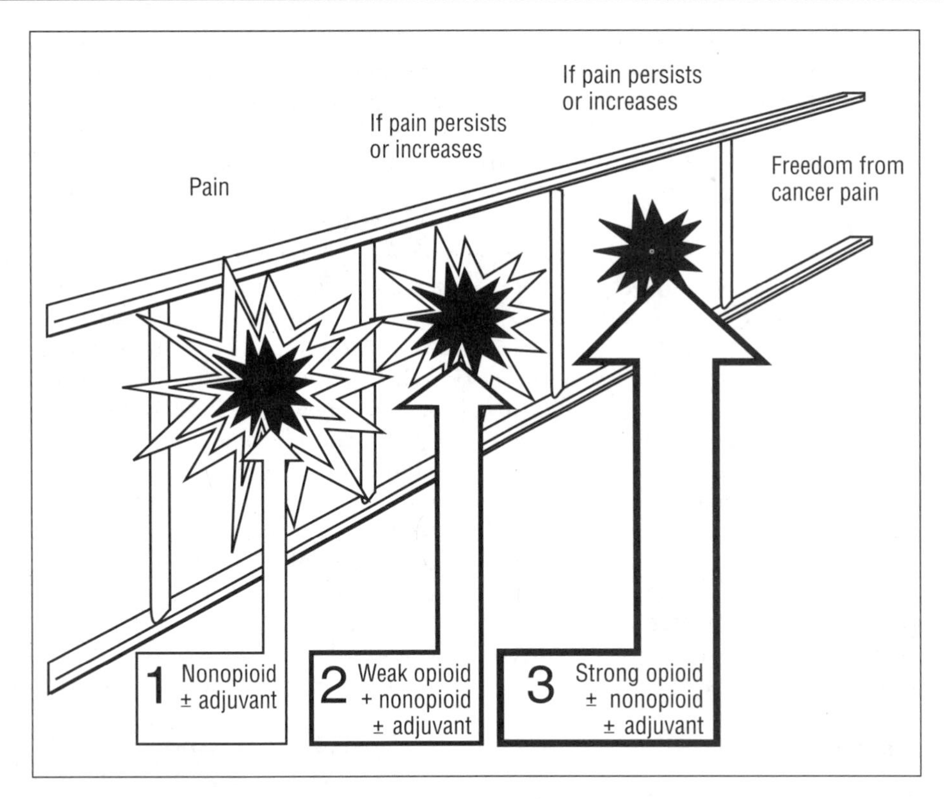

Fig 38-4. The WHO 3-step ladder for cancer pain relief.[15]

Selection of Drugs

Nonopioid Analgesics

The major group of nonopioid analgesics is the NSAIDs. Acetaminophen, although not technically an NSAID, is often included in this group because of its analgesic properties. Analgesia is thought to occur as a result of inhibition of the enzyme cyclooxygenase, which reduces the production of inflammatory mediators, predominantly prostaglandins, known to sensitize or activate peripheral nociceptors. Thus, the mode of action is peripheral, compared with the central action of opioids. It is therefore rational to administer opioids and nonopioids concurrently to take advantage of both modes of action. Additionally, the combination often provides greater pain relief than simply the effect of one analgesic added to the other.

Indications

A specific indication for NSAID use is pain associated with an inflammatory reaction surrounding a tumor. This is most obvious in cutaneous metastatic nodules or infiltration. A second specific indication is pain associated with metastases to bone.[16]

The synergism of NSAIDs with opioids is an additional indication for their use, and may allow a reduction in the opioid dose in patients suffering from undesirable side effects such as oversedation and mental cloudiness.

Selecting a Nonopioid Analgesic

A wide variety of NSAIDs is available for use (Table 38-3). Generally, claims of superior anti-inflammatory effect, pain relieving qualities, or safety profile have not been definitively established. Clinical experience has shown that no NSAID is consistently reliable for pain relief in all patients. Selection is therefore empirical; if one drug fails to produce the desired effect, try another. Each drug should be administered long enough to allow an adequate trial.

The only rational distinction among NSAIDs is based on differences in pharmacologic characteristics rather than therapeutic efficacy. For example, piroxicam has a long half-life and can be given once daily, a convenient dosing that encourages compliance. Nonacetylated salicylates are the drug of choice in patients at risk for bleeding disorders and in those receiving chemotherapy sparing effect on platelet aggregation.

Dosing and Routes of Administration

Dosing with NSAIDs has been evaluated mostly in patients with chronic nonmalignant painful medical conditions. Nevertheless, these studies are the basis for the doses recommended for the treatment of pain in cancer patients. One must therefore be thoughtful in using these doses in cancer patients, who are usually older, may have single or multiple organ compromise or failure, and may be receiving cytotoxic or other drugs whose effects are not complementary to those of NSAIDs. Under these circumstances, doses may need to be lower than recommended levels. Alternatively, doses may need to be higher if the desired effect is not achieved and there are no contraindications to increasing the dose. The cardinal pharmacologic principle regulating dosing with NSAIDs is the "ceiling effect": increasing the dose of a drug above a certain level will fail to provide additional pain relief but may indeed produce adverse effects. In general, NSAIDs produce analgesic effects at lower doses and

Table 38-3. Commonly Used Nonsteroidal Antiinflammatory Drugs

Generic Name and Class	Trade Name	Approx. Half-Life (h)	Dosing Schedule	Recommended Starting Dose (mg/day)	Maximum Recommended Dose (mg/day)
Salicylates					
Acetylsalicylic acid	Aspirin, etc.	3–12	q 4–6 h	2600	6000
Choline magnesium trisalicylate	Trilisate	8–12	q 8–12 h	1500 X 1 then 500 q 12	4000
Salsalate	Disalcid	8–12	q 8–12 h	1500 X 1 then 500 q 12	4000
Diflunisal	Dolobid, Dolobis	8–12	q 12 h	1000 X 1 then 500 q 12	1500
Acetic Acid Derivatives					
Indomethacin	Indocin, Indocid, Indomethine	4–5	q 8–12 h	75	200
Sulindac	Clinoril, Arthorobid	14	q 12 h	300	400
Tolmetin	Tolectin	1	q 6–8 h	600	2000
Ketorolac	Toradol	4–7	q 4–6 h	120	240
Suprofen		2–4	q 6 h	600	800
Fenamates					
Mefenamic acid	Ponstel, Ponstan, Ponstil, Namphen	2	q 6 h	4	1000
Meclofenamate sodium	Meclomen	2–4	q 6–8 h	150	400
Propionic Acid Derivatives					
Ibuprofen	Motrin, Advil, Nuprin, Rifen	3–4	q 4–8 h	1200	4200
Naproxen	Naprosyn, Naprosine, Proxen	13	q 12 h	500	1000
Fenoprofen	Nalfon, Fenopran, Nalgesic, Progesic	2–3	q 6 h	800	3200
Ketoprofen	Orudis, Alrheumat	2–3	q 6–8 h	150	300
Flurbiprofen	Ansaid	5–6	q 8–12 h	100	300
Diclofenac	Voltaren	2	q 6 h	75	200
Oxaprozin	Daypro	50–60	q 24 h	1200	1800
Oxicams					
Piroxicam	Feldene	45	q 24 h	20	40
Pyranocarboxylic Acids					
Etodolac	Lodine	7.3	q 6–8 h	800	1200
Naphthylalkanones					
Nabumetone	Relafen	22–30	q 12–24 h	1000	2000

Adapted from Patt et al.[18]

anti-inflammatory effects at higher doses.[17] Dose ranges for selected NSAIDs are given in Table 38-3.[18]

Three routes of administration are available for NSAIDs. Most must be given orally. Indomethacin is also available in rectal suppository form, and ketorolac, popular for postoperative pain, is available for intramuscular administration. Ketorolac is not approved in this country for intravenous use, but this route has been used extensively in Europe with no additional side effects.[19] Because it is less traumatic to the patient, intravenous administration is preferable to intramuscular injection.

Side Effects

The major toxic effects of NSAIDs occur in the kidneys and gastrointestinal (GI) tract; however, any organ system may be affected, and adverse reactions have been reported in the CNS, lung, and liver.[20] Patients with impaired renal function should be given NSAIDs with caution. A history of GI bleeding or concurrent dyspeptic symptoms probably indicates that NSAIDs should not be used. Patients with a remote history of GI bleeding or a vague history of peptic disease should be given cytoprotective and antiulcer therapy on a prophylactic basis if NSAIDs are used.

The threat of a bleeding diathesis is of particular concern in cancer patients because they frequently have compromised platelet levels and poorly functioning platelets secondary to chemotherapy or other anticancer drugs. Choline magnesium trisalicylate, salsalate, and diflunisal, all nonacetylated salicylates, are the NSAIDs of choice for treating patients with platelet or bleeding abnormalities. Choline magnesium trisalicylate is available in liquid form, making its administration possible for patients unable to swallow pills.

Opioids

A useful classification of opioids is based on their predominant pharmacologic action: 1) pure agonists, 2) mixed agonist/antagonists, and 3) partial agonists (Table 38-4). Although some opioids are categorized as "pure" agonists, all opioids have a dual action of producing analgesia (agonist) and reversing it (antagonist) to varying degrees.[21] The prototype agonist is morphine. The prototype antagonist is naloxone, a drug that will reverse analgesia and all the other pharmacologic actions of opioids and, in opioid-dependent patients, can cause an abstinence, or withdrawal, reaction. The predominant action of mixed agonist/antagonists and partial agonists is agonist but they also have a potentially significant antagonist action.

The practical significance of this classification relates to a switch in medication from one category to another. Patients who have been treated with pure agonists should not be switched to either mixed agonist/antagonists or partial agonists because of the possibility of precipitating a withdrawal reaction. However, patients who have been treated with mixed agonist/antagonists or partial agonists may be switched to pure agonists with impunity because there is no potential for a withdrawal reaction.

Another practical classification distinguishes weak from strong opioids based on their capacity to relieve mild, moderate, or severe pain (Table 38-5). Perhaps any narcotic could relieve any pain, but the side effects accompanying the necessary dosage make it impractical to use the weaker narcotics for severe pain.

Table 38-4. Pharmacologic Classification of Opioids

Classification	Opioid
Pure agonist	Propoxyphene Codeine Dihydrocodeine Oxycodone Hydrocodone Morphine Hydromorphone Methadone Levorphanol Meperidine
Mixed agonist/antagonist	Pentazocine Butorphanol Nalbuphine
Partial agonist	Buprenorphine

Mechanism of Action

Exogenous opioids act as ligands that bind to certain stereospecific and saturable receptors in the CNS and other tissues (eg, the large bowel).[22] These receptors also serve an endogenous opioid system: the endorphins, enkephalins, and dynorphins. There is reasonably firm evidence for four major categories of CNS receptors: mu, kappa, delta, and sigma. It is thought that these receptors mediate the various effects of the opioids. The affinity with which an opioid binds to one or more of these receptors may account for its characteristic action. For example, dysphoria and psychomimetic effects are associated with opioids with a stronger affinity for sigma receptors, whereas potent analgesia is associated with opioids with a stronger affinity for mu receptors.

Because all opioids act by binding to CNS receptors, combining a significant number of them in the treatment of pain is seldom advantageous. For

Table 38-5. Classification of Opioids Based on Analgesic Potency

Classification	Opioid
Weak opioid	Propoxyphene Codeine Oxycodone Hydrocodone
Strong opioid	Morphine Hydromorphone Methadone Levorphanol Meperidine Fentanyl

example, the combination of morphine, hydromorphone, and meperidine provides no therapeutic benefit over an adequate dose of any one of these drugs. Such polypharmacy is not infrequently practiced, probably because of a reluctance to simply increase the dose of a single opioid to an effective level, albeit one that may exceed the "usual" or "recommended" dose. Unfortunately, this untested practice has become traditional probably because of fear of sanction by state and federal regulatory agencies for prescribing one drug outside the usual or recommended dosage range. However, from the patient's perspective, it is less confusing and the results are the same if an adequate dose of a single agent is used.

The combining of drugs with a similar mechanism of action is rational when the objective is to take advantage of specific pharmacologic characteristics of each drug. For example, use of methadone, a drug with a long half-life whose dosing interval may be 6 hours, requires concomitant prescribing of a complementary short-acting drug, such as morphine or hydromorphone, for "breakthrough" pain which may occur before the end of 6 hours.

Taking advantage of synergistic action between opioids with a predominantly central site of action and analgesics with predominantly peripheral sites of action is also a rational therapeutic maneuver.

Trepidation Associated With Starting Opioids for Pain Treatment

The decision to initiate opioid therapy, especially a decision to use "strong" opioids, is usually associated with a feeling of trepidation on the part of the physician. Concern about side effects and developing tolerance, fear of creating an "addict," a misconception that there is a "ceiling effect" (ie, opioids will be ineffective when the pain gets very severe), and fear of sanctions by regulatory authorities are probably the most cogent reasons for this trepidation. Why these concerns and fears are overrated and unjustified will be discussed subsequently.

Unfortunately, owing to this trepidation, physicians tend to delay or reserve the use of strong opioids until the terminal phase of a patient's illness.[23] Pain of such severity that it can be relieved only by opioids obviously is an indication for their use regardless of the stage of the disease (localized or advanced). Frequently, the prescribing of analgesic drugs, using weak opioids singly or in combination with nonopioid analgesics, is practiced far beyond the point of usefulness of these drugs for relieving pain. The inconvenience to the patient of taking a large number of pills (polypharmacy) rather than the convenience of taking only a few (strong opioids) should not be overlooked. It is important to put trepidation aside and prescribe opioids whenever they are needed if cancer patients suffering pain are to be treated adequately.

The decision to initiate opioid therapy for pain should be made when: 1) the initial pain is so intense that it is obvious strong opioids will be required for relief, or 2) as pain increases in intensity during the progression of the patient's disease, nonopioid analgesics are no longer able to relieve it. In the first circumstance, the decision to initiate opioid analgesics should come easily because of the obvious intensity of the pain and the imperative to relieve it. In the second circumstance, the decision is less obvious because of the evolving and subtle nature of the increase in pain intensity.

The Initiation Process

A maxim of pain treatment using opioids is to start treatment with the weakest opioid possessing sufficient analgesic properties in order to minimize the possibility of undesirable side effects. Ongoing reassessment of the patient's pain relief is the most reliable procedure for determining when an opioid should be started. A weak opioid, as defined in Table 38-5, may be used alone or in combination with a nonopioid analgesic. Again, ongoing reassessment will indicate when the drug is no longer effective for relieving the pain. A clue that pain intensity is increasing, or tolerance is developing, is a decrease in the interval of effectiveness of a single dose of the medication. Most of these drugs are effective for 3 to 4 hours. If pain is controlled for only 2 to 2.5 hours, the dose should be increased or a change made to a stronger opioid.

Reluctance to start prescribing strong opioids often results in increasing the number of dose units of a weak opioid/nonopioid analgesic combination. The limiting factor in increasing the opioid dose in an opioid/nonopioid analgesic (usually acetaminophen or NSAID) combination is the amount of nonopioid present. Increasing the number of dose units of the combination to increase the dosage of the opioid will eventually increase the nonopioid portion to toxic levels. Strong opioids alone should be started long before toxic levels of the nonopioid are reached.

Opioid therapy is frequently delayed in patients with a possible long-term painful prognosis because of concerns about tolerance and physical and psychologic dependency (addiction). Prognosis and survival time should not be determining factors for initiating opioid therapy. Similarly, tolerance and physical dependence should not be a deterrent to possible long-term use. Experience with cancer patients suggests that clinical tolerance is unlikely to develop. Physical dependence on opioids is a normal pharmacologic phenomenon; the only consequence is a withdrawal reaction on abrupt discontinuation—a process that can be avoided simply by a gradual decrease in dosage as pain intensity decreases. Addiction seldom occurs when opioids are used for their legitimate medical purposes.[24] Therefore, the possibility of cancer patients becoming addicted to opioids is remote. It is not logical to postpone opioid use because of the possibility of long-term use and fear of tolerance, physical dependence, and an irrational fear of addiction.

Once the decision has been made to use an opioid, the next step is to choose the appropriate one. The choice begins with assessing the pain intensity. Mild to moderate pain requires only weak opioids. Severe pain requires strong opioids regardless of the potential duration of administration.

Weak Opioids

Propoxyphene

Propoxyphene is the only one of four stereoisomers of methadone to have analgesic activity; it binds to opioid receptors. Its analgesic potency is approximately 50% to 67% of that of codeine when given orally. Data are conflicting as to whether this drug is more effective than appropriate doses of aspirin, other NSAIDs, or acetaminophen. Nonetheless, it may be useful for patients with mild pain. It should not necessarily be considered a "step up" the analgesic ladder for those patients whose pain is no longer relieved by aspirin or acetaminophen, notwithstanding the fact that it is technically an opioid.

Codeine

Codeine, probably the most widely used opioid for treating cancer pain, is effective in controlling mild pain. The frequent combination of codeine and either aspirin or acetaminophen produces a greater analgesic effect than the mere sum of the two analgesics' effects. Continuing the use of codeine, alone or in combination, after it no longer relieves pain is commonly done to avoid prescribing a stronger opioid.

Oxycodone

Until recently, oxycodone was unavailable in the US except in combination with aspirin or acetaminophen (Percocet, Percodan, Tylox). Oxycodone is now available separately as a 5-mg tablet and as a liquid (1 and 20 mg/mL), making it useful for mild to moderate pain and alleviating concerns about reaching toxic levels of nonnarcotics with escalating doses of combination products.

Hydrocodone

Hydrocodone is used extensively in antitussive compounds. It is also used in fixed combination with acetaminophen for the treatment of mild to moderate pain; it is not available as a single-agent analgesic. No studies comparing its potency with those of other analgesics are available. It is generally considered slightly weaker than combination oxycodone products. A particular precaution is that some fixed-combination hydrocodone products (Anexsia 7.5/650, Vicodin ES) contain as much as 650 to 750 mg of acetaminophen in a single tablet, and toxic doses of acetaminophen will be reached more quickly if the number of tablets is increased or the interval of administration is decreased to avoid use of a stronger opioid.

Strong Opioids

Morphine

Morphine is the prototype for strong opioids: it is the most widely used opioid worldwide and the most extensively studied. However, despite the wealth of clinical experience and investigational data, there are probably more myths and misconceptions about morphine than about any other opioid.

Hydromorphone

Hydromorphone is readily absorbed from the GI tract and will control severe pain when given orally. It is more potent by weight than morphine, with 1.3 mg of hydromorphone being equianalgesic to 10 mg of morphine given intramuscularly. Because of biotransformation in the liver (first-pass effect), the oral dose of hydromorphone must be four to five times the parenteral dose to produce an equianalgesic effect. When given orally, hydromorphone achieves its peak effect slightly quicker than morphine and also has a slightly shorter duration of action. It may be necessary to administer hydromorphone at 3-hour intervals.

Methadone

Methadone is as potent an analgesic as morphine in comparable doses when administered intramuscularly. However, because of its favorable oral-to-parenteral ratio of 2:1 (first-pass effect is slight), the equianalgesic oral dose needs to be only twice the parenteral dose. The most important clinical consideration is the long half-life of methadone. Although the duration of analgesic effectiveness of a single oral dose is approximately 4 hours, the terminal elimination half-life varies from 13 to 51 hours. When doses are repeated every 4 hours, the drug accumulates and the blood concentration may reach toxic levels. Initial dosing must be determined carefully to avoid this complication. After the first 3 to 4 days, the interval of administration can be extended, which effectively reduces the 24-hour dosage while maintaining the analgesic level. Methadone may be effective when administered every 6 to 8 hours.

Methadone may be difficult to use in older patients and in cancer patients whose disease is progressing rapidly and who experience frequent changes in pain level. Some patients associate methadone with the treatment of heroin or other drug addiction and are afraid that methadone use will stigmatize them as being drug addicts.

Levorphanol

Levorphanol can be used orally to control severe pain. It is readily absorbed from the GI tract and has a favorable oral-to-parenteral ratio of approximately 1:1. Its half-life is approximately 11 hours; therefore, some accumulation occurs and dosing intervals of >4 hours may be possible.

Meperidine

Although extensively used for postoperative pain, meperidine is not recommended for the treatment of chronic pain. It is readily absorbed from the GI tract, but has an unfavorable oral-to-parenteral ratio of 4:1. Meperidine is the weakest of the "strong" opioids when compared with morphine. When given intramuscularly, a 75- to 100-mg dose of meperidine is equianalgesic to a 10-mg dose of morphine. When given orally, 300 mg is equianalgesic to 30 mg of morphine. The duration of action of meperidine is ≤3 hours, making frequent dosing necessary.

The most serious drawback to the chronic administration of meperidine is the accumulation of the metabolite normeperidine, which has a longer half-life than the parent compound. Normeperidine is a CNS stimulant and may cause tremors, muscle twitches, and seizures. Toxicity is more likely to occur if there is renal failure.

Fentanyl

A potent agonist, fentanyl is considered approximately 100 times more potent than morphine by weight. It has just recently been introduced as an analgesic for the treatment of chronic pain. Previously, its major use was as a general anesthetic. Physicians other than anesthesiologists have had limited experience with fentanyl in general, and specifically for chronic pain.

The pharmacology of fentanyl is helpful in understanding its use for chronic pain. In single intravenous doses, its duration of analgesia is 30 to 60 minutes; therefore, it is considered to have a short duration of action. However, since its use for chronic pain control is confined to transdermal administration, this pharmacodynamic information is irrelevant because the transdermal system delivers the drug continuously until the system is exhausted. The transdermal system operates like an intravenous infusion. In most patients, the system is effective for 72 hours, in some only for 48 hours.

With the transdermal system, the prescribed concentration of fentanyl in the blood is not reached for ≥12 hours after initiation of therapy. Therefore, doses of a rapidly acting opioid agonist must be given, either orally, rectally, or parenterally, during the first 12 or more hours for adequate pain control while fentanyl reaches its prescribed concentration. If the patient experiences an adverse effect of the drug and the drug is discontinued, he or she must be monitored for up to 24 hours following discontinuance because fentanyl is stored in subcutaneous fat and a 50% decline in the serum concentration of fentanyl may take ≥17 hours.

No systematic studies using fentanyl as an initial analgesic agent for chronic pain have been done. Patients with chronic pain should be treated initially with another short-acting agonist until a dose is established that controls the pain, then converted to transdermal fentanyl. This approach is recommended because of the difficulty titrating the dose using transdermal fentanyl alone (a consequence of the duration of delivery by the system).

Mixed Agonist/Antagonists and Partial Agonists

Opioids with mixed agonist/antagonist activity and partial agonists are not recommended for cancer patients with chronic pain. The incidence of psychomimetic reactions is higher than with pure agonists, and only pentazocine is available in the US for oral administration. Differential binding to specific opioid binding sites is thought to account for this characteristic of the drug.[21] Additionally, one should be cautioned not to switch to an agonist/antagonist or a partial agonist in patients being treated with a pure agonist because of the potential for precipitating a withdrawal reaction. The partial agonist buprenorphine will also precipitate a withdrawal reaction in patients who are tolerant to morphine-like agonists, and the respiratory depression caused by this drug is not easily reversed by naloxone.[25]

Pharmacologic Features of Opioids

As with all drugs, the pharmacokinetic and pharmacodynamic characteristics of opioids are of practical therapeutic importance. For opioids, pharmacokinetics is defined as what the body does to the drug before it reaches the opioid binding sites in the CNS, and pharmacodynamics is defined as what the opioid does to the body after it reaches the opioid binding sites in the CNS. Morphine will be discussed as representative of the class of strong opioids.

Pharmacokinetics

Morphine is readily absorbed from the GI tract and metabolized to morphine-3-glucuronide and morphine-6-glucuronide. Morphine-6-glucuronide is a potent analgesic, but morphine-3-glucuronide may antagonize its analgesic effect.[26] The specific role of these metabolites in analgesia remains to be determined.

Hepatic metabolism, through a first-pass effect (biotransformation), basically inactivates approximately two thirds of an orally administered dose; ie, two thirds of an oral dose does not have analgesic capabilities. Parenterally administered doses do not suffer from this first-pass effect because they reach binding sites before the liver reduces their effectiveness. Thus, clinicians often perceive parenterally administered opioids to be more effective than orally administered ones. The dose of oral opioids should be adjusted upward to compensate for the first-pass effect. If one keeps this pharmacokinetic principle in mind, success with oral administration of opioids will occur in the vast majority of patients.

Pharmacodynamics

Morphine primarily affects the CNS and the bowel. The CNS effects differ depending on whether individuals are experiencing pain.[27] Pain antagonizes the analgesic effects of opioids; therefore, patients in severe pain will require a higher opioid dose than is usually recommended in standard pharmacology textbooks and other references. Respiratory depression is also antagonized by pain.[27] As long as the increased dose does not excessively exceed the level necessary to control the pain, respiratory depression is exceedingly unlikely. Confusion about these points has often resulted in patients in pain receiving inadequate doses of morphine or other opioids.

Morphine's effects on the CNS are diverse and include analgesia, drowsiness, mood changes, decrease in mental acuity, nausea, vomiting, and alterations in the endocrine and autonomic nervous systems. In contrast to NSAIDs, there is no ceiling effect with morphine. Incremental increases in dose will always produce additional analgesia in patients whose pain is nociceptive or uncomplicated by other factors. The principle of "dosing to effect" should always be followed when using morphine; ie, increase the dose until the desired effect is achieved or undesirable side effects prevent further escalation. In general, side effects are encountered only at the onset of therapy and are transient.

Effects on the small and large intestine are caused by marked decrease or halting of propulsive contractions and peristaltic waves. Tolerance to bowel effects seldom occurs; therefore, it is extremely important to institute a bowel cleaning program when morphine is given, especially with long-term administration.

Morphine may also affect urinary bladder function, causing both urgency and difficulty with urination because of increased sphincter tone. There may be a drop in blood pressure due to peripheral arteriolar and venous dilatation.

Pharmacodynamics of other opioids are essentially the same as for morphine. Significant clinical differences are discussed with the specific opioids.

Dosing

Probably the most common error in dosing with opioids is underdosing.[1-3] The dose of morphine usually recommended for severe pain is 10 mg intramuscularly. This dose was determined by single-dose studies in postoperative patients.[28] However, pain associated with cancer and many chronic benign painful conditions is frequently much more severe than postoperative pain and will require doses higher than 10 mg. "The proper dose of morphine is whatever it takes to relieve the pain." Ten milligrams intramuscularly or an equianalgesic oral dose may be a reasonable starting dose, but pain relief should be evaluated 30 to 60 minutes after administration and the dose titrated upward until the pain is relieved. Rapid upward titration is possible because of the antagonistic effect of pain on the respiratory depression associated with opioids. So long as the patient is experiencing pain, respiratory depression as a possible complication of opioid administration should not be a deterrent to administering an adequate dose.

To titrate upward by the oral route, the patient is instructed to take a "breakthrough" dose of immediate-release morphine between the scheduled doses of immediate-release morphine whenever the pain returns. The duration of action of immediate-release morphine is approximately 4 hours. Therefore, the "breakthrough" dose will be taken any time between the 4-hour intervals of scheduled dosing. If the combination of scheduled and the breakthrough doses is inadequate to control the pain, the combined dose for the 24-hour period is used as a new scheduled dose in divided doses every 4 hours, and a new breakthrough dose is used that is 50% higher than the previous one.

To titrate upward by the intravenous route, morphine is administered until the pain is relieved or intolerable side effects occur, or it is determined that the patient has pain which is only partially responsive to opioids (neuropathic pain). Incremental doses (given as bolus or rapid infusions) range from 5 to 15 mg, based on an assessment of pain severity. The intravenous titration method avoids the titration intervals present with oral titration.

In a multicenter study, adequate morphine dosages for pain relief varied from 60 to 3,000 mg per 24 hours in divided doses.[29] These levels should not be considered upper or lower limits, but merely the wide range necessary to individualize dosing to adequately relieve pain. As mentioned earlier, there is no ceiling effect for morphine: an increase in dose will always produce a concomitant increase in pain relief. A possible exception may occur with neuropathic pain, when increases in opioid dose produce no corresponding increase in analgesia, but an increase in side effects. For nociceptive pain, there are anecdotal reports of patients receiving 36 to 50 *grams* of morphine over 24 hours who are alert and able to function satisfactorily.

Undertreatment of pain will occur if dosing intervals with immediate-release morphine exceed 4 hours. To obviate this problem, morphine is now available in a controlled-release form that extends its effectiveness to 12 hours. Combining this form with immediate-release morphine can produce near constant pain control. A method of pain control using this combination will be described subsequently.

Comparing Morphine With Other Opioids

The pharmacodynamics of other opioid drugs are similar to those of morphine, although an individual may experience more or fewer side effects with other drugs and the same drug may cause different side effects in different patients. For example, morphine may cause nausea and vomiting in one patient but not in another. These side effects may occur with any opioid, and a switch may be necessary in a given patient. However, there are pharmacologic differences among the opioids that will be discussed below.

Table 38-6 shows the oral-to-parenteral dose ratios and the equianalgesic doses for commonly used opioids. This table can be used to convert the dose of one opioid into that of another and to convert one route of administration to another. The reference standard is 10 mg of morphine given intramuscularly for treatment of severe pain.

Side Effects

Side effects of a drug are merely pharmacodynamic effects that in most situations are considered undesirable. This is not always true for opioids. Patients with diarrhea in addition to pain appreciate the constipating effect of the opioid that results in control of the diarrhea along with pain control. The same is true for the antitussive effects of opioids in patients with cough, and, in some cases, for their anxiolytic and sedative effects.

Side effects may be transient or persistent. Transient reactions that are usually associated with initiation of opioid therapy include sedation, mental clouding (including transient hallucinations), dizziness, urinary retention, nausea, vomiting, and itching. A careful pharmacodynamic evaluation should be made of these side effects before it is concluded that opioids in general or a particular opioid and route of administration must be abandoned. Symptoms may arise from multiple causes; for an opioid to be implicated, a definite relationship should be established.

Nausea and vomiting can be controlled with antinauseants; after a week or two, these often can be discontinued and the patient can remain on the oral narcotic free of nausea and vomiting. Patients with persistent problems urinating can be taught to catheterize themselves, and after several days urinate normally. Many of the transient side effects are dose dependent; once the dose is adjusted properly, the side effects are minimized or disappear.

Persistent side effects should be vigorously treated. Sedation can be countered with CNS stimulants such as dextroamphetamine sulfate or methylphenidate. Both are known to have a synergistic action with opioids and may not only correct the sedation but also enhance pain relief. Sedation as a side effect may be confused with prolonged sleep after prolonged sleep deprivation. Patients who have unrelieved pain for a significant period may have been unable to sleep for much of that time and be sleep-deprived. With adequate pain relief, they are able to sleep and may do so for an extended period; this "catching up" may be interpreted as oversedation.

The most consistent and persistent side effect is constipation. It occurs with all opioids, including weak ones, especially codeine, and with all routes of administration. A bowel cleaning program should be instituted immediately with the prescribing of narcotics, especially when chronic administration is anticipated. Since propulsion is the action blocked by the opioid, administering stool softeners alone is insufficient to prevent this side effect. A mild laxative in combination with a stool softener should be administered for effective relief. Failure to control constipation may cause nausea and vomiting. Patients are frequently labeled as "allergic" to an opioid if nausea and vomiting occur with initiation of opioid treatment, when in fact they are simply not moving their bowels as they should.

The intrinsic attributes of opioids may be confused with side effects. Tolerance and physical dependence are two attributes associated with long-term administration. In cancer patients, clinical tolerance occurs very slowly and for practical purposes not at all. Dose escalation for this reason is required infrequently[2]; if required, the escalation is usually due to disease progression causing an increase in pain intensity.

Physical dependence occurs but is of no consequence because it does not cause symptoms or undesirable effects until the opioid is no longer needed and the patient discontinues it. Abrupt discontinuation will produce the distressful symptoms of an abstinence or withdrawal reaction. This can be avoided by gradually reducing the opioid dose. Cancer patients taking opioids for pain relief welcome the discontinuation of these drugs when pain abates, and there is ample evidence that patients taking opioids for pain relief do not develop an addiction.[24,30] Additionally, addiction to a drug has been shown to involve more complex factors than merely exposure. The likelihood is remote of a cancer patient who takes opioids for pain becoming a drug abuser or typical street drug "addict."[31,32] Many clinicians have an irrational fear of this, and

Table 38-6. Oral-to-Parenteral Dose Ratios of Weak and Strong Opioids for Treatment of Mild to Severe Pain

Oral and Parenteral Opioid Analgesics for Moderate-to-Severe Pain

	Route*	Equianalgesic Dose+ (mg)	Duration (hr)	Plasma Half-life (hr)
A. Narcotic Agonists				
Morphine	IM	10	4-6	2-3.5
	PO	60	4-7	
Codeine	IM	130	4-6	3
	PO	200+	4-6	
Oxycodone	IM	15		—
	PO	30	3-5	
Heroin	IM	5	4-5	0.5
	PO	(60)	4-5	
Levorphanol	IM	2	4-6	12-16
(Levo-dromoran)	PO	4	4-7	
Hydromorphone	IM	1.5	4-5	2-3
(Dilaudid)	PO	7.5	4-6	
Oxymorphone	IM	1	4-6	2-3
(Numorphan)	PR	10	4-6	
Meperidine	IM	75	4-5	3-4
(Demerol)	PO	300+	4-6	12-16
Methadone	IM	10		15-30
(Dolophine)	PO	20		
B. Mixed Agonist-Antagonists				
Pentazocine	IM	60	4-6	2-3
(Talwin)	PO	180+	4-7	
Nalbuphine	IM	10	4-6	5
(Nubain)	PO	–		
Butorphanol	IM	2	4-6	2.5-3.5
(Stadol)	PO	–		
C. Partial Agonists				
Buprenorphine	IM	0.4	4-6	7
(Temgesic)	SL	0.8	5-6	

For these equianalgesic doses (see also comments) the time of peak analgesia ranges from 1.5 to 2 hours and the duration from 4 to 6 hours. Oxycodone and meperidine are shorter-acting (3-5 hours) and diflunisal and naproxen are longer-acting (8 to 12 hours).

* These are the recommended starting doses from which the optimal dose for each patient is determined by titration and the maximal dose limited by adverse effects.

Continued

Table 38-6 *Continued.* Oral-to-Parenteral Dose Ratios of Weak and Strong Opioids for Treatment of Mild to Severe Pain

Analgesics Commonly Used Orally for Mild-to-Moderate Pain

Drug	Dose* (mg)	Dose Range (mg)	Comments	Precautions
A. Non-Narcotics				
Aspirin	650	650	Often used in combination with opioid-type analgesics	Renal dysfunction; avoid in hematologic disorders and in combination with steroids
Choline magnesium trisalicylate	ND	1500-3000	Longer duration of action than aspirin	Minimal GI side effects; no effect on platelets
Acetaminophen	650	650	No significant antiinflammatory effects	Minimal GI side effects; no effect on platelets
Ibuprofen (Motrin)	ND	200-400	Antiinflammatory and analgesic effects	
Fenoprofen (Nalfon)	ND	200-400	Like ibuprofen	Like aspirin
Diflunisal (Dolobid)	ND	500-1000	Longer duration of action than ibuprofen; higher analgesic potential than aspirin	Like aspirin
Naproxen (Naprosyn)	550	250-500	Like diflunisal	Like aspirin
B. Morphine-Like Agonists				
Codeine	32-65	32-65	Often used in combination with nonopioid analgesics; biotransformed in part to morphine	Impaired ventilation; bronchial asthma; increased intracranial pressure
Oxycodone	5	5-10	Shorter acting; also in combination with nonopioid analgesics (Percodan, Percocet) which limits dose escalation	Like codeine
Meperidine (Demerol)	50	50-100	Shorter acting; biotransformed to normeperidine, a toxic metabolite	Normeperidine accumulates with repetitive dosing causing CNS excitation; not for patients with impaired renal function or receiving monoamine oxidase inhibitors
Propoxyphene HCl (Darvon) Propoxyphene napsylate (Darvon-N)	65-130	65-130	"Weak" narcotic; often used in combination with nonopioid analgesics; long half-life; biotransformed to potentially toxic metabolite (norpropoxyphene)	Propoxyphene and metabolite accumulate with repetitive dosing; overdose complicated by convulsions

ND = not determined.

Continued

Table 38-6 *Continued.* Oral-to-Parenteral Dose Ratios of Weak and Strong Opioids for Treatment of Mild to Severe Pain

Analgesics Commonly Used Orally for Mild-to-Moderate Pain

Drug	Dose* (mg)	Dose Range (mg)	Comments	Precautions
C. Mixed Agonist-Antagonists				
Pentazocine (Talwin)	50	50-100	In combination with nonopioids; in combination with naloxone to discourage parenteral abuse	May cause psychotomimetic effects; may precipitate withdrawal in opioid-dependent patients

For these equianalgesic doses (see also comments) the time of peak analgesia ranges from 1.5 to 2 hours and the duration from 4 to 6 hours. Oxycodone and meperidine are shorter-acting (3-5 hours) and diflunisal and naproxen are longer-acting (8 to 12 hours).

* These are the recommended starting doses from which the optimal dose for each patient is determined by titration and the maximal dose limited by adverse effects.

ND = not determined.

consequently many patients suffer needlessly because use of strong opioids is postponed or doses are inadequate for pain relief.

Most patients can be treated with oral opioids, even for the severest pain, if adequate attention is paid to treatment of side effects. Patience on the part of both the physician and patient in overcoming side effects can pay big dividends in optimum pain relief and cost containment.

Side effects occurring with oral administration, or with any other route of administration, are frequently misinterpreted as an allergy to the opioid. True allergies to opioids are extremely rare, and true allergic reactions such as skin eruptions and urticaria should be present before an allergy is diagnosed. A persistent, intolerable side effect may warrant discontinuation of a particular opioid, but this should not be diagnosed as allergy.

Routes of Administration

Oral

Opioids are effective pain relievers when given by mouth, and patients prefer this route of administration because of its effectiveness, ease of administration, and convenience. If healthcare professionals recognize and apply basic pharmacokinetic principles when treating pain with orally administered opioids, it will be apparent that the same pain control can be achieved with oral administration as with any other route. Transient, undesirable side effects that may occur with initiation of opioid treatment are infrequently caused by the route of administration alone, and a particular route should not be abandoned for that reason. Every effort should be made to aggressively treat side effects and make oral administration a success since parenteral and other routes of administration are more cumbersome and often more expensive.

Lack of effect with oral opioids is also given as a reason to change the route of administration. This situation requires careful pharmacodynamic evaluation.[33] Dose titration must be continued until some type of pharmacodynamic effect is achieved—pain is relieved or intolerable side effects develop—before the oral route can be declared ineffective. Hopefully, pain relief will occur before intolerable side effects. A seemingly high oral dose of opioid that produces neither pain relief nor side effects cannot be considered "dosing to effect," and therefore the oral route cannot be ruled ineffective on that basis alone.

Rectal and Other Body Orifices

Most analgesics given by these routes are effective but patients generally have an aversion to them, especially if the dose to be administered requires application of multiple suppositories or if treatment extends over a long interval. However, these routes are particularly useful if nausea and vomiting of short duration precludes oral administration. Rectal administration is the most commonly utilized of these routes; it is contraindicated in patients with a low platelet count. Pharmacists willing to compound tailor-made suppositories containing various drugs and in various doses are able to overcome some of the objections to rectal administration.

Drugs are readily absorbed via the vagina, and this route should be considered as an alternative to rectal administration in selected circumstances.

Parenteral

Parenteral routes include intramuscular, intravenous, transdermal, subcutaneous, and intraspinal administration. Pharmacokinetic principles are important to remember when using these routes. Intramuscular, intravenous, and subcutaneous routes are pharmacokinetically similar, whereas the transdermal and intraspinal routes are pharmacokinetically different. Claims of superiority for parenteral routes in the treatment of chronic cancer pain are anecdotal. This route is usually chosen not because it is superior but for various practical dosing considerations. The traditional intramuscular route of parenteral administration is falling more and more into disfavor because it is traumatic for the patient and produces less consistent results.

The most common reason for parenteral administration is the unavailability of the oral route. Persistent nausea and vomiting (for whatever reason), difficulty in or defective swallowing (eg, tracheoesophageal fistula), mental cloudiness or obtundation, and intestinal obstruction are common reasons patients cannot take pain medication orally. Another appropriate reason for parenteral administration occurs when pain intensifies to the extent that the dose required to control it becomes unusually large. The number of tablets required to achieve this dose may be so large that swallowing that number becomes impractical. Since the equianalgesic parenteral dose is smaller because of the pharmacokinetics of opioid administration by this route, it may be more practical to administer the drug parenterally.

Transdermal fentanyl is an attractive choice when the oral route is not available, because it is noninvasive, readily available, and easy to use. Being noninvasive, transdermal administration obviates the risk of infection inherent in many invasive routes. It can be used during temporary and prolonged unavailability of the oral route.

Invasive routes for opioid administration such as subcutaneous, intravenous, and intraspinal ones are, in general, employed for reasons of practicality and convenience rather than for efficacy of pain relief. The patient may be unable to receive the drug in a simpler manner, or it may be easier to administer the required dose by an invasive technique rather than a simpler route of administration. Devices for administering drugs by such routes range in sophistication from a simple syringe-driver administering a drug(s) subcutaneously to a totally implanted, computer-programmable infusion pump system administering a drug(s) via an intraspinal catheter. Unfortunately, controlled studies with these sophisticated techniques are not available, nor is there a consensus among experts in pain control as to when a specific technique is indicated. An important consideration in the use of these techniques is the level of expertise required of the caregiver as well as an increase in the support staff to administer and supervise the technique, as the degree of sophistication increases.

Physicians involved in the ongoing care of patients with cancer pain must understand the above issues when deciding to use more labor-intensive and sophisticated pain-relieving techniques. The emphasis should always be on simple pain-relieving techniques.

Adjuvant Drugs and Coanalgesics

Adjuvant drugs and coanalgesics may be defined as drugs that have a nonanalgesic primary pharmacologic action, but which in special situations have analgesic properties, enhance the pain-relieving properties of primary analgesics, or indirectly contribute to the overall relief of pain. This definition is broad and might be considered so broad as to include almost all categories of drugs. Additionally, the terms *adjuvant* and *coanalgesic* are arbitrary when used in this context. Although reports of therapeutic benefit from these drugs are often provocative,[34] most practitioners who treat pain patients recognize that drugs other than primary analgesics are useful; however, the specific indications for their use are often confusing. For practical purposes, the categories of drugs that fit this definition and that seem to produce the most useful results are tricyclic antidepressants, anticonvulsants, oral local anesthetics, corticosteroids, methotrimeprazine, and CNS stimulants.

Tricyclic Antidepressants

Tricyclic antidepressants are reported to be useful in a variety of neuropathic painful conditions of both malignant and nonmalignant origin.[34,35] Because pain associated with cancer may in part be secondary to nerve damage (neuropathic pain), the adjuvant use of these drugs with either nonopioid or opioid analgesics in the management of cancer patients with pain from any cause is justified, as long as no contraindication is present in a specific patient. This "first generation" antidepressant group has been demonstrated to be more effective in treating neuropathic pain than later generations.[36]

The dose required for treatment of neuropathic pain is much lower than for the treatment of depression. It is advisable to initiate therapy with a small dose. For example, in patients younger than 40 years, a single daily dose of amitriptyline 25 mg given around 9 pm is usually tolerated. For patients older than 40, a single daily dose of 10 mg is advisable given at the same time. Once the tolerability of this dose is determined, the dose can be increased incrementally, usually every other day. Should unacceptable side effects be experienced, the dose should be lowered to the previous amount that did not cause side effects. If one tricyclic is not tolerated, another should be tried.

A favorable side effect of these drugs is their sedative effect secondary to improvement in the sleep pattern. Patients usually experience this benefit immediately, while the beneficial effect on the pain may be delayed by a variable period after onset of therapy. However, the beneficial effect of these drugs on neuropathic pain usually occurs earlier than the time required for them to influence depression. The watchword for use of these drugs in patients with neuropathic pain is patience.

Anticonvulsants

Anticonvulsants have proven usefulness in patients with neuropathic pain who experience a sharp, shooting, or lancinating pain component. However, these drugs also may benefit patients who have neuropathic pain without this characteristic. Since the evidence for their effectiveness is anecdotal, empirical trials are justified in all patients who experience neuropathic pain. As with the use of antidepressants, anticonvulsants should be given at a low starting dosage and gradually increased to the therapeutic ranges used in treatment of convulsive disorders. Carbamazepine, phenytoin, valproate, and clonazepam are anticonvulsants currently used for treating this type of pain. Blood levels of carbamazepine and phenytoin should be monitored at regular intervals to prevent toxic accumulation.

Oral Local Anesthetics

Mexiletine, an orally active 1B antiarrhythmic agent structurally similar to lidocaine, has been reported to be effective in the treatment of neuropathic pain. Other drugs in this class have also been used for this purpose, but side effects reported with their use as antiarrhythmic drugs make them unattractive for treating neuropathic pain. Mexiletine should be considered as second-line treatment since clinical experience is limited. Its use should be considered only after adequate trials with combined antidepressant and anticonvulsant drugs have proved ineffective. Clinically, mexiletine is usually not considered a drug to supplant the above two categories of drugs but rather is given adjuvantly.

Corticosteroids

Clinical experience has proved corticosteroids to be useful in treating the pain associated with bone metastasis and tumor infiltration of neural structures. When corticosteroids are effective, pain relief is usually dramatic. Any corticosteroid may be used, but dexamethasone is a common choice because of its minimal effect on electrolytes and other metabolic functions. A dosage of 16 mg daily given in divided oral doses is usually effective. Short-term use is preferable because of potential metabolic side effects, but in some patients long-term use with vigorous treatment of the side effects may be necessary. The side effects of corticosteroids that are beneficial to the patient include an increase in appetite and improved sense of well being.

Methotrimeprazine

Methotrimeprazine is the only phenothiazine with demonstrated analgesic properties. It has proved useful in some patients with pain from advanced cancer when opioids have been problematic or in patients with pain and severe nausea or anxiety. It is usually administered parenterally and has the potential to cause hypotension. It should be used only when traditional analgesics are ineffective.

CNS Stimulants

Low-dose dextroamphetamine and methylphenidate are useful to counteract the sedative effects of opioids and other CNS depressants used to treat pain and other distressing symptoms of advanced cancer. These drugs should be administered in the early morning and again around noon only if necessary. Administering them after noon may interfere with sleeping at night. Alleviating sedation may allow the opioid dose to be increased, which alleviates more pain.

An Integrated Treatment Plan

Determining which drugs to use, singly or in combination, from the above compendium to achieve optimum pain relief for the cancer patient is the immediate challenge for the physician. The ultimate challenge, however, arises when this goal is made difficult by the unexpected seeming lack of responsiveness to these drugs in certain patients. Drug selection involves identifying an appropriate analgesic, or combination of analgesics, and combining it with an appropriate adjuvant(s), if indicated. The watchwords in this process are patience and persistence. Adequate pain control can be achieved in most patients using relatively simple techniques.

Elements of the process of selecting appropriate drugs include the following:

Avoiding Unnecessary Polypharmacy

Prescribing multiple opioids with identical mechanisms of action (binding on the opioid binding sites of the CNS) and choosing multiple opioids with no discernible pharmacokinetic or pharmacodynamic rationale have become traditions for physicians using strong opioids. This unfocused and unnecessary use of multiple opioids for pain treatment serves no therapeutic purpose and is confusing to the patient. However, if opioids are combined to take advantage of pharmacologic differences, such as differences in duration of effect, it is rational and desirable.

An example of polypharmacy without a purpose is combining opioids having a short duration of action, such as morphine and hydromorphone, and even additional similar opioids, in their "usual" or "recommended" doses to control pain as its intensity increases rather than simply increasing the dose of one of them to achieve adequate pain relief. This tradition probably developed because of physicians' fear of sanction by government disciplinary and regulatory agencies if doses beyond the usual or recommended ones are prescribed. Physicians should resist this fear and prescribe opioids in a simple manner that is not confusing to their patients. If short-duration opioids are effective and appropriate, the use of a single drug in an appropriate dose is much simpler for the patient to manage than a myriad of opioids whose mechanism of action is similar and whose combination offers no advantage for the patient.

Another example of polypharmacy, as mentioned earlier, is associated with the trepidation to begin the use of strong opioids for pain control. Polypharmacy use of acetaminophen and NSAIDs combined with nonopioid/weak opioid analgesics far beyond their effectiveness to relieve pain is excessive, resulting in inadequately relieved pain.

Rational Combining of Opioids

Combining opioids can be useful, and indeed desirable, if based on sound pharmacokinetic/pharmacodynamic principles of opioid use, for example, combining opioids with long and short half-lives. Opioids with long half-lives are desirable because they can be administered at longer intervals, for example every 6 hours, thus requiring fewer doses during a 24-hour interval. This is a convenience to the patient, and furthermore, has a positive psychologic effect because the patient is less often reminded of his or her infirmity. However, additional pain may occur, for whatever reason, between doses and require a supplemental opioid. An opioid with a short-acting half-life fulfills this need. Consistent pain relief is achieved by combining the two opioids. However, opioids with long half-lives are difficult to handle in patients whose pain intensity changes frequently because of the lag in reaching pain relief after a dose is changed. The long half-life of the drug eventually causes oversedation. This problem is especially prevalent in the elderly.

With the development of controlled-release morphine, problems associated with combining drugs with long and short half-lives have diminished. Controlled-release products do not have the problems inherent in opioids with long half-lives. Prolonged effectiveness with the controlled-release products is related to the release mechanism in the delivery system, which releases the morphine over 12 hours.

Adequate pain control frequently can be achieved with the 12-hour controlled-release regimen alone. Should "breakthrough" pain occur during this interval, for whatever reason, it can be treated with immediate-release morphine. By using a combination of controlled-release and immediate-release morphine, a treatment regimen analogous with that used in treating an insulin-dependent diabetic with long-acting and short-acting insulin can be devised.

The first consideration in devising this treatment regimen is to determine the amount of immediate-release morphine necessary to control the patient's pain over a 24-hour period. This 24-hour dosage is determined by multiplying the single dose necessary to relieve pain for a 4-hour period by the total number of doses required to maintain the pain-free state over a 24-hour interval. For example, if a patient requires 60 mg of immediate-release morphine to relieve pain effectively for 4 hours, six doses will be required to effectively relieve the pain for 24 hours. The dosage would be 6 x 60 = 360 mg/24 hours. This 24-hour dosage will be the amount of controlled-release morphine that will be administered in 12-hour divided doses. In the example cited, 180 mg is administered every 12 hours. If pain is controlled with the controlled-release morphine, no additional pain medication will be required. However, immediate-release morphine is always prescribed along with the controlled-release morphine in case of breakthrough pain, ie, pain occurring for whatever reason during the 12-hour interval that is not relieved by the controlled-release morphine. Breakthrough pain can be caused by trauma or simply a failure of the controlled-release morphine to control the pain for the full 12 hours. The breakthrough dose is usually one sixth of the total 24-hour dosage, but it should be titrated to meet the goal of adequate pain relief and not be arbitrarily determined. This procedure is analogous to prescribing short-acting insulin along with long-acting insulin to cover the contingency of needing more insulin during the interval long-acting insulin is thought to be adequate for blood sugar control.

After the patient starts taking controlled-release morphine, the number of breakthrough doses of immediate-release morphine required to maintain pain control serves as a monitor to determine when the dose of controlled-release morphine should be increased. When the number of doses of breakthrough medication exceeds two during the daytime 12-hour interval and one during the nighttime 12-hour interval, the dosage of controlled-release morphine should be increased. The dose of controlled-release morphine is increased by the amount of immediate-release morphine required by the patient in addition to the controlled-release morphine.

Any immediate-release, short-acting opioid can be used in conjunction with controlled-release morphine for treating breakthrough pain, but the use of immediate-release morphine obviates converting a non-morphine opioid breakthrough dosage to a morphine dosage when the controlled-release morphine dose needs to be increased. Also, keeping the number of different medications to a minimum simplifies the medication process.

This combination regimen has many advantages. It is convenient; ambulatory patients can carry their medications. Frequent dosing is unnecessary; therefore, patients are not conspicuous when taking medication. In addition, pain is controlled throughout the night; thus, neither pain nor the need to awake to take medicine interferes with sleep. For these reasons, all patients with persistent pain should be considered for this type of pain management. Figs 38-5A and 38-5B illustrate this method.

Consultation/Special Techniques

Patients who seemingly do not respond to simple measures for controlling pain are frequently considered to need some type of special technique to relieve it, as if there is some intrinsic relief inherent in the technique itself. Most often, a novel route of opioid administration, alone or in combination with a local anesthetic, or some type of neurostimulatory or neuroablative invasive procedure is thought to be the answer. These procedures require the expertise of specially trained physicians. The difficulty in applying these procedures lies in the selection of patients. Most reports alleging that a change in route of administration of the opioid or use of opioids in combination with local anesthetics or neurostimulatory or neuroablative procedures will produce superior pain control with fewer side effects for seemingly difficult pain problems are based on poorly controlled studies. The evidence is weak that patients were actually unresponsive to adequate simple pain treatment methods; ie, failure of pain relief after dosing to effect was not established. Most invasive techniques drastically alter the pharmacokinetics of opioids, and a comparison of equianalgesic doses between methods of treatment is difficult to ascertain. In addition, deafferentation procedures may indeed provide temporary relief, but in the long run, pain that may be more severe and even more difficult to treat than the original pain may appear and significantly decrease the quality of life.

When consulting with physicians who are expert in these types of procedures, the physician responsible for the long-term management of the patient's pain, and other distressing symptoms, should discuss what the long-term outcome is likely to be and what the medical, nursing, and other supportive requirements are for maintaining the system that is contemplated. The complications associated with the system and the likelihood of having to repeat the procedure to correct a malfunction in it should also be discussed. Another factor that should be considered when contemplating invasive and ablative procedures is the longevity of the patient. Some ablative procedures are only effective for a few months. If the patient's expected survival is less than the expected effectiveness of the procedure, the procedure is indicated. However, if anticipated survival exceeds the period of likely effectiveness of the procedure, undertaking the procedure is problematic, because as stated previously, emergence of a pain more severe than the original pain is a distinct probability.

The physician primarily responsible for the pain management of the patient should not assume that a pain-relieving procedure will solve a difficult pain management problem. The procedure may make the problem worse, and managing the system may be labor intensive, costly to the patient, and distressing to the patient and family.

Psychologic Issues in Cancer Pain Control

A myriad of psychologic issues is invariably associated with chronic pain. These issues relate to the effect of the pain on the cancer patient and the psychosocial consequences to the patient, family, and friends. Healthcare providers must recognize these issues and either address them or consult with appropriate professionals to ensure that the issues are addressed. It is unlikely that optimum pain relief will be achieved if the psychologic issues are not resolved.

The psychologic issues depend, to a large degree, on the patient's perceived responsibility to his or her family in meeting financial, interpersonal, advisory, intercessory, and other needs. Ensuring that these needs are met will hopefully make the family more functional and will allow for the maximum fulfillment of the potential of all its members during the patient's illness.

Barriers to Adequate Cancer Pain Control

Despite efforts to provide adequate information about specific methods of pain control, pain in cancer patients continues to be inadequately treated. Since most patients who are likely to be inadequately treated are those requiring opioid analgesics, the barriers relate to adequate and appropriate opioid use. These barriers involve both medical and extramedical factors that must be recognized and corrected if adequate pain relief is to be a reality for cancer patients. They fall into the following categories:

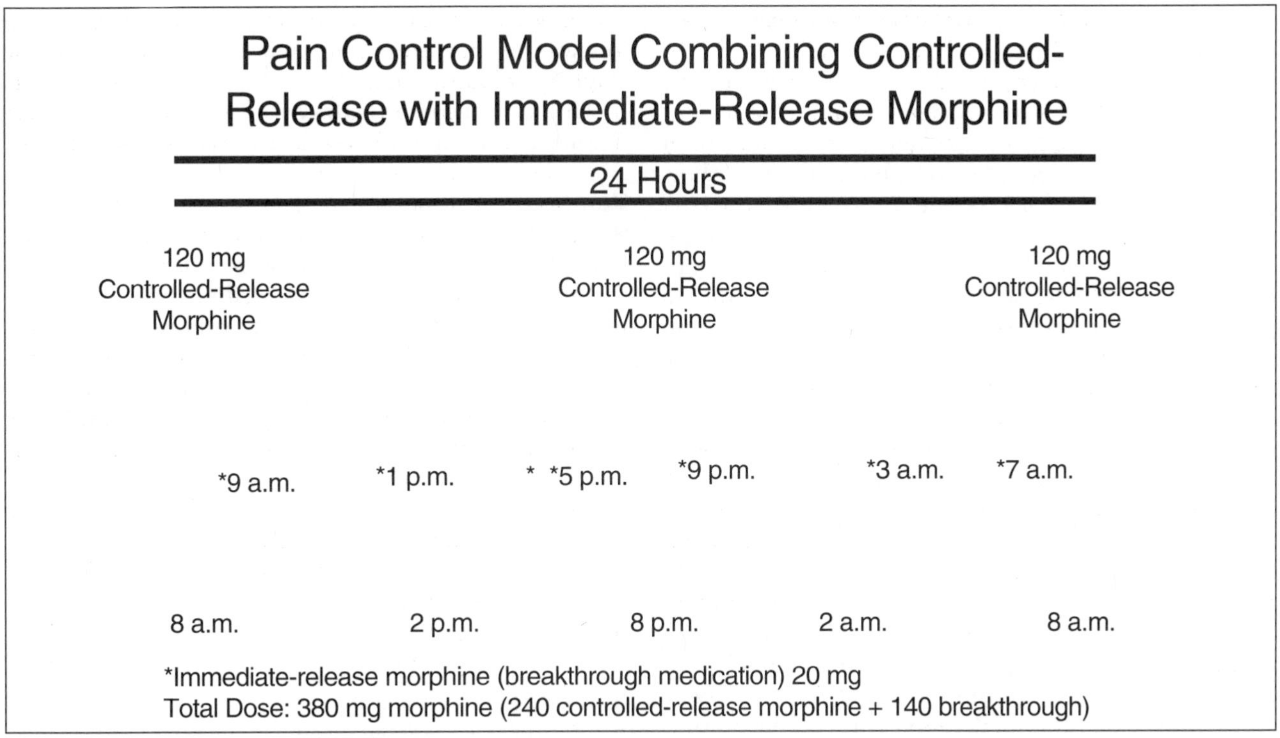

Pain Control Model Combining Controlled-Release with Immediate-Release Morphine

24 Hours

120 mg Controlled-Release Morphine		120 mg Controlled-Release Morphine		120 mg Controlled-Release Morphine

*9 a.m. *1 p.m. * *5 p.m. *9 p.m. *3 a.m. *7 a.m.

8 a.m. 2 p.m. 8 p.m. 2 a.m. 8 a.m.

*Immediate-release morphine (breakthrough medication) 20 mg
Total Dose: 380 mg morphine (240 controlled-release morphine + 140 breakthrough)

Fig 38-5A. Pain control model combining controlled-release with immediate-release morphine. Illustration of a patient receiving an inadequate dose of controlled-release morphine requiring multiple doses of breakthrough medication over 24 hours.

Pain Control Model Combining Controlled-Release with Immediate-Release Morphine

24 Hours

180 mg Controlled-Release Morphine		180 mg Controlled-Release Morphine		180 mg Controlled-Release Morphine

*4 p.m.

8 a.m. 2 p.m. 8 p.m. 2 a.m. 8 a.m.

*Immediate-release morphine (breakthrough medication) 30 mg
Total Dose: 390 mg morphine (360 controlled-release morphine + 30 breakthrough)

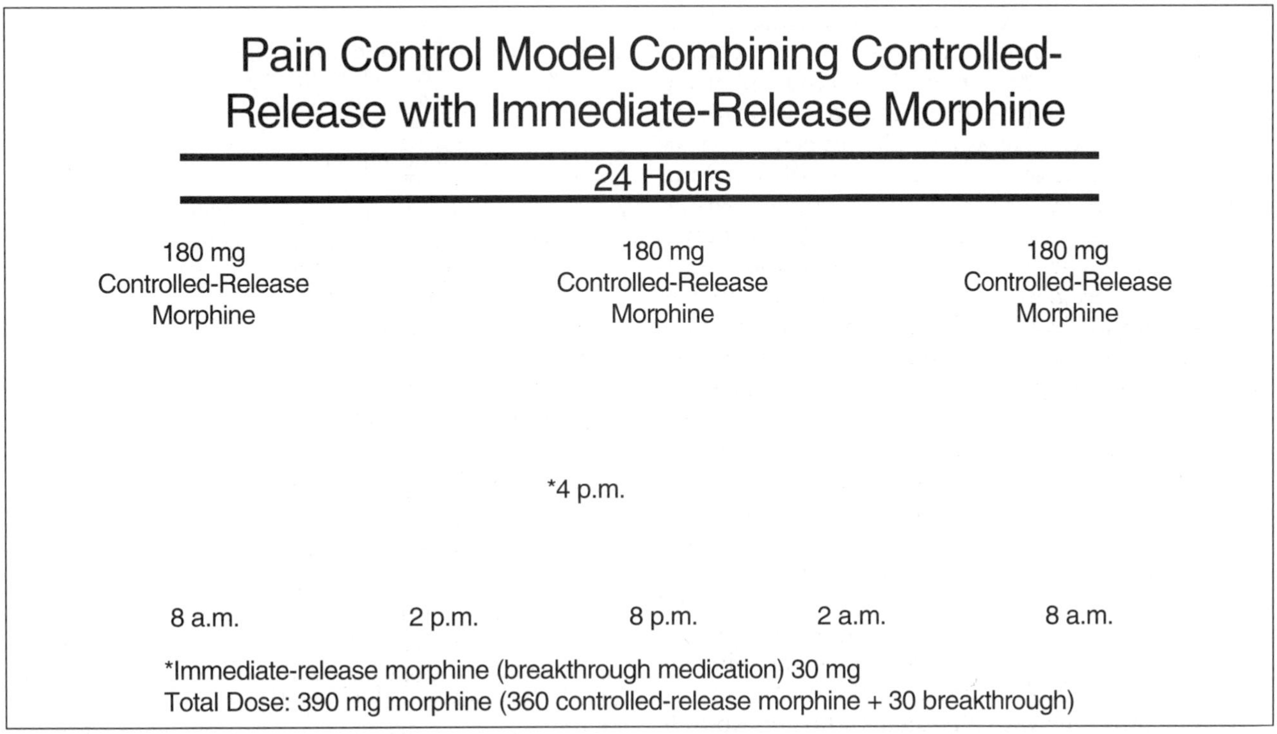

Fig 38-5B. Pain control model combining controlled-release with immediate-release morphine. Illustration of a patient receiving an adequate dose of controlled-release morphine requiring only an occasional dose of breakthrough medication over 24 hours. This patient can sleep through the night without interruption because of pain.

Cultural and Societal Barriers to Appropriate Use of Opioids

Prejudicial attitudes and misconceptions about the pharmacologic properties of opioids and societal confusion between the legitimate and illegitimate use of these drugs have existed for so long that they are thoroughly ingrained in our culture. Behavior on the part of members of a society, including healthcare professionals, that is rooted in the culture in which one lives is difficult to change. Such is the case with healthcare providers regarding the prescribing, dispensing, and administering of opioids, and, in many instances, the patient's willingness to take them. Behavior accepted and validated by a culture becomes instinctive, and deviation from this behavior requires a volitional decision that can produce angst and perhaps a sense of betrayal on the part of the person who decides to deviate. The undertreatment of pain with opioids seems to have attained this position.

There can be no question about the intent and desire of most healthcare professionals to relieve pain in their patients. A resolve to achieve this requires that the instinctive behavior described above be set aside and a volitional, rational decision to prescribe opioids based on scientific pharmacokinetic and pharmacodynamic principles be made.

Knowledge Deficits

There remain knowledge deficits resulting from a general unawareness of new information on opioid pharmacology learned from treating cancer patients in pain. Information on opioid dosing in most pharmacology textbooks was initially obtained using patients with postoperative pain as a model. In general, postoperative pain is less severe than the chronic pain of cancer and other chronic conditions. Other pharmacologic information about opioids was obtained from persons who volunteered to participate in opioid studies and who were not experiencing pain.

Now that modern treatment has extended the lives of cancer patients, many of them experience chronic pain of varying severity, and they serve as a new model for studying opioid pharmacology. Several salient facts have emerged:

- Pain is a natural "antagonist" to the analgesic effects of opioids; therefore, doses, in many cases seemingly high, must be used that overcome this effect.
- Pain similarly "antagonizes" respiratory depression; therefore, respiratory depression is not a deterrent to choosing an adequate dose of opioid to relieve pain.
- Psychologic dependence (addiction) on opioids seldom occurs in patients taking opioids for their legitimate pain-relieving qualities.
- There is no ceiling effect for dosing with opioids for patients with nociceptive pain. With each incremental dose increase, there will be an corresponding increase in pain relief.

This knowledge provides a rationale for prescribing opioids based on modern pharmacologic information.

Regulatory Barriers

State licensing and disciplinary boards and state and federal drug enforcement agencies continue practices that deter physicians from prescribing opioids appropriately and adequately, and pharmacists are reluctant to dispense opioids in certain cases in the name of preventing diversion of legal drugs to illegal uses. It is important that physicians, pharmacists, and other healthcare professionals work to establish proper guidelines for the use of opioids so that all involved clearly understand what the boundaries are. The goal of adequate availability of opioids for patients who need them for their legitimate medical purposes while preventing their diversion to illegal use must be achieved.

References

1. Edwards WT. Optimizing opioid treatment of postoperative pain. *J Pain Symptom Management.* 1990;5:S24-S36.
2. Foley KM. The treatment of cancer pain. *N Engl J Med.* 1985;313:84-95.
3. Marks RE, Sachar EJ. Undertreatment of medical inpatients with narcotic analgesics. *Ann Intern Med.* 1973;78: 173-181.
4. Jaffe JH. Misinformation: euphoria and addiction. In Hill CS Jr, Fields WS, eds. *Drug Treatment of Cancer Pain in a Drug-Oriented Society.* New York, NY: Raven Press; 1989. Advances in pain research and therapy; vol 11.
5. Hill CS Jr. Relationship among cultural, educational, and regulatory agency influences on optimum cancer pain treatment. *J Pain Symptom Management.* 1990;5:S37-S45.
6. Ferrell BR, Wisdom C, Wenzl C. Quality of life as an outcome variable in the management of cancer pain. *Cancer.* 1989;63(11 suppl):2321-2327.
7. Humphrey D. *Final Exit.* New York, NY: Dell Trade Paperback; 1992.
8. Fields HL. *Pain.* New York, NY: McGraw-Hill Book Co; 1987;133-169.
9. Arner S, Meyerson BA. Lack of analgesic effect of opioids on neuropathic and idiopathic forms of pain. *Pain.* 1988;33:11-23.
10. Arner S, Arner B. Differential effects of epidural morphine in the treatment of cancer-related pain. *Acta Anaesthesiol Scand.* 1985;29:32-36.
11. Foley KM. Pain syndromes in patients with cancer. *Med Clin North Am.* 1987;71:169-184.
12. Wong D, Whaley LF. *Clinical Handbook of Pediatric Nursing.* St Louis, Mo: CV Mosby Co; 1986.
13. Nemni SR. A psychophysical methodology for the development of measurement scales: the quantification of the qualities of cancer pain. Doctoral dissertation. Fort Worth, Tex: Texas Christian University; December 1988.

14. WHO Technical Report Series, No 804, 1990 (Cancer pain relief and palliative care: report of a WHO expert committee).

15. *Cancer Pain Relief.* 2nd ed. Geneva: World Health Organization; 1989.

16. Payne R. Pharmacologic management of bone pain in the cancer patient. *Clin J Pain.* 1989;5(suppl 2):S43-S50.

17. Waldman SD, Kilbride MJ. The nonsteroidal anti-inflammatory drugs: current concepts. *Pain Digest.* 1992; 2:289-294.

18. Patt RB, Szalados JE, Wu CL. Pharmacotherapeutic guidelines (appendix C). In: Patt RB, ed. *Cancer Pain.* Philadelphia, Pa: JB Lippincott Co; 1993:570-571.

19. Miller LJ, Kramer MA. Pain management with intravenous ketorolac. *Ann Pharmacother.* 1993;27:307-308.

20. Stambaugh JE Jr. Role of nonsteroidal anti-inflammatory drugs. In: Patt RB, ed. *Cancer Pain.* Philadelphia, Pa: JB Lippincott Co; 1993:105-117.

21. Houde RW. Analgesic effectiveness of the narcotic agonist/antagonists. *Br J Clin Pharmacol.* 1979;1(suppl 3):297s-308s.

22. Snyder SH. Drug and neurotransmitter receptors in the brain. *Science.* 1984;224:22-31.

23. Cleeland CS. Pain control: public and physicians' attitudes. In: Hill CS Jr, Fields WS, eds. *Drug Treatment of Cancer Pain in a Drug-Oriented Society. Advances in Pain Research and Therapy.* New York, NY: Raven Press; 1989(vol. 11):81-89.

24. Porter J, Jick H. Addiction rare in patients treated with narcotics. *N Engl J Med.* 1980;302:123.

25. Inturrisi CE. Management of cancer pain: pharmacology and principles of management. *Cancer.* 1989;63 (11 suppl):2308-2320.

26. Smith MT, Watt JA, Cramond T. Morphine-3-glucuronide a: potent antagonist of morphine analgesia. *Life Sci.* 1990;47:579.

27. Hanks GW, Twycross RG, Lloyd JW. Unexpected complication of successful nerve block. *Anaesthesia.* 1981;36: 37-39.

28. Twycross RG. The management of pain in cancer: a guide to drugs and dosages. *Oncology.* 1988;2:35.

29. Kaiko RF, Grandy RP, Oshlack B, et al. The United States experience with oral controlled-release morphine (MS Contin Tablets). *Cancer.* 1989;63(suppl 11):2348-2354.

30. Perry S, Heidrich G. Management of pain during debridement: a survey of US burn units. *Pain.* 1982;13:267.

31. Foley KM. Controversies in cancer pain: medical perspectives. *Cancer.* 1989;63(11 suppl):2257-2265.

32. Foley KM. The "decriminalization" of cancer pain. In: Hill CS Jr, Fields WS, eds. *Drug Treatment of Cancer Pain in a Drug-Oriented Society.* New York, NY: Raven Press; 1989: Advances in pain research and therapy; vol 11.

33. Portenoy RK, Foley KM, Inturrisi CE. The nature of opioid responsiveness and its implications for neuropathic pain: new hypotheses derived from studies of opioid infusions. *Pain.* 1990;43:273-286.

34. Bruera E, Ripamonti C. Adjuvants to opioid analgesics. In: Patt RB, ed. *Cancer Pain.* Philadelphia, Pa: JB Lippincott Co; 1993:143-159.

35. Max MB, Culnane M, Schafer SC, et al. Amitriptyline relieves diabetic neuropathy pain in patients with normal or depressed mood. *Neurology.* 1987;37:589-596.

36. McQuay HJ. Pharmacological treatment of neuralgic and neuropathic pain. *Cancer Surv.* 1988;7:141-159.

Glossary

Allodynia: Pain caused by a stimulus that ordinarily does not cause pain, eg, touch, pressure from clothes, and cold air blowing on the skin. As implied from the above, patients commonly perceive this sensation when the skin is stimulated.

Breakthrough pain: Pain that exceeds the pain control provided by an analgesic drug and occurs during the time the analgesic is usually providing pain relief.

Ceiling effect: The dose level of a drug beyond which increasing the dose does not produce an increase in pharmacodynamic effect of the drug. Increasing the dose after the maximum desired pharmacodynamic effect is achieved is likely to produce intolerable side effects or drug toxicity.

Central pain: Pain associated with a lesion of the central nervous system.

Coanalgesic: A drug whose use is primarily for conditions other than pain relief, but under special physiologic conditions relieves pain; eg, antidepressants and anticonvulsants may relieve neuropathic pain.

Dysesthesia: An unpleasant abnormal sensation, whether spontaneous or evoked.

Hypalgesia: Diminished sensitivity to noxious stimulation.

Hyperalgesia, primary: A state of increased pain sensation caused by a stimulus that ordinarily produces a pain of lesser degree, and occurs at the site of injury.

Hyperalgesia, secondary: A state of increased pain sensation as described under primary hyperalgesia, but occurring in apparently undamaged tissue, usually in tissue immediately surrounding the site of injury.

Incident pain: Pain occurring with movement, position, or other "incident," regardless of what the pain-producing incident is. Patient may be entirely free of pain when the "incident" is not happening, or the "incident" may serve to exacerbate a constant pain.

Neuropathic pain: Pain that occurs as a result of nerve damage, or pain due to functional abnormalities of the nervous system. Nerves may be considered "damaged" by merely cutting them.

Nociceptive pain: Pain caused by activation of nociceptors. Activation is usually by overt tissue damage. This is the pain most commonly experienced by patients and is represented by any condition that causes tissue damage.

Nociceptor: A peripheral nervous system receptor which is preferentially sensitive to a noxious (tissue damaging) stimulus.

Noxious: A noxious stimulus is a tissue-damaging stimulus.

Pain: An unpleasant sensory experience perceived as arising from a specific body region that is often associated with actual or potential tissue damage, or described in terms of such damage, and evokes various negative emotions, especially when chronic.

Paresthesia: An abnormal sensation, whether spontaneous or evoked. Contrast with dysesthesia, which is an "unpleasant" abnormal sensation.

Paraneoplastic syndromes: Painful syndromes occurring in the presence of malignancy, but apparently not directly caused by it. These syndromes usually affect the muscles, joints, or bones.

Postmastectomy syndrome: Pain occurring at the mastectomy site and usually the inner aspect of the extremity on the mastectomy side, which has characteristics of neuropathic pain (see Table 38-1).

Postthoracotomy syndrome: Pain occurring on the hemithorax of the thoracotomy site which has characteristics of neuropathic pain (see Table 38-1).

Trigger point: A circumscribed point of increased painful sensitivity on the skin and underlying muscular structures, which is detected by direct palpation and which reproduces the pain complained of by the patient.

39

PSYCHIATRIC COMPLICATIONS IN CANCER PATIENTS

Mary Jane Massie, MD, Ladd Spiegel, MD, Marguerite S. Lederberg, MD, Jimmie C. Holland, MD

Cancer is a group of diseases that for centuries has struck fear in the hearts of people. Its previously certain fatal outcome, absence of known cause or cure, and association with pain and disfiguring lesions made it particularly frightening and loathsome. Physicians long avoided telling patients they had cancer, believing the diagnosis would be too painful to hear. The press avoided printing the word and the family colluded with the physician to keep the diagnosis a secret from the patient.

Several factors have contributed to attitude changes in the United States. The American Cancer Society, founded in 1913, began to educate the public about early diagnosis and treatment. In the 1950s and the 1960s, physicians and patients became less pessimistic about cancer as radiation therapy and chemotherapy altered the pattern of outcome for several neoplasms in children and young adults. Clinicians began discussing more openly all aspects of the illness with patients and families.

The hospice movement in Europe and pioneering work of Dr. Elisabeth Kubler-Ross in the US led to a re-examination of and improvement in care for dying patients. Far more attention was given to symptom control, particularly pain. Patients who wished to discuss their fears of advanced cancer and death could do so because the situation's reality could be acknowledged.

Cancer's transition from a group of neglected and hopeless diseases to one of potential cures, increased treatment efforts, and extensive research generated more interest in the disease's psychosocial aspects. The field of psycho-oncology was developed to deal with the human dimensions of cancer and its impact on the psychologic and social functioning of patients, their families, and treating staff.

Psychologic Impact of Cancer

In the past physicians avoided realistically discussing the patient's diagnosis and prognosis. The "truth telling" debates in the 1960s and 1970s led to our current belief, supported by clinical studies, that compassionate honesty is helpful—not damaging—to both adult and pediatric patients.

Persons who receive diagnoses of cancer exhibit characteristic normal responses (Table 39-1). A period of initial disbelief, denial, or despair is common and generally lasts 2 to 5 days. Patients may state "this just can't be happening to me," "pathology must have mixed up my slides," "I knew it all along," or "there is no reason to take treatment, it won't work." The second phase, characterized by dysphoric mood, lasts 1 to 2 weeks. Patients often report having anxiety symptoms, depressed mood, anorexia, insomnia, and irritability. The ability to concentrate and to carry out usual daily activities is impaired, and intrusive thoughts of the illness and uncertainty about the future are present. Adaptation usually begins after several weeks as patients integrate new information, confront reality issues, find reasons for optimism, and resume activities.[1] Of course, adaptation continues for months after diagnosis.

The patient's perceptions of the disease, its manifestations, and the stigma commonly attached to cancer contribute to these responses. For adults, fear of a painful death is a primary concern. All patients fear

Mary Jane Massie, MD, Attending Psychiatrist, Memorial Sloan-Kettering Cancer Center and Associate Professor of Clinical Psychiatry, Cornell University Medical College, New York, New York

Ladd Spiegel, MD, Adjunct Attending Psychiatrist, Memorial Sloan-Kettering Cancer Center and Clinical Instructor of Psychiatry and Pediatrics, Cornell University Medical College, New York

Marguerite S. Lederberg, MD, Attending Psychiatrist, Memorial Sloan-Kettering Cancer Center and Associate Professor of Clinical Psychiatry, Cornell University Medical College, New York, New York

Jimmie C. Holland, MD, Chief, Psychiatry Service, Memorial Sloan-Kettering Cancer Center and Professor of Psychiatry, Cornell University Medical College, New York, New York

Table 39-1. Normal Responses to Crises Encountered With Cancer

Symptoms	Duration
Phase 1: Initial Response	
Disbelief or denial	2-5 days
("wrong diagnosis"; "mixed up slides")	
Despair	
("I knew it all along"; "no reason to take treatment")	
Phase 2: Dysphoria	
Anxiety	7-14 days
depressed mood	
anorexia	
insomnia	
irritability	
poor concentration	
disruption of daily activities	
Phase 3: Adaptation	
Adjusts to new information	>14 days but can extend for months
confronts the issues presented	
finds reasons for optimism	
"gets on" with activities	
(eg, new or revised treatment plan, other goals)	

the potential for disability, dependence, altered appearance, and changed body function. The new role of being sick or different involves a change in nearly every aspect of the adult's or child's life. The fear of being separated from or abandoned by family and friends is common.

Although such concerns are pervasive, the initial level of psychologic distress is highly variable and accounted for by three factors (Table 39-2): (1) medical (tumor type and site, stage at diagnosis, associated pain, treatment required, rehabilitation available, clinical course of illness, associated medical conditions); (2) patient-related (level of cognitive and psychologic development, ability to cope with stressful events, emotional maturity, ability to accept altered or unachieved life goals, prior experiences with cancer, concurrent life stresses, support of family and others); and (3) societal (attitudes toward cancer and treatment, stigma associated with diagnosis, health care policies).[2] Consideration of these factors enables the physician to better evaluate the patient.

Cancer treatment, often lengthy and arduous, necessitates flexibility in patterns of emotional adaptation. Beyond the initial adjustment, the possibility of cure changes the threat of death to a focus on uncertainty and management of treatment side effects. Simultaneously, the patient must also meet normal school, work, and family obligations, maintain confidence in the outcome and a sense of control, and manage financial burdens.

Pediatric Issues

Discussion of the diagnosis of cancer with the sick child is now a routine part of pediatric care. The diagnosis and prognosis, including the issue of death, needs to be discussed in a developmentally appropriate manner, on several occasions, with the participation of the family.[3] Pathologic patterns of communication in the family are diminished by efforts to reduce "keeping secrets." Compliance is enhanced by the child's sense of involvement in the treatment.

The effects of childhood cancer on the family include reactions of anger, grief, hostility, guilt, mourning for possible loss, and disbelief.[4] For most parents, the diagnosis of cancer in their child means

Table 39-2. Factors That Influence Patients' Psychologic Adaptation to Cancer

Medical

- Tumor site, stage at diagnosis
- Predicted outcome
- Symptoms, functional loss(es)
- Treatment(s) required
- Rehabilitation available
- Clinical course of illness
- Associated medical conditions

Patient-Related

- Level of cognitive and psychologic development
- Ability to cope with life crises
- Emotional maturity and ability to accept altered or unachieved life goals
- Prior experiences with cancer (family member's death from cancer)
- Concurrent life crises (divorce, grief, other illness)
- Support of family and others

Societal

- Attitudes towards cancer and treatment
- Stigma associated with diagnosis
- Health care policy (insurance for care, disability, protection from job discrimination)

"death" despite recent changes in prognosis of many neoplasms. An intellectual understanding that many medical advances have occurred does little to decrease parents' distress and fears; they must accept the rigors of treatment without any guarantee of success. The illness alters all aspects of family life. The parents' goals, wishes, and expectations for the ill child are forever changed. The diagnosis of cancer in a child will most likely aggravate existing family problems. However, contrary to popular belief, the likelihood of divorce is not increased, nor are couples brought closer together.[5]

Because parents must devote time to the child's clinic visits and hospitalizations, there may be inadvertent parental neglect of the siblings. Many concerns of siblings are strikingly similar to those of the sick child: symptoms of anxiety, social isolation, decreased self-esteem, and a sense of vulnerability to illness and injury are prominent. Numerous behavioral and school problems have been documented.[6]

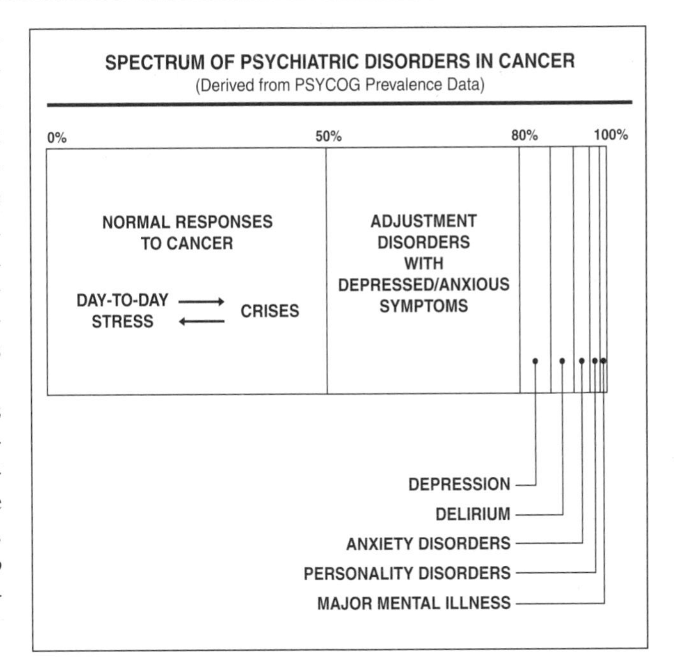

Fig 39-1. Prevalence of psychiatric disorders in 215 adult cancer patients indicated that slightly more than half were adjusting normally to the crisis of illness. Adjustment disorder with depressed and/or anxious mood was the most common psychiatric disorder diagnosed. From Derogatis et al.[7]

Prevalence of Psychiatric Disorders in Cancer Patients

The many myths about psychologic problems in cancer patients vary from "all patients are distressed and need psychiatric help" to "no one is upset and no one needs help." One of the first efforts in psychooncology was to obtain objective data on the type and frequency of emotional problems in cancer patients. Using criteria from the Diagnostic and Statistical Manual of Mental Disorders (DSM-III) classification of psychiatric disorders, the Psychosocial Collaborative Oncology Group at three cancer centers determined the prevalence of psychiatric disorders in 215 randomly assessed hospitalized and ambulatory adult patients with cancer (Fig 39-1).[7] Slightly more than half (53%) were adjusting normally to the crisis of illness. The remainder (47%) had sufficient distress to receive a diagnosis of a psychiatric disorder. Adjustment disorder with depressed and/or anxious mood was by far the most common diagnosis (68%). Major depressive disorder was next (13%), followed by organic mental disorder (8%), personality disorder (7%), and pre-existing anxiety disorder (4%). Nearly 90% of the psychiatric disorders (adjustment disorders, organic mental disorders, and major depression) were related to responses to disease or treatment. Only 11% represented prior psychiatric problems, such as personality and anxiety disorders. Comparable research in children is lacking, but clinical data appear to reflect a similar spectrum of problems. The physician who treats cancer patients can expect to find, for the most part, a group of psychologically healthy individuals who are responding to the stresses posed by cancer and its treatment.

Disorders in Cancer Patients with Pain

In the Psychosocial Collaborative Oncology Group Study, 39% of those who received a psychiatric diagnosis experienced significant pain. In contrast, only 19% of patients who did not receive a psychiatric diagnosis had significant pain. The psychiatric diagnosis of the patients was predominantly adjustment disorder with depressed or mixed mood (69%), but, of note, 15% of patients with significant pain had symptoms of a major depression.

Both data and clinical observation show that the psychiatric symptoms of patients who are in pain must initially be considered a consequence of uncontrolled pain. Acute anxiety, depression with despair (especially when the adult patient believes the pain means disease progression), agitation, irritability, lack of cooperation, anger, and inability to sleep may be the emotional or behavioral concomitants of pain. In a physically ill child, chronic pain may present with symptoms of apathy, withdrawal, and clinging behaviors. These symptoms are not labeled as a psychiatric disorder unless they persist after pain is adequately controlled. Clinicians should first assist in pain control and then reassess the patient's mental state after pain is controlled to determine whether or not the patient has a psychiatric disorder. Undertreatment of pain is a major problem in both adult and pediatric settings.[8] Aggressive pain management strategies, including narcotics, are essential to the emotional care of both physically ill children and adults. Long-term psychiatric sequelae are less likely in children whose pain is well treated. There is no evidence of increased risk of subsequent drug abuse in children receiving narcotic analgesia. In fact, pediatric patients associate the narcotic effects with the unpleasant aspects of the illness and seek to avoid them during the recovery phase.

Specific Psychologic Problems and Their Medical Management

While most adults and children adjust well to the stress of cancer, persistent, severe, or intolerable level of distress that prohibits the patient's usual functioning is not normal and requires evaluation, diagnosis, and management by a mental health professional. Seven psychiatric disorders occur frequently enough in cancer to warrant a description of their clinical picture. Three are direct responses to illness: adjustment disorders with anxiety and/or depression, major depressive disorder, and organic mental disorders. The remaining four—primary anxiety disorders, personality disorders, schizophrenia, and bipolar disorders—are pre-existing conditions that are often exacerbated by illness.

Adjustment Disorders

The most common psychiatric disorder diagnosed in adults and children with cancer is an adjustment disorder in reaction to the stress of illness. The characteristic symptoms are those of anxiety and depression. The key features of adjustment disorders are the unusual persistence of symptoms and undue interference with occupational or school functioning. When symptoms are severe, adjustment disorders are difficult to differentiate from major depression or generalized anxiety disorders. Regular patient follow-up often clarifies these diagnostic questions.

Treatment of Adjustment Disorders

Interventions are directed at helping the patient adapt to the stresses of cancer and resume successful coping. Individual psychotherapy focuses on clarifying the medical situation and the meaning of illness, and on reinforcing positive defense mechanisms. It is often desirable to include a spouse, partner, or family member to enhance support at home. Group therapy is often helpful, as are behavioral methods such as relaxation and hypnosis. The decision to prescribe psychotropic medication is based on the presence of a high level of distress or an inability to carry out daily activities. A therapeutic trial of benzodiazepines (eg, alprazolam, 0.25 mg po TID) may effectively control symptoms and facilitate other therapeutic interventions. Although the common fear of causing addiction to psychotropic drugs in both adult and pediatric cancer patients is unfounded, these drugs are underprescribed, and patients experience distress that could be controlled by judicious use of medication.

Major Depressive Disorder

The overlap of physical illness and symptoms of depression is widely recognized. Diagnosis of depression in physically healthy adults and children requires the presence of somatic complaints, insomnia, anorexia, fatigue, and weight loss. These symptoms, however, are common to both cancer and depression. In cancer patients, the diagnosis of depression must depend on dysphoric mood or appearance, apathy, crying, anhedonia, feelings of helplessness, decreased self-esteem, guilt, social withdrawal, and thoughts of "wishing for death" or suicide.

Depression has been studied in both adult and pediatric cancer patients using a range of assessment methods.[9,10] In general, the more narrowly the term is defined, the lower the prevalence of depression that is reported. Several studies utilizing patient self-report and observer ratings found major depression in approximately one fourth of hospitalized adult cancer patients.[9] This prevalence is similar to patients with other serious medical illnesses, suggesting that the level of illness, not the specific diagnosis, is the primary determinant.[11,12] Factors associated with higher prevalence of depression in cancer patients are: greater level of physical impairment, more advanced stages of illness, pancreatic cancer, pain, and prior history of depression.[13]

The clinical evaluation of the patient includes a careful assessment of symptoms and history of emotional problems, particularly previous depressive episodes, family history of depression or suicide, concurrent life stresses, and level of social support. Exploring the patient's understanding of the medical situation and meaning of illness is essential. The contribution of pain to depressive symptoms needs to be determined because no psychiatric disorder can be diagnosed with certainty until pain is controlled.[14]

Symptoms of depression can be produced by numerous commonly prescribed medications, including methyldopa, reserpine, barbiturates, diazepam, and propranolol. Of the many cancer chemotherapeutic agents, depressive symptoms are produced by relatively few: prednisone, dexamethasone, vincristine, vinblastine, procarbazine, asparaginase, amphotericin-B, tamoxifen, and interferon.[15] Many metabolic, nutritional, endocrine, and neurologic disorders produce depressive symptoms.[16] Adult cancer patients with abnormal levels of potassium, sodium, or calcium may become depressed, as can patients with a variety of nutritional deficiencies (folate, B_{12}).

Hypo- or hyperthyroidism and adrenal insufficiency can also produce depressive symptoms.

Suicidal ideation requires careful assessment to determine if it reflects depressive illness or expresses a wish to have ultimate control over intolerable symptoms. Adult cancer patients who are at higher risk are those with poor prognosis, advanced stages of illness, a prior psychiatric history or history of substance abuse, previous suicide attempts, or a family history of suicide. A recent death of a friend or partner, few social supports, depression with extreme hopelessness, poorly controlled pain, delirium, and recent information of a grave prognosis are significant risk factors.[17]

Treatment of Depressive Disorders

Prolonged and severe depression usually requires treatment that combines psychotherapy with somatic treatment—either medication or electroconvulsive therapy.

Pharmacologic treatments appropriate for use in adult cancer patients are: the tricyclic antidepressants (TCAs); heterocyclic antidepressants; atypical antidepressants; monoamine oxidase inhibitors (MAOIs); psychostimulants; lithium carbonate; and benzodiazepines.[18] Table 39-3 shows the starting dose and range of therapeutic daily doses for these classes.

Table 39-3. Antidepressant Medications Used in Cancer Patients

Drug Name	Starting Daily Dosage mg (PO)	Therapeutic Daily Dosage mg (PO)
Tricyclic antidepressants		
Amitriptyline	25	75-100
Doxepin	25	75-100
Imipramine	25	75-100
Desipramine	25	75-100
Nortriptyline	25	50-100
Heterocyclic antidepressants		
Maprotiline	25	50-75
Amoxapine	25	100-150
Atypical antidepressants		
Buproprion	15	200-450
Fluoxetine	20	20-60
Trazodone	50	150-200
Sertraline	50	50-150
Paroxetine	10	20-60
Monoamine oxidase inhibitors		
Isocarboxazid	10	20-40
Phenelzine	15	30-60
Tranylcypromine	10	20-40
Lithium carbonate	300	600-1,200
Psychostimulants		
Dextroamphetamine	2.5 at 8 am and noon	5-30
Methylphenidate	2.5 at 8 am and noon	5-30
Pemoline	18.75 in am and noon	37.5-150
Benzodiazepines		
Alprazolam	0.25-1.00	0.75-6.00

Adapted from Massie and Holland.[43]

Tricyclic Antidepressants

The tricyclic antidepressantss are used as the first-line antidepressants because of their established effectiveness, relative safety, and ease of administration. There are several reports of the efficacy of TCAs in depressed adults with cancer.[19-21] The precise mechanism by which the TCAs work is unknown, although there is pharmacologic evidence that they affect the monoamine neurotransmitter systems in the brain.

The various tricyclic compounds are largely similar in efficacy and side-effect profiles. The choice of an antidepressant depends on the patient's specific medical problems and the TCA's side-effect profile. The agitated depressed patient with insomnia may benefit from a TCA that has anticholinergic-mediated sedative effects, such as amitriptyline or doxepin. The patient with stomatitis secondary to chemotherapy or radiation therapy, slowed intestinal motility, or urinary hesitancy should receive a TCA with the least anticholinergic effects, such as desipramine or nortriptyline.

In debilitated patients, TCAs are started at low doses. At bedtime 10 to 25 mg can be given and increased by 25 mg every 1 to 2 days. Depressed cancer patients often show a therapeutic response to TCA at a lower total dose (25 to 125 mg/d) than physically healthy, depressed patients (150 to 300 mg/d). The precise mechanism(s) for this effect is unclear but may represent increased end-organ sensitivity to these compounds. Patients are usually maintained on a TCA for 4 to 6 months after symptoms improve, after which time the dose is gradually lowered and discontinued. Tricyclic antidepressants have been used successfully in children with cancer.[22] The effects on appetite and sleep are frequently immediate; the effects on mood may be delayed or not clinically apparent.

Imipramine, doxepin, nortriptyline, desipramine, and amitriptyline are frequently used in the management of neuropathic pain in cancer patients. The dosage is similar to the treatment of depression. Analgesic efficacy, if it occurs, is usually observed at a dose of 50 to 150 mg daily; higher doses are needed occasionally. Although the initial assumption was that analgesic effects resulted indirectly from the effect on depression, it is now clear that these TCAs have a separate specific analgesic action probably mediated through several neurotransmitters, most prominently norepinephrine and serotonin.[23]

Heterocyclic Antidepressants

If a patient does not respond to a trial of TCAs or cannot tolerate the side effects, a heterocyclic antidepressant (amoxapine or maprotiline) or an atypical antidepressant (bupropion, fluoxetine, trazodone, or sertraline) should be considered. The side effect profile of the heterocyclic compounds is similar to the TCAs. Maprotiline should be avoided in patients who are at high risk for seizures, as the incidence of seizures can be increased with this medication. Amoxapine has strong dopamine-blocking activity. Hence, patients who are taking other dopamine blockers (eg, antiemetics) have an increased risk of developing extrapyramidal symptoms and dyskinesias.

Atypical Antidepressants

The atypical antidepressants are generally considered to be less cardiotoxic than the TCAs.

Bupropion may be activating in medically ill patients. It should be avoided in patients with seizure disorders and brain tumors and those who are malnourished.

Fluoxetine, a selective inhibitor of neuronal serotonin uptake, has fewer sedative and autonomic effects than the TCAs. The most common side effects are mild nausea and a brief period of increased anxiety; hyponatremia is an uncommon adverse effect. Fluoxetine can cause appetite suppression, which usually lasts for a period of several weeks. Some cancer patients experience transient weight loss, but weight usually returns to baseline level.

Trazodone is strongly sedating and in low doses (100 mg at bedtime) is helpful in the treatment of the depressed cancer patient with insomnia. Effective antidepressant doses are often greater than 300 mg daily. Trazodone has been associated with priapism and should, therefore, be used with caution in male patients.

Lithium Carbonate

Patients who were receiving lithium carbonate prior to beginning cancer treatment should be maintained on their therapeutic dose. Maintenance doses of lithium may need adjustment in seriously ill patients in whom dehydration is a risk; serum levels should be monitored. Lithium should be prescribed with caution in patients receiving cisplatin because of both drugs' potential nephrotoxicity.

Several authors have reported a granulocyte-stimulating property of lithium in neutropenic cancer patients. However, the functional capabilities of these leukocytes have not been determined, and the stimulation effect appears to be transient.

Monoamine Oxidase Inhibitors

If a patient has responded well to an MAOI for depression prior to treatment for cancer, its continued use is warranted. Most psychiatrists are reluctant to initiate treatment with MAOIs in cancer patients because further dietary restriction, required with MAOI administration, is often poorly received. MAOIs are usually reserved for patients in whom a TCA has failed or has not been well tolerated.

Psychostimulants

In cancer patients, low doses of the psychostimulants (dextroamphetamine, methylphenidate, and pemoline) potentiate the analgesic effect of narcotics and promote a sense of well-being. Typically, patients are maintained for 1 to 2 months, after which approximately two thirds will be able to be withdrawn without a recurrence of depressive symptoms. Those who develop recurrence of depressive symptoms can be maintained for long periods of time (eg, up to 1 year). Tolerance may develop, and adjustment of the dose may be necessary.

Benzodiazepines

The triazalobenzodiazepine alprazolam is particularly useful in cancer patients who have mixed symptoms of anxiety and depression.

Electroconvulsive Therapy

Occasionally, electroconvulsive therapy (ECT) must be considered for adult cancer patients whose depression is resistant to other interventions and in whom it represents a life-threatening complication of cancer. When prominent psychotic features are present or treatment with antidepressants poses unacceptable side effects, ECT should be considered.

Organic Mental Disorders (Delirium)

Delirium, the second most common psychiatric diagnosis among cancer patients, is due both to the direct effects of cancer on the central nervous system (CNS) and the indirect CNS complications of the disease and treatment. Posner has reported that 15% to 20% of hospitalized cancer patients have cognitive function abnormalities unrelated to structural disease.[24] Approximately one fifth of psychiatric consultations are for assistance in the diagnosis and management of delirium.[1] Delirium is usually due to one or more causes: medications, electrolyte imbalance, failure of a vital organ or system, nutritional deficiencies, infections, vascular diseases, or hormone-producing tumors.[25]

Early symptoms of delirium are often unrecognized and, hence, undertreated. Any patient who shows acute onset of agitation, behavioral changes, impaired cognitive function, altered attention span, or a fluctuating level of consciousness should be evaluated for presence of delirium. As in adults, delirium is frequently underdiagnosed and undertreated in children. Predominant causes include the cumulative sedative effects of antihistamines, benzodiazepines, and analgesics. Children may exhibit symptoms of agitation, confusion, and fear. Treatment strategies include elimination of unnecessary sedating agents, with the exception of analgesics, verbal reassurance by a consistent companion, and low-dose neuroleptic treatment (eg, haloperidol).

Many drugs can cause acute confusional states. Confusion is a common adverse effect of opioids. Among the more than 280 chemotherapeutic agents now available for cancer, delirium has been associated with methotrexate (with intrathecal or intravenous administration), flurouracil, vincristine, vinblastine, bleomycin, carmustine (BCNU), cisplatin, asparaginase, procarbazine, cytosine arabinoside, ifosphamide, and corticosteriods. Other medications commonly prescribed for cancer patients that can cause confusional states are interleukin-2, amphotericin, and acyclovir.

Steroid compounds are a frequent cause of delirium. Psychiatric disturbances range from common minor mood disturbance to psychosis.[26] Characteristic symptoms include affective changes (emotional lability, euphoria, depressed mood), anxiety, fears, paranoid interpretation of events, suspiciousness, delusions, and hallucinations. More severe symptoms develop within 4 to 5 days of high-dose steroid treatment or with rapidly tapered doses, but psychiatric symptoms can also develop while patients are on maintenance dose. No relationship has been shown between the development of steroid-induced mental status changes and premorbid personality or psychiatric history.[27]

Treatment of Organic Mental Disorders (Delirium)

Organic mental disorders require corrective medical interventions, but interim symptomatic treatment may be necessary. Patients with "quiet" delirium do not require psychopharmacologic management. General care should include sensory stimulation to avoid deprivation effects, provision of familiar stimuli such as family, use of companions to ensure safety, and adequate nursing care.

Delirious adult and pediatric patients with psychotic symptoms or agitation respond to neuroleptic medication. Haloperidol is the most commonly prescribed medication because of its excellent safety record with little effect on heart rate, blood pressure, respiration, or cardiac output. Haloperidol can be given orally in tablet or concentrate, or parenterally (IM or IV). Peak plasma concentrations are achieved in 2 to 4 hours after an oral dose, and measurable plasma concentrations occur in 15 to 30 minutes after parenteral administration.

The initial dose of haloperidol for both adult and pediatric cancer patients is low, starting with 0.5 mg to 1.0 mg administered orally or 0.25 mg to 0.5 mg parenterally. The dose can be repeated at 30-minute intervals until symptoms are controlled. If psychotic symptoms are reduced but agitation remains, low-dose benzodiazepines can be added. Dystonic reactions, though uncommon, are treated with anticholinergic agents such as diphenylhydrazine or benzotropine.

Anxiety Disorders

The types of anxiety encountered in the oncology setting are: (1) episodes of acute anxiety related to the stress of cancer and its treatment, (2) anxiety related to medical illness, and (3) chronic anxiety disorders that antedate the cancer diagnosis and are exacerbated during treatment.

Situational anxiety is common, and most patients are anxious while waiting to hear their diagnosis; before stressful or painful procedures (bone marrow aspiration, chemotherapy administration, radiation therapy, wound debridement); prior to surgery; and while awaiting test results. Anxiety is expected at these times, and most patients manage with the reassurance and support from their physicians. At times further treatment is necessary. Extreme fearfulness, inability to cooperate or understand procedures, a prior history of panic attacks, needle phobia, or claustrophobia may require an anxiolytic medication (eg, lorazepam, 1.0 mg po TID, or alprazolam, 0.5 mg po TID) to reduce symptoms to a manageable level. Hypnotics (eg, triazolam, 0.125 to 0.25 mg po) are particularly useful during the perioperative period.

The differential diagnosis of anxiety in the cancer patient can be complex. Patients in severe pain may appear anxious or agitated and usually respond to adequate pain control with analgesics. The anxiety that accompanies respiratory distress, while eventually relieved by medical intervention, often requires an anxiolytic. Many patients on steroids experience insomnia and anxiety, which should be treated with benzodiazepines. Patients developing metabolic encephalopathy (delirium) can appear restless or anxious, and treatment with neuroleptics is often required as determination and correction (if possible) of the cause(s) is begun. Anxiety symptoms are also features of withdrawal from narcotics, benzodiazepines, and barbiturates. Since patients who abuse alcohol or drugs commonly underreport substance intake prior to admission, the physician needs to consider alcohol or drug withdrawal in all patients who develop otherwise unexplained anxiety symptoms during the first week of hospitalization. Other medical conditions that may have anxiety as a prominent feature or presenting symptom are hyperthyroidism, pheochromocytoma, carcinoid, and mitral valve prolapse.

Anxiety disorders that antedate the onset of cancer can compromise medical treatment. Phobias and panic disorders are the most common types. Occasionally patients have their first episode of panic while being treated in a medical setting. Psychiatric evaluation prior to undertaking cancer treatment is essential in patients with a history of panic disorder or phobia. Patients with claustrophobia may have extreme anxiety in the confined spaces of diagnostic scanning devices or radiation therapy treatment rooms. Patients with needle phobias report having avoided medical evaluations for years because of their fears. Patients with agoraphobia often are unable to tolerate hospital admission unaccompanied by a family member.

Phobias related to medical procedures are common in children with cancer. While careful attention to preparation of children in advance of painful procedures (eg, role-playing) may limit the incidence of anxiety, specific behavioral interventions, including relaxation training and distraction, may be indicated for specific symptoms.[28] Self-hypnosis is a highly effective treatment for both generalized anxiety and specific phobias in children and adolescents.

Post-traumatic stress disorder (PTSD) is a specific type of anxiety disorder due to the effects of traumatic experiences, including military combat, natural catastrophes, assault, rape, accidents, and life-threatening illness. Recall of prior painful or frightening treatment are common causes of PTSD in cancer patients, especially children. Illness can also exacerbate feelings about earlier traumas, noted particularly in cancer patients who are Holocaust survivors. In the adult and pediatric cancer patient, symptoms can develop at various stages of illness but are frequent at the time of diagnosis. Important variables in the disorder's development are the patient's personality traits, the biological vulnerability to stressful events, and the severity of the stressor. In general, pediatric and geriatric populations have more difficulty coping with stressful events and are at risk for PTSD. The underdeveloped emotional state of children prevents them from using various adaptive strategies, and the elderly are likely to have fixed coping mechanisms that minimize their flexibility in dealing with trauma.

In adults the typical presenting symptoms include periods of intrusive repetition of the stressful event (nightmares, flashbacks, and intrusive thoughts) along with denial, emotional numbness, and depression. A syndrome of recurrent nightmares, separation anxiety, and emotional blunting consistent with the diagnosis of PTSD has been reported in children being treated for cancer.[29] In both adults and children, use of denial is prominent and minimizes the painful event. The nonspecific emotional symptoms can make the diagnosis difficult to distinguish from a generalized anxiety disorder, depression, or panic disorder. Questions about intrusive phenomena help to determine the specific diagnosis. Many patients are relieved to understand their symptoms are an expected response to severe stress.

Treatment of Anxiety Disorders

Many patients with intermittent anxiety, simple phobias, or PTSD find relaxation therapy and distraction techniques helpful. Play therapy is generally indicated for children with PTSD. When the need for a diagnostic procedure or treatment is urgent, benzodiazepines should be used (eg, prior to venipuncture, intravenous chemotherapy administration, a scanning procedure, or radiation therapy treatment).

Benzodiazepines are the drugs of choice for both acute and chronic anxiety states. The most common side-effects—sedation and confusion—occur more frequently in older patients and in those with impaired liver function. Short-acting benzodiazepines, such as alprazolam, lorazepam, and oxazepam, are often prescribed. Oxazepam and lorazepam are metabolized by conjugation and excreted by the kidney and hence are better tolerated by patients with impaired hepatic function and by those taking other medications with sedative effects (eg, analgesics). Lorazepam reduces vomiting in cancer patients receiving emetogenic cancer chemotherapies.

Clonazepam has been found to be useful in patients with organic mental disorders or seizure disorders who develop symptoms of depersonalization or anxiety. This longer acting benzodiazepine is also useful for individuals who have end of dose failure with recurrence of anxiety symptoms. It is effective in patients with organic mood disorders with symptoms of mania and as an adjuvant analgesic in patients with neuropathic pain.

Table 39-4 lists the usual initial dose of benzodiazepines, approximate dose equivalent, half-life, and presence or absence of active metabolites. Dose schedule depends on the patient's tolerance and the anxiolytic's duration of action. When a long-acting benzodiazepine is used in patients with chronic anxiety, the dose should not exceed twice a day. The shorter-acting benzodiazepines are given three to four

Table 39-4. Commonly Prescribed Benzodiazepines in Cancer Patients

Drug	Approximate Dose Equivalent	Initial Dosage PO (mg)	Half Life (Hr)	Active Metabolite
Short to Intermediate Half-Life				
Alprazolam	0.5	0.25-0.5 TID	10-15	No
Chlordiazepoxide	10.0	10-25 TID	5-30	Yes
Clonazepam	1.0	0.5 BID	18-50	No
Lorazepam*	1.0	0.5-2.0 TID	10-20	No
Oxazepam	10.0	10-15 TID	5-15	No
Temazepam†	15.0	15-30 QHS	10-15	No
Triazolam†	0.25	0.125-0.25 QHS	1-5	No
Long Half-Life				
Clorazepate	7.5	7.5-15 BID	30-200	Yes
Diazepam	5.0	5-10 BID	20-70	Yes

*Lorazepam can also be administered intramuscularly; other benzodiazepines are erratically absorbed when given intramuscularly.

†Hypnotic agents.

Adapted from Massie and Holland.[43]

times a day. It is best to increase the dose before switching to another agent in patients with persistent symptoms.

Patients who experience severe anticipatory anxiety (ie, anxiety before chemotherapy administration) are given an anxiolytic the night before and immediately prior to the treatment. Patients with chronic anxiety states require anxiolytics daily or intermittently for months or years. Cancer patients, even those with chronic anxiety, usually do not take more medication than they absolutely require and eagerly discontinue medications as soon as their symptoms remit.

The most common side effects of the benzodiazepines are dose-dependent and include drowsiness, confusion, and motor incoordination. When the dose is lowered, uncomfortable sedation often disappears, while the antianxiety effects continue. Sedation is most common and most severe in patients with impaired liver function. Physicians should be aware of the synergistic effects of the benzodiazepines with other medications with CNS depressant properties, such as narcotics.

Low-dose neuroleptics are effective in patients with severe anxiety that is not controlled with maximal therapeutic doses of benzodiazepines. The low efficacy of the antihistamines for anxiety limits their general usefulness, although they are prescribed for control of anxiety in patients with respiratory impairment or other conditions where benzodiazepines are contraindicated.

Post-traumatic stress disorder is most often treated with TCAs, which appear to be effective in reducing the panic and depressive symptoms in most adult patients. In children, benzodiazepines are useful because of their effect on the often-noted anxiety and restlessness.

Personality Disorders

Patients (or families) with "difficult" personalities frustrate and anger those who treat them. The stress of cancer exaggerates their normally maladaptive coping strategies and they become even more difficult than usual. The disorders are recognizable by the exaggeration of common characteristics: the paranoid person who is suspicious and constantly threatens litigation; the obsessive person whose excessive attention to details of care is accompanied by repeated criticism; the dependent person who demands care far beyond objective needs and who may be dependent on alcohol or drugs; the patient with borderline disorder who is unable to conform to rules, who manipulates, divides, and may disturb other patients as well as staff; and the histrionic person who overdramatizes symptoms and distress. Since personality disorders are not felt by the patients to be a problem, management usually depends on helping staff to understand the pattern and to contain their behavior. Many of these patients benefit from consistent limit setting, applied in a quiet, firm, but kindly manner.[30]

Schizophrenia and Bipolar Disorders

Schizophrenia and bipolar disorders illness are rare in the general population and hence uncommon in cancer patients. However, when present, they require careful management to ensure the patient's cooperation with treatment and to prevent escalation of symptoms under stress. Previously prescribed neuroleptics should be continued—coordinating management with the anesthesiologist—when surgery is required because of potential paradoxical blood pressure reactions. Lithium should also be continued but may need to be stopped briefly during periods of fluid restriction.

Indications for Psychiatric Evaluation

Many mild to moderately severe psychiatric disorders are managed successfully by the oncologist and a sensitive staff. However, it is clear that cancer patients experience a significant number of psychiatric disorders requiring accurate diagnosis for precise and effective treatment. Once treatment is outlined, management may often be carried out by the physician with help of social workers or other mental health professionals. The more severe psychiatric problems require close collaboration between the oncologist and psychiatrist.

Table 39-5 outlines the indications for psychiatric consultation. Disorders directly related to illness, preexisting psychiatric disorders exacerbated by illness and major mental disorders have been described. Four additional indications warrant discussion:

Table 39-5. Indications for Psychiatric Evaluation

Disorders directly related to illness
- Adjustment disorders (reactive anxiety and depression)
- Major depression and suicidal risk
- Delirium from CNS complications

Pre-existing disorders exacerbated by illness
- Anxiety disorders
- Personality disorders

Major mental disorders
- Schizophrenia
- Bipolar affective disorder

Capacity to consent or to refuse treatment

Leaving against medical advice

Sexual dysfunction

Significant distress from conflict with family or staff

Adapted from Lederberg and Massie.[30]

Capacity to Consent to or Refuse Treatment

A psychiatric consultation may be needed when a patient refuses a procedure critical to survival or when the capacity to give informed consent is in question. Rarely is legal advice or a judge's decision necessary for emergency treatment. However, when elective treatment is planned for a mentally impaired patient with no family, court direction may be needed. An increasingly common concern is the patient who refuses a clearly life-sustaining treatment, such as dialysis, as part of a decision to forego all further treatment. Physicians and nurses often are not certain whether the patient is truly capable of assessing all the options. The presence of acute depression, which dulls mental processes and strongly biases decisions, poses a difficult and sometimes urgent reason for psychiatric consultation.[30]

Leaving Against Medical Advice

Requests to leave the hospital against advice are most commonly due to the presence of a confusional state secondary to illness or medication and as such often represent an acute danger to self, allowing for brief restraint and treatment following psychiatric evaluation. An acutely psychotic state or an exacerbated prior psychiatric disorder may also result in poor judgment. The cause of the behavior must be determined and a decision made as to whether the patient can be managed safely at home or whether he or she must remain in the hospital with a relative or companion. Often the severity of the patient's illness prevents safe transfer to a medical-psychiatric unit, but improvement occurs rapidly under the care of familiar medical staff, with one-to-one observation and low doses of a neuroleptic drug such as haloperidol.

Sexual Dysfunction

Infertility and sexual dysfunction are often unavoidable consequences of irradiation, surgery, and chemotherapy. In men, the opportunity for sperm banking before treatment can both arouse and assuage concerns about infertility. In women, psychologic preparation for the premature menopause and sterility associated with chemotherapy or the altered sexual function that results from gynecologic surgery is very useful in diminishing the inevitable adverse reactions. Soon after completion of treatment, patients are reluctant to bring up sexual problems, and physicians and staff are equally reluctant to ask about them. In later follow-up visits, the burden is on the oncologist to inquire into the sexual problems common with several tumor sites: colon, breast, testicular, gynecologic neoplasms, prostate, bladder, head and neck tumors, and Hodgkin's disease.

Significant Distress from Conflict with Family or Staff

Sometimes a case becomes imbued with persistent conflict. This may stem from the patient's personality, but it often involves the family's problems or, more rarely, the staff's inadvertent mishandling. A psychiatric consultant can provide an objective assessment that identifies and confronts the sources of the problematic behavior. Family meetings, possibly with the patient and selected staff members present, often help to ease family distress; similarly, staff conferences encourage a more concerted and effective approach to the family and patient.

Psychologic Interventions for Cancer Patients

The cornerstone of psychologic interventions in cancer is emotional support. Psychoeducational counseling focusing on advice and information about illness can be helpful to both patient and family and can be carried out by different members of the treatment team. Religious counseling is meaningful for many patients during the existential crisis created by cancer. A one-to-one visit by a "veteran" patient who has successfully negotiated the same cancer treatment often helps. Psychotherapy provided by a mental health professional usually consists of short-term, crisis-oriented supportive therapy to assist the patient to strengthen adaptive defenses and better cope with the problems of illness.

Group therapy, led either by professionals or cancer survivors, is useful in several ways. First, groups have an educational function in orienting and teaching patients. Second, groups encourage emotional learning and can relieve anxiety by allowing individuals to share similar problems and solutions. Third, the support they provide often becomes a voice for social awareness and change, giving participants a valuable sense of strength. Behavioral therapies emphasize self-regulatory interventions and are well-received by patients. Many learn relaxation exercises, visual imagery for distraction, and self-hypnotic suggestions. Although these techniques do not have antitumor effect, such techniques are particularly effective in reducing anticipatory nausea and vomiting in patients receiving chemotherapy.

Long-term Survivors and Cured Patients

Advances in cancer treatment have resulted in a rapidly growing population of over 5 million long-term survivors, many of them children and young adults. Psychiatric sequelae of cancer in both children and adults include those related to the direct effects of the disease, as well as those that are consequences of the treatments, of family factors, and the individual psychology of the person. Early studies of adults using measures such as marriage and level of education showed few psychologic effects, but recent investigators, using more refined measures, have shown more symptoms. However, the long-term adjustment of survivors of childhood cancer appears largely unimpaired.[31] Cured cancer patients have special medical and psychiatric concerns including fears of termination of treatment, preoccupation with disease recurrence and minor physical problems, a sense of greater vulnerability to illness (the Damocles syndrome), pervasive awareness of mortality and difficulty with re-entry into normal life (the Lazarus syndrome), persistent guilt (the survivor syndrome), difficult adjustment to physical losses and handicaps, a sense of physical inferiority, diminished self-esteem or confidence, perceived loss of job mobility, and fear of insurance discrimination (Table 39-6). Concerns about infertility, often submerged at the time of diagnosis and treatment, can reappear when patients consider marrying.

The survivor's intellectual functioning is a major concern. Children and adults with brain tumors are at risk from both their disease and treatment. Most have residual deficits, with mild-to-marked decline in IQ scores and a dementia-like syndrome. Children with acute lymphoblastic leukemia (ALL) who received more than 25 Gy of cranial irradiation scored lower

Table 39-6. Psychologic Problems of Cancer Survivors

Psychologic Problems of Cancer Survivors
Fears of termination of treatment
Preoccupation with disease recurrence
Preoccupation with minor physical problems
Persistent sense of vulnerability to illness and death (the Damocles syndrome)
Difficulty with re-entry into normal life (the Lazarus syndrome)
Persistent guilt (the survivor syndrome)
Adjustment to physical losses and handicaps
Diminished self-esteem or self-confidence
Perceived loss of job mobility
Awareness of insurance discrimination

Adapted from Lederberg and Massie.[30]

on a range of cognitive tests in several long-term follow-up studies.[32,33] As a consequence, CNS prophylaxis for ALL currently uses 18 Gy and/or intrathecal methotrexate. This regimen produces less cognitive impairment, and protocols are structured so that only children with high-risk leukemia receive this treatment.[34]

As the number of cancer survivors grows, more attention is being given to societal attitudes. The National Coalition of Cancer Survivorship is an outgrowth of the need for and value of support. The issues surrounding health and life insurance policies are a prime example of an area where research is needed to delineate problems and develop solutions. Many centers around the country are developing "survivor clinics" that incorporate a multidisciplinary approach to the cured child, adolescent, or adult.

Management of Grief

Grief is frequently encountered in the oncology setting, and staff management can affect the nature of bereavement and influence the family's long-term adjustment. Once death has occurred, grieving has acute and chronic components.[35] Reminders of the deceased precipitate waves of an overwhelming sense of loss, crying, and agitation. The intense distress of the first few months are characterized by social withdrawal, preoccupation with the deceased, diminished concentration, restlessness, depressed mood, anxiety, insomnia, and anorexia. The bereaved spouse or parent repeatedly recalls how the final days were handled, how the painful news of grave prognosis and death were conveyed, and how sensitively the final moments were managed. The surviving relatives or parents may search for fault and tend to blame both themselves and staff. The physician must recognize his or her special meaning to survivors and understand their reactions in this context. A meeting held 1 to 2 months after the death is a valuable setting where autopsy findings and any troubling questions can be discussed.

Over several months, grief usually diminishes in intensity. The duration of normal grieving is much more variable than originally assumed and often extends well beyond a year. Parents, for example, often report that they are "never the same again"; some never really recover. Older spouses from a long union often grieve acutely for 2 to 4 years or longer.[36]

Psychologic Problems in High-Risk Individuals

The current explosion of information about genetic contribution to the development of cancer has brought into existence a new population, people whose family history is such that they are clearly at high risk for certain cancers. Psychologically, it is useful to differentiate between people who are afraid they might be at risk and people who are afraid because they know they are at risk. The first group benefits from being educated about what, if any, is their increased risk. Some will remain excessively anxious even in the absence of objective reason and may be said to suffer from cancerophobia; they benefit from psychologic support and regular checkups with a trusted oncologist to prevent them from squandering time and resources consulting with numerous physicians.

Patients in the second group, those who are at increased genetic risk, benefit from the same education, but also need detailed genetic and psychologic counseling to help them make difficult decisions regarding marriage, child bearing, pre-natal testing, and further personal testing or medical interventions (eg, prophylactic mastectomy for the woman at genetic high risk of developing breast cancer).

Breast cancer is the most common cancer known to have a possible genetic component (up to 30% of cases), and high-risk surveillance programs that have medical/surgical, genetic counseling, and psychiatric evaluation components have been developed. Support groups have proven very helpful and have enabled many women who were too frightened to practice breast self-examination to begin to do it regularly.[37]

Stresses on Oncology Staff

Recent studies have helped clarify the picture of emotional reactions of patients and their relatives to cancer, but few studies have addressed the stresses on the oncologist and its effect on personal and professional life.[38-40] Studies show that, despite recent criticism of medicine as uncaring, patients still accept treatment largely because they trust their doctors and his or her recommendations.[41] The harried, stressed oncologist is compromised in his or her ability to give attention to the art of medicine, yet seldom is this human aspect of care more important than in oncology.

Most physicians generally tolerate work stresses well and have personality characteristics that are known to buffer stress: a strong commitment to work, a sense of control of their work without letting the magnitude of the problems become overwhelming, and a view of daily problems as a challenge.[42] However, physicians also have the characteristics that predispose them to chronic stress. Many work long hours, are chronically fatigued, and seek little recreation; many have trouble saying no to requests for additional work.

The practice of oncology carries specific additional strains. There is the uncertainty inherent in most treatment decisions and the repeated impact of patients' deaths. Some personal stress inevitably accompanies decisions about withholding or stopping life-sustaining treatment amid all the medical, social, and ethical ambiguities that abound in the current climate. Learning to discuss these issues with patients and families is difficult and painful.

The physician with symptoms of emotional fatigue or burnout notices he or she has less zest and enthusiasm for work; and depressed mood may ensue. The need for a few drinks after work or experimenting with drugs to relax are ominous signs. On the physical side, insomnia is common. Appetite change may lead to weight gain or weight loss. The stressed physician reports feeling exhausted and tired all the time. Headaches or somatic pains are indicators of distress. At this point, the physician may tune out and feel detached from his or her patients. This is an early sign of stress in house staff who say they feel less able to care and are cynical and pessimistic about the meaning of their work. They may begin to work longer hours and have a sense that "nobody can do it right but me" and "nobody works around here but me," when in fact they are less efficient and less effective.[40]

Monitoring symptoms of emotional fatigue and acknowledging stress are important for anyone working in oncology. Survival tactics must be instituted that include recognizing limitations, developing a comfortable perspective on self and work, accepting personal and medical inadequacies, using gallows humor to lighten the meaning of painful events, working a normal workday for a few weeks, stopping when others do, taking a long weekend, and regular exercise. When symptoms do not remit, psychiatric consultation should be sought.

Summary

The most common psychiatric complications in both adults and children with cancer are depression, anxiety, and delirium. It is important for patient comfort and quality of life to evaluate and to manage the psychologic distress in the patient with cancer. Psychotherapeutic, psychopharmacologic, and behavioral interventions can be tailored to the very ill patient's needs. Clinical observation and research has furthered our understanding of the problems of long-term survivors, cured patients, grieving families, individuals at high genetic risk of developing cancer, and oncology staff.

References

1. Massie MJ, Holland JC. Consultation and liaison issues in cancer care. Psychiatr Med. 1987;5:343-359.

2. Holland JC. Psychological aspects of cancer. In: Holland JF, Frei E, eds. *Cancer Medicine*. 2nd ed. Philadelphia, Pa: Lea & Febiger; 1982:1175-1203, 2325-2331.

3. Lewis M, Lewis DO, Schonfeld DJ. Dying and death in childhood and adolescence. In: Lewis M, ed. *Child and Adolescent Psychiatry: A Comprehensive Textbook*. Baltimore, Md: Williams & Williams; 1991:1051-1059.

4. Powazek M, Schijving J, Goff JR, et al. Psychosocial ramifications of childhood leukemia: one year post-diagnosis. In: Schulman JL, Kupat MJ, eds. *The Child With Cancer.* Springfield, Ill: Charles C Thomas Publisher; 1980:143-155.

5. Lansky SB, Cairns NU, Hassannein R, et al. Childhood cancer: parent discord and divorce. *Pediatrics.* 1978;62:184-188.

6. Kagen-Goodheart L. Reentry: living with childhood cancer. *Am J Orthopsychiatry.* 1977;47:651-658.

7. Derogatis LR, Morrow GR, Fetting J, et al. Prevalence of psychiatric disorders among cancer patients. *JAMA.* 1983; 249:751-757.

8. Weisman S, Schechter N. The management of pain in children. *Pediatr Rev*. 1991;12:237-243.

9. Bukberg J, Penman D, Holland JC. Depression in hospitalized cancer patients. *Psychosom Med.* 1984;46:199-212.

10. Massie MJ. Depression. In: Holland J, Rowland JR, eds. *Handbook of Psycho-Oncology: Psychological Care of the Patient with Cancer.* New York, NY: Oxford University Press; 1989:283-290.

11. Moffic H, Paykel ES. Depression in medical inpatients. *Br J Psychiatry.* 1975;126:346-353.

12. Schwab JJ, Bialow M, Brown JM, Holzer CE. Diagnosing depression in medical inpatients. *Ann Intern Med.* 1967; 67:695-707.

13. Holland JC, Hughes Korzun A, Tross S, et al. Comparative psychological disturbance in pancreatic and gastric cancer. *Am J Psychiatry.* 1986;143:982-986.

14. Massie MJ, Holland JC. The cancer patient with pain: psychiatric complications and their management. *Med Clin North Am.* 1987;71:243-258.

15. Young DF. Neurological complications of cancer chemotherapy. In: Silverstein A, ed. *Neurological Complications of Therapy: Selected Topics.* New York, NY: Futura Publishing; 1982:57-113.

16. Hall RCW, Popkin MK, Devaul RA, Faillace LA, Stickney SK. Physical illness presenting as psychiatric disease. *Arch Gen Psychiatry.* 1978;35:1315-1320.

17. Breitbart W. Suicide in cancer patients. In: Holland JC, Rowland JH, eds. *Handbook of Psycho-Oncology: Psychological Care of the Patient With Cancer.* New York, NY: Oxford University Press; 1989:291-299.

18. Massie MJ, Holland JC. Psychiatric complications of cancer pain. *J Pain Symptom Manage.* 1992;7:99-109.

19. Purohit DR, Navlakha PL, Modi RS, et al. The role of antidepressants in hospitalized cancer patients. *J Assoc Physicians India.* 1978;26:245-248.

20. Costa D, Mogos I, Toma T. Efficacy and safety of mianserin in the treatment of depression of women with cancer. *Acta Psychiatr Scand.* 1985;72:85-92.

21. Massie MJ, Lesko LM. Psychopharmacological management. In: Holland JC, Rowland JH, eds. *Handbook of Psycho-Oncology: Psychological Care of the Patient With Cancer.* New York, NY: Oxford University Press; 1989:470-491.

22. Pfefferbaum-Levin B, Kumor K, Cangir A, Choroszy M, Roseberry EA. Tricyclic antidepressants for children wtih cancer. *Am J Psychiatry.* 1983;140:1074-1076.

23. France RD. The future for antidepressants: treatment of pain. *Psychopathology.* 1987;20:99-113.

24. Posner JB. Neurologic complications in systemic cancer. *Dis Mon.* 1978;2:7-60.

25. Lipowsky ZJ. Delirium: acute brain failure in man. Springfield, Ill: Charles C Thomas Publisher; 1980.

26. Hall RCW, Popkin MK, Stickney SK, Gardner ER. Presentation of the steroid psychosis. *J Nerv Ment Dis.* 1979;167:229-236.

27. Stiefel FC, Breitbart WS, Holland JC. Corticosteroids in cancer: neuropsychiatric complications. *Cancer Invest.* 1989;7:479-491.

28. Redd WH, Jacobsen PB, Die-Trill M, Dermatis H, McEvoy M, Holland JC. Cognitive-attentional distraction in the control of conditioned nausea in pediatric cancer patients receiving chemotherapy. *J Consult Clin Psychol.* 1987;55:391-395.

29. Nir Y. Post-traumatic stress disorder in children with cancer. In: Pynoos RS, Eth S, eds. *Post-Traumatic Stress Disorder in Children.* Washington, DC: American Psychiatric Press; 1985:121-132.

30. Lederberg MS, Massie MJ. Psychosocial and ethical issues in the care of cancer patients. In: DeVita VT, Hellman S, Rosenberg SA, eds. *Cancer: Principles and Practice of Oncology.* 4th ed. Philadelphia, Pa: JB Lippincott Co; 1993:2448.

31. Greenberg HS, Kazak AE, Meadows AT. Psychological functioning in 8- to 16-year-old cancer survivors and their parents. *J Pediatr.* 1989;114:488-493.

32. Copeland DR, Fletcher JM, Pfefferbaum-Levine B, et al. Neuropsychological sequelae of childhood cancer in long-term survivors. *Pediatrics.* 1985;75:745-753.

33. Tamaroff M, Miller DR, Murphy ML, et al. Immediate and long-term post-therapy neuropsychologic performance in children with acute lymphoblastic leukemia treated without central nervous system radiation. *J Pediatr.* 1982; 101:524-529.

34. Anderson BL, Stehbens JA. Intellectual functioning of children with leukemia by age at diagnosis. Presented at the American Psychological Association Convention. 1985.

35. Osterweis M, Solomon F, Green M, eds. *Bereavement Reactions, Consequences and Care.* Washington, DC: National Academy Press; 1984.

36. Parkes CM, Weiss R. *Recovery From Bereavement.* New York, NY: Basic Books; 1983.

37. Kash KM, Holland JC, Halper MS, Miller DG. Psychological distress and surveillance behaviors of women with a family history of breast cancer. *JNCI.* 1992;84:24-30.

38. Mount BM. Dealing with our losses. *J Clin Oncol.* 1986; 4:1127-1134.

39. Kash K, Holland JC. Special problems of physicians and house staff. In: Holland JC, Rowland JH, eds. *Handbook of Psycho-Oncology: Psychological Care of the Patient With Cancer.* New York, NY: Oxford University Press; 1989:647-657.

40. Lederberg MS. Psychological problems of staff and their management. In: Holland JC, Rowland JH, eds. *Handbook of Psycho-Oncology: Psychological Care of the Patient With Cancer.* New York, NY: Oxford University Press; 1989:631-646.

41. Penman D, Holland JC, Bahna G, et al. Informed consent for investigational chemotherapy: patients' and physicians' perceptions. *J Clin Oncol.* 1984;2:849-855.

42. Kobasa SC, Pucceti MD. Personality and social resources in stress-resistance. *J Pers Soc Psychol.* 1983; 45:839-850.

43. Massie MJ, Holland JC. The cancer patient with pain: psychiatric complications and their management. *J Pain and Symptom Management.* 1992;7:99-109.

40

SEXUALITY AND CANCER

Barbara L. Andersen, PhD, and Margaret A. Lamb, PhD, RN

Cancer and cancer treatments produce significant sexual disruption, and this morbidity occurs across all sites of disease.[1] Many variables may increase the likelihood of psychologic and behavioral difficulties, but the magnitude of cancer treatment remains one of the most important. To the extent that cancer patients can be treated effectively with less radical therapies, their quality of life, including sexual functioning, will be enhanced.

This chapter details the sexual difficulties of cancer patients. A site-by-site review is provided so that the reader can easily locate the data for the group of interest. Since many health providers may not have extensive scientific or clinical backgrounds in sexuality, two supplementary topics are included. The first is a brief overview of "normal" sexual functioning, including sexual behavior, the sexual response cycle (desire, excitement, orgasm, and resolution), and common sexual dysfunctions. This introductory section provides the context for appreciating the similarities and differences between sexual dysfunctions of healthy individuals and those of cancer patients. Following the site review is a strategy for a routine assessment of sexuality appropriate for the history and physical examination. The acronym ALARM is used to facilitate recall of the major topics. Finally, a brief description of the PLISSIT[2] intervention model is presented.

Overview of Sexual Function and Dysfunction

Sexual Behavior

In the United States, the first large-scale study of sexual behavior was by Alfred Kinsey and colleagues.[3,4] Although many of their findings are dated, their focus on specific sexual behaviors is still used today in assessing sexuality. For example, in their interviews with thousands of women and men, they assessed the following activities across the lifespan: preadolescent heterosexual and homosexual play; masturbation; nocturnal sex emissions/dreams; heterosexual "petting"; premarital, marital, and extra-marital coitus; intercourse with prostitutes (for males only); homosexual contacts; animal contacts; and, finally, the "total sexual outlet," defined as the sum of the various activities that culminated in orgasm. Other topics now recognized as important to sexual development and, perhaps, the subsequent occurrence of sexual dysfunctions, such as incest and traumatic sexual experiences,[5] were not assessed. Our own studies of heterosexual adult women[6] have identified the following groupings of sexual behavior: preliminary foreplay (eg, kissing, embracing, undressing), intimate foreplay (eg, manual/oral genital stimulation), intercourse, anal stimulation, and masturbation. For heterosexual adults, the frequency of intercourse is a central sexual activity, as it is significantly correlated with sexual satisfaction and adjustment.[6] As intercourse may become difficult or impossible following cancer treatment, it may be important to assess the frequency of other sexual activities (eg, partner kissing, body touching) as well.

The Sexual Response Cycle

Sexual Desire

The second and third areas for assessment are the phases of the sexual response cycle—desire, excitement, orgasm, and resolution—and the corresponding sexual dysfunctions. Sexual desire is most often thought of as a biologic drive that is also hormonally mediated. Data is most consistent for the necessary (but not sufficient) role of androgens, probably testosterone, in male sexual desire.[7] For example, a dose-response relationship has been found between testosterone administration and cognitive sexual

---

Barbara L. Andersen, PhD, Professor, Department of Psychology and Department of Obstetrics and Gynecology, The Ohio State University, Columbus, Ohio

Margaret A. Lamb, PhD, RN, Associate Professor, Department of Nursing, University of New Hampshire, Durham, New Hampshire

responses and nocturnal erections.[8] Hormone/sexual behavior relationships for women are less clear, although estrogen, progesterone, and androgen have been studied. Regarding estrogen effects, it is clear that some amount of estrogen is necessary for normal vaginal lubrication, and receipt of estrogen replacement therapy following menopause may reduce the problematic symptoms (eg, lack of lubrication, atrophic vaginitis), which will allow sexual activity or functioning to proceed unimpaired.[9] In contrast, progesterone may actually have an inhibitory effect.[7] Finally, testosterone may have direct effects on sexual functioning; both Bancroft et al[10] and Schreiner-Engel et al[11] have found positive relationships between testosterone levels and frequency of masturbation and vaginal responses to erotic stimuli.

Psychologic conceptualizations view desire as an urge for sexual activity that may be triggered by internal cues (eg, fantasy) or external cues (eg, pornography, the presence of an interested partner).[12] Initially the term "inhibited sexual desire" was applied to individuals who chronically failed to initiate or respond to sexual cues.[13] In more recent diagnostic criteria, such as the DSM-IIIR[14] definition of hypoactive sexual desire, there are no specific behavioral, affective, or physiologic markers. Instead, low desire is linked to the absence of specific cognitions—sexual fantasies. Clinical descriptions of individuals complaining of low desire suggest a general disinterest in sexual activity. Such an attitude can be manifested behaviorally by never initiating sexual contact, avoiding sexual contexts, or refusing a partner's initiations. The latter are not presumed to be due to negative responses (ie, aversions) to interpersonal or genital contact, an important point to consider when ruling out an alternative diagnosis of sexual aversion disorder (see discussion below). Instead, individuals with low desire disorder are thought to be indifferent or neutral towards sexual activity. For some, sexual drive or urging seems not to occur, but for others there may be active efforts to stem it. Cognitively, individuals with low desire may report no sexual fantasies or other pleasant, arousing sexual cognition. Emotionally, they may describe themselves as not feeling "sexy" or sexual. In this context, disruption in the frequency, focus, intensity, or duration of sexual activity is probable, and secondary disruption of subsequent sexual responses may occur.

Problems with sexual desire disorder must be distinguished from sexual aversion disorder. The latter is usually defined as persistent or recurrent aversion to, or avoidance of, all or almost all, genital contact with a sexual partner. The behavioral reference of complete (or almost complete) absence of genital contact presumably signifies that all sexual activity and latter stages of the sexual response cycle are circumvented. Aside from specific genital avoidance, there may be wide variation, with some individuals preceding up to the point of genital exposure during sex but others avoidant of any situation construed as "sexual." Kaplan describes cases of men or women who have been asexual all of their adult life.[15] One etiologic basis for such extreme responses may be early traumatic sexual experiences (eg, incest, rape, forced participation in pornographic activities) which, unfortunately, were the individual's introduction to sexuality. Because of the commonality of anxiety (with resultant avoidance) as a contributor to many sexual dysfunctions, the diagnostician must decide when it is of sufficient magnitude to merit the designation of aversion disorder as opposed to being a contributor to other sexual dysfunctions.

Sexual Excitement/Arousal

The sexual excitement phase of the response cycle presumably begins with physical or psychologic sexual stimulation. The general physiologic responses are widespread vasocongestion, either superficial or deep, and myotonia, with either voluntary or involuntary muscle contractions. Other changes include heart rate and blood pressure increases and respiration becoming deeper and more rapid. For women, sexual excitement is also characterized by the appearance of vaginal lubrication, produced by vasocongestion in the vaginal walls leading to transudation of fluid. Other changes include a slight enlargement of the clitoris and uterus with engorgement. The uterus also rises in position with the vagina expanding and ballooning out. Maximal vasocongestion of the vagina produces a congested orgasmic platform in the lower one-third of the vaginal barrel. For men, the obvious physiologic response is penile erection. In addition, vasocongestion of the scrotum produces a smoothing out of skin ridges on the scrotal sac, and the testes are partially elevated toward the perineum due to the shortening of the spermatic cords. Psychologic descriptions of sexual arousal may yield reports of the individual's awareness of the physiologic sensations (eg, vaginal lubrication, pelvic warmth or "heaviness" for women and erection for men) and self reports of feeling excited.

Among healthy men, erectile disorder is diagnosed using one of two criteria. Either there is disruption of a predominant physiologic response—partial or complete failure in attaining or maintaining an erection—such that sexual activity is disrupted, or there is a lack of subjective feelings of sexual excitement and pleasure during sexual activity. These difficulties are usually recurrent. Historically, anxiety has been the hypothesized mechanism for arousal deficits. Dysfunctional attentional processes and negative affects have been the core of psychologic theories. Masters and Johnson[16] proposed both "spectatoring" as a distracting process (ie, the individual "watches" for his sexual response with a negative expectation that, for example, erection will be inadequate) and anxiety about performance (erectile) failure as the specific problem. Another model has been provided by Barlow,[17] and Beck,[18] which emphasizes the physiologic, cognitive, and emotional dysfunctions which lead to erectile failure. Supporting data indicate that men with erection difficulties underreport their levels of sexual arousal (relative to the magnitude of actual erectile response) if queried,[19] focus their attention on nonerotic rather than erotic cues,[20] and report negative (depressed) feelings[20] and a lack of control over their sexual responses.[21] This dysfunctional process is reiterated and "improved" on (ie, the individual becomes proficient at focusing on the wrong aspects of the sexual context—the consequences of not performing—with the continuation of erectile insufficiency), and avoids sexual contexts in the future.

Prior to the use of female arousal disorder as a diagnostic label, the majority of female sexual dysfunctions—particularly those appearing to have some impairment of sexual excitement—were classified under the generic label of frigidity and may have included women with difficulty with one or more phases of the sexual response cycle and/or accompanying negative affects, such as anxiety or aversion. Today, many see the diagnostic criteria for female arousal disorder as parallel to the criteria for male erectile dysfunction. That is, either there is disruption of a predominant physiologic response—lubrication-swelling of the genitals—until the "completion of sexual activity," or there is a lack of subjective feelings of sexual excitement and pleasure during sexual activity.

In contrast to the vast literature on sexual arousal among men, the literature on women is smaller and less focused on physiologic impairments to arousal. Studies have, however, addressed the physiologic, affective, and cognitive aspects of arousal. Data on the correspondence between physiologic measures and women's subjective reports of arousal, however, have been mixed,[22] which indicates that clinical presentations of a woman's reporting satisfactory physiologic response but without feelings of sexual arousal would not be uncommon. Also, such data raise issue with the advisability of relying only on verbal reports of lubrication or swelling when making diagnostic decisions about the presence of arousal deficits. The conceptual models discussed above for male arousal deficits have been applied to women, although with a less satisfactory fit. Nonpsychologic etiologic hypotheses for low arousal in women include postmenopausal changes (ie, concomitant of estrogen deprivation), and disruptive chronic conditions such as diabetes or cancer.

Orgasm

Masters and Johnson[23] proposed that orgasm is a reflex-like response that occurs once a plateau of excitement has been reached. The physiologic and behavioral indices of orgasm involve the whole body—facial grimaces, generalized myotonia of the muscles, carpopedal spasms, and contractions of the gluteal and abdominal muscles. For women, orgasm is also marked by rhythmic contractions of the uterus, the orgasmic platform, and the rectal sphincter. Men may perceive orgasm as a process consisting of two stages, emission and ejaculation. In the first, there is a sense of ejaculatory inevitability. The lag between these sensations and the second stage, ejaculation, is the result of contraction in the epididymis, vas deferentia, seminal vesicles, and prostate, which deposits the semen into the posterior urethra. At this same time the internal sphincter of the neck of the urinary bladder is closed. If it remains open (as with nerve damage), the ejaculate spills into the bladder (ie, retrograde ejaculation); the sensation of orgasm would continue although ejaculation is "dry." Attention is usually focused on these sensations (concentrated on sensations in the clitoris, vagina, and uterus for women and the penis, prostate, and seminal vesicles for men), and awareness of competing environmental stimuli is lessened. The subjective experience includes feelings of intense pleasure with a peaking and rapid, exhilarating release, regardless of the manner in which orgasm is achieved.[24]

Inhibited female orgasm has been defined as delayed or absent orgasm following an unimpaired sexual excitement phase which is "adequate in focus, intensity, and duration." Clinically, orgasmic dysfunction takes one of two forms. Some women have never experienced orgasm under any circumstances (the possible exception might be an occasional orgasm during sleep with erotic dreams). It is estimated that 5% to 10% of women have not experienced orgasm, with the percentages declining across the adult decades.[25-27] The latter finding has been interpreted to reflect the instrumental role of the accrual of sexual experience, per se, in facilitating a woman's orgasmic responsiveness. Other women are orgasmic but infrequently so or not in preferred circumstances (eg, orgasm does not occur with coitus). Many women, perhaps the majority, are not orgasmic during intercourse, and this is a normal sexual response pattern. Other clinical scenarios (eg, a woman becoming nonorgasmic after being so) are rare.

The parallel orgasmic dysfunction for men is inhibited male orgasm. As with women, the diagnosis presumes a normal excitement phase and sexual circumstances that are adequate in focus, intensity, and duration. Unlike the criteria for women, the diagnosis is usually restricted to orgasm failure with a woman during intercourse. The factors resulting in responsiveness in particular situations (eg, delayed ejaculation with a female partner but not with masturbation) are not elaborated. This is the least common dysfunction for men, perhaps only accounting for 3% to 8% of the men seeking treatment.[28] Delayed ejaculation is not unique to heterosexual couples. Delayed (or "retarded") ejaculation can occur in homosexual men as well.[29] Clinically, men may also have other sexual difficulties, such as low desire and/or arousal deficits. As with women, drugs such as tricyclics and MAO inhibitors will suppress ejaculation.[30]

A second orgasmic dysfunction found in men is premature ejaculation. A "premature" ejaculation is thought to be one occurring with minimal stimulation or before, upon, or shortly after penetration and before the man wishes it. Clinically, men may feel that they have no control over the timing of their ejaculations. This scenario is a common complaint of men seeking treatment, perhaps accounting for 20% to 40% of all cases.[28] Although data are not available, it is more likely that younger men (under 50 years of age) rather than older (over 50 years of age) will seek treatment since older men are aware that aging slows the ejaculation response.

Resolution

After orgasm and during the resolution phase, the anatomic and physiologic changes of excitement reverse. In women, vasocongestion diminishes, and the vagina shortens and narrows. In men, erection diminishes markedly. A filmy sheet of perspiration covers the body and the elevated heart rate and respiration from orgasm gradually return to normal. There are concomitant psychologic sensations of bodily relaxation and feelings of release and sexual contentment/satisfaction. If orgasm has not occurred, the same physiologic processes occur more slowly, and the psychologic responses are usually either neutral or negative (eg, continued sexual tension, disappointment at having not experienced orgasm).

Other Sexual Responses and Difficulties

Vaginismus is thought to be a relatively rare condition affecting women. The diagnostic term refers to a recurrent or persistent involuntary spasm of the lower portion of the vagina sufficient to interfere with intercourse. With the spasm, localized pain usually occurs. A confirming diagnosis is ordinarily made via a pelvic examination when the spasm can be visually or manually detected. The simplicity of the criteria belies the heterogeneity that can be found in clinical groups.[31] The spasm may occur not only during intercourse, but in other contexts, ranging from a woman inserting her own finger or a tampon into the vagina to a pelvic examination by a gynecologist. Vaginismus can also occur from imagined or anticipated penetration. Since the condition is generally disruptive to coitus, a woman seeking treatment may never have had intercourse, even if married. Alternatively, she may have a lengthy history of "managing" the problem more or less successfully. Some women desire sex and may be aroused by sexual activities that do not include penetration, while others report global disinterest, nonresponsiveness, and avoidance.

For women, it is important to rule out vaginismus as a cause of dyspareunia, which is defined for both men and women as recurrent or persistent *genital* (emphases added) pain occurring before, during, or after sexual intercourse. In addition to ruling out vaginismus, lack of lubrication may cause pain because vaginal dryness commonly produces friction and discomfort. There has been relatively little study of dyspareunia, and even fewer discussions or data from male samples. An exception is the Wabreks' essay[32] on the most common physical precipitant. They note that hypotheses for the pain can be narrowed by carefully questioning the patient about the location and timing of the pain as well as the sexual response cycle phase or sexual techniques that modulate the pain. Once physical factors are ruled out via clinical interview, medical history, and gynecologic or urologic physical examination, psychologic hypotheses are more viable.

Sexual Morbidity in Cancer Patients

Overview

There are many similarities between the sexual problems of healthy individuals and those with cancer, but we will highlight some obvious differences. First, the sexual problems of cancer patients typically have an acute onset, appearing immediately after treatment. Prior to their diagnosis, most cancer patients have had satisfactory sexual adjustment. The usual clinical pattern for the appearance of sexual problems following cancer treatment is that they begin as soon as intercourse is resumed. This suddenness and, for some, severity of difficulty is distressing. Further, if individuals have not been forewarned by their health care providers about the likelihood or nature of the problems, the distress may be heightened.

Second, sexual difficulties for cancer patients are usually pervasive, with major alterations in the frequency or range of sexual behavior and disruption of more than one phase of the sexual response cycle. Because of this, some patients may be concerned about maintaining *any* sexual activity. In contrast, the sexual difficulties of healthy individuals are more likely to be circumscribed, such as being most severe for one phase (eg, orgasmic disruption) with little or no impairment of the other phases.

Third, maintaining one's sexual self-esteem or sexual activity may be difficult because of other diseases or treatment side effects that are, in themselves, difficult to control. Fatigue or low energy and pain are two such disruptors. After treatment, many cancer patients report residual and activity-disrupting fatigue,[33] which may, in turn, lead to lowered sexual desire. Also, genital pain or other pains are deterrents to sexual desire and arousal during sexual activity.

Fourth, data suggest that the response cycle disruptions for cancer patients differ from those of healthy individuals. Disruption of sexual desire may be a primary problem, but more typically the loss is concomitant with arousal deficits. Also, many cancer patients maintain their sexual desire, and some even continue sexual relations when there are significant deterrents, such as dyspareunia.[34] This latter scenario underscores the importance of maintaining one's sexual life despite cancer. For cancer patients, difficulty with sexual excitement, both in terms of bodily response (erection or lubrication) and subjective feelings of arousal, is a common problem. Orgasmic dysfunction is common, either because of lowered excitement or specific impairment, and the difficulty is usually pervasive rather than situational, as is often the case for healthy individuals. For example, a woman who was orgasmic during intercourse prior to treatment for cervical cancer discovers that she is nonorgasmic, and, further, feels insufficiently aroused to even approach orgasm. Similarly, men with prostate cancer who are treated surgically may be unable to achieve erection. Problematic resolution responses among cancer patients are varied. Those who experience pain during intercourse often have residual discomfort. Those without pain but who have disruptions of desire, excitement, or orgasm may feel sexual tension, disappointment, or fear their sexual responsiveness is permanently changed.

Finally, the prognosis for sexual problems among healthy individuals is positive, whereas the sexual problems of cancer patients are likely to be difficult to treat and, perhaps, refractory. Prevention through provision of the least disruptive, but comparably curative treatment is the single most important strategy. For example, research has demonstrated that breast-saving treatments, as opposed to radical surgeries, result in significantly better psychologic and sexual adjustment. Similar findings are emerging for treatment of in situ vulvar disease, prostate cancer, and disease at other sites. Interventions to reduce the incidence and severity of problems would be most effective if delivered during the diagnostic, treatment, and early post-treatment periods. Interventions would have to be tailored to specific disease and treatment effects, and accurate and detailed explanations of the anticipated sexual disruptions would be central. This would enable patients to anticipate difficulties, and further information might provide specific strategies for managing their problems.

In the sections to follow we provide a site-specific review of sexual outcomes. To summarize the incidence and types of sexual problems, Tables 40-1 for men and 40-2 for women provide estimates of behavioral and sexual response cycle disruptions. These data are composites of the available studies. The methodology rating in each table categorizes the types and number of studies that contributed to the estimate. As can be seen, the majority of the research consists of retrospective studies of limited patient samples. The notable exception is the literature for women with breast or gynecologic cancer.

Breast Cancer

The most well-studied cancer patient group is that of women with breast cancer. Much of the early research was conducted with women who received modified radical mastectomy or, in some cases, radical mastectomy. The strongest data come from controlled longitudinal studies. In these studies, 30% to 40% reported significant sexual problems (eg, loss of desire, reduced frequency of intercourse, or reduction in excitement) 1 to 2 years posttreatment compared with 10% of women with benign disease receiving diagnostic biopsy.[35,36] Body image, a difficult concept to measure, was also significantly disrupted.

The most recent studies have come from clinical trials in which psychologic or behavioral endpoints have been examined along with disease endpoints in the comparison of modified radical mastectomy vs lumpectomy and radiotherapy. With few exceptions,[37] studies have reported a benefit with the less disfiguring treatment for women studied in the United States, England, the Netherlands, and Denmark.[38-40] For the lumpectomy patients, such differences include less alteration in body image and greater comfort with nudity and in discussing sexuality with one's partner, fewer changes in the frequency of intercourse, and a lower incidence of sexual dysfunction. In sum, quality of life data on sexual functioning supports improved outcome for lesser surgical therapies.

Colon and Rectum

Consistently better sexual outcomes are reported for those patients receiving an anterior resection rather than abdominoperineal resection (APR) of the rectum. For men, estimates of sexual dysfunction are less than 50% for anterior resection but significantly more than 50% (approaching 90% to 100%) for APR.[41-47] These differences may be due to the effects of greater denervation of the sympathetic nerves with APR as well as adjustment to having an abdominal stoma. These data are also consistent with other data that suggest a more difficult adjustment in general following APR.[47] Estimates for women come from much smaller samples, but, in general, they usually report more positive outcomes than for men regardless ot the surgical approach. One inves-

Table 40-1. Sexual Morbidity Estimates for Men

Site	Subgroup	Method Rating*	Area of Sexual Functioning Difficulty			
			No Sexual Activity (%)	Desire (%)	Excitement (%)	Orgasm (%)
Colon-rectum						
	Anterior resection	3	10-30	30-60	10-30	10-30
	Abdominoperineal resection	3	60-100	30-60	50-90	70-100
Bladder		3	30-50	30-70	50-90	25-35
Prostate						
	(A) Retropubic	3			85	78
	(B) Perineal	3			88	100
	A or B with hormonal therapy	3			100	100
	Radiotherapy	3			37	
	Interstitial therapy with lymphadenectomy	4			15-25	30
Testicular						
	Seminoma:					
	Orch + RT	4		12	15	10
	Nonseminoma:					
	Orch + RL ± chemo	4		15-20	5-15	20-40
	Orch + RL + RT ± chemo	4		50	24	55
Hodgkin's disease		2			20-30	

*Methodology rating scale for prior empirical literature: 1 = Randomized trials; 2 = Single group longitudinal investigations ± control(s); 3 = More than 3 retrospective studies; 4 = Only 1-2 retrospective studies.

Legend: Orch = orchiectomy; RT = radiation therapy; RL = retroperitoneal lymphadenectomy; chemo = chemotherapy.

tigation reported that 28% of the women had reduced desire, and 21% had dyspareunia.[43]

Bladder

Superficial bladder tumors are treated by transurethral resection and fulguration, which may result in minimal sexual disruption; however, documenting data are not available. Men and women undergoing repeated cystoscopies have been noted to report reduced sexual desire and may have pain with intercourse due to urethral irritation.[48]

Since the average bladder cancer patient is in his or her late 60s, lower frequencies of sexual activity and frequent lapses in functioning (eg, erectile failure) would be expected. Treatment for invasive bladder cancer has historically consisted of radical cystectomy with urinary diversion via an external conduit with ileal stoma. Twenty-six percent of the men studied by Bergman et al[49] and 50% of the men studied by Schover et al[50] reported stopping all sexual activity postoperatively. Of those attempting to remain sexually active, inadequately rigid or only brief erections occurred in almost all men (90%). Orgasm, if experienced, is reported by approximately one half of the patients as less intense and without ejaculate. Outcomes such as these have intensified efforts to modify surgical procedures and lower morbidity.

The sexual outcomes for women with bladder cancer have not been well studied. In many respects, they are similar to women with gynecologic cancer receiving an anterior pelvic exenteration in which the vagina is narrowed instead of removed. Schover and von Eschenbach[51] reported that approximately 25% of women cease sexual activity. Those continuing with activity report few sexual dysfunctions with the exception of dyspareunia, which was reported by 75% of the sexually active sample. Vaginal tightness and lack of lubrication appear to be the primary causes of the dyspareunia.

The recent steps which have been taken to improve sexual outcomes have included nerve-sparing cystoprostatectomy with urethrectomy, continent diver-

Table 40-2. Sexual Morbidity Estimates for Women

Site	Subgroup	Method Rating*	Area of Sexual Functioning Difficulty				
			No Sexual Activity (%)	Desire (%)	Excitement(%)	Orgasm (%)	Dyspareunia (%)
Breast							
	Modified radical mastectomy	2			30-40		
	Lumpectomy + RT +/– chemo	1			15-25		
Colon-rectum							
	Anterior resection	3		10-30		30-60	
	10-30			10-30			
	Abdominoperineal resection	3		60-100		30-60	
	50-90			70-100			
Bladder		4	25	10	0	0	75
Cervix, endometrial		2	15	30-50	25-50	25-40	30-50
	Surgery	2		30-40	25-35	25	30
	RT	2		30-50	35-45	35	40-60
	Surgery + RT	2		40-50	40-60	40	40-60
Vulva							
	In situ	4	33	15	36	28	8
	Invasive: vulvectomy	3	50	15	40	30	20
Hodgkin's disease		2	20	32			

*Methodology rating scale for prior empirical literature: 1 = Randomized trials; 2 = Single group longitudinal investigations ± control(s); 3 = More than 3 retrospective studies; 4 = Only 1-2 retrospective studies.

Legend: RT = radiation therapy; chemo = chemotherapy.

sions, and penile prosthesis surgery. Forty percent of men capable of erections prior to surgery retained their functioning with continent diversions to reduce urinary incontinence and obtain satisfactory voiding. Steven et al[52] modified the surgical procedure by leaving the apical prostatic capsule, making it possible to create an internal urinary diversion. Of the eight sexually active patients studied, erectile capacity was preserved in four, with three of these able to continue intercourse. Other authors have described related surgical procedures with intraabdominal reservoirs for urinary diversions that patients can empty with self-catheterization. Marshall et al[53] reported on 25 patients who underwent total neobladder reconstruction with the majority having urethral anastomosis. Sexual functioning was preserved in 71% of the patients. Mansson et al[54] compared two patient groups, one receiving the standard conduit diversion and the other with reservoir. Both groups had substantial sexual difficulties; however, the reservoir group had better overall adjustment. The latter finding was attributed to the absence of odor, leakage, and embarrassment, common problems for patients with urinary conduits. Boyd and Schiff[55] have reported 19 patients with diffuse transitional cell carcinoma who had undergone cystoprostatectomy with urethrectomy and had been implanted with inflatable penile prostheses. Sexual functioning was satisfactory with acceptable function and appearance for those in whom the glandular urethra could remain intact. When total urethrectomy was necessary, the glans penis would collapse, causing difficulties with orgasm and appearance. This again documents the improved outcomes following less radical procedures, aggressive reconstructive efforts, or both.

Male Genitalia

Prostate

Prostate treatments produce substantial sexual changes, but even the diagnostic biopsy may result in sexual difficulties. For example, approximately 24% of open perineal biopsy[56,57] and 32% of transurethral resection[58-61] patients report erectile failure. In addition, approximately 57% of the patients report a complete loss, or at least a reduced amount, of seminal fluid ejaculated.

The effect that radical prostatectomy has on sexual functioning varies depending upon several factors. These include preoperative potency, neurovascular bundle preservation, age, and clinical stage. Brendler and Walsh reported 69% preservation of potency in men who were preoperatively potent.[62] Furthermore, preservation of both neurovascular bundles was associated with 76% potency as compared with 60% of those who had only one neurovascular bundle preserved.[62] Patient age and recovery of sexual function has also been shown to be significantly correlated. Ninety one percent of men younger than age 50 recovered potency as compared with only 25% of men over age 50.[62] Advancing clinical stage is directly correlated with decreasing potency. This is directly related to both the extent of the tumor and the scope of the surgical procedure, which often entails the excision of one or both neurovascular bundles.[62] If hormone therapy and/or orchiectomy are included, virtually all the patients experience erectile failure and ejaculation difficulty.[63]

Some patients with local disease opt for supervoltage irradiation, which is also used for patients with regional disease. When patients with either limited or extracapsular extension have been treated with definitive courses, approximately 25% experience significant erectile difficulties.[64] Another treatment has been interstitial implantation (usually with a retropubic approach) of the prostate with iodine 125 (^{125}I) or gold (^{198}Au) combined with pelvic lymphadenectomy. The lowest estimates of sexual difficulties have been found with these treatments, with erectile difficulties in the range of 15% to 25% and the retrograde ejaculation in the range of 30%.[65-67]

Patients with metastatic disease or extensive regional spread are treated with regimens such as bilateral orchiectomy, estrogen administration, or both. The majority of patients who receive estrogen develop gynecomastia (the excessive development of male mammary glands), a troubling side effect. Ellis and Grayheck[68] estimated that erectile difficulties occur for 47% of the patients who receive orchiectomy alone, 22% for estrogen alone, and 73% for malaise, weight loss, anemia, and pain that patients with metastatic cancer experience.

Testis

This cancer accounts for only 0.5% of cancer in males, but it is the most common site for disease among those aged 15 to 35 years. There has been a surge of studies of the sexual and fertility outcomes for these men, perhaps for two reasons: (1) improvements in cure rates, particularly for disseminated tumors, have been achieved with chemotherapy, and (2) the disease strikes men in the prime of their procreating and sexual-functioning years. Thus, fertility status and sexuality are a major concern.

Testicular cancer is classified either as pure seminoma (accounting for roughly 40% of the cases) or as nonseminoma. Treatment for each differs, and each results in a different sexual outcome. Pure seminoma is radiosensitive, so the standard treatment consists of radical orchiectomy of the testicle (disease in both testicles is rare), followed by nodal irradiation. Chemotherapy is used for cases that fail to respond. Nonseminomas are treated with radical orchiectomy followed by chemotherapy. Retroperitoneal lymphadenectomy (RL) may be done between orchiectomy and chemotherapy. Since data indicate that RL has a significant negative impact on sexual functioning and fertility (due to permanent difficulty with ejaculation), clarification of the medical indications for RL is important. Only studies providing histopathology and treatment information will be reviewed because of their importance in predicting outcome.

Schover et al[69] provided a retrospective report on the sexual outcomes for 84 men who received orchiectomy and radiotherapy for seminoma. In terms of sexual behavior, 19% of the sample reported none or only low rates of sexual activity (ie, one episode of sexual activity less than once per month). In terms of disruption of the sexual response cycle, 12% of the sample reported low desire, 15% reported erectile dysfunction, and 10% reported difficulty with orgasm (particularly lowered intensity). These estimates are unexpected, since the mean age of this sample was 45 years. However, 45% of the sample also reported reduced semen volume, which has been hypothesized to occur from radiation scatter to the prostate and seminal vesicles. Correlational analyses suggested that higher radiation dosages to the periaortic field was predictive of greater erectile and orgasmic difficulties.

Three retrospective studies have provided data for nonseminoma patients: Bracken and Johnson,[70] Nijman et al,[71] and Schover and von Eschenbach.[72] In these studies, all patients received orchiectomy and RL, with or without other therapies. Reduced ejaculate volume (none in most cases) occurred in 90% to 100% of the men across studies and therapies. These data in combination with those for seminoma patients point to the instrumental role of RL in reducing or eliminating semen outflow. Sexual outcomes for patients receiving orchiectomy and retroperitoneal lymphadenectomy, with or without chemotherapy, appear similar. Sex life is affected by treatment for testicular cancer but major permanent sexual dysfunction is not common.[73] In a recent study by Aass and colleagues, 18% of men treated for testicular cancer stated that their sexual life was inferior to the pretreatment experience.[64] Dry ejaculation represents the principal sequelae after retroperitoneal surgery. The frequency of this side effect can be reduced by nerve sparing surgery. Donohue and colleagues reported that, now that nerve sparing techniques have been developed, the only long-term morbidity of retroperitoneal lymph node dissection—anejaculation—has been avoided.[74]

Penis

When the disease is confined to the organ, total penectomy leaves patients significantly impaired; however, stimulation of the remaining genital tissue, including the mons pubis, the perineum, and the scrotum, can produce orgasm for some.[75] Ejaculation can occur through the perineal urethrostomy, and the accompanying sensations of the bulbocavernosus and ischiocavernosus musculature. Patients with partial excisions can remain capable of erection, orgasm, and ejaculation.[70]

Female Genitalia

Cervix, Endometrium, and Ovary

Clinical studies have noted that signs and symptoms such as postcoital bleeding or pelvic pain may alert a woman to her gynecologic disease and need for medical care. The sexually disruptive effects of these early signs were reported by Andersen et al.[76] Forty-one women recently diagnosed with early stage cervical or endometrial cancer and a matched group of healthy women in no gynecologic distress were studied. Analyses indicated that prior to the onset of cancer signs and symptoms the gynecologic cancer patients reported similar patterns of sexual activity and responsiveness as the healthy sample. With the appearance of disease signs and symptoms (ie, fatigue, postcoital bleeding, vaginal discharge, pain), the women who would subsequently receive a cancer diagnosis reported four- to fivefold increases in the frequency of sexual dysfunctions. Since 75% of the women with cancer experienced a substantial change in sexual functioning, it is likely these problems influenced the women to seek medical consultation.

There have been many retrospective studies; however, the majority have been studies of patients with cervical cancer with the major focus on treatment alternatives of radical hysterectomy, radiotherapy, or combination treatment for those with early stage disease. The widespread belief that radiotherapy is the most disruptive treatment comes from the findings of poorly controlled studies. The only experiment to be conducted was that of Vincent et al in 1975.[77] Fifty women with early stage cervical disease were randomly assigned to receive either radical hysterectomy or radiotherapy. Analyses indicated that the changes in sexual desire and activity from pretreatment to 6 months posttreatment were comparable: estimates of diminished desire were obtained from 24% of the radiation therapy and 20% of the surgical patients. Decreased frequency of intercourse was reported by 29% of the radiation and 33% of the surgical patients. This experiment provided convincing evidence that, in general, the rates of sexual behavior disruption and dysfunction are comparable for the two major treatment options.

Other controlled longitudinal research by Andersen et al[34] has examined the nature and timing of sexual difficulties for women with early stage disease. Women with stage I or II cervical or endometrial disease were assessed prior to treatment and at 4-, 8-, and 12-months posttreatment. Their sexual outcomes were compared with data from two matched comparison groups—women diagnosed and treated for benign disease (eg, uterine fibroid treated with simple hysterectomy) and healthy women. Analyses indicated that the primary sexual behavior disrupted by the disease and treatment process for women with malignant or benign disease was the frequency of intercourse, declining from an average of 9.5 occasions per month to 6 to 7 occasions per month during the posttreatment period. The absence of change on other sexual behavior variables (eg, range of current sexual activities) other than intercourse would appear to indicate that disruption of the couples' behavioral repertoire during sexual activity did not occur. That is, when couples engaged in intercourse, albeit less often, the women reported having participated in the same sexual activities (eg, body caressing, oral-genital stimulation). It is important to note that there were no significant differences between groups in the percentage of women becoming sexually inactive, with the estimates ranging from 5% to 15% of all the assessments. The difficulty with sexual excitement for both disease groups was substantial. Following treatment, women with disease reported having fewer signs of sexual excitement and lower arousability for sexual activities with their partner. Both the evaluators and the women felt that significant arousal problems were experienced. As noted above, a likely reason for the arousal deficits was the occurrence of disruptors (eg, dyspareunia, due in part to radiation effects and/or induced menopause).

Vulva

This cancer typically occurs late in life; the average age of onset is 65 years. In contrast, the mean age for women with in situ disease is within the third or fourth decade. Despite the morbidity of surgery and other modalities used for treatment of the vulva, attention to the sexual or psychologic outcomes for women is recent, with the first substantive reports not appearing until 1983. Even though older than the "average" patient with cervical or ovary disease, there is no data to suggest that women with vulvar cancer will be less distressed by their genital distortion or sexual dysfunction.

In 1979 DiSaia and colleagues[78] provided encouraging observations for the beneficial impact on quality of life of the less radical surgical techniques for microinvasive disease. DiSaia contrasted the reports of sexual functioning of two women treated with radical vulvectomy versus 18 women treated with wide local excision. Not surprisingly, the reports of sexual functioning from the two samples showed that the excision patients reported experiencing orgasms and other sexual responses, whereas the radical vulvectomy patients became nonorgasmic. Since then, individualized (and, consequently, more conservative) approaches for treatment of the vulva have been advocated and evaluated.[79]

Andersen and Broffitt[6] have provided data on women treated with wide local excision and related treatments for in situ disease compared with a matched sample of gynecologically healthy women. Overall, it appears that in situ patients as a group are more likely to be sexually inactive at follow up, whether or not they have available sexual partners, than age-matched healthy counterparts. However, if the women have a sexual relationship, the rates of sexual dysfunction appear only slightly higher than those for healthy women. Additional analyses contrasting treatment methods (eg, surgery vs laser vs combined treatment) found no significant differences.

These outcomes contrast markedly with those for women with invasive disease. Prior to the adoption of lesser surgeries, many women were treated with radical or modified radical vulvectomy, with or without groin dissection. While these reports are limited by their small sample sizes (ranging from 9 to 25) and retrospective evaluations, the general trend of the data was consistent: at least 30% to 50% of patients become sexually inactive, and of the women remaining active, 60% to 70% have multiple sexual dysfunctions. For the women who become sexually inactive, many factors may be contributory. For some this is due to negative feelings (by the woman or her partner) about the physical changes of the body, and for others it may be due to severe dyspareunia, such as may occur with a narrowed introitus. When queried, the majority of women would have preferred to remain sexually active.[80]

Hodgkin's Disease

In the past few years the survival rate for this disease has dramatically improved; for example, five-year survival was 40% in 1960 compared to 79% in 1983-89.[81] (See Chapter 28.) This change has resulted from the use of complex chemotherapy protocols and extended field radiation. Unfortunately, infertility and sexual morbidity with these therapies is high. As long-term follow up data accumulate, other therapies with lesser morbidity may be found.

General survey[82] and interview and questionnaire assessments[83] indicate that decreased energy and interest in sexual activity, with resultant lowered activity levels, may be problems for at least 25% of men and women. Similar rates (32%) in loss of desire have also been reported for combined samples of Hodgkin's disease patients and non-Hodgkin's lymphoma patients.[33] Specific sexual dysfunctions (eg, erectile failure) have not been reported, but with treatment-induced ovarian failure, reports of dyspareunia would not be unexpected. Correlates of sexual disruption include continued low energy and depression. There is also data to suggest that Hodgkin's disease patients may be at greater risk for marital disruption, possibly due to the extended strain on families during the lengthy treatment period and the difficulties with impaired fertility.[82]

Data suggest that current treatment regimens result in permanent infertility for most patients. Hormonal studies of male Hodgkin's patients 12 months to 12 years after completion of combination chemotherapy with MOPP or MVPP have found azoospermia; testicular biopsies indicated complete loss of the germinal epithelium. Less than 10% of these patients achieve sperm densities of minimum range.[84,85] However, approximately one third of patients with advanced Hodgkin's disease have been found to manifest gonadal dysfunction prior to therapy.[86] For women, parallel decrements have been reported. With radiation only, a dose-response relationship appears to interact with age, such that younger women generally require a higher dose to produce permanent amenorrhea. In a study of 41 women with advanced Hodgkin's disease receiving MVPP (21 of whom also received MVPP as a maintenance therapy or had other agents because of relapse), Chapman et al[87,88] reported that only 17% of the women had functioning ovaries at a mean of 3 years after completing therapy. Also, ovarian failure (as reflected by amenorrhea) occurred after fewer cycles of therapy in older women. Hodgkin's disease per se does not appear to impair ovarian functioning: 27% of the women in the latter study conceived in the presence of active disease. In contrast to these data, a report on a trial of radiation therapy and TVVPP (thiotepa, vinblastine, vincristine, procarbazine, and prednisone) for 34 women that followed the women for a mean of 7 years has reported that 100% of the women less than 35 years at treatment and 50% of the women over 35 years continued to menstruate. One third of the sample subsequently became pregnant.[89]

One strategy designed to reduce or prevent gonadal toxicity stems from the research findings that prepubertal gonads are relatively more resistant to damage than pubertal or mature gonads. This resistance is most likely due to their inactive state. Hormonal manipulation geared towards suppressing gonadal activity during cytotoxic chemotherapy is currently being researched.

The prevention of testicular damage during cancer therapy is being investigated by the suppression of spermatogenesis. This suppression is achieved by using hypothalamic-releasing factors, specifically gonadotropin-releasing hormone (Gn-RH) antagonists.[90] Similarly for women, research is now being focused on decreasing the gonadal stimulation of the ovaries during cancer therapy to reduce or prevent ovarian failure. This is achieved by the use of oral estrogens, which produce negative feedback to the hypothalamic-pituitary axis, resulting in ovarian suppression.[86] The efficacy of gonadal suppression to reduce or prevent gonadal damage during chemotherapy remains unclear, since this research is still in the early phases.

Brief Assessment of Sexual Functioning

For cancer patients, the diagnostic period is a crisis.[91] Despite this, patients must process complex information and instructions as they undergo diagnostic studies and learn of treatment possibilities. Survival is a central concern. As this issue is clarified, concerns regarding impending treatments and their short- and long-term effects become paramount. This is the context in which assessment of the patient's previous sexual functioning and explanation of the sexual morbidity from the disease and treatment(s) becomes important. Assessment of a patient's predisease sexual functioning will: (1) enable the health care provider to individualize the explanation of the anticipated sexual difficulties for each patient (eg, disruption in fertility may be important to a heterosexual male but not to a homosexual male), (2) provide important baseline information for understanding any posttreatment sexual problems, and (3) establish a context and precedent for patients to voice their sexual concerns. Finally, a brief assessment and information about probable sexual difficulties will prevent many sexual problems that may occur from lack of information or confusion.

Table 40-3 provides a brief assessment model designed to assess both important sexual behaviors (eg, intercourse) and the sexual response cycle. The acronym ALARM used in this table refers to the assessment of the following: sexual *a*ctivities, *l*ibido/desire, *a*rousal and orgasm, *r*esolution, and any *m*edical history relevant to sexual functioning. Many other relevant areas, such as marital adjustment, are omitted; however, we assume assessment will be individualized within these central areas. Sample questions are provided for illustration. The examples used are for heterosexual individuals, and some modification would be necessary for gay/lesbian individuals.

Two important aspects of conducting a brief assessment like the one suggested here are to understand sexual behavior and sexual functioning in healthy individuals and to have the ability to discuss sexual functioning in a frank, open, and nonjudgmental manner. To the extent that the health care provider is informed, comfortable, and interested in addressing these concerns, cancer patients will begin to feel more hopeful and confident in coping with the sexual difficulties they may face.

A Model for Intervention Planning

Assessment of sexual functioning at the time of diagnosis and treatment planning will provide the context for delivery of treatment-specific information on possible sexual sequelae. It will also be the time to provide early guidance for continuing sexual activity through the treatment process or resuming activity should it be temporarily interrupted. Following treatment, more extensive intervention efforts may be needed. Many significant sexual problems will require referral to an expert in treating sexual dysfunction, but others might be dealt with by more limited efforts by oncology physicians or nurses. Provided below is a commonly used model, Annon's[2] PLISSIT model, for thinking about and planning treatment for the individual patient. The acronym refers to the following:

(P) Permission: The cancer patient is given *permission* to be sexual when undergoing or recovering from treatment or when living with the disease. Specifically, the health professional communicates acceptance and encouragement to voice sexual concerns related to the patient or the partner. For example, the professional could indicate that many people may lose their sexual desire when they are feeling ill, tired, or distressed from the cancer experience. Further, it is acceptable and potentially useful to share feelings of this sort with others, such as a member of the healthcare team or the partner.

(LI) Limited information: The cancer patient is provided with factual *information* about the effects of the disease and treatment on sexuality and fertility. In addition, basic information about sexuality may be necessary. Common areas of concern may be the capacity for continued performance (eg, full erections, ejaculation, orgasm), fertility or possible interferences, such as pain.

(SS) Specific suggestions: The cancer patient is provided with *specific strategies* for managing their sexual activity. Examples include setting the context for sex so that it is optimal for comfort and arousal (eg, choosing times when

Table 40-3. ALARM Model for the Assessment of Sexual Functioning and Sample Questions

(A) Activity: Frequency of current sexual activities (eg, intercourse, kissing, masturbation).
Example:
1. Prior to the appearance of any sign/symptoms of your illness, how frequently were you engaging in intercourse (specific weekly or monthly estimate)?
2. On occasions other than when having intercourse (or an equivalent intimate activity), do you share other forms of physical affection with your partner, such as kissing, hugging, or both on a daily basis?
3. In the recent past (eg, last 6 months) have you masturbated? If so, estimate how often this has occurred (specific weekly or monthly estimate).

(L) Libido/Desire: Desire for sexual activity and interest in initiating or responding to partner's initiations for sexual activity.
Example:
1. Prior to the appearance of your illness, would you have described yourself as generally interested in having sex?
2. Considering your current regular sexual relationship, who usually initiates sexual activity?
3. You indicated that your current frequency for intercourse is x times per week/month. Would you personally prefer to have intercourse more often, less often, or at the current frequency?

(A) Arousal and Orgasm: Occurrence of erection/lubrication and ejaculation/vaginal contractions, accompanied by feelings of excitement.
Example (for men):
1. When you are interested in having sexual activity, with your partner or alone, do you have any difficulty in achieving an erection? Do you feel emotionally aroused?
2. If there is erectile difficulty: When did this problem start, how often does it occur, are there particular circumstances for its occurrence (eg, with partner only), and what do you understand to be the cause for the difficulty?
3. During sexual activity, either alone or with a partner, do you have any difficulty with ejaculation, such as ejacalating "too soon" or only after an extended period of time?
4. If premature/delayed ejaculation is suggested: While it is difficult to estimate precisely, how long would you estimate that it takes on the average to ejaculate after intensive stimulation begins?

Example (for women):
1. When you are interested in engaging in sexual activity do you notice that your genitals become moist?
2. If post menopausal: Has there been any change in vaginal lubrication during sexual activity since the menopause? Are you currently taking hormonal replacement therapy?
3. If there is arousal deficit: Do you experience any pain with intercourse? How long have you had problems with becoming aroused during sexual activity, and are there particular circumstances during which you have felt more arousal than others?
4. During sexual activity, either alone or with a partner, can you experience a climax or orgasm?
5. If orgasm does not occur: Are you bothered at all by the absence of orgasm?

(R) Resolution: Feelings of release of tension following sexual activity and satisfaction with current sexual life.
Example:
1. Following intercourse or masturbation do you feel that there has been a release of sexual tension?
2. On a scale from 1 (indicating that it could not be worse) to 10 (indicating that it could not be better) how would you rate your current sexual life?
3. Do you have any feelings of discomfort or pain immediately after sexual activity?
4. If there is resolution difficulty: Describe the problems you are having after sexual activity, how long they have occurred, and your understanding of their cause or causes.

(M) Medical history relevant to sexuality: Current age and medical history (eg, Have you had diabetes? hypertension?), psychiatric history (eg, Have you had emotional difficulties in the past for which you have sought treatment?), and substance use history (eg, How much alcohol or drugs do you consume on weekly basis?), what do you drink (eg, beer? wine? alcohol?) which may have caused acute or chronic disruption of sexual activity or responses.

rested, emptying urinary pouches), ways to decrease discomfort or conserve energy (eg, different coital positions), or activities in lieu of intercourse (eg, body massage; masturbation).

(IT) Intensive therapy: Many cancer patients will require referral to *sexual therapy or psychotherapy* to manage sexual dysfunctions, permanent sexual disabilities, distress from the sexual changes, or marital distress. Such problems require mental health professionals experienced in many intervention strategies.

Appropriate members of the oncology team can discuss both the permission concept and the limited information component of the PLISSIT model with every cancer patient. Specific suggestions require expertise, which may or may not be available within the team. These efforts can now be augmented by two ACS patient teaching booklets. These are *Sexuality and Cancer: For the Man Who Has Cancer and His Partner* and *Sexuality and Cancer: For the Woman Who Has Cancer and Her Partner.* Both can be excellent supplements to the oncology team's important efforts to help women and men with cancer cope with changes in their sexual life.

References

1. Andersen BL. Sexual functioning morbidity among cancer survivors: present status and future research directions. *Cancer.* 1985;55:1835-1842.

2. Annon J. *The Behavioral Treatment of Sexual Problems, I.* Honolulu, HI: Kapiolani Health Services; 1974:1.

3. Kinsey AC, Pomeroy WB, Martin CE. *Sexual Behavior in the Human Male.* Philadelphia, Pa: WB Saunders Co; 1948.

4. Kinsey AC, Pomeroy WB, Martin CE, Gebhard PH. *Sexual Behavior in the Human Female.* Philadelphia, Pa: WB Saunders Co; 1953.

5. Fritz GS, Stoll K, Wagner NN. A comparison of males and females who were sexually molested as children. *J Sex Marital Ther.* 1981;7:54-59.

6. Andersen BL, Broffitt B. Is there a reliable and valid self report measure of sexual behavior? *Arch Sex Behav.* 1988; 17:509-525.

7. Bancroft J. Sexual desire and the brain. *Sex Marital Ther.* 1988;3:11-27.

8. O'Carroll R, Shapiro C, Bancroft J. Androgens, behavior, and nocturnal erections in hypogonadal men: the effect of varying the replacement dose. *Clin Endocrinol.* 1985;23:527-538.

9. Walling MK, Andersen BL, Johnson SR. Hormonal replacement therapy for postmenopausal women: sexual outcomes and related gynecologic effects. *Arch Sex Behav.* 1990;119:119-137.

10. Bancroft J, Sanders D, Davidson DW, Warner P. Mood, sexuality, hormones and the menstrual cycle. III: sexuality and the role of androgens. *Br J Psych.* 1983;125:310-315.

11. Schreiner-Engel P, Schiavi RC, Smith H, White D. Plasma testosterone and female sexual behavior. In: Hock Z, Lief HI, eds. *Proceedings of the 5th World Congress of Sexology.* Amsterdam: *Excerpta Medica;* 1982.

12. Leiblum SR, Rosen RC, eds. *Sexual Desire Disorders.* New York, NY: Guilford Press; 1988.

13. Lief HI. Inhibited sexual desire. *Med Asp Hum Sex.* 1977;7:94-95.

14. *Diagnostic and Statistical Manual of Mental Disorders.* (DSM-IV). Washington, DC: American Psychiatric Association; 1994.

15. Kaplan HS. Anxiety and sexual dysfunction. *J Clin Psych.* 1988;49:21-25.

16. Masters WH, Johnson VE. *Human Sexual Inadequacy.* Boston, Mass: Little, Brown; 1970.

17. Barlow DH. Causes of sexual dysfunction: the role of anxiety and cognitive interference. *J Consult Clin Psychol.* 1986;54:140-148.

18. Beck JG. Self-generated distraction in erectile dysfunction: the role of attentional processes. *Adv Behav Res Ther.* 1986;8:205-221.

19. Sakheim DK, Barlow DH, Abramson DJ, Beck JG. Distinguishing between organogenic and psychogenic erectile dysfunction. *Behav Res Ther.* 1987;25:379-390.

20. Abramson DJ, Barlow DH, Beck JG, Sakheim DK, Kelly JP. The effects of attentional focus and partner responsiveness on sexual responding: replication and extension. *Arch Sex Behav.* 1985;14:361-371.

21. Beck JG, Barlow DH, Sakheim DK. Sexual arousal and suppression patterns in functional and dysfunctional men. Presented at the annual convention of the American Psychological Association; August, 1982; Washington, DC.

22. Palace EM, Gorzalka BB. The enhancing effects of anxiety on arousal in sexually dysfunctional and functional women. *J Abnorm Psychol.* 1990;99:403-411.

23. Masters WH, Johnson VE. *Human Sexual Response.* Boston, Mass: Little, Brown; 1966.

24. Newcomb MD, Bentler PM. Dimensions of subjective female orgasmic responsiveness. *J Pers Soc Psychol.* 1983; 44:862-873.

25. Wakefield JC. Sex bias in the diagnosis of primary orgasmic dysfunction. *Am Psychol.* 1987;42:464-471.

26. Wakefield JC. Female primary orgasmic dysfunction: Masters and Johnson versus DSM-IIIR on diagnosis and incidence. *J Sex Research.* 1988;24:363-377.

27. Morokoff PJ. Sex bias and POD. *Am Psychol.* 1989;44: 73-75.

28. Spector IP, Carey MP. Incidence and prevalence of the sexual dysfunctions: a critical review of the empirical literature. *Arch Sex Behav.* 1990;19:389-408.

29. Wilensky M, Myers MF. Retarded ejaculation in homosexual patients: a report of nine cases. *J Sex Research.* 1987;23:85-105.

30. Nininger JE. Inhibition of ejaculation by amitriptyline. *Am J Psych.* 1990;135:750-751.

31. Lamont J. Vaginismus. *Am J Obstet Gynecol.* 1978; 131:632-636.

32. Wabrek AJ, Wabrek CJ. Dyspareunia. *J Sex Marital Ther.* 1975;1:234-241.

33. Devlen J, Maguire P, Phillips P, et al. Psychological problems associated with diagnosis and treatment of lymphomas. II: prospective study. *Br Med J.* 1987;295:955-957.

34. Andersen BL, Anderson B, deProsse C. Controlled prospective longitudinal study of women with cancer. I: sexual functioning outcomes. *J Consult Clin Psychol.* 1989; 57:683-691.

35. Maguire GP, Lee EG, Bevington DJ, et al. Psychiatric problems in the first year after mastectomy. *Br Med J.* 1978;1:963-965.

36. Morris T, Greer HS, White P. Psychological and social adjustment to mastectomy: a two-year follow-up study. *Cancer.* 1977;40:2381-2387.

37. Fallowfield LJ, Baum M, Maguire P. Effects of breast conservation on psychological morbidity associated with diagnosis and treatment of early breast cancer. *Br Med J.* 1986;293:1331-1334.

38. Beckmann J, Johansen L, Richardt C, et al. Psychological reactions in younger women operated on for breast cancer. *Danish Med Bull.* 1983;30:10-13.

39. Kemeny MM, Wellisch DK, Schain WS. Psychosocial outcome in a randomized surgical trial for treatment of primary breast cancer. *Cancer.* 1988;62:1231-1237.

40. Steinberg MD, Juliano MA, Wise L. Psychological outcome of lumpectomy versus mastectomy in the treatment of breast cancer. *Am J Psych.* 1985;142:34-39.

41. Aso R, Yasutami M. Urinary and sexual disturbances following radical surgery for rectal cancer, and pudendal nerve block as a countermeasure for urinary disturbance. *Am J Proctol.* 1974;6:60-70.

42. Bernstein WC, Bernstein EF. Sexual dysfunction following radical surgery for cancer of the rectum. *Dis Colon Rectum.* 1966;9:328-332.

43. Druss RG, O'Connor JF, Prudden JF, et al. Psychologic response to edectomy II. *Arch Gen Psych.* 1969;20:419-427.

44. Hellstrom P. Urinary and sexual dysfunction after rectosigmoid surgery. *Annales Chirurgiae et Gyunaecolgiea.* 1988;77:51-56.

45. Kinn AC, Ohman U. Bladder and sexual function after surgery for rectal cancer. *Dis Colon Rectum.* 1985;29:43-48.

46. Weinstein M, Roberts M. Sexual potency following surgery for rectal carcinoma. *Ann Surg.* 1977;185:295-300.

47. Williams NS, Johnston D. The quality of life after rectal excision for low rectal cancer. *Br J Surg.* 1983;70:460-462.

48. Schover LR, von Eschenbach AC, Smith DB, et al. Sexual rehabilitation of urologic cancer patients: a practical approach. *CA.* 1984;34:3-11.

49. Bergman B, Nilsson S, Petersen I. The effect on erection and orgasm of cystectomy, prostatectomy and vesiculectomy for cancer of the bladder: a clinical and electromyographic study. *Br J Urol.* 1979;51:114-120.

50. Schover LR, Evans R, von Eschenbach AC. Sexual rehabilitation and male radical cystectomy. *J Urol.* 1986; 136:1015-1017.

51. Schover LR, von Eschenbach AC. Sexual function and female radical cystectomy: a case series. *J Urol.* 1985; 134:465-468.

52. Steven K, Klarskov P, Jakobsen H, et al. Transpubic cystectomy and ileocecal bladder replacement after preoperative radiotherapy for bladder cancer. *J Urol.* 1986;135: 470-475.

53. Marshall FF, Mostwin JL, Radebaugh LC, Walsh PC, Brendler CB. Ileocolic neobladder post-cystectomy: continence and potency. *J Urol.* 1991;145:502-504.

54. Mansson A, Johnson G, Mansson W. Quality of life after cystectomy: comparison between patients with conduit and those with caeca reservoir diversion. *Br J Urol.* 1988;62:240-245.

55. Boyd SD, Schiff WM. Inflatable penile prostheses in patients undergoing cystoprostatectomy with urethrectomy. *J Urol.* 1989;141:60-62.

56. Dahlen CP, Goodwin WE. Sexual potency after perineal biopsy. *J Urol.* 1957;77:660-669.

57. Finkle AL, Moyers TG. Sexual potency in aging males. V: coital ability following open perineal prostatic biopsy. *J Urol.* 1960;84:649-653.

58. Finkle AL, Prian D. Sexual potency in elderly men before and after prostatectomy. *JAMA.* 1966;196:394.

59. Gold FM, Hotchkiss RS. Sexual potency following simple prostatectomy. *NY State J Med.* 1969;A:2987-2989.

60. Holtgrewer HL, Volk WL. Late results of transurethral prostatectomy. *J Urol.* 1964;91:51-55.

61. Madorsky ML, Ashamalla MG, Schussler I, et al. Postprostatectomy impotence. *J Urol.* 1976;1154:401-403.

62. Brendler CB, Walsh PC. The role of radical prostatectomy in the treatment of prostate cancer. *CA: Cancer J Clin.* 1992; 42:212-222.

63. Scott WW, Boyd HL. Combined hormonal control therapy and radical prostatectomy in the treatment of selected cases of advanced carcinoma of the prostate: a retrospective study based upon 25 years of experience. *J Urol.* 1969; 101:86-92.

64. Aass N, Grunfeld B, Kaaslhus O, Foss SD. Pre- and post-treatment sexual life in testicular cancer patients: a descriptive investigation. *Br J Cancer.* 1993;67:1113-1117.

65. Carlton CE, Hudgins PT, Guerriero WG, et al. Radiotherapy in the management of stage C carcinoma of the prostate. *J Urol.* 1976;116:206-210.

66. Fowler JE, Barzell W, Hilaris BS, et al. Complications of 125 iodine implantation and pelvic lymphadenectomy in the treatment of prostatic cancer. *J Urol.* 1979;121:447-451.

67. Herr HW. Preservation of sexual potency in prostatic cancer patients after pelvic lymphadenectomy and retropubic ^{125}I implantation. *J Urol.* 1979;121:621-623.

68. Ellis WJ, Grayheck JT. Sexual function in aging males after orchiectomy and estrogen therapy. *J Urol.* 1963; 89:895-899.

69. Schover LR, Gonzales M, von Eschenbach AC. Sexual and marital relationships. *Urology.* 1986;17:117-123.

70. Bracken RB, Johnson DE. Sexual function and fecundity after treatment for testicular tumors. *Urology.* 1976; 7:35-38.

71. Nijman JM, Koops HS, Oldhoff J, et al. Sexual function after bilateral retroperitoneal lymph node dissection for non-seminomatous testicular cancer. *Arch Androl.* 1987;18: 255-267.

72. Schover LR, von Eschenbach AC. Sexual and marital relationships after treatment for nonseminomatous testicular cancer. *Urology.* 1985;25:251-255.

73. Grigor KM, Donohue JP. Reproductive aspects of testicular germ cell cancer: General discussion. *Eur Urol.* 1993; 23:177-181.

74. Donohue JP, Thornhill JA, Foster RS, Rowland RG, Bihrle R. Primary retroperitoneal lymph-node dissection in clinical stage A non-seminomatous germ cell testis cancer. Review of the Indiana University experience. *Br J Urol.* 1993;71:329-335.

75. Witkin MH, Kaplan HS. Sex therapy and penectomy. *J Sex Marital Ther.* 1982;8:209-221.

76. Andersen BL, Lachenbruch PA, Anderson B, et al. Sexual dysfunction and signs of gynecologic cancer. *Cancer.* 1986;56:1880-1886.

77. Vincent CE, Vincent B, Greiss FC, et al. Some marital-sexual concomitants of carcinoma of the cervix. *South Med J.* 1975;68:551-558.

78. DiSaia PJ, Creasman WT, Rich WM. An alternate approach to early cancer of the vulva. *Am J Obstet Gynecol.* 1979;133:825-832.

79. Hacker NF. Alternate strategies in managing vulva cancer. *Cancer.* In press.

80. Andersen BL, Hacker NF. Psychosexual adjustment after vulvar surgery. *Obstet Gynecol.* 1983;62:457-462.

81. American Cancer Society. *Cancer Facts and Figures—1994.* Atlanta, Ga: American Cancer Society.

82. Fobair P, Hoppe RT, Bloom J, et al. Psychosocial problems among survivors of Hodgkin's disease. *J Clin Oncol.* 1986;4:805-814.

83. Cella DF, Tross S. Psychological adjustment to survival from Hodgkin's disease. *J Consult Clin Psychol.* 1986;54:616-622.

84. Waxman JH, Ahmen R, Smith D, et al. Failure to preserve fertility in patients with Hodgkin's disease. *Cancer Chemother Pharmacol.* 1987;19:159-162.

85. Whitehead E, Shaiet SM, Blackledge G, et al. The effects of Hodgkin's disease and combination chemotherapy on gonadal function in the adult male. *Cancer.* 1982;49:418-422.

86. Chapman RM, Sutcliffe SB. Protection of ovarian function by oral contraceptives in women receiving chemotherapy for Hodgkin's disease. *Blood.* 1981;58:849-851.

87. Chapman RM, Sutcliffe SB, Malpas JS. Cytotoxic-induced ovarian failure in women with Hodgkin's disease. I: hormone function. *JAMA.* 1979;242:1877-1881.

88. Chapman RM, Sutcliffe SB, Malpas JS. Cytotoxic-induced ovarian failure in women with Hodgkin's disease. II: effects on sexual function. *JAMA.* 1979;242:1882-1899.

89. Lacher MJ, Tooner K. Pregnancies and menstrual function before and after combined radiation (RT) and chemotherapy (TVPP) for Hodgkin's disease. *Cancer Investigation.* 1986;4:93-100.

90. Barton C, Waxman J. Effects of chemotherapy on fertility. *Blood Rev.* 1990;4:187-195.

91. Andersen BL, Anderson B, deProsse C. Controlled prospective longitudinal study of women with cancer. II: psychological outcomes. *J Consult Clin Psychol.* 1989;57:692-697.

41

METASTATIC TUMORS OF UNKNOWN ORIGIN: DIAGNOSTIC AND THERAPEUTIC IMPLICATIONS

Richard J. Steckel, MD, A. Robert Kagan, MD

Clinical Considerations

Metastases from an unknown primary tumor may first present clinically as lymph node masses in the neck, axilla, or inguinal area,[1,2] as one or more lung nodules on a chest radiograph, as gradual enlargement of the abdomen,[3] or as a symptomatic bone lesion.

When the presence of widespread metastatic disease is evident and the primary site of the tumor remains unknown, little purpose will be served in proceeding with further diagnostic steps (eg, the use of imaging examinations and other techniques to search vigorously for a primary tumor) when it seems likely that there will be no effective therapy even if the primary site can be located. Metastatic tumors for which curative, or reasonably effective palliative treatment is now available for some patients include lymphomas, laryngopharyngeal squamous cell carcinomas metastatic to lymph nodes in the upper two thirds of the neck, germinal cell malignancies, small cell lung carcinomas, hormone-dependent carcinomas originating in the breast, prostate, or endometrium, thyroid carcinomas, and some malignancies of neural crest origin. Several rare tumors that occur in infants and young children can also be treated effectively after they have become widely disseminated, but their sites of origin can usually be identified using a combination of histologic and clinical findings.[4]

Published data on the numbers of patients who present with metastatic disease and unknown primary tumors often underestimate the true frequency of this condition. Metastatic tumors in patients without identified primary tumors are often subsequently reclassified as "known" primary tumors on the basis of inconclusive evidence (eg, a suggestive histologic appearance from a biopsied metastasis or the identification of the suspected "primary tumor" on an imaging study or at autopsy). In other words, delayed reclassification of a patient's tumor from an *unknown* primary to a *known* primary is frequently based on "guilt by association," and not on positive identification of the actual tumor source.

When metastatic nodes in the upper neck containing squamous cell or poorly differentiated carcinoma are the only abnormal clinical findings in a patient, an occult primary tumor in the pharynx, larynx, or nasopharynx can usually be found by meticulous clinical examination. On the other hand, it is not rare for patients to come to the attention of the physician with a metastatic lymph node in the *lower* portion of the neck containing adenocarcinoma or an undifferentiated tumor. In this situation the critical question, once again, is how far to go in subjecting the patient to numerous diagnostic studies, including radiologic imaging examinations, in the hope of locating a primary site for the rare disseminated malignancy that may be amenable to palliation or cure.

Many extended diagnostic workups that are done to elucidate metastatic disease of unknown origin will ultimately fail to locate the primary tumor site. Furthermore, even if the primary tumor is found, these diagnostic studies will often not result in useful information for improving the length and/or quality of a patient's life.[5-9] In one study,[10] UCLA Hospital Tumor Registry data were examined for patients who were first seen at least 5 years previously with disseminated cancer from an unknown primary site (Table 41-1). Registry cases in this study were ascertained for the period 1968 through 1974. In patients for whom postmortem documents later became available, an autopsy report or a death certificate was examined to determine whether the primary site could be identified *after* the patient's death.

Richard J. Steckel, MD, Professor, Radiological Services and Radiation Oncology, UCLA School of Medicine and Director, Jonsson Comprehensive Cancer Center, Los Angeles, California

A. Robert Kagan, MD, Chief, Radiation Oncology, Southern California Kaiser Permanente Medical Group and Clinical Professor, Radiation Oncology, UCLA School of Medicine, Los Angeles, California

Table 41-1. Cancer Patients with Unknown Primary Tumors (1968-1974)

Presenting Site of Metastatic Cancer	No. of Cases	Patients Died (by Jan. 1979)	Autopsy Results Known	Primary Not Found at Autopsy
Abdominal mass	43	41	10	7
Bone	42	38	3	2
Cervical lymph node	42	37	5	4
Lung and/or pleura	39	37	6	4
Thoracic lymph node	11	11	2	0
Chest wall	7	7	1	0
Liver	29	28	2	1
Brain	19	15	2	1
Skin	6	5	1	0
Abdominal lymph node	5	4	0	0
Inguinal node	8	4	1	0
Eye	1	1	0	0
Peripheral soft tissue	3	3	1	1
Total	255	231	34	20*/34

*The 14 primary tumors that were identified at autopsy include seven that originated in the lung (none of the small-cell type); two in the pancreas; one each in the kidney, bladder, biliary ducts, and posterior mediastinum (a neurogenic malignancy); and one visceral Kaposi's sarcoma.

From Steckel and Kagan.[10]

Of approximately 7,000 new patients recorded in the UCLA Registry during the 6-year period of this study, 255 (approximately 4%) were found to have had metastatic cancer with a persistently unknown primary tumor at the last report date when the patient was still alive. Patient follow-up by the Registry during the entire period of this study was 98%. Of the 255 patients with unknown primary tumors, 231 (91%) had died by January 1979. However, autopsy results and death certificates were available for only 34 of the 231 patients. In 20 of these 34 patients the primary site could not be located *even at autopsy.* Of the remaining 14 autopsied patients, seven were found to have primary bronchogenic tumors (none was of the small cell type), two had metastatic tumors that originated in the pancreas, one each had primary tumors of the kidney, bladder, biliary ducts, and posterior mediastinum (the latter was a malignant neurogenic tumor), and one patient had visceral Kaposi's sarcoma. Therefore, in all of the documented patients who had persistent unknown primary tumors and in whom an autopsy led eventually to the identification of the primary tumor site, it is doubtful *even today* that prior knowledge of the site of origin of the patient's tumor would have had any influence on treatment or on survival!

Pathologic Contributions

Lymphoma in an enlarged node can sometimes be distinguished histochemically from an undifferentiated carcinoma by using special stains such as the one for leukocyte common antigen.[11] In a similar fashion, metastatic small cell endocrine tumors can sometimes be identified by staining histologic sections for S-100 antigen or neuron-specific enolase. Some germinal tumors that are metastatic from an occult primary tumor at a gonadal *or* an extragonadal site will stain for alpha feto-protein (AFP), human chorionic gonadotrophin (HCG), or both. The polymerase chain reaction (PCR) technique can now be used to identify the Epstein-Barr virus (EBV) genome in biopsied metastatic tumor tissue from an upper cervical lymph node that originates from an occult *nasopharyngeal* primary tumor.[12,13] Accordingly, the judicious use of biopsy information can often serve to guide subsequent diagnostic studies and to conserve time and costs.

When faced with an enlarged lymph node containing a poorly differentiated tumor, the most important distinction to be made histologically is between a diffuse lymphoma or a germinal cell tumor which *can* be treated effectively, and an undifferentiated carcinoma of unknown origin.[14] Patients with the latter type of tumor, when it has become widely disseminated, usually survive less than 6 months *regardless* of treatment. Even the subgroup of small cell carcinomas known as "poorly differentiated neuroendocrine tumors," for which aggressive systemic treatment has been recommended by some authors,[15] has a dismal prognosis with combination chemotherapy in most patients. Metastatic *adeno*carcinoma of unknown origin in lymph nodes is usually untreatable,[16,17] with the exception of isolated axillary adenopathy: some women who present with enlarged unilateral axillary nodes will be found subsequently to have a subclinical *breast* primary tumor. This can be detected by careful mammography after the metastatic axillary lymph node has been biopsied and tested for estrogen and progesterone receptors.[18-20]

Radiologic Contributions

Radiologic imaging examinations may contribute to the initial evaluation of metastatic lesions that appear at several body sites. While computed tomography (CT) is the most sensitive means to detect metastatic pulmonary lesions, lung nodules from an unknown primary tumor usually come to attention first as incidental findings on standard chest radiographs. A radionuclide bone scan is the most sensitive and versatile method to detect focal abnormalities in the presence of unexplained musculoskeletal symptoms, whereas radiographs of symptomatic areas are *more specific* for diagnosing metastatic bone lesions. CT and magnetic resonance imaging (MRI) may sometimes contribute additional diagnostic information after the "conventional" radiologic bone studies have been performed. Enlargement of the liver from suspected metastases or an increase in abdominal girth from malignant ascites may prompt a CT study of the abdomen. Focal liver metastases or mesenteric tumor deposits from a primary carcinoma in the female genital tract or the gastrointestinal tract can often be visualized on abdominal CT scans, even if the primary tumor site cannot be identified. The minimum diagnostic imaging studies that should be considered when a patient first presents with metastatic tumor and an unknown primary site are summarized in Table 41-2.

Radiologic imaging techniques may also guide percutaneous needle biopsies of metastatic lesions in the liver, lymph nodes, bones, lungs, or abdomen, to expedite a diagnosis in a person with a disseminated malignancy and an unknown primary tumor (see below). Radiologic examinations can also help to evaluate or prevent certain complications of metastatic disease that may be susceptible to palliative measures, such as obstructive jaundice from enlarged nodes in the porta hepatis, a superior vena cava syndrome, an impending pathologic fracture, or bowel obstruction.

Table 41-2. Diagnostic Imaging Recommendations for Patients with an Occult Primary Carcinoma

Presenting Site of Metastatic Disease	Minimum Imaging Studies Recommended (Chest Radiographs Are Always Indicated)
Abdominal mass	Abdominal CT scan
Hepatomegaly	Abdominal CT scan Consider barium enema/UGI series
Biliary tract (painless jaundice)	Percutaneous and/or endoscopic cholangio-pancreatogram
Malignant ascites	Abdominal CT scan Consider barium enema/UGI series
Malignant pleural effusion	Mammogram in women (if chest radiographs otherwise negative) Consider chest CT scan
Upper cervical lymph nodes	CT scan of upper airways Consider thyroid scan
Lower cervical lymph nodes	CT chest/abdomen Consider mammogram in women
Axillary lymph nodes (undifferentiated cancer)	Mammography in women (if chest radiographs are nondiagnostic)
Spinal epidural space (on myelogram or MRI)	Chest CT (if radiographs are nondiagnostic)
Bone	Radionuclide bone scan survey, with correlative radiographs CT of chest/abdomen (if chest radiographs are nondiagnostic) Consider ultrasound of prostate (men) or mammogram (women)
Lungs (multiple nodules)	CT abdomen/pelvis Consider BE/UGI series

From Kagan and Steckel.[21]

It is not uncommon for primary laryngopharyngeal tumors to present initially as metastatic squamous cell cancer involving the upper cervical lymph nodes. The primary source of the metastatic disease may sometimes be difficult to locate by clinical examination in these patients, even by direct endoscopy, when the tumor is small or predominantly submucosal. An area of submucosal thickening or a small primary tumor mass can sometimes be recognized in such cases with cross-sectional imaging techniques (CT

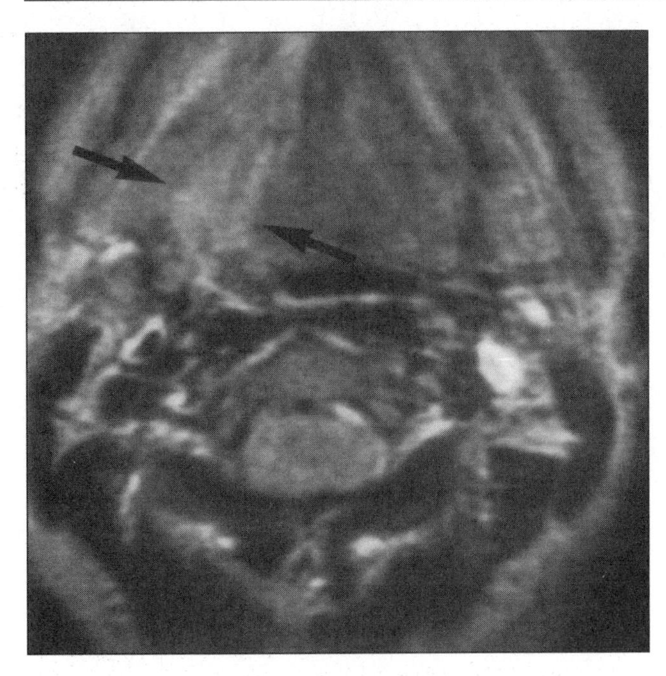

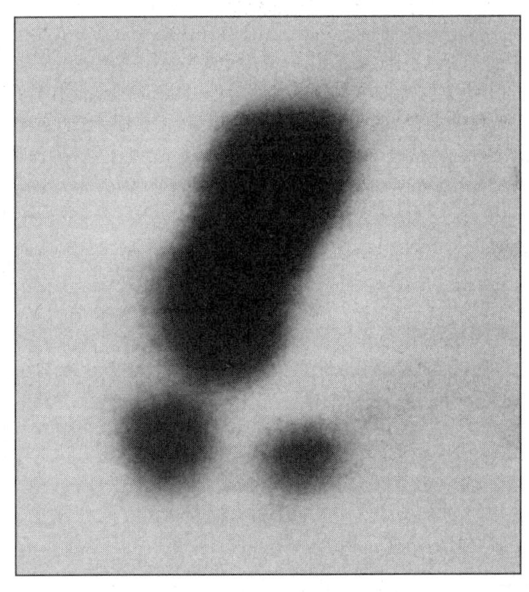

Fig 41-1. An occult squamous cell carcinoma of the right side of the tongue is visible as an area of increased signal on a T2-weighted MRI scan ***A***. In connection with a clinical study of positron emission tomography (PET) with radioactive fluorodeoxyglucose (FDG) for cancer, the same tongue tumor was visualized by PET as a large area of increased metabolic activity ***B***. In addition, two cervical lymph nodes involved by metastatic tumor were shown on the PET scan as smaller areas of metabolic hyperactivity posterior to the primary tongue lesion. These lymph nodes were not palpable, *nor* were they visible on the MRI scan (above).

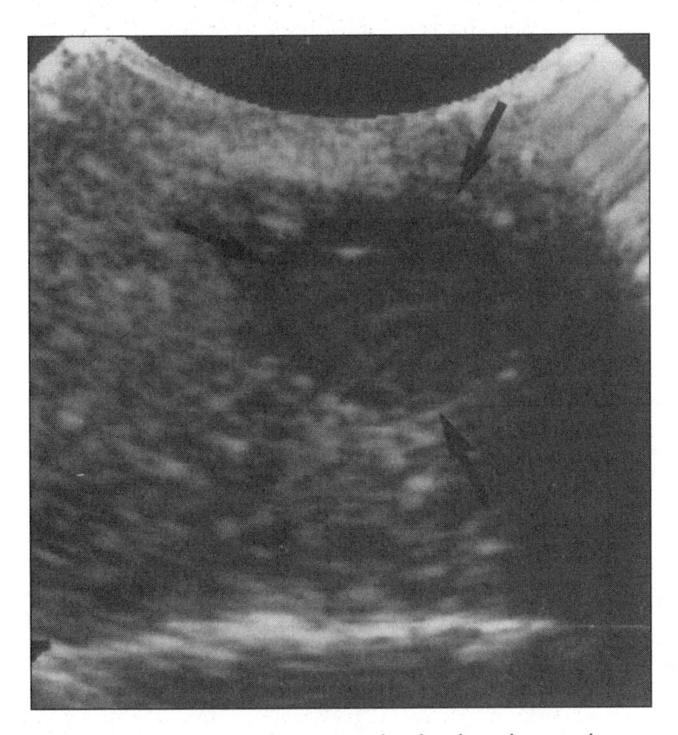

Fig 41-2. A young man who presented with enlarged inguinal lymph nodes was confirmed by biopsy of the nodes to have a seminoma. A nonpalpable (one-centimeter) primary tumor mass (arrows) was found subsequently in the left testicle by ultrasound examination. (Courtesy of Edward C. Grant, MD)

or MRI), even when prior endoscopy and "blind biopsies" have been negative (Fig 41-1). Similarly, a nonpalpable primary cancer can sometimes be found with a testicular ultrasound scan in a patient who presented first with a metastatic inguinal, abdominal, mediastinal, or lower neck mass (Fig 41-2).

Other metastatic cancers that may be treated for palliation include hormonally sensitive tumors of the breast, prostate, and endometrium. Careful diagnostic mammograms, or a CT or MRI scan of the pelvis, can assist in finding small primary tumors in these locations. Small carcinoids in the large or small bowel, with metastatic disease to the liver, can sometimes be identified with gastrointestinal contrast examinations. Islet cell primary tumors in the pancreas presenting as metastatic disease in the liver can be visualized using dynamic CT scans with contrast infusions. Ovarian primary carcinomas can often be identified with pelvic ultrasound examinations in women who are initially diagnosed with malignant ascites.

Conclusion

The exhaustive use of diagnostic studies to locate a primary source for a tumor that has already become widely disseminated may be a questionable practice at best, and at worst it may subject a patient with an incurable malignancy to potential harm. There must be a therapeutic purpose in mind to justify an active diagnostic approach. "Intellectual curiosity" alone is no justification for launching an aggressive search to locate a primary tumor in the presence of widespread metastatic disease when no useful therapeutic purpose can be served.

References

1. Guarischi A, Keane TJ, Elhakim T. Metastatic inguinal nodes from an unknown primary neoplasm: a review of 56 cases. *Cancer.* 1987;59:572-577.

2. Velez A, Walsh D, Karikusis CP. Treatment of unknown primary melanoma. *Cancer.* 1991;68:2579-2581.

3. Ringenberg QS, Doll DC, Loy TS, Yarbro JW. Malignant ascites of unknown origin. *Cancer.* 1989;64:753-755.

4. Kagan AR, Steckel RJ. Abdominal mass and cervical adenopathy in a child. *AJR.* 1979;132:643-645.

5. Devine KD. Cancer in the neck without obvious source. *Mayo Clin Proc.* 1978;53:644-650.

6. Nystrom JS, Weiner JM, Wolf RM, et al. Identifying the primary site in metastatic cancer of unknown origin: inadequacy of roentgenographic procedures. *JAMA.* 1979;241: 381-383.

7. Stewart JR, Tattersall MHN, Woods RL, et al. Unknown primary adenocarcinoma: incidence of overinvestigation and natural history. *BMJ.* 1979;1:1530-1533.

8. Brewin TB. The cancer patient: too many scans and x-rays? *Lancet.* 1981;2:1098-1099.

9. Steckel RJ, Kagan AR. Evaluation of the unknown primary neoplasm. *Radiol Clin North Am.* 1982;20:601-605.

10. Steckel RJ, Kagan AR. Diagnostic persistence in working up metastatic cancer with an unknown primary site. *Radiology.* 1980;134:367-369.

11. Horning SJ, Carrier EK, Rouse RV, Warnke RA, Michie SA. Lymphomas presenting as histologically unclassified neoplasms: characteristics and response to treatment. *J Clin Oncol.* 1989;7:1281-1287.

12. Feinmesser R, Miyazaki I, Cheung R, Freeman JL, Noyek AM, Dosch HM. Diagnosis of nasopharyngeal carcinoma by DNA amplification of tissue obtained by fine-needle aspiration. *N Engl J Med.* 1991;326:17-21.

13. Jacobs CD, Pinto AJ. Head and neck cancer with an occult primary tumor. *N Engl J Med.* 1991;326:58-59.

14. Greco FA, Hainsworth JD. Tumors of unknown origin. *CA.* 1992;42,2:96-115.

15. Remick SC, Ruckdeschel JC. Extrapulmonary and pulmonary small-cell carcinoma: tumor biology, therapy and outcome. *Med Pediatr Oncol.* 1992;20:89-99.

16. Lee NK, Byers RM, Abbruzzese JL, Wolf P. Metastatic adenocarcinoma to the neck from an unknown primary source. *Am J Surg.* 1991;162:306-309.

17. Wagener DJT, de Mulder PHM, Burghouts JT, Croles JJ. Phase II trial of cisplatin for adenocarcinoma of unknown primary site. *Eur J Cancer.* 1991;27,6:755-757.

18. Baron PL, Moore MP, Kinne DW, Cancela FC, Osborne MP, Petrek JA. Occult breast cancer presenting with axillary metastases. *Arch Surg.* 1990;125:210-214.

19. Ellerbroek N, Holmes F, Singletary E, Evans H, Oswald M, NcNeese M. Treatment of patients with isolated axillary nodal metastases from an occult primary carcinoma consistent with breast origin. *Cancer.* 1990;66:1461-1467.

20. Campana F, Fourquet A, Ashby MA, et al. Presentation of axillary lymphadenopathy without detectable breast primary (TON1b breast cancer): experience at Institut Curie. *Radiother Oncol.* 1989;15:321-325.

21. Kagan AR, Steckel RJ. Metastases from unknown primary tumors. *Invest Radiol.* 1988;23:545-547.

42

IDENTIFICATION AND CARE OF CANCER FAMILIES

Frederick P. Li, MD

There were about 1.2 million new diagnoses of cancer (other than carcinomas of the skin) in the United States in 1994, and approximately 538,000 deaths. Cigarette smoking is the dominant cause of cancer mortality, accounting for more than 165,000 deaths annually from cancers of the lung, oral cavity, bladder, and other sites.[1] For other common forms of cancer, such as carcinomas of the breast, colon, pancreas, kidney, and prostate, the causes remain uncertain. Studies of environmental carcinogens have often revealed small excess risks that are difficult to interpret, particularly when confirmatory studies produce discordant results. In contrast, a family history of cancer is a highly consistent risk factor for neoplasia in humans.[2]

Cancer Occurrence in Families

Virtually all cancers manifest a tendency to aggregate in families. Close relatives of a cancer patient can be considered to have an increased risk of that neoplasm, as well as of additional cancers in some instances. The excess risk of the cancer that has developed in a close relative is usually twofold to threefold above the baseline rate. However, susceptibility is much higher in certain families that are carriers of one of 200 single-gene traits that confer increased risk of neoplasia (Table 42-1).[3] The frequency of neoplastic manifestations approaches 100% for several rare hereditary disorders. Benign and malignant tumors are the sole manifestation of some predisposing inherited disorders, but are rarely featured in others. Several clinical characteristics have been described for hereditary cancers. These include specificity of the cancers by organ site or tissue; earlier age of occurrence than is usual for that neoplasm; multifocal cancers within the susceptible organ, including bilateral involvement of paired organs such as breast and kidney; and development of multiple primary cancers. However, these findings in individual patients need to be interpreted with caution. With improved cancer survival due to better treatments, more patients are at risk of developing multiple primary cancers. Furthermore, age at diagnosis of most cancers can be highly variable, and generally is not a reliable indicator of innate predisposition.[4]

Family aggregation of cancer can be due to both hereditary influences and shared exposure to environmental carcinogens. The possibility exists that every cancer arises as a consequence of complex interactions between host factors and environmental carcinogens. Carcinogens in experimental animals can produce different frequencies and types of tumors among different animal species and strains. As tools improve for studying genetically determined responses to carcinogenic exposures in humans, the role of host factors has become more evident. The multifactorial concept of human carcinogenesis is consistent with current knowledge about the fundamental molecular and cellular changes that convert a normal cell into a cancer cell.[5] The basic lesion in cancer appears to be alterations in the genetic control of cellular processes—that is, cancer at the molecular level is a genetic disease. Among the estimated 100,000 genes in the human genome, only a small fraction seems to be critically involved in cancer development. Many of these genes can be classified into two major groups: dominant oncogenes and tumor suppressor genes.[6] Multiple alterations of these genes appear to be required to produce cancer. These defects can be inherited, acquired through spontaneous mutation, or induced by environmental carcinogens.

Tumor suppressor genes have been discovered through clinical, epidemiologic, and molecular genetic studies of cancer families. Knudson's two-mutation hypothesis provides an important conceptual frame-

Frederick P. Li, MD, Professor of Medicine and Epidemiology, Head, Division of Cancer Epidemiology and Control, Dana-Farber Cancer Institute, Harvard Medical School and Harvard School of Public Health, Boston, Massachusetts

Table 42-1. Some Heritable Single-Gene Traits Associated With Cancer Development*

Organ System	Predisposing Genetic Disorder (Mode of Inheritance and Major Cancer Type)	Gene/Chromosome Locus
Digestive	Polyposis coli (AD; colon and rectum)	*APC*/5q
	Gardner's syndrome (AD; colon and rectum)	*APC*/5q
	Hereditary hemochromatosis (AD; liver cancer)	—
	Palmar-plantar hyperkeratosis (AD; esophagus)	—
	Hereditary pancreatitis (AD; pancreas)	—
	Fibrocystic pulmonary dysplasia (AD; lung)	—
	Debrisoquine genotype (AD; lung)	*CYPIID*/22q
Genitourinary	Wilms' tumor (AD; kidney)	*WT1*/11p
	von Hippel-Lindau syndrome (AD; renal carcinoma)	3p
Brain and endocrine	Retinoblastoma (AD; eyes)	*Rb*/13q
	Neurofibromatosis type 1 (AD; brain and nerves)	*NFI*/17q
	Neurofibromatosis type 2 (AD; brain and nerves)	22q
	Multiple endocrine neoplasia, type I (AD; parathyroid, pituitary, pancreatic islet)	11q
	Nevoid basal cell carcinoma syndrome (AD; medulloblastoma, skin)	9q
	Multiple endocrine neoplasia, type II (AD; medullary thyroid carcinoma, pheochromocytoma)	10p
Hematologic	Constitutional immunodeficiency, eg, X-linked lymphoproliferative syndrome (XL; lymphoma)	Xq
	Fanconi's anemia (AR; leukemia)	9q
Musculoskeletal	Multiple exostosis (AD; osteogenic sarcoma)	—
	Li-Fraumeni syndrome (AD; sarcoma, other)	*p53*

*Excluding familial site-specific cancers and weak associations based on isolated case reports.

AD = autosomal dominant, AR = autosomal recessive, XL = X-linked. Inheritance mode refers to disease pattern in pedigrees and not to molecular action of the gene.

Adapted from Li.[26]

work for studying these rare families to gain new understanding of human carcinogenesis.[6] The model postulates that at least two mutations are required to transform a normal cell into a cancer cell. At the molecular level, familial and sporadic (nonfamilial) forms of a cancer involve the same gene(s). In sporadic cancer, no mutation is inherited and two somatic mutations must occur within one cell. Hereditary cancer is due to a germinal mutation that has been inherited from one parent and propagated in all somatic cells of susceptible family members; a second mutation transforms the cell. The hypothesis implies that any somatic cell of cancer gene-carriers can be examined for the first mutation, and a comparison of tumor and somatic cells can reveal the second mutation. Thus, the complex carcinogenic process in the sporadic form of a cancer can be dissected into two components in the familial form. Laboratory studies reveal that in certain cancers the two mutations result in loss or inactivation of both alleles of one gene. Some of these genes act as tumor suppressors, the prototype of which is hereditary retinoblastoma.[6] For common cancers in humans, however, more than two hits are likely to be involved in cancer initiation, promotion, and progression.

Collection and Interpretation of Family History of Cancer

Physicians learned as medical students that the family history is part of the complete medical record. During clinical clerkships we were taught to inquire about the occurrence of neoplasia and other major diseases among close relatives. The information was obtained during the initial evaluation of every patient, and applied in considering the differential diagnosis and planning workup. However, collection of family history data is often neglected by busy practitioners, in part because its utility is not fully appreciated. In fact, the family history of cancer can lead to the identification of certain cancer-prone patients and to new knowledge of the fundamental biology of human cancers.

The term *family* is nonspecific and carries several meanings. A family might encompass relatives who share a common ancestry, or persons within a household including adopted children, in-laws, and spouses. Investigations of shared exposure to environmental carcinogens, such as passive exposure to cigarette smoking in the home, should extend to all persons in the household. For studies of genetic factors in cancer, however, the focus of attention is usually on relatives who share the same blood line. The study subjects can be the nuclear family, such as first-degree relatives (parents, siblings, and offspring), or include distant relatives in unusual family cancer aggregates. In routine medical practice, the family history can be obtained with the following question: who among your blood relatives has ever had a cancer? Even if no one has, the response should be recorded, and this part of the medical interview has been completed. When a positive response is elicited, additional data should be collected on the sex of the affected family member(s), the relationship to the respondent, age(s) at diagnosis, primary site and histology of each tumor, and disease outcome. A pedigree can be drawn to summarize the history of cancer in multiple members of a family.

Physicians are often asked by patients about the clinical implications of a family history of cancer. Unfortunately, cancer is a common disease over a lifetime among Americans, occurring in 1 of every 3 persons.[2] However, less than 1% of all cancers occur in childhood, and only 10% occur before 45 years of age; aggregates of cancers at early ages are much less likely to be due to chance association. Families with a single form of cancer in multiple relatives are more likely to have an inherited predisposition. Two relatives with the same rare cancer should prompt additional evaluation, whereas three or more cases of the common forms of cancer should be present before seeking consultation.[7] In families of research interest, confirmation of the medical history of family members should be sought through examinations of pathology reports, medical records, and death certificates. The family history reported by patients is accurate for site of cancer in only 80% of close relatives and 60% of distant relatives.[8] Analysis of the pedigree might reveal the presence of a known cancer syndrome or predisposing hereditary disorder. The information should be shared with the family, along with recommendations for future management.

Clinical Patterns of Cancers in Families

Many genes that predispose to cancer in humans are expressed in a single tissue and organ. This section summarizes the data on several illustrative site-specific familial cancers and cancer syndromes that have recently been shown to be due to inherited susceptibility genes.

Carcinoma of the Colon and Rectum

Many studies have described familial aggregation of cancers of the colon and rectum, the commonest internal neoplasm in the US and areas of Europe. The data suggest that close relatives of colon cancer cases have a threefold excess risk of this cancer when compared with control groups or population incidence rates.[9] Striking clusters of colon cancer in patterns suggesting autosomal dominant transmission with high penetrance have been reported. Affected relatives tend to have carcinomas of the right (proximal) colon at early ages. A recent proctosigmoidoscopy study of 34 families of patients with colorectal cancer or adenomatous polyp suggests that inherited susceptibility may have a major role in colon tumors in general.[10] The results of pedigree analysis favored the model of dominantly inherited susceptibility to colonic adenomas and cancer. The frequency of the susceptibility allele was reported to be 19% in the study. The finding implies that most patients with adenoma or carcinoma of the colon have inherent susceptibility to these disorders, but the results need to be confirmed.

Colorectal carcinoma develops in nearly all patients with dominantly inherited adenomatous polyposis coli (APC) and Gardner's syndrome (polyposis of the colon and stomach associated with osseous tumors of the jaw, skull and other sites, fibromas of the mesentary and skin, and, in rare instances, sarcoma and carcinoma of the ampulla of Vater).[10,11] The frequency of the APC mutant in the general population is on the order of 1 per 10,000 persons in the population. Colon cancers in polyposis gene carriers tend to arise at early ages, occasionally in teenagers, and at multiple foci in the bowel. Extensive efforts to identify the gene were unsuccessful until Herrera and coworkers in 1986 described a patient with polyposis, multiple malformations, mental retardation, and a constitutional deletion of chromosome 5q13-22.[11] This single case raised the possibility that the constellation of diseases, including colonic polyposis and carcinoma, resulted from loss of a polyposis-associated gene on chromosome 5q. Tests of this hypothesis by linkage analysis of affected families confirmed the location on chromosome 5q of the gene for both polyposis and Gardner's syndrome.[12] The APC gene has recently been isolated and is a tumor suppressor gene.[13] Inherited point mutations in polyposis patients have been found widely scattered throughout the gene. However, inherited APC mutations have not been detected in familial colon cancer without polyposis, suggesting additional hereditary "colon cancer genes."

Analyses of colon tumor tissue from unselected cases have revealed multiple genetic alterations. On average, colon carcinomas appear to have deletion of nearly 20% of all alleles in a nonrandom distribution.[14] These include chromosome 5q deletions in about 30% of carcinomas and adenomas that span the APC gene and a second colon cancer-associated gene, *MCC* (missing in colon cancer). Deletions of chromosome 17 involve the *p53* tumor suppressor gene, and deletions of chromosome 18 involve the *DCC* (deleted in colon cancer) gene.[15] In addition, activating mutations of *RAS* oncogene have been found in colon cancers and stool specimens, which might prove useful in the detection of colon adenoma and carcinoma.

Carcinoma of the Breast

According to epidemiologic studies, a family history of breast cancer is a consistent risk factor for the neoplasm. Other host factors include early menarche, late menopause, and nulliparity, whereas environmental influences such as alcohol and diet remain subjects of controversy.[16] In affected families, the risk may be transmitted through either parent, and males have been affected in some kindreds. The relative risk of breast cancer is reported to be approximately twofold to threefold among close relatives of cases, although most figures are not based on lifetime observation. Some breast cancer families manifest an autosomal dominant pattern with high penetrance, ie, a risk of breast cancer that approaches 50% among daughters of affected women in the family. Patients at highest risk have a family history of premenopausal, bilateral breast cancer affecting both mother and maternal grandmother, or both mother and sister. However, analyses of the genetic epidemiology of breast cancer have been complicated by several factors, including sex-dependent susceptibility, variable age at onset of disease, and genetic heterogeneity among affected families.

Cytogenetic analyses show that breast cancer cells are highly aneuploid, and karyotypes are difficult to interpret. Several chromosome regions show nonrandom losses, and several oncogenes have been shown to be activated by point mutation (*RAS*) or gene amplification (HER-2/*neu*). Recent data have identified at least three inherited single-gene defects that predispose to breast cancer. One is the ataxia-telangiectasia (*AT*) gene(s), which has been mapped to chromosome 11*q*.[17] In a follow-up study of obligate carriers of the *AT* gene, a fivefold excess of breast cancer was found when compared with controls. Second, germ line mutations in the *p53* tumor suppressor gene has been detected in some families with Li-Fraumeni syndrome, which features early-onset breast cancer.[18] Isolated breast cancer families without the syndrome can also have inherited *p53* mutations, but the frequency is probably less than 1%. A third gene, mapped to chromosome 17q but not yet isolated, has been identified by linkage analysis of families with breast cancer of early onset.[19] Available data suggest that the 17q gene can account for a substantial proportion of familial breast cancers in young women. Other forms of familial breast and ovarian cancers are attributable to this gene.

Carcinoma of the Prostate

Cancer of the prostate, though one of the commonest cancers in men, remains a disease of unknown cause. Prostatic cancer has been reported to have a familial tendency, but the importance of family history is only beginning to be quantified. A recent hospital-based study of male relatives of 691 consecutive patients with prostate cancer showed an odds ratio of around 2 for men with an affected first- or second-degree relative.[20] However, the odds ratio was 8.8 for those with both first- and second-degree relatives affected. The risk increases with the total number of affected family members. Familial prostate cancer, which tends to occur at an early age, accounts for a substantial proportion of the disease in younger men. The study represents the most complete analysis to date of familial prostate cancer. However, it was based on patients at a referral center that treats selected patients, and a confirmatory population-based study should be made.

Respiratory Tract

Tobacco smoking is the dominant cause of cancers of the upper and lower respiratory system. A few studies show that a family history of lung cancer also constitutes a risk factor for the neoplasm after adjustment for the effect of cigarette smoking.[21] Linkage studies of familial clusters of lung cancer have not been possible because of the high mortality associated with the tumor. Use of polymerase chain reaction to recover specific DNA sequences from paraffin-fixed tissues might permit examination of these families in future studies. Familial occurrence of lung cancer has been associated with genetically determined metabolism of carcinogens in cigarette smoke. Many carcinogens in tobacco smoke require metabolic activation within the target tissues, particularly through pathways of the cytochrome P-450 gene family. Early studies focused on aryl hydrocarbon hydroxylase (AHH), but its association with increased lung cancer risk remains tenuous. Current studies are examining another pathway within the P-450 gene system that is measured by the metabolism of the medication for hypertension, debrisoquine.[22] Available data suggest that lung and bladder cancers occur with higher frequency among smokers who are active metabolizers of debrisoquine. Although genetic influences have an etiologic role in lung cancer, the observation does not alter the fact that smoking cessation is the most effective solution to the lung cancer epidemic.[23]

Multiple Cancer Syndromes

Families have been reported with cancer syndromes of diverse anatomic sites and tissues that are attributed to inherited factors. These families generally have no predisposing clinical features, and they are identified primarily on the basis of statistical association. The diagnosis of these syndromes can be difficult in individual families encountered in the clinic. Aggregation of diverse cancers in a family, such as clusters of lung, bladder, and oral cancers, can result from cigarette smoking. In some families, breast, ovarian, and endometrial cancers might be due to shared reproductive and dietary risk factors.

Recent attention has focused on a familial cancer syndrome of breast cancer in young women, childhood sarcomas, and other neoplasms.[18] Analytical epidemiologic studies have shown that mothers of population-based series of children with sarcoma have an excess of breast cancer. Also, segregation analysis of 159 families of children with a soft tissue sarcoma at one institution found evidence for transmission of a dominant cancer susceptibility gene. To date, at least seven component cancers of the syndrome, now called Li-Fraumeni syndrome, have been reported: breast cancer, soft tissue sarcoma, osteosarcoma, acute leukemia, brain tumors, adrenocortical carcinoma, and gonadal germ cell tumors. Searches for the inherited cancer-predisposing gene have found inherited mutations in the *p53* tumor suppressor gene in several families. The finding provides opportunities for testing previously unaffected family members for this mutation, which predicts future high risk.

Cancer Prevention in Families

Knowledge of a strong family history of cancer can be applied to cancer prevention and early detection.[7] In families with a known predisposing gene, the risk of cancer can often be estimated and used in surveillance and genetic counseling. The emerging field of cancer chemoprevention offers opportunities to place cancer-prone individuals on treatments that might delay or prevent cancer development.[24]

Inherited precursor lesions of cancer can be useful in early diagnosis and surveillance, as exemplified by families with dysplastic nevus syndrome and susceptibility to melanoma.[25] The characteristics of dysplastic nevi include nevi that are larger than usual, both macular and papular components in individual lesions, borders that are often irregular and poorly defined, and pigmentation that range from tan to pink. Dysplastic nevi tend to arise most frequently on the trunk, and can be transmitted as an autosomal dominant trait that predisposes to melanoma. For affected kindreds, a thorough skin examination should be performed and suspicious pigmented lesions excised. Since ultraviolet radiation is an etiologic factor in melanoma, avoidance of sunlight exposure is important in predisposed families. When working or playing in sunlight, these individuals should use sunscreens.

Early cancer detection in cancer families can proceed even in the absence of discernible precursor lesions and biomarkers of a carrier state. In breast cancer, early detection has been demonstrated to reduce mortality rates. The single most effective screening procedure is mammography, which currently involves exposure to very little radiation. Targeted screening of mothers, sisters, and older daughters of patients with breast cancer can be an important approach to reducing mortality in breast cancer families. In families with germ line *p53* mutation, predictive testing of clinically healthy family members for the defect is feasible, but the risks and benefits need to be studied. The possibility of chemoprevention in women prone to breast cancer is being studied in a tamoxifen trial.[24]

Early detection of colorectal carcinomas is feasible in predisposed families. Emerging evidence suggests that inherited factors have a role in the development in a high proportion of colonic adenomas and carcinoma. In rare polyposis families, prophylactic colectomy is currently recommended when multiple polyps are found. Some polyposis patients are treated with total proctocolectomy with permanent ileostomy, particularly when multiple rectal polyps are detected. The lower rectum is spared in those who are free of rectal polyps, but postoperatively periodic proctoscopic examinations are required to detect cancer in the rectal stump and to remove new polyps.

Conclusion

Familial aggregation has been reported for virtually every form of cancer in humans.[2] Among cancer families, however, the level of excess risk is heterogeneous and ranges up to a thousandfold. Familial clusters of cancer are often due to inherited susceptibility, but environmental influences and chance association must also be considered. Inherited susceptibility to cancer is often manifest by occurrence of the same neoplasm among multiple blood relatives. These neoplasms tend to occur at earlier ages than usual, bilaterally in paired organs, and in multiple primary foci within the predisposed organ. Hereditary cancers can also develop as multiple primary tumors. Recent advances in molecular biology have greatly enhanced the importance of studying cancer families to identify tumor suppressor genes. Germ line mutations in these genes can be transmitted to subsequent generations and predispose to cancer among carriers in the family. Members of cancer families may benefit from genetic counseling and early disease detection. In familial cancers triggered by environmental carcinogens, patient education regarding avoidance of harmful exposures can help prevent or delay onset of neoplasia.[23]

References

1. Boring CC, Squires TS, Tong T, Montgomery S. Cancer Statistics, 1994. *CA Cancer J Clin.* 1994;44:7-26.

2. Li FP. Molecular epidemiology of familial cancers. In: Harlow E, ed. *Origins of Human Cancer: A Comprehensive Review.* Cold Spring Harbor, NY: Cold Spring Harbor Laboratory Press; 1991:211-218.

3. Mulvihill JJ, Miller RW, Fraumeni JF Jr, eds. *Genetics of Human Cancer.* New York, NY: Raven Press; 1977.

4. Schneider NR, Chaganti SR, German J, Chaganti RSK. Familial predisposition to cancer and age at onset of disease in randomly selected cancer patients. *Am J Hum Genet.* 1983;35:454-467.

5. Bishop JM. The molecular genetics of cancer. *Science.* 1987;235:305-311.

6. Knudson AG Jr. Hereditary cancer, oncogenes, and antioncogenes. *Cancer Res.* 1985;45:1437-1443.

7. Parry DM, Mulvihill JJ, Miller RW, Berg K, Carter CL. Strategies for controlling cancer through genetics. *Cancer Res.* 1987;47:6814-6817.

8. Love RR, Evans AM, Josten DM. The accuracy of patient reports of a family history of cancer. *J Chronic Dis.* 1985; 38:289-293.

9. Bale SJ, Chakravarti A, Strong LC. Aggregation of colon cancer in family data. *Genet Epidemiol.* 1984;1:53-61.

10. Cannon-Albright LA, Skolnick MH, Bishop T, Lee RG, Burt RW. Common inheritance of susceptibility to colonic adenomatous polyps and associated colorectal cancers. *N Engl J Med.* 1988;319:533-537.

11. Herrera L, Kakati S, Gibas L, Pietrzak E, Sandberg AA. Gardner syndrome in a man with an interstitial deletion of 5q. *Am J Med Genet.* 1986;25:473-476.

12. Bodmer WF, Bailey CJ, Bodmer J, et al. Localization of the gene for familial adenomatous polyposis on chromosome 5. *Nature.* 1987;328:614-616.

13. Weinberg RA. Tumor suppressor genes. *Science.* 1991;254:1138-1146.

14. Vogelstein B, Fearon ER, Kern SE, et al. Allelotype of colorectal carcinomas. *Science.* 1989;244:207-211.

15. Kinzler KW, Nilbert MC, Vogelstein B, et al. Identification of a gene located at chromosome 5q21 that is mutated in colorectal cancers. *Science.* 1991;251:1366-1370.

16. Sattin RW, Rubin GL, Webster LA, et al. Family history and the risk of breast cancer. *JAMA.* 1985;253:1908-1913.

17. Swift M, Morrell D, Massey RB, Chase CL. Incidence of cancer in 161 families affected by ataxia-telangiectasia. *N Engl J Med.* 1991;325:1831-1836.

18. Li FP, Garber JE, Friend SH, et al. Recommendations on predictive testing for germ line *p53* mutations among cancer-prone individuals. *J Natl Cancer Inst.* 1992;84:1156-1160.

19. Narod SA, Feunteun J, Lynch HT, et al. Familial breast-ovarian cancer locus on chromosome 17q12-q23. *Lancet.* 1991;338:82-83.

20. Steinberg GD, Carter BS, Beaty TH, Childs B, Walsh PC. Family history and the risk of prostate cancer. *Prostate.* 1990;17:337-347.

21. Ooi WL, Elston RC, Chen VW, Bailey-Wilson JE, Rothschild H. Increased familial risk for lung cancer. *J Natl Cancer Inst.* 1986;76:217-222.

22. Caporaso NE, Tucker MA, Hoover RN, et al. Lung cancer and the debrisoquine metabolic phenotype. *J Natl Cancer Inst.* 1990;82:1264-1272.

23. Schelling TC. Addictive drugs: the cigarette experience. *Science.* 1992;255:430-433.

24. Nayfield SG, Karp JE, Ford LG, Dorr FA, Kramer BS. Potential role of tamoxifen in prevention of breast cancer. *J Natl Cancer Inst.* 1991;83:1450-1459.

25. Greene MH, Clark WH Jr, Tucker MA, et al. Acquired precursors of cutaneous malignant melanoma: the familial dyplastic nevus syndrome. *N Engl J Med.* 1985;312:91-97.

26. Li FP. Familial cancer syndromes and clusters. *Curr Probl Cancer.* 1990;16(2):77-113.

INDEX

Page numbers followed by "f" represent figures; those followed by "t" represent tables.

C

D

E

G

H

N

U

CHARTERED DIVISIONS
OF THE
AMERICAN CANCER SOCIETY

Alabama Division, Inc.
504 Brookwood Boulevard
Homewood, Alabama 35209
(205) 879-2242

Alaska Division, Inc.
1057 West Fireweed Lane
Suite 204
Anchorage, Alaska 99503
(907) 277-8696

Arizona Division, Inc.
2929 East Thomas Road
Phoenix, Arizona 85016
(602) 224-0524

Arkansas Division, Inc.
901 North University
Little Rock, Arkansas 72207
(501) 664-3480

California Division, Inc.
1710 Webster Street
Oakland, California 94604
(510) 893-7900

Colorado Division, Inc.
2255 South Oneida
Denver, Colorado 80224
(303) 758-2030

Connecticut Division, Inc.
Barnes Park South
14 Village Lane
Wallingford, Connecticut 06492
(203) 265-7161

Delaware Division, Inc.
92 Read's Way, Suite 205
New Castle, Delaware 19720
(302) 324-4227

District of Columbia Division, Inc.
1875 Connecticut Avenue, NW
Suite 730
Washington, DC 20009
(202) 483-2600

Florida Division, Inc.
3709 West Jetton Avenue
Tampa, Florida 33629-5146
(813) 253-0541

Georgia Division, Inc.
2200 Lake Blvd.
Atlanta, Georgia 30319
(404) 816-7800

Hawaii Pacific Division, Inc.
Community Services Center Bldg.
200 North Vineyard Boulevard
Suite 100-A
Honolulu, Hawaii 96817
(808) 531-1662

Idaho Division, Inc.
2676 Vista Avenue
Boise, Idaho 83705-0386
(208) 343-4609

Illinois Division, Inc.
77 East Monroe
Chicago, Illinois 60603-5795
(312) 641-6150

Indiana Division, Inc.
8730 Commerce Park Place
Indianapolis, Indiana 46268
(317) 872-4432

Iowa Division, Inc.
8364 Hickman Road
Suite D
Des Moines, Iowa 50325
(515) 253-0147

Kansas Division, Inc.
1315 SW Arrowhead Road
Topeka, Kansas 66604
(913) 273-4114

Kentucky Division, Inc.
701 West Muhammad Ali Blvd.
Louisville, Kentucky 40201-1807
(502) 584-6782

Louisiana Division, Inc.
2200 Veterans' Memorial Blvd.
Suite 214
Kenner, Louisiana 70062
(504) 469-0021

Maine Division, Inc.
52 Federal Street
Brunswick, Maine 04011
(207) 729-3339

Maryland Division, Inc.
8219 Town Center Drive
Baltimore, Maryland 21236-0026
(410) 931-6850

Massachusetts Division, Inc.
247 Commonwealth Avenue
Boston, Massachusetts 02116
(617) 267-2650

Michigan Division, Inc.
1205 East Saginaw Street
Lansing, Michigan 48906
(517) 371-2920

Minnesota Division, Inc.
3316 West 66th Street
Minneapolis, Minnesota 55435
(612) 925-2772

Mississippi Division, Inc.
1380 Livingston Lane
Lakeover Office Park
Jackson, Mississippi 39213
(601) 362-8874

Missouri Division, Inc.
3322 American Avenue
Jefferson City, Missouri 65102
(314) 893-4800

Montana Division, Inc.
17 North 26th Street
Billings, Montana 59101
(406) 252-7111

Nebraska Division, Inc.
8502 West Center Road
Omaha, Nebraska 68124-5255
(402) 393-5800

Nevada Division, Inc.
1325 East Harmon
Las Vegas, Nevada 89119
(702) 798-6857

New Hampshire Division, Inc.
Gail Singer Memorial Bldg.
360 Route 101, Unit 501
Bedford, New Hampshire 03110-5032
(603) 472-8899

New Jersey Division, Inc.
2600 US Highway 1
North Brunswick, New Jersey 08902
(908) 297-8000

New Mexico Division, Inc.
5800 Lomas Blvd., NE
Albuquerque, New Mexico 87110
(505) 260-2105

New York State Division, Inc.
6725 Lyons Street
East Syracuse, New York 13057
(315) 437-7025

CHARTERED DIVISIONS OF THE AMERICAN CANCER SOCIETY *continued*

■ **Long Island Division, Inc.**
75 Davids Drive
Hauppauge, New York 11788
(516) 436-7070

■ **New York City Division, Inc.**
19 West 56th Street
New York, New York 10019
(212) 586-8700

■ **Queens Division, Inc.**
112-25 Queens Boulevard
Forest Hills, New York 11375
(718) 263-2224

■ **Westchester Division, Inc.**
30 Glenn Street
White Plains, New York 10603
(914) 949-4800

North Carolina Division, Inc.
11 South Boylan Avenue
Suite 221
Raleigh, North Carolina 27603
(919) 834-8463

North Dakota Division, Inc.
123 Roberts Street
Fargo, North Dakota 58102
(701) 232-1385

Ohio Division, Inc.
5555 Frantz Road
Dublin, Ohio 43017
(614) 889-9565

Oklahoma Division, Inc.
4323 NW 63rd, Suite 110
Oklahoma City, Oklahoma 73116
(405) 843-9888

Oregon Division, Inc.
0330 SW Curry
Portland, Oregon 97201
(503) 295-6422

Pennsylvania Division, Inc.
Route 422 & Sipe Avenue
Hershey, Pennsylvania 17033-0897
(717) 533-6144

■ **Philadelphia Division, Inc.**
1626 Locust Street
Philadelphia, Pennsylvania 19103
(215) 985-5400

Puerto Rico Division, Inc.
Calle Alverio #577
Esquina Sargento Medina
Hato Rey, Puerto Rico 00918
(809) 764-2295

Rhode Island Division, Inc.
400 Main Street
Pawtucket, Rhode Island 02860
(401) 722-8480

South Carolina Division, Inc.
128 Stonemark Lane
Westpark Plaza
Columbia, South Carolina 29210-3855
(803) 750-1693

South Dakota Division, Inc.
4101 Carnegie Place
Sioux Falls, South Dakota 57106-2322
(605) 361-8277

Tennessee Division, Inc.
1315 Eighth Avenue, South
Nashville, Tennessee 37203
(615) 255-1227

Texas Division, Inc.
2433 Ridgepoint Drive
Austin, Texas 78754
(512) 928-2262

Utah Division, Inc.
941 East 3300 S.
Salt Lake City, Utah 84106
(801) 483-1500

Vermont Division, Inc.
13 Loomis Street
Montpelier, Vermont 05602
(802) 223-2348

Virginia Division, Inc.
4240 Park Place Court
Glen Allen, Virginia 23060
(804) 527-3700

Washington Division, Inc.
2120 First Avenue North
Seattle, Washington 98109-1140
(206) 283-1152

West Virginia Division, Inc.
2428 Kanawha Boulevard East
Charleston, West Virginia 25311
(304) 344-3611

Wisconsin Division, Inc.
N19 W24350 Riverwood Drive
Waukesha, Wisconsin 53188
(414) 523-5500

Wyoming Division, Inc.
4202 Ridge Road
Cheyenne, Wyoming 82001
(307) 638-3331